TEXTBOOK OF
INFLUENZA

Textbook of
INFLUENZA

Karl G. Nicholson

MD, FRCP, FRCPath, MFPHM
Senior Lecturer in Infectious Diseases
Medical Directorate
Department of Infectious Diseases and Tropical Medicine
The Leicester Royal Infirmary
Leicester, UK

Robert G. Webster

PhD, FRS
Member and Chairman
Rose Marie Thomas Chair
Department of Virology and Molecular Biology
St Jude Children's Research Hospital
Memphis, Tennessee, USA

Alan J. Hay

PhD
Division of Virology
National Institute for Medical Research
The Ridgeway
Mill Hill, London, UK

**Blackwell
Science**

© 1998
Blackwell Science Ltd
Editorial Offices:
Osney Mead, Oxford OX2 0EL
25 John Street, London WC1N 2BL
23 Ainslie Place, Edinburgh EH3 6AJ
350 Main Street, Malden
  MA 02148 5018, USA
54 University Street, Carlton
  Victoria 3053, Australia
10, rue Casimir Delavigne
  75006 Paris, France

Other Editorial Offices:
Blackwell Wissenschafts-Verlag GmbH
  Kurfürstendamm 57
  10707 Berlin, Germany

Blackwell Science KK
  MG Kodenmacho Building
  7–10 Kodenmacho Nihombashi
  Chuo-ku, Tokyo 104, Japan

First published 1998
Reprinted 2000

Set by DP Photosetting, Aylesbury, Bucks
Printed and bound in Great Britain
by The Alden Group Ltd, Oxford and Northampton

The Blackwell Science logo is a
trade mark of Blackwell Science Ltd,
registered at the United Kingdom
Trade Marks Registry

DISTRIBUTORS

  Marston Book Services Ltd
  PO Box 269
  Abingdon
  Oxon OX14 4YN
  (*Orders*: Tel: 01235 465500
                Fax: 01235 465555)

USA
  Blackwell Science, Inc.
  Commerce Place
  350 Main Street
  Malden, MA 02148 5018
  (*Orders*: Tel: 800 759 6102
                      781 388 8250
                Fax: 781 388 8255)

Canada
  Login Brothers Book Company
  324 Saulteaux Crescent
  Winnipeg, Manitoba R3J 3T2
  (*Orders*: Tel: 204 837 2987)

Australia
  Blackwell Science Pty Ltd
  54 University Street
  Carlton, Victoria 3053
  (*Orders*: Tel: 03 9347 0300
                Fax: 03 9347 5001)

Catalogue records for this title
are available from the British Library
and the Library of Congress

ISBN 0-632-04803-4

The opinions expressed in this
publication do not necessarily
represent the views of Blackwell
Science

For further information on
Blackwell Science, visit our website:
www.blackwell-science.com

Contents

Colour plates fall between pp 288 and 289

List of Contributors

Fred Y. Aoki MD, *Professor of Medicine, Medical Microbiology, Pharmacology and Therapeutics; Head, Section of Clinical Pharmacology, University of Manitoba, 510-730 William Avenue, Winnipeg, Manitoba, Canada R3E 0W3*

William J. Bean Jr. *121 Irwin Avenue, Pittsburgh, Pennsylvania 15202, USA*

Pamuk Bilsel PhD, *385 Talbot Avenue #20, Pacifica, California 94044, USA*

Thomas M. Chambers PhD, *Associate Professor, Department of Veterinary Science, Maxwell H. Gluck Equine Research Center, University of Kentucky, Lexington, Kentucky 40546-0099, USA*

Peter M. Colman PhD, *Director, Biomolecular Research Institute, 343 Royal Parade, Parkville, Victoria 3052, Australia*

Janet M. Daly PhD, *Division of Virology, National Institute for Biological Standards and Control, Blanche Lane, South Mimms, Potters Bar, Hertfordshire, EN6 3QG, UK*

Peter C. Doherty PhD, FRS, *Chairman, Department of Immunology, St. Jude Children's Research Hospital, 332 North Lauderdale St, Memphis, Tennessee 38104, USA*

Vittorio Demicheli MD, MSc, *Institute of Medical Statistics, University of Pavia, 27100 Pavia, Italy*

David S. Fedson MD, *Pasteur Mérieux MSD, 8 rue Jonas Salk, 69367, Lyon Cedex 07, France*

Ian G.S. Furminger PhD, *Technical Director, Evans Medical, Evans House, Regent Park, Kingston Road, Leatherhead, Surrey KT22 7PQ, UK*

Adolfo García-Sastre PhD, *Mount Sinai School of Medicine, Department of Microbiology, 1 Gustave Levy Place , New York, NY 10029, USA*

Yuri Ghendon MD, PhD, *Professor of Virology, Moscow Institute for Viral Preparations, 1 Dubrovskaya Str. 15, Moscow 109088, Russian Federation*

Reinhard Glück PhD, *Head of Virology, Swiss Serum and Vaccine Institute Berne, CH-3001, Berne, Switzerland*

Christine M. Graham BSc, *National Institute for Medical Research, The Ridgeway, Mill Hill, London NW7 1AA, UK*

William C. Gruber MD, *Associate Professor of Pediatrics, Department of Pediatrics, Division of Infectious Diseases, Vanderbilt University School of Medicine, D-7235 Medical Center North, Nashville, Tennessee 37232-2581, USA*

Alan J. Hay PhD, *Division of Virology, National Institute for Medical Research, The Ridgeway, Mill Hill, London, NW7 1AA, UK*

Frederick G. Hayden MD, *Professor of Medicine and Pathology, Division of Epidemiology and Virology, University of Virginia School of Medicine, Charlottesville, Virginia, USA*

Virginia S. Hinshaw PhD, *Professor of Virology/ Dean of the Graduate School/Senior Research Officer, Graduate School, University of Wisconsin-Madison, 500 Lincoln Drive, Madison, Wisconsin 53706-1380, USA*

Toshihiro Ito DVM, PhD, *Associate Professor, Department of Veterinary Public Health, Faculty of Agriculture, Tottori University, 4-101, Minami, Koyama-cho, Tottori, 680, Japan*

Tom Jefferson OStJ, MSc, MRCGP, MFPHM, DRCOG, DTM&H, RAMC, *Edmund Parkes Professor of Preventive Medicine, Ministry of Defence, Army Medical Directorate, Building 21, Keogh Barracks, Ash Vale, Aldershot, Hampshire GU12 5RR, UK*

Yoshihiro Kawaoka DVM, PhD, *Professor of Department of Pathobiological Sciences, School of Veterinary Medicine, University of Wisconsin-Madison, 2015 Linden Drive West, Madison, Wisconsin 53706, USA*

Wendy A. Keitel MD, *Assistant Professor of Microbiology, Immunology and Medicine, Acute Viral Respiratory Disease Unit, Department of Microbiology, Baylor College of Medicine, One Baylor Plaza, Texas Medical Center, Houston, Texas 77030-3498, USA*

Robert M. Krug PhD, *Professor and Chairman, Department of Molecular Biology and Biochemistry, Rutgers University, Center for Advanced Biotechnology and Medicine, 679 Hoes Lane, Piscataway, New Jersey 08855-1179, USA*

Robert Lambkin MRPharmS, PhD, *Postdoctoral Fellow, Academic Virology and Retroscreen Ltd., Department of Medical Microbiology, St Bartholomew's and the Royal London School of Medicine and Dentistry, Turner Street, Whitechapel, London E1 2AD, UK*

Jane Leese FRCP, *Senior Medical Officer, Department of Health, Room 706, Wellington House, 135–155, Waterloo Road, London SE1 8UG, UK*

Arnold S. Monto MD, *Professor of Epidemiology, School of Public Health, University of Michigan, Ann Arbor, Michigan USA*

Jennifer A. Mumford PhD, *Head of Centre for Preventive Medicine, Animal Health Trust, Lanwades Park, Kentford, Newmarket, Suffolk CB7 5NH, UK*

Thomas Muster PhD, *Department of Dermatology, University of Vienna Medical School, Vienna, Austria*

Kristin L. Nichol MD, MPH, *Professor of Medicine, University of Minnesota, Chief of Medicine, Minneapolis VA Medical Center, One Veterans Drive, Minneapolis 55417, USA*

Karl G. Nicholson MD, FRCP, FRCPath, MFPHM, *Senior Lecturer in Infectious and Tropical Diseases, Department of Infectious Diseases and Tropical Medicine, The Leicester Royal Infirmary, Leicester LE1 5WW, UK*

Jonathan S. Nguyen-Van-Tam MBE, MFPHM, *Senior Lecturer in Public Health Medicine, University of Nottingham Medical School, Queen's Medical Centre, Nottingham NG7 2UH, UK*

Christopher W. Olsen DVM, PhD, *Assistant Professor of Public Health, Department of Pathobiological Sciences, School of Veterinary Medicine, University of Wisconsin-Madison, 2015 Linden Drive West, Madison, Wisconsin 53706, USA*

John S. Oxford PhD, *Professor of Virology, Academic Virology and Retroscreen Ltd., Department of Medical Microbiology, St Bartholomew's and the Royal London School of Medicine and Dentistry, Turner Street, Whitechapel, London E1 2AD, UK*

Andriani C. Patera PhD, *National Institute for Medical Research, The Ridgeway, Mill Hill, London NW7 1AA, UK*

Charles R. Penn MA, PhD, *Director of Research, Centre for Applied Microbiology and Research, Porton Down, Salisbury SP4 0JG, UK*

Pedro A. Piedra MD, *Assistant Professor, Department of Microbiology, Immunology and Pediatrics, Baylor College of Medicine, One Baylor Plaza, Texas Medical Center, Houston, Texas 77030-3498, USA*

Christopher W. Potter PhD, FRCPath, *Professor of Virology, University of Sheffield Medical School, Beech Hill Road, Sheffield S10 2RX, UK*

James S. Robertson BSc, PhD, *Division of Virology, National Institute for Biological Standards and Control, Blanche Lane, South Mimms, Potters Bar, Hertfordshire EN6 3QG, UK*

Rob W.H. Ruigrok, *Group Leader, EMBL Grenoble Outstation, c/o ILL, BP 156, 38042 Grenoble cedex 9, France*

Christoph Scholtissek Dipl. Chem. Dr. rer. nat., *Retired Professor for Biochemistry and Virology of the Faculty of Veterinary Medicine of the University of Giessen, Waldstrasse 53, D – 35440 Linden, Germany*

Claire A. Smith PhD, *National Institute for Medical Research, The Ridgeway, Mill Hill, London NW7 1AA, UK*

David A. Steinhauer PhD, *National Institute for Medical Research, The Ridgeway, Mill Hill, London NW7 1AA, UK*

Philip G. Stevenson DPhil MRCP, *Department of Immunology, St Jude Children's Research Hospital, 332 North Lauderdale St, Memphis, Tennessee 38104, USA*

Susan E. Tamblyn MD, DPH, FRCPC, *Medical Officer of Health, Perth District Health Unit, 653 West Grove Street, Stratford, Ontario, N5A 1L4, Canada*

David Brian Thomas MA, DPhil, *Senior Scientist, National Institute for Medical Research, The Ridgeway, Mill Hill, London NW7 1AA, UK*

John J. Treanor MD, *Associate Professor of Medicine, Infectious Diseases Unit, University of Rochester School of Medicine, 601 Elmwood Avenue, Rochester, NY 14642, USA*

David Tyrrell CBE, MD, DSc, FRCP, FRCPath, FRS, *Retired Director of MRC Common Cold Unit, Centre for Applied Microbiology and Research, Porton Down, Salisbury, Wiltshire SP4 0JG, UK*

John M. Watson FRCP, FFPHM, *Consultant Epidemiologist, PHLS Communicable Disease Surveillance Centre, 61 Colindale Avenue, London NW9 5EQ, UK*

Robert G. Webster PhD, FRS, *Rose Marie Thomas Chair, Department of Virology and Molecular Biology, St. Jude Children's Research Hospital, 332 N. Lauderdale, Memphis, Tennessee 38105-2794, USA*

Alfred Wegmann MD, *Swiss Serum and Vaccine Institute Berne, CH-3001, Berne, Switzerland*

Stephen A. Wharton PhD, *National Institute for Medical Research, The Ridgeway, Mill Hill, London NW7 1AA, UK*

Michael S. Williams BSc, *Biologics Consulting Group, 137 Kale Avenue, Sterling, Virginia 20164, USA*

Martin J. Wiselka MD, PhD, MRCP, *Consultant in Infectious Diseases, Department of Infectious Diseases and Tropical Medicine, Leicester Royal Infirmary, Infirmary Square, Leicester LE1 5WW, UK*

John M. Wood PhD, *Scientist, Division of Virology, National Institute for Biological Standards and Control, Blanche Lane, South Mimms, Potters Bar, Hertfordshire EN6 3QG, UK*

Maria Zambon MB, BCh, PhD, *Enteric and Respiratory Virus Laboratory, Central Public Health Laboratory, 61 Colindale Avenue, London NW9 5HT, UK*

Foreword

During the past few decades a series of books on clinical and laboratory aspects of influenza has appeared. They were published as, step by step, we moved forward from the days when influenza could be recognized and discussed solely in terms of its clinical and epidemic characteristics. I first put my foot on one of those steps when the virus had recently been grown in eggs and so I was involved in the excitement of studying exactly what disease it caused and what new serotype was causing the new epidemic. We were just beginning to discover what the particle looked like, how it was made, how to vaccinate, and so on. This was one of the first occasions on which our understanding of an epidemic infection grew alongside our understanding of the biology of the virus.

At that time the serious student or research worker could find all he or she needed, indeed almost all that was known, within a chapter in a comprehensive textbook of medical virology. Since that time it has become increasingly difficult to assimilate the burgeoning information by going to original papers or even reviews – some reviews are little better than a catalogue of references. So a whole book on the subject was very welcome.

Whether we start from bedside medicine or basic molecular biology or somewhere in between, what we need is a discriminating and up-to-date scholarly account of the key facts and leading ideas and how these link with each other and form an overall network of knowledge. It is, I believe, an axiom of clinical and biological science that the best thinkers and investigators have an up-to-date knowledge of the broad principles of what is going on in areas of research adjacent to those in which they themselves work and are expert. Obviously we cannot all be expert in all aspects of influenza; just to understand the nature and the possible significance of a new drug we might need to appreciate the relevance of X-ray crystallography and solving the structure of a viral neuraminidase as well as the importance of drug distribution and the pathogenesis of influenzal pneumonia.

This book was planned and written to meet such a need and because knowledge has grown so fast it takes us much further than did its predecessors. It can provide a sound analysis of individual topics as well as a grand panorama. Of course, it will not stand alone. The burgeoning Internet and Websites can be used to keep fully up-to-date and to supplement printed journals. But a book can still be the best way to build up a broad and accurate mental picture on which we can fill in extra details from our own experience and the research of others. Try this one!

David Tyrrell

Preface

As the world awaits the uncertainties of the next millenium with excitement and apprehension, we predict with certainty, on the basis of the history of pandemics during the past century, that another pandemic of influenza will occur sometime in the future. The events in Hong Kong during the past year, when six deaths occurred among 18 people hospitalized with influenza A H5N1 ('bird flu'), should alert us to the possibility that, despite medical and virological advances in recent years, a future pandemic could cause as many millions of deaths in young adults as the infamous Spanish flu of 1918–19. An even greater cumulative impact results from the annual morbidity, mortality and socioeconomic costs arising from constantly evolving strains of influenza A and B.

Since the last pandemic, major advances in molecular virology have been applied extensively to the study and prevention of influenza, and a new reference book has therefore become necessary. This textbook of influenza provides a comprehensive authoritative summary of clinical influenza and its scientific basis, and the wealth of information provided is highly relevant to clinical and molecular virologists, immunologists, clinicians, public health doctors, health economists and students in each discipline.

This book includes 41 chapters which provide a historical and clinical background and describe developments in most aspects of influenza. These range from basic research on the structure and function of viral genes and protein products, through evolution and ecology of influenza viruses, interspecies transmission, surveillance and molecular epidemiology, cellular and humoral immunity, laboratory diagnosis and vaccines, to therapeutics, health economics and control programmes. During the past 5 years, notable advances have taken place in the field of antiviral drugs, particularly neuraminidase inhibitors which have revealed great promise in the volunteer challenge studies and are currently being assessed in multinational phase III studies.

All of the chapters are original and have been written specifically for the book Each entry provides a comprehensive synopsis of the selected topic to inform a wide range of readers from students to specialists. Individual chapters are contributed by investigators widely acknowledged as experts in their field. Because each chapter has been written to be self-standing there is inevitably some overlap. While repetition has in most instances been kept to a minimum, we make no apologies for its existence, because each author brings a different perspective and it is felt that the alternative of flitting from one chapter to another to fully explore a topic would be irritating. Size limitations have not permitted each contribution to be exhaustive or allowed the citation of every significant publication in the field. Rather our goal has been to provide a core of essential information and relevant references to inform readers and equip them to explore the wider literature.

Inevitably there will be important developments in the field of influenza both during and after publication of the book. The outbreak of H5N1 influenza in Hong Kong is an example. We do not feel that this detracts from the value of the text as a treatise, particularly as much of the information provided is based on work confirmed by various laboratories, field workers or clinicians, and is unlikely to be altered substantially by subsequent work.

We have already found entries in this text extremely useful as a reference, as a teaching aid, and as a topic of general interest, and we trust that others will find it of equal value.

Karl G. Nicholson
Robert G. Webster
Alan J. Hay

Acknowledgements

Neither this book nor many of the recent developments in the field of influenza would have existed without the immense enthusiasm and determination of each of the contributors. We are enormously grateful to each and every one of them for providing scholarly well-researched chapters, and extensive references. We are also indebted to Rosemary Sumray, National Institute for Medical Research, Mill Hill, London for her prodigious efforts in compiling and revising manuscripts. We also wish to acknowledge the enthusiastic support of our publishers for their faith in us, particularly to Amanda Ryde, and also Linda Crossman, Editorial Manager, and Emma Hamilton, Editorial Assistant, for their sustained support and encouragement. Last, but by no means least, we acknowledge the support, understanding and tolerance provided by our wives and children.

Karl G. Nicholson
Robert G. Webster
Alan J. Hay

Section 1
Historical Introduction

CHAPTER 1

Chronicle of Influenza Pandemics

Christopher W. Potter

For those who lived through the influenza pandemics of 1957 and 1968, the prospect of such future episodes evokes concern and apprehension: for those who remember the pandemic of 1918-20, the emotion may be of horror and fear. It is the experience and knowledge of the severity of these and other pandemics, and the more common but less severe epidemics, which have made influenza the most studied of virus diseases, until the advent of the human immunodeficiency virus (HIV); led to the commissioning of an international network of laboratories by the World Health Organization (WHO) to monitor influenza virus variation and spread in attempts to anticipate future outbreaks; and has focused the concern of researchers, physicians, diagnostic laboratories, epidemiologists, pharmaceutical companies and health authorities. Despite this, our knowledge of many aspects remains fragmentary; all authorities predict that future pandemics will occur, but are unsure of when or the ability or will to implement measures to prevent the tragedies of the past (Glezen 1996). It is not surprising that influenza has been termed, 'the last great plague' (Smillie & Kilbourne 1963).

Two conditions must be satisfied for an outbreak of influenza to be classed as a pandemic. Firstly, the outbreak of infection, arising in a specific geographical area, spreads throughout the world; a high percentage of individuals are infected resulting in increased mortality rates. Secondly, a pandemic is caused by a new influenza A virus subtype, the haemagglutinin (HA) of which is not related to that of influenza viruses circulating immediately before the outbreak, and could not have arisen from those viruses by mutation (Web-ster & Laver 1975). Each influenza A virus subtype possesses one of 15 distinct HAs designated H1, H2, H3, and so on, which do not cross-react in serological tests (see Chapter 22): immunity to influenza is principally related to antibody to the HA, and the appearance of a new virus subtype with a different HA means that immunity acquired from past influenza infection confers no protection against the new virus subtype, and the spread of infection by the latter is unchecked.

The pandemics of influenza which have occurred since 1957 are clearly identified by both worldwide infection and analysis of the virus subtype responsible; however, prior to this the viruses concerned are unknown. Before 1933 when human influenza virus was first isolated, identification of pandemics was based solely on observations of a rapid worldwide spread, and morbidity and mortality figures, which suggested the emergence of a new virus serotype. But analysis of pandemics based on epidemiology alone, or analysis of concurrent virus strains alone, is not secure: in 1947 worldwide outbreaks of influenza suggested pandemic infection, but later analysis of the virus responsible showed that it arose by extensive mutation from previously circulating virus strains (see p. 12); and analysis of sera from elderly people indicated that a new virus subtype circulated in 1900, but there is little evidence of widespread influenza infection at that time (see p. 8).

Source material

Despite the reservations that must be imposed on the interpretation of much of the older literature,

numerous commentators have attempted to identify pandemics within the entire historic period;
inevitably, the earlier the records the less reliable
the information. The earliest reports of influenza
include an outbreak in 412 BC recorded by both
Hippocrates and Livy (Grmek 1893); speculation as
to the cause of the pestilence which devastated
Athens in 430 BC during the Peloponnesian war; an
epidemic of respiratory infection in the armies of
Charlemagne; several outbreaks of fever and
coughing in the Middle Ages to 1500; the sweating
sickness that debilitated French and English armies
during the Hundred Years War; and the outbreak at
the court of Mary Tudor in 1562: much of these are
curiosities without scientific substance, and their
debate is more suited to the coffee lounge than
seminar rooms.

The first description of an epidemic where
symptoms were clearly influenzal occurred in AD
1173–4 (Hirsch 1883); and although several reports
suggest influenza outbreaks during the 14th and
15th century, the next convincing report was by
Molineux (1694). Three epidemics in the 16th century have been interpreted as influenza (Patterson
1987; Beveridge 1991), whilst confidence that pandemic infection occurred at reported times during
the 17th century in America and Europe is shared
by some authors (Webster 1800; Hirsch 1883). From
the beginning of the 18th century, the quality and
quantity of data increased; and medical historians
are drawn to comment on the number of infected
persons, the countries involved and the possible
origins of the virus strains involved. Data from the
18th and 19th centuries have been analysed in four
comprehensive accounts (Hirsch 1883; Thompson
1890; Creighton 1894; Finkler 1899); these have been
extensively reviewed (Beveridge 1977; Pyle 1986;
Patterson 1987), and supplemented with primary
source material, including city death rates and
parish burial records (Patterson 1987). Since the
pandemic of 1889–92, data have been more reliable
and more thoroughly reviewed; and since 1957,
when the causal viruses were available for analysis,
the status of pandemics is not questioned. An
extensive literature describes the 1918–20 and later
pandemics.

Influenza pandemics

Pandemics before AD 1700

In assessing the data supporting the case for an
influenza pandemic, the observations and opinions
of several authors have been analysed; epidemics
which are cited by only one author were not considered pandemics, and evidence for a pandemic is
only considered where two or more authors,
reviewing the source material, separately agreed on
a possible pandemic occurring in a particular year.
This analysis is given in Table 1.1. The outbreak of
respiratory infections in 1173–74 is regarded as an
accurate description of influenza (Hirsch 1883), but
there is no support for a case that this was a pandemic; and reports of influenza between 1200 and
1500 are too meagre and vague to allow comment.
The severe outbreak of influenza in 1510 was
probably a pandemic with the infection first
appearing in Africa and spreading to Europe
(Beveridge 1991). However, although the Columbian Exchange (Crosby 1972) had been established,
the absence of comment of concomitant infection in
the Americas dictates reservation. In contrast, the
long time taken for boats to cross the Atlantic at this
time suggests that infection could have burnt out
before a journey was completed, and this would
have limited spread. The outbreak of 1557 was
possibly a pandemic, but the first influenza pandemic agreed by all authors occurred in 1580. This
pandemic originated in Asia during the summer of
that year, spread to Africa, and then to Europe
along two corridors from Asia Minor and North-
West Africa (Pyle 1986). The whole of Europe was
infected from south to north in a 6-month period,
and infection subsequently spread to America (Pyle
1986; Beveridge 1991). Illness rates were high; 8000
deaths were reported from Rome, and some Spanish cities were decimated (Beveridge 1991). In
Britain, there were two waves of infection, one in
the summer and the second in the autumn.

Pandemics of the 18th and 19th centuries

Records for the 17th century are too sparse to
permit deduction, but data from 1700 are more

Table 1.1 History of major influenza outbreaks.

Year	Epidemicity	Affected countries	First recognized (season)	Origin	Comments
1173–74	+	Europe—first convincing description of influenza epidemic			
1200–1500		Seven outbreaks recorded which cannot be evaluated under above headings			
1510	++	Europe, Africa	NK	Africa	—
1557	+	Europe, Japan	NK	NK	—
1580	+++	Europe, Africa, N. America	Summer	Asia	—
1600–99		Five to eight outbreaks recorded which cannot be evaluated under above headings			
1729–33	+++	Europe, N. & S. America, Russia	Spring	Russia	Two distinct waves, or two distinct epidemics; second more severe
1761–62	+	Europe, N. America	Winter	NK	—
1781–82	+++	Europe, China, India, N. America, Russia	Autumn	Russia/China	Two waves; second more severe
1788–90	+	Europe, N. America	NK	NK	Possibly related to 1781–82 pandemic
1799–1802	++	Europe, China, Brazil, Russia	Autumn	Russia/China	Authorities disagree (+ to +++)
1830–33	+++	Europe, N. America, Russia, India, China	Winter	China	Two waves; second more severe
1847–48	++	Europe, Russia, N. America?	Spring	Asia/Russia	Authorities disagree (+ to +++)
1857–58	+	Europe, N. & S. America	Autumn	Panama	—
1889–91	+++	All countries affected	Spring	Russia	Extensive seeding in spring/summer; winter pandemic. Later waves more severe
1900	+++	Europe, N. & S. America, Australia	NK	NK	Little clinical illness; new virus subtype indicated by serology
1918–20	+++	All countries affected	Spring	USA/China	Two distinct phases; second more severe
1946–48	+	All countries affected	—	Australia/China	Virus related to previous circulating strains
1957–58	+++	All countries affected	Winter/Spring	China	Two waves; second of equal or greater severity
1968–69	+++	All countries affected	Summer	China	In Europe, peak 1 year after USA
1977–78	+++	All countries affected	Summer	China/Russia	—

+, Epidemic; ++, probably pandemic; +++, pandemic; NK, not known.

informative. The first agreed influenza pandemic of this century began in 1729 (Hirsch 1883; Finkler 1899; Pyle 1986; Patterson 1987): the outbreak started in Russia in the spring months, spread westwards in expanding waves to embrace all Europe within a 6-month period (Pyle 1986), and encompassed the whole known world over a 3-year period with high death rates (see Table 1.1). Distinct waves of infection were recorded; the later were more severe than the first (Brown 1932; Beveridge 1977; Patterson 1987). The second wave in Europe in 1732, and the first recorded infections in North America in the same year (Webster 1800), could have arisen from earlier seeding (Patterson 1987). In contrast, one authority interpreted the data as indicating two distinct and unrelated outbreaks of influenza in 1729–30 and 1732–33: only the second was a true pandemic, originating in the USA, Russia or China, according to different observers, and then spreading to the Americas from Russia and Europe where illness and mortality rates were high (Beveridge 1991). Which interpretation is correct cannot be resolved from the available data; however, a single pandemic with milder episodes in 1729–30 and with extensive seeding, followed by more severe outbreaks without a clear pattern of spread from a single region and showing greater severity, is a pattern to be seen in future pandemics and is the favoured interpretation.

The next pandemic occurred after a gap of some 40 years in 1781–82 (Finkler 1899; Pyle 1986). Most authors agree that the outbreak began in China in the autumn, spread to Russia and from there westwards in widening circles to encompass the whole of Europe in a period of 8 months (Pyle & Patterson 1984). There is evidence of extensive seeding in both Russia and North America in the early months of the pandemic, followed by extensive outbreaks. The attack rate was reported to be high, particularly among young adults (Thompson 1890): at the peak of the pandemic, 30 000 fell ill each day in St Petersburg; two-thirds of the population of Rome became ill; and the outbreak is reported to have raged through Britain during the summer of 1782. Although the total attack rate was estimated at 10 million people, the death rate was relatively low (Patterson 1987).

Controversy surrounds the definition of the outbreak of influenza that occurred in 1799–1802. The contagion was first reported in Moscow in the autumn of 1799, spreading to involve all Russia by the spring of 1800 and finally to affect all of eastern Europe by the summer of 1800 (Pyle 1986; Patterson 1987). Further outbreaks were recorded in Europe in 1802 and 1803. Although infection rates were high, mortality was low (Patterson 1987). There was no record of influenza in North America at this time, and, as the Colombian Exchange was well established, this outbreak cannot be considered a pandemic (Patterson 1987). A second reviewer linked the above events to influenza in China and South America which occurred at the same time, and therefore concluded that the outbreak was a pandemic (Beveridge 1977). These differences cannot be resolved, and the outbreak is classified as a probable pandemic (see Table 1.1).

No disagreement exists among commentators for the pandemic of 1830–33 (Beveridge 1977; Pyle 1986; Patterson 1987), which has been ranked in terms of severity with the pandemic of 1918–1920 (Beveridge 1977). The pandemic began in the winter of 1830 in China, from where it spread southwards by sea to reach the Philippines, India and Indonesia, and across Russia into Europe. The contagion spread into North America to cause outbreaks in 1831–32, recurred in Europe at the same time and recurred again in Europe in 1832–33 (Pyle & Patterson 1984). All authors comment on the high attack rate of 20–25% of the population, but the mortality rate was not exceptionally high (Patterson 1987). One author suggests that the epidemic of 1832–33 was a separate pandemic, since both little infection was seen in the earlier period and the later outbreak was more lethal (Patterson 1987); however, the pattern of a more lethal outbreak in 1832 following a milder one in 1830 is the more likely interpretation (Patterson 1987), and the similarities with the pandemic of 1729–33 are remarkable (see above).

The outbreak of influenza in 1847–48 again provoked disagreement amongst modern reviewers: Beveridge (1977) classed it as a pandemic which began in March in Russia and then spread to Europe and North and South America; Patterson (1985) found no evidence of infection in America or South Asia and limited the extent of the outbreak to Europe and Russia. Primary sources fail to resolve these differences, and the outbreak is considered only a probable pandemic; however, attack rates were high, particularly among the young with more than 1 million cases in Russia, and a marked increase in mortality was recorded in London (Beveridge 1977; Pyle & Patterson 1984).

The pandemic of 1889–92

The influenza pandemic which began in 1889 is better documented than any of the previous episodes, and the first to be described as truly global; prior to this time, documentation is heavily biased by reports from Europe and North America and commentaries from other parts of the world are virtually absent. The history of the pandemic is

Fig. 1.1 The influenza pandemic of 1889–92. Point of origin (square) May 1889; lines of spread of the pandemic (arrows); number of months after May 1889 (0) when epidemic infection was recorded (number accompanies corresponding arrow); the site of some second-wave outbreaks (circles). (From the accounts of Pyle 1986; Patterson 1987; Beveridge 1991.)

based on sharply increased morbidity and mortality figures; and since communications and travel were relatively slow, the spread of infection was monitored without too much confusion: this spread has been fully described by Beveridge (1977) and Patterson (1987), and is shown in Fig. 1.1.

All authors agree that the years following the influenza outbreak in 1847–48 were virtually free of epidemic influenza until 1889 when the pandemic began (Patterson 1987). The origin of the pandemic is contentious, since some claims were probably other infections, such as malaria or dengue (Patterson 1987); however, the consensus of opinion is that the epidemic arose first in central Russia in the spring of 1889 and was largely confined to that area until late summer. From September to October 1889, the outbreak began to spread at the rate of travel: in the 3 months from October 1889, outbreaks were reported in widening circles to encompass the whole of Europe; in January 1890 the Mediterranean countries were fully involved, and at this time the outbreak had reached some parts of northern Africa; and infection crossed the ocean to North American ports in December 1889, and to South America in February 1890. The pandemic also reached Singapore and the Chinese

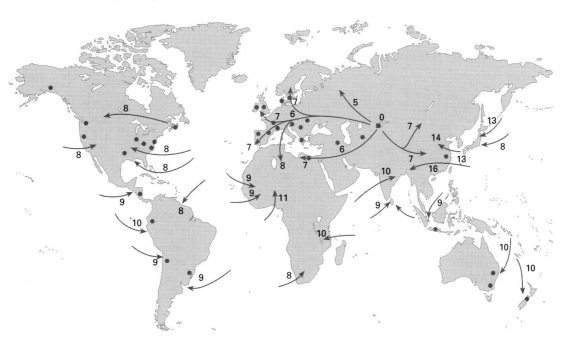

coast in February 1890 from where it spread inland to infect the Chinese nation which had been spared infection from central Russia by the barrier of the vast, uninhibited plains of that area. Infection reached India in February 1890, Australia and New Zealand in March 1890 and sub-Sahara Africa between January and May of that year. By the middle of 1890 the infection was clearly pandemic (see Fig. 1.1). The attack rate was estimated at between 25 and 50% of populations; and the global number of deaths was approximately 300 000 or 1.5 per thousand cases (Parsons 1893). Most of the deaths were seen in the elderly population (see Fig. 1.3) and were the result of secondary bacterial pneumonia; indeed, the frequency of pneumonia due to *Haemophilus influenzae* suggested to observers that this was the cause of the pandemic, and gave the organism its name (Parsons 1893).

The initial wave of infection in 1889–90 was followed by second and third waves in 1891 and 1892 (Frost 1919; Patterson 1976). These sprang up in various parts of the world, exhibiting no pattern of spread from a single focal point, often occurring in widely disparate parts of the world at the same time, and were probably outbreaks from virus seeded into the populations during the first wave: the location of some of these outbreaks is shown in Fig. 1.1. The mortality data suggest that the second wave was associated with a higher number of deaths, and the third wave was marked by a further increase in mortality (Parsons 1891, 1893; Frost 1919; Patterson 1987). The reason for this is obscure, but is recorded for earlier pandemics and would be seen in the future (see Table 1.1). Following the increase in mortality from 1890 to 1892, the mortality rate increased again in 1893 although no distinct influenza epidemic occurred (Parsons 1891; Frost 1919): this observation is not commented on by later reviewers.

It would be 40 years after this pandemic before human influenza viruses were isolated and studied in the laboratory, and therefore the nature of the virus which caused the pandemic of 1889–92 is unknown. However, the influenza A (H2) virus which caused the pandemic of 1957 is known, and studies with this virus and sera taken before 1957 from people who were alive in 1889 showed the presence of antibody to H2: younger persons did not have this antibody (Davenport *et al.* 1969; Masurel & Marine 1973). The interpretation placed on this finding is that an influenza A (H2) virus caused the pandemic of 1889 and then disappeared at the turn of the century: the virus re-emerged in 1957 to cause a pandemic in a world population most of whom had no previous contact with the virus and no immunity. This cyclical theory is tenable for the origin of pandemic viruses: a limited number of viruses circulate in humans to cause pandemics, disappear and then reappear decades later in a non-immune world. The theory has also been used to explain why the first waves of many pandemics have a lower attack rate in the elderly than the young; the former would have some immunity as a result of earlier exposure to the virus in their youth. In contrast, there is no evidence that an influenza virus can survive for years cryptically in nature, then to re-emerge; but this is not an essential element of the cyclical theory (see p. 4).

The pandemic of 1898–1901

The influenza pandemic which began in 1898 has excited little attention from reviewers: Patterson (1987) reported the spread of the pandemic; Pyle (1986) commented briefly on an increase in deaths in Massachusetts in 1900; but Beveridge (1977, 1991) ignored the event. Interest is mainly retrospective, since there is now evidence that the outbreak was caused by a new influenza A virus subtype. That influenza was active at the time is recognized from mortality figures which increased from 1898 to reach a peak in London in 1900 (Jordan 1927), and similar increases in mortality occurred in Australia (Burnet & Clark 1942) and North America (Frost 1919). The origins of the pandemic cannot be deduced from the data, but recognition of epidemics in the above countries and in Alaska, the Pacific Islands, Sweden, north-west Europe, Italy, France, Japan and Turkey at the same time indicate the worldwide distribution of infection (Patterson 1987). The outbreaks were mainly mild (Patterson 1987); indeed, interest stems almost entirely from studies of sera collected before 1968 from individuals alive at the beginning of the century: this indicated the presence of antibodies to influenza A (H3), which was unknown until shown to be the cause of the pandemic of 1968 (Davenport *et al.* 1969; Masurel & Marine 1973). Interpretation based on the age of those with antibody was that influenza A (H3) had been active at the time of the 1898-1901 pandemic, but not after approximately 1920. The observation gives support to the cyclical theory for influenza pandemics (see above): an influenza A (H3) subtype virus emerged in 1898 to cause the pandemic of the following 3 years; was later replaced by a virus which caused the 1918–22 pandemic; but remained cryptic in nature, or recurred, to cause the pandemic of 1968.

The pandemic of 1918–20

When the history of the influenza pandemic of 1918-20 is read, the emotive language used by reviewers will be seen to be fully justified: statements include, 'the greatest medical holocaust in history' (Waring 1971); 'the pandemic ranks with the plague of Justinian and the Black Death as one of the three most destructive human epidemics', and 'influenza killed more people in a few months than all the armies of the 1914/18 war in four years' (Walters 1978). At a more personal level, the epidemic, 'struck terror into the hearts of people' (Sage 1985), causing 'deaths in the hospital exceeding 25% per night during the peak' (Starr 1976); people endured visits 'down to the morgue to look at the boys laid out in long rows' (Grist 1979). The pandemic has been extensively chronicled (Crosby 1976; Beveridge 1977); the impact on North America (Jordan 1927; Crosby 1976; Pyle 1986), India (Gill 1928), Africa (Patterson & Pyle 1983), Australia (Burnet & Clark 1942), and Europe (MacNeal 1919; Crosby 1976) has been detailed; and a large literature describes the events in countries, towns and military camps and personal experiences (Walters 1978; Grist 1979). Much will never be known because of the propaganda surrounding the 1914–18 war in Europe, the Russian Revolution and the lack of reports from many countries including the Middle and Far East and South America.

The origin of the pandemic is not known. Reviewers have commented on a possible origin in China, since many Chinese labourers were migrating from China where influenza was recorded, to the USA and Europe in 1918 (Burnet & Clark 1942; Crosby 1976; Walters 1978). Conversely, documentary evidence indicates that the first outbreaks occurred at approximately the same time in North America at Detroit, South Carolina and San Quentin Prison in March 1918, and reviewers accept that this evidence supports a theory for the origin of the pandemic in the USA (Patterson 1977; Crosby 1989). From here the pandemic can be traced in place and time, and this is shown in Fig. 1.2.

From the three above sites in the USA, the infection spread eastwards as young Americans were drawn to the army and naval training establishments of the American Expeditionary Force (AEF), and to the war in Europe. Although large numbers of cases were recorded, the infection appeared no more virulent than had been seen in the past; however, an increase in deaths among young adults, and some unusual pathological features of some of these fatal cases, was observed and reported, but not appreciated at the time (Crosby 1976). All authors agree that infection was transmitted by ship by the AEF personnel to military depots at Bordeaux, France in April 1918. From here, infection spread to the British Expeditionary Force (BEF) and other forces involved in the war in April/May 1918, and in the same months reached Italy and Spain: the latter country highlighted the pandemic which now carries the name 'Spanish Influenza'. This period also saw outbreaks in Germany, and the pandemic was clearly influencing the course of the war. In June, the disease arrived in Britain, and from there was transmitted by the BEF to Murmansk and Russia, where it spread with great rapidity (see Fig. 1.2). Infection reached North Africa in May 1918 and circled Africa to affect Bombay and Calcutta and then China, New Zealand and the Philippines in June 1918. In each country infection spread quickly for a few weeks and then sharply declined; however, North America, the possible origin of the pandemic, remained virtually free of influenza from June to August 1918, despite large numbers of infected people arriving by boat at the east coast ports. The events

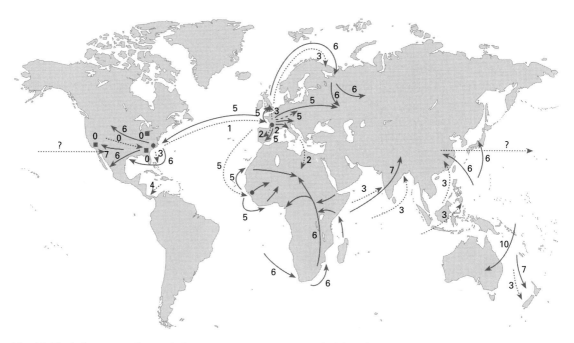

Fig. 1.2 The influenza pandemic of 1918–20. First outbreaks (squares) March 1918; lines of spread of first wave of the pandemic (dashed arrows), and lines of spread of second wave (full arrows); number of months after March 1918 (0) when epidemic infection was recorded (number accompanies corresponding arrow); focal points where onset of second wave was recorded (circles). (From the accounts of Gill 1928; Crosby 1976; Beveridge 1977; Pyle & Patterson 1984; Pyle 1986; Patterson 1987.)

of March–July 1918, outlined above were not viewed as exceptional; pandemics of influenza had occurred before, and the number of deaths recorded were comparable with past experience: in contrast, the events which were to follow remain unique to the history of influenza.

Three events occurred in August 1918 which were so closely related in time that some authors have suggested that they were unconnected; this is most unlikely, but how they are related is not known. Firstly, in August 1918, influenza broke out on a boat travelling from England to Freetown, Sierra Leone; on landing, the affected crew were taken to a local hospital and as a result influenza broke out amongst dock workers and later in other parts of the town. Within a few cycles of infection, it was apparent that the disease had become more virulent, with a 10-fold increase in the death rate amongst cases. Secondly, the influenza epidemic in Europe saw the emergence from Brest, one of the main ports of France serving the needs of the war,

of a markedly more virulent form of influenza which rapidly spread to all of Europe; and from England travelled with an army and naval contingent to Archangel from where it spread throughout Russia. Finally, a ship arriving at Boston, USA from Europe unleashed on that city, and subsequently the whole country, the more lethal form of influenza (see Fig. 1.2); however, with hindsight, it has been suggested that this may have arisen from earlier seeding infection (Glezen 1996). The pandemic reached Australia in January 1919 having been held at bay for some months by quarantine restrictions (Burnet & Clark 1942). Infection spread through Africa from Freetown to other ports, and from there by lines of communication to cause in a few weeks 1.5–2.0 million deaths (Patterson & Pyle 1983); India was infected in October 1918 and the epidemic there resulted in 7 million deaths; the epidemic in North America caused approximately 600 000 deaths; in England and Wales the official deaths numbered 200 000

(Beveridge 1991) and a similar proportion of the populations of other European countries and Australia died, again within a few weeks; and the death rate in Samoa and Alaska was 25% of the population (Beveridge 1991; Ghendon 1994). Many countries experienced second (1918–19) and third waves (1919–20) of the more virulent form of infection. No figures exist for many parts of the world, but the pandemic is estimated to have infected 50% of the world's population; 25% suffered a clinical infection and the total mortality was 40–50 million: the often quoted figure of 20 million deaths is palpably too low (Crosby 1976).

For many doctors and pathologists of the day, the 'Spanish Influenza' presented unique features (Crosby 1976). Patients commonly experienced a sudden onset of severe headache, back pain, fever, epistaxis, anorexia, nausea and vomiting, cough, general aching pains in muscles and joints and a fever of 102–104°F. For most, the symptoms lasted 2–4 days; and, except for the frequent symptom of epistaxis, the symptoms were the well-recognized symptoms of influenza (Nicholson 1992). Many patients recovered completely after the acute attack, but in some cases the fall in temperature was marked by a period of remission after which the temperature rose again with symptoms consistent with a secondary bacterial pneumonia seen following influenza in other outbreaks; many patients died of this complication. The Spanish Influenza, in some patients, followed a different course unique to experienced experts of the day: following the onset of the above acute symptoms, there was clear evidence of tracheobronchitis and bronchiolitis, shortage of breath and the appearance of mahogany spots around the mouth which would extend and coalesce into a violaceous heliotrope cyanosis until, 'a white man could not be discriminated from a coloured' (Grist 1979). A peculiar stench emanated from many patients. With increasing cyanosis patients begin to gasp for breath; blood-stained fluid would froth from the mouth; patients would become delirious, and death would follow from suffocation (MacNeal 1919; Nuzum *et al.* 1976; Starr 1976; Walters 1978; Grist 1979): with rigor mortis, bloody fluid would gush from the mouth and nostrils. The time from hospital admission to death

could be as short as a few hours to 2–3 days. Postmortem examination would not show the signs of secondary bacterial pneumonia; rather, the lungs contained up to a litre of bloodstained, frothy and fibrin-free fluid; petechial and confluent haemorrhages were seen in the lining of the trachea and bronchi; and the lung tissue exhibited intense inflammatory changes with marked local adenopathy (Crosby 1976; Nuzum *et al.* 1976). Deaths were mainly seen in the 20–40-year age group (Collins 1951), and this is distinct from the experience of all other recorded influenza pandemics (Fig. 1.3). Lastly, the death rate seen in the second (August 1918–19) and third (1919–20) waves of the pandemic was approximately 1.5% of all clinical cases of influenza; in all other influenza pandemics, the figure was 10-fold less.

Sera from persons who lived through the 1918–20 pandemic and born before 1933 contain antibody to an influenza A (H1) virus similar to a virus later identified as the cause of swine influenza (Shope 1931). More recently, nine RNA fragments approximately 200 nucleotides long were recovered from the lung tissue of an American serviceman who died from influenza in 1918: these sequences were from genes which code for five different influenza virus proteins. When transcribed to DNA using the reverse transcriptase-polymerase chain reaction (RT-PCR) technique and sequenced these

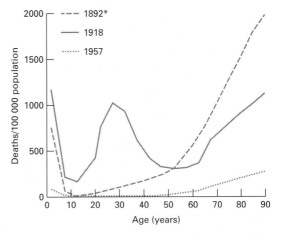

Fig. 1.3 Deaths from pneumonia and influenza in USA in three influenza pandemics. *Massachusetts only. (Adapted from Dauer & Serfling 1961.)

showed close similarity to the influenza virus isolated by Shope (Taubenberger *et al.* 1997). Thus, the antibody studies and the sequence data indicate that the 1918–20 pandemic was caused by an influenza A (H1) virus which is closely related to the virus later found in pigs, and which remains an infection of this species to the present time.

The 'non-pandemic' of 1946–48

Pandemics of influenza which occurred after 1933 can be accurately identified, since the viruses responsible can be isolated and analysed, and the spread of infection accurately monitored. The outbreak of influenza in 1946–47, which was originally considered a pandemic (Kilbourne 1977), was caused by a new influenza A virus, since the virus HA did not crossreact with antibody against previously circulating virus strains: this satisfied one of the two criteria for a pandemic (Webster & Laver 1975). The outbreak was first recognized in Australia in 1946 (Beveridge 1977), though some authors suggest that the virus originated in China (Langmuir 1961; Pyle 1986); and the infection spread to cover the world (Beveridge 1991): this satisfied the second requirement for a pandemic. In addition, vaccination against the earlier virus strain conferred no protection against infection by the new strain (Pyle 1986). However, later commentators, perhaps some with hindsight, pointed out that the epidemic was not truly global (Stuart-Harris 1953; Langmuir & Schoenbaum 1976); that worldwide spread was slow, and not explosive as seen previously (Langmuir 1961); that the pattern of spread was distinct from that of previous pandemics (Pyle 1986); and that the outbreak was relatively mild with low mortality (Kilbourne 1977; Ghendon 1994). The question was resolved when the virus which caused the outbreak was shown to have arisen by extensive mutation from previously circulating influenza (H1) strains, and therefore the epidemic was not a pandemic by definition (Noble 1982). It is possible that, without the data from virus analysis, the 1946–47 outbreak would be classed as a pandemic; and this councils caution in judging historical pandemics from evidence of spread of infection alone.

The pandemic of 1957–58

The influenza virus which caused the 1957–58 pandemic originated in the Yunan Province of China in February 1957 (Pyle 1986); it caused extensive infection in China during March, reached Hong Kong in April, and then spread rapidly to Singapore, Taiwan and Japan (Fukumi 1959). At this point the WHO, which had set up the extensive network of laboratories in 1947 to monitor influenza worldwide, became aware of the outbreak caused by a new influenza virus subtype (Chu *et al.* 1957). A special meeting of authorities on influenza held in May 1957, accurately predicted subsequent events, apart from an early epidemic in Japan: the outbreak would spread quickly to the Southern Hemisphere causing severe epidemics during the winter, and would spread and seed itself in the Northern Hemisphere where latter epidemics would occur in the winter of that region. The spread of the pandemic is shown in Fig. 1.4. Infection spread to India, Australia and Indonesia in May; to Pakistan, Europe, North America and the Middle East in June; to South Africa, South America, New Zealand and the Pacific Islands in July; and to Central, West and East Africa, eastern Europe and the Caribbean in August (Dunn 1958; Payne 1958). Two major land routes of spread were firstly, across Russia to Scandinavia and Eastern Europe (Payne 1958; Langmuir 1961); and secondly, from a large conference held at Grinnel, Iowa involving 1800 young persons from 43 states and several foreign countries, which drew individuals from epidemic areas to initiate an outbreak of 200 cases during the conference and allowed much dissemination from infected individuals returning home (see Fig. 1.4). Except for these two events, infection was transmitted mainly along sea lanes; transmission by aeroplanes was not a major method of spread (Pyle 1986). Thus, within approximately 6 months, the pandemic had spanned the globe. In most countries infection was first seen in ports, then urban areas and later in rural areas; infection was first seen in schoolchildren, then preschool children and adults (Jordan 1961).

Most detailed studies of the pandemic come from North America and Europe where infection was

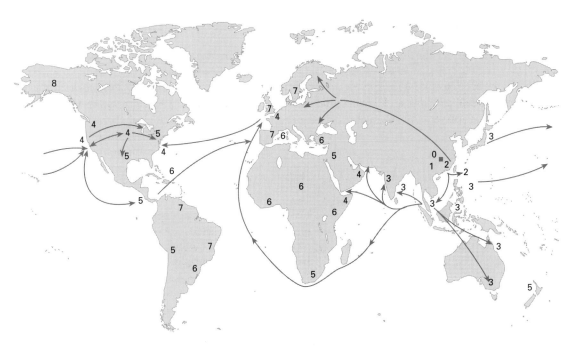

Fig. 1.4 The influenza pandemic of 1957–58. Point of origin (square) February 1957; lines of spread of the pandemic (arrows); number of months after February 1957 (0) when epidemic infection was recorded (number accompanies corresponding arrow). (Adapted from Payne 1958.)

seeded from June 1957, and where the first outbreaks started in September with the peak in October of that year; epidemics coincided with the opening of the winter school term (Payne 1958). A second wave of infection was observed early in 1958, which broke out in numerous regions including Europe, North America, the former USSR and Japan (Payne 1958): the two waves of infection were similar in severity in some countries (Dauer & Serfling 1961), but greater for the second wave in others (McDonald 1958): together, the pandemic affected some 40–50% of people, of which 25–30% experienced clinical disease. The course of infection was clinically typical (Nicholson 1992), with most deaths due to secondary bacterial pneumonia. The mortality rate was estimated at approximately 1/4000; these occurred predominantly in the very young and very old (see Fig. 1.3). Deaths due to the pandemic were calculated at approximately 80 000 in the USA (Dauer & Serfling 1961), and a similar

number, adjusted for population, occurred in many other countries; thus, the total death rate probably exceeded 1 million people.

The influenza virus subtype which caused the 1957–58 pandemic differed from previous recognized influenza viruses in both the HA and neuraminidase (NA) surface glycoproteins, and could not have arisen from previously circulating virus strains. The evidence suggests that this influenza A (H2) virus was a reassortant resulting from a dual infection with a human and avian influenza virus (Webster & Laver 1972; Scholtissek *et al.* 1978b) which possibly took place in a pig (Scholtissek *et al.* 1985), since both the HA and NA were probably derived from an avian origin whilst the other genes were derived from a human virus (Scholtissek *et al.* 1978b; Kawaoka *et al.* 1989). The result was a new virus subtype capable of infecting humans: since immunity is principally dependent upon serum antibody to the virus HA, and to a lesser extent the NA, immunity acquired by past influenza infection had no value in protecting people, and infection spread throughout the world. In contrast, sera taken from elderly people before the pandemic was shown to have antibody against the H2 of the new virus strain: this suggests that they had experienced infection by this virus in the past, and offers an explanation for the lower attack rate in older people (Payne 1958). By matching the presence of antibody to age, epidemiologists have estimated that an influenza A (H2) virus probably caused the pandemic of 1898–92 (Davenport *et al.* 1969; Masurel & Marine 1973), and again indicates that the influenza viruses which cause pandemics in humans may disappear and then reappear when immunity has disappeared from the world with the death of previously infected people (see above). Where the virus may persist in the interim period is unknown. We remain ignorant as to which of the above two explanations for the origin of pandemics is correct; however, the two theories are not incompatible. It is arguable that a variety of reassortants may arise at any time, and that the same serotype may emerge at different times: given that only a few subtypes can cause pandemic infection and that antibody acquired during previous infection may be a selective factor which determines when a particular subtype can cause a pandemic, the cyclical occurrence of subtypes would follow.

The pandemic of 1968–70

The outbreak of influenza which began in China in July 1968, first reported in the London *Times*, spread to Hong Kong in the same month to initiate an epidemic of 500 000 cases (Chang 1969; Cockburn *et al.* 1969); the epidemic was quickly shown to be caused by a new virus subtype, designated influenza A (H3). By August infection had spread to Taiwan, the Philippines, Singapore and Vietnam; and by September to India, Australia and Iran. This pattern of spread from a focal point in China closely resembled the pattern of the 1957–58 pandemic; however, from this point differences were observed (Cockburn *et al.* 1969). Infection failed to spread in Japan, and a significant epidemic did not occur in that country until January 1969. Infection entered North America in September via California from troops returning from Vietnam, and after extensive seeding, spread from East to West throughout the country (Sharrar 1969); the epidemic built up to a peak in December 1968 when mortality was as high as in the 1957–58 pandemic. Influenza was first

diagnosed in the UK and much of Europe from September 1968, but spread slowly with extensive seeding as a mild outbreak to peak with greatest mortality in December 1969; however, this epidemic was reported to be relatively mild (Roden 1969; Stuart-Harris 1979). Why the experience of North America and Europe, with peak mortality rates a year apart, was so distinct is not known. Finally the epidemic reached South America and South Africa in mid-1969.

The global spread of infection in 1968, and analysis which showed that this epidemic was caused by a new virus subtype, defined the outbreak as a pandemic. The NA antigen was similar to the earlier virus, and, since antibodies to this glycoprotein confer partial protection against clinical disease though not virus infection (Johansson *et al.* 1989), this may explain the relative mildness of the pandemic. In contrast, the HA was probably derived by reassortment from an avian source (Scholtissek *et al.* 1978b; Kawaoka *et al.* 1989) against which the population had no immunity. Antibody to the HA of the 1968–69 virus was identified in sera collected before 1968 from elderly persons alive during the 1898–1900 pandemic (Masurel 1969), suggesting that the two pandemics were caused by related viruses. This reiterates the cyclical theory of influenza pandemics: again there is no information as to where the virus survived in the intervening 70 years, but this is not essential to the theory since the virus may have recurred (see above).

The pandemic of 1977–78

From the end of May 1977, outbreaks of influenza were recorded in three Chinese provinces, and the virus responsible was rapidly recognized as the influenza A (H1) subtype and distinct from the influenza viruses which had circulated from 1968 to that time (Kung *et al.* 1978). In November, further outbreaks were recorded in China, Taiwan, the Philippines, Siberia, Singapore and parts of Russia (Zhdanov *et al.* 1978); in January, outbreaks were recorded in North America, the UK, a number of central European countries and Japan; by February, epidemics were reported from other parts of North America, Scandinavia, the southern countries of

Europe and the Middle East; by March, the outbreak had reached Australia and central America; and by June South America and New Zealand were affected. All the outbreaks were described as mild and occurred almost exclusively to persons under 20 years of age. Analysis of the virus strain which caused the pandemic showed it to be closely related to the influenza A (H1) viruses which circulated from 1947 to 1957: this explains why infections were concentrated in the young, since persons aged 20 years or more had experienced the infection earlier and possessed some immunity.

This worldwide outbreak of influenza, originating in China and encompassing the globe within 10 months, may be classed as a pandemic since it satisfies both criteria of the definition; however, the outbreak challenges current perceptions of an influenza pandemic. Firstly, the spread of the outbreak was certainly global, but infection was limited to young persons and therefore was not all embracing. It could be argued that the pandemics of 1957 and 1968 had the highest attack rates in younger persons, since the elderly had antibodies acquired from childhood infection with related virus strains in 1989–92 and 1898–1901, respectively: in 1977, the situation was in principal no different, but a larger proportion of people had previously acquired antibody and were immune. Secondly, the virus was not derived from a previously circulating strain, but was nearly identical to virus strains circulating from 1947 to 1957 (Scholtissek *et al.* 1978a); indeed, knowing the speed and extent of antigenic drift which occurs in influenza A viruses, it is difficult to understand how the virus had remained so stable in the intervening decades, and to suggest that the outbreak was not part of the natural pattern of influenza pandemics. Lastly, in all the pandemics that had taken place since the influenza A virus was isolated in 1933, the previously circulating virus subtype had disappeared with the emergence of the new subtype; however, in the present case, influenza A (H3) strains continued to cause epidemics in parallel with the new influenza A (H1) strains, and this situation of dual circulation of the two virus subtypes continues to the present day (1998). The feature of pandemics that the previously circulating

serotype disappears with the emergence of a new subtype, is not part of the definition of a pandemic; but if the 1977 outbreak is to be classed as a pandemic, this behaviour is a departure from previous pandemic experience. In contrast, if the 1977 outbreak is not to be classed as a pandemic, the definition of a pandemic should be extended.

Conclusion

Although the study of influenza pandemics is of absorbing interest to epidemiologists and medical historians, it also serves to underline the importance of this disease in periodically causing great morbidity, significant mortality and to be socially and economically disruptive. In addition, the repeating pattern of pandemics, and our accepted inability to predict or contain them, indicates that pandemics will occur in the future. It is therefore important to analyse the past for information that might help in the future.

Origin of pandemics

Table 1.1 records 10 pandemics, agreed by all reviewers, that have occurred in the past 400 years, and two probable pandemics in 1799–1802 and 1847–48. Of these 12 episodes, the point of origin is suggested as China/Russia/Asia for all 11 where data were available. This analysis clearly indicates that the next pandemic will probably originate in this area, and this view is supported by many authorities; however, some reservations should attend this conclusion. Firstly, attention has been drawn to the xenogenic attitude of many commentators — the wish to identify the origin of a pandemic as somewhere else (Crosby 1976; Pyle & Patterson 1984) — and the loud voices of Europe and North America who seek evidence of origin in the silent spaces of Eastern countries, particularly China (Beveridge 1977; Glezen 1996). This is particularly true of the pandemics of 1918 when the first outbreaks were recorded in North America (Crosby 1976), 1889 when the early outbreaks were in Russia (Patterson 1987) and the epidemic of 1947 when the causal virus was first isolated in Australia (Beveridge 1977); in all cases, authorities have argued for an earlier origin in China (Burnet & Clark 1942; Walters 1978). Secondly, the areas of China/Russia/Asia cover some one-third of inhabited lands of the planet, and to identify this area as the origin of pandemic influenza lacks rigour. Finally, the most plausible theory for the origin of pandemic influenza viruses is reassortment of human and avian viruses in pigs (see Chapter 13). It is China where one-quarter of the population of the earth live, and where ducks, pigs and humans live in the closest proximity and the highest density, that the reassortment is most likely to occur; thus, to incriminate China as the origin of past and future pandemics is convenient. China may, and probably is, the origin of most pandemics (Shortridge & Stuart-Harris 1982), but the historical record need not be distorted to support this theory, since reassortant viruses could arise elsewhere.

Season of pandemics

Of the 12 agreed and probable pandemics recorded in Table 1.1, there is no apparent season that coincides with the start of a pandemic, though numerically spring/summer starts are more frequent than autumn/winter (Pyle & Patterson 1984). Given the above theories for the mechanism underlying the emergence of new pandemic influenza viruses, there does not appear to be any reason why season should be a determining factor.

Climate for pandemics

Although the origin of pandemics may not be related to a particular season, the effects of climate on the spread of pandemics have been commented on by numerous authors. Epidemic spread during the spring and summer months were slow in 1889 and accurately predicted to be relatively slow in the Northern Hemispheres in 1957 and 1968; however, the distinct history of the 1968 pandemic in North America and Europe is unexplained, and suggests that more subtle factors are involved than just season. Authors have drawn attention to the importance of low temperatures (Jordan 1961; Davey & Reid 1972), high relative humidity (Jordan 1927) or a combination of these factors for the

spread of pandemic infection (Gill 1928; Noble 1982). It can be assumed that these are but two of the climatic factors which influence spread (Jordan 1927). A second factor for transmission is crowding, which can also be influenced by the above: people crowd in cold weather (Jordan 1927), children crowd in schools—where outbreaks frequently begin (Davey & Reid 1972)—and families crowd in winter months (Beveridge 1977). A further consideration is the survival of the virus since this affects transmission: the influenza virus survives best at low temperatures and high humidity, which again relates to the climatic factors mentioned above (Schulman & Kilbourne 1961). Finally, spread may be clinically inapparent in summer months but extensive seeding can occur during this time (Beveridge 1977). Outbreaks often begin in schools, spreading to adults in their families: the elderly, without contact with young children, are less likely to be affected, at least in the first waves (McDonald 1958; Jordan 1961).

Waves of infection

A common characteristic of pandemics is several waves of infection (Patterson 1987), and that second and subsequent waves are frequently more severe than the initial wave (see Table 1.1): the pandemic of 1918–20 is a dramatic example. The reasons for this are not known. It has been suggested that with increasing cycles of human infection, the virus may become more virulent (Beveridge 1977), but this is unlikely. More probably, it is the later waves which affect the older, and more susceptible who have escaped infection in initial outbreaks which concentrate in children and their immediate families, and who may have residual immunity due to previous exposure, that influences the statistics; however, the experience of 1918–20 is an exception to this.

Timing of pandemics

The interval of time between the 12 pandemics listed in Table 1.1 varies from a decade (1889–1900 and 1957–68) to 50 years (1729/33–1781/82): the interval has not significantly increased or decreased with the passage of time suggesting that increased population, travel, and so on are not determining factors. Alternatively, if analysis is based solely on the 10 agreed pandemics (see Table 1.1), the interval between pandemics in the period from 1700 to 1889 is 50–60 years and for the period since 1889 is 10–40 years; the interval may therefore be shortening, and if more recent experience is to be a guide, the next pandemic will be before 2008 counting from 1968, or 2017 if the pandemic of 1977 is accepted. Failure attends attempts to find a recurring pattern, as suggested by the cyclic theory, that would be predictive; either a pattern cannot be seen because of mistakes in recognizing past pandemics and the inclusion of non-pandemics, or no pattern exists. If pandemics occur in cycles the best fit for a cycle is to recognize that the pandemic of 1957 by influenza virus A (H2) and 1968 by influenza A (H3) are 11 years apart and these match to the pandemics of 1889 by influenza A (H2) and 1900 by influenza A (H3) with the same time interval; assuming that the influenza A (H1) pandemic of 1918–20 is the third point in the cycle, the pandemics since 1847 show a fit with time, with intervals of approximately 10, 20 and 40 years between the three points: this suggests that the next pandemic should have occurred in about 1988. This failed prediction ignores the pandemic of 1977: if this episode is included in the analysis, the time intervals between pandemics given above are distorted, and at best suggests the next pandemic will occur in about 2017. It should be evident from the above that speculation as to the date of the next pandemic is unrewarding.

References

Beveridge, W.I.B. (1977) *Influenza: The Last Great Plague.* Heinemann, London.

Beveridge, W.I.B. (1991) The chronicle of influenza epidemics. *Hist Phil Life Sci* **13**, 223–35.

Brown, M.W. (1932) Early epidemics of influenza in America. *J Med Records* **135**, 449–51.

Burnet, F.M. & Clark, E. (1942) *Influenza.* Macmillan, London.

Chang, W.K. (1969) National influenza experience in Hong Kong, 1968. *Bull WHO* **41**, 349–51.

Chu, C.M., Shao, C. & Hou, C.C. (1957) Studies of strains of influenza virus isolated during the epidemic in 1957 in Changchun. *Voprosy Virusologii* **2**, 278–81.

Cockburn, W.C., Delon, P.J. & Ferreira, W. (1969) Origin and progress of the 1968–89 Hong Kong influenza epidemic. *Bull WHO* **41**, 345–53.

Collins, S.D. (1951) Trends on epidemics of influenza and pneumonia, 1918–51. *Public Health Rep* **66**, 1487–516.

Creighton, C. (1894) *A History of Epidemics in Britain.* Cambridge University Press, London.

Crosby, A.W. (1972) *The Columbian Exchange: Biological and Cultural Consequences of 1492.* Greenwood Press, Westford, CT.

Crosby, A.W. (1976) *Epidemic and Peace, 1918.* Greenwood Press, Westford, CT.

Crosby, A.W. (1989) *America's Forgotten Pandemic: The Influenza of 1918.* Cambridge University Press, Cambridge.

Dauer, C.C. & Serfling, R.E. (1961) Mortality from influenza. 1957–58 and 1959–60. *Am Rev Resp Dis* **83**, 15–28.

Davenport, F.M., Minuse, E., Hennessy, A.V. & Francis, T. (1969) Interpretations of influenza antibody patterns of man. *Bull WHO* **41**, 453–60.

Davey, M.L. & Reid, D. (1972) Relationship of air temperature to outbreaks of influenza. *Br J Prevent Soc Med* **26**, 28–32.

Dunn, F.L. (1958) Pandemic influenza in 1957. *J Am Med Assoc* **166**, 1140–8.

Finkler, D. (1899) Influenza in twentieth century practice. In: Shipman, T.L. (ed.) *An International Encyclopaedia of Modern Medical Science*, pp. 21–32, abstract 12. Sampson Law & Marston, London.

Frost, W.H. (1919) The epidemiology of influenza. *J Am Med Assoc* **73**, 313–18.

Fukumi, H. (1959) Summary report of the Asian influenza epidemic in Japan, 1957. *Bull WHO* **20**, 187–98.

Ghendon, Y. (1994) Introduction to pandemic influenza through history. *Eur J Epidemiol* **10**, 451–3.

Gill, C.A. (1928) *The Genetics of Epidemics.* Baillière Tindall, London.

Glezen, W.P. (1996) Emerging infections: pandemic influenza. *Epidemiol Rev* **18**, 65–76.

Grist, N.R. (1979) Pandemic influenza 1918. *Br Med J* **ii**, 1632–3.

Grmek, M.D. (1893) *Les Maladies a l'Aube de la Civilization Accidentale.* Payot, Paris.

Hirsch, A. (1883) *Handbook of Geographical and Historical Pathology.* New Sydenham Society, London.

Johansson, B.E., Bucher, D.J. & Kilbourne, E.D. (1989) Purified influenza virus haemagglutinin and neuraminidase are equivalent in stimulating antibody response, but induce contrasting types of immunity to infection. *J Virol* **63**, 1239–46.

Jordan, E.O. (1927) *Epidemic Influenza: A Survey.* American Medical Association, Chicago.

Jordan, W.S. (1961) Mechanism of spread of Asian influenza. *Am Rev Resp Dis* **83**, 29–35.

Kawaoka, Y., Krauss, S. & Webster, R.G. (1989) Avian-to-human transmission of the PB$_1$ gene of influenza A viruses in the 1957 and 1958 pandemics. *J Virol* **63**, 4603–8.

Kilbourne, E.D. (1977) Influenza pandemics in perspective. *J Am Med Assoc* **237**, 1225–8.

Kung, H.C., Jen, K.F., Yuan, W.C., Tien, S.F. & Chu, C.M. (1978) Influenza in China in 1977: recurrence of influenza virus A subtype H1N1 *Bull WHO* **56**, 913–18.

Langmuir, A.D. & Schoenbaum, S.C. (1976) The epidemiology of influenza. *Hosp Pract* **11**, 49–56.

Langmuir, A.D. (1961) Epidemiology of Asian influenza. *Am Rev Resp Dis* **83**, 2–18.

MacNeal, W.J. (1919) The influenza epidemic of 1918 in the American Expeditionary Forces in France and England. *Arch Int Med* **23**, 657–88.

Masurel, N. & Marine, W.M. (1973) Recycling of Asian and Hong Kong influenza A virus haemagglutinin in man. *Am J Epidemiol* **97**, 44–9.

Masurel, N. (1969) Serological characteristics of a 'new' serotype of influenza A virus: the Hong Kong strain. *Bull WHO* **41**, 461–8.

McDonald, J.C. (1958) Asian influenza in Great Britain 1957-58. *Proc Roy Soc Med* **51**, 1016–18.

Molineux, T. (1694) Dr Molineux's historical account of the late general coughs and colds; with some observations on other epidemic distemper. *Phil Trans Roy Soc Lond* **18**, 105–9.

Nicholson, K.G. (1992) Clinical features of influenza. *Sem Resp Infect* **7**, 26–37.

Noble, G.R. (1982) Epidemiological and clinical aspects of influenza. In: Beare, A.S. (ed.) *Basic and Applied Influenza Research*, pp. 11–50, CRC Press, Boca Raton.

Nuzum, J.W., Pilot, I., Stangl, F.A. & Bovar, B.E. (1976) 1918 pandemic influenza and pneumonia in a large civil hospital. *Illinois Med J* **150**, 612–16.

Parsons, H.F. (1891) The influenza epidemics of 1889–90 and 1891 and their distribution in England and Wales. *Br Med J* ii, 303–10.

Parsons, H.F. (1893) Further Report and Papers on Epidemic Influenza, 1889–92, Local Government Board. Eyre and Spottiswood, London.

Patterson, K.D. & Pyle, G.F. (1983) The diffusion of influenza in sub-Sahara Africa during the 1918–19 pandemic. *Soc Sci Med* **17**, 1299–307.

Patterson, K.D. (1985) Pandemic and epidemic influenza 1830–1848. *Soc Sci Med* **21**, 571–80.

Patterson, K.D. (1987) *Pandemic Influenza 1700–1900: A Study in Historical Epidemiology*. Rowman & Littlefield, New Jersey.

Payne, A.M.-M. (1958) Symposium on the Asian influenza epidemic, 1957. *Proc Roy Soc Med* **51**, 1009–15.

Pyle, G.F. & Patterson, K.D. (1984) Influenza diffusion in European history: patterns and paradigms. *Ecol Dis* **2**, 173–84.

Pyle, G.F. (1986) *The Diffusion of Influenza: Patterns and Paradigms*. Rowan & Littlefield, New Jersey.

Roden, A.T. (1969) National experience with Hong Kong influenza in the UK, 1968–69. *Bull WHO* **41**, 375–80.

Sage, M.W. (1985) Pittsburgh plague—1918: an oral history. *Home Healthcare Nurse* **13**, 49–54.

Scholtissek, C., Burger, H., Kistner, O. & Shortridge, K.F. (1985) The nucleoprotein as a possible major factor in determining host specificity of influenza H3N2 viruses. *Virology* **147**, 287–94.

Scholtissek, C., von Hoyningen, V. & Rott, R. (1978a) Genetic relatedness between the new 1977 epidemic strains (H1N1) of influenza and human influenza strains isolated between 1947 and 1857. *Virology* **89**, 613–17.

Scholtissek, C., Rhode, W., von Hoyningen, V. & Rott, R. (1978b) On the origins of the human influenza virus subtypes H2N2 and H3N2. *Virology* **87**, 13–20.

Schulman, J.L. & Kilbourne, E.D. (1961) Experimental transmission of influenza virus infection in mice. II. Some factors affecting the incidence of transmitted infection. *J Exp Med* **118**, 267–75.

Sharrar, R.G. (1969) National influenza experience in the USA 1968-69. *Bull WHO* **41**, 361–6.

Shope, R.E. (1931) Swine influenza. III. Filtration experiments and aetiology. *J Exp Med* **54**, 373–80.

Shortridge, K.F. & Stuart-Harris, C.H. (1982) An influenza epicentre? *Lancet* ii, 812–13.

Smillie, W.G. & Kilbourne, E.D. (1963) *Preventative Medicine and Public Health*, pp. 192–7. Macmillan, New York.

Starr, I. (1976) Influenza in 1918: recollections of the epidemic in Philadelphia. *Ann Int Med* **85**, 516–18.

Stuart-Harris, C.H. (1953) *Influenza*. Edward Semple, London.

Stuart-Harris, C.H. (1979) Epidemiology of influenza in man. *Br Med Bull* **35**, 3–8.

Taubenberger, J.K., Reid, A.H., Krafft, A.E. *et al.* (1997) Initial genetic characterization of the 1918 'Spanish' influenza virus. *Science* **275**, 1793–6.

Thompson, E.S. (1890) *Influenza*. Pervical, London.

Walters, J.H. (1978) Influenza 1918: the contemporary perspective. *Bull NY Acad Med* **54**, 855–64.

Waring, J.I. (1971) *A History of Medicine in South Carolina, 1900-70*, p. 33. South Carolina Medical Association.

Webster, N. (1800) *A Brief History of Epidemic and Pestiential Diseases*, Vol. 2, Section 12, pp. 39–58. Woodall, London.

Webster, R.G. & Laver, W.G. (1972) The origin of pandemic influenza. *Bull WHO* **47**, 449–52.

Webster, R.G. & Laver, W.G. (1975) Pandemic variation of influenza viruses. In: Kilbourne, E.D. (ed.) *The Influenza Viruses and Influenza*, pp. 269–314. Academic Press, New York.

Zhdanov, V.M., Lvov, D.K., Zakstelskaya, L.Y. *et al.* (1978) Return of epidemic A1 (H1N1) influenza virus. *Lancet* **i**, 294–5.

CHAPTER 2

Discovery of Influenza Viruses

David Tyrrell

As we have seen, good clinical observation and epidemiological recording had indicated that there was a distinctive disease commonly known as influenza. Its comings and goings could not be predicted. Some observers thought it was related to climate or other more mysterious 'influences' but in certain circumstances it seemed to behave as a communicable disease spreading across a country, from human to human, though at times it seemed to be associated with similar illnesses in animals, such as horses. However, there was no clinical observation, such as the exanthems of smallpox or chickenpox, that could be used to distinguish it from other febrile infections with respiratory tract symptoms, particularly in individual cases. However, in characteristic outbreaks there was a high incidence particularly noticeable among young adults. Patients were prostrated with high fever and muscle aches. Pneumonia might supervene and there was a low but distinct mortality which was not seen in common respiratory catarrhal conditions. Thus influenza cases and outbreaks could be recognized and distinguished from the general run of colds and allied illnesses but there were relatively few such influenza epidemics in the latter half of the 19th century and therefore little to study.

In the 1880s and 1890s it became possible to culture bacteria and using the new methods organisms such as *Vibrio cholerae* were discovered and shown to cause epidemic diseases such as cholera. So investigators looked for a characteristic bacterium as the cause of influenza—there was ample opportunity since there was a worldwide epidemic of influenza in 1889 after which epidemics were

more frequent and severe. Many different organisms were found in respiratory secretions. One candidate was a bacillus found by Pfeiffer. Even though it was not found in all cases or in all outbreaks it was widely believed to cause the syndrome and this is commemorated in its present name of *Haemophilus influenzae*. It is worth remembering that by the early 1900s the concept of pathogenic filterable viruses was established. They were recognized as causes of diseases as varied as tobacco mosaic disease, rinderpest of cattle and fowl plague. They were detected by a standard set of experiments in which bacteria were removed by filtration and then the disease was reproduced by inoculating experimental animals or plants. Thus filtered respiratory secretions from cases of influenza were inoculated into laboratory animals, but these attempts were unsuccessful, or at least unconvincing. At the end of World War I a pandemic in three waves of influenza swept across the world, killing young and old in many different communities (Medical Research Committee 1919, Ministry of Health, 1920). In certain places, in spite of the terrible dislocation of life, detailed pathological and bacteriological studies were made. It was observed that the characteristic severe pneumonia, which was responsible for so much of the mortality, showed a remarkable histopathological picture— there was a hyaline membrane lining the alveoli, and intra-alveolar haemorrhage—though in many cases there was also inflammation as found in bacterial pneumonia and indeed bacteria were both seen and cultured. But in outbreaks in different localities different invading bacteria were found, for instance pneumococci in one area and haemolytic streptococci and *Haemophilus* in another, but sometimes there were cases in which no bacteria could be seen or cultured.

Hunting for a virus

As the epidemic subsided there was a common belief that it must have been due to a rapidly spreading virus which had not yet been detected, and that the bacteria were secondary invaders. Yet some thought that *H. influenzae* could be the cause while others had claimed to grow a 'virus' in so-called Noguchi cultures in which cubes of rabbit kidney in ascitic fluid were sealed with paraffin and inoculated with drops of clinical material. The 'virus' appeared as a visible cloud of small particles visible under the light microscope (Medical Research Committee 1919; Topley & Wilson 1929). These methods were later discredited. Animal inoculations were done but were unconvincing. But there were serious disagreements throughout the 1920s and as late as 1929 the problem seemed insoluble to a distinguished bacteriologist like W. Scott and an authoritative textbook of bacteriology stated that there was general agreement that the existence of a virus had not 'been satisfactorily demonstrated' (Topley & Wilson 1929). But the social dislocation and mortality had been so terrible that it was felt that something ought to be done about it. The sight or story of healthy young men being struck down and dying within a day or two aroused fear and panic in some but it was also a spur to research organizations to tackle the problem of finding the cause of the disease before it struck again.

In 1922 the Medical Research Council (MRC), who had already expressed themselves as dissatisfied with the state of bacteriology in Britain, announced a policy to encourage research on viruses. They were already supporting work at St Bartholomew's Hospital on the diagnosis of smallpox and they decided to develop further work at the newly founded National Institute for Medical Research (NIMR) which was housed in an old chest hospital at Holly Hill, Hampstead (Thomson 1987). They wished to see advances in the methods for studying viruses and recruited a varied group of individuals. One was a volunteer who came up to the laboratory after attending to his business in central London. He was a skilled amateur microscopist, Barnard, who developed ultraviolet light microscopes with which he visualized the larger virus particles such as those of smallpox. Then there was Elford, a physicist who refined methods such as ultrafiltration through collodion membranes and ultracentrifugation so that they could be used to determine the size of infectious virus particles.

Dog distemper and other viruses

The MRC also wanted work to be done on a specific virus infection and they were in fact approached through the *Field* magazine to study distemper of dogs which was affecting up to 50% of puppies at the time. With the request came a generous offer of funds without which they could not have completed the research. Thus the Council agreed to take on the project at the NIMR and after the initial stages the project was run by Dr (later Sir Patrick) Laidlaw. He was a very able man who had worked with the director, the great Sir Henry Dale; however, he was very modest and retiring and liked to work by supporting and encouraging younger members of his department. Because the disease was so highly infectious it was necessary to set up special facilities in which to house, breed and in due course experiment on the animals. Thus, land was acquired at Mill Hill, at that time outside the London conurbation, and suitable quarters were built and a strict isolation regime was set up in which the animal technicians and scientific staff wore protective clothing and were decontaminated on entering and leaving the unit. Such work was vehemently opposed by some dog lovers. However, there was a story that in country areas ferrets caught the disease when there was an outbreak among dogs. Experiments showed that ferrets were indeed highly susceptible and suffered a clear-cut disease. This made them a useful and relatively convenient animal with which to detect and study the virus. In due course a vaccination procedure was developed and handed over to Wellcome Laboratories to develop into a commercial product.

The MRC also recruited from St Bartholomew's Hospital a brilliant young man with biological leanings, Christopher Andrewes, whose father was Professor of Pathology in the Medical School and who had made a study of influenza during the pandemic (1920). Although medically trained, the young Dr Andrewes was more interested in laboratory research and natural history (Tyrrell 1991). After preliminary work at the NIMR he then spent 2 years at the Rockefeller Institute in New York City studying rheumatic fever. He worked for a while on cancer viruses and in the USA on a virus of rabbits. When he returned to the UK he co-operated with Elford and began to prove that virus infectivity was carried on particles of different sizes. It had been shown that antigens and antibodies reacted with each other in quantitatively predictable ways, but there was a view at the time that viruses were in some way different. With a visiting worker, Burnet from Australia, he studied some model systems that were available in the Institute and showed that virus neutralization obeyed simple quantitative laws. Thus, these studies began to reveal the characteristics of viruses, not by negative criteria—such as that they could not be seen with a microscope and could not be cultivated in the media used for growing bacteria—but positively, by their size and ability to react with specific antisera. Dale had specially invited Burnet to come to enhance his team and he also studied the growth of viruses in embryonated eggs (Burnet & Ferry 1934) Later in life he received the Nobel Prize—and Dale was justified in thinking that it was more important to gather good staff than to build bigger laboratories.

Common colds and swine influenza

In 1930 Andrewes was 'stranded' in New York because his father had suffered a mild stroke while visiting the city and he needed to wait with his son until he was well enough to undertake the journey home. To fill in time he visited Dochez at the College of Physicians and Surgeons to see his experiments to show that common colds could be transmitted to human beings and chimpanzees, held in strict isolation, by intranasal inoculation of filtered nasal secretions. Dochez also claimed to have transmitted the cold virus through serial passages in cultures of chopped suspended chick

embryo tissue. When Andrewes returned to London he tried to repeat Dochez's results using volunteers—Bart's Hospital medical students (Andrewes 1965). The MRC could not afford to have isolation facilities set up and although he produced colds with nasal secretions from cold sufferers he could not produce colds with cultured material—even some brought by Dochez from New York by sea—and, because some colds may have been picked up as the volunteers went about their business in London, the results seemed likely to continue to be negative or inconclusive so the project was dropped in 1932 (Andrewes 1965).

Meanwhile in the USA a young physician, Richard Shope, was working on the problem of influenza in pigs. He came from Iowa and had intended to study forestry but he became interested in the study of infectious diseases. He was a genial and friendly person but he had an independent and enquiring mind, quite willing to follow an unusual idea. There had been some evidence that outbreaks of influenza in swine had occurred in the Middle West states at about the time of the human pandemic and in subsequent winters. This resurrection of an old idea stimulated work at the Princeton branch of the Rockefeller Institute in New York where Shope was employed. Using the methods of the day he showed that bacteria-free filtrates produced a mild illness if inoculated intranasally into young pigs but the full-blown disease was produced if they were also given the bacterium *Haemophilus influenzae suis*—the pig equivalent of the human organism—and this work was published in the prestigious *Journal of Experimental Medicine* in 1931 (Shope 1931).

Finally there was a young bacteriologist at NIMR who was working under Laidlaw; his name was Wilson Smith. He was a northerner with a stern face and manner and a dry sense of humour. He had had a difficult childhood and was known to be very careful, reliable and hard working.

Human influenza—and serendipity

All these somewhat disconnected strands came together in 1933 when there was a sharp epidemic of influenza in the London area. It was decided to try to prove the presence of an influenza virus by transmitting disease to animals. Wilson Smith collected throat washings from cases including colleagues and himself and, while Andrewes was laid low by the virus, he inoculated his washings by various routes including the intranasal routes used by Shope and Dochez. He used ferrets since they were available for the distemper work (Figs 2.1 and 2.2). There was also a story emanating from the Wellcome Laboratories that their ferrets had just caught

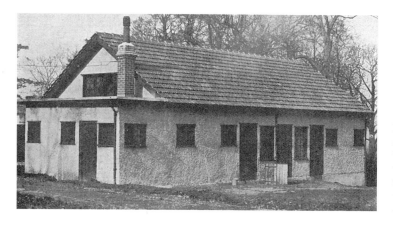

Fig. 2.1 The house designed for the study of distemper in dogs. This was used to house ferrets in isolation for the first successful transmission of influenza at Mill Hill, London, UK. (From: *The Field Distemper Fund, Report for June 1925.*)

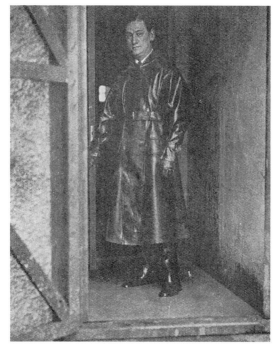

Fig. 2.2 An attendant at the door of the building, wearing rubber clothing which was washed down with disinfectant when the attendant went in and out and before going from one infected animal to another. There is a bath of disinfectant at the entrance. (From: *The Field Distemper Fund, Report for June 1925.*)

influenza (though it finally turned out to be distemper). The only illnesses were in, but only in, the ferrets; they developed high fever, nasal discharge and sneezing, and were obviously unwell. The work was dislocated by influenza infections in the staff and by distemper in the NIMR ferrets and the two viruses may well have been mixed up. In the end the issue was clarified by isolating a virus from Wilson Smith which he may well have caught from a ferret but which would have been freed from distemper virus because that virus would not have grown in his throat (Andrewes 1984). So finally it was concluded that there was a filterable virus present, which could be transmitted serially from ferret to ferret and rendered them immune to reinfection. This was seen as an important advance when the results were published in 1933 (Smith *et al.* 1933). The detailed study of pathology or epidemiology was not able to provide any more understanding until the causative agent could be detected and studied in the laboratory. There was even a cartoon of Andrewes and other doctors on horseback behind a pack of ferrets bounding in pursuit of a retreating virus to the cry of 'Yoicks and Tally Ho' (Fig. 2.3) — he enjoyed that and had it hung on his wall.

Andrewes and Shope kept in touch and exchanged news, ideas, viruses and other reagents. They shared

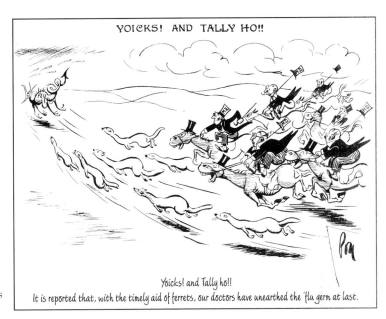

YOICKS! AND TALLY HO!!

Yoicks! and Tally ho!!
It is reported that, with the timely aid of ferrets, our doctors have unearthed the 'flu germ at last.

Fig. 2.3 The cartoon resulting from the first reports of the infection of ferrets, published in the *Evening News* in 1933.

an enthusiasm for life and science, they loved the outdoors and both had a boyish sense of humour (Andrewes 1979). They corresponded on much else besides science often in hilarious terms and continued thus until Shope died. When confirming the NIMR work Shope had found it easier to infect ferrets if he anaesthetized them (Shope 1934) and then it was found that mice, which had seemed to be resistant could be infected under anaesthesia and would develop lung lesions—here was another step forward (Andrewes *et al.* 1934). Mice, being small and easy to handle, could be used to titrate virus and to measure antibody by neutralization tests.

The news was quickly passed from London to New York but it appeared that Francis had just made the same observation and was under pressure to publish at once. Cables were exchanged and it was agreed to press on with publication of the English results and then Francis would publish his. These discoveries created some excitement but their greatest importance was that they provided a means by which influenza viruses could be detected and studied in any reasonably well-equipped research laboratory. Further studies confirmed that the virus grown was a major cause of epidemics. A new recruit to the laboratory, Stuart-Harris, was doing a routine 'round' to check

on the clinical status of the animals when a ferret sneezed at him and shortly after he developed an influenza-like illness which was accompanied by a rising titre of antibodies and virus was recovered from his throat by animal inoculation; this virus was mouse adapted as was the virus given to the ferret (Smith & Stuart-Harris 1936). Thus Koch's postulates were fulfilled—by accident. Stuart-Harris also went out to groups such as army camps where influenza outbreaks were reported, and he documented the illnesses and tested patients for virus. The results showed that the epidemics were often caused by influenza viruses, but there were also outbreaks in which no virus was found which were slightly different clinically and which he called febrile catarrh (later shown to be due to adenovirus infection). In his Linacre lecture, Laidlaw was able to report a remarkably wide-ranging account of the basic facts about the influenza A virus and he paid tribute to the youthful energy, enthusiasm and hard work of the workers on both sides of the Atlantic (Laidlaw 1935).

Types of influenza viruses

The Rockefeller Institute and Hospital with the Laboratories of the International Division of the

Rockefeller Foundation stood on the banks of the East River on Manhattan Island in central New York City. Here work on the influenza virus was taken up and vigorously pursued. T. Francis Jr confirmed independently the susceptibility of ferrets to influenza (Francis & Magill 1935) and recovered a virus from specimens collected in Puerto Rico (PR8) which has been used ever since along with that isolated by Wilson Smith (WS) as a prototype influenza A virus strain (Francis & Magill 1935). Francis, and independently Magill, detected a new type of influenza virus, using ferrets and mice as before (Francis 1940). This had no antigenic relationship to the previous strains, which were called type A while the new one was called type B. The nomenclature was proposed in a joint paper from the New York and Hampstead groups. In this it was suggested that possible new serotypes be sent to one or other of the laboratories for verification — perhaps the germ of the idea of influenza virus reference centres (Horsfall *et al.* 1940).

Of fertile eggs and haemagglutinins

Meanwhile the search for better ways of growing and studying the viruses went on. Burnet had a long-standing interest in using the chick embryo to propagate and detect viruses (Burnet & Ferry 1934) and at NIMR it was shown that influenza viruses would infect such embryos and also grow in cultures of chopped tissue suspended in Tyrode's solution (Smith 1935). In New York they passed virus in such flasks up to 70 times (Magill & Francis 1936). This method had been initiated by the Maitlands in Manchester in the 1920s and had been developed and studied by Li and Rivers at the Rockefeller (Maitland & Maitland 1928). Francis found that viruses could be passaged apparently indefinitely in these cultures and used as a source of new virus, though it still had to be detected by inoculation into animals. Burnet, back in Australia, found that influenza viruses could be isolated by inoculation into the amniotic cavity of the embryo and, after isolation, could be grown to high titre by inoculation into the allantoic cavity. Using this new source of virus it was quickly shown by Mclelland and Hare in Canada and by Hirst in New York City

that the virus would agglutinate red cells. Other workers saw agglutinated red cells when they were harvesting allantoic fluid but blamed it on dirty glassware or some such technical fault. However, once again 'fortune favoured the prepared mind' and an important advance was made for influenza virus research and indeed for the whole of virology. In a short paper Hirst showed it could be used as a method of detecting and titrating virus and antibodies against it (Hirst 1941). He followed this up with detailed papers published in 1942. The method was remarkably simple since agglutination could be detected by the pattern of red cells settling at the bottom of a test tube. Anti-influenza haemagglutinin (HI or haemagglutination inhibiting) antibodies, proved to have very similar specificities to neutralizing antibodies and were shown to be well correlated with immunity, both naturally acquired and induced by vaccination or other experimental procedures.

Hirst also noticed that the haemagglutination was not permanent, but that it disappeared after a while, leaving the cells inagglutinable and the virus free in the surrounding medium. He concluded that there must be an enzyme on the surface of the virus which was able to destroy the receptor on the surface of the red cells. Thus was recognized the second major component of the virus surface — the neuraminidase — which was explored in more depth in Australia.

Early influenza virus vaccines

There were several early attempts to vaccinate against influenza virus infection. At NIMR it was shown that animals could be inoculated with virus parenterally without becoming sick and that they developed antiviral antibodies (Smith *et al.* 1935). The American scientists did similar experiments and also used tissue culture passaged virus as well as mouse lung. Attempts were made to apply this to humans. The allantoic cavity provided a source of relatively high titre and uncontaminated virus which made a good starting material for the production of vaccines, which began to be studied widely at the end of the war. Experience gained by work on inactivated influenza viruses also paved the way for Salk's pioneering development of the first poliovirus vaccine.

Basic virus structure and function

Until the 1950s influenza viruses were the only human viruses that could be studied in a relatively simple way and where it was possible to start analysing basic biological phenomena like attachment to cells, reaction with antibody, and the nature of the virus enzyme, the only one known. One of the first individuals to start thinking deeply about the nature of the influenza virus was L. Hoyle. He was a solitary character, who worked first in Manchester and was then employed by the Public Health Laboratory Service to run a small laboratory in the Midlands. However, he found time to study the composition of the influenza virus particle. His first work, in the 1930s, was to investigate the nature of the complement fixing antigen discovered by Wilson Smith. He concluded that it was a soluble antigen, but also part of the virus particle (Hoyle & Fairbrother 1937). Wilson Smith also studied the virus particle further and later on showed that it apparently contained antigens derived from the cell, but it was not clear whether these antigens were an integral part of the particle or 'scaffolding left by careless builders'.

World influenza centres

As soon as the war was over Andrewes returned to NIMR and it was clear by then that a major problem in developing a successful vaccination programme was that the influenza viruses, which caused most of the epidemics, changed antigenically at irregular intervals and in unpredictable directions, and seemed to spread around the world. He therefore proposed to the newly formed World Health Organization (WHO) that there should be a world influenza centre at NIMR linked with national laboratories which were looking for influenza epidemics and sending viruses to London where they could be compared with each other and with reference strains, so that antigenically novel epidemic strains could be identified and quickly passed to vaccine manufacturers. It is a remarkable

fact that this concept and that basic organization are still in operation and indeed the idea of a chain of WHO linked laboratories for reference and research has been extended to a number of other topics of international interest and importance, such as endocrinology.

The influenza viruses of animals and birds were also investigated at the centre and at veterinary research centres. It is an odd historical fact that the first influenza virus was actually cultivated early in the century and long before the events related here. Fowl plague, the highly lethal epidemic disease of domestic birds, was studied as a fulminating systemic virus infection. But, as pointed out by Waterson, it was demonstrated to be associated with the cellular fraction of the blood rather than the plasma (Waterson & Wilkinson 1978) and Burnet had grown it in eggs quite unaware that he was working with an influenza virus (Burnet & Ferry 1934). It was not until 1955 that Schaeffer and his colleagues in Tuebingen showed that the antigen in the nucleus of infected cells crossreacted with that of influenza viruses of mammals and then that the virus was in fact an influenza virus of birds. However, the systematic analysis of influenza viruses in wildlife was only possible once the basic methods of egg propagation and serology were widely applied.

Influenza C viruses

It was the use of egg isolation methods that revealed the presence of another type of influenza virus in humans. They are called influenza C viruses and they were discovered independently by two groups studying the aetiology of respiratory disease using chick embryo inoculation to propagate the virus and haemagglutination to detect its presence (Taylor 1951). As is typical in the story of the discovery of infectious agents it was the most tricky strains which were recognized last, for these agents do not grow particularly well in eggs, the haemagglutination is not easy to detect (the tests have to be run at refrigerator temperature) and the disease produced is a mild nondescript common cold which occurs sporadically and not in recognizable epidemics. Indeed they are sufficiently different at the biological level to be regarded as belonging to a different virus group or subgroup, but their existence became known for the practical reason that they were picked up using methods which had been developed in the study of the 'typical' influenza viruses.

Conclusion

I hope it has become clear in this sketch that it has been the introduction of an appropriate and powerful technique that has led to rapid and valuable advances in knowledge and understanding though this has only happened when the environment and support for research were right and imaginative and industrious individuals seized opportunities and openings when they appeared. I am also impressed by the combination of friendly co-operation and vigorous competition across the Atlantic which marked the initial period of discovery — something that I also experienced in the 'breakthrough' years of work on rhinoviruses and coronaviruses.

References

Andrewes, C.H. (1965) Early research work on colds. In: *The Common Cold*, pp. 51–55. Weidenfeld & Nicolson, London.

Andrewes, C.H. (1979) Richard Edwin Shope. In: *Biographical Memoirs*, 50th edn, pp. 353–75. National Academy of Sciences of the United States, Washington DC.

Andrewes, C.H. (1984) Influenza A in ferrets, mice and pigs. In: Stuart-Harris, C.H. & Potter, C.W (eds) *The Molecular Virology and Epidemiology of Influenza*, pp. 1–3. Academic Press, London.

Andrewes, C.H., Laidlaw, P.P. & Smith, W. (1934) The susceptibility of mice to the viruses of human and swine influenza. *Lancet* **ii**, 859–62.

Burnet, F.M. & Ferry, J.D. (1934) The differentiation of the viruses of fowl plague and Newcastle disease: experiments using the technique of choroallantoic inoculation of the developing egg. *Br J Exp Pathol* **15**, 56–64.

Francis, T. Jr (1940) A new type of virus from epidemic influenza. *Science* **92**, 405–6.

Francis, T. Jr & Magill, T.P. (1935) Immunological studies with the virus of influenza. *J Exp Med* **62**, 505–16.

Hirst, G.K. (1941) The agglutination of red cells by allantoic fluid of chick embryos infected with influenza virus. *Science* **94**, 22–3.

Horsfall, F.L. Jr, Lennette, E.H., Rickard, E.R., Andrewes, C.H., Smith, W. & Stuart-Harris, C.H. (1940) The nomenclature of influenza. *Lancet* **ii**, 413.

Hoyle, L. & Fairbrother, R.W. (1937) Antigenic structure of influenza virus; the preparation of elementary body suspensions and the nature of the complement fixing antigen. *J Hygiene (Cambridge)* **37**, 512–19.

Laidlaw, P.P. (1935) Epidemic influenza: a virus disease. *Lancet* **i**, 1118–24.

Magill, T.P. & Francis, T. Jr (1936) Studies with human influenza virus cultivated in artificial medium. *J Exp Med* **63**, 803–11.

Maitland, H.B. & Maitland, M.C. (1928) Cultivation of vaccinia virus without tissue culture. *Lancet* **ii**, 596–7.

Medical Research Committee (1919) *Special Report Series. Studies of influenza in hospitals in the British Army in France*. Medical Research Committee, London.

Ministry of Health (1920) *Reports on Public Health and Medical Subjects, no. 4. Report on the pandemic of influenza 1918–19*. His Majesty's Stationery Office, London.

Shope, R.E. (1931) Swine influenza. III. Filtration experiments and aetiology. *J Exp Med* **54**, 373–85.

Shope, R.E. (1934) The infection of ferrets with swine influenza virus. *J Exp Med* **62**, 49–61.

Smith, W. (1935) Cultivation of the virus of influenza. *Br J Exp Pathol* **16**, 508–12.

Smith, W., Andrewes, C.H. & Laidlaw, P.P. (1933) A virus obtained from influenza patients. *Lancet* **ii**, 66–8.

Smith, W., Andrewes, C.H. & Laidlaw, P.P. (1935) Influenza: experiments on the immunization of ferrets and mice. *Br J Exp Pathol* **16**, 291–302.

Smith, W. & Stuart-Harris, C.H. (1936) Influenza infection of man from the ferret. *Lancet* **ii, 121–3**.

Taylor, R.M. (1951) A further note on 1233 ('influenza C') virus. *Archiv gesamte Virusforschung* **4**, 485–500.

Thomson, A.L. (1987) Preventive medicine: infections and infestations. In: *Half a Century of Medical Research*. Vol. 2: *The Programme of the Medical Research Council (UK)*, pp. 108–36. Medical Research Council, London.

Topley, W.W.C. & Wilson, G.S. (1929) Acute respiratory infections. In: *Principles of Bacteriology and Immunity*, pp. 1081–109. Edward Arnold, London.

Tyrrell, D.A.J. (1991) Christopher Howard Andrewes. In: *Biographical Memoirs of Fellows of the Royal Society*, 37th edn, pp. 35–68. The Royal Society, London.

Waterson, A.P. & Wilkinson, L. (1978) Work on the influenzas and other common virus diseases of animals and man. In: *An Introduction to the History of Virology*, pp. 135–46. Cambridge University Press, Cambridge.

Section 2
Virus Structure
and Replication

CHAPTER 3

Structure of Influenza A, B and C Viruses

Rob W.H. Ruigrok

General description

Influenza viruses are negative-strand RNA viruses with a segmented genome. The eight RNA segments of influenza A and B viruses and seven segments of influenza C viruses (McGeoch *et al.* 1976; Desselberger *et al.* 1980) are independently encapsidated by the viral nucleoprotein (NP) and each segment is associated with a polymerase complex. The subviral particle consisting of viral RNA (vRNA), NP and polymerase complex is called a ribonucleoprotein (RNP) particle. The eight

(or seven) RNP particles are located inside a shell of M1 protein which lines the viral lipid membrane; see Fig. 3.1. The lipid membrane is derived from the plasma membrane of the infected cell during the budding process (Kates *et al.* 1962). Embedded in the membrane are three proteins: two spike glycoproteins, the haemagglutinin (HA) and neuraminidase (NA), and a membrane-channel protein, M2 (Zebedee & Lamb 1988). The HA is a trimer of identical subunits which contains the receptor binding activity at the tip of the molecule, and the membrane fusion activity which is activated by the

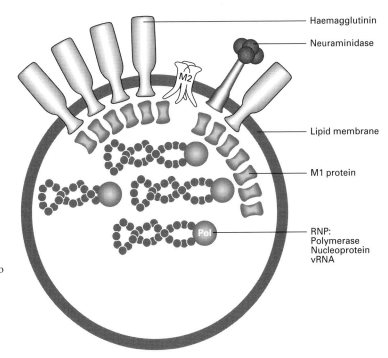

Fig. 3.1 Schematic drawing of influenza virus. The drawing is not to scale and only four of the ribonucleoproteins (RNPs) are represented. The RNP complement per virion and the interactions between the viral components are discussed in the text.

Haemagglutinin

Neuraminidase

Lipid membrane

M1 protein

RNP:
Polymerase
Nucleoprotein
vRNA

low pH in the endosome during entry into the cell (Wharton *et al.* 1989). The neuraminidase is a tetramer of identical subunits which contains the receptor destroying activity necessary for release of newly formed virus from the surface of the infected cell (Colman 1989). M2 forms a tetrameric membrane channel (Sugrue & Hay 1991; Pinto *et al.* 1992). This channel probably allows acidification of the interior of the virus while it passes through the acidic endosome, which is thought to be needed for the release of the RNP particles into the cytoplasm after the membrane fusion step (Bukrinskaya *et al.* 1982; Hay *et al.* 1985; Wharton *et al.* 1990; Martin & Helenius 1991). The structures and functions of the HA, NA and M2 are described in Chapter 7.

Electron micrographs of thin sections of influenza virus show that the inside of the lipid membrane is thicker and darker than the outside; this is probably caused by the M1 protein lining the membrane (Nermut 1972; Schulze 1972; Oxford & Hockley 1987). This can also be seen in cryoelectron micrographs of virus which show not only the outside of the virus but also its inside (see below) (Booy *et al.* 1985; Fujiyoshi *et al.* 1994). In cryoelectron micrographs one would expect that, if influenza virus were a filled sphere, the density, i.e. the darkness, would increase towards the middle of the virus. Since this is not the case it suggests that M1 only lines the inside of the membrane and does not form a matrix to fill the virus. When influenza virus is negatively stained with sodium silicotungstate (SST) or phosphotungstic acid (PTA), the stain sometimes enters the virus particle and shows the M1 layer inside the viral membrane. There are two major types of M1 protein arrangement that can be distinguished: a fingerprint of fine lines (Nermut 1972; Schulze 1972; Wrigley 1979; Ruigrok *et al.* 1989) that are spaced some 40 Å apart (Fig. 3.2, bottom); and a coiled structure that consists of the same kind of lines but in which the lines are in pairs (Fig. 3.2, top) (Nermut & Frank 1971; Murti *et al.* 1980; Ruigrok *et al.* 1989). The lines in both kinds of structures consist of subunits that are spaced at about 40 Å along the lines (Ruigrok *et al.* 1989). The coiled structure was observed in the earliest micrographs of negatively stained virus (Hoyle *et al.* 1961; Apostolov & Flewett 1965) and was inter-

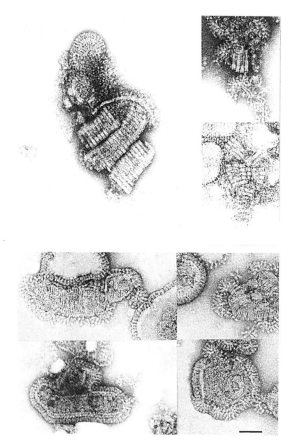

Fig. 3.2 Influenza virus M1 protein. Electron micrographs of influenza A/X31 virus negatively stained with sodium silicotungstate. Stain has penetrated the viral membrane and outlines the M1 layer underneath the membrane. Two M1 polymer types can be seen: 'coils' (top) and 'fingerprints' (bottom). The bar represents 500 Å.

preted to be the nucleocapsid. The only arguments that the coils are not an RNP complex but an M1 polymer are the morphological arguments given above. It has not been possible to isolate intact coils and immunogold labelling of intact coils inside virus with anti-M1, anti-NP or antipolymerase antibodies was not possible, probably because of protection by the viral membrane (Murti *et al.* 1992). In some images of negatively stained virus, as in the picture of the elongated virus particle in Fig. 3.2, bottom left, going from the outside to the inside of the particle one can observe the spike layer, the membrane, a dark stain-filled line and then the M1 layer. The M1 molecules closest to the membrane are clearly outlined and seem slightly elongated. Schulze (1972) determined a width for the M1 layer of 60 Å (in agreement with unpublished measurements by R. Ruigrok and A. Barge). Electron microscopy of isolated M1 revealed a small rod with a length of 55 Å and a diameter of 30 Å (A. Barge and R. Ruigrok, unpublished results), and images like that of the elongated virion in Fig. 3.2 suggest that M1 is touching the membrane with one of its short sides, as drawn in Fig. 3.1. There are several reports that have suggested that M1 is embedded into the viral membrane (Bucher *et al.* 1980; Gregoriades & Frangione 1981), but since the size of M1 in the virus is very similar to the size of free M1, any membrane insertion cannot be very extensive. Recently, Kretzschmar *et al.* (1996) have shown that mutations in the four hydrophobic regions that were thought to be responsible for membrane insertion had no effect on membrane association of M1 when expressed in eukaryotic cells. The interaction of M1 with RNP is discussed below.

Since the genome of the influenza viruses is segmented, the nucleocapsid is also segmented and, up to now, it has not been possible to isolate a superstructure containing all eight RNPs. RNA makes up about 10–12% of the weight of the RNP (Pons *et al.* 1969; Krug 1971; Compans *et al.* 1972; Jennings *et al.* 1983), which means that each monomer of NP is bound to 20–26 nucleotides of RNA (Compans *et al.* 1972; Jennings *et al.* 1983). NP binds to the phosphate-sugar backbone of the RNA in a sequence non-specific manner and, in doing so, prevents RNA secondary structure formation and exposes the nucleotide bases to the outside. The polymerase can thus transcribe the vRNA without requiring dissociation of NP from the RNA (Baudin *et al.* 1994). The polymerase consists of three subunits, PB1, PB2 and PA, the functions of which are described in Chapter 4. One polymerase complex is bound to one end of each RNP rod (Murti *et al.* 1988). In the RNP, the polymerase binds to both the 3′ and 5′ ends of the vRNA (Hagen *et al.* 1994; Cianci *et al.* 1995; Klumpp *et al.* 1997) and holds these ends together in a circular structure. This circle is then supercoiled into

a rod-like structure (Pons *et al.* 1969; Compans *et al.* 1972; Heggeness *et al.* 1982; Jennings *et al.* 1983; Klumpp *et al.* 1997). Figure 3.3 shows electron micrographs of RNPs negatively stained with SST (top) or shadowed with platinum (middle). The particles are rather flexible and often show loops at one or both ends; the turns of the supercoil can be

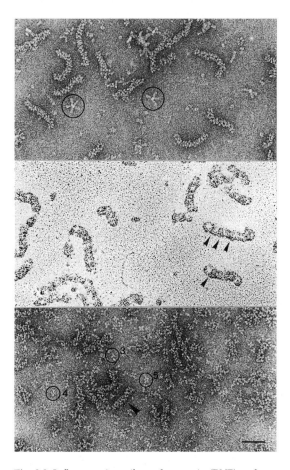

Fig. 3.3 Influenza virus ribonucleoprotein (RNP) and RNA-free nucleoprotein (NP) self-polymers. Electron micrographs of influenza A/PR/8/34 RNP negatively stained with sodium silicotungstate (top) and rotary shadowed with platinum (middle). Some contaminating rosettes of haemagglutinin in the top picture are encircled and the arrowheads in the middle picture indicate turns of the supercoil. The bottom picture shows negatively stained NP free of RNA. The arrowhead indicates an NP self-polymer that is indistinguishable from intact RNP and the circles with numbers 3, 4 and 5 indicate trimers, tetramers and pentamers of NP. The bar represents 500 Å.

seen in the shadowed image. The lengths of the RNPs reflect the lengths of the vRNAs that they contain and three length classes have been recognized: the longest probably containing RNA segments 1–3; the middle length class containing segments 4–6; and the shortest containing segments 7 and 8 (Compans *et al.* 1972). The isolated NP monomer is a rod of 62 Å by 35 Å with a constriction in the middle (Ruigrok & Baudin 1995). NP self-polymerizes into various structures, the smallest being trimers and tetramers and the largest having the same morphology as intact RNP (Fig. 3.3, bottom). Thus, the morphology of RNP is defined by the protein (Pons *et al.* 1969; Ruigrok & Baudin 1995).

Differences between A, B and C viruses

The structures of influenza A and B viruses are very similar although the B viruses may be somewhat more regular (see below). The main difference between A and B viruses is in the membrane channel spanning the lipid envelope: in the case of the A viruses it is the M2 protein (Zebedee & Lamb 1988), encoded by a spliced mRNA of gene segment 7, which also codes for M1 (Lamb *et al.* 1981); and in the case of B viruses it is the NB protein (Betakova *et al.* 1996; Brassard *et al.* 1996) which is encoded by RNA segment 6 in an overlapping reading frame in the same mRNA that codes for NA (Shaw *et al.* 1983). A good candidate for the influenza C virus membrane channel is CM2, encoded by RNA segment 6 (Hongo *et al.* 1997). This segment also codes for M1 which is translated from a spliced mRNA (Yamashita *et al.* 1988), but it is not yet clear how translation of CM2 is initiated.

Another difference between A and B viruses is the size of their genomes; 14 639 nucleotides for a particular B virus compared to 13 588 nucleotides for A/PR/8/34. This difference is not reflected in the size of the proteins but B-virus RNAs have longer non-coding sequences. These non-coding sequences may contain type-specific signals for packaging into newly formed virus.

The major difference between the A and B viruses on the one hand and the C viruses on the other is that influenza C virus has only one surface glycoprotein (Compans *et al.* 1977; Herrler *et al.*

1979, 1981) and contains only seven RNA segments (Desselberger *et al.* 1980). The single influenza C glycoprotein harbours the fusion and receptor binding activities, which are contained in the HA of the A and B viruses (Herrler *et al.* 1981; Kitame *et al.* 1982), plus the receptor destroying activity which is associated with the NA of A and B viruses. This receptor destroying activity is not a neuraminidase as for A and B (Kendal 1975), but is an esterase (Herrler *et al.* 1985). The single influenza C glycoprotein has the same gross morphology as HA of A and B viruses and can be organized into a hexagonal surface lattice (Flewett & Apostolov 1967; Apostolov & Flewett 1969; Compans *et al.* 1977; Herrler *et al.* 1981; Hewat *et al.* 1984); see Fig. 3.4.

Heterogeneity of influenza virus

Influenza virus particles are notoriously variable. The most objective way to study virus morphology is by cryoelectron microscopy (cryoEM) of virus suspensions in vitrified water (Booy *et al.* 1985), which avoids possible preparation artefacts due to staining or air-drying of the virus. In cryoEM the ring of spikes and the inside of the virus particles are revealed. A typical cryomicrograph of a preparation of purified influenza A/X31 virus can be seen in Fig. 3.5. There are virus particles with

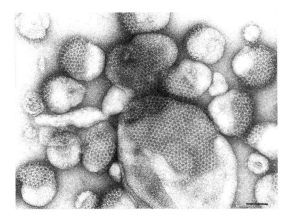

Fig. 3.4 Influenza C virus hexagonal surface lattice. Electron micrograph of influenza C/Taylor/1233/47 virus negatively stained with uranyl acetate. The bar represents 500 Å. (Reprinted from Hewat *et al.* 1984, with permission from Academic Press.)

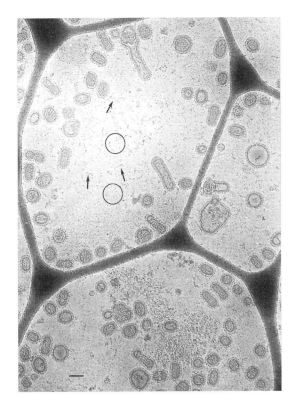

Fig. 3.5 Purified but heterogeneous influenza A virus preparation. Cryoelectron micrograph of influenza A/X31 virus. The arrows indicate free ribonucleoprotein and some free spikes are encircled. The bar represents 1000 Å. (Reprinted from Booy *et al.* 1985, with permission from Academic Press.)

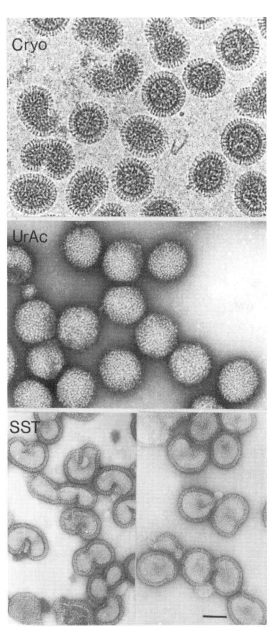

Fig. 3.6 Electron micrographs of influenza B virus. Top, cryoelectron micrograph; middle, after negative staining with uranyl acetate; bottom, after negative staining with sodium silicotungstate. The bar represents 1000 Å.

different shapes and sizes although most of the longer and bigger particles are relatively empty. In the background free RNP and spikes can be observed. In this context, 'purified virus' does not mean that all the virus particles have the same size and shape, but that on a polyacrylamide gel only viral proteins can be seen. The smaller virus particles are filled with RNP particles and often seem to be slightly elongated. A cryoEM picture of influenza B/Yamagata/16/88 virus is shown in Fig. 3.6 ('Cryo'). In B-virus preparations there seems to be less variation in size and shape and more particles appear round. However, some deformed kidney-shaped particles can also be seen. When influenza virus is prepared in a more classical way for EM, by negative staining with uranyl acetate (Fig. 3.6,

UrAc), all virus particles appear round, a particular and reproducible effect of uranyl acetate. Negative staining with SST (Fig. 3.6, SST, left) sometimes leads to all the virus particles looking kidney shaped, as seen after staining with PTA, but sometimes the virions are better preserved as shown in Fig. 3.6 (SST, right). These artefacts of the negative staining procedure strongly reinforce the impression of the variability of influenza virus (Ruigrok & Hewat 1991).

Characterization of homogeneous virus suspensions and stoichiometry of viral proteins

Suspensions of heterogeneous virus cannot be used for the determination of the weight of a typical influenza virion nor for the determination of the stoichiometry of the viral proteins. Therefore, the virus was purified to near homogeneity by consecutive sucrose gradient purification steps. Since it was easier to obtain homogeneous preparations of

influenza B virus, perhaps because B virus is more regular than A virus (see above), influenza B/Hong Kong/8/73 was extensively characterized using four independent biophysical techniques: small-angle neutron scattering (SANS), scanning transmission electron microscopy (STEM), cryoEM and hydrodynamic analysis. The results of these measurements are given in Table 3.1 which shows that the average diameter of an influenza virus particle is about 1270 Å. The number of spikes per virion was estimated by counting the number of spikes (38 ± 2) that could be seen in the halo coming out of the viral membrane in a cryoEM picture and assuming close packing of the spikes on the virus surface. However, the resulting value of 530 spikes per virion only holds if only one row of spikes is counted and is possibly an overestimation of the real number. Mass determinations by STEM on intact and spikeless virus led to estimates of 400–450 spikes per virion. In one experiment the NA was removed from influenza B virus by protease digestion leading to an estimate of about 50 NA

Table 3.1 Weights and diameters of influenza virus particles.

Strain	Diameter (Å)	Weight of intact virion (10^6 Da)	Weight of spikeless virion (10^6 Da)	Number of spikes per virion
A/X31 (A/PR/8/34 × A/Hong Kong/68)	1275 ± 162 (UrAc)* 1275 ± 173 (CryoEM)†			
A/X49 (A/PR/8/34 × A/England/864/75)		161 ± 17 (STEM)¶	75 ± 17 (STEM)	420 (STEM)
B/Singapore/222/79		182 ± 19 (STEM)	87 ± 17 (STEM)	463 (STEM)
B/Hong Kong/8/73	1363 ± 163 (UrAc)* 1275 ± 100 (CryoEM)† 1270 ± 70 (CryoEM)‡ (2x) 635 ± 4 (Rs)§ 1180 (SANS)	178 ± 22 (STEM) 176 ± 20 (SANS)** 202 ± 13††	95 ± 24 (STEM)	405 (STEM) 530 (CryoEM) 400 (SANS)

* Measurements from electron micrographs of pure but not homogeneous virus negatively stained with uranyl acetate (Ruigrok & Hewat 1991).

†, ‡ Independent measurements from cryoelectron micrographs of virus in vitrified water († Ruigrok & Hewat 1991, pure but not homogeneous; ‡ Booy *et al.* 1985, homogeneous suspension).

§ Stokes (or hydrodynamic) radius measured by light scattering (Mellema *et al.* 1981), ± standard deviation (s.d.) of the mean.

¶ Mass measurement of virus by electron scattering using scanning transmission electron microscopy (Ruigrok *et al.* 1984a). The value given here is the measured value ± s.d. of the population. See remark on possible correction in the text.

** Mass determination by small-angle neutron scattering (Cusack *et al.* 1985); see remarks on possible errors in the text.

†† Derived from the sedimentation coefficient (650 ± 23 S), diffusion coefficient ($3.35 ± 0.03 \times 10^{-8}$ cm^{2}s^{-1}) and partial specific volume of 0.767 ml/g (Ruigrok, 1985).

tetramers per virus particle (R. Ruigrok, unpublished results), in agreement with an earlier estimate by Bucher and Palese (1975), although the NA content per virion is thought to vary between strains. SANS gives rise to a circular scattering pattern which was interpreted by building a spherical shell model of the virus. This model gives estimates of the amounts of protein or lipid in each shell, indicating a total of 400 spikes per virion (Cusack *et al.* 1985).

Mass determinations by SANS and STEM are subject to certain systematic errors. The mass determined by SANS is directly dependent on the concentration of the virus in suspension which could not be determined better than within 7%, giving an average virus weight of between 164 and 188 MDa (1 MDa is 10^6 Da). The value determined by STEM may be underestimated by about 7% due to multiple electron scattering by thick samples (analogous to a correction calculated for the mass determination of vesicular stomatitis virus, Thomas *et al.* 1985), which

would lead to a revised value of 191 MDa. These corrections would influence only the absolute values but not the percentage weight of spikes.

The percentage weight of the viral lipid was determined chemically; see Table 3.2 for values and references. To calculate the stoichiometry of the viral proteins, a total virus weight of 190 MDa for influenza B virus was used. We assumed that each virus particle contains a full set of genome segments, that each NP monomer binds to 23 nucleotides and that each RNP contains one set of polymerase subunits (Murti *et al.* 1988). Adding the percentages of all the components leaves 17% of the viral weight for the M1 protein. An earlier estimate of the amount of M1 needed to make a closely packed shell inside the lipid membrane mentions 1500–2000 copies of M1 per virion (Nermut 1972). However, the packing of M1 does not seem to be very dense and a shell made up of units with a 40 by 40 Å spacing could be built with about 1100 monomers (Ruigrok *et al.* 1989). Obviously, if the

Table 3.2 Stoichiometry of components of influenza B/Hong Kong/8/73 virus. A total weight of influenza B virus of 190 MDa is assumed, of which about 20% is lipid* and 2.5% is RNA (total genome is 14 639 nt corresponding to 4.5 MDa).

RNA segment	Encoded protein	Molecular weight of protein in (kDa)†	Number of copies per virion	Percentage of 190 MDa
1	PB2	86	8	0.36
2	PB1	83	8	0.35
3	PA	80	8	0.34
4	HA	64 (70)	350–400 trimers	38–44
5	NP	56	630‡	19
6	NA	51 (60)	50 tetramers	6
	NB	12	15 monomers§	0.1
7	M1	27	1100	17
8	NS1	31	—	
	NS2	13	—	

* 24%, Blough *et al.* (1967); 20%, Blough and Merlie (1970); 19%, Klenk *et al.* (1972) — all for influenza A viruses; 20% for influenza B virus (Ruigrok 1985).

† Predicted from the mRNA coding sequence; between brackets an estimate of the molecular weight of the external domain of the glycoprotein taking into account its glycosylation.

‡ Assuming a full genomic complement per virion and 23 nucleotides per nucleoprotein monomer.

§ Brassard *et al.* (1996). This number is similar to the amount of M2 in influenza A virus particles: 14–68 monomers (Zebedee & Lamb 1988). It is likely that the NB protein also forms tetramers, in analogy to M2.

virus in the homogeneous preparation does not on average contain a full set of RNPs (see discussion below), this would influence the percentage weight of M1. The M1 content of a purified virus preparation may vary between preparations and between different strains (Kendal *et al.* 1977; Oxford *et al.* 1981). This may be due to the degree of homogeneity of the virus in the preparation since the homogeneous virus preparations that were used for the biophysical measurements had a higher infectious titre per milligram of viral protein, a higher HA content and a lower M1 content than the starting suspension of purified, non-homogeneous virus (Ruigrok *et al.* 1985). Furthermore, as shown in Fig. 3.4 many of the larger or more irregular virus particles are empty of RNP and this would influence the percentage weight of M1.

The number of copies of the proteins per virus particle given in Table 3.2 is lower than normally given (Lamb 1989). Most reviews on the composition of influenza virus are based on an earlier review by Compans and Choppin (1975) who assumed a total protein content of 200 MDa, which would correspond to a virus weight of 260 MDa. Another difference with earlier estimates of stoichiometries is the percentage of spikes. The more traditional view is that the spike content is only about 20%, based on quantification of radiolabel on polyacrylamide gels (Compans *et al.* 1970), although another estimate using the same method gave 38% HA (Laver 1964).

Complement of RNP per virus particle

A preparation of purified influenza virus contains about equal amounts of the RNA segments (McGeoch *et al.* 1976). However, a central question is whether each individual virus particle contains a full complement of RNPs and whether or not a unique virus structure exists. There are arguments for and against the different points of view (for a more extensive discussion see Enami *et al.* 1991 and Duhaut & McCauley 1996). Arguments against a unique structure include the observation that virus suspensions, in which a small amount of aggregation has been induced, have a higher infectious titre than non-aggregated virus (Hirst & Pons 1973).

Incorporation of foreign genes in reverse genetics experiments have suggested that a virus particle could contain at least nine segments (Enami *et al.* 1991; Neumann & Hobom 1995). However, these viruses are not stable and may not be free from helper virus. Enami *et al.* (1991) suggested that each virus particle might package as many as 10 or 11 RNP particles. If this were true it would increase the genome mass by 10–15 MDa (weight of RNA plus NP) which, for a virus of 190 MDa that contains 45–50% spikes and 20% lipid (Table 3.2), would allow no weight for M1.

On the other hand, mixed infections never lead to stable viruses that contain two HA or NA subtypes (Laver & Downie 1976) suggesting that there is only one copy of each gene per virion. Smith and Hay (1982) suggested an RNP selection mechanism based on the comparison of the genome of released virus and the vRNA composition in the infected cell. Recently Duhaut and McCauley (1996) found that cells infected with defective virus strains, which had predominantly a single defective RNA, contained more or less equal amounts of the eight intact vRNAs and an excess of the defective RNA. However, in newly formed virus there was specifically less of the vRNA corresponding to the defective RNA, which is consistent with a selective packaging model. Similar conclusions can be drawn from work by Bergmann and Muster (1995) who constructed mutants in the NA gene which resulted in a reduced amount of this gene in infected cells but not in newly formed virus. Recent work indicates that at least part of the packaging selection may reside in the non-coding sequences which are specific for each RNA segment (Odagiri & Tashiro 1997).

The two points of view could be united by the assumption of a selective RNP packaging mechanism which, however, allows for some freedom and, consequently, a virus structure which is flexible enough to accommodate different amounts of RNPs. This interpretation would also agree with the mass determinations on homogeneous virus suspensions. The STEM mass determination method was found to have a random internal error of about 6–7%, which corresponds to the spread in the mass determination of human adenovirus type

5, which has a unique structure (Ruigrok *et al.* 1984b). The larger standard deviation in the mass of influenza virus (10–12% for intact virus and 20–25% for spikeless virus; Table 3.1) and in particular the same absolute spread in mass values of intact and spikeless virus, suggest that there is a real variation in mass even in these very homogeneous virus suspensions, in particular in the RNP plus M1 content.

Interaction between viral proteins

The structure of any macromolecular assembly such as a virus must include a description of the interactions between the constituent proteins. Interactions between viral proteins are indicated when a mutation in one protein can be suppressed by a mutation in another protein, such as the ts81 mutation in fowl plague virus NP that is suppressed by a mutation in the PB2 protein (Mandler *et al.* 1991), or when, for example, inhibition of influenza A virus growth by antibodies against M2 can be overcome by a mutation in M1 (Zebedee & Lamb 1989). It has been suggested that NS2 is a structural protein and interacts with M1 on the basis of biochemical experiments (Yasuda *et al.* 1993), but compensatory mutations such as described above have not yet been described. Furthermore, there is as yet no functional rationale for M1–NS2 interaction.

The RNPs are functional units where each of the components is necessary for function *in vivo* and *in vitro* and in reverse genetics experiments (Luytjes *et al.* 1989; Huang *et al.* 1990; Kimura *et al.* 1992; de la Luna *et al.* 1993; Mena *et al.* 1994). Inside the virus particle interactions between RNP and M1 are likely, as suggested by the inhibition of transcription activity *in vitro* by M1 (Zvonarjev & Ghendon 1980; Ye *et al.* 1989; Elster *et al.* 1994). Recently, the atomic structure of an N-terminal portion of M1 was determined, suggesting how M1 may interact with the RNA in the RNP (Sha & Luo 1997). The positively charged residues between lysine 95 and arginine 105, that make up the RNA binding domain of M1 (Watanabe *et al.* 1996; Elster *et al.* 1997) and also its nuclear localization signal (Ye *et al.* 1995), are exposed on a platform made up of α-helices and are lined up to bind to the negatively charged phosphate-sugar backbone of the RNA.

As mentioned above, the glycoprotein of influenza C virus forms a hexagonal network on the viral surface. It is possible that this occurs due to the absence of tetrameric NA molecules, which could disturb possible hexagonal packing of HA on the surface of A and B viruses, rather than reflecting an essential structural difference between the two types of viruses. On rare occasions, regularly packed spikes have been observed in influenza A virus preparations, hexagonal for HA and cubic for NA (Wrigley *et al.* 1986) but only on irregularly shaped particles. Apart from these rare cases of regular packing of spikes on the virus surface, it has been reported that NA on the influenza A virus surface is found in discrete patches, in contrast to HA which is more evenly distributed (Murti & Webster 1986).

Enveloped viruses bud at cell membranes in a process whereby non-viral proteins are eliminated. Direct interaction between the glycoproteins and the viral core has been shown by cryoEM for Sindbis virus (Cheng *et al.* 1995) and for Semliki Forest virus (Fuller *et al.* 1995) and by coexpression of the matrix protein and glycoprotein for HIV (Cosson 1996). Budding of vesicular stomatitis virus also requires interaction between the cytoplasmic tails of the single glycoprotein and the core, even if the external domain is absent (Metsikkö & Simons 1986). It would seem logical therefore that there also exists an interaction between the conserved cytoplasmic tails of the glycoproteins and M1 of influenza virus. Two reports of *in vitro* coexpression of M1 and the spike proteins under the control of a T7 promotor failed to show any interaction between M1 and HA or NA (Kretzschmar *et al.* 1996; Zhang & Lamb 1996) whereas another report demonstrated a stronger interaction with NA than with HA (Enami & Enami 1996). Influenza virus particles can form in the absence of HA (Pattnaik *et al.* 1986) although these particles seem to contain double the amount of NA. Using reverse genetics, Jin *et al.* (1994) showed that virus could form with HA lacking its cytoplasmic tail, although a revertant virus was isolated suggesting a selective advantage for the presence of the tail. However, the absence of the cytoplasmic tail of NA affects the incorporation of NA into virus and virus morphology (Mitnaul *et al.* 1996). Recently, Jin *et al.* (1997) compared viruses that lacked the HA or NA cytoplasmic tails with virus that lacked both cytoplasmic tails. The results suggested that the effects of the absence of the HA tail on virus production and morphology were minor, the effects of the absence of the NA tail were stronger, but the absence of both tails led to greatly reduced virus production and to an aberrant virus morphology. They suggested that the presence of both tails is important but that the absence of one could be partly compensated by the presence of the other. These results are in agreement with those from Lin and Air (1993) who were able to isolate a virus which lacked most of the coding part of segment 6 RNA. However, the part of the RNA that codes for the transmembrane and cytoplasmic tail of NA was never lost (Yang *et al.* 1997) suggesting that this part of the molecule is necessary for the virus life cycle.

If our estimate of the stoichiometry of viral proteins is accurate, there would be as many monomers of the spikes as copies of M1. That could mean that each HA or NA interacts with three or four M1 molecules, respectively, and that a virus-like, regular organization of M1 is needed for M1–spike tail interaction. Finally, experiments by Naim and Roth (1993) suggest that, although the cytoplasmic tails may be important for the production of infectious virus, the structure of the transmembrane domain is more important for the incorporation of the spikes into virus. It is possible that the transmembrane parts of the spikes have an influence on the structure of the lipid membrane, allowing it to interact with M1, or vice versa.

Budding

M1 seems to be the key player in the structure of influenza virus being involved in interactions with RNP, lipid and possibly the spikes. M1 is produced in the cell as a soluble protein which becomes insoluble the moment it takes its part in virus budding. For the matrix protein of vesicular stomatitis virus it has been shown that the soluble protein may polymerize around polymerization initiation sites (Gaudin *et al.* 1995) and it was suggested that these sites may be the starting points for virus budding. The same scenario may be proposed for the budding of influenza virus. The fact that M1 can self-associate into several morphologically distinct polymers inside the virus particle (see Fig. 3.2) may suggest that the M1 polymer shape is influenced by the structure of a hypothetical initiation site. The M2 tetramer, the cytoplasmic tails of the glycoproteins or the small proportion of M1 molecules that have a zinc ion bound (Elster *et al.* 1994) could be involved in initiation of M1 polymerization.

Acknowledgements

I thank Annie Barge and Florence Baudin for help with preparing the figures, Elizabeth Hewat and Frank Booy for allowing me to use their micrographs and John McCauley, Stephen Cusack and Yves Gaudin for discussions and critical comments on the text.

References

Apostolov, K. & Flewett, T.H. (1965) Internal structure of influenza virus. *Virology* **26**, 506–508.

Apostolov, K. & Flewett, T.H. (1969) Further observations on the structure of influenza viruses A and C. *J Gen Virol* **4**, 365–370.

Baudin, F., Bach, C., Cusack, S. & Ruigrok, R.W.H. (1994) Structure of influenza virus RNP. I. Influenza virus nucleoprotein melts secondary structure in panhandle RNA and exposes the bases to the solvent. *EMBO J* **13**, 3158–65.

Bergmann, M. & Muster, T. (1995) The relative amount of an influenza A virus segment in the viral particle is not affected by a reduction in replication of that segment. *J Gen Virol* **76**, 3211–5.

Betakova, T., Nermut, M.V. & Hay, A.J. (1996) The NB protein is an integral component of the membrane of influenza B virus. *J Gen Virol* **77**, 2689–94.

Blough, H.A. & Merlie, J.P. (1970) The lipids of incomplete influenza virus. *Virology* **40**, 685–92.

Blough, H.A., Weinstein, D.B., Lawson, D.E.M. & Kodicek, E. (1967) The effect of vitamin A on myxoviruses. II. Alterations in the lipids of influenza virus. *Virology* **33**, 459–66.

Brassard, D.L., Leser, G.P. & Lamb, R.A. (1996) Influenza B virus NB is a component of the virion. *Virology* **220**, 350–60.

Booy, F.P., Ruigrok, R.W.H. & van Bruggen, E.F.J. (1985) Electron microscopy of influenza virus. A comparison of negatively stained and ice-embedded particles. *J Mol Biol* **184**, 667–76.

Bucher, D.J. & Palese, P. (1975) The biologically active proteins of influenza virus, neuraminidase. In: Kilbourne, E.D. (ed.) *Influenza Virus and Influenza*, pp. 83–123. Academic Press, New York.

Bucher, D.J., Kharitonenkov, I.G., Zakomirdin, J.A., Grigoriev, V.B., Klimenko, S.M. & Davis, J.F. (1980) Incorporation of influenza virus M-protein into liposomes. *J Virol* **36**, 586–90.

Bukrinskaya, A.G., Vorkunova, N.K., Kornilayeva, G.V., Narmanbetova, R.A. & Vorkunova, G.K. (1982) Influenza virus uncoating in infected cells and effect of rimantadine. *J Gen Virol* **60**, 49–59.

Cheng, R.H., Kuhn, R.J., Olson, N.H., Rossman, M.G., Choi, H.K. & Baker, T.S. (1995) Nucleocapsid and glycoprotein organization in an enveloped virus. *Cell* **80**, 621–30.

Cianci, C., Tiley, L. & Krystal, M. (1995) Differential activation of the influenza virus polymerase via template RNA binding. *J Virol* **69**, 3995–9.

Colman, P.M. (1989) Neuraminidase: Enzyme and antigen. In: Krug, R.M. (ed.) *The Influenza Viruses*, pp. 175–218. Plenum Press, New York & London.

Compans, R.W. & Choppin, P.W. (1975) Reproduction of myxoviruses. In: Fraenkel-Conrat, H. & Wagner, R.R. (eds) *Comprehensive Virology* 4, pp. 179–252. Plenum Press, New York & London.

Compans, R.W., Klenk, H.D., Caliguiri, L.A. & Choppin, P.W. (1970) Influenza virus proteins. I. Analysis of polypeptides of the virion and identification of spike glycoproteins. *Virology* **42**, 880–9.

Compans, R.W., Content, J. & Duesberg, P. (1972) Structure of the ribonucleoprotein of influenza virus. *Virology* **10**, 795–800.

Compans, R.W., Bishop, D.H.L. & Meier-Ewert, H. (1977) Structural components of influenza C viruses. *J Virol* **21**, 658–65.

Cosson, P. (1996) Direct interaction between the envelope and matrix proteins of HIV. *EMBO J* **15**, 5783–8.

Cusack, S., Ruigrok, R.W.H., Krijgsman, P.C.J. & Mellema, J.E. (1985) Structure and composition of influenza virus. A small-angle neutron scattering study. *J Mol Biol* **186**, 565–82.

de la Luna, S., Martin, J., Portela, A. & Ortin, J. (1993) Influenza virus naked RNA can be expressed upon transfection into cells co-expressing the three subunits of the polymerase and the nucleoprotein from simian virus 40 recombinant viruses. *J Gen Virol* **74**, 535–9.

Desselberger, U., Racianello, V.R., Zazra, J.J. & Palese, P. (1980) The 3'- and 5'-terminal sequences of influenza A, B and C viruses are highly conserved and show partial inverted complementarity. *Gene* **8**, 315–28.

Duhaut, S.D. & McCauley, J.W. (1996) Defective RNAs inhibit the assembly of influenza virus genome segments in a segment-specific manner. *Virology* **216**, 326–37.

Elster, C., Fourest, E., Baudin, F., Larsen, K., Cusack, S. & Ruigrok, R.W.H. (1994) A small percentage of influenza virus M1 protein contains zinc but zinc does not influence *in vitro* M1–RNA interaction. *J Gen Virol* **75**, 37–42.

Elster, C., Larsen, K., Gagnon, J., Ruigrok, R.W.H. & Baudin, F. (1997) Influenza virus M1 protein binds to RNA through its nuclear localization signal. *J Gen Virol* **78**, 1589–96.

Enami, M. & Enami, K. (1996) Influenza haemagglutinin and neuraminidase glycoproteins stimulate the membrane association of the matrix protein. *J Virol* **70**, 6653–7.

Enami, M., Sharma, G., Benham, C. & Palese, P. (1991) An influenza virus containing nine different RNA segments. *Virology* **185**, 291–8.

Flewett, T.H. & Apostolov, K. (1967) A reticular structure in the wall of influenza C virus. *J Gen Virol* **1**, 297–304.

Fujiyoshi, Y., Kume, N.P., Sakata, K. & Sato, S.B. (1994) Fine structure of influenza A virus observed by electron cryo-microscopy. *EMBO J* **13**, 318–26.

Fuller, S.D., Berriman, J.A., Butcher, S.J. & Gowen, B.E. (1995) Low pH induces swivelling of the glycoprotein heterodimers in the Semliki Forest virus spike complex. *Cell* **81**, 715–25.

Gaudin, Y., Barge, A., Ebel, C. & Ruigrok, R.W.H. (1995) Aggregation of VSV M protein is reversible and mediated by nucleation sites. Implications for viral assembly. *Virology* **206**, 28–37.

Gregoriades, A. & Frangione, B. (1981) Insertion of influenza M protein into the viral lipid bilayer and localization of site of insertion. *J Virol* **40**, 323–8.

Hagen, M., Chung, T.D., Butcher, J.A. & Krystal, M. (1994) Recombinant influenza virus polymerase: requirement of both 5' and 3' viral ends for endonuclease activity. *J Virol* **68**, 1509–15.

Hay, A.J., Wolstenholme, A.J., Skehel, J.J. & Smith, M.H. (1985) The molecular basis of the specific anti-influenza action of amantadine. *EMBO J* **4**, 3021–4.

Heggeness, M.H., Smith, P.R., Ulmanen, I., Krug, R.M. & Choppin, P.W. (1982) Studies on the helical nucleocapsid of influenza virus. *Virology* **118**, 466–70.

Herrler, G., Compans, R.W. & Meier-Ewert, H. (1979) A precursor glycoprotein in influenza C virus. *Virology* **99**, 49–56.

Herrler, G., Nagele, A., Meier-Ewert, H., Bhown, A.S. & Compans, R.W. (1981) Isolation and structural analysis of influenza C virion glycoproteins. *Virology* **113**, 439–51.

Herrler, G., Rott, R., Klenk, H.D., Müller, H.P., Shukla, A.K. & Schauer, R. (1985) The receptor-destroying enzyme of influenza C virus is neuraminidate-O-acetylesterase. *EMBO J* **4**, 1503–6.

Hewat, E.A., Cusack, S., Ruigrok, R.W.H. & Verwey, C. (1984) Low resolution structure of the influenza C glycoprotein determined by electron microscopy. *J Mol Biol* **175**, 175–93.

Hirst, G.K. & Pons, M.W. (1973) Mechanism of influenza recombination. II. Virus aggregation and its effect on plaque formation by so-called noninfective virus. *Virology* **56**, 620–31.

Hongo, S., Sugawara, K., Muraki, Y., Kitame, F. & Nakamura, K. (1997) Characterization of a second protein (CM2) encoded by RNA segment 6 of influenza C virus. *J Virol* **71**, 2786–92.

Hoyle, L., Horne, R.W. & Waterson, A.P. (1961) The structure and composition of the myxoviruses. II. Components released from the influenza virus particle by ether. *Virology* **13**, 448–59.

Huang, T.S., Palese, P. & Krystal, M. (1990) Determination of influenza virus proteins required for genome replication. *J Virol* **64**, 5669–73.

Jennings, P.A., Finch, J.T., Winter, G. & Robertson, J.S. (1983) Does the higher order structure of the influenza virus ribonucleoprotein guide sequence rearrangements in influenza virus RNA? *Cell* **34**, 619–27.

Jin, H., Leser, G.P. & Lamb, R.A. (1994) The influenza virus haemagglutinin cytoplasmic tail is not essential for virus assembly or infectivity. *EMBO J* **13**, 5504–15.

Jin, H., Leser, G.P., Zhang, J. & Lamb, R.A. (1997) Influenza virus haemagglutinin and neuraminidase cytoplasmic tails control particle shape. *EMBO J* **16**, 1236–47.

Kates, M., Allison, A.C., Tyrell, D.A. & James, A.T. (1962) Origin of lipids in influenza virus. *Cold Spring Harbor Symp Quant Biol* **27**, 293–301.

Kendal, A.P. (1975) A comparison of influenza C with prototype myxovirus receptor-destroying activity (neuraminidase) and structural polypeptides. *Virology* **65**, 87–99.

Kendal, A.P., Calphin, J.C. & Palmer, E.L. (1977) Replication of influenza virus at elevated temperatures: Production of virus-like particles with reduced matrix protein content. *Virology* **76**, 186–95.

Kimura, N., Nishida, M., Nagata, K., Ishihama, A., Oda, K., & Nakada, S. (1992) Transcription of a recombinant influenza virus RNA in cells that can express the influenza virus RNA polymerase and nucleoprotein genes. *J Gen Virol* **73**, 1321–8.

Kitame, F., Sugawara, K., Ohwada, K. & Homma, M. (1982) Proteoolytic activation of haemolysis and fusion by influenza C virions. *Archiv Virol* **73**, 357–61.

Klenk, H.D., Rott, R. & Becht, H. (1972) On the structure of the influenza virus envelope. *Virology* **47**, 579–91.

Klumpp, K., Ruigrok, R.W.H. & Baudin, F. (1997) Roles of the influenza virus polymerase and nucleoprotein in forming a functional RNP structure. *EMBO J* **16**, 1248–57.

Kretzschmar, E., Bui, M. & Rose, J.K. (1996) Membrane association of influenza virus matrix protein does not require specific hydrophobic domains or the viral glycoproteins. *Virology* **220**, 37–45.

Krug, R.M. (1971) Influenza viral RNPs newly synthesized during the latent period of viral growth in MDCK cells. *Virology* **44**, 125–36.

Lamb, R.A. (1989) Genes and proteins of the influenza viruses. In: Krug, R.M. (ed.) *The Influenza Viruses*, pp. 1–87. Plenum Press, New York & London.

Lamb, R.A., Lai, C.J. & Choppin, P.W. (1981) Sequences of mRNAs derived from genome RNA segment 7 of influenza virus: colinear and interrupted mRNAs code for overlapping proteins. *Proc Natl Acad Sci USA* **78**, 4170–4.

Laver, W.G. (1964) Structural studies on the protein subunits from three strains of influenza virus. *J Mol Biol* **9**, 109–24.

Laver, W.G. & Downie, J.C. (1976) Influenza virus recombination. I. Matrix protein markers and segregation during mixed infection. *Virology* **70**, 105–17.

Lin, C. & Air, G.M. (1993) Selection and characterization of a neuraminidase-minus mutant of influenza virus and its rescue by cloned neuraminidase genes. *Virology* **194**, 403–7.

Luytjes, W., Krystal, M., Enami, M., Parvin, J.D. & Palese, P. (1989) Amplification, expression, and packaging of a foreign gene by influenza virus. *Cell* **59**, 1107–13.

Mandler, J., Müller, K. & Scholtissek, C. (1991) Mutants and revertants of an avian influenza A virus with temperature-sensitive defects in the nucleoprotein and PB2. *Virology* **181**, 512–9.

Martin, K. & Helenius, A. (1991) Nuclear transport of influenza virus ribonucleoproteins: The viral matrix protein (M1) promotes export and inhibits import. *Cell* **67**, 117–30.

McGeoch, D., Fellner, P. & Newton, C. (1976) Influenza virus genome consists of eight distinct RNA species. *Proc Natl Acad Sci USA* **73**, 3045–9.

Mellema, J.E., Andree, P.J., Krijgsman, P.C.J. *et al.* (1981) Structural investigations of influenza B virus. *J Mol Biol* **151**, 329–36.

Mena, I., de la Luna, S., Albo, C. *et al.* (1994) Synthesis of biologically active influenza virus core proteins using a vaccinia virus-T7 RNA polymerase expression system. *J Gen Virol* **75**, 2109–14.

Metsikkö, K. & Simons, K. (1986) The budding mechanism of spikeless vesicular stomatitis virus particles. *EMBO J* **5**, 1913–20.

Mitnaul, L.J., Castrucci, M.R., Murti, K.G. & Kawaoka, Y. (1996) The cytoplasmic tail of influenza virus neuraminidase (NA) affects incorporation into virions, virion morphology, and virulence in mice but is not essential for virus replication. *J Virol* **70**, 873–9.

Murti, K.G. & Webster, R.G. (1986) Distribution of haemagglutinin and neuraminidase on influenza virions as revealed by immunoelectron microscopy. *Virology* **149**, 36–43.

Murti, K.G., Bean, W.J. & Webster, R.G. (1980) Helical ribonucleoproteins of influenza virus: an electron microscopic analysis. *Virology* **104**, 224–9.

Murti, K.G., Webster, R.G. & Jones, I.M. (1988) Localization of RNA polymerases on influenza viral ribonucleoproteins by immunogold labelling. *Virology* **164**, 562–6.

Murti, K.G., Brown, P.S., Bean, W.J. & Webster, R.G. (1992) Composition of the helical internal components of influenza virus as revealed by immunogold labelling/ electron microscopy. *Virology* **186**, 294–9.

Naim, H.Y. & Roth, M.G. (1993) Basis for selective incorporation of glycoproteins into the influenza virus envelope. *J Virol* **67**, 4831–41.

Nermut, M.V. (1972) Further investigation on the fine structure of influenza virus. *J Gen Virol* **17**, 317–31.

Nermut, M.V. & Frank, H. (1971) Fine structure of influenza A2 (Singapore) as revealed by negative staining, freeze-drying and freeze-etching. *J Gen Virol* **10**, 37–51.

Neumann, G. & Hobom, G. (1995) Mutational analysis of influenza virus promotor elements *in vivo*. *J Gen Virol* **76**, 1709–17.

Odagiri, T. & Tashiro, M. (1997) Segment specific non-coding sequences of the influenza virus genome RNA are involved in the specific competition between defective interfering RNA and its progenitor RNA segment at the virion assembly step. *J Virol* **71**, 2138–45.

Oxford, J.S. & Hockley, D.J. (1987) Orthomyxoviridae. In: Nermut, M.V. & Steven, A.C. (eds) *Animal Virus Structure*, pp. 213–32. Elsevier, Amsterdam.

Oxford, J.S., Corcoran, T. & Hugentobler, A.L. (1981) Quantitative analysis of the protein composition of influenza A and B viruses using high resolution SDS polyacrylamide gels. *J Biol Standard* **9**, 483–91.

Pattnaik, A.K., Brown, D.J. & Nayak, D.P. (1986) Formation of influenza virus particles lacking haemagglutinin on the viral envelope. *J Virol* **60**, 994–1001.

Pinto, L.H., Holsinger, L.J. & Lamb, R.A. (1992) Influenza virus M2 protein has ion channel activity. *Cell* **69**, 517–28.

Pons, M.W., Schulze, I.T., Hirst, G.K. & Hauser, R. (1969) Isolation and characterization of the ribonucleoprotein of influenza virus. *Virology* **39**, 250–9.

Ruigrok, R.W.H. (1985) *Structural studies on influenza virus.* PhD thesis, State University of Leiden, The Netherlands.

Ruigrok, R.W.H. & Baudin, F. (1995) Structure of influenza virus RNP. II. Purified, RNA-free influenza ribonucleoprotein forms structures that are indistinguishable from the intact viral ribonucleoprotein particles. *J Gen Virol* **76**, 1009–14.

Ruigrok, R.W.H. & Hewat, E.A. (1991) Comparison of negatively stained and frozen hydrated samples of influenza viruses A and B and of vesicular stomatitis virus. *Micron Microsc Acta* **22**, 423–34.

Ruigrok, R.W.H., Andree, P.J., Hooft van Huysduynen, R.A.M. & Mellema, J.E. (1984a) Characterization of three highly purified influenza virus strains by electron microscopy. *J Gen Virol* **65**, 799–802.

Ruigrok, R.W.H., Nermut, M.V. & Andree, P.J. (1984b) The molecular mass of adenovirus type 5 as determined by means of scanning transmission electron microscopy (STEM). *J Virol Meth* **9**, 69–78.

Ruigrok, R.W.H., Krijgsman, P.C.J., de Ronde-Verloop, F.M. & de Jong, J.C. (1985) Natural heterogeneity of shape, infectivity and protein composition in an influenza A (H$_3$N$_2$) preparation. *Virus Res* **3**, 69–76.

Ruigrok, R.W.H., Calder, L.J. & Wharton, S.A. (1989) Electron microscopy of the influenza virus submembranal structure. *Virology* **173**, 311–6.

Schulze, I.T. (1972) The structure of influenza virus. II. A model based on the morphology and composition of subviral particles. *Virology* **47**, 181–96.

Sha, B. & Luo, M. (1997) Structure of a bifunctional membrane-RNA binding protein, influenza virus matrix protein. *Nat Struct Biol* **4**, 239–44.

Shaw, M.W., Choppin, P.W. & Lamb, R.A. (1983) A previously unrecognized influenza B virus glycoprotein from a bicistronic mRNA that also encodes the viral neuraminidase. *Proc Natl Acad Sci USA* **80**, 4879–83.

Smith, G.L. & Hay, A.J. (1982) Replication of the influenza virus genome. *Virology* **118**, 96–108.

Sugrue, R.J. & Hay, A.J. (1991) Structural characteristics of the M2 protein of influenza A viruses: evidence that it forms a tetrameric channel. *Virology* **180**, 617–24.

Thomas, D., Newcomb, W.W., Brown, J.C. *et al.* (1985) Mass and molecular composition of vesicular stomatitis virus: a STEM analysis. *J Virol* **54**, 598–607.

Watanabe, K., Handa, H., Mizumoto, K. & Nagata, K. (1996) Mechanism for inhibition of influenza virus RNA polymerase activity by matrix protein. *J Virol* **70**, 241–7.

Wharton, S.A., Weis, W., Skehel, J.J. & Wiley, D.C. (1989) Structure, function, and antigenicity of the haemagglutinin of influenza virus. In: Krug, R.M. (ed.) *The Influenza Viruses*, pp. 153–74. Plenum Press, New York & London.

Wharton, S.A., Hay, A.J., Sugrue, R.J., Skehel, J.J., Weis, W.I. & Wiley, D.C. (1990) Membrane fusion by influenza viruses and the mechanism of action of amantadine. In: Laver, W.G. & Air, G.M. (eds) *Use of X-ray Crystallography in the Design of Antiviral Agents*, pp. 1–12. Academic Press, Orlando.

Wrigley, N.G. (1979) Electron microscopy of influenza virus. *Br Med Bull* **35**, 35–8.

Wrigley, N.G., Brown, E.B. & Skehel, J.J. (1986) Electron microscopy of influenza virus. In: Harris J.R. (ed) *Electron Microscopy of Proteins. 5 Viral Structure*, pp. 103–63. Academic Press Inc., London.

Yamashita, M., Krystal, M. & Palese, P. (1988) Evidence that the matrix protein of influenza C virus is encoded for by a spliced mRNA. *J Virol* **62**, 3348–55.

Yang, P., Bansal, A., Liu, C. & Air, G.M. (1997) Hemagglutinin specificity and neuraminidase coding capacity of neuraminidase-deficient influenza viruses. *Virology* **229**, 155–65.

Yasuda, J., Nakada, S., Kato, A., Toyoda, T. & Ishihama, A. (1993) Molecular assembly of influenza virus: association of the NS2 protein with virion matrix. *Virology* **196**, 249–55.

Ye, Z., Baylor, N.W. & Wagner, R.R. (1989) Transcription-inhibition and RNA-binding domains of influenza A virus matrix protein mapped with anti-idiotypic antibodies and synthetic peptides. *J Virol* **63**, 3586–94.

Ye, Z., Robinson, D. & Wagner, R.R. (1995) Nucleus-targeting domain of the matrix protein (M1) of influenza virus. *J Virol* **69**, 1964–70.

Zebedee, S.L. & Lamb, R.A. (1988) Influenza virus M2 protein: monoclonal antibody restriction of virus growth and detection of M2 in virions. *J Virol* **62**, 2762–72.

Zebedee, S.L. & Lamb, R.A. (1989) Growth restriction of influenza A virus by M2 protein antibody is genetically linked to the M1 protein. *Proc Natl Acad Sci USA* **86**, 1061–5.

Zhang, J. & Lamb, R.A. (1996) Characterization of the membrane association of the influenza virus matrix protein in living cells. *Virology* **225**, 255–66.

Zvonarjev, A.Y. & Ghendon, Y.Z. (1980) Influence of membrane (M) protein on influenza virion transcription activity *in vitro* and its susceptibility to rimantadine. *J Virol* **33**, 583–6.

CHAPTER 4

The Virus Genome and its Replication

Alan J. Hay

The family *Orthomyxoviridae* includes three genera, the influenza A, B and C viruses. B and C viruses are largely restricted to man, whereas the majority of influenza A viruses infect avian species and only a few antigenic subtypes infect man and other animals, in particular pigs and horses (see Chapter 10). A fourth genus, *Thogotavirus*, includes tick-transmitted orthomyxoviruses (Pringle 1996). This chapter describes briefly the general features of the genetic make-up of influenza viruses, the protein products they encode and the process of virus replication. The structure and function of certain virus proteins, including the haemagglutinin (HA), the neuraminidase (NA) and the M2, NB and NS1 proteins, are considered in detail in Chapters 5–8. With a few exceptions, the corresponding genes and protein products and the mechanisms involved in virus replication are similar for the three types of influenza virus. The influenza A viruses have been the most thoroughly investigated and are best understood—thus the discussion will predominantly reflect information derived from the study of these viruses.

The virus genome

The RNA genome is single-stranded, of negative polarity (i.e. complementary to mRNA) and segmented, most segments encoding single gene products. The genomes of A and B viruses comprise eight segments whereas that of influenza C comprises seven segments. A single RNA segment of influenza C encodes a haemagglutinin-esterase fusion (HEF) protein which possesses both the receptor binding and membrane fusion activities of

the haemagglutinin and the receptor destroying activity of the neuraminidase, which are encoded by separate gene segments of influenza A and B viruses. The lengths of the genome segments and the proteins they encode are listed in Table 4.1. With the exception of the smallest segments, in particular M and NS, they encode single gene products. There is relatively little redundancy. The short noncoding sequences at each end include the sequences of 11–13 nucleotides at the 5′ ends and 9–12 nucleotides at the 3′ ends which are highly conserved between the seven or eight different RNA segments of the genome and which are similar for A, B and C viruses (Skehel & Hay 1978; Desselberger *et al.* 1980; Stoeckle *et al.* 1987).

The three largest genes code for the components of the RNA polymerase, PB1, PB2 and PA of influenza A (Horisberger 1980) and their equivalents in B and C viruses (Yamashita *et al.* 1989). Segment 4 (in terms of length) encodes the haemagglutinin (HA) of influenza A and B viruses and the HEF protein of influenza C. Segment 5 encodes the nucleoprotein, the major structural component associated with the virus RNA to form the ribonucleoprotein (RNP). Segment 6 of A and B viruses encodes the virus neuraminidase (NA); there is no equivalent RNA segment in influenza C, the corresponding function being fulfilled by the HEF protein. This segment of influenza B viruses also encodes the NB protein. The two proteins, NA and NB, are translated from overlapping reading frames of the bicistronic mRNA; NB initiates at the first AUG, four nucleotides before the AUG which initiates translation of the NA in a +1 reading frame (Shaw *et al.* 1983). Only 300 nucleotides encode the

Table 4.1 Influenza genes and their products.

Genome segment	Influenza A		Influenza B		Influenza C	
	RNA segment length	Polypeptide length	RNA segment length	Polypeptide length	RNA segment length	Polypeptide length
PB2	2341	759	2396	770	2365	774
PB1	2341	757	2386	752	2363	754
PA	2233	716	2308	726	2183	704
HA	1778	566	1882	584	2071	654
NP	1565	498	1842	560	1809	565
NA	1413	454	1557	466 (NA)	—	—
				100 (NB)		
M	1027	252 (M1)	1188	248 (M1)	1180	242 (M1)
		97 (M2)		109 (BM2)		139 (CM2)
NS	890	230 (NS1)	1098	281 (NS1)	934	286 (NS1)
		121 (NS2)		122 (NS2)		122 (NS2)

The data listed are for influenza viruses A/PR/8/34 (all segments); B/AA/1/66 (segments 1, 2, 3, 5, 7 and 8: De Borde *et al.* 1988); B/Lee/40 (segments 4 and 6: Krystal *et al.* 1982; Shaw *et al.* 1982); C/JJ/50 (segments 1, 2, 3 and 6: Yamashita *et al.* 1988, 1989); C/California/78 (segments 4, 5 and 7: Nakada *et al.* 1984a,b; Buonagurio *et al.* 1986).

100 amino acid NB, whereas the sequence of 1398 nucleotides encoding the 466 amino acid NA occupies most of the mRNA transcript. NB, like the NA, is an integral membrane protein and is a component of the virus envelope (Betakova *et al.* 1996; Brassard *et al.* 1996). On the basis of similarities in structure and ion channel activity it has been suggested that NB has an analogous function in virus uncoating to that of the M2 product of the M gene of influenza A viruses (see Chapter 7).

The two smallest segments of A and B (segments 7 and 8) and C (segments 6 and 7) viruses also encode two proteins (Fig. 4.1). The coding strategies of the M genes of the three viruses differ both in terms of the mechanisms involved and in terms of the functions of the secondary products. The principal product in terms of amount, the M1 or matrix protein, which is the major internal structural component of the virus particle (see chapter 3), is translated from the full-length (colinear) mRNA transcript of A and B segment 7; in contrast, it is the product of a spliced mRNA of influenza C segment 7, translation terminating at a codon introduced at the splice junction (Yamashita *et al.* 1988; Hongo *et al.* 1994). The CM2 protein is synthesized from the full-length mRNA; translation initiates at an internal AUG initiation codon in a +1 reading frame overlapping that encoding M1. Which of three AUG codons between nucleotides 730 and 748 is used has yet to be determined, as has the amino acid sequence at the N terminus of the protein. The function of the CM2 integral membrane protein is not known, although on the basis of structural similarities it has been proposed that it performs a function similar to that of the M2 protein of influenza A viruses (Hongo *et al.* 1997). The BM2 protein of influenza B is also translated from the full-length bicistronic mRNA of the M gene and initiates at an internal AUG codon which overlaps the termination codon for M1 in a pentanucleotide, UAAUG (Horvath *et al.* 1990). In contrast to the M2 protein of influenza A and C viruses, which are integral membrane proteins, BM2 is a soluble cytoplasmic protein, the function of which is unknown. Furthermore, neither A nor C viruses appear to encode an equivalent protein. The M2 ion channel is translated from a spliced mRNA of the M gene of influenza A such that the first nine amino acids are shared with the M1 protein and the bulk of the molecule is translated in a +1 reading frame from a sequence of 263 nucleotides close to the 3' end of the transcript and overlapping the sequence encoding the M1 product (Inglis & Brown 1981; Lamb *et al.* 1981). The M2 protein forms a homotetrameric

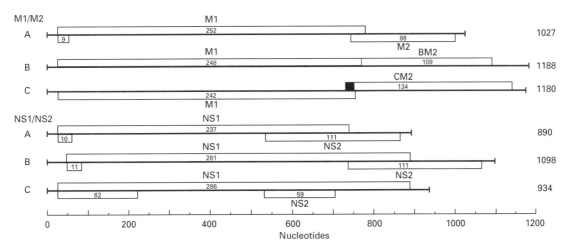

Fig. 4.1 Schematic representation of the coding regions (positive sense) of the M and NS genes of influenza A, B and C viruses. The lengths of the genome segments are indicated on the right. The positions of initiation and termination of translation are indicated in relation to the scale at the bottom and the number of amino acids encoded are shown within the boxes. The products of the full-length (colinear) mRNAs are shown above the lines and the products of spliced mRNAs below the lines. The influenza BM1 and BM2 proteins are translated from a bicistronic mRNA, the initiation codon for BM2 overlapping the termination codon for M1 in the pentanucleotide UAAUG, nucleotides 769–773 (Horvath *et al*. 1990). Translation of CM2 of influenza C from the full-length mRNA does not initiate at the first AUG; which of three internal AUGs between nucleotides 731 and 748 is used has not been determined (Hongo *et al*. 1994). M1 of influenza C is translated from a spliced mRNA; translation initiates at the first AUG (nucleotides 26–28) and terminates at a UGA codon (nucleotides 752–754) generated by the splice (Yamashita *et al*. 1988). M2 of influenza A and NS2 of influenza A, B and C viruses are products of both exons of the spliced mRNAs (Lamb & Lai 1980; Lamb *et al*. 1981; Briedis & Lamb 1982). The short N-terminal regions are therefore identical in sequence to those of the corresponding M1/NS1 proteins and the remainder of the molecule is translated in the +1 reading frame from the second exon. Influenza A M2 and influenza A and B NS2 coding sequences overlap the termination sites of the corresponding product of the full-length mRNA and terminate close to the end of the transcript (Nakada *et al*. 1986). The first exon of influenza C spliced NS mRNA encodes approximately half of the polypeptide (62 amino acids) and translation of the second exon terminates upstream of the termination site for NS1, which is close to the end of the transcript (Nakada *et al*. 1986). The details shown relate to the M and NS genes of A/PR/8/34, B/AnnArbor/1/66 and C/AnnArbor/1/50.

proton channel which participates with the HA in uncoating the infecting virus RNP during endocytosis, and can modulate the pH of the *trans* Golgi (see Chapter 7).

The smallest RNA segments of the three types of virus each encode two products using a similar strategy to that of the M gene of influenza A. The major product, the nonstructural RNA-binding NS1 protein, is translated from the full-length mRNA, while NS2 is translated from a spliced mRNA. The mRNAs of A and B NS2 proteins contain a short 5′ leader sequence, which encodes 10 and 11 amino acids, respectively, corresponding to the N termini of the NS1 products, spliced to approximately 360 nucleotides at the 3′ end of the transcript which encode a further 111 amino acids in the +1 reading frame, which overlaps the termination site for NS1 (Fig. 4.1; Lamb & Lai 1980; Briedis & Lamb 1982). The spliced mRNA of the influenza C NS gene contains a longer 5′ terminal region which encodes about half of the polypeptide, and translation in a +1 reading frame terminates upstream of the termination site for NS1, which is located close to the 3′ end of the transcript (Fig. 4.1; Nakada *et al*. 1986). Various regulatory roles of influenza A and B NS1 proteins are discussed in detail in Chapter 8. The function of the NS2 protein is not well understood; it has been shown to be associated with the M1 protein in virus particles (Yasuda *et al.* 1993; Ward *et al.* 1995) and to be involved in facilitating the exit of progeny vRNPs from the nucleus of virus-infected cells.

Like other negative-strand RNA viruses, the virion contains a transcriptase which initiates replication by transcribing the infecting genome into mRNA—a process referred to as primary transcription. Two notable features of influenza virus replication are that transcription and replication of the genome occur in the nucleus of the virus-infected cell and that the transcriptase uses the ends of host cell pre-mRNAs to prime the synthesis of viral mRNAs by a 'cap-snatching' mechanism.

Virus entry

The initial phase of virus infection involves the delivery of transcriptionally active virus RNPs to the nucleus of infected cells to initiate the expression and replication of the virus genome. The major glycoprotein spike on the virus, the HA of A and B viruses and the HEF protein of influenza C, attaches to sialic acid-containing glycoprotein and glycolipid receptors on the cell surface. The specificity of recognition may differ. In particular, the HAs of A and B viruses bind *N*-acetylneuraminic acid (sialic acid) whereas the HEF glycoprotein of influenza C binds to the modified sialic acid, 9–O-acetyl N-acetylneuraminic acid (Rogers *et al.* 1986; Herrler & Klenk 1991). This difference in binding specificity is reflected in the corresponding specificities of the receptor-destroying enzymes, the neuraminidase (NA) of A and B viruses which cleaves the terminal sialic acid residue from the receptor, and the acetyl-esterase activity of the HEF of influenza C which removes the 9–O-acetyl moiety from the terminal sialic acid (Herrler *et al.* 1985). Furthermore, the fine specificity of receptor binding may depend on the glycosidic linkage between the terminal sialic acid and penultimate galactose residues. For example, human influenza A viruses preferentially bind sialic acid residues attached to galactose by an α2→6 linkage whereas avian and equine viruses exhibit a preference for sialic acid attached by an α2→3 linkage (Rogers & Paulson

1983; Connor *et al.* 1994). Following attachment the virus enters the cell by receptor-mediated endocytosis via clathrin-coated pits. The acid pH, between 5 and 6, of endosomes activates the processes which promote the uncoating and entry of the virus RNP into the cytoplasm. It triggers a structural change in the HA which induces fusion between the virus membrane and the endosome membrane to liberate the internal core (see Chapter 5). Secondly, prior to this fusion event, H^+ flows through the M2 channel in the membrane of influenza A viruses to cause an acid-induced dissociation of the M1 (matrix) protein from the virion RNP, which is essential for subsequent migration of free RNPs from the cytoplasm to the nucleus (see Chapter 7; Whittaker *et al.* 1996b). Inhibition of either event by artifically increasing endosome pH or specifically blocking the M2 channel with amantadine prevents infection (Hay 1992).

RNA transcription and replication

Entry of the virus RNPs into the nucleus through nuclear pores involves the normal cellular machinery, and components with which NP interacts have been identified (Whittaker *et al.* 1996b; Wang *et al.* 1997). The initial phase of transcription (primary transcription) of the genome into mRNAs is catalysed by the virion RNA polymerase attached to the infecting virus RNPs (Hay *et al.* 1977b). Only after subsequent synthesis of virus proteins does replication of the virus RNA ensue. Synthesis of the viral mRNAs is primed by 5'-capped (m^7Gppp Nm-containing) fragments, 10-13 nucleotides in length, of newly synthesized host cell pre-mRNAs and transcription terminates prior to the end of the template at a stretch of 5–7 uridylate (U) residues which appears to serve as a template for reiterative copying of poly(A) tails (Bouloy *et al.* 1978; Krug *et al.* 1979; Krug 1981; Plotch *et al.* 1979, 1981; Hay *et al.* 1977a; Skehel & Hay 1978; Robertson *et al.* 1981). The viral mRNAs are therefore incomplete transcripts with additional sequences attached to both ends. To replicate the genome RNAs, exact complementary template cRNAs are synthesized without priming (Hay *et al.* 1977b, 1982).

The transcription complex of influenza A viruses

consists of a trimeric polymerase comprising PB1, PB2 and PA proteins together with the NP in association with the RNA template. The PB1 component is the transcriptase *per se* which catalyses nucleotide addition in the initiation and elongation of the RNA transcript (Ulmanen *et al.* 1981; Biswas & Nayak 1994; Romanos & Hay 1984; Asano *et al.* 1995). The PB2 component is a cap-dependent endonuclease which serves both to bind the capped RNA and to cleave it to generate the primers of viral mRNA synthesis (Ulmanen *et al.* 1981; Blaas *et al.* 1982; Shi *et al.* 1995). The PA component is required for vRNA replication (Nakagawa *et al.* 1996) but its actual role is less well understood. Virion RNPs are super-coiled rod-shaped structures in which both the 5′ and 3′ ends of the virus RNAs are associated with the polymerase complex (see Chapter 3). The significance of this arrangement was demonstrated by the template requirements for the formation of an active transcriptase complex from recombinant polymerase subunits expressed by recombinant vaccinia viruses (Hagan *et al.* 1994; Tiley *et al.* 1994; Cianci *et al.* 1995), which indicated the following sequence of interactions in initiating synthesis of viral mRNAs.

1 Interaction of the conserved 5′ end of the template vRNA with the polymerase complex is required to activate the cap-binding function of PB2 to 'snatch' a host cell pre-mRNA.

2 Interaction of the conserved 3′ end of the template is then required to activate endonucleolytic cleavage of the bound cell mRNA to generate the 10–13 nucleotide primer which initiates transcription, usually at the penultimate 3′ C residue of the template. Interaction of the common sequence at the 5′ ends of the mRNA transcripts with the polymerase complex selectively protects the viral mRNAs from a similar endonucleolytic cleavage (Shih & Krug 1996a). The structural relationship between the partially complementary 5′ and 3′ ends of the vRNAs during initiation of transcription is still unclear (Klumpp *et al.* 1997). Mutational analyses of the transcriptional promoters have indicated, however, that they may form a partially double-stranded structure in which the ends are single-stranded and nucleotides 10–13 or 15 at the 3′ end form a duplex with nucleotides 11–14 or 16 at

the 5′ end which is stabilized by RNA–protein and protein–protein interactions (Fodor *et al.* 1994; Flick *et al.* 1996; Kim *et al.* 1997).

3 The primer, at the 5′ end of the mRNA, is released from PB2 after transcription of some 11–15 nucleotides (Braam *et al.* 1983).

4 Continued association of the 5′ end of the template vRNA with the transcriptase appears to be responsible for preventing elongation of the transcript to the end of the template; transcription terminates at the stretch of 5–7 uridylate residues some 20 nucleotides from the 5′ end, and polyadenylate (poly(A)) is added, apparently by a process of reiterative copying of the oligo U sequence (Luo *et al.* 1991; Li & Palese 1994). In the absence of viral protein synthesis this process perpetuates (Hay *et al.* 1977b). The factors required to cause the virion polymerase to switch from the primed synthesis of incomplete polyadenylated transcripts to unprimed initiation of complete transcripts are still poorly understood. Free nucleoprotein can promote readthrough of the transcription termination/polyadenylation signal, presumably by association with the nascent transcript (Beaton & Krug 1986; Shapiro & Krug 1988). Although it is apparent that the virion enzyme is involved in production of the cRNA template it is possible that different types of polymerase complex are involved in vRNA replication. Dissection of the transcription/replication activities of the different polymerase components expressed in established cell lines has shown that PB1 alone, in the presence of NP, is sufficient for unprimed transcription of a model viral RNA template (Nakagawa *et al.* 1996). Coexpression of PA and PB1 together with NP in another cell-line supported replication as well as transcription of RNA template (Nakagawa *et al.* 1995, 1996), whereas co-expression of all three polymerase subunits, PB1, PB2 and PA, in a third cell line was required for primed synthesis of viral mRNAs as well as unprimed transcription and replication (Kimura *et al.* 1992).

Regulation of gene expression

Regulation of virus gene expression involves the interaction of an array of host cell and viral factors and operates at various levels from the selective synthesis of vRNAs to regulation of mRNA translation. Only the more notable features are mentioned here. Superficially, the production of virus proteins is regulated with respect to the time they are required during replication and in relation to the relative amounts of the structural components required for assembly into virions. The relative synthesis of the different proteins during infection is largely determined by the relative amounts of the corresponding mRNAs (Hay 1977b; Shapiro *et al.* 1987). Two phases of gene expression, *early* and *late*, are readily distinguished. The *early* phase follows primary transcription and represents an initial stage of vRNA replication and amplification of mRNA production. It is characterized by the preferential synthesis of the NP and NS1 proteins and is the direct consequence of selective replication of the vRNA templates from which their mRNAs are transcribed (Skehel 1972; Hay *et al.* 1977b; Smith & Hay 1982; Shapiro *et al.* 1987). This reflects the prominent roles of these proteins in the regulation of transcription and replication of viral RNAs. During the *late* phase, principally concerned with the production of virion structural components, the vRNAs are synthesized in more equivalent amounts as required for progeny genomes, and preferential transcription of mRNAs is directed towards greater production of e.g. the HA and M1 proteins and reduced synthesis of NS1. The delayed synthesis of the M1 protein may also be related to its ability to inhibit vRNA transcription and mediate vRNP export out of the nucleus.

Regulation of mRNA splicing is also important in controlling the relative amounts of the products of full-length and spliced mRNAs of the M and NS genes. The extent of NS1 mRNA splicing, at a steady-state level of about 10%, is determined largely by a combination of the rate of splicing, which is controlled by *cis*-acting sequences in the NS1 mRNA, and the rate of export of the NS1 mRNA out of the nucleus (Alonso-Caplen & Krug 1991; Nemeroff *et al.* 1992). On the other hand, the production of the influenza A M2 ion channel protein at later times during infection is controlled by both viral and cellular proteins which together enhance the level of M2 mRNA (Valcárcel *et al.*

1991). Association of the viral polymerase complex with the 5′ terminal sequence of the M1 mRNA transcript blocks the more distal, stronger alternative 5′ splice site (which if used, generates a mRNA with a reading frame for only nine amino acids) and secondly, interaction of the cellular splicing factor SF2/ASF with a purine-rich splicing enhancer sequence in the 3′ exon activates the weaker more proximal M2 5′ splice site to increase production of M2 mRNA (Shih *et al.* 1995; Shih & Krug 1996b). Furthermore, inhibition of M1 mRNA splicing by the NS1 protein is reduced at later times during infection (Lu *et al.* 1994). In contrast to the relatively small proportion of spliced influenza A M mRNA, the majority of influenza C virus M mRNA is spliced to produce the M1 mRNA, reflecting the greater requirement for M1 than for the CM2 translation product of the full-length message (Hongo *et al.* 1994).

A major viral factor which regulates events at a post-transcriptional level is the RNA-binding protein NS1, discussed in detail in Chapter 8. On the one hand, the protein binds specifically to a stem-bulge structure of small nuclear RNA (snRNA) splicing factors, in particular the U6 snRNA, in order to block mRNA splicing (Fortes *et al.* 1994; Lu *et al.* 1994; Qiu *et al.* 1995), and to poly(A) RNA to inhibit the export of mRNA out of the nucleus (Alonso-Caplen *et al.* 1992; Fortes *et al.* 1994; Qiu & Krug 1994). The precise roles of these activities is unclear, although one consequence of trapping cellular pre-mRNAs in the nucleus of infected cells may be to increase the pool of potential primers for viral mRNA synthesis. However, although the NS1 protein of influenza B virus possesses an equivalent RNA binding domain, it lacks an effector domain present in NS1 of influenza A viruses (Qian *et al.* 1994) and as a consequence does not exhibit these two inhibitory activities in cells expressing the protein (Wang & Krug 1996). On the other hand, by binding to dsRNA, NS1 of both influenza A and B viruses blocks activation of the dsRNA-activated protein kinase (PKR) (Lu *et al.* 1995) which regulates the activity of the translation factor eIF2 and as a consequence reduces inhibition of translation. Virus infection also activates a cellular protein P58 which inhibits phosphorylation of eIF2 by PKR (Lee *et al.* 1992). In addition to combatting the more general effects of virus-induced shut-off of host cell protein synthesis, the NS1 protein can act as a specific enhancer of the initiation of translation of viral mRNAs (Enami *et al.* 1994; de la Luna *et al.* 1995). Furthermore, the 5' untranslated regions of the viral mRNAs, which contain information for the selective translation of viral over cellular mRNAs (Garfinkel & Katze 1993), may also provide the basis for preferential synthesis of certain virus proteins. Thus, like other viruses, influenza virus encodes a variety of mechanisms for regulating the selective synthesis of virus proteins during infection (Katze *et al.* 1986a,b).

Transport and assembly of virus components

Virus assembles at the plasma membrane of infected cells by a process of budding whereby the RNP–M1 core acquires a membrane derived from regions of the plasma membrane modified to contain almost exclusively virus membrane proteins.

The components of the transcription/replication complex, PB1, PB2, PA and NP each contain a karyophilic signal necessary for transport from their site of synthesis in the cytoplasm to the nucleus where they assemble into functional complexes and nucleocapsids destined for assembly into progeny virus particles. Furthermore, a sequence at the N terminus of NP has been shown to interact with nuclear pore docking proteins which may also facilitate translocation of infecting virus RNPs across the nuclear membrane (Wang *et al.* 1997). Regions of the three polymerase components which interact to form the trimeric complex have been mapped; PB1 is the core subunit of the assembly and N and C terminal regions interact with the PA and PB2 subunits, respectively (Gonzalez *et al.* 1996; Toyoda *et al.* 1996). The polymerase complex is associated with the termini of viral RNAs in RNPs (Klumpp *et al.* 1997). The mechanisms whereby these nucleocapsids are exported from the nucleus and a complement of genome (RNP) segments is assembled for packaging into progeny virus particles are poorly understood. M1 present in the nucleus has been shown to be required for vRNP export (Martin & Helenius 1991) and association of cytoplasmic M1 with vRNPs prevents re-entry (Whittaker *et al.* 1996a). The NS2 protein which is incorporated into virus particles has recently been more aptly renamed 'nuclear export protein' since it mediates export of vRNPs by acting as an adaptor between the viral RNP–M1 complexes and nucleoporins of the nuclear export machinery (P. Palese, personal communication).

The integral membrane proteins of the virus envelope, the HA, NA, M2 and NB proteins of influenza A and B viruses and the HEF and CM2 proteins of influenza C, are synthesized in association with the endoplasmic reticulum and inserted into the membrane by a signal recognition particle-dependent mechanism. During transport to the apical surface of epithelial cells via the Golgi apparatus, the proteins assemble into their mature multimeric structures and are modified by the addition of carbohydrate side chains and fatty acyl groups. In influenza A virus-infected cells the ionic environment of the exocytic pathway has been shown to be modified by the M2 proton channel; in particular, reduction in the acidity of the *trans* Golgi Network is necessary to prevent inactivation of the HAs of certain avian strains (Sugrue *et al.* 1990; Ciampor *et al.* 1992; Ohuchi *et al.* 1994; Takeuchi & Lamb 1994). The HAs of pathogenic avian influenza A viruses have a sequence of basic amino acids joining HA_1 and HA_2 which is readily cleaved by endoproteases, such as furin, within the *trans* Golgi Network (Stieneke-Grober *et al.* 1992) and as a consequence they become susceptible to low pH-induced structural alteration. From the correlation between the pH-modulating activity of the M2 proteins and the pH lability of the HAs of these viruses it is evident that this is an important function of their M2 proteins (Grambas *et al.* 1992). It is not clear, however, what advantage modification of pH or of the concentration of other ions within the exocytic pathway by M2 (or NB) might have for viruses with HAs which are cleaved only after insertion into the plasma membrane.

The virus membrane proteins are incorporated into areas of the plasma membrane from which cellular proteins become largely excluded. In addition to interacting with vRNPs and facilitating their egress from the nucleus, the M1 protein is associated with the plasma membrane and presumably forms the basis for interactions, still largely unknown, whereby the vRNPs assemble and bud from the plasma membrane of infected cells. The nature of interactions between the cytoplasmic domains of the integral membrane proteins and the M1–RNP complexes are poorly understood, as discussed in Chapter 3. The ion channel activity of M2 does not appear to be involved since inhibition by amantadine does not directly affect this stage of virus replication (Hay 1992). However, observations that antibodies against the N-terminal external domain of M2 can reduce virus production (Hughey *et al.* 1995) and that amino acid changes either within the C terminal cytoplasmic domain of M2 or within M1 abolish this effect of antibody interaction (Zebedee & Lamb 1989), indicate that interactions between M2 and M1 are important in assembling virus structure just as indirect structure–function interactions are involved in disassembly during virus infection.

References

Alonso-Caplen, F.V. & Krug, R.M. (1991) Regulation of the extent of splicing of influenza virus NS1 mRNA: role of the rates of splicing and of the nucleocytoplasmic transport of NS1 mRNA. *Mol Cell Biol* **11**, 1092–8.

Alonso-Caplen, F.V., Nemeroff, M.E., Qiu, Y. & Krug, R.M. (1992) Nucleocytoplasmic transport: the influenza virus NS$_1$ protein regulates the transport of spliced NS$_2$ mRNA and its precursor NS$_1$ mRNA. *Genes Dev* **6**, 255–67.

Asano, Y., Mizumoto, K., Maruyama, T. & Ishihama, A. (1995) Photoaffinity labelling of influenza virus RNA polymerase PB1 subunit with 8-azido GTP. *J Biochem (Tokyo)* **117**, 677–82.

Beaton, A.R. & Krug, R.M. (1986) Transcription antitermination during influenza viral template RNA synthesis requires the nucleocapsid protein and the absence of a 5' capped end. *Proc Natl Acad Sci USA* **83**, 6282–6.

Betakova, T., Nermut, M.V. & Hay, A.J. (1996) The NB protein is an integral component of the membrane of influenza B virus. *J Gen Virol* **77**, 2689–94.

Biswas, S.K. & Nayak, D.P. (1994) Mutational analysis of the conserved motifs of influenza A virus polymerase basic protein 1. *J Virol* **68**, 1819–26.

Blaas, D., Patzelt, E. & Kuechler, E. (1982) Cap-recognizing protein of influenza virus. *Virology* **116**, 339–48.

Bouloy, M., Plotch, S.J. & Krug, R.M. (1978) Globin mRNAs are primers for the transcription of influenza viral RNA *in vitro*. *Proc Natl Acad Sci USA* **75**, 4886–90.

Braam, J., Ulmanen, I. & Krug, R.M. (1983) Molecular model of a eucaryotic transcription complex: functions and movements of influenza P proteins during capped RNA-primed transcription. *Cell* **34**, 609–18.

Brassard, D.L., Leser, G.P. & Lamb, R.A. (1996) Influenza B virus NB glycoprotein is a component of virions. *Virology* **220**, 350–60.

Briedis, D.J. & Lamb, R.A. (1982) Influenza B virus genome: sequences and structural organization of RNA segment 8 and the mRNAs coding for the NS$_1$ and NS$_2$ proteins. *J Virol* **42**, 186–93.

Buonagurio, D.A., Nakada, S., Fitch, W.M. & Palese, P. (1986) Epidemiology of influenza C virus in man: multiple evolutionary lineages and low rate of change. *Virology* **153**, 12–21.

Ciampor, F., Bayley, P.M., Nermut, M.V., Hirst, E.M., Sugrue, R.J. & Hay, A.J. (1992) Evidence that the amantadine-induced, M$_2$-mediated conversion of influenza A virus haemagglutinin to the low pH conformation occurs in an acidic *trans* Golgi compartment. *Virology* **188**, 14–24.

Cianci, C., Tiley, L. & Krystal, M. (1995) Differential activation of the influenza virus polymerase via template RNA binding. *J Virol* **69**, 3995–9.

Connor, R.J., Kawaoka, Y., Webster, R.G. & Paulson, J.C. (1994) Receptor specificity in human, avian, and equine H2 and H3 influenza virus isolates. *Virology* **205**, 17–23.

DeBorde, D.C., Donabedian, A.M., Herlocher, M.L., Naeve, C.W. & Maassab, H.F. (1988) Sequence comparison of wild-type and cold-adapted B/Ann Arbor/1/66 influenza virus genes. *Virology* **163**, 429–43.

de la Luna, S., Fortes, P., Beloso, A. & Ortin, J. (1995) Influenza virus NS1 protein enhances the rate of translation initiation of viral mRNAs. *J Virol* **69**, 2427–33.

Desselberger, U., Racaniello, V.R., Zazra, J.J. & Palese, P. (1980) The 3' and 5' terminal sequences of influenza A, B and C virus RNA segments are highly conserved and show partial inverted complementarity. *Gene* **8**, 315–28.

Enami, K., Sato, T.A., Nakada, S. & Enami, M. (1994) Influenza virus NS1 protein stimulates translation of the M1 protein. *J Virol* **68**, 1432–7.

Flick, R., Neumann, G., Hoffmann, E., Neumeier, E. & Hobom, G. (1996) Promoter elements in the influenza vRNA terminal structure. *RNA* **2**, 1046–57.

Fodor, E., Pritlove, D.C. & Brownlee, G.G. (1994) The influenza virus panhandle is involved in the initiation of transcription. *J Virol* **68**, 4092–6.

Fortes, P., Beloso, A. & Ortin, J. (1994) Influenza virus NS$_1$ protein inhibits premRNA splicing and blocks mRNA nucleocytoplasmic transport. *EMBO J* **13**, 704–12.

Garfinkel, M.S. & Katze, M.G. (1993) Translational control by influenza virus. *J Biol Chem* **268**, 22 223–6.

Gonzalez, S., Zurcher, T. & Ortin, J. (1996) Identification of two separate domains in the influenza virus PB1 protein involved in the interaction with the PB2 and PA subunits: a model for the viral RNA polymerase structure. *Nucl Acids Res* **24**, 4456–63.

Grambas, S., Bennett, M.S. & Hay, A.J. (1992) Influence of amantadine resistance mutations on the pH regulatory function of the M_2 protein of influenza A viruses. *Virology* **191**, 541–9.

Hagen, M., Thomas, D.Y., Chung, J., Butcher, A. & Krystal, M. (1994) Recombinant influenza virus polymerase: requirements of both 5′ and 3′ viral ends for endonuclease activity. *J Virol* **68**, 1509–15.

Hay, A.J. (1992) The action of adamantanamines against influenza A viruses: inhibition of the M2 ion channel protein. *Sem Virol* **3**, 21–30.

Hay, A.J., Abraham, G., Skehel, J.J., Smith, J.C. & Fellner, P. (1977a) Influenza virus messenger RNAs are incomplete transcripts of the genome RNAs. *Nucl Acids Res* **4**, 4197–209.

Hay, A.J., Lomniczi, B., Bellamy, A.R. & Skehel, J.J. (1977b) Transcription of the influenza virus genome. *Virology* **83**, 337–55.

Hay, A.J., Skehel, J.J. & McCauley, J. (1982) Characterization of influenza virus RNA complete transcripts. *Virology* **116**, 517–22.

Herrler, G. & Klenk, H.D. (1991) Structure and function of the HEF glycoprotein of influenza C virus. *Adv Virus Res* **40**, 213–34.

Herrler, G., Rott, R., Klenk, H.D., Muller, H.P., Shukla, A.K. & Schauer, R. (1985) The receptor-destroying enzyme of influenza C virus is neuraminate-O-acetyl esterase. *EMBO J* **4**, 1503–6.

Hongo, S., Sugawara, K., Nishimura, H., Muraki, Y., Kitame, F. & Nakamura, K. (1994) Identification of a second protein encoded by influenza C virus RNA segment 6. *J Gen Virol* **75**, 3503–10.

Hongo, S., Sugawara, K., Muraki, Y., Kitame, F. & Nakamura, K. (1997) Characterization of a second protein (CM2) encoded by RNA segment 6 of influenza C virus. *J Virol* **71**, 2786–92.

Horisberger, M.A. (1980) The large P proteins of influenza A viruses are composed of one acidic and two basic polypeptides. *Virology* **107**, 302–5.

Horvath, C.M., Williams, M.A. & Lamb, R.A. (1990) Eukaryotic coupled translation of tandem cistrons: identification of the influenza B virus BM2 polypeptide. *EMBO J* **9**, 2639–47.

Hughey, P.G., Roberts, P.C., Holsinger, L.J., Zebedee, S.L., Lamb, R.A. & Compans, R.W. (1995) Effects of antibody to the influenza A virus M2 protein on M2 surface expression and virus assembly. *Virology* **212**, 411–21.

Inglis, S.C. & Brown, C.M. (1981) Spliced and unspliced RNAs encoded by virion RNA segment 7 of influenza virus. *Nucl Acids Res* **9**, 2727–40.

Katze, M.G., DeCorato, D. & Krug, R.M. (1986a) Cellular mRNA translation is blocked at both initiation and elongation after infection by influenza virus or adenovirus. *J Virol* **60**, 1027–39.

Katze, M.G., Detjen, B.M., Safer, B. & Krug, R.M. (1986b) Translational control by influenza virus: suppression of the kinase that phosphorylates the alpha subunit of initiation factor eIF-2 and selective translation of influenza viral mRNAs. *Mol Cell Biol* **6**, 1741–50.

Kim, H.-J., Fodor, E., Brownlee, G.G. & Seong, B.L. (1997) Mutational analysis of the RNA-fork model of the influenza A virus vRNA promoter *in vivo*. *J Gen Virol* **78**, 353–7.

Kimura, N., Nishida, M., Nagata, K., Ishihama, A., Oda, K. & Nakada, S. (1992) Transcription of a recombinant influenza virus RNA in cells that can express the influenza virus RNA polymerase and nucleoprotein genes. *J Gen Virol* **73**, 1321–8.

Klumpp, K., Ruigrok, R.W.H. & Baudin, F. (1997) Roles of the influenza virus polymerase and nucleoprotein in forming a functional RNP structure. *EMBO J* **16**, 1248–57.

Krug, R.M. (1981) Priming of influenza viral RNA transcription by capped heterologous RNAs. *Curr Top Microbiol Immunol* **93**, 125–49.

Krug, R.M., Broni, B. & Bouloy, M. (1979) Are the 5′ ends of influenza viral mRNAs synthesized *in vivo* donated by host mRNAs? *Cell* **18**, 329–34.

Krystal, M., Elliott, R.M., Benz, E.W. Jr, Young, J.F. & Palese, P. (1982) Evolution of influenza A and B viruses: conservation of structural features in the haemagglutinin genes. *Proc Natl Acad Sci USA* **79**, 4800–4.

Lamb, R.A. & Lai, C.J. (1980) Sequence of interrupted and uninterrupted mRNAs and cloned DNA coding for the two overlapping nonstructural proteins of influenza virus. *Cell.* **21**, 475–85.

Lamb, R.A., Lai, C.J. & Choppin, P.W. (1981) Sequences of mRNAs derived from genome RNA segment 7 of influenza virus: colinear and interrupted mRNAs code for overlapping proteins. *Proc Natl Acad Sci USA* **78**, 4170–4.

Lee, T.G., Tomita, J., Hovanessian, A.G. & Katze, M.G. (1992) Characterization and regulation of the 58 000-dalton cellular inhibitor of the interferon-induced, dsRNA-activated protein kinase. *J Biol Chem* **267**, 14 238–43.

Li, X. & Palese, P. (1994) Characterization of the polyadenylation signal of influenza virus RNA. *J Virol* **68**, 1245–9.

Lu, Y., Quian, X.Y. & Krug, R.M. (1994) The influenza virus NS_1 protein: a novel inhibitor of pre-mRNA splicing. *Genes Dev* **8**, 1817–28.

Lu, Y., Wambach, M., Katze, M.G. & Krug, R.M. (1995) Binding of the influenza virus NS1 protein to double-stranded RNA inhibits the activation of the protein kinase that phosphorylates the eIF-2 translation initiation factor. *Virology* **214**, 222–8.

Luo, G., Luytjes, W., Enami, M. & Palese, P. (1991) The polyadenylation signal of influenza virus RNA involves a stretch of uridines followed by the RNA duplex of the panhandle structure. *J Virol* **65**, 2861–7.

Martin, K. & Helenius, A. (1991) Nuclear transport of influenza virus ribonucleoproteins: the viral matrix protein (M$_1$) promotes export and inhibits import. *Cell* **67**, 117–30.

Nakada, S., Creager, R.S., Krystal, M., Aaronson, R.P. & Palese, P. (1984a) Influenza C virus haemagglutinin: comparison with influenza A and B virus haemagglutinins. *J Virol* **50**, 118–24.

Nakada, S., Creager, R.S., Krystal, M. & Palese, P. (1984b) Complete nucleotide sequence of the influenza C/California/78 virus nucleoprotein gene. *Virus Res* **1**, 433–41.

Nakada, S., Graves, P.N. & Palese, P. (1986) The influenza C virus NS gene: evidence for a spliced mRNA and a second NS gene product (NS$_2$ protein). *Virus Res* **4**, 1–11.

Nakagawa, Y., Kimura, N., Toyoda, T. *et al.* (1995) The RNA polymerase PB2 subunit is not required for replication of the influenza virus genome but is involved in capped mRNA synthesis. *J Virol* **69**, 728–33.

Nakagawa, Y., Oda, K. & Nakada, S. (1996) The PB1 subunit alone can catalyse cRNA synthesis, and the PA subunit in addition to the PB1 subunit is required for viral RNA synthesis in replication of the influenza virus genome. *J Virol* **70**, 6390–4.

Nemeroff, M.E., Utans, U., Kramer, A. & Krug, R.M. (1992) Identification of *cis*-acting intron and exon regions in influenza virus NS1 mRNA that inhibit splicing and cause the formation of aberrantly sedimenting presplicing complexes. *Mol Cell Biol* **12**, 962–70.

Ohuchi, M., Cramer, A., Yey, M., Ohuchi, R., Garten, W. & Klenk, H.-D. (1994) Rescue of vector-expressed fowl plague virus haemagglutinin in biologically active form by acidotropic agents and coexpressed M$_2$ protein. *J Virol* **68**, 920–6.

Plotch, S.J., Bouley, M. & Krug, R.M. (1979) Transfer of 5′-terminal cap of globin mRNA to influenza viral complementary RNA during transcription *in vitro*. *Proc Natl Acad Sci USA* **76**, 1618–22.

Plotch, S.J., Bouley, M., Ulmanen, I. & Krug, R.M. (1981) A unique cap (m^{7}GpppXm)-dependent influenza virion endonuclease cleaves capped RNAs to generate the primers that initiate viral RNA transcription. *Cell* **23**, 847–58.

Pringle, C.R. (1996) Virus taxonomy 1996—a bulletin from the Xth International Congress of Virology in Jerusalem. *Arch Virol* **141**, 2251–6.

Qian, X.-Y., Alonso-Caplen, F. & Krug, R.M. (1994) Two functional domains of the influenza virus NS$_1$ protein are required for regulation of nuclear export of mRNA. *J Virol* **68**, 2433–41.

Qiu, Y. & Krug, R.M. (1994) The influenza virus NS$_1$ protein is a poly A-binding protein that inhibits the nuclear export of mRNAs containing poly (A). *J Virol* **68**, 2425–32.

Qiu, Y., Nemeroff, M.E. & Krug, R.M. (1995) The influenza virus NS1 protein binds to a specific region in human U6 snRNA and inhibits U6–U2 and U6–U4 snRNA interactions during splicing. *RNA* **1**, 304–16.

Robertson, J.S., Schubert, M. & Lazzarini, R.A. (1981) Polyadenylation sites for influenza mRNA. *J Virol.* **38**, 157–63.

Rogers, G.N. & Paulson, J.C. (1983) Receptor determinants of human and animal influenza virus isolates: differences in receptor specificity of the H3 haemagglutinin based on species of origin. *Virology* **127**, 361–73.

Rogers, G.N., Herrler, G., Paulson, J.C. & Klenk, H.-D. (1986) Influenza C virus uses 9-O-acetyl-*N*-acetylneuraminic acid as a high affinity receptor determinant for attachment to cells. *EMBO J* **5**, 1359–65.

Romanos, M.A. & Hay, A.J. (1984) Identification of the influenza virus transcriptase by affinity-labelling with pyridoxal 5′-phosphate. *Virology* **132**, 110–17.

Shapiro, G.I. & Krug, R.M. (1988) Influenza virus RNA replication *in vitro*: synthesis of viral template RNAs and virion RNAs in the absence of an added primer. *J Virol* **62**, 2285–90.

Shapiro, G.I., Gurney, T. Jr & Krug, R.M. (1987) Influenza virus gene expression: control mechanisms at early and late times of infection and nuclear-cytoplasmic transport of virus-specific RNAs. *J Virol* **61**, 764–73.

Shaw, M.W., Lamb, R.A., Erickson, B.W., Briedis, D.J. & Choppin, P.W. (1982) Complete nucleotide sequence of the neuraminidase gene of influenza B virus. *Proc Natl Acad Sci USA* **79**, 6817–21.

Shaw, M.W., Choppin, P.W. & Lamb, R.A. (1983) A previously unrecognized influenza B virus glycoprotein from a bicistronic mRNA that also encodes the viral neuraminidase. *Proc Natl Acad Sci USA* **80**, 4879–83.

Shi, L., Summers, D.F., Peng, Q. & Galarza, J.M. (1995) Influenza A virus RNA polymerase subunit PB$_2$ is the endonuclease which cleaves host cell mRNA and functions only as the trimeric enzyme. *Virology* **208**, 38–47.

Shih, S.-R. & Krug, R.M. (1996a) Surprising function of the three influenza viral polymerase proteins: selective protection of viral mRNAs against the cap-snatching reaction catalysed by the same polymerase proteins. *Virology* **226**, 430–5.

Shih, S.-R. & Krug, R.M. (1996b) Novel exploitation of a nuclear function by influenza virus: the cellular SF2/ASF splicing factor controls the amount of the essential viral M2 ion channel protein in infected cells. *EMBO J* **15**, 5415–27.

Shih, S.-R., Nemeroff, M.E. & Krug, R.M. (1995) The choice of alternative 5′ splice sites in influenza virus M1 mRNA is regulated by the viral polymerase complex. *Proc Natl Acad Sci USA* **92**, 6324–8.

Smith, G.L. & Hay, A.J. (1982) Replication of the influenza virus genome. *Virology* **118**, 96–108.

Skehel, J.J. (1972) Polypeptide synthesis of influenza virus-infected cells. *Virology* **56**, 394–9.

Skehel, J.J. & Hay, A.J. (1978) Nucleotide sequences at the 5' termini of influenza virus RNAs and their transcripts. *Nucl Acids Res* **5**, 1207–19.

Stieneke-Grober, A., Vey, M., Angliker, H. *et al.* (1992) Influenza virus haemagglutinin with multibasic cleavage site is activated by furin, a subtilisin-like endoprotease. *EMBO J* **11**, 2407–14.

Stoeckle, M.Y., Shaw, M.W. & Choppin, P.W. (1987) Segment-specific and common nucleotide sequences in the noncoding regions of influenza B virus genome RNAs. *Proc Natl Acad Sci USA* **84**, 2703–7.

Sugrue, R.J., Bahadur, G., Zambon, M.C., Hall, S.M., Douglas, A.R. & Hay, A.J. (1990) Specific structural alteration of the influenza haemaglutinin by amantadine. *EMBO J* **9**, 3469–76.

Takeuchi, K. & Lamb, R.A. (1994) Influenza virus M_2 protein ion channel activity stabilizes the native form of fowl plague virus haemagglutinin during intracellular transport. *J Virol* **68**, 911–19.

Tiley, L.S., Hagen, M., Matthews, J.T. & Krystal, M. (1994) Sequence-specific binding of the influenza virus RNA polymerase to sequences located at the 5' ends of the viral RNAs. *J Virol* **68**, 5108–16.

Toyoda, T., Adyshev, D.M., Kobayashi, M., Iwata, A. & Ishihama, A. (1996) Molecular assembly of the influenza virus RNA polymerase: determination of the subunit-subunit contact sites. *J Gen Virol* **77**, 2149–57.

Ulmanen, I., Broni, B.A. & Krug, R.M. (1981) Role of two of the influenza virus core P proteins in recognizing cap 1 structures (m^7GpppNm) on RNAs and initiating viral RNA transcription. *Proc Natl Acad Sci USA* **78**, 7355–9.

Valcárcel, J., Portela, A. & Ortin, J. (1991) Regulated M1 mRNA splicing in influenza virus-infected cells. *J Gen Virol* **72**, 1301–8.

Wang, W. & Krug, R.M. (1996) The RNA-binding and effector domains of the viral NS1 protein are conserved to different extents among influenza A and B viruses. *Virology* **223**, 41–50.

Wang, P., Palese, P. & O'Neill, R.E. (1997) The NPI-1/NPI-3 (Karyopherin α) binding site on the influenza A virus nucleoprotein NP is a nonconventional nuclear localization signal. *J Virol* **71**, 1850–6.

Ward, A.C., Castelli, L.A., Lucantoni, A.C., White, J.F., Azad, A.A. & Macreadie, I.G. (1995) Expression and analysis of the NS2 protein of influenza A virus. *Arch Virol* **140**, 2067–73.

Whittaker, G., Bui, M. & Helenius, A. (1996a) Nuclear trafficking of influenza virus ribonucleoproteins in heterokaryons. *J Virol* **70**, 2743–56.

Whittaker, G., Bui, M. & Helenius, A. (1996b) The role of nuclear import and export in influenza virus infection. *Trends Cell Biol* **6**, 67–71.

Yamashita, M., Krystal, M. & Palese, P. (1988) Evidence that the matrix protein of influenza C virus is coded for by a spliced mRNA. *J Virol* **62**, 3348–55.

Yamashita, M., Krystal, M. & Palese, P. (1989) Comparison of the three large polymerase proteins of influenza A, B, and C viruses. *Virology* **171**, 458–66.

Yasuda, J., Nakada, S., Kato, A., Toyoda, T. & Ishihama, A. (1993) Molecular assembly of influenza virus: association of the NS2 protein with virion matrix. *Virology* **196**, 249–55.

Zebedee, S.L. & Lamb, R.A. (1989) Growth restriction of influenza A virus by M2 protein antibody is genetically linked to the M1 protein. *Proc Natl Acad Sci USA* **86**, 1061–5.

CHAPTER 5

Structure and Function of the Haemagglutinin

David A. Steinhauer and Stephen A. Wharton

Influenza virus infection is initiated by binding of virus particles to host cell surface receptors followed by receptor-mediated internalization. Fusion of the viral and endosomal membranes then allows for the transfer of viral nucleocapsids into the cytoplasm. Both the binding and the fusion functions are provided by the influenza virus haemagglutinin (HA) glycoprotein. The HA is also the primary target for neutralizing antibodies and is therefore the viral component of primary concern for vaccine design and development. The crystal structure has been determined to atomic resolution for the native HA, for the HA bound to a number of different receptor analogues, for proteolytic fragments of HA which have gone through the conformational changes required for mediating membrane fusion, and for HA complexed with neutralizing antibody. As such, the influenza virus HA provides a good model for studies on enveloped virus membrane glycoproteins regarding host cell entry and virus neutralization. Most of the structural studies have been done with the HA of A/Aichi/2/68, an H3 subtype influenza A virus, and this chapter will focus on the Aichi HA.

Structure of the native HA

The HA of A/Aichi/2/68 virus is a type I membrane glycoprotein with an N-terminal signal sequence, a membrane-anchor domain near the C-terminus, and a short cytoplasmic tail. Cleavage of the signal sequence results in a 550 amino acid polypeptide chain which forms homotrimers of approximately 220 kDa. The HA is post-translationally modified by the addition of N-linked carbohydrates at seven asparagine residues of each monomer and by covalent attachment of palmitic acid to three cysteine residues in the cytoplasmic tail region. The precursor form of the molecule (HA_0) is post-translationally cleaved into two subunits, HA_1 (328 residues) and HA_2 (221 residues), which are linked by a single disulphide bond between residues 14_1 and 137_2 (HA_1 residue 14 and HA_2 residue 137). This proteolytic processing of precursor HA_0 activates the membrane fusion potential of the HA and is therefore required for virus infectivity (Klenk et al. 1975; Lazarowitz & Choppin 1975; Skehel & Waterfield 1975; Huang et al. 1980; White et al. 1981). At present the high resolution structure of HA_0 is unknown. HA_0 and cleaved HA are indistinguishable by electron microscopy and both structures have receptor binding activity. In addition, most neutralizing monoclonal antibodies have similar reactivities to uncleaved and cleaved HA, suggesting that these structures are similar in the membrane-distal domain. However, in the structure of cleaved native HA described below the C-terminus of HA_1 and the N-terminus of HA_2 are separated by over $20\,\text{Å}$, demonstrating that a conformational change accompanies HA_0 cleavage.

Treatment of virus particles with the protease bromelain results in cleavage of HA at position 175 of HA_2, 10 residues from the membrane-anchor domain, and releases the ectodomain of HA as a soluble trimer which is commonly referred to as BHA (Brand & Skehel 1972). The crystal structure of BHA was first determined by Wilson et al. (1981), and has now been refined to a resolution of $2.15\,\text{Å}$ (Watowich et al. 1994). Plate 5.1 (facing p. 288) shows an α-carbon tracing of the structure of the BHA trimer and of one of the monomers. It is over 130 Å from the membrane-proximal region to the distal tip and ranges in radius from about 15 to 40 Å. Residues of the HA_2 subunit (shown in red) compose the backbone of the fibrous stem of the molecule. The interior of the stem region is characterized by a long triple-stranded coiled coil which splays open slightly towards the bottom where the HA_2 N-terminal domain, the 'fusion peptide', resides (shown in white). The fusion peptide is linked via two antiparallel β-strands to a shorter α-helix, which together with the long helix of the coiled coil and a connecting region make up the hairpin loop-like structure prominent in each monomer. The membrane-distal 'head' of the molecule is a globular domain rich in β-structure and is made up entirely of residues of the HA_1 subunit (shown in blue). This membrane-distal domain contains the receptor binding site at the tip of each monomer and is the region of the molecule generally recognized by neutralizing antibodies. At present there is no high resolution structural information regarding the protein C-terminal to the bromelain cleavage site, which includes the membrane-anchor domain and the cytoplasmic tail.

Receptor binding

A number of studies in the 1940s and 1950s provided evidence that influenza virus binds to 5-*N*-acetyl neuraminic acid (sialic acid)-containing constituents on the host cell surface (reviewed by Gottschalk 1959). When the structure of BHA was reported in 1981 (Wilson *et al.* 1981) it was noted that a shallow depression at the membrane-distal tip of each monomer was lined with amino acids which had been conserved since the emergence of H3 subtype viruses in humans in 1968, while residues surrounding the conserved pocket had varied during the antigenic drift of viruses prevalent from year to year. This suggested that the conserved pocket might form the binding site for sialic acid. Further evidence for this was provided by studies on receptor binding specificity (Rogers *et al.* 1983). Viruses with leucine at position 226 of HA_1, which is at the edge of the pocket, were shown to bind

preferentially to red blood cells derivitized to contain sialic acid with α-(2,6) linkages to galactose, while viruses with glutamine at this position were more specific for α-(2,3)-linked sialic acid.

X-ray crystallography studies on BHA complexed with receptor analogues have now shown that sialic acid is situated in the receptor binding site as depicted in Fig. 5.1 (Weis *et al.* 1988; Watowich *et al.* 1994; Eisen *et al.* 1997). A number of hydrogen bonds are formed among conserved residues and also between several of these residues and sialic acid (shown in red). The 'back' of the binding site is formed by His 183_1 and Tyr 195_1, and the side chains of Glu 190_1 and Leu 194_1 which protrude down from a short α-helix. Tyr 98_1 and Trp 153_1 are situated at the bottom of the depression and the 'sides' of the pocket are defined by residues $224_1–228_1$ and $134_1–138_1$. One of the carboxylate oxygens, the acetamido nitrogen, and the glycerol 8- and 9-hydroxyl groups of sialic acid appear to point into the pocket and form hydrogen bonds with conserved amino acids, while the 4-hydroxyl points out into solution. In agreement with the crystallographic model, proton-nuclear magnetic resonance (NMR) solution studies of BHA or intact virus complexed with receptor analogues have shown that an upfield chemical shift of the *N*-acetyl methyl resonance occurs in the presence of HA. This is most likely due to the methyl group being situated above the six-member ring of the Trp 153_1 side chain (Sauter *et al.* 1989, 1992; Hanson *et al.* 1992). In these studies, the binding affinities of sialic acid derivatives were also evaluated. It was shown that substitutions for the 2-carboxylate inhibited or abolished binding, and that affinity for HA was also reduced by the replacement of the 7- and 9-hydroxyls with larger groups or by substitution of the 5-acetamido side chain with either amido or *N*-benzylcarbonyl groups. In contrast, substitution of longer chains for the 4-hydroxyl group, which points out into solution, showed little effect on binding affinity. Studies measuring the inhibitory effects of sialic acid derivatives on erythrocyte binding by virus also demonstrated the importance of the glycerol side chain, the acetamido group, and the 2-carboxylate for binding (Kelm *et al.* 1992). The nature of the

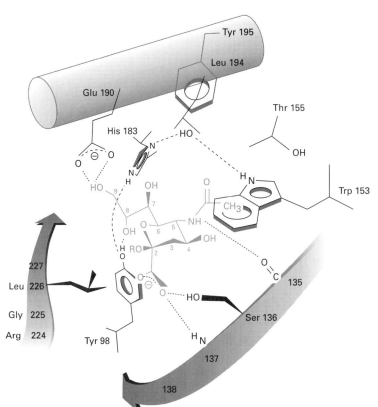

Fig. 5.1 Diagrammatic representation showing sialic acid (grey) and conserved amino acids of the receptor binding site. Hydrogen bonds are indicated by the dashes.

glycosidic linkage to sialic acid is also a factor in binding, as the β-anomer of methylsialic acid binds with much lower affinity than the α-anomer (Sauter *et al*. 1989) and is considerably less effective as an inhibitor of virus-erythrocyte binding (Pritchett *et al*. 1987).

It is well known that some virus strains bind preferentially to terminal sialic acids attached with α-(2,3) linkages while others favour binding to α-(2,6)-linked sialic acid; however, the structural basis for this binding specificity is not fully understood. Although it is not the exclusive determinant of binding specificity, the effects of variation at position $HA_1 226$ have been particularly well documented (Rogers *et al*. 1983, 1985; Daniels *et al*. 1987; Matrosovich *et al*. 1993; Connor *et al*. 1994), with glutamine at this position favouring binding to α-(2,3)-linked and leucine to α-(2,6)-linked sialic acid. The crystal structure of Aichi HA complexed with pentasaccharides containing either α-(2,3)- or α-(2,6)-

linked sialic acid reveal potential differences in the manner in which receptors with these linkages may bind to HA (Eisen *et al*. 1997; Plate 5.2, facing p. 288). Whereas the position of the terminal sialic acid is virtually superimposible in these structures the α-(2,6)-linked oligosaccharides were shown to bind in a folded conformation with the third saccharide positioned directly above the terminal sialic acid and the fourth and fifth sugars extending out of the pocket to the right side of the small helix (Plate 5.2, red). The α-(2,3)-linked molecule (Plate 5.2, green) was seen to adopt an extended conformation and exit from the left side of the pocket towards the trimer interface. Modelling of these oligosaccharide conformations into the structure of HA with glutamine at HA_1 position 226 suggests that the α-(2,3)-linked molecule might make more extensive contact with the glutamine 226_1 and provides one possible explanation for the receptor specificity which is observed (Eisen *et al*. 1997).

Dissociation constants for binding of α-methylsialic acid to HA have been measured at between 2 and 3 mmol using various assays (Sauter *et al.* 1989, 1992; Weinhold & Knowles 1992; Charych *et al.* 1993). This is a relatively low binding affinity compared to the tight binding of virus to host cells, which is thought to be due to the co-operative interaction of multiple HA and cell surface receptor molecules. One example of the effects of co-operative binding is illustrated by studies in which a surface plasmon resonance assay was used to measure binding of HA rosettes (average of 8 HA trimers/rosette) to a glycoprotein-coated surface (Takemoto *et al.* 1996). The dissociation constant for rosette binding was estimated to be approximately 100 nmol, an affinity about four orders of magnitude higher than those reported for α-methylsialic acid. It is also known that α_2-macroglobulin, a component of equine and guinea-pig sera which contains multiple sialic acid moieties, is a potent inhibitor of influenza infection (Pritchett & Paulson 1989). Thus, one approach for developing antiviral compounds designed to block influenza attachment to host cells has involved the synthesis of multivalent sialic acid analogues (Matrosovich *et al.* 1990; Glick *et al.* 1991; Sabesan *et al.* 1991; Spaltenstein & Whitesides 1991). Another approach is based on the use of monovalent sialic acid analogues which bind HA with high affinity (Toogood *et al.* 1991; Weinhold & Knowles 1992; Watowich *et al.* 1994). One strategy for achieving this is to use compounds capable of extending the region of contact with the HA. This has been demonstrated in X-ray crystallography studies in which the structure of BHA complexes with several high affinity receptor analogues was determined at resolution as high as 2.15 Å (Watowich *et al.* 1994). The improved resolution achieved in these studies shows that the sialic acid binding site is part of a series of hydrophilic pockets which form a groove along the surface of the molecule. A hydrophobic channel extends down from the sialic acid binding site towards Arg 224_1. The structure of BHA complexes with two of the high affinity analogues, which contain a naphthyl group attached to sialic acid via a short flexible linker, show that the substituents extend down this hydrophobic channel sig-nificantly increasing the areas of contact to HA (Watowich *et al.* 1994). The study of HA binding to natural receptors and to receptor analogues should continue to provide the basis for the design and development of potential antiviral drugs.

Membrane fusion

Structure of the HA at the pH of membrane fusion

Following cell attachment and internalization, the HA mediates fusion between the viral and endosomal membranes. Cellular proton pumps progressively acidify the endosomal compartments and at a specific pH, usually between 5.0 and 6.0 depending on the virus strain, the HA is induced to undergo irreversible conformational changes which are requisite for fusion activity (for recent reviews see Hughson 1995; Skehel *et al.* 1995; White 1995). These conformational changes have been analysed by a number of different techniques. For example, electron microscopy (EM) studies reveal that at the pH of fusion the membrane-distal domains of the HA spike appear more disordered and the stalk region more elongated (Doms *et al.* 1985; Ruigrok *et al.* 1986a). Proteolysis experiments have shown that while the native HA is resistant to degradation by a number of different proteases such as trypsin, endoproteinase Lys C, and proteinase K, at the pH of fusion the HA becomes susceptible to digestion by such enzymes (Skehel *et al.* 1982; Doms *et al.* 1985; Bizebard *et al.* 1995). In addition, several monoclonal antibodies have been characterized which can clearly distinguish between the native and low pH conformation of the molecule (Daniels *et al.* 1983b; Webster *et al.* 1983; Jackson & Nestorowicz 1985; White & Wilson 1987; Vareckóvá *et al.* 1993; Wharton *et al.* 1995). One of the consequences of the acid-induced structural rearrangements is that the aminoterminal domain of HA_2, which is buried in the interior of the native HA trimer (white in Plate 5.1), becomes extruded. This hydrophobic domain is highly conserved among influenza A viruses and is thought to play an intricate role in fusion, possibly through interactions with the target membrane (see below), and it is commonly referred to as the 'fusion peptide'.

Prior to the availability of high resolution structural information, evidence for the extensive nature of the molecular rearrangements of HA which accompany fusion came as a result of studies on viruses resistant to the antiviral drug amantadine (Daniels *et al.* 1985). At millimolar concentrations this compound inhibits influenza replication by raising the pH of endosomes, and mutant viruses resistant to the drug were shown to have an elevated pH of membrane fusion activity. Sequence analysis of the HA genes of several such mutants revealed that the substitutions responsible for this phenotype were distributed at domain interfaces throughout the structure of the native HA, such as those in and around the fusion peptide or at regions where subunits or monomers contact one another (Fig. 5.2). The positions of the mutations indicated that local destabilization of any of a number of these domain interfaces can lead to an elevated fusion pH. These results and those obtained in studies on receptor binding, proteolysis and antibody reactivity suggested that the acid-induced conformational changes involve rearrangement of a number of intact domains, with a significant amount of secondary and tertiary structure remaining unchanged.

Incubation of soluble BHA at the pH of fusion causes the membrane-distal domains to become detrimerized and, in the absence of lipid or detergents, results in the formation of aggregates due to the association of the extruded fusion peptides. These characteristics have made it necessary to work with proteolytic fragments for high resolution X-ray crystallography studies on the fusion pH HA. Digestion of low pH BHA aggregates with the endoproteinase Lys C results in cleavage at HA_1 position 27 and solubilizes the membrane-distal 'tops' of HA_1 (structure C in Plate 5.3). The observations that these HA_1 tops retain receptor binding activity and reactivity to a number of neutralizing monoclonal antibodies suggested that the structure of this domain remains similar to that of native HA, and this was confirmed by X-ray crystallography

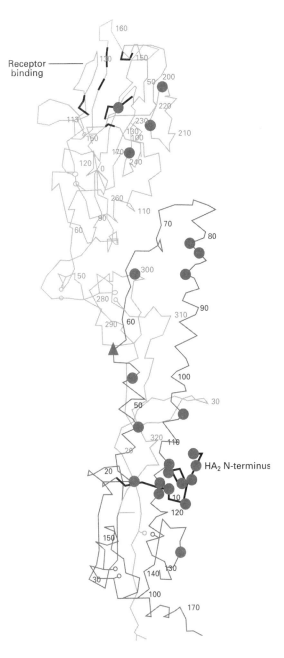

Fig. 5.2 Locations in the haemagglutinin structure of positions at which amino acid substitutions have been documented which affect the pH of membrane fusion. Circles indicate positions where changes caused an increase in fusion pH and the triangle shows the position of a mutant which has a lower pH of fusion. The fusion phenotypes were originally documented in the following references (Daniels *et al.* 1985; Doms *et al.* 1986; Gething *et al.* 1986; Wharton *et al.* 1986; Daniels *et al.* 1987; Steinhauer *et al.* 1991; Lin *et al.* 1997).

studies on the structure of Lys C tops complexed with the Fab of a monoclonal antibody, HC19 (Bizebard *et al.* 1995; Plates 5.3 and 5.4). As well as having implications concerning the mechanism of virus neutralization, these studies demonstrated that at the pH of fusion the structure of the detrimerized HA membrane-distal domains is virtually indistinguishable from that of the homologous domains in the native HA (Plates 5.3 and 5.4). The residues N-terminal to $HA_1 43$ and C-terminal to $HA_1 309$ (indicated by hatched lines in Plate 5.3), which form the HA_1 components of the stem structure in native HA are disordered. This suggests that the residues between $HA_1 27$ and $HA_1 43$ could provide a flexible link tethering the membrane-distal domains to the trimeric components of the fusion pH HA described below. Exactly where the membrane-distal domains are situated during the fusion process is unknown.

The rearrangements which occur in the stem region of HA at fusion pH have been derived primarily from the crystal structure of a thermolytic fragment of low pH HA (Bullough *et al.* 1994). As described above, treatment of low pH BHA aggregates with Lys C or with trypsin releases HA_1 tops due to cleavage at the lysine residue at position 27 of HA_1 (represented by structure C in Plate 5.3). The remaining aggregates can be solubilized by subsequent digestion with thermolysin, which removes the fusion peptide by cleavage first at position 23 and then 37 of HA_2. This results in a soluble trimeric product (TBHA$_2$) containing HA_2 residues 38–175 disulphide-linked to residues 1–27 of HA_1 (Daniels *et al.* 1983a; Ruigrok *et al.* 1988; structure E in Plate 5.3). The crystal structure of TBHA$_2$ shows that the conformational changes which accompany fusion include two major rearrangements of the stem region of the molecule which are detailed in Plate 5.3. One of the rearrangements involves the extended chain region (orange) which links the top of the long helix (yellow) to the shorter helix (red) in the native HA. At the pH of fusion this linking region also becomes helical, resulting in an extended coiled coil formed by residues from all three domains (yellow, orange and red). This extension of the coiled coil had been predicted based on structural studies using synthetic peptides (Carr & Kim 1993) and based on the observation that these three domains contained an almost unbroken register of heptad repeat motifs which are characteristic of coiled coils (Ward & Dopheide 1980). The other prominent rearrangement shown by the TBHA$_2$ structure involves the refolding of residues 106–112 of HA_2, which in the native HA form part of the coiled coil just membrane-distal to where the fusion peptide is situated (Plate 5.3a, green). At the pH of fusion this region forms a loop (Plate 5.3b, green) which reorients by approximately 180° the bottom of the long helix (dark blue) and residues C-terminal to it along with the disulphide-linked fragment of HA_1. HA_2 residues 163–175 are disordered which suggests that this region might be flexible at fusion pH.

Thermal denaturation studies (Ruigrok *et al.* 1988), and the observation that HA_2 residues 38–175 expressed in *Escherichia coli* fold directly into the low pH conformation (Chen *et al.* 1995), indicate that native HA is a metastable molecule which when triggered to induce fusion folds into a lower energy state. Mutant studies have shown that changes which increase the stability of the native HA conformation can result in inhibition of membrane fusion activity. For example, covalent cross-linking of the membrane-distal domains through the introduction of novel disulphide bonds leads to an inhibition of the acid-induced conformational changes, including the extrusion of fusion peptides which are located over 100 Å from the mutations, and blocks membrane fusion capacity (Godley *et al.* 1992; Kemble *et al.* 1992). Another study has demonstrated that a lysine to isoleucine substitution at HA_2 residue 58 leads to an acid-stable phenotype with a fusion pH 0.7 below that of wild-type HA (Steinhauer *et al.* 1991). This position in the native HA structure (triangle in Fig. 5.2) is located in the extended chain region of HA_2 (orange in Plate 5.3a) which is rearranged during fusion and the crystal structure of this mutant shows that the substitution results in the displacement of the main chain by nearly 4 Å and the orientation of the isoleucine side chain towards the interior of the molecule (Planchart AJP *et al.* in preparation). The use of compounds designed to stabilize the native HA conformation would seem to offer another reasonable approach for the development of anti-viral drugs and a number of inhibitors which appear to function in such a fashion have now been characterized (Bodian *et al.* 1993; Luo *et al.* 1997).

The interaction between HA and membranes and its role in promoting membrane fusion

One of the consequences of the acid-induced conformational changes of HA is that the fusion peptide is relocated from its position at the interior of the native structure to the tip of the newly formed extended coiled coil, a distance of over 100 Å. This could be the mechanism for putting this hydrophobic domain into a position to interact with the target endosomal membrane. Studies using photoactivatable lipids in the target membrane have shown that this indeed can happen (Tsurudome *et al.* 1992; Durrer *et al.* 1996). However, in the absence of target membrane the fusion peptide inserts into the viral envelope (Ruigrok *et al.* 1986b; Weber *et al.* 1994; Wharton *et al.* 1995). It is not clear whether this latter interaction also has a role in the fusion process or merely results in the inactivation of the fusion potential of the HA. However, it indicates that although the HA in the low pH conformation is very stable and remains trimeric, it possesses quite a degree of flexibility with regard to its orientation and association with lipid membranes (see below).

Mere interaction of the fusion peptide with the target membrane is not sufficient to bring about membrane fusion. Mutant HA molecules made by site-specific mutagenesis that have amino acid substitutions or deletions in the fusion peptide region of the HA can still undergo the low pH-induced conformational change and interact with target membranes but cannot fuse them (Steinhauer *et al.* 1995). The nature of the aminoterminal residue of the HA_2 is particularly important in determining fusion phenotype with only a glycine (the natural residue) or an alanine being fusogenic (Gething *et al.* 1986; Walker & Kawaoka 1993; Steinhauer *et al.* 1995). A deletion of this residue results in the HA being non-fusogenic (Garten *et al.* 1981; Steinhauer *et al.* 1995).

Synthetic peptides of the fusion peptide can also fuse membranes and have been used to study more directly the interaction of this region with membranes (Wharton *et al.* 1988; Rafalski *et al.* 1991; Steinhauer *et al.* 1995). The validity of using such a model system was illustrated by the fact that synthetic peptides with various amino acid substitutions or deletions always had the same fusion properties as the corresponding HA molecules with homologous sequences in the fusion peptide (Gething *et al.* 1986; Wharton *et al.* 1988; Steinhauer *et al.* 1995). By comparing the results obtained with fusogenic and non-fusogenic peptides, the structural requirements for promoting membrane fusion can be determined. Various spectroscopic methods using peptides and liposomes have shown that the secondary structure of the peptides is important. Although the peptides contain up to 40% α-helix and there is a loose correlation between fusogenicity and helical content, recently the importance of the presence of β-sheet has been realized (Gray *et al.* 1996). Some toxins which act by forming pores in target membranes do so in a β-sheet structure (Song *et al.* 1996). Fusogenic and non-fusogenic peptides seem to adopt similar orientations in the membrane although there appear to be differences in the ability to form hydrogen bonds with the phospholipids in the bilayer (Gray *et al.* 1996). It is not clear if the peptides interact with membranes and promote fusion as monomers, trimers or larger oligomers and this would have relevance when discussing models of membrane fusion (see below).

EM has been used to study the orientation of HA in the membrane (Wharton *et al.* 1995). An antibody was identified that binds specifically to HA in the low pH conformation via the 106_2–112_2 loop that is located at one end of the structure (Plate 5.3b green). Electron microscopic images of complexes of the antibody with various preparations of HA associated with membranes clearly show that the 106_2–112_2 loop is located at the membrane distal end of the molecule. This finding has two implications. Firstly, the long coiled coil of HA_2 (Plate 5.3) must become inverted in relation to the membrane as a consequence of the low pH conformational change. Whether this results from a tilting of the whole molecule or an unwinding, inversion and rewinding of the coiled coil is at present unclear. Secondly, in the final structure the fusion peptide and the membrane anchor are at the same end of the molecule. After fusion this would have to be the case as the target and viral membrane would be contiguous.

Taken together, these results suggest a possible mechanism of membrane fusion. Initially, the fusion peptide is relocated to the top of the coiled coil where it interacts with the target membrane. Then the stalk of the HA becomes inverted relative to the viral membrane, possibly as a result of the formation of the 106_2–112_2 loop. This would bring the target and viral membranes closer together. When they are sufficiently close as to overcome the repulsive forces of hydration, the destabilizing effect of the fusion peptide in the correct configuration causes the membranes to fuse. However, there are many aspects of the fusion process that are unclear and many models have been proposed (e.g. see White 1995). Many questions remain to be answered, for example: (i) What are the lipidic intermediates of fusion (see Lindau & Almers 1995 or Chernomordik *et al.* 1995 for reviews)? (ii) What happens to the HA_1 globular domains? (iii) Is it the HA bound to receptor that mediates fusion? (iv) How many HA molecules are involved at the site of fusion? There is evidence that the concerted action of many HA molecules forms a pore-like structure that then dilates and results in fusion (reviewed in White *et al.* 1996). The difficulty of studying the fusion process is that the intermediates are transitory, therefore ways of stopping the process at different stages must be sought to enable biochemical analysis.

Structure of HA complexed with a neutralizing antibody

Influenza virus HA is the primary target of neutralizing antibodies. Influenza can evade the host immune system because viruses can be selected which have mutations in the HA resulting in molecules that no longer bind antibody. Such mutations generally occur in the globular domain of HA_1 around the conserved receptor binding site (see Wiley & Skehel 1987). EM studies of several monoclonal antibody-BHA complexes demonstrated that the antibodies bind specifically to sites on the molecule where they select for mutations which confer resistance (Wrigley *et al.* 1983). This was supported by X-ray crystallography studies which showed that the amino acid substitution in an escape mutant resulted in only very localized changes in structure (Knossow *et al.* 1984) and was confirmed when the structure of an HA-Fab complex was determined by X-ray crystallography (Bizebard *et al.* 1995). This complex was comprised of a proteolytic fragment, Lys C tops ($HA_1$28–328), produced after low pH treatment of the HA, associated with the Fab of a neutralizing antibody, HC19. Plate 5.4a shows a complex of HC19 Fab associated with HA. Sequencing studies on mutants resistant to neutralization by this antibody revealed changes at positions 131_1, 157_1 or 158_1 which are located close to the receptor binding site. As discussed above, the globular domain of the fragment of HA_1 has the same structure as in the native molecule. However, there are some significant changes in the regions of the Fab that interact with the HA when compared to the uncomplexed molecule. In the complex, the H3 complimentarity-determining region (CDR) loop moves about 10 Å to protrude into the 'right hand' side of the receptor binding site of the HA (Plate 5.4b). This means that this loop is able to make additional hydrogen bonds with the HA (an extra four out of a total of 10). The position of the H3 CDR loop (yellow) would overlap with that of sialic acid bound in the site, so clearly the neutralization of infectivity by this antibody is caused by an inhibition of receptor binding. It is not clear whether other antibodies that bind farther away from the receptor binding site also inhibit receptor binding by steric hindrance, perhaps by other regions of the immunoglobulin or whether other mechanisms are involved. For descriptions of the molecular interactions between antibodies and viral antigens as well as the structural basis of why neutralization escape mutants bind antibody less efficiently see Colman (1994) or Bizebard *et al.* (1995).

References

Bizebard, T., Gigant, B., Rigolet, P. *et al.* (1995) Structure of influenza virus haemagglutinin complexed with a neutralizing antibody. *Nature* **376**, 92–4.

Bodian, D.L., Yamasaki, R.B., Buswell, R.L., Stearns, J.F., White, J.M. & Kuntz, I.D. (1993) Inhibition of the fusion-inducing conformational change of influenza haemagglutinin by benzoquinones and hydroquinones. *Biochemistry* **32**, 2967–78.

Brand, C.M. & Skehel, J.J. (1972) Crystalline antigen from the influenza virus envelope. *Nature New Biol* **238**, 145–7.

Bullough, P.A., Hughson, F.M., Skehel, J.J. & Wiley, D.C. (1994) The structure of influenza haemagglutinin at the pH of membrane fusion. *Nature* **371**, 37–43.

Carr, C.M. & Kim, P.S. (1993) A spring-loaded mechanism for the conformational change of influenza haemagglutinin. *Cell* **73**, 823–33.

Charych, D.H., Nagy, J.O., Spevac, W. & Bednarski, M.D. (1993) Direct colourimetric detection of a receptor-ligand interaction by a polymerized assembly. *Science* **261**, 585–8.

Chen, J., Wharton, S.A., Weissenhorn, W. *et al.* (1995) A soluble domain of the membrane-anchoring chain of influenza virus haemagglutinin (HA$_2$) folds in *Escherichia coli* into the low-pH-induced conformation. *Proc Natl Acad Sci USA* **92**, 12205–9.

Chernomordik, L., Kozlov, M.M. & Zimmerberg, J. (1995) Lipids in biological membrane fusion. *J Membr Biol* **146**, 1–14.

Colman, P.M. (1994) Influenza virus neuraminidase: structure, antibodies, and inhibitors. *Protein Sci* **3**, 1687–96.

Connor, R.J., Kawaoka, Y., Webster, R.G. & Paulson, J.C. (1994) Receptor specificity in human, avian, and equine H2 and H3 influenza virus isolates. *Virology* **205**, 17–23.

Daniels, R.S., Douglas, A.R., Skehel, J.J., Waterfield, M.D., Wilson, I.A. & Wiley, D.C. (1983a) Studies of the influenza virus haemagglutinin in the pH 5 conformation. In: Laver, W.G. (ed.) *The Origin of Pandemic Influenza Viruses*, pp. 1–7. Elsevier, New York.

Daniels, R.S., Douglas, A.R., Skehel, J.J. & Wiley, D.C. (1983b) Analyses of the antigenicity of influenza haemagglutinin at the pH optimum for virus-mediated membrane fusion. *J Gen Virol* **64**, 1657–62.

Daniels, R.S., Downie, J.C., Hay, A.J. *et al.* (1985) Fusion mutants of the influenza virus haemagglutinin. *Cell* **40**, 431–9.

Daniels, R.S., Jeffries, S., Yates, P. *et al.* (1987) The receptor binding and membrane fusion properties of influenza virus variants selected using antihaemagglutinin monoclonal antibodies. *EMBO J* **6**, 1459–65.

Doms, R.W., Gething, M.-J., Henneberry, J., White, J.M. & Helenius, A. (1986) Variant influenza virus haemagglutinin that induces fusion at elevated pH. *J Virol* **57**, 603–13.

Doms, R.W., Helenius, A. & White, J.M. (1985) Membrane fusion activity of the influenza virus haemagglutinin. *J Biol Chem* **260**, 2973–81.

Durrer, P., Galli, C., Hoenke, S. *et al.* (1996) H+-induced membrane insertion of influenza virus haemagglutinin involves the HA2 amino-terminal fusion peptide but not the coiled coil region. *J Biol Chem* **271**, 13417–21.

Eisen, M.B., Sabesan, S., Skehel, J.J. & Wiley, D.C. (1997) Binding of the influenza A virus to cell-surface receptors: structure of five haemagglutinin-sialyloligosaccharide complexes determined by X-ray crystallography. *Virology* **232**, 19–31.

Garten, W., Bosch, F.X., Linder, D., Rott, R. & Klenk, H.-D. (1981) Proteolytic activation of the influenza haemagglutinin: the structure of the cleavage site and the enzymes involved in cleavage. *Virology* **115**, 361–74.

Gething, M.-J., Doms, R.W., York, D. & White, J.M. (1986) Studies on the mechanism of membrane fusion: site-specific mutagenesis of the haemagglutinin of influenza virus. *J Cell Biol* **102**, 11–23.

Glick, G.D., Toogood, P.L., Wiley, D.C., Skehel, J.J. & Knowles, J.R. (1991) Ligand recognition by influenza virus. The binding of bivalent sialosides. *J Biol Chem* **266**, 23660–9.

Godley, L., Pfeifer, J., Steinhauer, D. *et al.* (1992) Introduction of intersubunit disulphide bonds in the membrane-distal region of the influenza haemagglutinin abolishes membrane fusion activity. *Cell* **68**, 635–45.

Gottschalk, A. (1959) The chemistry of virus receptors. In: Burnet, F.M. & Stanley W.M. (eds) *The Viruses*, pp. 51–61. Academic Press, New York.

Gray, C., Tatulian, S.A., Wharton, S.A. & Tamm, L.K. (1996) Effect of the N-terminal glycine on the secondary structure, orientation, and interaction of the influenza haemagglutinin fusion peptide with lipid bilayers. *Biophys J* **70**, 2275–86.

Hanson, J.E., Sauter, N.K., Skehel, J.J. & Wiley, D.C. (1992) Proton nuclear magnetic resonance studies of the binding of sialosides to intact influenza viruses. *Virology* **189**, 525–33.

Huang, R.T.C., Wahn, K., Klenk, H.-D. & Rott, R. (1980) Fusion between cell membranes and liposomes containing the glycoprotein of influenza virus. *Virology* **104**, 294–302.

Hughson, F.M. (1995) Structural characterization of viral fusion proteins. *Curr Biol* **5**, 265–74.

Jackson, D.C. & Nestorowicz, A. (1985) Antigenic determinants of influenza virus haemagglutinin. *Virology* **145**, 72–83.

Kelm, S., Paulson, J.C., Rose, U. *et al.* (1992) Use of sialic acid analogues to define functional groups involved in binding to the influenza virus haemagglutinin. *Eur J Biochem* **205**, 147–53.

Kemble, G.W., Bodian, D.L., Rose, J., Wilson, I.A. & White, J.M. (1992) Intermonomer disulphide bonds impair the fusion activity of influenza virus haemagglutinin. *J Virol* **66**, 4940–50.

Klenk, H.-D., Rott, R., Orlich, M. & Blodorn, J. (1975) Activation of influenza A viruses by trypsin treatment. *Virology* **68**, 426–39.

Knossow, M., Daniels, R.S., Douglas, A.R., Skehel, J.J. & Wiley, D.C. (1984) Three-dimensional structure of an antigenic mutant of the influenza virus haemagglutinin. *Nature* **311**, 678–80.

Lazarowicz, S.G. & Choppin, P.W. (1975) Enhancement of the infectivity of influenza A and B viruses by proteolytic cleavage of the haemagglutinin polypeptide. *Virology* **68**, 440–65.

Lin, Y.P., Wharton, S.A., Martin, J., Skehel, J.J., Wiley, D.C. & Steinhauer, D.A. (1997) Adaptation of egg-grown and transfectant influenza viruses for growth in mammalian cells: selection of haemagglutinin mutants with elevated pH of membrane fusion. *Virology* **233**, 402–10.

Lindau, M. & Almers, W. (1995) Structure and function of fusion pores in exocytosis and ectoplasmic membrane fusion. *Curr Opin Cell Biol* **7**, 509–17.

Luo, G., Torri, A., Harte, W.E. *et al.* (1997) Molecular mechanism underlying the action of a novel fusion inhibitor of influenza A virus. *J Virol* **71**, 4062–70.

Matrosovich, M.N., Gambaryan, A.S., Tuzikov, A.B. *et al.* (1993) Probing of the receptor-binding sites of the H1 and H3 influenza A and influenza B virus haemagglutinins by synthetic and natural sialosides. *Virology* **196**, 111–21.

Matrosovich, M.N., Mochalova, L.V., Marinina, V.P., Byramova, N.E. & Bovin, N.V. (1990) Synthetic polymeric sialoside inhibitors of influenza virus receptor-binding activity. *FEBS Letts* **272**, 209–12.

Pritchett, T.J., Brossmer, R., Rose, U. & Paulson, J.C. (1987) Recognition of monovalent sialosides by influenza virus H3 haemagglutinin. *Virology* **160**, 502–6.

Pritchett, T.J. & Paulson, J.C. (1989) Basis for potent inhibition of influenza virus infection by equine and guinea pig alpha-2-macroglobulin. *J Biol Chem* **264**, 9850–8.

Rafalski, M., Ortiz, A., Rockwell, A. *et al.* (1991) Membrane fusion activity of the influenza virus haemagglutinin: interaction of HA2 N-terminal peptides with phospholipid vesicles. *Biochemistry* **30**, 10211–20.

Rogers, G.N., Daniels, R.S., Skehel, J.J. *et al.* (1985) Host-mediated selection of influenza virus receptor variants. Sialic acid-alpha-2, 6-Gal-specific clones of A/duck/Ukraine/1/63 revert to sialic acid-alpha-2, 3-Gal wild type *in ovo*. *J Biol Chem* **260**, 7362–7.

Rogers, G.N., Paulson, J.C., Daniels, R.S., Skehel, J.J., Wilson, I.A. & Wiley, D.C. (1983) Single amino acid substitutions in influenza haemagglutinin change receptor binding specificity. *Nature* **304**, 76–8.

Ruigrok, R.W.H., Aitken, A., Calder, L.J. *et al.* (1988) Studies on the structure of influenza virus haemagglutinin at the pH of fusion. *J Gen Virol* **69**, 2785–95.

Ruigrok, R.W.H., Martin, S.R., Wharton, S.A., Skehel, J.J., Bayley, P.M., Wiley, D.C. (1986a) Conformational changes in the haemagglutinin of influenza virus which accompany heat-induced fusion of virus with liposomes. *Virology* **155**, 484–97.

Ruigrok, R.W.H., Wrigley, N.G., Calder, L.J. *et al.* (1986b) Electron microscopy of the low pH structure of influenza virus haemagglutinin. *EMBO J* **5**, 41–9.

Sabesan, S., Duus, J.O., Domaille, P., Kelm, S. & Paulson, J.C. (1991) Synthesis of cluster sialoside inhibitors for influenza virus. *J Am Chem Soc* **113**, 5865–6.

Sauter, N.K., Bednarski, M.D., Wurzberg, B.A. *et al.* (1989) Hemagglutinins of two influenza virus variants bind to sialic acid derivatives with millimolar dissociation constants: a 500-Mhz proton nuclear magnetic resonance study. *Biochemistry* **28**, 8388–96.

Sauter, N.K., Hanson, J.E., Glick, G.D. *et al.* (1992) Binding of influenza virus haemagglutinin to analogues of its cell-surface receptor, sialic acid: analysis by proton nuclear magnetic resonance spectroscopy and X-ray crystallography. *Biochemistry* **31**, 9609–21.

Skehel, J.J., Bayley, P.M., Brown, E.B. *et al.* (1982) Changes in the conformation of influenza virus haemagglutinin at the pH optimum of virus-mediated membrane fusion. *Proc Natl Acad Sci USA* **79**, 968–72.

Skehel, J.J., Bizebard, T., Bullough, P.A. *et al.* (1995) Membrane fusion by influenza haemagglutinin. In: *Cold Spring Harbor Symposia on Quantitative Biology*, Vol. LX, pp. 573–80. Cold Spring Harbor Laboratory Press.

Skehel, J.J. & Waterfield, M.D. (1975) Studies on the primary structure of the influenza virus haemagglutinin. *Proc Natl Acad Sci USA* **72**, 93–7.

Song, L., Hobaugh, M.R., Shustak, C., Cheley, S., Bayley, H. & Gouaux, J.E. (1996) Structure of staphylococcal alpha-haemolysin, a heptameric transmembrane pore. *Science* **274**, 1859–66.

Spaltenstein, A. & Whitesides, G.M. (1991) Polyacrylamides bearing alpha-sialoside groups strongly inhibit agglutination of erythrocytes by influenza virus. *J Am Chem Soc* **113**, 686–7.

Steinhauer, D.A., Wharton, S.A., Skehel, J.J., Wiley, D.C. & Hay, A.J. (1991) Amantadine selection of a mutant influenza virus containing an acid-stable haemagglutinin glycoprotein: evidence for virus-specific regulation of pH of an intracellular compartment involved in glycoprotein transport. *Proc Natl Acad Sci USA* **88**, 11525–9.

Steinhauer, D.A., Wharton, S.A., Skehel, J.J. & Wiley, D.C. (1995) Studies of the membrane fusion activities of fusion peptide mutants of influenza virus haemagglutinin. *J Virol* **69**, 6643–51.

Takemoto, D.K., Skehel, J.J. & Wiley, D.C. (1996) A surface plasmon resonance assay for the binding of influenza virus haemagglutinin to its sialic acid receptor. *Virology* **217**, 452–8.

Toogood, P.L., Galliker, P.K., Glick, G.D. & Knowles, J.R. (1991) Monovalent sialosides that bind tightly to influenza A virus. *J Med Chem* **34**, 3138–40.

Tsurudome, M., Gluck, R., Graf, R., Falchetto, R., Schaller, U. & Brunner, J. (1992) Lipid interactions of the haemagglutinin HA2 NH2-terminal segment during influenza virus-induced membrane fusion. *J Biol Chem* **267**, 20225–32.

Varecková, E., Mucha, V., Ciampor, F., Betakova, T. & Russ, G. (1993) Monoclonal antibodies demonstrate accessible HA2 epitopes in minor subpopulation of native influenza virus haemagglutinin molecules. *Arch Virol* **130**, 45–56.

Walker, J.A. & Kawaoka, Y. (1993) Importance of conserved amino acids at the cleavage site of the haemagglutinin of a virulent avian influenza A virus. *J Gen Virol* **74**, 311–14.

Ward, C.W. & Dopheide, T.A.A. (1980) Influenza virus haemagglutinin. Structural predictions suggest that fibrillar appearance is due to the presence of a coiled coil. *Aust J Biol Sci* **33**, 441–7.

Watowich, S.J., Skehel, J.J. & Wiley, D.C. (1994) Crystal structures of influenza virus haemagglutinin in complex with high-affinity receptor analogs. *Structure* **2**, 719–31.

Weber, T., Paesold, G., Galli, C., Mischler, R., Semenza, G. & Brunner, J. (1994) Evidence for H+-induced insertion of influenza haemagglutinin HA2 N-terminal segment into viral membrane. *J Biol Chem* **269**, 18353–8.

Webster, R.G., Brown, L.E. & Jackson, D.C. (1983) Changes in the antigenicity of the haemagglutinin molecule of H3 influenza virus at acidic pH. *Virology* **126**, 587–99.

Weinhold, E. & Knowles, J.R. (1992) Design and evaluation of a tightly binding fluorescent ligand for influenza A haemagglutinin. *J Am Chem Soc* **114**, 9270–5.

Weis, W.I., Brown, J.H., Cusack, S., Paulson, J.C., Skehel, J.J. & Wiley, D.C. (1988) Structure of the influenza virus haemagglutinin complexed with its receptor, sialic acid. *Nature* **333**, 426–31.

Wharton, S.A., Calder, L.J., Ruigrok, R.W.H., Skehel, J.J., Steinhauer, D.A. & Wiley, D.C. (1995) Electron micro-scopy of antibody complexes of influenza virus haemagglutinin in the fusion pH conformation. *EMBO J* **14**, 240–6.

Wharton, S.A., Martin, S.R., Ruigrok, R.W.H., Skehel, J.J. & Wiley, D.C. (1988) Membrane fusion by peptide analogues of influenza virus haemagglutinin. *J Gen Virol* **69**, 1847–57.

Wharton, S.A., Skehel, J.J. & Wiley, D.C. (1986) Studies of influenza haemagglutinin-mediated membrane fusion. *Virology* **149**, 27–35.

White, J.M. (1995) Membrane fusion: the influenza paradigm. In: *Cold Spring Harbor Symposia on Quantitative Biology*, Vol. LX, pp. 581–8. Cold Spring Harbor Laboratory Press.

White, J.M., Danieli, T., Henis, Y.I., Melikyan, G. & Cohen, F.S. (1996) Membrane fusion by the influenza haemagglutinin: the fusion pore. *Soc Gen Physiol Ser* **51**, 223–9.

White, J.M., Matlin, K. & Helenius, A. (1981) Cell fusion by Semliki Forest, influenza and vesicular stomatitis viruses. *J Cell Biol* **89**, 674–9.

White, J.M. & Wilson, I.A. (1987) Antipeptide antibodies detect steps in a protein conformational change: low-pH activation of the influenza virus haemagglutinin. *J Cell Biol* **105**, 2887–96.

Wiley, D.C. & Skehel, J.J. (1987) The structure and function of the haemagglutinin membrane glycoprotein of influenza virus. *Ann Rev Biochem* **56**, 365–94.

Wilson, I.A., Skehel, J.J. & Wiley, D.C. (1981) Structure of the haemagglutinin membrane glycoprotein of influenza virus at 3 angstroms resolution. *Nature* **289**, 366–73.

Wrigley, N.G., Brown, E.B., Daniels, R.S., Douglas, A.R., Skehel, J.J. & Wiley, D.C. (1983) Electron microscopy of influenza haemagglutinin-monoclonal antibody complexes. *Virology* **131**, 308–14.

CHAPTER 6

Structure and Function of the Neuraminidase

Peter M. Colman

Introduction

Neuraminidases (sialidases) catalyse the cleavage of glycosidic linkages adjacent to N-acetyl-neuraminic acid (Neu5Ac, sialic acid — see Fig. 6.1). Sialic acid is commonly the terminal sugar residue on oligosaccharide side chains of glycoconjugates and it is an integral part of the influenza virus receptor. The viral enzyme thus destroys its own receptor (Hirst 1942). The presence of such enzyme activity on the surface of virions seems contrary to requirements for viral attachment to cells. The clearest demonstration for a biological role for the enzyme is in studies by Palese and Compans (1976) who observed that when virus was cultured in the presence of enzyme inhibitors it was restricted to a single replication cycle by virtue of the progeny being immobilized at the surface of infected cells. This work indicated that the enzyme had no role in attachment, fusion, replication, assembly or budding of virus, although it is likely that the inhibitors used did not enter cells, making it difficult to rule out some intracellular role for neuraminidase. The discovery of more potent neuraminidase inhibitors (von Itzstein et al. 1993) which have antiviral activity in animals and man has led to a better understanding of the role of the enzyme in the viral life cycle, and especially of the balanced relationship between cellular attachment and receptor removal.

Structural studies of neuraminidase in complex with specific monoclonal antibodies provided the first atomic resolution images of any viral antigen-antibody interaction (Colman et al. 1987). These data have provided a foundation for understanding the antibody-binding characteristics of both shifted and drifted strains of influenza. They have also given insight into the basis on which active sites on viral antigens can be preserved in the face of selection pressure in an immune population.

This chapter concentrates on structural aspects of the influenza neuraminidase which have led to:
1 the discovery of novel, potent enzyme inhibitors (in clinical trial at the time of writing);
2 an appreciation of all forms of antigenic variation; and
3 an understanding of the relationship between the protein's antigenic and enzymatic properties.

Chemical structure and morphology

Influenza virus neuraminidase is a tetrameric glycoprotein of molecular mass 240 kDa. Electron microscopy of negatively stained material (Wrigley et al. 1973) has shown that the protein has a mushroom-shaped morphology. A hydrophobic stalk peptide is responsible for membrane anchoring and a globular head contains the enzyme active site and the antigenic sites of the molecule. The globular head can be liberated from virions by proteolysis without destroying either antigenicity or enzyme activity, and crystals prepared from such material (Laver 1978) were the basis for the subsequent screening of different antigenic variants for crystals suitable for structural studies by X-ray diffraction (Varghese et al. 1983; Laver et al. 1984).

Amino acid sequencing and gene sequencing (reviewed in Colman 1989) showed that the membrane anchor is near the N-terminus (residues 7–35), and that the protease cleavage site discovered

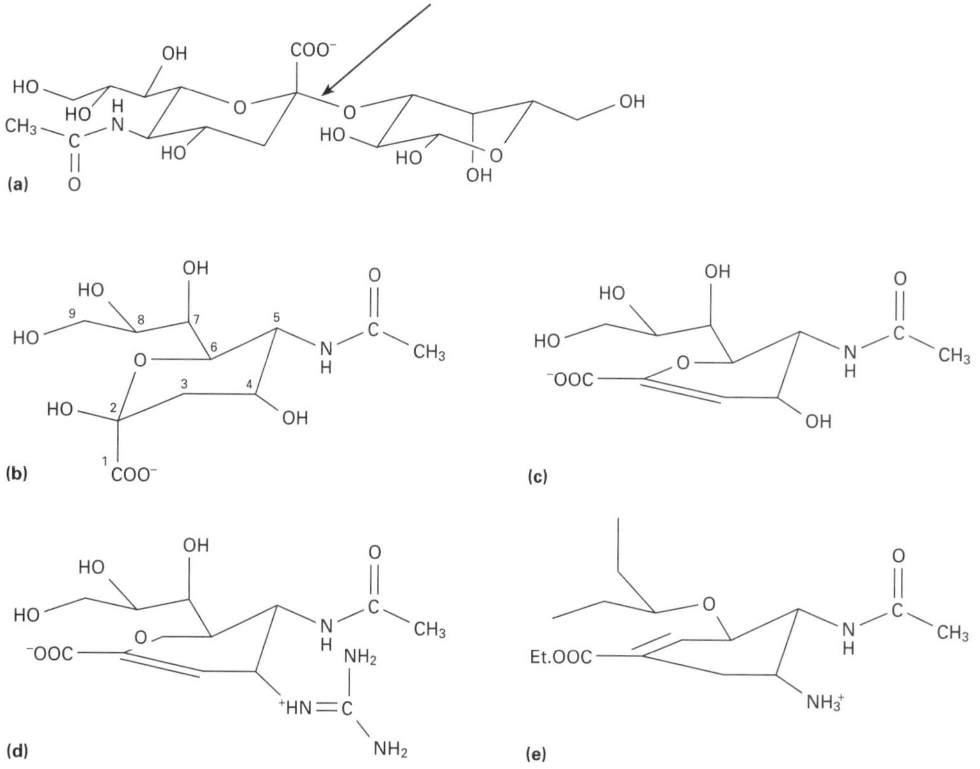

Fig. 6.1 (a) α-2,3-Sialyl galactose, showing the bond cleaved by the action of neuraminidase; (b) α-sialic acid (Neu5Ac); (c) Neu5Ac2en; (d) 4-guanidino-Neu5Ac2en; (e) GS4104.

by Laver (1978) is near residue 80. The polypeptide is approximately 470 amino acids in length, varying slightly from strain to strain. Here we use the numbering system of the N2 protein, the strain whose three-dimensional structure was the first to be determined (Varghese *et al.* 1983).

The number of sites at which N-linked glycosylation could occur (reviewed in Colman 1989) is also quite variable, but typically there are a few (three in the N2 subtype) such sites in the stalk region (residues 36–78) and a similar number (five in the N2 subtype) in the head region (79–469). The greater density of carbohydrate in the stalk might reflect a need for proteolytic protection.

More than 60 influenza virus neuraminidase sequences have currently been deposited in databases. These represent both type A and type B strains of influenza, and include within the A strains more than half of the nine neuraminidase subtypes. Viruses infecting humans, birds, horses and a whale are included. Among these sequences, only one carbohydrate attachment site is conserved. The sequence Asn146-X-Thr is found in all of these sequences bar one, and that is the neurovirulent strain A/WSN/33, where the sequence is Arg-X-Thr. The loss of carbohydrate at this site has recently been shown to correlate with the acquired neurovirulence of this particular influenza strain (Li *et al.* 1993). The reason for its preservation on other strains of virus is unclear. Analysis of the carbohydrate composition of N2 neuraminidase of A/Tokyo/3/67 (Ward *et al.* 1983) revealed that the uncommon residue, N-acetylgalactosamine, is part of the carbohydrate at Asn146, but not of any other carbohydrate within the neuraminidase head, nor of any of the characterized carbohydrates of the haemagglutinin.

The sequence collection also reveals that a number of cystine residues, known from the three-dimensional structure to be in disulphide bonds, are conserved structural features. Within the head region of the molecule, these disulphide bridges are 92–417, 124–129, 183–230, 232–237, 278–291, 280–289, 318–337 and 421–447. In addition to these 16 conserved amino acids, the sequence collection of the head regions contains another 49 invariant positions, about half of which are known from the three-dimensional structure to be in the catalytic site or immediately adjacent to it.

Sequence comparisons show that within the globular head regions any two neuraminidase subtypes are of the order of 45% identical, and that any two A and B strains are of the order of 30% identical (Colman 1989). Sequence variation within subtypes may be as low as a few per cent.

Three-dimensional structure and catalytic activity

X-ray crystallography of two N2 strains provided the first high-resolution three-dimensional image of the molecule (Colman *et al.* 1983; Varghese *et al.* 1983). The enzyme subunit is comprised of six β-sheets of four antiparallel strands, the sheets being arranged like the blades of a propeller (Plate 6.1; see plate section facing p. 288). Four subunits are arranged with circular four-fold symmetry to form the tetrameric particle (100 Å × 100 Å × 60 Å) seen in the electron microscope. The N-terminus of the crystalline material (residue 78) is located very close to this four-fold symmetry axis. Presumably, this defines the lower surface (proximal to the viral membrane) of the tetramer. At this point (residue 78) the four 'stalk' peptides are close to each other and in a position to form the *c.* 60 Å-long filamentous structure which connects the heads to the transmembrane segment (residues 7–35).

The catalytic site of the protein is a strain-invariant pocket (Plate 6.2; see plate section facing p. 288) into which Neu5Ac (Fig. 6.1) binds (Colman *et al.* 1983; Burmeister *et al.* 1992; Varghese *et al.* 1992). The pocket is located centrally on the propeller axis at the N-terminal ends of the central strands of the six β-sheets. It is lined by an unusually large number of potentially charged amino acid side chains, five arginyl residues (118, 152, 224, 292, 371), four glutamyl residues (119, 227, 276, 277) and one

aspartyl residue (151). Neu5Ac is bound in this pocket in the α-anomer in a half-chair configuration, so that the carboxylate moiety of the sugar, axial in the chair conformation, is equatorial and located between three of the arginyl residues (118, 292, 371) referred to above. The glycerol side chain is hydrogen bonded to glutamate 276 and the *N*-acetyl side chain sits in a hydrophobic pocket formed by Trp178 and Leu134. The 4-hydroxyl side chain of Neu5Ac is hydrogen bonded to Glu227 and in an ionic interaction with Glu118. The floor of the active site contains the invariant Tyr406 and Glu277, both in close proximity to the ring oxygen atom of the substrate (Plate 6.2; see plate section facing p. 288). The transition state analogue, Neu5Ac2en (Fig. 6.1), binds isosterically in the site, its tighter binding with respect to Neu5Ac deriving in part from the equatorial presentation of the carboxylate. The 4-hydroxyl side chain is not only unbalanced with respect to charge on the protein, but it also occupies a pocket which is partly filled with water molecules. Replacing this hydroxyl with a guanidinyl side chain improves binding by nearly four orders of magnitude (see below), and the resulting compound, 4-guanidino-Neu5Ac2en (Fig. 6.1), now known as zanamivir, has antiviral properties which are discussed elsewhere in this volume (Chapter 36).

The structure of the catalytic centre, in the presence and absence of inhibitors and substrate analogues, has given some insight into the mechanism of action. Ring distortion, from chair to half-chair, is likely to precede bond cleavage. A theoretical study of glycosidic bond cleavage has shown that if the reaction is initiated from the half-chair conformation then cleavage proceeds without the development of stable intermediates (Smith 1997). Asp151 is well positioned to function as the proton donor in the reaction, but the pH profile of the enzyme activity suggests that this role may be an indirect one, possibly via a water molecule. Tyr406 and Glu277 are appropriately located to stabilize any developing positive charge on the carboxonium cation intermediate (Chong *et al.* 1992).

The β-propeller fold is conserved across influenza neuraminidase subtypes as expected (Tulip *et al.* 1991; Burmeister *et al.* 1992) and, surprisingly, has also been observed in bacterial neuraminidases which are soluble, monomeric enzymes. The bacterial neuraminidases have no sequence homology with influenza neuraminidase, but there are pronounced similarities in the type and arrangement of amino acids in the catalytic site (reviewed in Taylor 1996). Similarly, the haemagglutinin–neuraminidase protein of paramyxoviruses has no measurable sequence similarity with the influenza enzyme, but a model has been proposed which illustrates that the propeller fold for that protein is consistent with a conserved catalytic site with similar features to influenza neuraminidase (Colman *et al.* 1993). The preservation of the tri-arginyl cluster and analogues of Glu277, Tyr406 and Asp151 in all known three-dimensional structures of neuraminidases supports the proposed role of these residues in catalysis. Other active site amino acids are important for engaging the substrate and this is achieved in different ways in the viral and bacterial enzymes.

Antigenic variation and antibody binding

Amino acid substitutions which distinguish different strains within a subtype of influenza virus have been mapped to the three-dimensional structure of neuraminidase as a means of identifying possible sites on the antigen to which antibodies might bind. The resulting definition of antigenic sites is imprecise, and the understanding of what structural changes give new strains a survival advantage in the wild is incomplete, but there is a general view that a small number of amino acid sequence changes which are scattered around the surface of the antigen is required for the appearance of a new epidemic-causing strain.

Before discussing structural aspects of antigenic variation, salient data from structural studies of antibodies with neuraminidase (Colman *et al.* 1987; Tulip *et al.* 1992a; Malby *et al.* 1994) and other antigens will be briefly summarized. A central issue to consider is how the functional active site of the neuraminidase enzyme is preserved across all strains in the face of antibody responses in the host population.

In many respects complexes between antibodies and protein antigens resemble other protein–protein interactions (Colman 1988). The size of the interacting surfaces on the two molecules is not less than about $700\,\text{Å}^2$ and more than a dozen or so amino acids from each of the participating molecules participate in forming atomic contacts across the interface. Hydrogen bonds, ionic interactions and hydrophobic interactions may all be found in a given complex. The surfaces in contact are complementary in shape (Lawrence & Colman 1993) and chemical character (McCoy *et al.* 1997). However, the contributions to the free energy of binding are probably not evenly distributed across the interface. These contributions depend on the atomic environment of all interface atoms, and therefore include intra- and intermolecular interactions within the interface.

The issue of size of the antibody binding site is a critical one. The surface area of the enzyme active site of neuraminidase is less than $600\,\text{Å}^2$. Like other enzyme active sites, it is also an invaginated region of the molecule. If the lower limit for surface-area contact of an antibody with an antigen is larger than the functional (enzyme) site on the virus then amino acid variation which is part of the antibody binding site but not part of the functional site will always be a possibility (Colman *et al.* 1983). In this way, functionally viable antigenic variants may arise. A structure of an antibody fragment complexed with influenza haemagglutinin further illustrates this point (Bizebard *et al.* 1995). Other methods for hiding functional sites from antibody surveillance include locating them on highly invaginated structures which antibodies might not easily reach (Colman *et al.* 1983). This hypothesis was especially popular for rhinoviruses where the receptor binding region is a canyon-like depression on the viral surface (Rossmann *et al.* 1985), but a recent study has shown that antibody can penetrate the canyon (Smith *et al.* 1996b). Thus, even in this case, the antibody footprint size has been called upon to explain the preservation of receptor binding activity in the face of host–antibody interactions.

By definition, antigens within a particular subtype crossreact with antibodies raised against other members of the subtype, and the mapping of intrasubtype variation to the structure makes clear that there remain between members of the subtype 'large areas' of constant structure to which an antibody, in theory, might bind (illustrated in Colman 1992). 'Large areas' in this context means surface patches of the order of $700\,\text{Å}^2$ and comprising a dozen or more amino acids, which is approximately the minimum size of an antibody binding site on a protein antigen as discussed above. Intersubtype variation, on the other hand, is characterized by the absence of crossreacting antibodies, and comparison of the three-dimensional structures of N2 and N9 subtype neuraminidases illustrates that they share no such 'large areas' of identical structure for binding by a common antibody (Tulip *et al.* 1991).

Monoclonal variants of neuraminidase, selected by culturing virus in the presence of a particular antineuraminidase antibody, are typically characterized by a single amino acid sequence change with respect to wild-type virus (see e.g. Webster *et al.* 1987). The type of stereochemical substitution which occurs in these experiments ranges from the subtle (e.g. Ser to Ala) to the severe (e.g. Ile to Arg), but in all cases a clear growth advantage is conferred on the variant. Three-dimensional structures of the variants differ from that of wild-type only at the site of the substitution (Varghese *et al.* 1988; Tulip *et al.* 1991). Why should one amino acid substitution within an antibody binding surface involving a dozen or more amino acids make such a difference? Protein–protein interactions are usually characterized by large surface areas as described here for antibody–antigen interactions, and various studies now suggest that not all parts of the surface contribute equally to the energy of the interaction (see e.g. Clackson & Wells 1995). The loss of a single hydrogen bond within the binding interface might cost 4 kcal/mol of binding energy and this could have the effect of reducing the binding affinity by a factor of nearly 1000, sufficient to explain the selective advantage enjoyed by the variant over the wild-type.

The picture which emerges from monoclonal variants is that an antibody–antigen complex may be abrogated by small changes to the antigen.

However, examples are known of non-homologous amino acid substitutions being tolerated within the binding interface. The antineuraminidase antibody selects a variant in which Ile368 is changed to Arg, and that variant shows 10-fold reduction with respect to wild-type neuraminidase in binding to the monoclonal antibody NC41 (Webster *et al.* 1987). Furthermore, the three-dimensional structure of the complex between NC41 and the Ile368 to Arg mutant has been determined (Tulip *et al.* 1992b) and shows that the larger arginyl side chain is accommodated because of a compensating movement of an amino acid on the light chain of the antibody with respect to its position in the complex with wild-type antigen.

Prediction of the outcome of amino substitutions within an antibody–antigen interface is not yet possible without knowledge of the structural context within the interface of the substituted residue.

Drug discovery

Over the 30 years since 1966, there have been three attempts to discover inhibitors of neuraminidase with a view to assessing their activity as anti-influenza drugs. The first was a screening programme, the second was centred around derivatives of the transition state analogue Neu5Ac2en, and the third continues as a structure-based approach which has so far yielded two clinical candidates.

Edmond *et al.* (1966) set out to synthesise analogues of Neu5Ac, but resorted to screening in the face of synthetic difficulties. Of the compounds they investigated, N-substituted oxamic acids were the most potent. They showed no antiviral activity on virus grown in whole embryonated eggs, and this was attributed to breakdown of the compounds to inactive products.

The synthesis of the transition state analogue Neu5Ac2en by Meindl and Tuppy (1969) was a landmark in the search for potent neuraminidase inhibitors. It initiated a programme of chemical derivation of the compound which failed to yield molecules that were significantly more active than Neu5Ac2en itself (Meindl *et al.* 1974) but which did enable Palese and Compans (1976) to demonstrate the mode of action of the inhibitor in limiting viral replication in tissue culture to a single cycle. Electron microscopy showed that the most potent of these derivatives, the trifluoro-acetyl analogue, caused progeny virions to be immobilized at the surface of infected cells through interactions with the cell surface and with other virions (Palese & Compans 1976). The failure of this inhibitor to produce an antiviral effect in mice (Palese & Schulman 1977) was attributed to rapid degradation or excretion of the molecule, and cast doubts over the appropriateness of the Neu5Ac2en framework, and of the validity of neuraminidase as a target for therapy; after all, neuraminidase inhibitors could not stop infection.

The description of the three-dimensional structure of the enzyme (Varghese *et al.* 1983) and of its invariant catalytic pocket (Colman *et al.* 1983) revitalized the search for new and more potent inhibitors. This was now driven by considerations of the active site structure and of the binding mode of Neu5Ac and Neu5Ac2en into the site (Varghese *et al.* 1992). Those interactions are described above and discussed in more detail in Colman (1994). The introduction of positively charged substituents at the 4-position was governed by the presence of two conserved carboxylates (glutamates 118 and 227) adjacent to the 4-hydroxyl moiety of the substrate. An amino (NH2) probe of the active site using GRID (Goodford 1985) confirmed this approach (reviewed in Colman 1994). The 4-amino- and 4-guanidino- derivatives of Neu5Ac2en are approximately two and four orders of magnitude, respectively, more potent influenza neuraminidase inhibitors than Neu5Ac2en itself (von Itzstein *et al.* 1993).

The discovery of zanamivir and its potent antiviral properties in man has led to a search for other molecules with similar activity. Two general classes of molecule have been investigated to date: those based on the Neu5Ac2en framework with different substituents, particularly at the C6 (glycerol) position; and benzoic acid and carbocyclic frameworks. A number of 6-carboxamide analogues of zanamivir have been synthesized (Sollis *et al.* 1996) and found to be selectively active against type A influenza neuraminidase. The poor activity against the type B enzyme seems to be related to very subtle active site differences in the glycerol binding pocket which impose a higher energy barrier on a conformational change in the side chain of Glu276 (Smith *et al.* 1996a) which is required to accommodate the carboxamides. This conformational change allows Glu276 to form a salt link with Arg224 and exposes a hydrophobic pocket for interaction with lipophilic substituents on the carboxamide.

Although none of the benzoic acid derivatives described so far have high activity as enzyme inhibitors (reviewed in Luo *et al.* 1996), a carbocyclic compound (GS4104, Fig. 6.1e) with inhibitory activity comparable to zanamivir has recently been reported (Kim *et al.* 1997). Like zanamivir, GS4104 is the result of a structure-based approach to drug design. The discovery of other compounds derived from consideration of the neuraminidase active site structure seems likely.

Although consideration of the target structure has driven the discovery of considerably more potent inhibitors, subtleties in the details of the target and ligand structures, together with unknown dynamic aspects of the ligand–target interaction, require that the process of structure-based drug design remains firmly rooted in experiment. Two examples illustrate this point.

1 The predicted orientation of the guanidino moiety in the interaction of 4-guanidino-Neu5Ac2en with neuraminidase requires hydrogen bonding to Glu119 (von Itzstein *et al.* 1993), but the observation is an ionic interaction (Varghese *et al.* 1995). If the prediction is computed with the enzyme structure held rigid, it results in a configuration consistent with experiment (Varghese *et al.* 1995).

2 Though the active sites of type A and B neuraminidase are very similar, a small difference in these structures in the neighbourhood of Glu276 seems to affect the free movement of the side chain of that amino acid, which in turn results in certain analogues of Neu5Ac2en with carboxamide substitutions at C6 showing selective activity towards type A neuraminidase (see above).

Drug resistance

The introduction of a new antiviral agent is expected to lead to the appearance of resistant strains of the virus. This is the case even when the target site of the drug is a hitherto invariant site. Antibodies are not able to put the neuraminidase active site under selection pressure because of: (i) the large surface area of interaction which they require; (ii) the small surface area of the active site; and (iii) the possibility of single amino acid sequence substitutions, near to but outside of the active site, being sufficient to abolish antibody binding. Antibodies are expected to make interactions with neuraminidase that the substrate does not, and for that reason enzymatically viable antigenic variants can arise.

Zanamivir makes interactions with the enzyme which the natural substrate does not, and therein lies the possibility of drug-resistant strains emerging.

Resistant variants have been selected in tissue culture by growing virus in the presence of the inhibitor. Two types of variant have been observed so far, those with mutations in the sialic acid binding pocket of the haemagglutinin (McKimm-Breschkin *et al.* 1996a), and those with mutations in the enzyme site of the neuraminidase (Blick *et al.* 1995). These variants do not arise rapidly; they require multiple passaging of virus with the drug, unlike amantidine-resistant variants which arise rapidly in culture and in patients (Hay *et al.* 1985; Hayden *et al.* 1991). The haemagglutinin variants are drug dependent, reverting to wild-type when the drug is removed, but the neuraminidase variants are not. On the basis of red-cell elution assays, it is suspected, but not yet proven, that the haemagglutinin variants have reduced binding affinity for the receptor, allowing elution of progeny even though the neuraminidase is inactivated by the inhibitor (McKimm-Breschkin *et al.* 1996a). In the absence of the inhibitor, the neuraminidase is active and these variants might not attach sufficiently well to cells to penetrate, because the balance between binding and destruction of the receptor has been shifted. This may be an explanation for the drug dependence of the haemagglutinin variants.

The most common neuraminidase variant selected in these experiments is Glu119 to Gly (Blick *et al.* 1995; Staschke *et al.* 1995; Gubareva *et al.* 1996). The variant is still sensitive to the drug in plaque assays but only at concentrations 1000 times that needed to suppress wild-type growth. The mutant has been studied crystallographically in the presence and absence of the inhibitor and found to be structurally identical to wild-type apart from the absence of the side chain at position 119, the presence of water molecules in the space formerly occupied by the side chain, and a concomitant small change in the active site solvent structure (Blick *et al.* 1995). There is disagreement in the literature about the properties of this variant. Blick *et al.* (1995) and McKimm-Breschkin *et al.* (1996b) find the variant to have the same specific activity as wild-type but a reduced stability, whereas Staschke *et al.* (1995) report the specific activity to be 5% of wild-type.

It is generally but not universally true that the more potent neuraminidase inhibitors are better inhibitors of multicycle replication in tissue culture, and are better antiviral agents in animals. However, some wild strains of influenza fail the tissue culture test, even though their neuraminidases are inhibited and they are sensitive to the drug in animals (Woods *et al.* 1993). Selection of variants by the drug in tissue culture may give rise to such a phenotype which would not then be expected to be clinically relevant. The only important measure of resistance is in infected patients being treated with drug. To date, no clinically derived variants have been isolated from patients undergoing treatment with zanamivir.

References

Bizebard, T., Gigant, B., Rigolet, P. *et al.* (1995) Structure of influenza virus haemagglutinin complexed with a neutralizing antibody. *Nature* **376**, 92–4.

Blick, T.J., Tiong, T., Sahasrabudhe, A. *et al.* (1995) Generation and characterisation of an influenza virus neuraminidase variant with decreased sensitivity to the neuraminidase-specific inhibitor 4-guanidino-Neu5Ac2en. *Virology* **214**, 475–84.

Burmeister, W.P., Ruigrok, R.W.H. & Cusak, S. (1992) The 2.2 Å resolution crystal structure of influenza B neuraminidase and its complex with sialic acid. *EMBO J* **11**, 49–56.

Chong, A.K., Pegg, M.S., Taylor, N.R. & von Itzstein, M. (1992) Evidence for a sialosyl cation transition-state complex in the reaction of sialidase from influenza virus. *Eur J Biochem* **207**, 335–43.

Clackson, T.A. & Wells, J.A. (1995) A hot spot of binding energy in a hormone-receptor interface. *Science* **267**, 383–6.

Colman, P.M. (1988) Structure of antibody-antigen complexes: implications for immune recognition. *Adv Immunol* **43**, 99–132.

Colman, P.M. (1989) Influenza virus neuraminidase: enzyme and antigen. In: Krug, R.M. (ed.) *The Influenza Viruses*, pp. 175–218. Plenum Press, New York.

Colman, P.M. (1992) Structural basis of antigenic variation: studies of influenza virus neuraminidase. *Immunol Cell Biol* **70**, 209–14.

Colman, P.M. (1994) Influenza virus neuraminidase: structure, antibodies, and inhibitors. *Protein Sci* **3**, 1687–96.

Colman, P.M., Varghese, J.N. & Laver, W.G. (1983) Structure of the catalytic and antigenic sites in influenza virus neuraminidase. *Nature* **303**, 41–4.

Colman, P.M., Laver, W.G., Varghese, J.N. *et al.* (1987) The three dimensional structure of a complex of antibody with influenza virus neuraminidase. *Nature* **326**, 358–63.

Colman, P.M., Hoyne, P.A. & Lawrence, M.C. (1993) Sequence and structure alignment of paramyxovirus haemagglutinin-neuraminidase (HN) with influenza virus neuraminidase. *J Virol* **67**, 2972–80.

Edmond, J.D., Johnston, R.G., Kidd, D., Rylance, H.J. & Sommerville, R.G. (1966) The inhibition of neuraminidase and antiviral action. *Br J Pharmacol Chemother* **27**, 415–26.

Goodford, P.J. (1985) A computational procedure for determining energetically favourable binding sites on biologically important macromolecules. *J Med Chem* **28**, 849–57.

Gubareva, L.V., Bethell, R.C., Hart, G.J., Murti, K.G., Penn, C.R. & Webster, R.G. (1996) Characterization of mutants of influenza A virus selected with the neuraminidase inhibitor 4-guanidino-Neu5Ac2en. *J Virol* **70**, 1818–27.

Hay, A.J., Wostenholme, A.J., Skehel, J.J. & Smith, M.H. (1985) The molecular basis of the specific anti-influenza action of amantidine. *EMBO J* **4**, 3021–4.

Hayden, F.G., Sperber, S.J., Belshe, R.B., Clover, R.D., Hay, A.J. & Pyke, S. (1991) Recovery of drug-resistant influenza A virus during therapeutic use of rimantidine. *Antimicrobial Agents Chemother* **35**, 1741–7.

Hirst, G.K. (1942) Adsorption of influenza haemagglutinins and virus by red blood cells. *J Exp Med* **76**, 195–209.

Kraulis, P.J. (1991) MOLSCRIPT: a program to produce both detailed and schematic plots of protein structures. *J Appl Cryst* **24**, 946–50.

Kim, C.U., Willard, L., Williams, M.A. *et al.* (1997) Influenza neuraminidase inhibitors possessing a novel hydrophobic interaction in the enzyme active site: design, synthesis, and structural analysis of carbocyclic sialic acid analogues with potent anti-influenza activity. *J Am Chem Soc* **119**, 681–90.

Laver, W.G. (1978) Crystallisation and peptide maps of neuraminidase heads from H2N2 and H3N2 influenza virus strains. *Virology* **86**, 78–87.

Laver, W.G., Colman, P.M., Webster, R.G., Hinshaw, V.S. & Air, G.M. (1984) Influenza virus neuraminidase with haemagglutinin activity. *Virology* **137**, 314–23.

Lawrence, M.C. & Colman, P.M. (1993) Shape complementarity at protein–protein interfaces. *J Mol Biol* **234**, 946–50.

Li, S., Schulman, J., Hamura, S. & Palese, P. (1993) Glycosylation of neuraminidase determines the neurovirulence of influenza A/WSN/33 virus. *J Virol* **67**, 6667–73.

Luo, M., Air, G.M. & Brouillette, W.J. (1996) Design of aromatic inhibitors of influenza virus neuraminidase. In: Brown, L.E., Hampson, A.W. & Webster, R.G. (eds) *Options for the Control of Influenza III*, pp. 702–12. Elsevier, Amsterdam.

McCoy, A.J., Chandana Epa V. & Colman, P.M. (1997) Electrostatic complementarity at protein/protein interfaces. *J Mol Biol* **268**, 570–84.

McKimm-Breschkin, J.L., Blick, T.J., Sahasrabudhe, A.V. *et al.* (1996a) Generation and characterisation of variants of the NWS/G70C influenza virus after *in vitro* passage in 4-amino-Neu5Ac2en and 4-guanidino-Neu5Ac2en. *Antimicrobial Agents Chemother* **40**, 40–6.

McKimm-Breschkin, J.L., McDonald, M., Blick, T.J. & Colman, P.M. (1996b) Mutation in the influenza virus neuraminidase gene resulting in decreased sensitivity to the neuraminidase inhibitor 4-guanidino-Neu5Ac2en leads to instability of the enzyme. *Virology* **225**, 240–2.

Malby, R.L., Tulip, W.R., Harley, V.R. *et al.* (1994) The structure of a complex between the NC10 antibody and influenza virus neuraminidase and comparison with the overlapping binding site of the NC41 antibody. *Structure* **2**, 733–46.

Meindl, P. & Tuppy, H. (1969) 2-Deoxy-2,3-dehydrosialic acids. I. Synthesis and properties of 2-deoxy-2,3-dehydro-*N*-acetylneuraminic acids and their methyl esters. *Monatshefte Chem* **100**, 1295–1306.

Meindl, P., Bodo, G., Palese, P., Schulman, J. & Tuppy, H. (1974) Inhibition of neuraminidase activity by derivatives of 2-deoxy-2,3-dehydro-*N*-acetylneuraminic acid. *Virology* **58**, 457–63.

Palese, P. & Compans, R.W. (1976) Inhibition of influenza virus replication in tissue culture by 2-deoxy-2,3-dehydro-N-trifluoro-acetyl-neuraminic acid (FANA): mechanism of action. *J Gen Virol* **33**, 159–63.

Palese, P. & Schulman, J.L. (1977) Inhibitors of viral neuraminidase as potential antiviral drugs. In: Oxford, J.S. (ed.) *Chemoprophylaxis and Virus Infections of the Upper Respiratory Tract*, Vol. 1, pp. 189–205. CRC Press, Boca Raton, Florida.

Rossmann, M.G., Arnold, E., Erikson, A.E. *et al.* (1985) Structure of a human common cold virus and its relationship to other picornaviruses. *Nature* **317**, 145–53.

Smith, B.J. (1997) A conformational study of 2-oxanol: insight into the role of ring distortion on enzyme catalysed glycosidic bond cleavage. *J Am Chem Soc* **119**, 2699–706.

Smith, P.W., Sollis, S.L., Howes, P.D. *et al.* (1996a) Novel inhibitors of sialidases related to GG167; structure-activity, crystallographic and molecular dynamics studies with 4-H-pyran-2-carboxylic acid-6-carboxamides. *Bioorganic Med Chem Lett* **6**, 2931–6.

Smith, T.J., Chase, E.S., Schmidt, T.J., Olson, N.H. & Baker, T.S. (1996b) Neutralising antibody to human rhinovirus 14 penetrates the receptor-binding canyon. *Nature* **383**, 350–4.

Sollis, S.L., Smith, P.W., Howes, P.D., Cherry, P.C. & Bethell, R.C. (1996) Novel inhibitors of influenza sialidase related to GG167; synthesis of 4-amino and guanidino-4H-pyran-2-carboxylic acid-6-propylamides; selective inhibitors of influenza A virus sialidase. *Bioorganic Med Chem Lett* **6**, 1805–8.

Staschke, K.A., Colacino, J.M., Baxter, A.J. *et al.* (1995) Molecular basis for the resistance of influenza viruses to 4-guanidino-Neu5Ac2en. *Virology* **214**, 642–6.

Taylor, G. (1996) Sialidases: structures, biological significance and therapeutic potential. *Curr Opin Struct Biol* **6**, 830–7.

Tulip, W.R., Varghese, J.N., Baker, A.T. *et al.* (1991) Refined atomic structures of N9 subtype influenza virus neuraminidase and escape mutants. *J Mol Biol* **221**, 487–97.

Tulip, W.R., Varghese, J.N., Laver, W.G., Webster, R.G. & Colman, P.M. (1992a) Refined crystal structure of the influenza virus N9 neuraminidase-NC41 Fab complex. *J Mol Biol* **227**, 122–48.

Tulip, W.R., Varghese, J.N., Webster, R.G., Laver, W.G. & Colman, P.M. (1992b) Crystal structures of two mutant neuraminidase-antibody complexes with amino acid substitutions in the interface. *J Mol Biol* **227**, 149–59.

Varghese, J.N., Laver, W.G. & Colman, P.M. (1983) Structure of the influenza virus glycoprotein antigen neuraminidase at 2.9 Å resolution. *Nature* **303**, 35–40.

Varghese, J.N., Webster, R.G., Laver, W.G. & Colman, P.M. (1988) Structure of an escape mutant of glycoprotein N2 neuraminidase of influenza virus A/Tokyo/3/67 at 3 Å. *J Mol Biol* **200**, 201–3.

Varghese, J.N., McKimm-Breschkin, J.L., Caldwell, J.B., Kortt, A.A. & Colman, P.M. (1992) The structure of the complex between influenza virus neuraminidase and sialic acid, the viral receptor. *Proteins Struct Funct Genet* **14**, 327–32.

Varghese, J.N., Epa, V.E. & Colman, P.M. (1995) Three-dimensional structure of the complex of 4-guanidino-Neu5Ac2en and influenza virus neuraminidase. *Protein Sci* **4**, 1081–7.

von Itzstein, M., Wu, W-Y., Kok, G.B. *et al.* (1993) Rational design of potent sialidase-based inhibitors of influenza virus replication. *Nature* **363**, 418–23.

Ward, C.W., Murray, J.M., Roxburgh, C.M. & Jackson, D.C. (1983) Chemical and antigenic characterisation of the carbohydrate side chains of an Asian (N2) influenza virus neuraminidase. *Virology* **126**, 370–5.

Webster, R.G., Air, G.M., Metzger, D.W. *et al.* (1987) Antigenic structure and variation in an influenza N9 neuraminidase. *J Virol* **61**, 2910–6.

Wrigley, N.G., Skehel, J.J., Charlwood, P.A. & Brand, C.M. (1973) The size and shape of influenza virus neuraminidase. *Virology* **51**, 525–9.

Woods, J.M., Bethel, R.C., Coates, A.V. *et al.* (1993) 4-guanidino-2,4-dideoxy-2,3-dehydro-*N*-acetylneuraminic acid is a highly effective inhibitor both of the sialidase and of growth of a wide range of influenza A and B viruses *in vitro*. *Antimicrobial Agents Chemother* **37**, 1473–9.

CHAPTER 7

Functional Properties of the Virus Ion Channels

Alan J. Hay

Introduction

In the understanding of biochemical processes elucidation of functional activities is facilitated by the use of selective inhibitors of key reactions. So it was for the M2 protein of influenza A viruses and its function in virus replication. The anti-influenza A activity of amantadine and related compounds was discovered around 1960 (Davies *et al.* 1964) and early studies indicated that their action was directed against a stage in virus entry into cells (Kato & Eggers 1969). However, it was not until the advent of nucleic acid sequencing and mutational analysis that characterization of amantadine-resistant mutants identified the M2 product of the M gene as the target of selective drug action (Hay *et al.* 1985). Investigations of the consequences of inhibiting M2 activity provided the first clues that the M2 protein may function as an ion channel (Hay 1989; Sugrue *et al.* 1990) and this was subsequently confirmed by direct electrophysiological measurement (Pinto *et al.* 1992; Tosteson *et al.* 1994; Chizhmakov *et al.* 1996a).

The replication of influenza B and C viruses is not selectively inhibited *in vivo* or *in vitro* by adamantane derivatives or other inhibitors of M2 and no selective inhibitor has yet been discovered which may be used to identify proteins which perform an equivalent function to that of M2 in influenza A virus replication. The NB protein of influenza B (Williams & Lamb 1986; Betakova *et al.* 1996; Brassard *et al.* 1996) and the CM2 protein of influenza C (Hongo *et al.* 1997) do, however, share a number of features in common with M2; in particular they are small oligomeric integral membrane proteins, orientated with a short N-terminal

M2 protein (influenza A)

MSLLTEVETPTRNGWECSCSDSSDP*LVIAASIIGILHFILWIL*DRLFFKCIYRRLKYGLKRGPSTEGBPESMREEYRQEQQNAVDVDDGHFVNIELE

NB protein (influenza B)

MNNATFNYTNVNPISHIRG*SVIITICVSFTVILTVFGYIA*KIFTNRNNCTNNAIGLCKRIKCSGCEPFCNKRDDTSSPRTGVDIPSFILPGLNLSESTPN

CM2 protein (influenza C)

MGRMAMKWLVVIIYFSITSQPASACNLKTCLNLF*NNTDAVTVHCFNENQGYMLTLASLGLGIITMLYLLV*KIIIELVNGFVLGRWERWCGDIKTTIMPEIDSMEKDIALFRERLDLGEDAPDETDNSPIPFSNDGIFE

1   10   20   30   40   50   60   70   80   90   100   110   120   130

Fig. 7.1 Amino acid sequences of the M2 protein of A/chicken/Germany/27 (H7N7), the NB protein of B/Panama/45/90 and the CM2 protein of C/Yamagata/1/88. Potential sites of N-linked glycosylation are indicated in bold and hydrophobic sequences thought to form the membrane spanning domains are underlined. The 97 amino acid sequence of M2 is translated from a spliced mRNA of the M gene (Lamb *et al.* 1981; see Chapter 4). The locations of single amino acid substitutions which confer resistance to amantadine and related compounds are indicated in bold italics. The 100 amino acid sequence of the NB protein is encoded by the bicistronic mRNA of the neuraminidase gene; translation of NB is initiated seven nucleotides before initiation of NA translation in a different reading frame (Shaw *et al.* 1983). The amino acid sequence of CM2 is translated from the unspliced mRNA of the M gene; the site of translation initiation has not been established with certainty and the sequence shown starts from the initiation codon at nucleotides 731–733 of the colinear transcript (Hongo *et al.* 1994).

domain external to the membrane (Fig. 7.1), and are minor components of the virus envelope. Their potential ion channel functions are being studied directly by electrophysiological means.

The M2 protein of influenza A viruses

Analyses of the drug susceptibility of reassortants between amantadine-sensitive and amantadine-resistant viruses showed that the principal determinant of susceptibility to amantadine and related inhibitors is the M gene (Lubeck *et al.* 1978; Hay *et al.* 1979; Belshe *et al.* 1988), but that for certain pathogenic avian strains, such as fowl plague virus, the haemagglutinin (HA) is also influential, for reasons discussed below (Scholtissek & Faulkner 1979; Hay *et al.* 1986). Thus, with few exceptions, the resistance of mutants selected either following passage of virus in cell culture in the presence of drug, or following treatment of animals, birds or humans with amantadine or rimantadine, has been shown to be due to single amino acid changes within the transmembrane domain of M2, predominantly at residues 27, 30, 31 or 34, depending on the virus (Hay *et al.* 1985; Belshe *et al.* 1988; reviewed by Hay 1996).

The M2 protein is a homotetramer of 97 amino acid subunits, translated from a spliced mRNA of the M gene (Lamb *et al.* 1981: see Chapter 4; Holsinger & Lamb 1991; Sugrue & Hay 1991). The membrane spanning domain comprises the hydrophobic sequence of amino acids 25–43 (Fig. 7.1). The initial deduction, from the locations of amino acid changes which confer resistance, was therefore that amantadine interacts with this region of a pore formed by the M2 protein (Sugrue & Hay 1991). This is supported by neutron diffraction studies which indicated that amantadine interacted with the equivalent region of a 25-residue peptide (amino acids 22–46, including the transmembrane domain) incorporated into a lipid bilayer (Duff *et al.* 1994). Furthermore, truncated mutant channels, lacking most of either the N-terminal external domain or the C-terminal cytoplasmic domain, exhibit a similar drug sensitivity to that of the wild-type protein (A. Philips, N. Mulrine, I. Chizhmakov & A. Hay, unpublished results).

Roles of M2 in virus replication

Two roles for the M2 channel in virus replication, both of which are related to the functionality of the haemagglutinin, were identified by their susceptibility to inhibition by amantadine, one in the uncoating of the virus ribonucleoprotein (RNP) during virus entry and the other in modulating the pH of the *trans* Golgi of virus-infected cells (reviewed in Hay 1992). Structural interactions of M2 with other virus proteins, such as M1, which may be involved in virus assembly are not affected by the channel-blocking action of amantadine (Zebedee & Lamb 1989; Hughey *et al.* 1995).

Modification of trans Golgi pH

The first indication that M2 may act as an ion channel came from the observation that amantadine caused low-pH inactivation of the HA of certain pathogenic avian viruses, e.g. fowl plague virus, during transport from its site of synthesis in the endoplasmic reticulum to the plasma membrane of virus-infected cells (Sugrue *et al.* 1990a). Unlike the HAs of human influenza viruses, the fusion activity of these HAs is proteolytically activated by proteases such as furin within the *trans* Golgi (Stieneke-Grober *et al.* 1992), consequently rendering them susceptible to an irreversible structural change on exposure to low (fusion) pH. The HA, itself acting as a pH probe, and the cytochemical pH probe DAMP were used to demonstrate that inhibition of M2 by amantadine caused a drop in the pH of the *trans* Golgi below that required to trigger the change in conformation of HA, an effect reversed by proton ionophores such as monensin (Steinhauer *et al.* 1991; Ciampor *et al.* 1992a; Grambas & Hay 1992). The function of M2 during cotransport with HA (Ohuchi *et al.* 1994; Takeuchi & Lamb 1994) is therefore to reduce the acidity of *trans* Golgi vesicles, by conducting the outward flow of H^+, and consequently to prevent exposure of the acid-sensitive HA to an adverse low pH. The importance of this function of M2 for these viruses is emphasized by the correlation between the activity of M2 and the pH stability of the HA (Grambas *et al.* 1992) and explains the influence of properties of their HAs on their sensitivity to amantadine.

Virus uncoating

The role of M2 common to different subtypes of influenza A viruses is involved, in concert with the membrane-fusing activity of the HA, in effecting the uncoating of the virus RNP during entry into cells. On the one hand, the low pH in late endosomes triggers the conformational change in the HA which causes the virus membrane to fuse with the endosome membrane to release the nucleocapsid of the virus into the cytoplasm. On the other hand, it is perceived that, prior to this event, H^+ flow through the M2 channel in the virus membrane to promote a low pH-induced dissociation of the M1 protein from the virus RNP, which is necessary to allow entry of RNPs into the nucleus and initiation of replication. Inhibition of M2 by amantadine blocked the release of free RNPs causing the retention of RNP–M1 complexes in the cytoplasm (Bukrinskaya *et al.* 1982; Martin & Helenius 1991). A similar effect was produced on infection of cells expressing the M1 protein. Association of M1 in the cytoplasm with the incoming virus RNPs blocked their entry into the nucleus; this was reversed by brief acidification of the cytoplasm, which dissociated the bound M1 and permitted subsequent entry of the virus RNPs into the nucleus (Bui *et al.* 1996). Efficient removal of M1 from RNPs of detergent solubilized virus occurs at pH below 6 in isotonic solution (Zhirnov 1990). Furthermore, the specific reduction by amantadine and enhancement by the H^+ ionophore monension of the rate of membrane fusion *in vitro* between virus and liposomes provides further evidence for the involvement of H^+ transfer by M2 in the entry process (Bron *et al.* 1993; Wharton *et al.* 1994). Purified M2, incorporated into lipid vesicles containing a pH probe, was shown to promote the translocation of H^+ across the membrane (Schroeder *et al.* 1994) in a manner analogous to that proposed for M2 in the virion and observed for M2 in the *trans* Golgi or plasma membrane of virus-infected or M2-transfected cells (Ciampor *et al.* 1992b; Hay *et al.* 1993).

Ion channel activity of M2

Ion channel activity of the M2 protein has been demonstrated directly by electrophysiological measurements of ionic currents across:
- the plasma membrane of oocytes of *Xenopus laevis* expressing M2, following microinjection of mRNA (Pinto *et al.* 1992);
- the plasma membrane of mammalian cells, transiently or stably transfected with M2 cDNA to express M2 (Wang *et al.* 1994; Chizhmakov *et al.* 1996a); or
- planar lipid bilayers into which purified M2 had been incorporated (Tosteson *et al.* 1994).

In all three systems ion currents were specifically blocked by amantadine, demonstrating that inhibition of ion channel activity of M2 is the basis of its anti-influenza A activity. Differences between the experimental systems used have, however, led to different conclusions, in particular as regards the ions that pass through the channel.

Using a two-electrode voltage clamp procedure it was concluded that M2 expressed in the surface membrane of *Xenopus* oocytes forms cation channels with high permeability for Na^+, which are activated (i.e. changed from closed to open state) by low pH, less than 7 (Pinto *et al.* 1992; Wang *et al.* 1995). Substitution of histidine 37 within the transmembrane domain by alanine, glycine or glutamic acid abolished low pH activation and appeared to render the mutant channels permanently open at high external pH (pH 8), indicating that histidine 37 is directly involved in activation of the channel (Pinto *et al.* 1992; Wang *et al.* 1995). As for other cation channels, H^+ can also pass through the M2 channel and cause a measurable reduction in the pH of the ooplasm in response to reduced external pH (Shimbo *et al.* 1996). On the basis of these observations it was suggested that the counterflow of Na^+ ions, by maintaining electroneutrality, permits permeation of sufficient H^+ into the virion to cause the low-pH disassembly of M1–RNP and subsequent release of free RNPs following endocytosis. The demonstration that purified M2 reconstituted into lipid bilayers formed cation channels with similar characteristics of pH dependence and Na^+ permeability (Tosteson *et al.* 1994;

Shimbo *et al.* 1996) confirmed that the M2 protein alone (in the absence of other ion channels) could account for the ion channel activity of M2 observed in *Xenopus* oocytes. Analyses of the amantadine sensitivity of mixed oligomers formed during co-expression in *Xenopus* oocytes of wild-type M2 and an amantadine-resistant (S3IN) mutant protein indicated that the homotetramer forms the active M2 channel (Sakaguchi *et al.* 1997).

Patch-clamp measurements of mouse erythro-leukaemia (MEL) cells, which are much smaller than *Xenopus* oocytes and allow control of the internal as well as the external medium, showed that M2 expressed in these cells formed a proton channel with high selectivity for H^+ and relatively low permeability for other physiological cations and anions including Na^+, K^+ and Cl^- (Chizhmakov *et al.* 1996a). Permeability for H^+ was 10^7 times greater than that for Na^+, and H^+ current could be measured using buffers containing only the membrane-impermanent cation N-methyl-D-glucamine (NMDG) and anions, N-2-hydroxyethylpiperazine-N'-2-ethanesulphonic acid (HEPES) or 2'-(N-morpholino) ethansulphonic acid (MES), and were not affected by inclusion of Na^+, K^+ or Cl^-. H^+ current, i.e. flow of H^+ through the channel, which is small at neutral or alkaline pH due to the low H^+ concentration increased as external pH was reduced in response to the increase in the electrochemical gradient, reaching saturation at pH~4. The apparent dissociation constant for interaction of H^+ with sites on M2 during permeation through the channel was approximately $10\,\mu M$ (pH 5) and is consistent with its function in the pH range 5–6 present within endosomes and the *trans* Golgi of virus-infected cells (Grambas & Hay 1992). Activation of the channel was also solely dependent on H^+ and occurred as pH was reduced from pH 8 to 6.5, with an apparent dissociation constant for H^+ binding of approximately $0.1\,\mu M$ (Chizhmakov *et al.* 1996a,b). Differences have been observed in the activation characteristics of M2 channels of viruses which differ in their pH of fusion, in particular in response to changes in internal and external pH (Chizhmakov *et al.* 1998a); however, it has not yet been possible to explain either the mechanism whereby amino acid differences within the trans-

membrane domain cause the change or the significance of the difference in channel activation in terms of the different pH stabilities of the HAs. Studies of other mutant proteins in this system have shown that substitution of histidine 37 by alanine caused an increase in permeability of M2 to Na^+ indicating that this amino acid residue is important in determining the proton selectivity of the channel (N. Mulrine & A. Hay, unpublished observations). The toxicity of this mutant protein (H37A), suppressed by rimantadine during selection of transfected cells, emphasizes the relative noncytotoxicity of wild-type M2 channels. Deletion mutants lacking most of the N-terminal external domain or most of the C-terminal internal domain have properties similar to those of the full-length protein. A 'minimal channel' peptide comprising mainly the transmembrane domain (amino acids 22–46) has been shown to form amantadine-sensitive proton channels in planar lipid bilayers (Duff & Ashley 1992).

Despite differences in interpretation of data obtained for M2 expressed in *Xenopus* oocytes and in MEL cells it is evident that the M2 channel can transfer H^+ across membranes with the H^+ electrochemical gradient and has properties consistent with its role in modifying virion and *trans* Golgi pH during virus infection. As yet we understand little regarding the mechanism of H^+ transfer, its regulation or block by amantadine (and related compounds). Inhibition is specific and irreversible, whereas channel activity of drug-resistant mutants is completely refractory to amantadine or rimantadine. The kinetics of inhibition indicate binding of one molecule of drug per channel. The available data are inconsistent with drug simply occluding the channel, as for certain non-competitive blockers of other ion channels, and indicate that block is the result of a drug-induced allosteric change in the channel, which may also irreversibly trap the drug (Wang *et al.* 1993; Chizhmakov *et al.* 1996b).

The NB protein of influenza B viruses

The NB protein (100 amino acids) is encoded within the neuraminidase (NA) gene of influenza B and is translated from the first initiation codon of the mRNA, four nucleotides before the AUG codon which initiates translation of the NA (Shaw *et al.* 1983). Like M2 it is synthesized in virus-infected cells in amounts comparable with the amounts of other structural components, but is incorporated into virus particles in relatively small amounts (Betakova *et al.* 1996; Brassard *et al.* 1996). NB forms dimers, but its multimeric nature has yet to be established; two N-linked polylactosaminoglycan side chains are attached to residues 3 and 7 near the N-terminus (Williams & Lamb 1988).

Ion channel activity of NB

The ion channel activity of NB has been studied in systems similar to those used to study M2. Purified, *Escherichia coli*-expressed NB reconstituted into artificial lipid bilayers formed cation-permeable channels at pH between 5.5 and 6.5, which were blocked by antibody against the C-terminal portion of the protein, while at a lower pH of 2.5 the channels were more permeable to Cl^- than to Na^+ (Sunstrom *et al.* 1996). Using a pH probe incorporated into membrane vesicles derived from the membrane of *E. coli* expressing NB, Ewart *et al.* (1996) showed that the protein was permeable to H^+. Studies in *Xenopus* oocytes proved inconclusive in discriminating an NB channel activity (Shimbo *et al.* 1995).

MEL cells expressing NB were used to compare directly the ion channel properties of NB with those of M2. Although there are similarities in proton permeability of the two proteins there are some notable differences in channel activity (Chizhmakov *et al.* 1998b). Activation of the NB proton channel requires Na^+ (at concentrations greater than 5 mM); no H^+ current flowed through NB in response to a large pH gradient when measurements were done in the presence of only the impermeable ions NMDG and HEPES/MES, conditions which elicited full activity of M2. Secondly, external pH below 5.5 activated a Cl^- permeability. The two activities were studied separately, proton currents in chloride-free sodium glutamate solutions and chloride currents in sodium-free NMDG chloride or choline chloride solutions. NB proton currents were similar to M2 proton currents in their response to changes in pH gradient, their depen-

dence on membrane potential, and their saturation at high external H^+ concentrations (the apparent dissociation constant for H^+ of 10 µM (pH 5) was similar to that of M2). The Cl^- currents activated slowly in response to a drop in pH below 5.5 and exhibited very strong outward rectification, i.e. outward current (corresponding to inward flow of the negative chloride ion) was much greater than inward current. In normal physiological solutions (below pH 5.5) NB is permeable to both H^+ and Cl^-; it is not yet clear, however, whether a single NB channel is permeable to both ions or whether two different molecular entities account for separate permeabilities to H^+ and Cl^-.

It is therefore apparent that during endocytosis NB in the virion has the inherent ability to transfer H^+ across the virion membrane to promote low pH disassembly of the internal structure, similar to that of M2 which is blocked by amantadine. The reason why NB possesses a Cl^- flux, absent in the case of M2, is not understood, although inward cotransport of Cl^- would potentiate flow of H^+ into the virion.

The CM2 protein of influenza C viruses

The CM2 protein (139 amino acids) of influenza C is translated from the full-length mRNA of the M gene whereas the M1 protein is translated from a spliced mRNA (Yamashita *et al.* 1988; Hongo *et al.* 1994). There is presently no information as to its function. However, as pointed out above, it shares a number of structural features in common with the M2 and NB proteins (Fig. 7.1) which are consistent with the notion that it performs an analogous ion transfer function. Like M2, CM2 is an acylated phosphoprotein which forms disulphide-linked tetramers; like NB, N-linked polylactosaminoglycan side chains are associated with the N-terminal domain (Williams & Lamb 1988; Sugrue *et al.* 1990b; Hongo *et al.* 1997). On the basis of these structural similarities it has been proposed that CM2 may also function as an ion channel in virus uncoating. However, studies of *in vitro* dissociation of the M1–RNP complex have indicated that M1 of influenza C virus dissociates at neutral pH in contrast to M1 of A and B viruses which dissociate only when exposed to a pH of below 6 (Zhirnov 1990; Zhirnov & Grigoriev 1994). Thus a requirement for a H⁺ transfer activity of CM2 in the virus is less compelling.

Concluding remarks

Influenza A and B viruses (and probably influenza C) possess ion channels, M2 and NB (and CM2?), respectively, which play an essential role in the initiation of infection. The common functional activity of M2 and NB is their proton permeability, which is perceived to conduct protons into the virion during endocytosis to promote an acid-induced dissociation of the M1 (matrix) protein from the virus RNP to allow its entry into the nucleus. However, the M2 and NB channels differ in certain key respects, e.g. NB requires Na⁺ for activation of its proton permeability and it possesses an H⁺-activated Cl⁻ permeability, whereas M2, under the same conditions, forms an H⁺-activated proton channel. Reasons for these differences are not clear; however, there are some notable differences between influenza A and B viruses. At the cellular level, the M2 channel has been shown to have a dual role, at least in certain pathogenic avian viruses, in that in addition to its accessory role in virus uncoating, it is also required to regulate *trans* Golgi pH to 'chaperone' the cleaved HA to the cell surface. At the level of virus–host interaction, whereas influenza B viruses infect only man, influenza A viruses are essentially avian viruses and differences in the sites of replication and environments encountered during virus transmission may require differences in channel properties in order to protect the integrity of the infectious particle. This raises interesting questions regarding the evolution of the different coding strategies and the different ion permeabilities of the proteins of the two viruses and whether they impose limitations on their ability to infect different host species.

References

Belshe, R.B., Hall Smith, M., Hall, C.B., Betts, R. & Hay, A.J. (1988) Genetic basis of resistance to rimantadine emerging during treatment of influenza virus infection. *J Virol* **62**, 1508–12.

Betakova, T., Nermut, M.V. & Hay, A.J. (1996) The NB protein is an integral component of the membrane of influenza B virus. *J Gen Virol* **77**, 2689–94.

Brassard, D.L., Leser, G.P. & Lamb, R.A. (1996) Influenza B virus NB glycoprotein is a component of virions. *Virology* **220**, 350–60.

Bron, R., Kendal, A.P., Klenk, H.D. & Wilschut, J. (1993) Role of the M2 protein in influenza virus membrane fusion: effects of amantadine and monensin on fusion kinetics. *Virology* **195**, 808–11.

Bui, M., Whittaker, G. & Helenius, A. (1996) Effect of M1 protein and low pH on nuclear transport of influenza virus ribonucleoproteins. *J Virol* **70**, 8391–401.

Bukrinskaya, A.G., Vorkunova, N.K., Kornilayeva, G.V., Narmanbetova, R.A. & Vorkunova, G.K. (1982) Influenza virus uncoating in infected cells and effect of rimantadine. *J Gen Virol* **60**, 49–59.

Chizhmakov, I.V., Geraghty, F.M., Ogden, D.C., Hayhurst, A., Antoniou, M. & Hay, A.J. (1996a) Selective proton permeability and pH regulation of the influenza virus M2 channel expressed in mouse erythroleukaemia cells. *J Physiol* **494**, 329–36.

Chizhmakov, I.V., Ogden, D.C., Geraghty, F.M., Betakova, T., Skinner, A. & Hay, A.J. (1996b) Characteristics of the influenza A virus M2 proton channel. In: Brown, L.E., Hampson, A. W. & Webster, R. G. (eds) *Options for the Control of Influenza III*, pp. 343–50. Elsevier Science B.V., Amsterdam.

Chizhmakov, I.V., Ogden, D.C., Geraghty, F.M. *et al.* (1998a) Differences in activation of the M2 proton channels of two influenza viruses and identification of the amino acids involved (submitted for publication).

Chizhmakov, I.V., Ogden, D.C., Betakova, T. & Hay, A.J. (1998b) The NB protein of influenza B virus elicits both a Na⁺-activated proton conductance and a H⁺-activated chloride conductance when expressed in mouse erythroleukaemia cells (submitted for publication).

Ciampor, F., Bayley, P.M., Nermut, M.V., Hirst, E.M.A., Sugrue, R.J. & Hay, A.J. (1992a) Evidence that the amantadine-induced, M2-mediated conversion of influenza A virus haemagglutinin to the low pH conformation occurs in an acidic *trans* Golgi compartment. *Virology* **188**, 14–24.

Ciampor, F., Thompson, C.A., Grambas, S. & Hay, A.J. (1992b) Regulation of pH by the M2 protein of influenza A viruses. *Virus Res* **22**, 247–58.

Davies, W.L., Grunert, R.R., Haff, R.F. *et al.* (1964) Antiviral activity of 1-adamantanamine (amantadine). *Science* **144**, 862–3.

Duff, K.C. & Ashley, R.H. (1992) The transmembrane domain of influenza A M2 protein forms amantadine-sensitive proton channels in planar lipid bilayers. *Virology* **190**, 485–9.

Duff, K.C., Gilchrist, P.J., Saxena, A.M. & Bradshaw, J.P. (1994) Neutron diffraction reveals the site of amantadine blockade in the influenza A M2 ion channel. *Virology* **202**, 287–93.

Ewart, G.D., Sutherland, T., Gage, P.W. & Cox, G.B. (1996) The Vpu protein of human immunodeficiency virus type 1 forms cation-selective ion channels. *J Virol* **70**, 7108–15.

Grambas, S. & Hay, A.J. (1992) Maturation of influenza A virus haemagglutinin—estimates of the pH encountered during transport and its regulation by the M2 protein. *Virology* **190**, 11–18.

Grambas, S., Bennett, M.S. & Hay, A.J. (1992) Influence of amantadine resistance mutations on the pH regulatory function of the M2 protein of influenza A viruses. *Virology* **191**, 541–9.

Hay, A.J. (1989) The mechanism of action of amantadine and rimantadine against influenza viruses. In: Notkins A.L. & Oldstone, M.B.A. (eds) *Concepts in Viral Pathogenesis*, Vol. III, pp. 361–7. Springer Verlag, New York.

Hay, A.J. (1992) The action of adamantanamines against influenza A viruses: inhibition of the M2 ion channel protein. *Sem Virol* **3**, 21–30.

Hay, A.J. (1996) Amantadine and rimantadine—mechanisms. In: Richman, D.D. (ed.) *Antiviral Drug Resistance*, pp. 43–58. John Wiley & Sons, Ltd, Chichester, England.

Hay, A.J., Kennedy, N.T.C., Skehel, J.J. & Appleyard, G. (1979) The matrix protein gene determines amantadine sensitivity of influenza viruses. *J Gen Virol* **42**, 189–91.

Hay, A.J., Wolstenholme, A.J., Skehel, J.J. & Smith, M.H. (1985) The molecular basis of the specific anti-influenza action of amantadine. *EMBO J.* **4**, 3021–4.

Hay, A.J., Zambon, M.C., Wolstenholme, A.J., Skehel, J.J. & Smith, M.H. (1986) Molecular basis of resistance of influenza A viruses to amantadine. *J Antimicrobiol Chemother* **18** (Suppl. B), 19–29.

Hay, A.J., Thompson, C.A., Geraghty, F.M., Hayhurst, A., Grambas, S. & Bennett, M.S. (1993) The role of the M2 protein in influenza A virus infection. In: Hannoun, C., Kendal, A.P., Klenk, H.D. & Ruben, F.L. (eds) *Options for Control of Influenza II*, pp. 281–8. Excerpta Medica, Amsterdam.

Holsinger, L.J. & Lamb, R.A. (1991) Influenza virus M2 integral membrane protein is a homotetramer stabilized by formation of disulphide bonds. *Virology* **183**, 32–43.

Hongo, S., Sugawara, K., Nishimura, H., Muraki, Y., Kitame, F. & Nakamura, K. (1994) Identification of a second protein encoded by influenza C virus RNA segment 6. *J Gen Virol* **75**, 3503–10.

Hongo, S., Sugawara, K., Muraki, Y., Kitame, F. & Nakamura, K. (1997) Characterization of a second protein (CM2) encoded by RNA segment 6 of influenza C virus. *J Virol* **71**, 2786–92.

Hughey, P.G., Roberts, P.C., Holsinger, L.J., Zebedee, S.L., Lamb, R.A. & Compans, R.W. (1995) Effects of antibody to the influenza A virus M2 protein on M2 surface expression and virus assembly. *Virology* **212**, 411–21.

Kato, N. & Eggers, H.J. (1969) Inhibition of uncoating of fowl plague virus by 1-adamantanamine hydrochloride. *Virology* **37**, 632–41.

Lamb, R.A., Lai, C.-J. & Choppin, P.W. (1981) Sequences of mRNAs derived from genome RNA segment 7 of influenza virus: colinear and interrupted mRNAs code for overlapping proteins. *Proc Natl Acad Sci USA* **78**, 4170–4.

Lubeck, M.D., Schulman, J.L. & Palese, P. (1978) Susceptibility of influenza A viruses to amantadine is influenced by the gene coding for M protein. *J Virol* **28**, 710–16.

Martin, K. & Helenius, A. (1991) Nuclear transport of influenza virus ribonucleoproteins: the viral matrix protein (M1) promotes export and inhibits import. *Cell* **67**, 117–30.

Ohuchi, M., Cramer, A., Vey, M., Ohuchi, R., Garten, W. & Klenk, H.-D. (1994) Rescue of vector-expressed fowl plague virus haemagglutinin in biologically active form by acidotropic agents and coexpressed M$_2$ protein. *J Virol* **68**, 920–6.

Pinto, L.H., Holsinger, L.J. & Lamb, R.A. (1992) Influenza virus M$_2$ protein has ion channel activity. *Cell* **69**, 517–28.

Sakaguchi, T., Tu, Q., Pinto, L.H. & Lamb, R.A. (1997) The active oligomeric state of the minimalistic influenza virus M2 ion channel is a tetramer. *Proc Natl Acad Sci USA* **94**, 5000–5.

Scholtissek, C. & Faulkner, G.P. (1979) Amantadine-resistant and -sensitive influenza A strains and recombinants. *J Gen Virol* **44**, 807–15.

Schroeder, C., Ford, C.M., Wharton, S.A. & Hay, A.J. (1994) Functional reconsitution in lipid vesicles of influenza virus M2 protein expressed by baculovirus: evidence for proton transfer activity. *J Gen Virol* **75**, 3477–84.

Shaw, M.W., Choppin, P.W. & Lamb, R.A. (1983) A previously unrecognized influenza B virus glycoprotein from a bicistronic mRNA that also encodes the viral neuraminidase. *Proc Natl Acad Sci USA* **80**, 4879–83.

Shimbo, K., Brassard, D.L., Lamb, R.A. & Pinto, L. (1995) Viral and cellular small integral membrane proteins can modify ion channels endogenous to *Xenopus* oocytes. *Biophys J* **69**, 1819–29.

Shimbo, K., Brassard, D.L., Lamb, R.A. & Pinto, L. (1996) Ion selectivity and activation of the M$_2$ ion channel of influenza virus. *Biophys J* **70**, 1335–46.

Steinhauer, D.A., Wharton, S.A., Skehel, J.J., Wiley, D.C. & Hay, A.J. (1991) Amantadine selection of a mutant influenza virus containing an acid-stable haemagglutinin glycoprotein: evidence for virus-specific regulation of the pH of glycoprotein transport vesicles. *Proc Natl Acad Sci USA* **88**, 11525–9.

Stieneke-Grober, A., Vey, M., Angliker, H. *et al.* (1992) Influenza virus haemagglutinin with multibasic cleavage site is activated by furin, a subtilisin-like endoprotease. *EMBO J* **11**, 2407–14.

Sugrue, R.J. & Hay, A.J. (1991) Structural characteristics of the M2 protein of the influenza A viruses: evidence that it forms a tetrameric channel. *Virology* **180**, 617–24.

Sugrue, R.J., Bahadur, G., Zambon, M.C., Hall, S.M., Douglas, A.R. & Hay, A.J. (1990a) Specific structural alteration of the influenza haemagglutinin by amantadine. *EMBO J* **9**, 3469–76.

Sugrue, R.J., Belshe, R.B. & Hay, A.J. (1990b) Palmitoylation of the influenza A virus M2 protein. *Virology* **179**, 51–6.

Sunstrom, N.A., Premkumar, L.S., Premkumar, A., Ewart, G., Cox, G.B. & Gage, P.W. (1996) Ion channels formed by NB, an influenza B virus protein. *J Membr Biol* **150**, 127–32.

Takeuchi, K. & Lamb, R.A. (1994) Influenza virus M2 protein ion channel activity stabilizes the native form of fowl plague virus haemagglutinin during intracellular transport. *J Virol* **68**, 911–19.

Tosteson, M.T., Pinto, L.H., Holsinger, L.J. & Lamb., R.A. (1994) Reconstitution of the influenza virus M_2 ion channel in lipid bilayers. *J Membr Biol* **142**, 117–26.

Wang, C., Takeuchi, K., Pinto, L.H. & Lamb, R.A. (1993) Ion channel activity of influenza A virus M_2 protein: characterization of the amantadine block. *J Virol* **67**, 5585–94.

Wang, C., Lamb, R.A. & Pinto, L.H. (1994) Direct measurement of the influenza A virus M_2 protein ion channel activity in mammalian cells. *Virology* **205**, 133–40.

Wang, C., Lamb, R.A. & Pinto, L.H. (1995) Activation of the M_2 ion channel of influenza virus: a role for the transmembrane domain histidine residue. *Biophys J* **69**, 1363–71.

Wharton, S.A., Belshe, R.B., Skehel, J.J. & Hay, A.J. (1994) Role of virion M2 protein in influenza virus uncoating: specific reduction in the rate of membrane fusion between virus and liposomes by amantadine. *J Gen Virol* **75**, 945–8.

Williams, M.A. & Lamb, R.A. (1986) Determination of the orientation of an integral membrane protein and sites of glycosylation by oligonucleotide-directed mutagenesis: influenza B virus NB glycoprotein lacks a cleavable signal sequence and has an extracellular NH_2-terminal region. *Mol Cell Biol* **6**, 4317–28.

Williams, M.A. & Lamb, R.A. (1988) Polylactosaminoglycan modification of a small integral membrane glycoprotein, influenza B virus NB. *Mol Cell Biol* **8**, 1186–96.

Yamashita, M., Krystal, M. & Palese, P. (1988) Evidence that the matrix protein of influenza C virus is coded for by spliced mRNA. *J Virol* **62**, 3348–55.

Zebedee, S.L. & Lamb, R.A. (1989) Growth restriction of influenza A virus by M2 protein antibody is genetically linked to the M1 protein. *Proc Natl Acad Sci USA* **86**, 1061–5.

Zhirnov, O.P. (1990) Solubilization of matrix protein M1/M from virions occurs at different pH for orthomyxo- and paramyxoviruses. *Virology* **176**, 274–9.

Zhirnov, O.P. & Grigoriev, V.B. (1994) Disassembly of influenza C viruses distinct from that of influenza A and B viruses requires neutral-alkaline pH. *Virology* **200**, 284–91.

CHAPTER 8

Unique Functions of the NS1 Protein

Robert M. Krug

Historical background

In 1971, a virus-specific protein of about 26 kDa was identified in extracts from influenza virus-infected cells (Lazarowitz *et al.* 1971). Because this protein was present in infected cells, but was not incorporated into virions, it was named non-structural protein, or NS protein. This name was subsequently changed to the NS1 protein, because of the subsequent discovery of a second virus-specific protein that also appeared to be non-structural. The NS1 protein was shown to be localized in the nucleus (Lazarowitz *et al.* 1971; Compans 1973; Krug & Etkind 1973), but little progress in elucidating its function was made for almost 20 years. Several groups of investigators isolated viruses with temperature-sensitive mutations in the NS1 gene (Wolstenholme *et al.* 1980; Koennecke *et al.* 1981; Shimizu *et al.* 1982; Hatada *et al.* 1990). However, the phenotypes at the non-permissive temperature were difficult to interpret. With most, though not all, of these mutant viruses, the synthesis of virus-specific proteins at later times of infection at the non-permissive temperature was greatly reduced relative to that at the permissive temperature, even though virus-specific RNA synthesis, including viral mRNA synthesis, was not significantly reduced. It was not clear how a defect in the NS1 protein, or in fact in any virus-specific protein, could cause such a phenotype. Other evidence indicated that the NS1 protein is not involved in virion RNA synthesis. Thus, an *in vitro* system that synthesizes virion RNA was not affected by the removal of endogenous NS1 protein (Shapiro & Krug 1988); and the replication of a recombinant influenza virus genome segment did not require the NS1 protein (Huang *et al.* 1990). Consequently, the actual function of the NS1 protein remained unknown.

Functions of the NS1 protein

Inhibition of nuclear export of poly(A)-containing mRNA

Finally, research in the early 1990s demonstrated that the NS1 protein is an unique post-transcriptional regulator that has several activities. The first surprising finding was obtained in transient transfection experiments: the NS1 protein inhibits the nuclear export of poly(A)-containing spliced mRNAs (Alonso-Caplen *et al.* 1992; Qiu & Krug 1994; Fortes *et al.* 1994; Qian *et al.* 1994). This inhibition by the NS1 protein occurred even when the cells were transfected with a DNA directly encoding the spliced form of the target mRNA, indicating that the NS1 protein acted directly on mRNA export and that the inhibition of mRNA export was independent of the splicing process (Alonso-Caplen *et al.* 1992; Qiu & Krug 1994; Qian *et al.* 1994). The inhibition of nuclear export of poly(A)-containing mRNAs is apparently mediated, at least in part, by the specific binding of the NS1 protein to poly(A) (Qiu & Krug 1994). This *in vitro* specificity is exhibited *in vivo*: the NS1 protein inhibits the nuclear export of mRNAs only when they contain a poly(A) tail produced by the cellular cleavage/polyadenylation system (Qiu & Krug 1994). In contrast, the NS1 protein does not inhibit the nuclear export of histone mRNA whose 3' end is generated by cleavage without the subsequent addition of poly(A).

Functional domains of the NS1 protein

As a consequence of the discovery of one function of the NS1 protein, it became possible to map the functional domains of the protein (Qian *et al.* 1994). A series of mutations were introduced that were approximately evenly spaced throughout the 237 amino acid protein. The mutated NS1 proteins were assayed for their ability to inhibit the nuclear export of poly(A)-containing mRNA and to bind to poly(A) *in vitro*. This analysis identified two functional domains that are required for the inhibition of nuclear export of mRNA *in vivo* (Fig. 8.1). A sequence near the amino end (amino acids 19–38) comprises the RNA binding domain, and is also required for dimerization of the protein. The NS1 protein exists as a dimer *in vivo* and *in vitro*, and it is almost certainly the dimer that binds to the RNA target (Nemeroff *et al.* 1995). The second functional domain, which is located in the carboxyl half of the molecule (amino acids 134–161), is not required for RNA binding, but is nonetheless required for function *in vivo* (Qian *et al.* 1994). This domain is presumed to be an effector domain that interacts with host nuclear proteins to inhibit nuclear RNA export.

Inhibition of pre-mRNA splicing

Subsequently, transient transfection experiments established that the NS1 protein also inhibits pre-mRNA splicing *in vivo* (Fortes *et al.* 1994; Lu *et al.* 1994), a function that also requires both the RNA binding and effector domains (Lu *et al.* 1994). In addition, the NS1 protein inhibits *in vitro* splicing catalysed by nuclear extracts from uninfected cells, indicating that it acts directly on the splicing machinery (Lu *et al.* 1994; Qiu *et al.* 1995). The mode

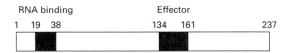

Fig. 8.1 The functional domains of the NS1 protein of influenza A virus as determined by mutational analysis. The domain required for dimerization of the NS1 protein is coincident with the RNA binding domain. (From Qian *et al.* 1994, with permission from American Society of Microbiology.)

by which the NS1 protein inhibits pre-mRNA splicing is novel. This inhibition is mediated by the specific binding of the NS1 protein to one of the five human spliceosomal small nuclear RNAs (snRNAs), U6 snRNA (Qiu *et al.* 1995). This snRNA plays a central role in the interactions that the five spliceosomal snRNAs undergo with each other and with the pre-mRNA during splicing (reviewed in Nilsen 1994; Sharp 1994). Initially U6 snRNA is in the form of a hydrogen-bonded complex with U4 snRNA. Subsequently, after dissociation from U4 snRNA, U6 snRNA interacts with the 5′ splice site of the pre-mRNA and also with three different sequences in U2 snRNA. It has been postulated that this U6-U2 snRNA complex plays a direct catalytic role in splicing (Madhani & Guthrie 1992). The ability of U6 snRNA to undergo these interactions is blocked by the NS1 protein, which binds to a specific stem-bulge in this snRNA (Qiu *et al.* 1995; Fig. 8.2). This U6 binding site includes two sequences that play critical roles in splicing: the U6 nucleotides that form one of the helices (helix II) with U2 snRNA; and the invariant U6 sequence (ACAGAG) that plays a critical role in 5′ splice site selection (reviewed in Nilsen 1994). In the presence of the NS1 protein (except at high concentrations), pre-mRNAs form spliceosomes, but subsequent catalytic steps in splicing are inhibited (Qiu *et al.* 1995). Mutational analysis of the NS1 protein, as well as RNA competition experiments, indicates that U6 snRNA and poly(A) most likely share the same, or similar, binding sites on the protein (Qiu & Krug 1994; Lu *et al.* 1995; Qiu *et al.* 1995).

One experiment has related the splicing results obtained in this *in vitro* system to events in infected cells (Lu *et al.* 1995). Unfortunately, it has not been possible to make a meaningful analysis of the splicing of host pre-mRNAs in influenza virus-infected cells themselves, because all host polymerase II transcripts are degraded in the nucleus of infected cells, this being due at least in part to the cleavage of their 5′ ends by the viral cap-dependent endonuclease (Katze & Krug 1984; Krug *et al.* 1989). As an alternative approach, it was demonstrated that the NS1 protein synthesized during infection is specifically associated with U6 snRNA molecules (Lu *et al.* 1995). This specific NS1 protein–U6

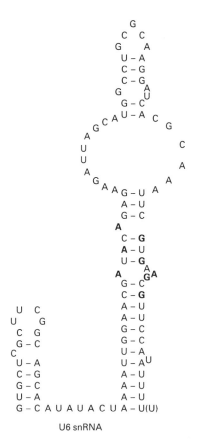

Fig. 8.2 Binding site of the NS1 protein on U6 snRNA, as determined by chemical modification/interference experiments. The U6 snRNA structure shown is that originally proposed by Rinke *et al.* (1985). The bases at which chemical modification causes interference to the binding of the NS1 protein are shown in bold. (From Qiu *et al.* 1995, with permission from Cambridge University Press.)

snRNA interaction suggests that the NS1 protein inhibits splicing in infected cells.

Subsequently, the NS1 protein was shown to bind to a second snRNA, a minor species called U6atac snRNA (Wang & Krug 1997). This snRNA, which is the counterpart of U6 snRNA, is involved in the splicing of a small number of pre-mRNAs that possess AU (or AT at the genomic level) and AC at the 5' and 3' ends of their introns, respectively (Jackson 1991; Hall & Padgett 1994, 1996; Nilsen 1996; Tarn & Steitz 1996a,b). Other than U5 snRNA, a different set of snRNAs participate in the splicing of AT-AC introns: U11, U12, U4atac and U6atac

instead of U1, U2, U4 and U6. The sequence conservation between U6atac snRNA and human U6 snRNA is less than that between human and yeast U6 snRNAs (Brow & Guthrie 1988; Tarn & Steitz 1996a). It was therefore surprising that the NS1 protein binds to only U6atac snRNA among the four snRNAs that are specific for AT-AC splicing (Wang & Krug 1997). The binding site is a specific stem-bulge near the 3' end of U6atac snRNA, the sequence of which differs significantly from the sequence of the stem-bulge to which the NS1 protein binds in U6 snRNA (Qiu *et al.* 1995; Wang & Krug 1997). As a result of the binding of the NS1 protein to this U6atac stem-bulge, AT-AC splicing is inhibited (Wang & Krug 1997). Although the U6atac and U6 snRNAs most likely bind to similar sites on the NS1 protein, U6atac snRNA binds with 5–10-fold lower affinity than human U6 snRNA. It is remarkable that the NS1 protein specifically targets the two snRNAs which serve analogous functions in the two different types of mammalian spliceosomes, particularly considering the sequence diversity of these two snRNAs.

Sequestering double-stranded RNA away from the PKR kinase

Another post-transcriptional function of the NS1 protein is mediated by its binding to a third RNA target, double-stranded RNA (dsRNA). *In vitro* experiments established that the NS1 protein binds dsRNA (Hatada & Fukuda 1992; Lu *et al.* 1995). As a consequence, the activation of the dsRNA-activated protein kinase (PKR) is blocked, so that the phosphorylation of the α subunit of the eukaryotic translation initiation factor 2 (eIF2) and the consequent inhibition of translation do not occur (Lu *et al.* 1995). It can be presumed that the NS1 protein carries out the same function in influenza virus-infected cells, particularly as studies indicate that PKR is initially activated during infection (Katze 1992). Such activation can be attributed to the production of virus-specific RNA molecules containing double-stranded regions. The potential for the formation of such 'dsRNA' molecules stems from the presence of both positive-sense and negative-sense RNAs that are synthesized in the nucleus during infection (Krug *et al.* 1989). At subsequent times of infection PKR is suppressed by processes requiring viral gene expression, thereby maintaining high levels of protein synthesis (Katze 1992). One of these virus-specific gene products could be the NS1 protein, which is predominantly in the nucleus (Lazarowitz *et al.* 1971; Compans 1973; Krug & Etkind 1973). The NS1 protein would sequester viral 'dsRNA' molecules in the nucleus, thereby blocking the activation of PKR in the cytoplasm. In addition, influenza virus mounts a second attack against PKR: activating a 58 kDa cellular protein that inhibits the phosphorylation of eIF2α by PKR, including already-activated PKR (Lee *et al.* 1990, 1992). Another virus, vaccinia virus, also utilizes a two-pronged attack against PKR (Akkaraju *et al.* 1989; Beattie *et al.* 1991; Watson *et al.* 1991; Beattie *et al.* 1995).

Does the NS1 protein have other effects on translation? A small fraction of the NS1 protein in infected cells appears to be associated with polyribosomes (Compans 1973; Krug & Etkind 1973), and it is conceivable that this NS1 protein population could be binding to one or more polyribosome-associated RNAs. In addition, it has been reported that the NS1 protein stimulated the translation of either a few specific viral mRNAs (Enami *et al.* 1994) or many viral mRNAs (Luna *et al.* 1995), and that this stimulation apparently required, at least in part, sequences in the 5' untranslated regions of the viral mRNAs. However, it can be argued that these effects on translation could result from the activity of the NS1 protein in blocking activation of PKR. Both of the studies cited above employed transfection experiments, which have been shown to result in the activation of PKR that is directed against only the plasmid-derived mRNAs (Kaufman & Murtha 1987). The NS1 protein would be expected to block this activation, thereby increasing the rate of initiation of the translation of the plasmid-derived mRNAs. In fact, one of the studies cited above (Luna *et al.* 1995) showed that the the major effect of the NS1 protein was to increase the rate of translation initiation of the plasmid-derived mRNAs in the transfected cells. In addition, evidence indicates that a partial, rather than a complete, blockage of the activation of PKR by the NS1 protein would favour the translation of viral over cellular mRNAs, because influenza viral mRNAs are better initiators of translation (Katze *et al.* 1984, 1986). In addition, it has been reported that an oligoribonucleotide corresponding to the 5' untranslated region binds to a small extent to the NS1 protein (Park & Katze 1995). However, the significance of this binding is unclear. Unlike all other RNAs that bind specifically to the NS1 protein (Lu *et al.* 1995), the binding of this oligoribonucleotide is not blocked by dsRNA (Park & Katze 1995). Further, viral mRNAs that contain this 5' untranslated region do not bind to the NS1 protein (Qiu & Krug 1994), indicating that covalent attachment of the 5' untranslated region to the body of the viral mRNA eliminates all detectable binding. Further experiments are needed to clarify the precise role that the NS1 protein, a predominantly nuclear protein (Lazarowitz *et al.* 1971; Compans 1973; Krug & Etkind 1973), plays in translation that occurs in the cytoplasm of infected cells.

The structure of the RNA binding domain

The NS1 protein binds with similar dissociation constants to three RNAs: poly(A), a specific stem-bulge in U6 snRNA, and dsRNA (Qiu & Krug 1994; Lu *et al.* 1995; Qiu *et al.* 1995). In addition, it binds with a higher dissociation constant (lower affinity) to a specific stem-bulge in the minor snRNA, U6atac snRNA (Wang & Krug 1997). Both mutational analysis of the protein and RNA competition experiments suggest that all these RNAs share the same (or similar) binding sites on the protein (Qiu & Krug 1994; Lu *et al.* 1995; Qiu *et al.* 1995; Wang & Krug 1997). As noted above, the NS1 protein functions as a dimer when it binds to these RNAs (Nemeroff *et al.* 1995). Clearly, structural studies of NS1–RNA complexes are needed to obtain a definitive picture of how the NS1 protein dimer binds to its several RNA targets. Such studies were facilitated by the demonstration that a fragment of the NS1 protein containing the first 73 N-terminal amino acids (NS1(1–73)) possesses all the RNA binding and dimerization activities of the full-length protein (Qian *et al.* 1995).

As the first step in such an analysis, both nuclear

magnetic resonance and X-ray crystallography have shown that the dimeric NS1 RNA binding domain (NS1(1–73)) in the absence of RNA adopts a novel six-helical chain fold (Chien *et al.* 1997; Liu *et al.* 1997; Plate 8.1, facing p. 288). No proteins in the protein database exhibit significant structural homology with the NS1 dimer. However, portions of a few proteins exhibit significant structural homology with the NS1 monomer: the monomer of the Rop protein of the ColE1 plasmid of *E. coli*, a dsRNA-binding protein (Banner *et al.* 1987; Eberle *et al.* 1991; Predki *et al.* 1995); and homeodomains from transcription factors, some of which bind RNA as well as DNA (Kissinger *et al.* 1990; Dubnau & Struhl 1996; Rivera-Pomar *et al.* 1996). The majority of RNA-binding proteins bind to RNA via β-sheets (Nagai *et al.* 1990; Hoffman *et al.* 1991; Wittekind *et al.* 1992; Schindelin *et al.* 1993, 1994; Schnuchel *et al.* 1993; Newkirk *et al.* 1994; Oubridge *et al.* 1994; Bycroft *et al.* 1995; Castiglione Morelli *et al.* 1995; Kharrat *et al.* 1995). In contrast, the NS1 protein undoubtedly belongs to the much smaller group of proteins that bind to their specific RNA targets via one or more α-helices. This NS1 structure suggests several potential binding sites for RNA, which await experimental verification.

Mechanism of action of the effector domain

In contrast to the RNA binding domain, very little is known about how the effector domain of the NS1 protein functions. The initial identification of the effector domain was based on the loss of *in vivo* function (in nuclear export assays) in the NS1 protein caused by point mutations in the region extending from amino acids 134 to 161 (Qian *et al.* 1994; Fig. 8.1). Subsequently, a gain of function assay was designed using chimeric molecules in which portions of the carboxyl end of the NS1 protein were covalently linked to the Rev protein of human immunodeficiency virus-1 (HIV-1). The Rev protein facilitates the nuclear export of unspliced and partially spliced HIV-1 pre-mRNAs that encode virus structural proteins (Emerman *et al.* 1989; Felber *et al.* 1989; Hammarskjold *et al.* 1989; Malim *et al.* 1989a; Cullen 1995). In the absence of

the Rev protein, HIV-1 pre-mRNAs containing splice sites are retained in the nucleus because they are bound to spliceosomes where they undergo splicing. Like the NS1 protein, the Rev protein has essentially two functional domains as defined by mutational analysis: an RNA binding domain near the N-terminus that specifically interacts with a RNA target in the viral pre-mRNA (called the Rev response element, or RRE); and an effector domain, which is in the carboxyl half of the molecule, that is required for the *in vivo* activity of nuclear mRNA export (Daly *et al.* 1989; Malim *et al.* 1989a,b; Zapp & Green 1989; Venkatesh & Chinnadurai 1990; Malim *et al.* 1991; Cullen 1995). Rev protein molecules shuttle between the nucleus and cytoplasm; this suggests that they transport nuclear RRE-containing RNA molecules to the cytoplasm and then return to the nucleus to pick up more of the same RNA molecules for transport (Kalland *et al.* 1994; Meyer & Malim 1994; Richard *et al.* 1994; Stauber *et al.* 1995).

Because the Rev protein functions as an oligomer (Olsen *et al.* 1990; Malim & Cullen 1991; Cole *et al.* 1993), it was postulated that the NS1 effector domain in a NS1–Rev chimera would be able to inhibit nuclear RNA export mediated by Rev protein molecules that are not covalently linked to the NS1A protein sequence (Qian *et al.* 1996; Chen *et al.* 1997). The wild-type Rev sequence in the NS1–Rev chimera would oligomerize with other wild-type Rev molecules in *trans*, and the resulting mixed oligomers would be retained in the nucleus. This would occur only if the nuclear retention activity of the NS1 effector domain in these mixed oligomers is dominant over the nuclear transport activity of the Rev effector domain.

This experimental approach established that the sequence of the NS1 protein extending from amino acids 79 to 231 constitutes the independent effector domain of this protein (Chen *et al.* 1997). Thus, this NS1 amino acid sequence functions with the heterologous Rev RNA binding domain, to cause RRE-containing RNA to be retained in the nucleus, even in the presence of the Rev effector domain that by itself facilitates the nuclear export of RRE-containing RNA. Indeed, the complexes that are formed in the nucleus between the Rev protein molecules and the NS1–Rev chimera containing this NS1 sequence are retained in the nucleus and do not shuttle (Chen *et al.* 1997). Consequently, the NS1A effector domain is indeed dominant over the Rev effector domain in controlling the nuclear export of this RNA. A shorter NS1A sequence lacks effector domain function, as removal of 16 amino acids from either end of this NS1A sequence eliminates nuclear retention activity in the NS1–Rev chimera. Though the entirety of this NS1A sequence is required for independent effector domain function (Chen *et al.* 1997), the only point mutations that inactivate effector domain function are localized in one portion of this sequence, extending from amino acids 134 to 161, as is the case for the nuclear export function of the full-length NS1 protein itself (Qian *et al.* 1994; Chen *et al.* 1997). Perhaps the amino acids from 134 to 161 constitute the region that primarily interacts with the host proteins involved in nuclear RNA export, whereas the other amino acids in the independent effector domain are needed primarily to maintain the proper fold of the polypeptide. The host nuclear proteins that functionally interact with the effector domain of the NS1 protein have not yet been identified.

The NS1 protein of influenza B viruses lacks a similar effector domain

The NS1 protein of influenza B viruses (NS1B protein) shares only some of the properties of the NS1 protein of influenza A viruses (NS1A protein). One of the two functional domains of the NS1A protein, the RNA binding domain, is preserved in the NS1B protein, even though there is little or no sequence homology between the two proteins (Briedis & Lamb 1982). The NS1B protein specifically binds to the same RNA targets as the NS1A protein (Qiu & Krug 1994; Lu *et al.* 1995; Qiu *et al.* 1995; Wang & Krug 1996). For both the NS1A and NS1B proteins, the binding to U6 snRNA causes an inhibition of pre-mRNA splicing *in vitro*, and the binding to dsRNA blocks the activation of the PKR kinase *in vitro* (Lu *et al.* 1994, 1995; Wang & Krug 1996). As is the case with the NS1A protein (Qian *et al.* 1995), a polypeptide containing an N-terminal sequence of the NS1B protein possesses all the RNA

binding activity of the full-length protein and exists in the form of a dimer (Wang & Krug 1996). Initial structural studies indicate that this N-terminal polypeptide, comprising the RNA binding domain of the NS1B protein, probably has a structure similar to that of the RNA binding domain of the influenza B protein described above (unpublished experiments). Thus, although the RNA binding domains of the NS1A and NS1B proteins have little or no sequence homology (Briedis & Lamb 1982), they most likely share a structural homology. The attainment of this structural homology requires amino acid sequences of different lengths: the minimum length of the N-terminal NS1A polypeptide that possesses RNA binding activity is 73 amino acids, whereas the corresponding NS1B polypeptide is 93 amino acids. The conservation of the RNA binding domain of the NS1 protein among influenza A and B viruses strongly suggests that this domain is required for the replication of all influenza A and B viruses.

In contrast, the NS1B protein lacks an effector domain that functions in the inhibition of pre-mRNA splicing and the nuclear export of poly(A)-containing mRNA. Thus, in cells transfected with a plasmid encoding the NS1B gene neither pre-mRNA splicing nor the nuclear export of mRNA was inhibited (Wang & Krug 1996). It can be concluded that this type of effector domain is not required for the replication of influenza B viruses. In fact, this type of effector domain is absent from the NS1 protein of a naturally occurring influenza virus A strain that contains a deletion of over 100 amino acids from its carboxyl end (Norton *et al.* 1987). This shortened NS1A protein has the RNA binding activity of the full-length NS1A protein, but fails to inhibit pre-mRNA splicing and the nuclear export of poly(A)-containing mRNA *in vivo* (Wang & Krug 1996). Nonetheless, a functional effector domain is apparently preserved in the overwhelming majority of naturally occurring NS1A proteins, which are full length (Wang & Krug 1996). Why has this effector domain been preserved in the NS1A proteins of all these influenza A viruses, in light of the ability of at least one influenza A virus to exist in nature without this NS1 protein domain? These results lead to another unanswered question:

what is the function of the large carboxyl region of NS1B proteins, particularly in light of the existence of a laboratory B virus variant with a truncated NS1 protein lacking the carboxyl region (Norton *et al.* 1987)?

Conclusions

Three functions of the NS1 protein of influenza A viruses (NS1A protein) have been identified:
1 the inhibition of the nuclear export of poly(A)-containing mRNA (Alonso-Caplen *et al.* 1992; Fortes *et al.* 1994; Qian *et al.* 1994; Qiu & Krug 1994);
2 the inhibition of pre-mRNA splicing (Fortes *et al.* 1994; Lu *et al.* 1994; Qiu *et al.* 1995; Wang & Krug 1997); and
3 the inhibition of the activation of PKR by the sequestering of dsRNA (Lu *et al.* 1995).

Of these three, the role of the latter function in influenza virus-infected cells is the most evident. As already discussed, during infection 'dsRNA' molecules are produced that activate PKR (Katze 1992). As one of the two ways that this activation would be prevented, the NS1 protein would bind to dsRNA and sequester it away from PKR (Lu *et al.* 1995). Efficient blocking of PKR kinase activation assumes even more importance during influenza-virus infection of its vertebrate host, where virus infection induces the synthesis of interferon that in turn induces the synthesis of increased amounts of PKR kinase (reviewed in Katze 1992; Rhoads 1993; Samuel 1993). Therefore, binding of dsRNA may be the function of the NS1 protein that is absolutely required for the replication of all influenza A and B viruses. Perhaps this *in vivo* function of the NS1 protein does not require its effector domain.

Why would the nuclear export function of the NS1A protein be advantageous to influenza A virus? One advantage can be postulated: because of the inhibition of the nuclear export of poly(A)-containing mRNA, cellular pre-mRNAs and mRNAs would be trapped in the nucleus. Consequently, all of these cellular capped RNAs would be accessible to the viral cap-dependent endonuclease for the production of the capped RNA primers that are needed for viral mRNA synthesis (Krug *et al.* 1989). Because all the sequestered cel-

lular RNAs would lose their 5′ caps, they would be susceptible to degradation. In fact, cellular pre-mRNAs and mRNAs are completely degraded in the nuclei at early times after influenza A virus infection (Katze & Krug 1984). These nuclear events would not be expected to occur in cells infected by influenza B viruses whose NS1 proteins lack effector domains like those in A-type viruses, so that the pattern of cellular and viral gene expression in cells infected by influenza B viruses would probably be different.

Subsequent actions of the NS1 protein in influenza virus-infected cells depend on whether the NS1A protein also blocks the nuclear export of viral mRNAs in these cells. Transient transfection experiments in uninfected cells have established that the NS1A protein inhibits the nuclear export of all mRNAs that contain poly(A) tails produced by the cellular cleavage and polyadenylation enzymes (Qiu & Krug 1994). However, the poly(A) tails of viral mRNAs synthesized in infected cells are produced by a different mechanism: reiterative copying by the viral transcriptase of a short stretch of U residues in the virion RNA template (Robertson *et al.* 1981; Krug *et al.* 1989). If the NS1 protein does not block the nuclear export of viral mRNAs that are produced by this mechanism, then the NS1 protein would selectively block the nuclear export of cellular, and not viral, mRNAs, so that the NS1 protein could function unaltered throughout infection.

Alternatively, if the NS1 protein also blocked the nuclear export of viral mRNAs, then at a subsequent time of infection the NS1 protein would have to lose its ability to block the nuclear export of poly(A)-containing mRNAs to allow the nuclear export of viral mRNAs. At present it is not known how the NS1 protein might lose this function, but several explanations have been proposed; e.g. changes in the phosphorylation of the NS1 protein that might inactivate the nuclear retention function of the NS1 protein (Vogle *et al.* 1993; Qiu & Krug 1994).

The role that the NS1A protein-mediated inhibition of pre-mRNA splicing plays in infected cells has not yet been established. The demonstration of a specific NS1A protein–U6 snRNA interaction in infected cells suggests that inhibition of pre-mRNA splicing by the NS1 protein does in fact occur in infected cells (Lu *et al.* 1995). Because the NS1A protein targets a specific snRNA in both the major (GU-AG introns) and minor (AT-AC introns) spliceosomes (Qiu *et al.* 1995; Wang & Krug 1997), all known pre-mRNA splicing systems would be inhibited. Indeed, influenza A virus has certainly devised an effective strategy for shutting down pre-mRNA splicing, but it is currently not clear how this would benefit virus gene expression. In addition, some mechanism has to operate to inactivate this function of the NS1A protein to allow the splicing of the viral M1 and NS1 mRNAs to occur at the appropriate times of infection (Krug *et al.* 1989; Shih *et al.* 1995). One of the major challenges will be to elucidate how the inhibition of pre-mRNA splicing by the NS1A protein serves an important role in influenza virus gene expression.

Acknowledgements

The research carried out in the author's laboratory was supported by a US National Institutes of Health grant (AI 11772—merit award) to the author, who thanks all the investigators who worked in his laboratory and were responsible for obtaining many of the results that are discussed in this chapter. The author also thanks his collaborators: Michael Katze, Arnold Rabson, Gaetano Montelione and Helen Berman.

References

Akkaraju, G.R., Whitaker-Dowling, P., Younger, J.S. & Jagus, R. (1989) Vaccinia specific kinase inhibitory factor prevents translation inhibition by double-stranded RNA in rabbit reticulocyte lysate. *J Biol Chem* **264**, 10321–5.

Alonso-Caplen, F.V., Nemeroff, M.E., Qiu, Y. & Krug, R.M. (1992) Nucleocytoplasmic transport: the influenza virus NS1 protein regulates the transport of spliced NS2 mRNA and its precursor NS1 mRNA. *Genes Dev* **6**, 255–67.

Banner, D.W., Kokkinidis, M. & Tsernoglou, D. (1987) Structure of the ColEI rop protein at 1.7 Å resolution. *J Mol Biol* **196**, 657–75.

Beattie, E., Tartaglia, J. & Paoletti, E. (1991) Vaccinia virus-encoded eIF2α homologue abrogates the antiviral effects of interferon. *Virology* **183**, 419–22.

Beattie, E., Denzler, K.L., Tartaglia, J., Perkus, M.E., Paoletti, E. & Jacobs, B.L. (1995) Reversal of the interferon-sensitive phenotype of a vaccinia virus lacking E3L by expression of the reovirus S4 gene. *J Virol* **69**, 499–505.

Briedis, D. & Lamb, R.A. (1982) Influenza B virus genome: sequences and structural organization of RNA segment 8 and the mRNAs coding for the NS1 and NS2 proteins. *J Virol* **42**, 186–93.

Brow, D.A. & Guthrie, C. (1988) Spliceosomal RNA U6 is remarkably conserved from yeast to mammals. *Nature* **334**, 213–8.

Bycroft, M., Grünert, S., Murzin, A.G., Proctor, M. & St. Johnston, D. (1995) NMR solution structure of a dsRNA binding domain from *Drosophila* staufen protein reveals homology to the N-terminal domain of ribosomal protein S5. *EMBO J* **14**, 3563–71.

Castiglione Morelli, M.A., Steir, G., Gibson, T. *et al.* (1995) The KH module has an αβ fold. *FEBS Lett* **258**, 193–8.

Chen, Z., Li, Y. & Krug, R.M. (1998) Novel features of the nuclear export of HIV-1 Rev protein-RNA complexes revealed by the inhibitory activities of chimeras containing Rev and influenza virus NS1 protein sequences. *Virology* (in press).

Chien, C.-Y., Tejero, R., Huang, Y. *et al.* (1997) A novel RNA-binding motif in influenza A virus non-structural protein 1. *Nat Struct Biol* **4**, 891–5.

Cole, J.L., Gehman, J.D., Shafer, J.A. & Kuo, L.C. (1993) Solution oligomerization of the Rev protein of HIV-1: implications for function. *Biochem* **32**, 11769–75.

Compans, R.W. (1973) Influenza virus proteins. II. Association with components of the cytoplasm. *Virology* **51**, 56–70.

Cullen, B.R. (1995) Regulation of HIV gene expression. *AIDS* **9** (Suppl. A), S19–S32.

Daly, T.J., Cook, K.S., Gray, G.S., Malone, T.E. & Rusche, J.R. (1989) Specific binding of the HIV-1 recombinant Rev protein to the Rev-responsive element *in vitro*. *Nature* **342**, 816–9.

Dubnau, J. & Struhl, G. (1996) RNA recognition and translational regulation by a homeodomain protein. *Nature* **379**, 694–9.

Eberle, W., Pastore, A., Sander, C. & Rosch, P. (1991) The structure of ColE1 rop in solution. *J Biomol NMR* **1**, 71–82.

Emerman, M., Vazeux, R. & Peden, K. (1989) The rev gene product of the human immunodeficiency virus affects envelope-specific RNA localization. *Cell* **57**, 1155–65.

Enami, K., Sato, T.A., Nakada, S. & Enami, M. (1994) Influenza virus NS1 protein stimulates the translation of the M1 protein. *J Virol* **68**, 1432–7.

Felber, B.K., Hadzopoulou-Cladaras, M., Cladaras, C., Copeland, T. & Pavlakis, G.N. (1989) Rev protein of human immunodeficiency virus type 1 affects the stability and transport of viral mRNA. *Proc Natl Acad Sci USA* **86**, 1495–9.

Fortes, P., Beloso, A. & Ortin, J. (1994) Influenza virus NS1 protein inhibits premRNA splicing and blocks mRNA nucleocytoplasmic transport. *EMBO J* **13**, 704–12.

Hall, S.L. & Padgett, R.A. (1994) Conserved sequences in a class of rare eukaryotic nuclear introns with non-consensus splice sites. *J Mol Biol* **239**, 357–65.

Hall, S.L. & Padgett, R.A. (1996) Requirement of U12 snRNA for *in vivo* splicing of a minor class of eukaryotic nuclear premRNA introns. *Science* **271**, 1716–8.

Hammarskjold, M.L., Heimer, J., Hammarskjold, B., Sangwan, I., Albert, L. & Rekosh, D. (1989) Regulation of human immunodeficiency virus *env* expression by the rev gene product. *J Virol* **63**, 1959–66.

Hatada, E. & Futada, R. (1992) Binding of influenza A virus NS1 protein to dsRNA *in vitro*. *J Gen Virol* **73**, 3325–9.

Hatada, E., Hasegawa, M., Shimizu, K., Hatanaka, M. & Fukuda, R. (1990) Analysis of influenza A virus temperature-sensitive mutants with mutations in RNA segment 8. *J Gen Virol* **71**, 1283–92.

Hoffman, D.W., Querry, C.C., Golden, B.L., White, S.W. & Keene, J.D. (1991) RNA-binding domain of the A protein component of the U1 small nuclear ribonucleoprotein analysed by NMR spectroscopy is structurally similar to ribosomal proteins. *Proc Natl Acad Sci USA* **88**, 2495–9.

Huang, T.-S., Palese, P. & Krystal, M. (1990) Determination of influenza virus proteins required for genome replication. *J Virol* **64**, 5669–73.

Jackson, I.J. (1991) A reappraisal of nonconsensus mRNA splice sites. *Nucl Acids Res* **19**, 3795–8.

Kalland, K.-H., Szilvay, A.M., Brokstad, K.A., Saetrevik, W. & Haukenes, G. (1994) The human immunodeficiency virus type 1 Rev protein shuttles between the cytoplasm and nuclear compartments. *Mol Cell Biol* **14**, 7436–44.

Kaufman, R.J. & Murtha, P. (1987) Translational control mediated by eukaryotic initiation factor-2 is restricted to specific mRNAs in transfected cells. *Mol Cell Biol* **7**, 1568–71.

Katze, M.G. (1992) The war against the interferon-induced dsRNA activated protein kinase: can virus win? *J Interferon Res* **12**, 241–8.

Katze, M.G. & Krug, R.M. (1984) Metabolism and expression of RNA polymerase II transcripts in influenza virus infected cells. *Mol Cell Biol* **4**, 2198–2206.

Katze, M.G., Chen, Y.-T. & Krug, R.M. (1984) Nuclear-cytoplasmic transport and VAI RNA-independent translation of influenza viral messenger RNAs in late adenovirus-infected cells. *Cell* **37**, 483–90.

Katze, M.G., Detjen, B.M., Safer, B. & Krug, R.M. (1986) Translation control by influenza virus: suppression of the kinase that phosphorylates the alpha subunit of initiation factor eIF-2 and selective translation of influenza viral mRNA. *Mol Cell Biol* **6**, 1741–50.

Kharrat, A., Macias, M.J., Gibson, T.J., Nilges, M. &

Pastore, A. (1995) Structure of the dsRNA binding domain of *E. coli* RNase III. *EMBO J* **14**, 3572–84.

Kissinger, C.R., Liu, B.S., Martin-Blanco, E., Kornberg, T.B. & Pabo, C.O. (1990) Crystal structure of an engrailed homeodomain-DNA complex at 2.8 Å resolution: a framework for understanding homeodomain-DNA interactions. *Cell* **63**, 579–90.

Koennecke, I., Boschek, C.B. & Scholtissek, C. (1981) Isolation and properties of a temperature-sensitive mutant (ts412) of the influenza A virus recombinant with a ts lesion in the gene coding for the nonstructural protein. *Virology* **110**, 16–25.

Krug, R.M. & Etkind, P.E. (1973) Cytoplasmic and nuclear virus-specific proteins in influenza virus-infected MDCK cells. *Virology* **56**, 334–48.

Krug, R.M., Alonso-Caplen, F.V., Julkunen, I. & Katze, M.G. (1989) Expression and replication of the influenza virus genome. In: Krug, R.M. (ed.) *The Influenza Viruses*, pp. 89–152. Plenum Press, New York.

Lazarowitz, S.G., Compans, R.W. & Choppin, P.W. (1971) Influenza virus structural and nonstructural proteins in infected cells and their plasma membranes. *Virology* **46**, 830–43.

Lee, T.G., Tomia, J., Hovanessian, A.G. & Katze, M.G. (1990) Purification and partial characterization of a cellular inhibitor of the interferon-induced 68 000 Mr protein kinase from influenza virus-infected cells. *Proc Natl Acad Sci USA* **87**, 6208–12.

Lee, T.G., Tomia, J., Hovanessian, A.G. & Katze, M.G. (1992) Characterization and regulation of the 58 000-dalton cellular inhibitor of the interferon-induced, dsRNA activated protein kinase. *J Biol Chem* **267**, 14238–43.

Liu, J., Lynch, P.A., Chien, C.-Y., Montelione, G.T., Krug, R.M. & Berman, H.M. (1997) Crystal structure of the unique multifunctional RNA-binding domain of the influenza virus NS1 protein. *Nat Struct Biol* **4**, 896–9.

Lu, Y., Qian, X. & Krug, R.M. (1994) The influenza virus NS1 protein: a novel inhibitor of premRNA splicing. *Genes Dev* **8**, 1817–28.

Lu, Y., Wambach, M., Katze, M.G. & Krug, R.M. (1995) Binding of the influenza virus NS1 protein to double-stranded RNA inhibits the activation of the protein kinase that phosphorylates the eIF-2 translation initiation factor. *Virology* **214**, 222–8.

Luna, S., Fortes, P., Beloso, A. & Ortin, J. (1995) Influenza virus NS1 protein enhances the rate of translation initiation of viral mRNAs. *J Virol* **69**, 2427–33.

Madhani, H.D. & Guthrie, C. (1992) A novel base-pairing interaction between U2 and U6 snRNAs suggests a mechanism for the catalytic activation of the spliceosome. *Cell* **71**, 803–17.

Malim, M.H. & Cullen, B.R. (1991) HIV-1 structural gene expression requires the binding of multiple Rev monomers to the viral RRE: implications for HIV-1 latency. *Cell* **65**, 241–8.

Malim, M.H., Hauber, J., Lee, S.-Y., Maizel, J.V. & Cullen, B.R. (1989a) The HIV-1 rev trans-activator acts through a structured target sequence to activate nuclear export of unspliced viral mRNA. *Nature* **338**, 254–7.

Malim, M.H., Bohnlein, S., Hauber, J. & Cullen, B.R. (1989b) Functional dissection of the HIV-1 Rev trans-activator-derivation of a trans-dominant repressor of Rev function. *Cell* **58**, 205–14.

Malim, M.H., McCarn, D.F., Tiley, L.S. & Cullen, B.R. (1991) Mutational definition of the human immunodeficiency virus type 1 Rev activation domain. *J Virol* **65**, 4248–54.

Meyer, B. & Malim, M.H. (1994) The HIV-1 Rev trans-activator shuttles between the nucleus and the cytoplasm. *Genes Dev* **8**, 1538–47.

Nagai, K., Oubridge, C., Jessen, T.H., Li, J. & Evans, P.R. (1990) Crystal structure of the RNA-binding domain of the U1 small nuclear ribonucleoprotein A. *Nature* **348**, 515–20.

Nemeroff, M.E., Qian, X. & Krug, R.M. (1995) The influenza virus NS1 protein forms multimers *in vitro* and *in vivo*. *Virology* **212**, 422–8.

Newkirk, K., Feng, W., Jian, W. *et al.* (1994) Solution NMR structure of the major cold shock protein (CspA) from *Escherichia coli*: identification of a binding epitope for DNA. *Proc Natl Acad Sci USA* **91**, 5114–8.

Nilsen, T.W. (1994) RNA–RNA interactions in the spliceosome: unraveling the ties that bind. *Cell* **78**, 1–4.

Nilsen, T.W. (1996) A parallel spliceosome. *Science* **273**, 1813.

Norton, G.P., Tanaka, T., Tobita, K. *et al.* (1987) Infectious influenza A and B virus variants with long carboxyl terminal deletions in the NS1 polypeptides. *Virology* **156**, 204–13.

Olsen, H.S., Cochrane, A.W., Dillon, P.J., Nalin, C.M. & Rosen, C.A. (1990) Interaction of the human immunodeficiency virus type 1 Rev protein with a structured region in env mRNA is dependent on multimer formation mediated through a basic stretch of amino acids. *Genes Dev* **4**, 1357–64.

Oubridge, C., Ito, N., Evans, P.R., Teo, C.-H. & Nagai, K. (1994) Crystal structure at 1.92 Å resolution of the RNA-binding domain of the U1A spliceosomal protein complexed with an RNA hairpin. *Nature* **372**, 432–8.

Park, Y.W. & Katze, M.G. (1995) Translational control by influenza virus. Identification of *cis*-acting sequences and *trans*-acting factors which may regulate selective viral mRNA translation. *J Biol Chem* **270**, 28433–9.

Predki, P.F., Nayak, L.M., Gottlieb, M.B.C. & Regan, L. (1995) Dissecting RNA–protein interactions: RNA–RNA recognition by Rop. *Cell* **80**, 41–50.

Qian, X., Alonso-Caplen, F. & Krug, R.M. (1994) Two functional domains of the influenza virus NS1 protein are required for regulation of nuclear export of mRNA. *J Virol* **68**, 2433–41.

Qian, X., Chien, C., Lu, Y., Montelione, G.T. & Krug, R.M. (1995) An amino-terminal polypeptide fragment of the influenza virus NS1 protein possesses specific RNA binding activity and largely helical backbone structure. *RNA* **1**, 948–56.

Qian, X.Y., Chen, Z.Y., Zhang, J., Rabson, A.B. & Krug, R.M. (1996) New approach for inhibiting Rev function and HIV-1 production using the influenza virus NS1 protein. *Proc Natl Acad Sci USA* **93**, 8873–7.

Qiu, Y. & Krug, R.M. (1994) The influenza virus NS1 protein is a poly (A)-binding protein that inhibits nuclear export of mRNAs containing poly (A). *J Virol* **68**, 2425–32.

Qiu, Y., Nemeroff, M.E. & Krug, R.M. (1995) The influenza virus NS1 protein binds to a specific region in human U6 snRNA and inhibits U6-U2 and U6-U4 snRNA interactions during splicing. *RNA* **1**, 304–16.

Rhoads, R.E. (1993) Regulation of eukaryotic protein synthesis by initiation factors. *J Biol Chem* **268**, 3017–20.

Richard, N., Iacampo, S. & Cochrane, A. (1994) HIV-1 Rev is capable of shuttling between the nucleus and cytoplasm. *Virology* **204**, 123–31.

Rinke, J., Appel, B., Digweed, M. & Luhrmann, R. (1985) Localization of a base-paired interaction between small nuclear RNAs U4 and U6 in intact U4/U6 ribonucleoprotein particles by psoralen cross-linking. *J Mol Biol* **185**, 721–31.

Rivera-Pomar, R., Niessing, D., Schmidt-Ott, U., Gehring, W.J. & Jackle, H. (1996) RNA binding and translational suppression by bicoid. *Nature* **379**, 746–9.

Robertson, J.S., Schubert, M. & Lazzarini, R.A. (1981) Polyadenylation sites for influenza virus mRNA. *J Virol* **38**, 157–63.

Samuel, C.E. (1993) The eIF-2a protein kinases, regulators of translation in eukaryotes from yeasts to humans. *J Biol Chem* **268**, 7603–6.

Schindelin, H., Marahiel, M.A. & Heinemann, U. (1993) Universal nucleic acid-binding domain revealed by crystal structure of the *B. subtilis* major cold-shock protein. *Nature* **364**, 164–8.

Schindelin, H., Jiang, W., Inouye, M. & Heinemann, U. (1994) Crystal structure of CspA, the major cold shock protein of *Escherichia coli*. *Proc Natl Acad Sci USA* **91**, 5119–23.

Schnuchel, A., Wiltscheck, R., Czisch, M. *et al.* (1993) Structure in solution of the major cold-shock protein from *Bacillus subtilis*. *Nature* **364**, 169–71.

Shapiro, G.I. & Krug, R.M. (1988) Influenza virus RNA replication *in vitro*: synthesis of viral template RNAs and virion RNAs in the absence of an added primer. *J Virol* **62**, 2285–90.

Sharp, P.A. (1994) Split genes and RNA splicing. *Cell* **77**, 805–15.

Shih, S., Nemeroff, M.E. & Krug, R.M. (1995) The choice of alternative 5′ splice sites in influenza virus M1 mRNA is regulated by the viral polymerase complex. *Proc Natl Acad Sci USA* **92**, 6324–8.

Shimizu, K., Mullinix, M.G., Channock, R.M. & Murphy, B.R. (1982) Temperature-sensitive mutants of influenza A/Udorn/72 (H3N2) virus. I. Isolation of temperature-sensitive mutants some of which exhibit host-dependent temperature sensitivity. *Virology* **117**, 38–44.

Stauber, R., Gaitanaris, G.A. & Pavlakis, G.N. (1995) Analysis of trafficking of Rev and transdominant Rev proteins in living cells using green fluorescent protein fusions: transdominant Rev blocks the export of Rev from the nucleus to the cytoplasm. *Virology* **213**, 439–49.

Tarn, W. & Steitz, J.A. (1996a) A novel spliceosome containing U11, U12, and U5 snRNPs excises a minor class (AT-AC) intron *in vitro*. *Cell* **84**, 801–11.

Tarn, W.-Y. & Steitz, J.A. (1996b) Highly diverged U4 and U6 small nuclear RNAs required for splicing rare AT-AC introns. *Science* **273**, 1824–32.

Venkatesh, L.K. & Chinnadurai, G. (1990) Mutants in a conserved region near the carboxy terminus of HIV-1 Rev identify functionally important residues and exhibit a dominant negative phenotype. *Virology* **178**, 327–30.

Vogle, U., Kunerl, M. & Scholtissek, C. (1993) Influenza A virus late mRNAs are specifically retained in the nucleus in the presence of a methyltransferase or a protein kinase inhibitor. *Virology* **198**, 227–33.

Wang, W. & Krug, R.M. (1996) The RNA-binding and effector domains are conserved to different extents among influenza A and B viruses. *Virology* **223**, 41–50.

Wang, W. & Krug, R.M. (1998) U6atac snRNA, the highly divergent counterpart of U6 snRNA, is the specific target that mediates inhibition of AT-AC splicing by the influenza virus NS1 protein. *RNA* **4**, 55–64.

Watson, J.C., Chang, H.W. & Jacobs, B.L. (1991) Characterization of a vaccinia virus-encoded double-stranded protein that may be involved in inhibition of the double-stranded RNA-dependent protein kinases. *Virology* **185**, 206–16.

Wittekind, M., Gorlach, M., Freidrichs, M., Dreyfuss, G. & Mueller, L. (1992) ^{1}H, ^{13}C, and ^{15}N NMR assignments and global folding pattern of the RNA-binding domain of the human hnRNP C proteins. *Biochem* **31**, 6254–65.

Wolstenholme, A.J., Barrett, T., Nichol, S.T. & Mahy, B.W.J. (1980) Influenza virus-specific RNA and protein syntheses in cells infected with temperature-sensitive mutants defective in the genome segment encoding nonstructural proteins. *J Virol* **35**, 1–7.

Zapp, M.L. & Green, M.R. (1989) Sequence-specific RNA binding by the HIV-1 Rev protein. *Nature* **342**, 714–6.

CHAPTER 9

Genetic Manipulation of Influenza Viruses

Thomas Muster and Adolfo García-Sastre

Influenza A viruses are segmented negative-strand RNA viruses. These viruses contain a lipid envelope in which the haemagglutinin (HA), neuraminidase (NA) and M2 proteins are anchored. The matrix protein M1 forms a protein layer beneath the envelope. The core of the virus, which is inside the M1 protein layer, consists of ribonucleoprotein (RNP) complexes, which contain genomic RNA molecules associated with the nucleoprotein (NP) and the viral polymerase subunits PB1, PB2 and PA. In addition to the eight viral structural proteins that form the virus, two nonstructural proteins (NS1 and NS2) are encoded by the genome (Lamb 1989). According to some reports the NS2 is also present in virions (Richardson & Akkina 1991; Yasuda *et al.* 1993). The genome consists of eight different RNA molecules. Since the RNAs are of negative polarity, they have to be transcribed into mRNA before the viral proteins can be synthesized. This transcription is performed by the incoming viral polymerase, an RNA-dependent RNA polymerase, which is also responsible for the replication of the viral RNA segments.

Introduction of mutations into the genome of influenza virus

The genetic manipulation of influenza viruses first became possible by treating viruses with mutagens such as 5-fluorouracil or nitrosoguanidine (Mahy 1983). The segmented nature of the genome of influenza viruses permits the genetic reassortment of two different influenza A virus strains, which takes place when the same cell is infected with the two different influenza viruses. Many functions and properties of the influenza virus genes were analysed by genetically reassorting mutagenized viruses with viruses capable of complementing for a particular phenotype. Following the selection of progeny reassortant viruses, the gene segment responsible for complementation of a particular function of the mutant virus was identified. This technique contributed considerably to our understanding of viral replication and to vaccine development. For example, it was shown that a temperature-sensitive (ts) neuraminidase virus mutant failed to exclude neuraminic acid from its envelope at non-permissive temperatures, thus leading to the formation of viral aggregates from infected cells during budding (Palese *et al.* 1974). Genes of influenza viruses determining host range phenotype were also identified by reassortment experiments (Almond 1977). Although this system remains a powerful technique for studying viral genes and for generating vaccine strains, only random mutations can be generated after treatment with mutagens.

A major obstacle to the development of techniques that allow the site-specific mutagenesis of influenza virus genes is the fact that the naked RNA of negative-strand viruses is not able to initiate infection when it is transfected into host cells. All types of viruses have to use the translation machinery of the host cell in order to achieve synthesis of the viral proteins. As a result, viruses need to present their genomic information as mRNA once they are inside their host cells. The genome of positive-strand RNA viruses is directly recognized as mRNA and DNA viruses can utilize cellular enzymes to generate viral mRNA. Therefore, the naked genomic RNA or DNA of these viruses is infectious. However, the situation is more complex in the case of negative-strand RNA viruses, in which the host cell does not provide the enzymes capable of transcribing the viral genomic RNA into mRNA. The genomic RNA of negative-strand RNA viruses has to be transcribed by an RNA-dependent polymerase, which is provided by the incoming virus. In addition, the RNA needs to be encapsidated with the NP in form of RNP complexes, in order to be recognized and transcribed by the viral polymerase.

Reverse genetics techniques that permit the site-specific genetic manipulation of negative-strand viruses were first established by P. Palese's group (García-Sastre & Palese 1993). In the initial experiment, *in vitro* reconstituted NA-specific RNPs were transfected into cells which had been previously infected with a helper influenza A virus (Enami *et al.* 1990). Specifically, the RNPs were generated *in vitro* by transcribing synthetic RNA from cDNA in the presence of purified NP protein and viral polymerase proteins. Methods such as DEAE-dextran transfection and electroporation were used to transfect RNP complexes into host cells (Luytjes *et al.* 1989; Li *et al.* 1995). Amplification and transcription of the transfected RNPs was supported in *trans* by viral proteins provided by the helper virus. The subsequent reassortment of the amplified synthetic RNPs with the RNPs of the helper virus yielded transfectant viruses containing the cDNA-derived NA segment (Fig. 9.1a).

An alternative method of introducing site-specific mutations into the influenza virus genome is based on the intracellular reconstitution of RNP complexes derived from plasmid-based expression vectors. In this system, influenza virus RNA transcripts are derived from plasmids which are transfected into cells. Genomic or antigenomic viral transcripts are generated via a cellular polymerase promoter at the 5′ end of the viral gene (Neumann *et al.* 1994), and a ribozyme sequence that generates the desired 3′ end by autocatalytic cleavage. Cotransfection with plasmids expressing the viral polymerase proteins PB1, PB2, and PA and NP protein results in the encapsidation, transcription

and replication of the expressed viral RNAs. The cotransfected cells are then infected with helper influenza virus, which takes up the intracellularly reconstituted RNPs (Fig. 9.1b). In contrast to the RNP transfection system this plasmid-based transfection system eliminates the need for purification of the viral NP and polymerase proteins which is required for *in vitro* reconstitution of RNP complexes (Pleschka *et al.* 1996).

It should be noted that both the RNP transfection technology and the plasmid-based reverse genetics system rely on the use of a helper virus which provides the remaining genetic backbone for the transfected gene segments. Therefore, it is essential to use a selection method to distinguish between transfectant viruses — containing the genetically manipulated and transfected RNA segment — and parental helper viruses. Several systems have been established to select for reassortant viruses containing the cDNA-derived gene segments. For example, a synthetic NA gene enabling the influenza virus to grow in the absence of exogenous proteases was transfected into cells that had previously been infected with a protease-dependent helper virus strain. The subsequent selection in the absence of proteases resulted in viruses in which the helper virus NA segment was exchanged with the synthetic RNA (Enami *et al.* 1990). Cloned NA genes could also be rescued by a NA-deficient mutant virus which needs exogenous neuraminidase to grow in tissue culture (Liu & Air 1993). In other experiments, viruses containing cDNA-derived HA RNA segments were rescued. In this case, the selection was performed in the presence of a neutralizing antiserum specific for the HA protein of the helper virus but not for the HA protein encoded by the transfected synthetic HA segment (Enami & Palese 1991). Antibody-based methods for positive selection of transfectant viruses were also used (Horimoto & Kawaoka 1994). Selection of transfectant influenza viruses containing genetically manipulated HA RNA segments was also possible by using a host-restricted influenza virus strain as helper virus (Grassauer *et al.* 1997). A host-restricted influenza virus strain was also used as helper virus to successfully rescue cDNA-derived

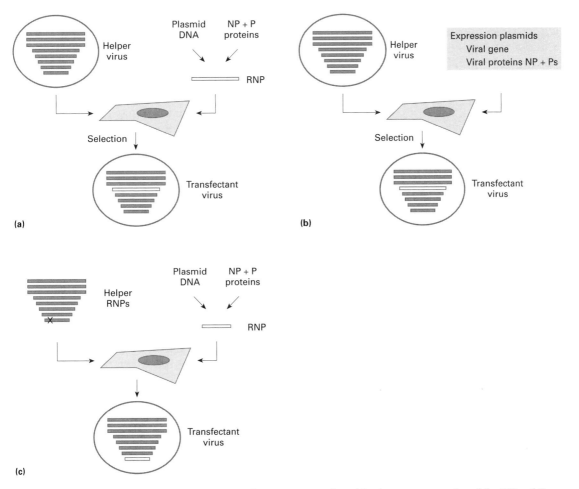

Fig. 9.1 Reverse genetics systems to rescue genetically manipulated influenza viruses. (a) Biologically active ribonucleoprotein (RNP) complexes are formed *in vitro* by incubating plasmid-derived RNA with purified viral nucleoprotein (NP) and polymerase (P) proteins. The reconstituted RNPs are transfected into cells that have previously been infected with an influenza helper virus. Upon selection, transfectant viruses containing the *in vitro*-derived RNP are obtained. (b) Expression plasmids coding for the NP and P proteins and a viral gene segment are cotransfected into cells. In this case, RNPs are reconstituted *in vivo* upon expression of the NP and P proteins and viral RNA in the cells. The cells are then infected with an influenza helper virus. Subsequently, selection for transfectant viruses containing the plasmid-derived RNP is performed. (c) RNPs are purified from influenza virus. After specifically destroying one of the RNPs, the remaining seven RNPs are cotransfected with the complementing *in vitro*-reconstituted RNP. Viruses containing the *in vitro*-derived RNP can be obtained by direct plaque formation, in the absence of a selection system.

PB2 genes into transfectant viruses (Subbarao *et al.* 1993). Other rescue or selection systems involved the use of ts mutants and drug-sensitive strains as helper viruses (Enami *et al.* 1991; Yasuda *et al.* 1994; Castrucci & Kawaoka 1995; Li *et al.* 1995). In addition, transfectant influenza B viruses were

also rescued following RNP transfection of genetically manipulated HA genes (Barclay & Palese 1995).

Recently, Enami (1997) has reported a technique which eliminates the need for a helper virus and thus the need for a selection system to obtain genetically manipulated influenza viruses. Influenza virus RNPs were purified and treated with RNaseH in the presence of a cDNA of the NS gene. This specifically digested the NS RNP. The NS-depleted RNPs were then cotransfected into cells with an *in vitro* reconstituted NS–RNP complex. Cells were then overlaid with agar, and recombinant viruses containing the cotransfected NS–RNP complex were obtained by direct plaque formation (Fig. 9.1c). Theoretically, this system could be used to genetically manipulate all eight influenza A virus gene segments.

The establishment of reverse genetics techniques to genetically manipulate influenza virus genomes, as well as other negative-strand RNA virus genomes, has revolutionized the field of research into this group of viruses.

The use of these technologies to generate live attenuated influenza virus vaccines, to express foreign antigens by transfectant influenza virus vectors and to analyse important functions of influenza virus proteins and RNAs will be discussed below.

Development of live attenuated influenza virus vaccines by reverse genetics

The generation of attenuated viruses containing defined and genetically stable mutations is one field of application of reverse genetics technology. These attenuated viruses might possibly be used as live vaccines to efficiently induce protective immune responses against wild-type viruses. One strategy for attenuating a pathogenic virus is the introduction of mutations into the non-coding regions of the viral genome. These non-coding regions usually contain *cis*-acting signals, which are required for the efficient replication, transcription, translation and packaging of the viral genome. Therefore, the viral non-coding regions are promising targets for the introduction of attenuating mutations. For example, each of the poliovirus vaccine Sabin strains has attenuating mutations in the 5′ non-coding region of the viral genome. These mutations were shown to decrease virus replication in neurones (Minor 1992; Brown & Lewis 1993). Similarly, the attenuation of Sindbis virus neuro-

virulence was possible by introducing defined mutations into the non-coding regions of the genome (Kuhn *et al*. 1992).

Generation of an attenuated transfectant influenza virus by specifically mutating the non-coding sequences of one of the viral genes was first reported by Muster *et al*. (1991). The NA/B-NS transfectant influenza A virus was engineered to contain an NA gene whose non-coding regions were replaced by the corresponding non-coding sequences of the NS gene of an influenza B virus. These influenza B virus-derived non-coding sequences were not efficiently recognized by the influenza A virus polymerase, resulting in altered levels of replication of the chimeric NA gene in NA/B-NS virus-infected cells. Thus, a five- to six-fold reduction in the NA-specific RNA levels was found in NA/B-NS infected cell. The same reduction was also found in purified viral particles. As a result, preparations of this virus contained a higher proportion of defective particles (lacking the NA gene) as compared to preparations of the wild-type virus (Luo *et al*. 1992). The NA/B-NS virus appeared to be attenuated in mice as indicated by a dramatic increase in its LD_{50}. Moreover, mice inoculated with a non-lethal dose of the NA/B-NS virus were subsequently protected against infection by wild-type influenza virus.

Other transfectant viruses whose NA genes contained only parts of the non-coding sequences of the NS gene of influenza B virus were made. For example, the NA gene of the transfectant virus NA/Y was generated by exchanging a computer-predicted stem structure in the non-coding region of the gene for the corresponding domain of the NS gene of influenza B virus (Bergmann & Muster 1995). In contrast to the NA/B-NS virus the amount of NA-specific genomic RNA was reduced in NA/Y virus-infected cells but not in purified viral particles. However, this virus was also effectively attenuated in mice as indicated by a 3 log increase in its LD_{50}. The results with the NA/B-NS and NA/Y transfectant viruses suggest that the introduction of mutations into the non-coding sequences is a promising strategy for obtaining a live attenuated virus vaccine against influenza.

Other strategies for attenuating influenza viruses

by genetic manipulation involve the generation of mutations in the coding regions of viral genes. In the past, attenuated influenza viruses were obtained by extensively passing the virus at low temperature (for a review see Kendal *et al.* 1981). As a result of adaptation to growth at low temperature, viruses which had lost their ability to replicate at $39\,^{\circ}C$ were obtained. The replication of such cold-adapted (*ca*) viruses is only slightly restricted in the cooler upper respiratory tract, but highly restricted in the warmer lower respiratory tract, the major site of disease-associated pathology. Sequence comparison between the wild-type and *ca* viruses revealed silent mutations and amino acid changes in the coding regions of several gene segments. Most amino acid changes were found to be the result of point mutations (Klimov *et al.* 1992; Herlocher *et al.* 1993, 1996). The attenuating mutations of the *ca* A/Leningrad/134/47/57 virus did not revert upon reisolation of the virus from vaccinated children (Klimov *et al.* 1995). However, the genetic instability of point mutations and the level of immunogenicity still represent potential problems for the use of *ca* strains as vaccines. These strains could be made safer by changing the codons containing the attenuating single point mutations into codons that would need two or three nucleotide changes in order to revert to the wild-type amino acid sequence. Other approaches to obtaining genetically manipulated stable and more immunogenic attenuated viruses might involve insertions, deletions or the introduction of multiple mutations into the same gene segment. For example, sequential addition of ts missense mutations into the PB2 gene of transfectant influenza A viruses resulted in an increase in their temperature sensitivity and attenuation properties. The ts phenotype was stable after replication in the upper respiratory tract of immunocompromised mice for two in three transfectants containing double mutations (Subbarao *et al.* 1995). Castrucci *et al.* (1992) obtained attenuated viruses when foreign amino acid sequences were inserted into the stalk region of the NA. Insertion and expression of immunomodulatory proteins such as cytokines might also be used in order to attenuate influenza viruses. Partial or complete deletion of a viral gene which mediates a specific function represents another possibility for attenuation of a virus. Recently, by introducing a frame shift mutation, we rescued an influenza A/PR8/32 virus with a 112 amino acid deletion of the C-terminal part of the NS1 protein. The plaque size of this transfectant virus on Madin–Darby canine kidney (MDCK) cells was significantly reduced as compared to the wild-type virus (Egorov *et al.* 1997). However, the replication properties of this virus in mice and ferrets remain to be analysed.

Although it is likely that transfectant influenza viruses containing insertions, deletions or multiple mutations will be stably attenuated, it has been shown that even deletion mutants could phenotypically revert through the acquisition of intragenic or extragenic suppressor mutations (Snyder *et al.* 1990; Treanor *et al.* 1991). Therefore, one needs to analyse whether the attenuated viruses retain their phenotype after extensive passages in tissue culture, mice or ferrets, the latter animals representing an accepted animal model for influenza viruses. Viruses reisolated from vaccinees also need to be analysed.

In this regard, Parkin *et al.* (1997) succeeded in engineering a stable live attenuated influenza A virus candidate vaccine. Importantly, this strain retained its attenuated phenotype after replication in nude mice, growth at non-permissive temperature and several passages in ferrets. The attenuated influenza virus strain was obtained by introducing a combination of mutations into the PB2 polymerase subunit of the virus. First, single amino acid changes, which were associated with ts phenotypes or which could potentially affect the cap-binding function of PB2, were introduced into the viral genome. These changes were generated using codons that required more than one nucleotide change to allow reversion to the wild-type PB2. Each of the mutations had only a limited effect on viral replication in tissue culture. In order to increase the level of attenuation, viruses containing several combinations of the single mutations were generated. Two mutants which were highly attenuated in the respiratory tracts of mice and ferrets and which had low reactogenicity in ferrets were obtained. In addition, both mutants had a ts phenotype. Animals immunized with the attenuated mutants were protected from wild-type virus-induced disease. Finally, the ts and attenuated phenotype of one of the two mutant viruses appeared to be stable, suggesting that this variant is suitable for human clinical trials. These studies demonstrated that the genetic manipulation of the influenza virus PB2 gene allows the generation of tailor-made genetically stable, attenuated and immunogenic influenza viruses.

Influenza virus as a vector for foreign antigens

Most viruses are able to elicit strong and long-lasting immune responses against their expressed antigens. Thus, it seems logical to consider viral vectors for vaccination purposes. Attenuated live viruses can be used to express protective antigens of other pathogens for which no safe attenuated strains are available. For example, chimeric canarypox virus expressing HIV antigens has been used in human clinical trials. Specifically, it has been shown that immunization with a canarypox virus vector expressing the HIV-1 gp160 protein followed by a boosting immunization with purified gp160 protein can elicit a cytotoxic T-cell as well as a B-cell immune response against HIV-1 in humans (Pialoux *et al.* 1995; Fleury *et al.* 1996). The development of methods to genetically manipulate the genome of influenza virus has also made it possible to use influenza virus as a vector for foreign antigens (for reviews see García-Sastre & Palese 1995a; Palese *et al.* 1996, 1997). Different properties of influenza virus suggest that it might be a useful vaccine vector. Firstly, different subtypes of influenza virus are available. Since antibodies against these different subtypes show no or little crossreactivity, pre-existing immunity to the vector in the host can be circumvented. Effective booster immunizations with different subtype influenza viruses expressing the same antigens should also be possible. Secondly, influenza viruses induce strong cellular and humoral systemic and mucosal immune responses. Moreover, influenza viruses are non-integrating, non-oncogenic viruses. In addition, attenuated influenza viruses are available that have been shown to be safe and protective in humans (Alexandrova *et al.* 1984; Wright *et al.* 1986; Rudenko *et al.* 1993).

One method of expressing foreign sequences by transfectant influenza viruses is based on grafting epitopes into various positions of the viral protein (Fig. 9.2a). One site which has been found to tolerate insertions of foreign antigens is the antigenic site B of the HA molecule. Antigenic site B consists of an exposed loop structure located on top of the HA and is known to be highly immunogenic. Immunizations with chimeric viruses containing foreign B-cell epitopes inserted into the antigenic site B elicited neutralizing antisera in mice (Li *et al.* 1993a; Muster *et al.* 1994). For example, antisera were induced which neutralized genetically divergent HIV-1 isolates when mice were immunized with a transfectant influenza virus expressing the highly conserved HIV-1 gp41 epitope ELDKWA (Muster *et al.* 1993, 1994). In addition to the neutralizing systemic immune response, intranasal immunizations of mice induced long-lasting local immune responses in the genital and intestinal mucosae, the main portals for entry of HIV-1 (Muster *et al.* 1995). By inserting the HIV-epitope sequence ELDKWAS into HAs belonging to different subtypes effective booster immunizations were made possible. Specifically, the HIV-specific epitope sequence was inserted into HAs belonging to the H1 and H3 subtypes. Ferrets were primed with the H1-ELDKWA virus and then boosted with the H1- or the H3-ELDKWA virus. Booster immunizations with the H3 subtype resulted in ELDKWA-specific titres up to 32-fold higher than those obtained by booster immunizations with the same (H1) subtype (Ferko *et al.* 1997).

The antigenic site B of the HA of transfectant influenza viruses has also been used to express B-cell epitopes derived from a malaria parasite. A transfectant influenza virus expressing a B-cell epitope from *Plasmodium yoelii* was able to induce protective antibody responses in mice against this malaria parasite (Rodrigues *et al.* 1994). Transfectant influenza viruses expressing a B-cell epitope from the outer membrane protein F of *Pseudomonas aeruginosa* were also able to induce antibodies against *P. aeruginosa* in immunized mice (Gilleland *et al.* 1997). These results suggest that influenza virus vectors are good inducers of antibody-mediated immunity against different pathogens.

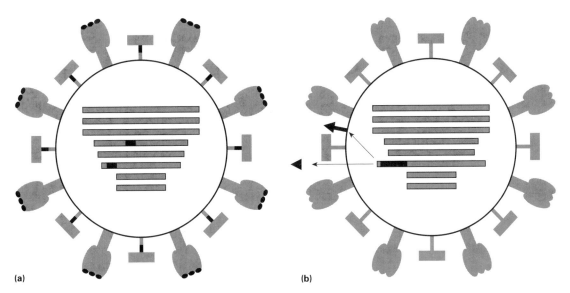

Fig. 9.2 Influenza virus as a vector for foreign antigens. (a) Epitope grafting. The foreign epitope is expressed as part of the viral protein. CD8+ T-cell-mediated immunity against foreign pathogens is induced when the corresponding T-cell epitopes are expressed in the stalk region of the neuraminidase, or in the antigenic sites B or E of the haemagglutinin proteins. B-cell-mediated immunity against foreign epitopes is induced when the foreign epitope is expressed in the antigenic site B, which forms an exposed loop on top of the haemagglutinin molecule.

(b) Expression of foreign polypeptides. Gene segments that code both for an essential viral protein and for a foreign polypeptide are constructed. Expression of the foreign sequence is achieved via the use of bicistronic genes or of a polyprotein with autocatalytic protease activity. The foreign polypeptide can either be expressed in a soluble form or be anchored into the viral membrane. The figure schematically represents an influenza A virus with its eight RNA segments and the haemagglutinin and neuraminidase surface glycoproteins. Black boxes and objects correspond to the foreign sequences.

In addition, transfectant influenza virus vectors are potent inducers of cellular immune responses. Transfectant viruses expressing a murine CD8+ T-cell HIV-epitope were able to induce cytotoxic T lymphocyte (CTL) responses against this epitope in immunized mice (Li *et al.* 1993a). As with the B-cell epitopes, the CTL epitope was inserted into the antigenic site B of the HA. Insertion of CD8+ T-cell epitopes into the stalk region of the NA also resulted in viruses that stimulated strong cytotoxic T-cell responses against the inserted epitope. Transfectant influenza viruses expressing T-cell epitopes were able to protect immunized animals against challenge with the foreign pathogen (Li *et al.* 1993c; Castrucci *et al.* 1994).

The induction of neutralizing antibodies against one viral vector makes it difficult, if not impossible, to use the same vector to boost the induced cellular immune response, since the vector will not be able to reinfect the same recipient. One possible way of avoiding this problem is to use two different viral vectors expressing the same foreign antigen for the priming and boosting immunizations. Particularly remarkable have been experiments involving combined immunizations of mice with recombinant influenza and vaccinia vectors expressing the same CTL epitope. Mice immunized with an influenza virus vector and boosted with a vaccinia virus vector expressing the same antigen were able to generate specific CD8+ T cells against the expressed antigen which represented approximately 1% of the spleen cells (Murata *et al.* 1996). This unique protocol of immunization generated a protective cellular immune response against the murine malaria parasite *Plasmodium yoelii* (Li *et al.* 1993c; Rodrigues *et al.* 1994). Interestingly, the order of administration of the recombinant viruses was found to be crucial for eliciting an effective secondary cellular immune response. This finding was not limited to a particular CTL epitope, since a comparable specific CD8+ T-cell response was induced in mice immunized with a combination of influenza and vaccinia virus expressing different H-2K^d- and H-2K^k-restricted epitopes (Murata *et al.* 1996). Finally, expression of more than one CTL epitope by influenza virus vectors did not decrease the efficiency of the immune response induced against each individual epitope (Isobe *et al.* 1995). These results strongly suggest that influenza virus vectors expressing CTL epitopes will induce effective cellular immune responses against different pathogens, especially if used in combination with a different vector expressing the same epitopes, such as recombinant vaccinia viruses.

Epitope grafting of a foreign sequence into an influenza virus protein may result in a non-functional chimeric viral protein, and make the rescue of a viable transfectant virus impossible. A different strategy for expressing foreign sequences by transfectant influenza viruses involves the engineering of gene segments containing an additional open reading frame (Fig. 9.2b). García-Sastre *et al.* (1994) constructed a viral RNA segment which encoded both a truncated form of gp41 of HIV and the NA. In this case, cap-independent translation of the second open reading frame was mediated by an internal ribosomal entry site (IRES) element. This approach was used to rescue a transfectant influenza virus which expressed a truncated form of gp41 of HIV-1. The gp41-derived polypeptide was expressed in the plasma membrane of infected cells. Interestingly, when the ectodomain of the gp41 polypeptide was fused with the transmembrane and cytoplasmic domains of the influenza virus HA, this polypeptide was also incorporated into viral particles (García-Sastre *et al.* 1994).

In a different approach, the CAT coding sequence was fused in frame to the viral NA coding sequences of the NA gene of a transfectant virus. Upon expression of the chimeric polyprotein, cleavage into the two CAT and NA polypeptides was mediated by an autoproteolytic protease sequence inserted between the CAT and NA open reading frames. As a result, an active form of the CAT protein was detected in cells infected with this transfectant virus. Importantly, the expression of the CAT gene was maintained after several passages in tissue culture (Percy *et al.* 1994). These results demonstrate that transfectant influenza viruses can be used to express foreign proteins and polypeptides of up to 200 amino acids in length.

Analysis of viral functions

Reverse genetics techniques to genetically manipulate influenza viruses have also been used to study the functions of *cis*- and *trans*-acting elements in viral replication. For this purpose, transfectant viruses containing mutations in different domains of the viral RNA or proteins were generated. The phenotypic characteristics of these transfectant viruses were then studied.

Analysis of non-coding sequences

The coding sequences of the eight different influenza virus genes are flanked by short non-coding sequences. It has been shown that these non-coding sequences contain signals needed for transcription, replication and packaging of the gene (Luytjes *et al.* 1989). However, it is not clear whether each viral gene is selectively incorporated into a virus particle, resulting in viruses with the correct complement of the eight genes, or whether the packaging of the different eight viral genes in virus particles is a random process. In the latter case, the virus needs to package an average of more than eight segments in order to generate a reasonable percentage of virus particles containing at least one copy of each gene. By generating a transfectant influenza virus which contained nine different RNA segments, Enami *et al.* (1991) were able to show that influenza viruses can package more than eight segments. This supports the random packaging model of the viral genes.

In a random packaging model, the relative amount of a viral gene in infected cells will be reflected in the viral progeny. While it is accepted that in the viral particle equimolar amounts of each RNA are present in virus preparations, there are controversial data regarding the relative amounts of the genomic RNAs in the infected cells (Smith &

Hay 1982; Enami *et al.* 1985). In this regard, the NA/B-NS transfectant virus, which contains multiple mutations in the non-coding sequences of the NA gene, showed reduced levels of the NA RNA in both infected cells and viral particles (Luo *et al.* 1992). However, other transfectant influenza viruses were found to have wild-type NA RNA levels in virus particles, while these levels were reduced in infected cells (Bergmann & Muster 1995). A selective packaging process has also been suggested by competition experiments involving defective RNA segments (Nayak *et al.* 1989; Duhaut & McCauley 1996; Odagiri & Tashiro 1997). Additional investigations are required to elucidate the mechanism by which influenza virus packages its RNA segments.

The effect on viral replication of mutations at the non-coding ends of the genes has also been analysed in transfectant influenza viruses. The terminal 12 and 13 nucleotide positions at the 3' and 5' ends of the viral RNA are highly conserved among the eight influenza virus genes of different viral strains (Desselberger *et al.* 1980). Important nucleotide positions within the conserved 3' and 5' ends which influence RNA transcription have been characterized by genetic and biochemical studies (Parvin *et al.* 1989; Yamanaka *et al.* 1991; Li & Palese 1992; Seong & Brownlee 1992a,b; Piccone *et al.* 1993; Li & Palese 1994; Neumann & Hobom 1995). It has become clear that sequences complementary within these ends are crucial for optimal transcription *in vitro* (Fodor *et al.* 1994, 1995; Pritlove *et al.* 1995) and *in vivo* (Luo *et al.* 1991; Flick *et al.* 1996; Kim *et al.* 1997). In addition, these ends are also needed for activation of the endonuclease activity of the influenza virus polymerase which is required for cap-priming of the viral mRNA (Hagen *et al.* 1994; Cianci *et al.* 1995). Experiments involving transfectant influenza viruses have demonstrated that the non-conserved regions of the viral genes also play an important role in viral gene expression. It has been shown that either a combination of deletions in the non-conserved non-coding region or the substitution of the NA non-coding region by the corresponding regions of other viral segments resulted in a reduced NA-specific RNA synthesis (Zheng *et al.* 1996). Similar results were obtained by Bergmann and Muster (1996) when they analysed influenza viruses which contained multiple mutations in the non-conserved residues of the NA gene. Interestingly, it appears that synergistic effects of the terminal sequences are needed for efficient viral RNA production. This might be explained by the fact that the overall structure of the terminal ends is important for efficient recognition and transcription by the viral polymerases. Mutations and deletions in the non-conserved terminal sequences may be responsible for changes in this structure which disrupts *cis*-acting signals. These data show that the promoter of the influenza A virus is not restricted to the conserved residues of the terminal region.

Analysis of coding regions

Transfectant viruses containing mutations in the coding regions of their genes have been used to study protein functions. The role of specific protein domains or single amino acids within a viral protein in virus host range and tropism, and viral growth, morphology, assembly and drug resistance have been analysed.

For example, a transfectant influenza virus was constructed to define the mutation responsible for the neurovirulent phenotype of influenza A/WSN/33 (WSN) virus in mice. Reassortant viruses between WSN virus and a non-neurovirulent influenza virus revealed that the WSN NA gene confers upon the latter virus the ability to grow in the absence of a protease in MDBK cells (Schulmann & Palese 1977). In addition, it was shown by Sugiura and Ueda (1979) that the WSN NA is required for the neurovirulence of the WSN strain. The WSN NA lacks a glycosylation site at amino acid position 130, which is conserved in other influenza virus neuraminidases. On the basis of these observations, a transfectant WSN virus was engineered in which the missing glycosylation site was restored. This Glyc+ mutant virus failed to replicate in mouse brain, demonstrating that the absence of this glycosylation site is required for the neurovirulence of the WSN virus (Li *et al.* 1993b).

Other transfectant viruses containing insertions or deletions of amino acid residues in the stalk region of the NA showed that the length of the stalk region can also affect viral host tropism (Castrucci & Kawaoka 1993; Luo *et al.* 1993).

Transfectant viruses also allowed the definition of the role of the viral M proteins in the growth properties of influenza A viruses. Previous studies based on fast-growing reassortant viruses indicated that the virus growth rate can be modulated by the M gene. This gene encodes two viral proteins, M1 and M2. A transfectant virus coding for the M1 protein of a fast-growing influenza virus strain and the M2 protein of a slow-growing virus was generated. The resulting transfectant virus retained the fast-growing properties, which indicates that the M1 protein plays an important role in the control of the growth rate of influenza viruses (Yasuda *et al.* 1994).

Transfectant viruses containing deletions in the cytoplasmic tails of their surface proteins were created in order to study viral assembly and morphogenesis. The interaction between viral proteins leading to virus particle formation is poorly understood. It is assumed that during viral budding, internal viral proteins interact with the external viral envelope proteins HA, NA and M2, which are inserted in the plasma membrane of the host cell, leading to viral particle formation. The cytoplasmic domains of these surface glycoproteins are good candidates for these interactions. In order to understand the role of the cytoplasmic tails on viral replication, transfectant viruses containing deletions in these protein domains were made. For example, a transfectant influenza virus lacking the C-terminal Glu in the cytoplasmic domain of the M2 protein was rescued, but attempts to rescue viruses lacking five or 10 M2 C-terminal residues failed. These data suggest that the cytoplasmic tail of M2 plays an important role in viral replication. However, the specific functional role of this domain and potential interaction sites with other viral proteins remain to be defined (Castrucci & Kawaoka 1995). It has also been found that specific amino acid substitutions at the cytoplasmic tail of the NA protein of transfectant influenza viruses affect the packaging levels of the NA protein into virions (Bilsel *et al.* 1993). However, the cytoplasmic tail of this protein is not

essential for its packaging into virus particles, since a transfectant virus lacking the NA tail was rescued and found to be able to incorporate the NA protein into the envelope (García-Sastre & Palese 1995b; Mitnaul *et al.* 1996). Furthermore, it was found that a transfectant influenza virus that contains a cytoplasmic tail minus mutant HA assembles and replicates efficiently (Jin *et al.* 1994). Interestingly, it was possible to obtain transfectant influenza viruses of the H3 subtype, but not of the H1 subtype, in which the conserved palmitylation sites within the HA cytoplasmic and transmembrane domains were eliminated (Zürcher *et al.* 1994; Jin *et al.* 1996). Transfectant influenza viruses that lack the cytoplasmic tail of both the HA and the NA were also obtained. Although these transfectants have a comparable protein composition to the wild-type virus, viral particle production in infected cells was reduced 10-fold. The viral particles appeared to be greatly elongated and of extended irregular shape (Jin *et al.* 1997). Thus, although the cytoplasmic tails of the NA and HA proteins of influenza viruses appear not to be essential for virus viability, they play an important role in virus morphogenesis.

Other HA transfectant viruses have provided evidence for a correlation of haemagglutinin cleavability and virulence of an avian influenza A virus (Horimoto & Kawaoka 1994), or confirmed the mutation responsible for acquisition of resistance to a haemagglutinin-specific inhibitor of influenza A virus (Luo *et al.* 1996). Bergmann *et al.* (1992) rescued transfectant viruses containing NA gene segments which were generated via non-homologous RNA recombination, suggesting that, in addition to reassortment- and mutational-based mechanisms of virus variability, recombination between influenza virus RNA genes may contribute to the evolutionary changes of the virus.

Future directions

Reverse genetics techniques allowing the genetic manipulation of influenza viruses represent powerful tools for studying these viruses and for generating recombinant influenza viruses with potential applications in clinical settings. These techniques involve the use of helper influenza viruses and/or treated RNPs. However, it is likely that simplified transfection methods allowing coexpression in mammalian cells of all eight influenza virus genes and viral NP and polymerase proteins from plasmids will also result in the generation of recombinant viruses. Such systems have been successfully used to rescue genetically manipulated negative-strand RNA viruses of the non-segmented paramyxovirus and rhabdovirus groups (Schnell *et al.* 1994; Collins *et al.* 1995; Garcin *et al.* 1995; Lawson *et al.* 1995; Radecke *et al.* 1995; Whelan *et al.* 1995; Hoffman & Banerjee 1997). In these cases, it was possible to express the viral genome or antigenome from a single plasmid. Due to the segmented nature of the genome of influenza viruses, more than one plasmid will be required to express the eight viral RNA segments. This might decrease the probability that all required expression plasmids will be transfected into the same cell. However, Bridgen and Elliot (1996) successfully established a rescue system for the three-segmented negative Bunyamwera virus. In addition, Mena *et al.* (1996) showed that it was possible to coexpress all 10 influenza virus proteins and a viral reporter gene from 11 plasmids. This resulted in viral particle formation in the transfected cells. Therefore, an entirely plasmid-based method to rescue recombinant influenza viruses should be possible. In any case, transfectant influenza viruses generated by reverse genetics methods have great potential for use in the future not only as live influenza virus vaccines, but also as effective vaccines against other human diseases such as AIDS, malaria and cancer.

References

Alexandrova, G.I., Polezhaev, F.I., Budilovsky, G.N. *et al.* (1984) Recombinant cold-adapted attenuated influenza A vaccines for use in children: reactogenicity and antigenic activity of cold-adapted recombinants and analysis of isolates from the vaccinees. *Infect Immun* **44**, 734–9.

Almond, J. (1977) A single gene determines the host range of influenza virus. *Nature* **270**, 617–8.

Barclay, W.S. & Palese, P. (1995) Influenza B viruses with site-specific mutations introduced into the HA gene. *J Virol* **69**, 1275–9.

Bergmann, M. & Muster, T. (1995) The relative amount of an influenza A virus segment present in the viral particle can be unaffected by a reduction in replication of that segment. *J Gen Virol* **76**, 3211–5.

Bergmann, M. & Muster, T. (1996) Mutations in the non-conserved noncoding sequences of the influenza A virus segments affect viral vRNA formation. *Virus Res* **44**, 23–31.

Bergmann, M., García-Sastre, A. & Palese, P. (1992) Transfection-mediated recombination of influenza A virus. *J Virol* **66**, 7576–80.

Bilsel, P., Castrucci, M.R. & Kawaoka, Y. (1993) Mutations in the cytoplasmic tail of influenza A virus neuraminidase affect incorporation into virions. *J Virol* **67**, 6762–7.

Bridgen, A. & Elliot, R.M. (1996) Rescue of a segmented negative-strand RNA virus entirely from cloned complementary DNAs. *Proc Natl Acad Sci USA* **93**, 15400–4.

Brown, F. & Lewis, B.P. (1993) Poliovirus attenuation: molecular mechanisms and practical aspects. *Dev Biol Stand* **78**, 1–187.

Castrucci, M.R. & Kawaoka, Y. (1993) Biologic importance of neuraminidase stalk length in influenza A virus. *J Virol* **67**, 759–64.

Castrucci, M.R. & Kawaoka, Y. (1995) Reverse genetics system for generation of an influenza A virus mutant containing a deletion of the carboxyl-terminal residue of M2 protein. *J Virol* **69**, 2725–8.

Castrucci, M.R., Bilsel, P. & Kawaoka, Y. (1992) Attenuation of influenza A virus by insertion of a foreign epitope into the neuraminidase. *J Virol* **66**, 4647–53.

Castrucci, M.R., Hou, S., Doherty, P.C. & Kawaoka, Y. (1994) Protection against lethal lymphocytic choriomeningitis virus (LCMV) infection by immunization of mice with an influenza virus containing an LCMV epitope recognized by cytotoxic T lymphocytes. *J Virol* **68**, 3486–90.

Cianci, C., Tiley, L. & Krystal, M. (1995) Differential activation of the influenza virus polymerase via template RNA binding. *J Virol* **69**, 3995–9.

Collins, P.L., Hill, M.G., Camargo, E., Grosfeld, H., Chanock, R.M. & Murphy, B.R. (1995) Production of infectious human respiratory syncytial virus from cloned cDNA confirms an essential role for the transcription elongation factor from the 5′ proximal open reading frame of the M2 mRNA in gene expression and provides a capability for vaccine development. *Proc Natl Acad Sci USA* **92**, 11563–7.

Desselberger, U., Racaniello, V.R., Zazra, J.J. & Palese, P. (1980) The 3′ and 5′ terminal sequences of influenza A, B and C virus RNA segments are highly conserved and show partial inverted complementarity. *Gene* **8**, 315–28.

Duhaut, S.D. & McCauley, J.W. (1996) Defective RNAs inhibit the assembly of influenza virus genome segments in a segment specific manner. *Virology* **216**, 326–37.

Egorov, A., Brandt, S., Sereinig, S., Alexandrova, G., Katinger, H. & Muster, T. (1997). Generation of influenza A transfectant viruses containing deletions of the C-terminal part of the NS1 protein. In: 10th International Conference on Negative Strand Viruses, Dublin, Ireland. Abstract 108.

Enami, M. (1997) Improved technique to genetically manipulate influenza virus. In: *Frontiers of RNA Virus Research*, p. 19. The Oji International Seminar in Natural Science, Kyoto, Japan.

Enami, M. & Palese, P. (1991) High efficiency formation of influenza virus transfectants. *J Virol* **65**, 2711–3.

Enami, M., Fukuda, R. & Ishihama, A. (1985) Transcription and replication of eight RNA segments of influenza virus. *Virology* **142**, 68–77.

Enami, M., Luytjes, W., Krystal, M. & Palese, P. (1990) Introduction of site-specific mutations into the genome of influenza virus. *Proc Natl Acad Sci USA* **87**, 3802–5.

Enami, M., Sharma, G., Benham, G. & Palese, P. (1991) An influenza virus containing nine different RNA segments. *Virology* **185**, 291–8.

Ferko, B., Egorov, A., Romanova, J. *et al.* (1997) Influenza virus as a vector for mucosal immunization. In: *Frontiers of RNA Virus Research*, p. 18. The Oji International Seminar in Natural Science, Kyoto, Japan.

Flick, R., Neumann, G., Hoffmann, E., Neumeier, E. & Hobom, G. (1996) Promoter elements in the influenza vRNA terminal structure. *RNA* **2**, 1046–57.

Fleury, B., Janvier, G., Pialoux, G. *et al.* (1996) Memory cytotoxic T lymphocyte response in human immunodeficiency virus type 1 (HIV-1)—negative volunteers immunized with a recombinant canarypox expressing gp160 of HIV-1 and boosted with a recombinant gp160. *J Infect Dis* **174**, 734–8.

Fodor, E., Pritlove, D.C. & Brownlee, G.G. (1994) The influenza panhandle is involved in the initiation of transcription. *J Virol* **68**, 4092–6.

Fodor, E., Pritlove, D.C. & Brownlee, G.G. (1995) Characterization of the RNA-fork model of virion RNA in the initiation of transcription in influenza A virus. *J Virol* **69**, 4012–9.

García-Sastre, A. & Palese, P. (1993) Genetic manipulation of negative-strand RNA virus genomes. *Annu Rev Microbiol* **47**, 765–90.

García-Sastre, A. & Palese, P. (1995a) Influenza virus vectors. *Biologicals* **23**, 171–8.

García-Sastre, A. & Palese, P. (1995b) The cytoplasmatic tail of the neuraminidase protein of influenza virus does not play an important role in the packaging of this protein into viral envelopes. *Virus Res* **37**, 37–47.

García-Sastre, A., Muster, T., Barclay, W.S., Percy, N. & Palese, P. (1994) Use of a mammalian internal ribosomal entry site element for expression of a foreign protein by a transfectant influenza virus. *J Virol* **68**, 6254–61.

Garcin, D., Pelet, T., Calain, P. *et al.* (1995) A highly recombinogenic system for the recovery of infectious Sendai paramyxovirus from cDNA; generation of a novel copy-back nondefective interfering virus. *EMBO J* **14**, 6087–94.

Grassauer, A., Egorov, A., Ferko, B., Klima, A., Katinger, H. & Muster, T. (1997) Rescue of a host-restricted influenza A virus by cloned haemagglutinin genes. In: 10th International Conference on Negative Strand Viruses 1997, Dublin, Ireland, Abstract 109.

Gilleland, H.E., Gilleland, L.B., Staczek, J. *et al.* (1997) Chimeric influenza viruses incorporating epitopes of outer membrane protein F as a vaccine against pulmonary infection with *Pseudomonas aeruginosa*. *Behring Inst Mitt* **98**, 291–301.

Hagen, M., Chung, T.D.Y., Butcher, J.A. & Krystal, M. (1994) Recombinant influenza virus polymerase: requirement of both 5' and 3' ends for endonuclease activity. *J Virol* **68**, 1509–15.

Herlocher, M.L., Maassab, H.F. & Webster, G.R. (1993) Molecular and biological changes in the cold-adapted 'master strain' A/AA/6/60 (H2N2) influenza virus. *Proc Natl Acad Sci USA* **90**, 6032–6.

Herlocher, M.L., Clavo, A.C. & Maassab, H.F. (1996) Sequence comparisons of A/AA/6/60 influenza viruses: mutations which may contribute to attenuation. *Virus Res* **42**, 11–25.

Horimoto, T. & Kawaoka, Y. (1994) Reverse genetics provides direct evidence for a correlation of haemagglutinin cleavability and virulence of an avian influenza A virus. *J Virol* **68**, 3120–8.

Hoffman, M.A. & Banerjee, A.K. (1997) An infectious clone of human parainfluenza virus type 3. *J Virol* **71**, 4272–7.

Isobe, H., Moran, T., Li, S. *et al.* (1995) Presentation by a major histocompatibility complex class I molecule of nucleoprotein peptide expressed in two different genes of an influenza virus transfectant. *J Exp Med* **181**, 203–13.

Jin, H., Leser, G.P. & Lamb, R.A. (1994) The influenza virus haemagglutinin cytoplasmatic tail is not essential for virus assembly or infectivity. *EMBO J* **22**, 5504–15.

Jin, H., Subbarao, K., Bagai, S. *et al.* (1996) Palmitylation of the influenza virus haemagglutinin (H3) is not essential for virus assembly or infectivity. *J Virol* **70**, 1406–14.

Jin, H., Leser, G.P., Zhang, J. & Lamb, R.A. (1997) Influenza virus haemagglutinin and neuraminidase cytplasmic tails control particle shape. *EMBO J* **16**, 1236–47.

Kendal, A.P., Maassab, H.F., Alexandrova, G.I. & Ghendon, Y.Z. (1981) Development of cold-adapted recombinant live, attenuated influenza A vaccines in the U.S.A. and U.S.S.R. *Antiviral Res* **1**, 339–65.

Kim, H.-J., Fodor, E., Brownlee, G.G. & Seong, B.L. (1997) Mutational analysis of the RNA-fork model of the influenza A virus vRNA promoter *in vivo*. *J Gen Virol* **78**, 353–7.

Klimov, A.I., Cox, N.J., Yotov, W.V., Rocha, E., Alexandrova, G.I. & Kendal, A.P. (1992) Sequence changes in the live attenuated, cold-adapted variants of influenza A/Leningrad/134/57 (H2N2) virus. *Virology* **186**, 795–7.

Klimov, A.I., Egorov, A.Y., Gushchina, M.I. *et al.* (1995) Genetic stability of cold-adapted A/Leningrad/134/47/57 (H2N2) influenza virus: sequence analysis of live cold-adapted reassortant vaccine strains before and after replication in children. *J Gen Virol* **76**, 1521–5.

Kuhn, R.J., Griffin, D.E., Zhang, H., Niesters, H.G.M. & Strauss, J.H. (1992) Attenuation of Sindbis virus neurovirulence by using defined mutations in non-translated regions of the genome RNA. *J Virol* **66**, 7121–7.

Lamb, R.A. (1989) Genes and proteins of the influenza viruses. In: Krug, R.M. (ed.) *The Influenza Viruses*, pp. 1–67. Plenum Press, New York.

Lawson, N.D., Stillman, E.A., Whitt, M.A. & Rose, J.K. (1995) Recombinant vesicular stomatitis viruses from DNA. *Proc Natl Acad Sci USA* **92**, 4477–81.

Li, X. & Palese, P. (1992) Mutational analysis of the promoter required for influenza virus virion RNA synthesis. *J Virol* **66**, 4331–8.

Li, X. & Palese, P. (1994) Characterization of the polyadenylation signal of influenza virus RNA. *J Virol* **68**, 1245–9.

Li, S., Polonis, V., Isobe, H. *et al.* (1993a) Chimeric influenza virus induces neutralizing antibodies and cytotoxic T cells against human immundeficiency virus type 1. *J Virol* **67**, 6659–66.

Li, S., Schulmann, J., Itamura, S. & Palese, P. (1993b) Glycosylation of neuraminidase determines the neurovirulence of influenza A/WSN/33 virus. *J Virol* **67**, 6667–73.

Li, S., Rodrigues, M., Rodrigues, D. *et al.* (1993c) Priming with recombinant influenza virus followed by administration of recombinant vaccinia virus induces CD8+ T cell-mediated protective immunity against malaria. *Proc Natl Acad Sci USA* **90**, 5214–8.

Li, S., Xu, M. & Coelingh, K. (1995) Electroporation of ribonucleoprotein complexes for rescue of the nucleoprotein and matrix genes. *Virus Res* **37**, 153–61.

Liu, C. & Air, G.M. (1993) Selection and characterization of a neuraminidase-minus mutant of influenza virus and its rescue by cloned neuraminidase genes. *Virology* **194**, 403–7.

Luytjes, W., Krystal, M., Enami, M., Parvin, J.D. & Palese, P. (1989) Amplification, expression, and packaging of a foreign gene by influenza virus. *Cell* **59**, 1107–13.

Luo, S., Chung, J. & Palese, P. (1993) Alterations of the stalk of the influenza virus neuraminidase: deletions and insertions. *Virus Res* **29**, 141–53.

Luo, G., Luytjes, W., Enami, M. & Palese, P. (1991) The polyadenylation signal of influenza virus RNA involves a stretch of uridines followed by the RNA duplex of the panhandle structure. *J Virol* **65**, 2861–7.

Luo, G., Bergmann, M., García-Sastre, A. & Palese, P. (1992) Mechanism of attenuation of a chimeric influenza A/B transfectant virus. *J Virol* **66**, 4679–85.

Luo, G., Colonno, R. & Krystal, M. (1996) Characterization of a haemagglutinin-specific inhibitor of influenza A virus. *Virology* **226**, 66–7.

Mahy, B.W.J. (1983) Mutants of influenza virus. In: Palese, P. & Kingsbury, D.W. (eds) *Genetics of Influenza Viruses*, pp. 192–242. Springer-Verlag, New York.

Mena, I., Vivo, A., Perez, E. & Portela, A. (1996) Rescue of a synthetic chloramphenicol acetyltransferase RNA into influenza virus-like particles obtained from recombinant plasmids. *J Virol* **70**, 5016–24.

Minor, P.D. (1992) The molecular biology of poliovaccines. *J Gen Virol* **74**, 3065–77.

Mitnaul, L.J., Castrucci, M.R., Murti, K.G. & Kawaoka, Y. (1996) The cytoplasmatic tail of influenza A virus neuraminidase (NA) affects NA incorporation into virions, virion morphology, and virulence in mice but is not essential for virus replication. *J Virol* **70**, 873–9.

Murata, K., García-Sastre, A., Tsuji, M. *et al.* (1996) Characterization of *in vivo* primary and secondary CD8+ T cell responses induced by recombinant influenza and vaccinia viruses. *Cell Immunol* **173**, 96–107.

Muster, T., Subbarao, E.K., Enami, M., Murphy, B.R. & Palese, P. (1991) An influenza A virus containing influenza B virus 5′ and 3′ noncoding regions on the neuraminidase gene is attenuated in mice. *Proc Natl Acad Sci USA* **88**, 5177–81.

Muster, T., Steindl, F., Purtscher, M. *et al.* (1993) A conserved neutralizing epitope on gp41 of HIV-1. *J Virol* **67**, 6642–7.

Muster, T., Guinea, R., Trkola, A. *et al.* (1994) Cross-neutralizing activity against divergent human immunodeficiency virus type 1 isolates induced by the gp41 sequence ELDKWAS. *J Virol* **68**, 4031–4.

Muster, T., Ferko, B., Klima, A. *et al.* (1995) Mucosal model of immunization against human immunodeficiency virus type 1 with a chimeric influenza virus. *J Virol* **69**, 6678–86.

Nayak, D.P., Chambers, T.M. & Akkina, R.K. (1989) Structure of defective interfering RNAs of influenza virus and their role in interference. In: Krug, R.M. (ed.) *The Influenza Viruses*, pp. 269–311. Plenum Press, New York.

Neumann, G. & Hobom, G. (1995) Mutational analysis of influenza virus promoter elements *in vivo*. *J Gen Virol* **76**, 1709–17.

Neumann, G., Zobel, A. & Hobom, G. (1994) RNA polymerase I-mediated expression of influenza viral RNA molecules. *Virology* **202**, 477–9.

Odagiri, T. & Tashiro, M. (1997) Segment-specific noncoding sequences of the influenza virus genome RNA are involved in the specific competition between defective interfering RNA and its progenitor RNA segment at the virion assembly step. *J Virol* **71**, 2138–45.

Palese, P., Tobita, K., Ueda, M. & Compans, R.W. (1974) Characterization of temperature sensitive influenza virus mutants defective in neuraminidase. *Virology* **61**, 397–410.

Palese, P., Zheng, H., Engelhardt, O.G., Pleschka, S. & García-Sastre, A. (1996) Negative-strand RNA viruses: genetic engineering and applications. *Proc Natl Acad Sci USA* **93**, 11354–8.

Palese, P., Zavala, F., Muster, T., Nussenzweig, R.S. & García-Sastre, A. (1997) Development of novel influenza virus vaccines and vectors. *J Infect Dis* **176** (Suppl. 1): S45–9.

Parvin, J.D., Palese, P., Honda, A., Ishihama, A. & Krystal, M. (1989) Promoter analysis of influenza virus RNA polymerase. *J Virol* **63**, 5142–52.

Parkin, N.T., Chiu, P. & Coelinghi, K. (1997) Genetically engineered live attenuated influenza A virus vaccine candidates. *J Virol* **71**, 2772–8.

Percy, N., Barclay, W.S., García-Sastre, A. & Palese, P. (1994) Expression of a foreign protein by influenza A virus. *J Virol* **68**, 4486–92.

Pialoux, G., Excler, J.-L., Rivière, Y. *et al.* (1995) A prime-boost approach to HIV preventive vaccine using a recombinant canarypox virus expressing glycoprotein 160 (MN) followed by a recombinant glycoprotein 160 (MN/LAI). *Aids Res Hum Retrovir* **11**, 373–81.

Piccone, M.E., Fernandez-Sesma, A. & Palese, P. (1993) Mutational analysis of the influenza virus vRNA promoter. *Virus Res* **28**, 99–112.

Pleschka, S., Jaskunas, R., Engelhardt, O.G., Zürcher, T., Palese, P. & García-Sastre, A. (1996) A plasmid-based reverse genetics system for influenza A virus. *J Virol* **70**, 4188–92.

Pritlove, D.C., Fodor, E., Seong, B.L. & Brownlee, G.G. (1995) *In vitro* transcription and polymerase binding studies of the termini of influenza A virus cRNA: evidence for a cRNA panhandle. *J Gen Virol* **76**, 2205–13.

Radecke, F., Spielhofer, P., Schneider, H. *et al.* (1995) Rescue of measles virus from cloned DNA. *EMBO J* **14**, 5773–84.

Richardson, J.C. & Akkina, R.K. (1991) NS2 protein of influenza virus is found in purified virus and phosphorylated in infected cells. *Arch Virol* **116**, 69–80.

Rodrigues, M., Li, S., Murata, K, Rodrigues, D. *et al.* (1994) Influenza and vaccinia viruses expressing malaria CD8+ T and B cell epitopes. *J Immunol* **153**, 4636–48.

Rudenko, L.G., Slepushkin, A.N., Monto, A.S. *et al.* (1993) Efficacy of live attenuated and inactivated influenza vaccines in schoolchildren and their unvaccinated contacts in Novgorod, Russia. *J Infect Dis* **168**, 881–7.

Schnell, M.J., Mebatsion, T. & Conzelmann, K.-K. (1994) Infectious rabies viruses from cloned cDNA. *EMBO J.* **13**, 4195–4203.

Schulmann, J.L. & Palese, P. (1977) Virulence factors of influenza A virus. WSN virus neuraminidase required for plaque production in MDBK cells. *J Virol* **24**, 170–6.

Seong, B.L. & Brownlee, G.G. (1992a) A new method for reconstituting influenza polymerase and RNA *in vitro*: a study of the promoter elements for cRNA and vRNA synthesis *in vitro* and viral rescue *in vivo*. *Virology* **186**, 247–60.

Seong, B.L. & Brownlee, G.G. (1992b) Nucleotides 9–11 of the influenza A virion RNA promoter are crucial for activity *in vitro*. *J Gen Virol* **73**, 3115–24.

Smith, G.L. & Hay, A.L. (1982) Replication of the influenza virus genome. *Virology* **118**, 96–108.

Snyder, M.H., London, W.T., Maassab, H.F., Chanock, R.M. & Murphy, B.R. (1990) A 36 nucleotide deletion mutation in the coding region of the NS1 gene of an influenza A virus RNA segment 8 specifies a temperature-dependent host range phenotype. *Virus Res* **15**, 69–84.

Subbarao, E.K., Kawaoka, Y. & Murphy, B.R. (1993) Rescue of an influenza A virus wild-type PB2 gene and a mutant derivative bearing a site-specific temperature-sensitive and attenuating mutation. *J Virol* **67**, 7223–8.

Subbarao, E.K., Park, E.J., Lawson, C.M., Chen, A.Y. & Murphy, B.R. (1995) Sequential addition of temperature-sensitive missense mutations into the PB2 gene of influenza A transfectant virus can effect an increase in temperature sensitivity and attenuation and permits the rational design of a genetically engineered live influenza A virus vaccine. *J Virol* **69**, 5969–77.

Sugiura, A. & Ueda, M. (1979) Neurovirulence of influenza virus in mice. I. Neurovirulence of recombinants between virulent and avirulent strains. *Virology* **101**, 440–9.

Treanor, J.T., Buja, R. & Murphy, B.R. (1991) Intragenic suppression of a deletion mutation of the nonstructural gene of an influenza A virus. *J Virol* **65**, 4204–10.

Whelan, S.P.J., Ball, L.A., Barr, J.N. & Wertz, G.T.W. (1995) Efficient recovery of infectious vesicular stomatitis virus entirely from cDNA clones. *Proc Natl Acad Sci USA* **92**, 8388–92.

Wright, P.F., Johnson, P.R. & Karzon, D.T. (1986) In: *Options for the Control of Influenza*, pp. 243–53. Liss, New York.

Yamanaka, K., Ogasawara, N., Yoshikawa, H., Ishihama, A. & Nagata, K. (1991) *In vivo* analysis of the promoter structure of the influenza virus RNA genome using a transfection system with an engineered RNA. *Proc Natl Acad Sci USA* **88**, 5369–73.

Yasuda, J., Nakata, S., Kato, A., Toyoda, T. & Ishihama, A. (1993) Molecular assembly of influenza virus: association of the NS2 protein with virion matrix. *Virology* **196**, 249–55.

Yasuda, J., Bucher, D.J. & Ishihama, A. (1994) Growth control of influenza A virus by M1 protein: analysis of transfectant viruses carrying the chimeric M gene. *J Virol* **68**, 8141–6.

Zheng, H., Palese, P. & García-Sastre, A. (1996) Non-conserved nucleotides at the 3' and 5' ends of an influenza A virus RNA play an important role in viral replication. *Virology* **217**, 242–51.

Zürcher, T., Luo, G. & Palese, P. (1994) Mutations at palmitylation sites of the influenza virus haemagglutinin affect virus formation. *J Virol* **68**, 5748–54.

Section 3
Evolution and Ecology of Influenza Viruses

CHAPTER 10

Evolution and Ecology of Influenza Viruses: Interspecies Transmission

Robert G. Webster and William J. Bean Jr

The natural reservoirs of influenza A viruses are the aquatic birds of the world (Hinshaw & Webster 1982; Webster *et al.* 1992). Influenza B viruses are restricted to humans while influenza C viruses have been isolated from humans and pigs. Influenza-like viruses belonging to the genus *Thogoto*-like viruses have been isolated from ticks (Nuttall *et al.* 1995) and an unclassified influenza-like virus has been isolated from Atlantic salmon (Dannevig *et al.* 1995). This chapter concentrates on influenza A viruses.

Extensive surveillance of humans, lower animals and birds has revealed only one additional subtype of influenza A in the past 10 years, H15 (Röhm *et al.* 1996), suggesting that there may be a finite number of distinct influenza A viruses in nature. Each of the haemagglutinin (HA) subtypes of influenza A viruses are found in birds, three subtypes in humans (H1, H2, H3), two in pigs (H1, H3), and two in horses (H3, H7). Periodically, influenza viruses infect other species including sea mammals, mink, etc., but have not established stable lineages in these species.

Natural reservoirs

Influenza A viruses are ubiquitous in ducks and other aquatic birds throughout the world and have been isolated from waterfowl in Russia (Lvov & Zhdanov 1987), China (Shortridge 1982; Guo *et al.* 1983), Japan (Yamane *et al.* 1978), Europe (Hannoun & Devaux 1980; Ottis & Bachmann 1980), North America (Slemons *et al.* 1974; Hinshaw *et al.* 1978), and Australia (MacKenzie *et al.* 1984). Both wild and domestic ducks are infected and the available evidence is that different duck species are suscep-

tible. The full extent of different aquatic bird species that may serve as reservoirs of influenza viruses has not been resolved and potentially include all orders of aquatic birds. Members of the order Procellariiformes (shearwaters), Pelecaniformes (cormorants), Anseriformes (swans, geese, ducks), Galliformes (turkeys, quail), Ciconiiformes (herons, ibis), Gruiformes (rails, coots) and Charadriiformes (gulls, turnstones) all contain families from which influenza viruses have been isolated. Influenza viruses have irregularly been isolated from a very limited number of Passeriformes (starlings, myna), but have not been found in Columbiformes (pigeons), Psittaciformes (parrots) or other orders of birds.

The majority of studies on influenza in aquatic birds has been done on wild ducks. These studies establish that influenza viruses replicate preferentially in the cells lining the intestinal tract, cause no disease signs and are excreted in high concentrations in the faeces (up to $10^{8.7}$ 50% egg infectious doses/g) (Webster *et al.* 1978). Avian influenza viruses have been isolated from freshly deposited faecal material and from unconcentrated lake water. This information indicates that waterfowl have a very efficient way to transmit viruses, i.e. via faecal material in the water supply and up to 30% of juvenile ducks can be shedding influenza viruses prior to migration. The virus shedding continues during migration and serves to spread the viruses to domestic avian species by contamination of the water supply.

In wild ducks in the Northern Hemisphere, influenza viruses predominate in August and September. Juvenile birds are infected as they congregate in marshalling areas in Canada prior to migration, when up to 30% of birds hatched that year are shedding influenza viruses. This annual epidemic of influenza in wild ducks that causes no disease signs must affect the majority of juvenile birds. During southern migration from Canada the birds continue to shed virus, and by the time they reach the lower Mississippi in November the frequency falls to 1.6–2% (Webster *et al.* 1976), in December and January in Louisiana it falls to 0.4% (Stallknecht *et al.* 1990a). Samples collected from wild ducks as they arrive back in Canada after spring migration show a 0.25% isolation rate (R. Webster 1976, unpublished data), which is sufficient to indicate that influenza viruses are brought back by the ducks.

Longitudinal studies of wild ducks in Canada from 1976 to 1997 revealed the following: (i) a high percentage (up to 30%) of juvenile birds have influenza virus infection when the birds congregate before migration in July/August; (ii) none of the birds show any symptoms of infection; and (iii) multiple subtypes of influenza virus are enzootic. These and other studies established that all of the 15 HA and the nine known NA subtypes of influenza viruses are found in wild ducks.

The avirulent nature of avian influenza infection in ducks may be the result of adaptation to this host over many centuries, creating a reservoir that ensures perpetuation of the virus. This speculation strongly suggests that ducks occupy a unique and very important position in the natural history of influenza viruses. Influenza viruses of avian origin have been implicated in outbreaks of influenza in mammals such as seals (see Chapter 15) and pigs (see Chapter 13), as well as in domestic poultry, especially turkeys (see Chapter 12).

A systematic study of shorebirds and gulls at Delaware Bay on the east coast of the USA revealed that influenza A viruses are prevalent in spring (May and June; up to 30%) and autumn (September and October; up to 8%) (Kawaoka *et al.* 1988). Most of the different HA and neuraminidase (NA) subtypes have been isolated. The predominant subtypes of influenza viruses in these birds differ from those in ducks suggesting that the gene pool of influenza viruses in shorebirds and gulls is different from that in ducks.

The predominant subtype of influenza virus circulating in aquatic birds differs from flyway to flyway and from year to year. A comparison of prevalence rates for the HA and NA subtypes between Germany and North America show different patterns of dominance. In North America, H3, H4 and H6 were the predominant subtypes in wild ducks whereas in Europe, H1, H2 and H4 were the prevalent subtypes in these aquatic birds (Süss *et al.* 1994). Studies from 1976 to 1990 in North America established that H3, H4 or H6 and N2, N6 or N8 were present in wild ducks every year (Sharp *et al.* 1993). This information implies that species other than ducks serve as reservoirs for the remaining HA and NA subtypes of influenza viruses in North America. One possibility is that the H1 and H2 subtypes are perpetuated in ducks in Europe and they are periodically introduced into North America. Phylogenetic analysis does not support this idea for the North American and European influenza virus subtypes having evolved as separate lineages (see below). Thus, the actual reservoirs of the majority of influenza subtypes in nature has not yet been resolved.

The vast majority of influenza A viruses from aquatic birds are non-pathogenic. The exception is A/Tern/South Africa/61 (H5N3) that was isolated from an outbreak of disease in terns (Becker 1966). Among the 15 subtypes of influenza A virus, two (H5, H7) have the potential to become highly pathogenic in domestic avian species including chickens and turkeys. This acquisition of virulence is associated with mutations and insertion of basic amino acids in the HA (see Chapter 12). It is interesting to note that the H5 and H7 strains that are pathogenic in domestic chickens do not cause lethality in ducks. Thus, the A/Chicken/Pennsylvania/1370/83 (H5N2) virus that has 100% lethality in chickens causes no disease signs in ducks, again suggesting the unique position of ducks in the ecology of influenza A viruses.

How are influenza A viruses perpetuated in aquatic birds?

There is convincing evidence that all 15 subtypes of influenza A viruses are perpetuated in the aquatic bird population. There is no evidence that influenza viruses persist for extended periods in individual animals. This indicates that some mechanism has evolved for maintaining influenza viruses in aquatic birds.

The maintenance of influenza virus in the aquatic bird population differs from the maintenance of influenza virus in humans in that a larger number of susceptible juveniles are introduced yearly after spring hatching. After the annual autumn epidemic of influenza virus in juvenile ducks, it is unlikely that many remain uninfected. The majority of infected birds are presumably immune to reinfection with the predominant influenza subtype. This may influence the changes in the subtype predominating in a particular flyway from year to year.

Several possibilities have been suggested for the perpetuation of influenza viruses in the aquatic bird population of the world.

Continuous circulation in aquatic bird species

The detection of small numbers of influenza viruses in wild ducks throughout the winter months in North America and Japan, and detection of virus in ducks as they arrive back in Canada at the beginning of the breeding season, support this notion.

Circulation between different avian species

Since influenza viruses are prevalent in shorebirds in the spring and in wild ducks in the autumn, there may be transmission between these species. About half of the influenza viruses isolated from gulls and shorebirds will experimentally infect ducks (Kawaoka *et al.* 1990). However, sampling of shorebirds in Alberta, Canada, during August and September failed to reveal any influenza viruses in shorebirds and gulls when they were prevalent in ducks.

Preservation in water or ice

When wild ducks are present in August and September, influenza viruses can be isolated from lake water without concentration. It is possible that influenza viruses are preserved frozen in lake water and reinfect ducks in the spring. Tests of lake water in the winter and spring have so far failed to detect influenza viruses. The infectivity of influenza viruses in water is dependent on the virus strain tested and the salinity, pH and temperature of the water; at 17°C some strains remain infectious for longer times (Stallknecht *et al.* 1990b), raising the possibility of persistence of influenza virus in water when the ducks are absent.

Persistence in individual animals

Although virus shedding from the intestinal tract in some ducks can continue for up to 2–4 weeks, there is no evidence that continued shedding occurs.

Continuous circulation in subtropical and tropical regions

There is increasing evidence that in the tropical and subtropical regions of the world, influenza viruses of humans are isolated all year round (Reichelderfer *et al.* 1989), whereas in temperate climates, influenza is a winter disease and the virus is infrequently isolated in the summer months. Influenza viruses have been isolated all year round from domestic ducks in Hong Kong (Shortridge 1982). Although surveillance studies for influenza viruses in wild ducks and shorebirds have not been done in tropical regions, the possibility has to be considered that influenza virus perpetuation is in tropical regions of the world and that migrating aquatic birds transport viruses from the tropical regions to the temperate regions during spring migration.

At this time the most convincing data support the first alternative, i.e. that there is continuous circulation of influenza viruses in wild ducks or other aquatic birds with very low levels of detectable virus while the birds are in their overwintering sites in the subtropics.

Interspecies transmission

Periodically influenza viruses in the aquatic bird reservoir transmit to swine, horses, domestic poultry and sea mammals (Webster *et al.* 1992) and cause infections that vary in severity from inapparent to severe with major disease outbreaks. In lower animals the entire virus is more often transmitted to the new host. Here we will consider a number of examples.

Interspecies transmission to lower animals and birds

In March 1989, a severe outbreak of respiratory diseases occurred in horses in the Jilin and Heilongjiang provinces of north-east China (Guo *et al.* 1990). Morbidity was 81% and mortality was as high as 20% in some herds. A second outbreak occurred in April 1990 in the Heilongjiang province with 41% morbidity and no mortality. Both outbreaks were caused by influenza viruses of the H3N8 subtype that were antigenically distinguishable from the prototype A/Equine/Miami/1/63 (H3N8) strain (Guo *et al.* 1992).

Serological studies done on acute and convalescent horse sera indicated that this H3N8 influenza virus was not present in China before 1989. Antigenic and sequence analyses along with phylogenetic evidence of the influenza viruses isolated from horses in north-east China in 1989 and 1990 suggest that these viruses were of avian origin. The viruses were antigenically most closely related to H3 viruses of avian origin. Direct comparison of the nucleotide sequences of all eight influenza A virus genes against a wide array of isolates showed that all of the eight genes of the A/Eq/Jilin/89 (H3N8) are similar to those of avian viruses. Phylogenetic analyses of the eight genes of Eq/Jilin/89 showed that they are not derived from the currently circulating equine 2 (H3N8) viruses. It is not known if this H3N8 influenza virus has become established in horses in China.

A second example of emergence of an influenza virus from the aquatic birds reservoir was the appearance of a highly pathogenic H5N2 influenza virus in domestic chickens in Mexico (Horimoto *et al.* 1995). In October of 1993, there was decreased egg production and increased mortality among Mexican chickens, in association with serological evidence of an H5N2 influenza virus. First isolated from chickens in May of 1994, after spreading widely in the country, the virus caused a mild respiratory syndrome in specific-pathogen free chickens. Within months the H5N2 virus became lethal in poultry. Phylogenetic analysis of the HA of H5 avian influenza viruses, including the Mexican isolates, indicated that the epidemic virus had originated from the introduction of a single virus of the North American lineage into Mexican chickens. This sequence of events demonstrates the stepwise acquisition of virulence by an avian influenza virus in nature.

A third example is the introduction of avian influenza viruses into pigs in Europe and is dealt with in Chapter 13.

Additionally, studies on the interspecies transmission of influenza viruses in Hong Kong in 1993 established that two different groups of H1N1 viruses were cocirculating among pigs that originated in southern China. One group belonged to the classic swine lineage, and the other to the Eurasian avian lineage. These studies showed that an avian influenza virus containing all gene segments from the avian reservoir had spread to pigs in southern China (Guan *et al.* 1996). Phylogenetic analysis indicates that the genes of the avian influenza H1N1 viruses form an Asian sublineage of the Eurasian avian lineage, suggesting that these viruses are an independent introduction into pigs in Asia. It remains to be determined whether these avian H1N1 viruses will become established in the pig population of Asia.

The available evidence indicates that the pig may be the mixing vessel for reassortment of human and avian influenza viruses. The infrequent transmission of avian influenza viruses to pigs may be the initial limiting step in interspecies transmission to humans. The establishment and spread of these viruses in pigs also appears to be limiting. A remaining question is whether subtypes other than H1N1 will transmit from the avian reservoir to pigs.

Interspecies transmission to humans

The available evidence indicates that the pandemics of human influenza of this century originated from the Eurasian avian lineage and transmitted via the pig to humans after reassorting with the currently circulating human strain. It is now known that swine influenza viruses (H1N1 and H3N2) transfer relatively frequently to humans. However, in 1977 when one of five soldiers at Fort Dix died of swine influenza, a national vaccine programme was initiated (Top & Russell 1977). It is now recognized that the majority of transfers of influenza virus from pigs to humans are benign and cause no disease signs in humans, but in the immunosuppressed and in pregnant women there are occasional fatalities (Rota *et al.* 1989). The critical issue is the ability to transmit from human to human and to date these viruses lack this property.

Epidemiological evidence supports the proposition that the Asian/57 (H2N2), Hong Kong/68 (H3N2) and the Russian/77 (H1N1) influenza pandemic strains all originated from China. Phylogenetic studies suggest that the catastrophic 'Spanish' influenza of 1918 may also be of Eurasian origin (Gorman *et al.* 1991) and raises the question of whether the precursors of this disastrous outbreak was of American or Asian origin. The phylogenetic evidence suggests that a totally new H1N1 virus of avian origin (not a reassortant) could have transmitted to humans from pigs. Since the high mortality associated with the catastrophic 1918 epidemic occurred in the second year of spread of this virus (Crosby 1976), it is possible that this virus originated in Asia and spread to North America before it acquired the property of high lethality in humans. Partial sequencing of four gene segments of influenza virus from an archival lung sample from a soldier who died in 1918 reveals that the virus is genetically similar to swine influenza viruses (Taubenberger *et al.* 1997). The virus did not possess a series of basic amino acids at the cleavage site of the HA and the reason for high virulence remains unresolved.

Both the Asian/57 (H2N2) and Hong Kong/68 (H3N2) pandemics originated by reassortment. In 1957 the Asian pandemic virus acquired three gene segments (PB1, HA and NA) from the avian influenza gene pool in wild ducks by genetic reassortment and kept five other genes from the circulating human strain (Kawaoka *et al.* 1989)

(Fig. 10.1). After the Asian strain appeared, the H1N1 strains disappeared from humans. In 1968 the Hong Kong pandemic virus acquired two genes (PB1 and HA) from the duck reservoir by reassortment and kept six genes from the virus circulating in humans.

The origin of the H1N1 Russian 1977 influenza virus is a mystery. This virus appeared in Anshan, northern China, in May of 1977 and subsequently spread to the rest of the world; it is identical in all genes to the virus that caused a human influenza epidemic in 1950 (Nakajima *et al.* 1978). Where was this virus for 27 years? The possible explanations include preservation in a frozen state, preservation in an animal reservoir, or retention in an integrated, as yet undetected form in the genetic material of a human or lower animal. The animal reservoir option is unlikely, for the accumulation of mutations would have continued. There is no evidence for integration of influenza genetic material into the host genome, leaving the most likely explanation that in 1977 the H1N1 virus was reintroduced to humans from a frozen source. It is possible that the re-emergence of this virus represents an escape from a laboratory.

Selective pressures affecting the evolution of influenza viruses in different hosts

The selective pressures that influence the evolution of the influenza viruses are the same ones that drive the evolution of any virus. For long-term survival, any virus must maintain the ability to transmit to new susceptible hosts in competition with other viruses. The unique structure and adaptability of the influenza viruses have, however, provided mechanisms for both long-term and short-term survival in diverse hosts with remarkably different disease forms and transmission modes. These differences in ecology correlate with remarkable differences in the evolutionary patterns seen in the different hosts. In addition, the individual viral RNA genome segments follow largely independent evolutionary paths due to their ability to reassort and the differing selective pressures affecting them.

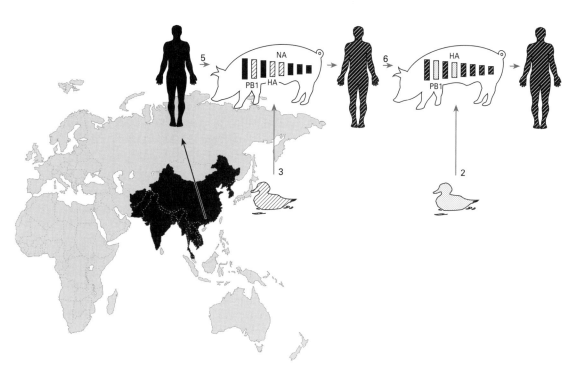

Fig. 10.1 Postulated evolution of recent human pandemic influenza viruses. The Asian/57 (H2N2) and Hong Kong/ 68 (H3N2) originated in Asia. Phylogenetic studies indicate that the Asian/57 (H2N2) influenza virus obtained five gene segments from the influenza virus circulating in humans and three gene segments (PB1, HA, NA) from a Eurasian avian influenza virus. It is postulated that reassortment occurred in the pig and that the reassortant transmitted to humans. Similarly, the Hong Kong/68 (H3N2) pandemic virus obtained six gene segments from the Asian/57 virus circulating in humans and two gene segments (PB1 and HA) from a Eurasian avian influenza virus; reassortment is postulated to have occurred in pigs.

Differences in the evolution patterns of the influenza virus genes in birds and mammals

As discussed previously, waterfowl and other birds are believed to be the primary host for all of the influenza A virus strains that have been introduced into mammals. Multiple examples of each of the genome segments of influenza virus isolates from various waterfowl species as well as those of virus isolated from mammals, have been sequenced and analysed to determine their evolutionary relationships. For each of the genome segments, multiple coexisting lineages of viruses infecting waterfowl have been found. These lineages include those specific for geographical regions, those found in North America typically being distinct from those of Eurasia. The genome segments from certain viruses of gulls also form their own lineages and have apparently diverged from those infecting other birds after becoming adapted to their specific host. Simplified phylogenetic trees for the genome segments coding for the internal and non-structural virus proteins, and for two representatives of the HA genes, are shown in Fig. 10.2.

The influenza viruses isolated from mammals are of two classes: (i) those that are closely related to avian virus and appear to have been only transiently established in the mammalian host; and (ii) those that have become established in a mammalian

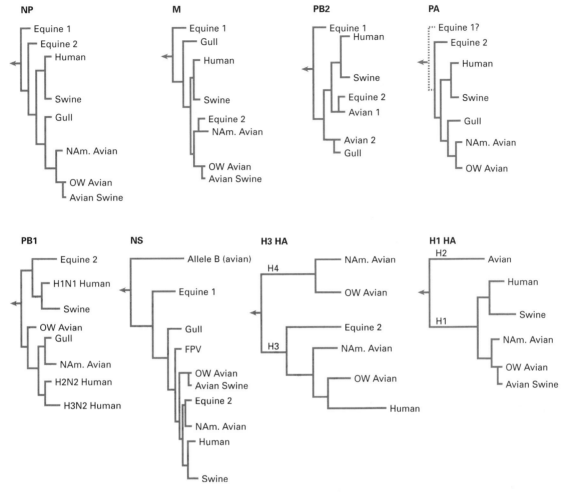

Fig. 10.2 Generalized phylogenies (cladograms) of influenza virus genes. Nucleotide phylogenies represented are taken from the references given in Webster *et al.* 1992. Phylogenies were determined with PAUP software version 2.4 (David Swofford, Illinois Natural History Survey), which uses a maximum-parsimony algorithm to find the shortest trees. The horizontal distance is proportional to the minimum number of nucleotide differences needed to join the gene sequences (no scale is given). Vertical lines are used for spacing branches and labels. The arrow at the left of each tree represents the node connecting the influenza B virus homologue. Equine 1 is represented by the Eq/Prague/56 (H7N7) virus isolate. Equine 2 is represented by recent H3N8 equine viruses. Unless noted otherwise, human represents human H1N1, H2N2 and H3N2 viruses; Swine, classic swine viruses (i.e. those related to Sw/Iowa/15/30); Gull, H13 gull viruses; FPV, fowl plague viruses; NAm. Avian, North American avian viruses; OW Avian, Old World or Eurasian avian viruses; Avian Swine, avian-like H1N1 swine viruses. There are two distinct avian lineages in the PB2 tree, Avian 1 and Avian 2, which contain Eurasian and North American avian viruses, respectively. (From Webster *et al.* 1992, with permission from American Society for Microbiology.)

host and have diverged progressively from the avian virus ancestor.

The established mammalian virus lineages include those isolated from horses, swine and humans. Each of the mammalian virus lineages

shows a progressive accumulation of mutations and a good correlation of its date of isolation and its position on its respective branch of the phylogenetic tree (Fig. 10.3). This consistent relationship is not seen among the avian viruses and if there is a

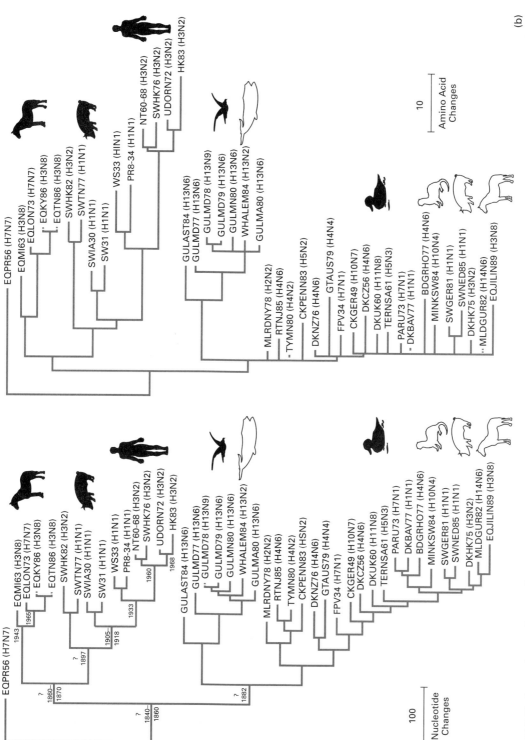

(a)

(b)

Fig. 10.3 Phylogenetic trees for 41 influenza A virus nucleoprotein genes rooted to influenza B virus nucleoprotein (B/Lee/40). (a) Nucleotide tree. Horizontal distance is proportional to the minimum number of nucleotide differences to join nodes and nucleoprotein sequences. Vertical lines are for spacing branches and labels. Animal symbols (black) denote the five host-specific lineages. Animal symbols (white) denote viruses in that lineage that have transmitted to other hosts. (b) Amino acid tree. A table of abbreviations for virus isolates shown in these trees may be found in Gorman *et al.* 1990, with permission from American Society for Microbiology.)

progressive accumulation of mutations in avian viruses with time, the time frame must be greater than the period covered by the available virus isolates.

Genome segments maintained in the avian reservoir appear to be in evolutionary stasis

The evolutionary stability of the genome RNAs of the avian viruses is shown in Fig. 9.3. In this diagram, the phylogenetic relationships were calculated from the nucleic acid sequences of the nucleoprotein gene, but the distances shown represent amino acid changes. The remarkable lack of amino acid changes among the viruses isolated from waterfowl is clearly evidence suggesting that these virus genes in the avian host are subject to stringent stabilizing selection. This conservation of phenotype (evolutionary stasis) suggests that the virus and host have reached a long established adaptive optimum and any change in the coding sequence of the RNA is likely to be deleterious.

Introduction of the virus into a mammalian host leads to a rapid, progressive accumulation of mutational changes

The striking difference in the evolutionary patterns of avian and mammalian influenza viruses are exemplified in the evolutionary relationships of the H3 and H4 HA genes (Bean *et al*. 1992). After introduction of the H3 HA gene into humans, there was rapid progressive evolution of the gene which contrasts with much slower evolution in avian species.

Additionally, most of the coding changes in the avian lineages have occurred in the terminal branches, while in the mammalian lineages the terminal and internal branches have similar ratios of coding and non-coding changes (Bean *et al*. 1992). This suggests fundamental differences in the evolution of the avian and mammalian viruses. While the mammalian virus hosts continuously select for new phenotypes, and consequently repeatedly eliminates their predecessors, the long-term survival of

the avian viruses appears to favour those that have not changed, and selection is primarily negative. As with the nucleoprotein gene described above, this conservation of phenotype probably reflects a long-established adaptive optimum for the virus HA in the avian host. The very close relationship between the first H3 HA genes in humans and some of the Eurasian avian viruses, clearly indicates its origin and suggests that only a few changes were required for its adaptation to humans.

In contrast, the H3 equine viruses have no known close relatives so their origin cannot be accurately placed. However, like the human H3 gene it also has shown a continuous accumulation of mutations with time.

The accumulation of mutations in the HA gene of human and equine viruses is undoubtedly driven by antibody pressure which, as discussed above, is largely absent in the waterfowl population. However, the internal proteins also have a dramatically increased mutation rate in humans and other mammals when compared to that in waterfowl. One possibility is that selection on the HA protein results in the periodic fixing of random mutations in non-selected genes resulting in the observed accumulation of mutations. Such an accumulation of mutations would be expected to lead to a decrease in fitness of the virus. Shu *et al*. (1993) has shown that the human influenza A virus nucleoprotein genes have been accumulating mutations at an essentially constant rate for more than 50 years, during which time there has been no observed decrease in fitness.

The apparent low rate of nucleotide substitutions in the avian influenza viruses and the lack of strong positive selection, may provide an explanation for the continued survival of multiple lineages of avian viruses and for their stability. If long-term survival favours those that have not changed, then virus populations in environments that undergo relatively few replication cycles would be more likely to yield progeny that do not have deleterious mutations. Those replicating in other environments or mutants in the original population might have a temporary selective advantage in a particular host or environment, but the accumulation of mutations in these subpopulations would be deleterious in other circumstances. Thus, the original population (perhaps often in a very small minority) would have a selective advantage as hosts or environmental conditions change.

Conclusion and outlook

With the realization that a future pandemic of influenza in humans is inevitable and perhaps imminent, we can look at what we know about the ecology and evolution of influenza viruses and utilize this in our planning for this event. Phylogenetic analysis of influenza viruses have revealed (i) all mammalian lineages originate from influenza viruses in aquatic birds; (ii) there is geographical separation of avian influenza virus lineages into Eurasian and American; (iii) influenza virus in their aquatic bird reservoir are in evolutionary stasis; (iv) after transfer to mammals there is rapid evolution; and (v) the human pandemics of this century have mainly occurred in South-East Asia and involves reassortment. This process probably occurs in pigs, for they possess receptors for both avian and human influenza viruses. Prediction of the subtype is not possible but there is a hypothesis based on seroarcheology that only H1, H2 and H3 subtypes can infect humans. This idea may be an oversimplification for the circulation of H7 influenza viruses in horses and the periodic transmission and infection of mammals (seals, mink) with H7 and other subtypes, gives no assurance that H2 will be the next predicted subtype.

Given the existence in the aquatic bird reservoir of all known influenza A subtypes, we must accept the fact that influenza is not an eradicable disease. Prevention and control are the only realistic goals. If we assume that people, pigs and aquatic birds are the principal variables associated with the interspecies transfer of influenza virus and the emergence of new human pandemic strains, it is important to maintain surveillance in these species. Live-bird markets that house a wide variety of avian species together (chickens, ducks, turkeys, pheasants, guinea fowl and occasionally pigs) for sale directly to the public provide outstanding conditions for genetic mixing and spreading of influenza viruses; monitoring of the birds in these

markets for influenza viruses will provide information that is relevant for both agricultural and human health. If pigs are the mixing vessel for influenza viruses, surveillance of influenza in this population may provide an early warning system for humans.

Acknowledgements

We thank Dayna Baker for manuscript preparation. This work was supported by Public Health Service research grant AI-29680 and AI-08831 from the National Institutes of Health CORE grant CA-21765 and American Lebanese Syrian Associated Charities (ALSAC).

References

Bean, W.J., Schell, M., Katz, J. *et al.* (1992) Evolution of the H3 influenza virus haemagglutinin from human and non-human hosts. *J Virol* **66**, 1129–38.

Becker, W.B. (1966) The isolation and classification of tern virus: influenza virus A/Tern/South Africa/61. *J Hygiene* **64**, 309–20.

Crosby, A.W. (1976) Flu and the American expeditionary force. In: *Epidemic and Peace 1918*, pp. 145–70. Greenwood Press, Westport, CT.

Dannevig, B.H., Falk, K. & Namork, E. (1995) Isolation of the casual virus of infectious salmon anaemia (ISA) in a long-term cell line from Atlantic salmon head kidney. *J Gen Virol* **76**, 1353–9.

Gorman, O.T., Bean, W.J., Kawaoka, Y., Donatelli, I., Guo, Y. & Webster, R.G. (1991) Evolution of influenza A virus nucleoprotein genes: implications for the origin of H1N1 human and classical swine viruses. *J Virol* **65**, 3704–14.

Guan, Y., Shortridge, K.F., Krauss, S., Li, P.H., Kawaoka, Y. & Webster, R.G. (1996) Emergence of avian H1N1 influenza viruses in pigs in China. *J Virol* **70**, 8041–6.

Guo, Y., Guo, Z., Pan, X., Guo, C., Wang, M. & Lu, X. (1990) Etiologic and seroepidemiology surveys of an equine influenza epidemic in North-east China. *Chin J Exp Clin Virol* **3**, 318–22.

Guo, Y., Min, W., Fengen, J., Ping, W. & Jiming, Z. (1983) Influenza ecology in China. In: Laver, W.G. (ed.) *The Origin of Pandemic Influenza Viruses*, pp. 211–23. Elsevier, New York.

Guo, Y., Wang, M., Kawaoka, Y., Gorman, O., Ito, T. & Saito, T. (1992) Characterization of a new avian-like influenza A virus from horses in China. *Virology* **188**, 245–55.

Hannoun, C. & Devaux, J.M. (1980) Circulation enzootique permanente de virus grippaux dans la baie de la Somme. *Comp Immunol Microbiol Infect Dis* **3**, 177–83.

Hinshaw, V.S. & Webster, R.G. (1982) The natural history of influenza A viruses. In: Beare, A.S. (ed.) *Basic and Applied Influenza Research*, pp. 79–104. CRC Press, Boca Raton.

Hinshaw, V.S., Webster, R.G. & Turner, B. (1978) Novel influenza A viruses isolated from Canadian feral ducks: including strains antigenically related to swine influenza (Hsw1N1) viruses. *J Gen Virol* **41**, 115–27.

Horimoto, T., Rivera, E., Pearson, J. *et al.* (1995) Origin and molecular changes associated with emergence of a highly pathogenic H5N2 influenza virus in Mexico. *Virology* **213**, 223–30.

Kawaoka, Y., Chambers, T.M., Sladen, W.L. & Webster, R.G. (1988) Is the gene pool of influenza viruses in shorebirds and gulls different from that in wild ducks? *Virology* **163**, 247–50.

Kawaoka, Y., Krauss, S. & Webster, R.G. (1989) Avian-to-human transmission of the PB1 gene of influenza A virus in the 1957 and 1968 pandemics. *J Virol* **63**, 4603–8.

Kawaoka, Y., Yamnikova, S., Chambers, T.M., Lvov, D.K. & Webster, R.G. (1990) Molecular characterization of a new haemagglutinin, subtype H14, of influenza A virus. *Virology* **179**, 759–67.

Lvov, D.K. & Zhdanov, V.M. (1987) Circulation of influenza virus genes in the biosphere. *Sov Med Rev Virol* **1**, 129–52.

Mackenzie, J.S., Edwards, E.C., Holmes, R.M. & Hinshaw, V.S. (1984) Isolation of ortho- and paramyxoviruses from wild birds in Western Australia, and the characterization of novel influenza A viruses. *Aust J Exp Biol Med Sci* **62**, 89–99.

Nakajima, K., Desselberger, U. & Palese, P. (1978) Recent human influenza A (H1N1) viruses are closely related genetically to strains isolated in 1950. *Nature (London)* **274**, 334–9.

Nuttall, P.A., Morse, M.A., Jones, L.D. & Portela, A. (1995) Adaptation of members of the Orthomyxoviridae family to transmission by ticks. In: Gibbs, A.J., Calisher, C.H. & Garcia-Arenal, F. (eds) *Molecular Basis of Virus Evolution*, pp. 416–25. Cambridge University Press, London.

Ottis, K. & Bachmann, P.A. (1980) Occurrence of Hsw 1N1 subtype influenza A viruses in wild ducks in Europe. *Arch Virol* **63**, 185–90.

Reichelderfer, P.S., Kendal, A.P., Shortridge, K.F. *et al.* (1989) Influenza surveillance in the Pacific Basin. Seasonality of virus occurrence: a preliminary report. In: Doraisingham, S., Ling, A.E. & Chan, Y.C. (eds) *Current Topics in Medical Virology*, pp. 412–38. World Scientific, Singapore.

Röhm, C., Zhou, N., Süss, J., Mackenzie, J. & Webster, R.G. (1996) Characterization of a novel influenza haemagglutinin, H15: criteria for determination of influenza A subtypes. *Virology* **217**, 508–16.

Rota, P.A., Rocha, E.P., Harmon, M.W. *et al.* (1989) Laboratory characterization of a swine influenza virus isolated from a fatal case of human influenza. *J Clin Microbiol* **27**, 1413–16.

Sharp, G.B., Kawaoka, Y., Wright, S.M., Turner, B., Hinshaw, V. & Webster, R.G. (1993) Wild ducks are the reservoir for only a limited number of influenza A subtypes. *Epidemiol Infect* **110**, 161–76.

Shortridge, K.F. (1982) Avian influenza A viruses of southern China and Hong Kong ecological aspects and implications for man. *Bull WHO* **60**, 129–35.

Shu, L., Bean, W.J. & Webster, R.G. (1993) Evolution of the human influenza A virus nucleoprotein from 1933 to 1988. *J Virol* **67**, 2723–9.

Slemons, R.D., Johnson, D.C., Osborn, J.S. & Hayes, F. (1974) Type A influenza viruses isolated from wild free-flying ducks in California. *Avian Dis* **18**, 119–25.

Stallknecht, D.E., Shane, S.M., Kearney, M.T. & Zwank, P.J. (1990b) Persistence of avian influenza viruses in water. *Avian Dis* **34**, 406–11.

Stallknecht, D.E., Shane, S.M., Zwank, P.J., Senne, D.A. & Kearney, M.T. (1990a) Avian influenza viruses from migratory and resident ducks of coastal Louisiana. *Avian Dis* **34**, 398–405.

Süss, J., Schäfer, J., Sinnecker, H. & Webster, R.G. (1994) Influenza virus subtypes in aquatic birds of eastern Germany. *Arch Virol* **135**, 101–14.

Taubenberger, J.K., Reid, A.H., Krafft, A.E., Bijwaard, K.E. & Fanning, T.G. (1997) Initial genetic characterization of the 1918 'Spanish' influenza virus. *Science* **275**, 1793–6.

Top, F.H. Jr & Russell, P.K. (1977) Swine influenza A at Fort Dix, New Jersey (January–February 1967). IV. Summary and speculation. *J Infect Dis* **136**, S376–80.

Webster, R.G., Morita, M., Pridgen, C. & Tumova, B. (1976) Ortho- and paramyxoviruses from migrating feral ducks: characterization of a new group of influenza A viruses. *J Gen Virol* **32**, 217–25.

Webster, R.G., Yakhno, M.A., Hinshaw, V.S., Bean, W.J. & Murti, K.G. (1978) Intestinal influenza: replication and characterization of influenza viruses in ducks. *Virology* **84**, 268–78.

Webster, R.G., Bean, W.J., Gorman, O.T., Chambers, T.M. & Kawaoka, Y. (1992) Evolution and ecology of influenza A viruses. *Microbiol Rev* **56**, 152–79.

Yamane, N., Odagisi, T. & Arikawa, J. (1978) Isolation of orthomyxoviruses from migrating and domestic ducks in Northern Japan in 1976–79. *Jpn J Med Sci Biol* **31**, 407–15.

CHAPTER 11

Genetic Reassortment of Human Influenza Viruses in Nature

Christoph Scholtissek

The human influenza A viruses existing today have emerged from an avian influenza A virus ancestor from about 100 years ago (Gammelin *et al.* 1990; Gorman *et al.* 1990; see also Chapters 10 and 12). However, influenza virus pandemics existing long before that time have been described. Therefore, it has been suggested that crossing the species barrier of influenza A viruses from birds to humans might occur from time to time as a rare event. Each time an avian virus arrives in a mammalian species and forms a stable lineage, it comes under a strong selection pressure to change so that centuries later reassortment of the segmented genome of such an ancient virus with that of a more recent isolate might not be compatible any more. Correspondingly, the human influenza B and C types seem to be such survivors although derived originally from an avian influenza A virus ancestor a long time ago (Gammelin *et al.* 1990). Individual genes of influenza A viruses might have quite different 'ages'. Thus, of the 15 haemagglutinin (HA) subtypes which have emerged and survived (Röhm *et al.* 1996), only three were found with human influenza A viruses. Similarly, of the nine different neuraminidase (NA) subtypes isolated up to now, only two are from human viruses (Schild *et al.* 1980). Of the non-structural (NS) protein genes two different 'alleles' were described (Scholtissek & von Hoyningen-Huene 1980; Treanor *et al.* 1989; Ludwig *et al.* 1991). So far only one has been found in human influenza A viruses. All these genes can reassort freely in nature if an organism becomes infected simultaneously with two such influenza A viruses.

Such subtypes have not been discerned within influenza B and C viruses, respectively. Only by more sensitive methods such as sequencing, etc., can different lineages be recognized. These two latter virus types do not have a significant animal reservoir from which individual genes might be introduced by reassortment. Thus, natural reassortment within the types B and C, respectively, is almost completely restricted to double infections of humans.

This chapter describes how far genetic reassortment between human influenza viruses occurs in nature and how far this reassortment contributes to genetic diversity.

Influenza A viruses

H1N1 viruses with internal genes of H3N2 strains

Historically three major influenza A virus subtypes have circulated in the human population; in the last decade of the 19th century an H2N2 virus and in the first decade of this century an H3 virus (which possibly had a N8 NA) were involved in epidemics. These data were obtained by serological 'archaeology'. From about 1910 until 1957 H1N1 viruses prevailed and were replaced by an H2N2 virus in 1957. In 1968 this subtype combination was substituted again by an H3N2 virus (Kilbourne 1987). While the H1N1 virus was introduced from an avian reservoir without reassortment (Gammelin *et al.* 1990; Gorman *et al.* 1990), the replacement in 1957 and 1968 were antigenic shifts in which only three or two genes, respectively, were replaced by reassortment with an avian influenza A virus (Scholtissek *et al.* 1978a; Kawaoka *et al.* 1989). In 1977 there was a re-emergence of an H1N1 virus which had already circulated in the human population in 1950 (Kendal *et al.* 1978; Nakajima *et al.* 1978; Scholtissek *et al.* 1978b). It is still an enigma how this virus from 1950 remained almost unchanged for about 27 years (Young *et al.* 1979; Buonagurio *et al.* 1986b). After the reintroduction of the H1N1 virus in 1977 the H3N2 subtype continued to circulate until the present day. Thus, since 1977 we have the unusual situation of cocirculation of two subtypes in the human population. Therefore it was not too surprising when both H3N2 and H1N1 viruses were isolated from a single person (Kendal *et al.* 1979). Such double infections of humans can create reassortants which have occurred and which have indeed caused epidemics. They have been isolated from humans in various influenza seasons in different years and different geographical regions, mainly between 1978 and 1981. In all these reassortants the genes for the surface antigens, the M and NS genes, were derived from the H1N1 parent, while the genes of the nucleocapsid were partially or, in most isolates, totally taken over from the H3N2 parent (Young *et al.* 1979; Bean *et al.* 1980; Nakajima *et al.* 1981; Cox *et al.* 1983; Xu *et al.* 1993a). Non-reassorted H1N1 viruses have always cocirculated during that time. After 1981 isolation of reasorted H1N1 viruses became seldom, the last one was found in 1988 (Cox *et al.* 1989; Xu *et al.* 1993b). At no time were corresponding reassorted human H3N2 viruses isolated.

There was no significant difference in the severity of epidemics or difference in the pathogenicity of naturally occurring reassortant and non-reassortant H1N1 viruses (Xu *et al.* 1993a). There is evidence of various independent formations and introductions of such reassortant H1N1 viruses, however, these reassortants did not establish stable lineages. Thus, although reassortment of this kind contributes to genetic diversity, the reassortants so far have no advantage over the non-reassortant parent H1N1 or H3N2 viruses, respectively.

Human H1N2 reassortant viruses

H1N2 reassortants with an NA derived from human H3N2 viruses were first isolated from pigs in 1978, 1980 and 1989/90 in Japan carrying the H1

from classical swine virus (Sugimura *et al.* 1980; Nerome *et al.* 1983, 1985; Yasuhara *et al.* 1983; Ouchi *et al.* 1996). Similar reassortants were obtained in France in 1987 and 1988. However, these reassortants contained an H1 of the avian-like swine virus circulating in northern Europe at that time (Gourreau *et al.* 1994; see also Chapter 13).

Between December 1988 and March 1989, 19 human isolates of H1N2 influenza A virus were isolated from sporadic cases in six Chinese cities (Guo *et al.* 1990). A genetic analysis revealed that only the HA gene was derived from the prevailing human H1N1 virus, while all the other genes, including the NA gene, were introduced from the prevailing human H3N2 strain (Guo *et al.* 1992; Li *et al.* 1992). Up to now such reassortants were isolated only in China in one influenza season and they did not spread further to other countries. These isolates also do not seem to have an advantage over the cocirculating parent viruses.

It is assumed that the H1N2 reassortants were created during double infection of humans by the two parent strains. However, since pigs are regarded to function, specifically in the region of southern China, as 'mixing vessels' for the creation of new human reassortant viruses (for a review see Scholtissek 1990), it cannot be excluded that H1N2 reassortants might have emerged first in pigs, possibly by some kind of backcross, and from there they could have been reintroduced into humans.

Artificial vaccine reassortants in humans and camels

Although the reassortants of human influenza A viruses (H1N1) were produced artificially in the laboratory in the former Leningrad in order to be used as killed vaccine in the human population, they will be described here because they seem to play a significant role in Middle Asia.

Reassortants between the human A/PR/8/34 (H1N1) and A/USSR/90/77 (H1N1) viruses were prepared in Leningrad and were used as ultraviolet (UV) light inactivated vaccine in Mongolia in 1978/ 79. After administration of these vaccines several children became sick with typical symptoms of influenza. Thereafter during various influenza seasons H1N1 viruses were isolated. Four such isolates were analysed genetically. Three of them turned out to be derived from this vaccine reassortant strain. Two of them even carried the HA of the PR8 strain. Since 12% of convalescent sera collected between 1985 and 1994 in different places in Mongolia from more than 200 mainly young patients contained HA-inhibiting antibodies against the PR8 strain, laboratory contaminations can be fairly well excluded (Anchlan *et al.* 1996).

Furthermore, between 1979 and 1983 13 H1N1 influenza A isolates were obtained from diseased camels in different locations in Mongolia. The genetic analyses of several of them demonstrated that these isolates were also almost identical with the vaccine strain prepared in Leningrad in 1978 and used in the Mongolian population in Ulaan-baatar. Experimental infection of camels with these isolates led to typical symptoms of influenza. This is remarkable in so far as ruminants normally do not range among natural hosts for influenza A viruses (Yamnikova *et al.* 1993). Thus, we have to assume that from the UV light inactivated vaccine live reassortants were created by multiplicity reactivation, which spread first in the human Mongolian population and purely by accident also had the capacity to infect camels and cause severe epizootics in this new host (Yamnikova *et al.* 1993).

Reassortment among influenza B viruses

Influenza B viruses are different from A viruses in so far as there is no animal reservoir of these B viruses (Kilbourne 1987). Influenza B viruses were introduced into the human population much earlier than influenza A viruses, possibly also from an avian influenza A ancestor (Gammelin *et al.* 1990). Therefore the former viruses are adapted to humans much better than the human A viruses and correspondingly their mutational and evolutionary rates to change are only about half of those of influenza A viruses (Yamashita *et al.* 1988; Kanegae *et al.* 1990; Cox & Bender 1995). Although influenza B viruses have not been divided into subtypes by serological means (in spite of the fact that there are clear differences among strains) it is known that

such 'subtypes', as defined by the level of significant differences in sequence of various genes, can cocirculate at the same time in the same geographical region (see Fig. 11.1b; Yamashita *et al.* 1988; Kanagae *et al.* 1990; Rota *et al.* 1990, 1992; Kinnunen *et al.* 1992). Thus, during the influenza season of 1988/89 all influenza B viruses isolated in the USA were related to the prototype B/Victoria/2/87, while in Asia this virus cocirculated with B/Yamagata/16/88-like viruses (Rota *et al.* 1990). In the 1990/91 season the Yamagata-like B viruses predominated worldwide (Rota *et al.* 1992).

When relatively easy techniques also became available to analyse other genes routinely, reassortants between these two independent lineages were discovered (Xu *et al.* 1993a). These reassortant strains seem not to have any advantage over their parent viruses since they do not seem to form their own lineage (Xu *et al.* 1993a; Cox & Bender 1995).

Reassortment among influenza C viruses

Influenza C viruses are different from influenza A and B viruses in that their RNA genome consists of seven segments. The properties of the two glyco-

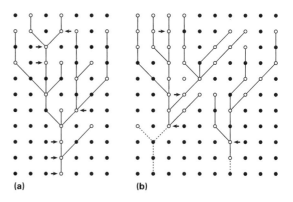

Fig. 11.1 (a) Model topology of influenza A (H3N2) haemagglutinin evolution. (b) Model topology of influenza B haemagglutinin evolution from 1985 to 1995. Open circles represent known intermediates. Closed circles represent hypothetical intermediates. Distances between virus isolates do not describe nucleotide differences. Dotted lines represent hypothetical pathway. Only vaccine strains are identified by arrows. (From Cox & Bender 1995, with permission from Academic Press.)

proteins of the latter two viruses are combined in the one surface glycoprotein, which has both hae-magglutinating and enzymatic activities (HE). The receptor-destroying enzyme is an esterase with a different specificity as NA. The influenza C type is not divided into immunologically discernable subtypes. These viruses cause only mild respiratory illness, mainly in children (Kilbourne 1987). Phy-logenetically they are more distantly related to influenza A viruses than influenza B viruses (Gammelin *et al.* 1990). They even seem better adapted to humans than influenza B viruses because the rates to change are extremely low (Buonagurio *et al.* 1986a). In this property they rather resemble avian influenza A viruses (Gam-melin *et al.* 1990; Gorman *et al.* 1990). Except for an occasional isolation from pigs (Guo & Desselberger 1984) a reservoir of these viruses in the animal kingdom does not seem to exist.

The epidemiology of influenza C viruses differs markedly from that of A viruses. Although two genetically closely related lineages of influenza A viruses can cocirculate for a relatively short time (see Fig. 11.1a; Cox & Bender 1995), usually changes within a major lineage accumulate with time. With influenza C viruses such a major lineage cannot be recognized and variants from multiple evolu-tionary pathways cocirculate (Buonagurio *et al.* 1985; Matsuzaki *et al.* 1994). In this and other respects influenza B viruses are located between the A and C types (Cox & Bender 1995).

Since many different lineages of influenza C viruses cocirculate it is not surprising that reas-sortment frequently occurs in nature. This was first recognized by Buonagurio *et al.* (1986a) when they compared sequences of the HE and NS genes of various strains isolated between 1947 and 1983. Final evidence was obtained when influenza C viruses isolated from the same outbreak in the same area in Japan were genetically analysed in all seven genes individually (Peng *et al.* 1994, 1996). Thus, with influenza C viruses reassort-ment contributes to a much larger extent to genetic diversity when compared to influenza A and B viruses. However, as with the latter two virus types, dominant reassortant lineages seem not to emerge.

Conclusion

It remains an enigma as to which mechanism an influenza A virus can dominantly replace another one such as happened during the pandemics of 1957 and 1968 and when the avian-like north Eur-opean swine virus replaced the classical swine virus in Italy in the 1980s (see Chapter 13). In other instances this replacement does not happen, for example, after the re-emergence of the H1N1 virus in 1977. Since that time both the H1N1 and H3N2 viruses cocirculate in the human population. It has been shown recently that even within one A sub-type two genetically distinct lineages can cocircu-late for a while (see Fig. 11.1a; Cox & Bender 1995). With influenza B and C viruses a few or many genetically distinct lineages, respectively, were found to cocirculate at the same time in the same region. Therefore it is not surprising that humans can become infected doubly with viruses of two different lineages during corrresponding influenza seasons creating reassortants among viruses of the same type, for which ample evidence has been presented. Although such reassortants contribute to genetic diversity of human influenza viruses, it is surprising that such reassortants have not yet dominantly replaced other cocirculating viruses or that they had no significantly different properties when compared with the parent viruses. Therefore it is more remarkable that such a reassortant, which is relatively harmless in the human population, after crossing the species barrier to another mam-mal can cause epizootics, for example in camels in Mongolia (Yamnikova *et al.* 1993). A similar exam-ple of this kind was the sudden appearance of an avian reassortant virus which killed hundreds of seals along the New England coast of the USA in 1979 (Bean *et al.* 1981). From laboratory experiments it has been known for some time that artificial reassortants, which had lost pathogenic properties for their original host, can cross the species barrier being highly pathogenic for animals which are normally not natural hosts for influenza A viruses (Scholtissek *et al.* 1979; Reinacher *et al.* 1983). Thus, until recently reassortment within a given species might be without consequences for that species but not necessarily for another species which might become susceptable to the new virus. Therefore it seems to be advisable to analyse human viruses genetically to watch out for the appearance of reassortants and how far such reassortants might present in other species with markedly different properties. This also holds true for reassortants which might be prepared and used in future as live vaccines in humans.

Acknowledgements

I thank Mrs Margot Seitz and Miss Mary Scarth for help during the preparation of the manuscript and for typing.

References

Anchlan, D., Ludwig, S., Nymadawa, P., Mendsaikhan, J. & Scholtissek, C. (1996) Previous H1N1 influenza A viruses circulating in the Mongolian population. *Arch Virol* **141**, 1553–69.

Bean, W.J., Cox, N.J. & Kendal, A.P. (1980) Recombination of human influenza A viruses in nature. *Nature* **284**, 638–40.

Bean, W.J., Hinshaw, V.S. & Webster, R.G. (1981) Genetic characterization of an influenza virus from seals. In: Bishop, D.H.L. & Compans, R.W. (eds) *The Replication of Negative Strand Viruses*, pp. 363–7. Elsevier-North Holland, New York.

Buonagurio, D.A., Nakada, S., Desselberger, U., Krystal, M. & Palese, P. (1985) Non-cumulative sequence changes in the hemagglutinin genes of influenza C virus isolates. *Virology* **146**, 221–32.

Buonagurio, D.A., Nakada, S., Fitch, W.M. & Palese, P. (1986a) Epidemiology of influenza C virus in man: multiple evolutionary lineages and low rate of change. *Virology* **153**, 12–21.

Buonagurio, D.A., Nakada, S., Parvin, J.D., Krystal, M., Palese, P. & Fitch, W.M. (1986b) Evolution of human influenza A viruses over 50 years: rapid, uniform, rate of change in NS gene. *Science* **232**, 980–2.

Cox, N.J. & Bender, C.A. (1995) The molecular epidemiology of influenza viruses. *Sem Virol* **6**, 359–370.

Cox, N.J., Bai, Z.S. & Kendal, A.P. (1983) Laboratory-based surveillance of influenza A (H1N1) and A (H3N2) viruses in 1980–1981: antigenic and genomic analyses. *Bull WHO* **61**, 143–52.

Cox, N.J., Black, R.A. & Kendal, A.P. (1989) Pathways of evolution of influenza A (H1N1) viruses from 1977 to 1986 as determined by oligonucleotide mapping and sequencing studies. *J Gen Virol* **70**, 299–313.

Gammelin, M., Altmüller, A., Reinhardt, U. *et al.* (1990) Phylogenetic analysis of nucleoprotein suggests that human influenza A viruses emerged from a 19th-century avian ancestor. *Molec Biol Evol* **7**, 194–200.

Gorman, O.T., Bean, W.J., Kawaoka, Y. & Webster, R.G. (1990) Evolution of the nucleoprotein gene of influenza A virus. *J Virol* **64**, 1487–97.

Gourreau, J.M., Kaiser, C., Valette, M., Douglas, A.R., Labie, J. & Aymard, M. (1994) Isolation of two H1N2 influenza viruses from swine in France. *Arch Virol* **135**, 365–82.

Guo, Y. & Desselberger, U. (1984) Genome analysis of influenza C viruses isolated in 1981/82 from pigs in China. *J Gen Virol* **65**, 1857–72.

Guo, Y., Xu, X. & Cox, N.J. (1992) Human influenza A (H1N2) viruses isolated from China. *J Gen Virol* **73**, 383–8.

Guo, Y., Xu, X., Cox, N.J. *et al.* (1990) Occurrence of a new subtype of influenza A (H1N2) viruses and studies on its origin. *Chin J Exp Clin Virol* **4**, 133–46.

Kanegae, Y., Sugita, S., Endo, A. *et al.* (1990) Evolutionary pattern of the hemagglutinin gene of influenza B viruses isolated in Japan: Cocirculating lineages in the same epidemic season. *J Virol* **64**, 2860–5.

Kawaoka, Y., Krauss, S. & Webster, R.G. (1989) Avian to human transmission of the PB1 gene of influenza A virus in the 1957 and 1968 pandemics. *J Virol* **63**, 4603–8.

Kendal, A.P., Lee, D.T., Parish, H.S., Noble, G.R. & Dowdle, W.R. (1979) Laboratory based surveillance of influenza virus in the United States during the winter of 1977–78. II. Isolation of mixture of A/Victoria- and A/USSR-like viruses from a single person during an epidemic in Wyoming, USA, January 1978. *Am J Epidemiol* **111**, 462–8.

Kendal, A.P., Noble, G.R., Skehel, J.J. & Dowdle, W.R. (1978) Antigenic similarity of influenza A (H1N1) viruses from epidemics in 1977–78 to 'Scandinavian' strain isolated in epidemics of 1950–51. *Virology* **89**, 632–6.

Kilbourne, E.D. (ed). (1987) *Influenza*. Plenum Medical, New York.

Kinnunen, L., Ikonen, N., Pöyry, T. & Pyhälä, R. (1992) Evolution of influenza B/Victoria/2/87-like viruses: Occurrence of a genetically conserved virus under conditions of low epidemic activity. *J Gen Virol* **73**, 733–6.

Li, X.S., Zhao, C.Y., Gao, H.M. *et al.* (1992) Origin and evolutionary characteristics of antigenic reassortant influenza A (H1N2) viruses isolated from man in China. *J Gen Virol* **73**, 1329–37.

Ludwig, S., Schultz, U., Mandler, J., Fitch, W.M. & Scholtissek, C. (1991) Phylogenetic relationship of the nonstructural (NS) genes of influenza A viruses. *Virology* **183**, 566–77.

Matsuzaki, Y., Muraki, Y., Sugawara, K. *et al.* (1994) Cocirculation of two distinct groups of influenza C virus in Yamagata city, Japan. *Virology* **202**, 792–802.

Nakajima, K., Desselberger, U. & Palese, P. (1978) Recent human influenza A (H1N1) viruses are closely related genetically to strains isolated in 1950. *Nature* **274**, 334–9.

Nakajima, S., Cox, N.J. & Kendal, A.P. (1981) Antigenic and genetic analyses of influenza A H1N1 viruses from different regions of the world, February 1978 to March 1980. *Infect Immun* **32**, 287–94.

Nerome, K., Sakamoto, S., Yano, N. *et al.* (1983) Antigenic characteristics and genomic composition of a naturally occurring recombinant influenza virus isolated from a pig in Japan. *J Gen Virol* **64**, 2611–20.

Nerome, K., Yoshioka, Y., Sakamoto, S., Yasuhara, M. & Oya, A. (1985) Characterization of a 1980-swine recombinant influenza virus possessing H1 hemagglutinin and N2 neuraminidase similar to that of the earliest Hong Kong (H3N2) viruses. *Arch Virol* **86**, 197–211.

Ouchi, A., Nerome, K., Kanegae, Y. *et al.* (1996) Large outbreaks of swine influenza in southern Japan caused by reassortant (H1N2) influenza viruses: Its epizootic background and characterization of the causative viruses. *J Gen Virol* **77**, 1751–9.

Peng, G., Hongo, S., Kimura, H. *et al.* (1996) Frequent occurrence of genetic reassortment between influenza C virus strains in nature. *J Gen Virol* **77**, 1489–92.

Peng, G., Hongo, S., Muraki, Y. *et al.* (1994) Genetic reassortment of influenza C viruses in man. *J Gen Virol* **75**, 3619–22.

Reinacher, M., Bonin, J., Narayan, O. & Scholtissek, C. (1983) Pathogenesis of neurovirulent influenza A virus infection in mice. Route of entry of virus into brain determines infection of different population of cells. *Lab Invest* **49**, 686–92.

Röhm, C., Zhou, N., Süss, J., Mackenzie, J. & Webster, R.G. (1996) Characterization of a novel influenza hemagglutinin, H15: criteria for determination of influenza A subtypes. *Virology* **217**, 508–16.

Rota, P.A., Hemphill, M.L., Whistler, T., Regnery, H.L. & Kendal, A.P. (1992) Antigenic and genetic characterization of the haemagglutinins of recent cocirculating strains of influenza B virus. *J Gen Virol* **73**, 2737–42.

Rota, P.A., Wallis, T.R., Harmon, M.W., Rota, J.S., Kendal, A.P. & Nerome, K. (1990) Cocirculation of two distinct evolutionary lineages of influenza type B virus since 1983. *Virology* **175**, 59–68.

Schild, G.C., Newman, R.W., Webster, R.G., Major, D. & Hinshaw, V.S. (1980) Antigenic analysis of influenza A virus surface antigens: consideration for the nomenclature of influenza virus. *Arch Virol* **63**, 171–84.

Scholtissek, C. (1990) Pigs as 'mixing vessels' for the creation of new pandemic influenza A viruses. *Med Principles Pract* **2**, 65–71.

Scholtissek, C. & von Hoyningen-Huene, V. (1980) Genetic relatedness of the gene which codes for the nonstructural (NS) protein of different influenza A strains. *Virology* **102**, 13–20.

Scholtissek, C., Rohde, W., von Hoyningen, V. & Rott, R. (1978a) On the origin of the human influenza virus subtypes H2N2 and H3N2. *Virology* **87**, 13–20.

Scholtissek, C., Vallbracht, A., Flehmig, B. & Rott, R. (1979) Correlation of pathogenicity and gene constellation of influenza A viruses. II. Highly neurovirulent recombinants derived from non-neurovirulent or weakly neurovirulent parent virus strains. *Virology* **95**, 492–500.

Scholtissek, C., von Hoyningen, V. & Rott, R. (1978b) Genetic relationship between the new 1977 epidemic strains (H1N1) of influenza and human influenza strains between 1947 and 1957 (H1N1). *Virology* **89**, 613–17.

Sugimura, T., Yonemochi, H., Ogawa, T., Tanaka, Y. & Kumagai, T. (1980) Isolation of a recombinant influenza virus (Hsw1N2) from swine in Japan. *Arch Virol* **66**, 271–4.

Treanor, J.J., Snyder, M.H., London, W.T. & Murphy, B.R. (1989) The B allele of the NS gene of avian influenza viruses, but not the A allele, attenuates a human influenza A virus for squirrel monkeys. *Virology* **171**, 1–9.

Xu, X., Guo, Y., Rota, P., Hemphill, M., Kendal, A.P. & Cox, N. (1993a) Genetic reassortment of human influenza virus in nature. In: Hannoun, C., Kendal, A.P., Klenk, H.D. & Ruben, F.L. (eds) *Options for the Control of Influenza II*, pp. 203–7. Excerpta Medica, Amsterdam.

Xu, X., Rocha, E.P., Regnery, H.L., Kendal, A.P. & Cox, N.J. (1993b) Genetic and antigenic analyses of influenza A (H1N1) viruses (1986–91). *Virus Res* **28**, 37–55.

Yamashita, M., Krystal, M., Fitch, W.M. & Palese, P. (1988) Influenza B virus evolution: cocirculating lineages and comparison of evolutionary pattern with those of influenza A and C viruses. *Virology* **163**, 112–22.

Yamnikova, S.S., Mandler, J., Bekh-Ochir, Z.H. *et al.* (1993) A reassortant H1N1 influenza A virus caused fatal epizootics among camels in Mongolia. *Virology* **197**, 558–63.

Yasuhara, H., Hirahara, T., Nakai, M. *et al.* (1983) Further isolation of a recombinant virus (H1N2), formerly (Hsw1N2) from a pig in Japan in 1980. *Microbiol Immunol* **27**, 43–50.

Young, J.F., Desselberger, U. & Palese, P. (1979) Evolution of human influenza A viruses in nature: Sequential mutations in the genome of new H1N1 isolates. *Cell* **18**, 73–83.

Young, J.F. & Palese, P. (1979) Evolution of human influenza A viruses in nature: recombination contributes to genetic variation of H1N1 strains. *Proc Natl Acad Sci USA* **76**, 6647–51.

CHAPTER 12

Avian Influenza

Toshihiro Ito and Yoshihiro Kawaoka

The first avian influenza (AI) virus was isolated in 1902, although it was not identified as a member of influenza A virus family until 1955 (Schafer 1955). Influenza viruses have been isolated from domestic poultry suffering from highly pathogenic avian influenza ('fowl plague') and from apparently healthy wild birds, including waterfowl. Antigenic and genetic studies strongly suggest that the 1957 Asian and 1968 Hong Kong pandemic strains were generated by genetic reassortment between human and avian viruses (Webster & Laver 1972; Scholtissek et al. 1978). The AI viruses have also caused outbreaks of influenza in mammals, such as seals (Webster et al. 1981), whales (Hinshaw et al. 1986), mink (Klingeborn et al. 1985), pigs in Europe (Scholtissek et al. 1983), and horses (Guo et al. 1992). Therefore, AI viruses are important not only because they cause economic losses in poultry but also because they can cause influenza outbreaks in humans and other mammals by either directly transmitting to these animals or by contributing viral genes to viruses in these species.

Ecology

Natural reservoirs

Slemons et al. (1974) were the first to find that apparently healthy wild ducks harbour influenza viruses and shed them in faeces. Longitudinal studies on wild ducks in Canada established that influenza A viruses are perpetuated in apparently healthy feral ducks (Hinshaw & Webster 1982). Each of the nine different neuraminidase (NA) subtypes and 14 of the 15 haemagglutinin (HA)

subtypes of influenza viruses have been isolated from wild ducks; viruses of the H13 subtype has so far been isolated only from seabirds. In wild ducks in the Northern Hemisphere, influenza viruses predominate in August and September. Juvenile birds are infected as they congregate in marshalling areas prior to migration, and up to 30% of the birds hatched each year shed influenza viruses in their faeces. Virus shedding continues during early migration, but the frequency of virus isolation falls to a very low level (<0.01%) by November. Although certain subtypes of influenza viruses predominate in wild ducks in a particular flyway, there are differences in predominant viruses from one flyway to another and from year to year (Hinshaw et al. 1985). The avirulent nature of AI infection in ducks may be the result of virus adaptation to this host over many centuries, creating a reservoir that perpetuates the viruses without endangering its host. This notion, when coupled with phylogenetic studies of influenza virus genes, can be extended to suggest that wild waterfowl represent a reservoir of all influenza A viruses and play a unique and very important role in the natural history of influenza viruses (Fig. 12.1).

Persistence in nature

In wild ducks, influenza viruses replicate preferentially in the cells that line the intestinal tract, cause no disease signs, and are excreted in high concentrations in the faeces. AI viruses have been isolated from faecal material and from unconcentrated lake water (Hinshaw et al. 1980b). Laboratory studies showed that viruses retained infectivity in

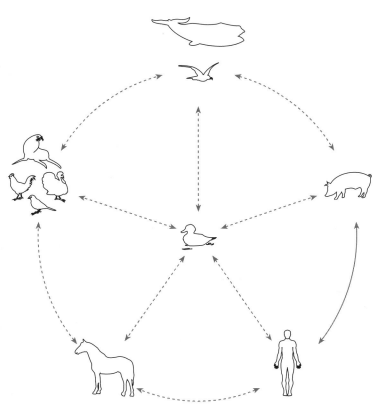

Fig. 12.1 The 'wheel of flu'. The working hypothesis is that wild aquatic birds are the primordial reservoir of all influenza viruses for avian and mammalian species. Transmission of influenza has been demonstrated between pigs and humans and between seals and humans (solid lines). There is excellent circumstantial evidence for transmission of influenza between wild ducks and turkeys (Halvorson *et al*. 1983) and the other species shown (Webster *et al*. 1981; Scholtissek *et al*. 1983; Hinshaw *et al*. 1986) (dotted lines), but formal evidence for transmission has not yet been established. (From Murphy & Webster 1996, with permission from Lippincott Raven Publishers.)

faecal material for as long as 30 days at 4°C and for 7 days at 20°C (Webster *et al*. 1978). This information indicates that waterfowl have a very efficient mode of transmitting their viruses, that is, via faecal material in water supplies. If one then considers that a large number of susceptible young ducks gather each year on Canadian lakes, it is easy to understand how many birds are exposed to and infected by virus shed into the lake water. This type of transmission would explain the high incidence of virus infection in Canadian ducks, particularly juveniles, who would otherwise never have been exposed to influenza viruses. Transmission via faeces also provides a way for ducks to spread their viruses to other birds, domestic and feral, as they migrate through an area.

How influenza viruses persist in ducks from year to year is not clear. Because ducks can shed the virus for up to 30 days (Hinshaw *et al*. 1980a), very few passages would be required to maintain the virus in the population. It is conceivable that AI

viruses remain viable in the frozen lakes over the winter until the birds return. In autumn in central Alaska when the most of the ducks have migrate south, viruses could still be isolated from the lake water (Ito *et al*. 1995), but not from frozen ice of lakes in winter. Another possibility is that other species such as shore birds transmit the viruses between species and from one hemisphere to another (Sharp *et al*. 1993). However, this possibility could not account for all of the viruses in ducks because viruses maintained in ducks and shore-birds do not completely overlap (see below).

Different gene pool in other species of birds

Influenza viruses have also been isolated from sea birds including gulls, terns, shearwaters, guillemots, sandpipers and ruddy turnstones (Becker 1966; Hinshaw & Webster 1982). A systematic study of shore birds on the east coast of the USA revealed that influenza A viruses are prevalent in spring (May–June) and autumn (September–October). Up to 30% of birds contain viruses during spring migration, and most of the different HA and NA subtypes including H13 have been isolated. The majority of these viruses are non-pathogenic in chickens and ducks, but the original isolate from terns in South Africa (A/Tern/SA/61 (H5N3)) (Becker 1966) is highly pathogenic for domestic poultry. Biological (Kawaoka *et al.* 1988) and epidemiological (Sharp *et al.* 1993) studies suggested that the influenza virus gene pool in shorebirds overlaps to some extent but not completely with that in ducks.

Influenza viruses have been isolated less frequently from passerine birds; however, studies during the highly pathogenic H7N7 outbreak in Australia in 1986 established that starlings and sparrows are susceptible to infection and could potentially spread AI (Cross 1986; Nestorowicz *et al.* 1987).

These studies have established that there is a vast reservoir of influenza A viruses in aquatic birds. In wild ducks, particularly, there is excellent circumstantial evidence for transmission of influenza viruses from migrating ducks to domestic poultry (Halvorson *et al.* 1983). Because influenza A viruses are ubiquitous in aquatic birds, it is essential that the poultry industry take step to minimize the likelihood of introduction of viruses from wild to domestic species.

Antigenic variability

Why is the antigenicity of AI viruses so highly conserved in nature? There are several possible explanations: (i) laboratory studies have shown that the antibody response of ducks to AI viruses is weak and short-lived. Ducks appear to be readily reinfected with the same virus within 2 months of the initial infection (Hinshaw *et al.* 1980a; Kida *et al.* 1980); (ii) even if ducks produce neutralizing antibody, the serum antibodies may not be effective at inhibiting viral replication in the intestinal tract, the site in ducks where these viruses preferentially replicate (Webster *et al.* 1978); and (iii) every year, large numbers of susceptible ducks are added to the population; over

30% of the annual duck population consists of juvenile birds that hatched that year.

Representatives of each of the known subtypes of influenza A virus have been identified from aquatic birds (Hinshaw *et al.* 1981). Sometimes, two or more antigenically distinct influenza viruses have been isolated from cloacal samples of wild ducks. Moreover, genetic reassortment has been demonstrated experimentally when ducks were infected with two antigenically distinct viruses (Hinshaw *et al.* 1980a). Therefore, it is not surprising that viruses with almost every possible combination of antigenic subtypes have been recovered from aquatic birds in nature.

Evolution

Genetic conservation

The result of genetic analyses of AI viruses can be summarized as follows: (i) multiple lineages of viruses cocirculate; (ii) nucleotide variation rates of AI viruses are lower than those of mammalian viruses; and (iii) viruses in the old and new world are genetically distinct. AI virus gene pools may have partitioned due to the geographical separation of waterfowl populations through separate flyways, breeding and overwintering grounds. The subdivision of host populations provides a great deal of heterogeneity to the virus populations and helps maintain multiple lineages of viruses.

Evidence for an avian origin of the influenza viruses

There is much evidence to suggest that waterfowl is the original host for all influenza viruses in other animals. Influenza viruses in wild waterfowl populations are ubiquitous; infection in nearly always asymptomatic, and large amounts of virus are shed by infected birds (Webster *et al.* 1978). In addition there is considerable genetic diversity in AI viruses; viruses of all 15 HA and all nine NA subtypes persist and circulate in the avian host reservoir. The very high level of conservation observed among the proteins of AI viruses suggests that an adaptive optimum has nearly been achieved. Therefore, AI viruses and their waterfowl hosts can be considered a classic example of an optimally adapted system. The very low levels of evolution observed for AI virus proteins suggests that many centuries would have been required to generate the current genetic diversity and distinct separation of avian virus HA and NA subtypes. In contrast, evolution of viral proteins in non-avian hosts typically shows a rapid accumulation of mutations away from avian-like forms (Gorman *et al.* 1991; Ludwig *et al.* 1995). In addition, genetic and phylogenetic analyses have shown that every gene that has appeared in the mammalian virus gene pools over the past century has an avian origin (Kawaoka *et al.* 1989; Gorman *et al.* 1990a,b; Ito *et al.* 1991; Bean *et al.* 1992). These results reveal that all of the gene lineages currently circulating in both mammals and poultry originated from AI viruses in wild waterfowl.

Host-range restriction

Host-range restriction exists among influenza viruses. AI viruses replicate poorly in primates (Murphy *et al.* 1982; Snyder *et al.* 1987; Beare & Webster 1991) and, although influenza viruses isolated from ducks replicate well in ducks (mainly in the intestinal tract), human viruses do not (Webster *et al.* 1978; Kida *et al.* 1980). The importance of HA and NA in the restriction of influenza virus replication has been demonstrated in avian systems; reassortant viruses containing the HA or NA gene from a human virus and the rest of the genes from a duck virus do not replicate in ducks (Hinshaw *et al.* 1983). The contributions of other gene segments to virus replication in birds have not been established; although nucleoprotein has been implicated for its contribution to host range restriction (Scholtissek *et al.* 1985), no direct evidence by reassortment experiments has been obtained. In fact, the molecular basis of host range restriction has been studied only for HA.

Although all influenza viruses recognize oligosaccharide that contains terminal sialic acid, the receptor specificity of HA differs among influenza viruses. Most of these viruses preferentially bind the sialic acid-α2,3-galactose (SAα2,3Gal) linkage, whereas human influenza viruses preferentially bind the SAα2,6Gal linkage on cell surface sialyloligosaccharides (Rogers & Paulson 1983; Rogers *et al.* 1983). Baum and Paulson (1990) have shown that epithelial cells in the human trachea, a virus replication site in humans, contain SAα2,6Gal, but not SAα2,3Gal linkages. Conversely, epithelial cells in duck intestine, where avian viruses replicate, contain SAα2,3Gal, but not SAα2,6Gal linkages (T. Ito and Y. Kawaoka, unpublished data). Together, these findings suggest that the receptor specificity of HA and the availability of the receptor may be important for host-range restriction of influenza viruses.

Pathogenicity

Although chickens and turkeys are usually considered to be somewhat similar in their susceptibility to influenza viruses, there is some experimental evidence that certain influenza viruses affect different avian species with different degree of severity (Narayan *et al.* 1969b). Experimental infection of virulent H5 influenza viruses (Alexander *et al.* 1986; Kawaoka *et al.* 1987) revealed that: (i) Tern/SA/61 (H5N3), Turkey/Ont/66 (H5N9), Chick/Penn/83 (H5N2) and Turkey/Ire/ 83 (H5N8) viruses are highly pathogenic for turkeys; (ii) Turkey/Ont/66 (H5N9) virus is less virulent for chickens than turkeys; (iii) Turkey/Ire/ 83 virus is highly pathogenic for quail, but the other viruses are not; (iv) in general, higher mortality is observed by intramuscular inoculation of the virus than by intranasal inoculation; and (v) all of these viruses are non-pathogenic for ducks, although a relatively high titre of viruses can be recovered from many of their organs, including blood. Ducks do not show any signs of disease. Pathogenicity also differs with the dose of virus; FPV/Rostock/34 (H7N1) virus requires only 1 EID_{50} of virus to kill adult chickens, whereas Turkey/Ireland/83 (H5N8) virus requires 104 EID_{50} of virus. These studies indicate that highly virulent influenza viruses vary in their host range and in their degree of virulence.

Turkey/Ont/7732/66 (H5N9) virus, which is highly pathogenic for turkeys but not for quail, becomes lethal for quail after several passages in this bird (Tashiro *et al.* 1987), suggesting that mutants are selected during virus replication in quail. The mechanism by which Turkey/Ont/7732/66 (H5N9) virus acquires virulence for quail is not clear, but the authors of the study claim that the variant virus replicates a little faster than the parent virus in quail embryo cells, and that this might account for the acquisition of virulence in quails. By the same token, avirulent H4N8 influenza virus acquires virulence by passage in chickens (Brugh 1986). This virus was originally isolated from a severe influenza outbreak in chickens. However, the virus did not kill chickens that had been experimentally infected via the intranasal route, indicating that this virus is less virulent than the H5 and H7 viruses. Researchers isolated a pathogenic variant of the virus and found that it kills 100% of chickens after intravenous inoculation. The selected virus produced plaques on chick embryo fibroblast cells in the absence of trypsin. Pathogenic variants from avirulent H5N2 influenza viruses that are related to the original avirulent Chick/Penn/83 (H5N2) viruses have been isolated by the same procedure (Brugh 1988; Ohuchi *et al.* 1989). Virulent AI viruses can also be selected in 14-day-old embryonated eggs from avirulent viruses (Brugh & Beck 1992; Horimoto *et al.* 1995). These studies suggest that acquisition of virulence might not be such a rare event in nature and that virulent viruses are readily generated from avirulent viruses in nature.

Signs

Disease signs vary, depending on, among other things, the species and age of poultry, strains of virus and accompanying bacterial infections. Typical clinical signs of highly pathogenic AI in chickens or turkeys include: decreased egg production, respiratory signs, rales, excessive lacrimation, sinusitis, cyanosis of unfeathered skin especially of the combs and wattles, oedema of the head and face, ruffled feathers, diarrhoea and nervous disorder (Plate 12.1, facing p. 288) (Alexander *et al.* 1978; Easterday & Tumova 1978). Sometimes these signs may not be observed, especially if the virulent strain causes early death.

Pathology

Gross lesion

Haemorrhagic, necrotic, congestive and transudative changes are characteristically observed in infections by highly virulent viruses (Uys & Becker 1967). Haemorrhagic changes are often severe in the oviducts and intestines. Yellowish necrotic foci are observed in internal organs (liver, spleen, kidney and lung) as the disease progresses. Sinusitis has been observed in a variety of species of poultry. In ducks, sinusitis seem to be common in the presence of other micro-organisms, such as *Mycoplasma* (Roberts 1964).

Histopathology

Histopathological information on AI infection is limited to cases where severe disease and obvious gross changes have occurred. Some of the changes caused by highly virulent viruses are common, and they frequently include oedema, haemorrhage, and foci of perivascular lymphoid cuffing and necrosis. Necrotic foci are observed in the spleen, liver, lung, kidney, intestine, pancreas and brain. The characteristics of these foci can differ among causative agents; multiple focal necrosis is prominent with Ty/Ont/7732/66 (H5N9) virus but not with Ty/Ont/6213/66 (H5N9) virus (Narayan *et al.* 1969a; Rouse *et al.* 1971). Necrotic foci in visceral organs are recognized by acidophilic changes and by heterophilic infiltration of swollen parenchymal cells with marginated nuclei.

Sometimes, despite high titres of virus, there are no lesions in the lung (Uys & Becker 1967). However, encephalitis (perivascular lymphoid cuffing, vascular-glial and neurone degeneration) develops in the cerebrum and cerebellum. Alteration in myocardial tissue has also been observed in some of the highly virulent virus infections (McKenzie *et al.* 1972).

Transmission

In natural infections of poultry with AI viruses, the mechanisms of virus transmission between birds are not fully understood. We do know that the speed of transmission differs considerably among viruses. Narayan *et al.* (1969a) showed transmission of virulent AI virus between turkeys caged together but not when the birds were placed about 1 m off the floor of the same room. In contrast, Bankowski and Conrad (1966) reported that transmission of virus occurred even between turkeys in adjacent pens. Alexander *et al.* (1986) systematically examined the variation of transmissibility and showed that transmissibility of virulent influenza virus varies depending on the species of poultry and/or the strain of virus. They found that Chick/Scot/59 (H5N1) and Tern/SA/61 (H5N3) viruses are less transmissible in chickens and turkeys than are other virulent viruses, that Turkey/Ont/66 (H5N9) and Turkey/Ire/83 (H5N8) viruses transmit well among turkeys but not among chickens, and that all of the virulent viruses they examined were less transmissible among quail than among chickens and turkeys.

Generally, virulent influenza viruses seem to be less transmissible from infected to susceptible birds than are avirulent viruses. This is probably due to the extremely rapid death that usually follows infection with virulent viruses and to the less stable HA of virulent influenza viruses. These viruses have cleaved HA, which is more readily inactivated by exposure to low pH (Scholtissek 1985). Evidence for vertical transmission of influenza viruses in poultry is scant; although viruses have been detected in eggs laid by experimentally infected birds (Narayan *et al.* 1969a; Bean *et al.* 1985), suggesting that there is the potential for such spread. There is no evidence, however, that these infected eggs will hatch. Similarly, turkey hens can be infected when artificially inseminated with semen experimentally contaminated with influenza virus (Samadieh & Bankowski 1971), yet 2- or 7-day-old poults hatched from their eggs are all negative for virus at day 18 even though virus could be recovered from 1-day-old poults (Samadieh & Bankowski 1971). In this study, poults hatched from surviving eggs infected at day 6 or 10 were also negative for virus. Virus concentrations as high as 10 million infec-

tious units per gram of faeces are shed by chickens infected with A/Chick/Penn/83 (H5N2) (Bean *et al.* 1985); lower concentrations of virus are shed in respiratory secretions. During epidemics of AI in poultry, humans, infected birds, and contaminated egg flats and cages are all possible sources for introduction of the virus to susceptible poultry flocks. During the 1983–84 outbreak in Pennsylvania, the insides of the affected houses were heavily contaminated with virus, and virus was isolated from all surfaces tested as well as from flies (Bean *et al.* 1985).

Passerine birds may also play a role in disseminating influenza virus during outbreaks of disease.

During the epidemic of a highly virulent influenza virus (A/Chicken/Victoria/1/85 [H7N7]) in 1985 in Australia, a virulent virus was isolated from a starling. Moreover, serological evidence for infection of sparrows by an H7N7 virus was also obtained (Cross 1986). Experimental infections of sparrows and starlings with highly virulent H7N7 viruses showed that the virus replicated well in these birds. In fact, it killed 100% of starlings and approximately 30% of sparrows infected (Nestrowicz *et al.* 1987). These results indicate that passerine birds can serve as mechanical and biologic vectors for highly virulent influenza viruses during an outbreak.

Economic loss

In domestic poultry, AI viruses have caused considerable economic losses. For example, the costs to eradicate a highly pathogenic H5N2 AI virus responsible for outbreaks in 1983–84 (destruction of over 17 million birds) were approximately US$61 million. Viruses of low pathogenicity in the laboratory can occasionally cause severe disease in the field, where exacerbation may occur. The importance of such infections can be best assessed in monetary terms. In Minnesota in 1978, over 140 turkey flocks were infected with influenza viruses of low pathogenicity resulting in estimated losses of over US$4 million (Poss *et al.* 1982).

Molecular basis of pathogenicity

Identification of genes involved in virulence

Disease resulting from influenza virus infection is a complex event that involves both viral and host gene products. Because of their segmented genome, influenza viruses can be reassorted *in vitro* to examine the gene(s) involved in determining their virulence. Using genetic reassortment, Bean and Webster (1978) showed that the genes encoding HA, NA, one of the polymerase, and nucleoprotein were required for virulence. Ogawa and Ueda (1981), using virulent and avirulent AI viruses, further showed that the HA gene was a key determinant and M gene was also involved in virulence. The genes associated with virulence varied with the virus pairs studied; extensive studies by Rott *et al.* have led to the concept that pathogenicity is polygenic and depends on an optimal gene constellation (Rott *et al.* 1976, 1979).

One of the differences between virulent and avirulent influenza viruses is plaque-forming ability; virulent viruses produce plaques without added trypsin, whereas avirulent viruses require trypsin to form plaques. Bosch *et al.* (1979) have shown that plaque-forming ability correlates with HA cleavage in tissue culture. The HA of virulent influenza is cleaved in the absence of trypsin, whereas the HA of avirulent viruses is not. These results suggest that there may be a difference between the HAs of virulent and avirulent viruses, which supports the genetic reassortment data, indicating that the HA gene is a key determinant.

Importance of basic amino acids and a glycosylation site near the HA cleavage site for virulence

Virulent viruses of the H5 and H7 subtypes cause systemic lethal infection in poultry, whereas avirulent viruses cause local infection in the respiratory or intestinal tract, or both (i.e. for reviews, see Webster & Rott 1987; Klenk & Rott 1988; Webster & Kawaoka 1988). This difference in tissue tropism is determined by HA cleavability, which in turn is regulated by the amino acid sequence upstream of the HA cleavage site, and by the presence or absence of a neighbouring carbohydrate side chain (Kawaoka & Webster 1988b, 1989; Ohuchi *et al.* 1989; Li *et al.* 1990; Vey *et al.* 1992). Only virulent-type HAs containing multiple basic residues are cleaved by intracellular proteases (e.g. furin, Stieneke-Grober *et al.* 1992; and PC6, Horimoto *et al.* 1994), which are ubiquitously expressed in most organs.

Most influenza A viruses have arginine (R) at the carboxylterminus of HA1 and glycine (G) at the aminoterminus of HA2. Among the H5 strains, glutamine (Q), which is located proximately upstream of the HA1 carboxylterminus, is also conserved (Kawaoka & Webster 1988a). Between the glutamine (Q) and glycine (G) residues lies a region designated the connecting peptide. This region varies in its sequence composition and in the number of amino acids it contains, depending on the H5 strain. All naturally isolated avirulent H5 viruses have four amino acids in the connecting peptide, for example, A/Turkey/Minnesota/1550/80 (H5N2) has Q-R-E-T-R\G (E, glutamic acid; T, threonine). If the four residues of the connecting peptide are basic amino acids, the virus retains its avirulence provided a carbohydrate side chain is nearby, as revealed by studies of A/Chicken/Pennsylvania/1/83 (H5N2) which has the connecting peptide sequence Q-K-K-K-R\G (K, lysine) (Kawaoka *et al.* 1984). Conversely, in the absence of a carbohydrate side chain, the same number of basic residues will support high levels of virulence, as exemplified by A/Chicken/Scotland/59 (H5N1) which has Q-R-K-K-R\G. For viruses to retain virulence in the presence of a nearby carbohydrate side chain, they must have additional amino acids in its connecting peptide (e.g. A/Turkey/Ireland/83 (H5N8) with Q-R-K-R-K-K-R\G). Previous studies with HA cleavage mutants have established the following minimal sequence requirement for the virulence phenotype of H5 viruses: Q-R/K-X-R/K-R\G (X = non-basic residue) in the absence of a neighbouring carbohydrate side chain. If the carbohydrate moiety is present, virulence is maintained only if two amino acids are inserted (Q-X-X-R/K-X-R/K-R\G), or if the conserved glutamine at position 5 or the proline at position 6 is altered (i.e.

B(X)-X(B)-R/K-X R/K-R\G (B = basic residue)) (Kawaoka & Webster 1988b, 1989; Ohuchi *et al.* 1989; Horimoto & Kawaoka 1994).

Vaccines for poultry

Efficacious vaccines for AI in domestic poultry have been prepared and tested in chickens and turkeys (Brugh *et al.* 1979; Brugh & Stone 1986). The products most widely tested are inactivated AI vaccines, which are administered in oil emulsion by injection. Naturally occurring avirulent strains of AI are efficacious against experimental challenge with classical 'fowl plaque' virus (Beard & Easter-day 1973). However, the possibility of reassort-ments with AI viruses present in poultry and the development of a strain with increased pathogeni-city has dissuaded investigators from using live attenuated vaccines. The inactivated oil emulsion vaccines have the disadvantage of not being amenable to mass inoculation. Also, according to US Department of Agriculture (USDA) regulations, broilers cannot be injected with oil emulsion vac-cines within 42 days of slaughter and since broiler chickens are usually ready for processing at 6–7 weeks of age, they cannot be vaccinated by this method. Moreover, field studies with inactivated AI oil emulsion vaccines have shown that these vaccines do not provide full protection; although they do reduce virus shedding and limit symptom severity (Halvorson *et al.* 1986; McCapes & Ban-kowski 1986). The efficacy of AI inactivated vac-cines could be greatly improved if the products were standardized and contained sufficient anti-gen. A simple test is available for standardization, and sufficient antigen in the vaccine has been shown to abolish virus shedding and symptoms after experimental challenge with highly patho-genic A/Chicken/Pennsylvania/83 (H5N2) (Wood *et al.* 1985). Genetically engineered vaccines, where the HA gene is expressed in vaccinia virus (Sutter *et al.* 1994), fowl poxvirus (Taylor *et al.* 1988; Beard *et al.* 1991; Trypathy & Schnitzlein 1991; Webster *et al.* 1991; Boyle & Heine 1993), or retroviruses (Hunt *et al.* 1988), have also shown to be efficacious. Direct DNA inoculations have demonstrated that *in vivo* transfections can be used to elicit protective immune responses. The direct inoculation of an H7 HA-expressing DNA protected chickens against lethal H7 influenza virus challenge (Fynan *et al.* 1993; Robinson *et al.* 1993). Such vaccines could overcome the problems of mass vaccination, low antigen contact, and the use of oil emulsion.

Acknowledgements

Work in our laboratory is supported by Public Health Service Research Grants AI-29599 and AI-33898 from the National Institutes of Health, National Institute of Allergy and Infectious Dis-eases; Cancer Centre Support (CORE) grant CA-21765; and American Lebanese Syrian Associated Charities.

References

Alexander, D.J., Allan, W.H., Parsons, D. & Parsons, G. (1978) The pathogenicity of four avian influenza A viruses for fowls, turkeys and ducks. *Res Vet Sci* **24**, 242–7.

Alexander, D.J., Parsons, G. & Manvell, R.J (1986) Experimental assessment of the pathogenicity of eight avian influenza A viruses of H5 subtype for chickens, turkeys, ducks and quail. *Avian Pathol* **15**, 647–62.

Bankowski, R.A. & Conrad, R.D. (1966) A new respiratory disease of turkeys caused by virus. In: *Proceedings of the 13th World Poultry Congress.* Kiev, p. 371.

Baum, L.G. & Paulson, J.C. (1990) Sialyloligosaccharides of the respiratory epithelium in the selection of human influenza virus receptor specificity. *Acta Histochem Suppl* **40**, 35–8.

Bean, W.J & Webster, R.G. (1978) Phenotypic properties associated with influenza genome segments. In: Mahy, B.J and Barry, R.D. (eds) *Negative Strand Viruses and the Host Cell.* Academic Press, London.

Bean, W.J., Kawaoka, Y., Wood, J.M., Pearson, J.E. & Webster, R.G. (1985) Characterization of virulent and avirulent A/Chicken/Pennsylvania/83 influenza A viruses: potential role of defective interfering RNAs in nature. *J Virol* **54**, 151–60.

Bean, W.J., Schell, M., Katz, J *et al.* (1992) Evolution of the H3 influenza virus hemagglutinin from human and non-human hosts. *J Virol* **66**, 1129–38.

Beard, C.W. & Easterday, B.C. (1973) A/Turkey/Oregon/71, an avirulent influenza isolate with the hemaggluti-nin of fowl plague virus. *Avian Dis* **17**, 173–81.

Beard, C.W., Schnitzlein, W.M. & Tripathy, D.N. (1991) Protection of chickens against highly pathogenic avian influenza virus (H5N2) by recombinant fowlpox viruses. *Avian Dis* **35**, 356–9.

Beare, A.S. & Webster, R.G. (1991) Replication of avian influenza viruses in humans. *Arch Virol* **119**, 37–42.

Becker, W. (1966) The isolation and classification of tern virus influenza virus A/Tern/South Africa/1961. *J Hygiene* **64**, 309.

Bosch, F.X., Orlich, M., Klenk, H.D. & Rott, R. (1979) The structure of the hemagglutinin, a determinant for the pathogenicity of influenza viruses. *Virology* **95**, 197–207.

Boyle, D.B. & Heine, H.G. (1993) Recombinant fowlpox virus vaccines for poultry. *Immunol Cell Biol* **71**, 391–7.

Brugh, M. (1986) Highly pathogenic virus recovered from mildly or non-pathogenic H4N8 and H5N2 avian influenza virus isolates. In: Easterday, B.C., Alexander, D.J. & Beard, C.W. (eds) *Proceedings of the 2nd International Symposium on Avian Influenza*, pp. 309–13. US Animal Health Association, Athens, Georgia.

Brugh, M. (1988) Highly pathogenic virus recovered from chickens infected with mildly pathogenic 1986 isolates of H5N2 avian influenza virus. *Avian Dis* **32**, 695–703.

Brugh, M., Beard, C.W. & Stone, H.D. (1979) Immunization of chickens and turkeys against avian influenza with monovalent and polyvalent oil emulsion vaccines. *Am J Vet Res* **40**, 165, 169.

Brugh, M. & Beck, J.R. (1992) Recovery of minority subpopulations of highly pathogenic avian influenza virus. In: Easterday, B.C. & Beard, C.W. (eds) *Proceedings of the 3rd International Symposium on Avian Influenza*, pp. 166–74. University of Wisconsin-Madison, Madison, Wisconsin.

Brugh, M. & Stone, H.D. (1986) Immunization of chickens against influenza with hemagglutinin specific (H5) oil emulsion vaccine. In: Easterday, B.C., Alexander, D.J. & Beard, C.W. (eds) *Proceedings of the 2nd International Symposium on Avian Influenza*, pp. 283–92. US Animal Health Association, Athens, Georgia.

Cross, G.M. (1986) The status of avian influenza in Australia. In: Easterday, B.C., Alexander, D.J. & Beard, C.W. (eds) *Proceedings of the 2nd International Symposium on Avian Influenza*, pp. 96–103, US Animal Health Association, Athens, Georgia.

Easterday, B.C. & Tumova, B. (1978) Avian influenza. In: Hofstad, M.S. *et al.* (eds) *Biester and Schwarte: Disease of Poultry*, 7th edn, pp. 549–73. Iowa State University Press, Ames.

Fynan, E.F., Robinson, H.L. & Webster, R.G. (1993) Use of DNA encoding influenza hemagglutinin as an avian influenza vaccine. *DNA Cell Biol* **12**, 785–9.

Gorman, O.T., Bean, W.J., Kawaoka, Y., Donatelli, I., Guo, Y.J. & Webster, R.G. (1991) Evolution of influenza A virus nucleoprotein genes: implications for the origins of H1N1 human and classical swine viruses. *J Virol* **65**, 3704–14.

Gorman, O.T., Bean, W.J., Kawaoka, Y. & Webster, R.G. (1990a) Evolution of the nucleoprotein gene of influenza A virus. *J Virol* **64**, 1487–97.

Gorman, O.T., Donis, R.O., Kawaoka, Y. & Webster, R.G. (1990b) Evolution of influenza A virus PB2 genes: implications for evolution of the ribonucleoprotein complex and origin of human influenza A virus. *J Virol* **64**, 4893–902.

Guo, Y., Wang, M., Kawaoka, Y. *et al.* (1992) Characterization of a new avian-like influenza A virus from horses in China. *Virology* **188**, 245–55.

Halvorson, D.A., Karunakaran, D., Abraham, A.S., Newman, J.A., Sivanandan, V. & Poss, P.E. (1986) Efficacy of vaccine in the control of avian influenza. In: Easterday, B.C., Alexander, D.J. & Beard, C.W. (eds) *Proceedings of the 2nd International Symposium on Avian Influenza*, pp. 264–70, US Animal Health Association, Athens, Georgia.

Halvorson, D., Karunakaran, D., Senne, D. *et al.* (1983) Epizootiology of avian influenza—simultaneous monitoring of sentinel ducks and turkeys in Minnesota. *Avian Dis* **7**, 77–85.

Hinshaw, V.S., Bean, W.J., Geraci, J., Fiorelli, P., Early, G. & Webster, R.G. (1986) Characterization of two influenza A viruses from a pilot whale. *J Virol* **58**, 655–6.

Hinshaw, V.S., Bean, W.J., Webster, R.G. & Sriram, G. (1980a) Genetic reassotment of influenza A viruses in the intestinal tract of ducks. *Virology* **102**, 412–19.

Hinshaw, V.S. & Webster, R.G. (1982) The natural history of influenza A viruses. In: Beard, A.S. (ed.) *Basic and Applied Influenza Research*. CRC Press, Boca Raton, Florida.

Hinshaw, V.S., Webster, R.G., Naeve, C.W. & Murphy, B.R. (1983) Altered tissue tropism of human–avian reassortant influenza viruses. *Virology* **128**, 260–3.

Hinshaw, V.S., Webster, R.G. & Rodriguez, R.J (1981) Influenza A viruses: combinations of hemagglutinin and neuraminidase subtypes isolated from animals and other sources. *Arch Virol* **67**, 191–201.

Hinshaw, V.S., Webster, R.G. & Turner, B. (1980b) The perpetuation of orthomyxoviruses and paramyxoviruses in Canadian waterfowl. *Canad J Microbiol* **26**, 622–9.

Hinshaw, V.S., Wood, J.M., Webster, R.G., Deibel, R. & Turner, B. (1985) Circulation of influenza viruses and paramyxoviruses in waterfowl originating from two different areas of North America. *Bull WHO* **63**, 711–19.

Horimoto, T. & Kawaoka, Y. (1994) Reverse genetics provides direct evidence for a correlation of hemagglutinin cleavability and virulence of an avian influenza A virus. *J Virol* **68**, 3120–8.

Horimoto, T. & Kawaoka, Y. (1995) Molecular changes in virulent mutants arising from avirulent avian influenza viruses during replication in 14-day-old embryonated eggs. *Virology* **206**, 755–9.

Horimoto, T., Nakayama, K., Smeekens, S.P. & Kawaoka, Y. (1994) Proprotein-processing endoproteases PC6 and furin both activate hemagglutinin of virulent avian influenza viruses. *J Virol* **68**, 6074–8.

Hunt, L.A., Brown, D.W., Robinson, H.L., Naeve, C.W. & Webster, R.G. (1988) Retrovirus-expressed hemagglutinin protects against lethal influenza virus infections. *J Virol* **62**, 3014–19.

Ito, T., Gorman, O.T., Kawaoka, Y., Bean, W.J & Webster, R.G. (1991) Evolutionary analysis of the influenza A virus M gene with comparison of the M1 and M2 proteins. *J Virol* **65**, 5491–8.

Ito, T., Okazaki, K., Kawaoka, Y., Takada, A., Webster, R.G. & Kida, H. (1995) Perpetuation of influenza A viruses in Alaskan waterfowl reservoirs. *Arch Virol* **140**, 1163–72.

Kawaoka, Y., Chambers, T.M., Sladen, W.L. & Webster, R.G. (1988) Is the gene pool of influenza viruses in shorebirds and gulls different from that in wild ducks? *Virology* **163**, 247–50.

Kawaoka, Y., Krauss, S. & Webster, R.G. (1989) Avian-to-human transmission of the PB1 gene of influenza A virus in the 1957 and 1968 pandemics. *J Virol* **63**, 4603–8.

Kawaoka, Y., Naeve, C.W. & Webster, R.G. (1984) Is virulence of H5N2 influenza viruses in chickens associated with loss of carbohydrate from the hemagglutinin? *Virology* **139**, 303–16.

Kawaoka, Y., Nestorowicz, A., Alexander, D.J & Webster, R.G. (1987) Molecular analyses of the hemagglutinin genes of H5 influenza viruses: origin of a virulent turkey strain. *Virology* **158**, 218–27.

Kawaoka, Y. & Webster, R.G. (1988a) Molecular mechanism of acquisition of virulence in influenza virus in nature. *Microbiol Path* **5**, 311–18.

Kawaoka, Y. & Webster, R.G. (1988b) Sequence requirements for cleavage activation of influenza virus hemagglutinin expressed in mammalian cells. *Proc Natl Acad Sci USA* **85**, 324–8.

Kawaoka, Y. & Webster, R.G. (1989) Interplay between carbohydrate in the stalk and the length of the connecting peptide determines the cleavability of influenza virus hemagglutinin. *J Virol* **63**, 3296–300.

Kida, H., Yanagawa, R. & Matsuoka, Y. (1980) Duck influenza lacking evidence of disease signs and immune response. *Infect Immun* **30**, 547–53.

Klenk, H.D. & Rott, R. (1988) The molecular biology of influenza virus pathogenicity. *Adv Virus Res* **34**, 247–81.

Klingeborn, B., Englund, L., Rott, R., Juntti, N. & Rockborn, G. (1985) An avian influenza A virus killing a mammalian species—the mink. Brief report. *Arch Virol* **86**, 347–51.

Li, S.Q., Orlich, M. & Rott, R. (1990) Generation of seal influenza virus variants pathogenic for chickens, because of hemagglutinin cleavage site changes. *J Virol* **64**, 3297–303.

Ludwig, S., Stitz, L., Planz, O., Van, H., Fitch, W.M. & Scholtissek, C. (1995) European swine virus as a possible source for the next influenza pandemic? *Virology* **212**, 555–61.

McCapes, R.H. & Bankowski, R.A. (1986) Use of avian influenza vaccines in California turkey breeders—medical rationale. In: Easterday, B.C., Alexander, D.J., & Beard, C.W. (eds) *Proceedings of the 2nd International Symposium on Avian Influenza*, pp. 271–8. US Animal Health Association, Athens, Georgia.

McKenzie, B.E., Easterday, B.C. & Will, J.A. (1972) Light and electron microscopic changes in the myocardium of influenza-infected turkeys. *Am J Pathol* **69**, 239–54.

Murphy, B.R. & Webster, R.G. (1996) Orthomyxoviruses. In: Fields, Knipe, Howley *et al. Virology*, pp. 1397–1446. Lippincott-Raven Publishers, Philadelphia.

Murphy, B.R., Hinshaw, V.S., Sly, D.L. *et al.* (1982) Virulence of avian influenza A viruses for squirrel monkeys. *Infect Immun* **37**, 1119–26.

Narayan, O., Lang, G. & Rouse, B.T. (1969a) A new influenza A virus infection in turkeys. IV. Experimental susceptibility of domestic birds to virus strain Turkey/Ontario/7732/1966. *Arch Gesamte Virusforsch* **26**, 149–65.

Narayan, O., Lang, G. & Rouse, B.T. (1969b) A new influenza A virus infection in turkeys. V. Pathology of the experimental disease by strains Turkey/Ontario/7732/1966. *Arch Gesamte Virusforsch* **26**, 166–82.

Nestorowicz, A., Kawaoka, Y., Bean, W.J. & Webster, R.G. (1987) Molecular analysis of the hemagglutinin genes of Australian H7N7 influenza viruses: role of passerine birds in maintenance or transmission? *Virology* **160**, 411–18.

Ogawa, T. & Ueda, M. (1981) Genes involved in the virulence of an avian influenza virus. *Virology* **113**, 304–13.

Ohuchi, M., Orlich, M., Ohuchi, R. *et al.* (1989) Mutations at the cleavage site of the hemagglutinin after the pathogenicity of influenza virus A/Chick/Penn/83 (H5N2). *Virology* **168**, 274–80.

Poss, P.E., Halvorson, D.A. & Karunakaran, D. (1982) Economic impact of avian influenza in domestic fowl in the United States. In: *Proceedings of the 1st International Symposium on Avian Influenza*, pp. 100–11, Carter Comp., Richmond, Virginia.

Roberts, D.H. (1964) The isolation of an influenza A virus and a *Mycoplasma* associated with duck sinusitis. *Vet Rec* **76**, 470.

Robinson, H.L., Hunt, L.A. & Webster, R.G. (1993) Protection against a lethal influenza virus challenge by immunization with a haemagglutinin-expressing plasmid DNA. *Vaccine* **11**, 957–60.

Rogers, G.N. & Paulson, J.C. (1983) Receptor determinants of human and animal influenza virus isolates: differences in receptor specificity of the H3 hemagglutinin based on species of origin. *Virology* **127**, 361–73.

Rogers, G.N., Paulson, J.C., Daniels, R.S., Skehel, J.J., Wilson, I.A. & Wiley, D.C. (1983) Single amino acid substitutions in influenza haemagglutinin change receptor binding specificity. *Nature* **304**, 76–8.

Rott, R., Orlich, M. & Scholtissek, C. (1976) Attenuation of pathogenicity of fowl plague virus by recombination with other influenza A viruses nonpathogenic for fowl: non-exclusive dependence of pathogenicity on hemagglutinin and neuraminidase of the virus. *J Virol* **19**, 54–60.

Rott, R., Orlich, M. & Scholtissek, C. (1979) Correlation of pathogenicity and gene constellation of influenza A viruses. III. Non-pathogenic recombinants derived from highly pathogenic parent strains. *J Gen Virol* **44**, 471–7.

Rouse, B.T., Lang, G. & Narayan, O. (1971) A new influenza A virus infection in turkeys. VII. Comparative immunology. *Canad J Comp Med* **35**, 44–51.

Samadieh, B. & Bankowski, R.A. (1971) Transmissibility of avian influenza A viruses. *Am J Vet Res* **32**, 939–45.

Schafer, W. (1955) Vergleichende sero-immunologische Untersuchungen uber die Viren der Influenza und klassischen Geflugelpest. *Z Naturforsch* **10b**, 81.

Scholtissek, C. (1985) Stability of infectious influenza A viruses at low pH and at elevated temperature. In: *Vaccine*, Vol. 3, 3rd edn. Butterworths, London.

Scholtissek., C., Burger., H., Bachmann., P.A. & Hannoun, C. (1983) Genetic relatedness of hemagglutinins of the H1 subtype of influenza A viruses isolated from swine and birds. *Virology* **129**, 521–3.

Scholtissek, C., Burger, H., Kistner, O. & Shortridge, K.F. (1985) The nucleoprotein as a possible major factor in determining host specificity of influenza H3N2 viruses. *Virology* **147**, 287–94.

Scholtissek, C., Rohde, W., von Hoyningen, V. & Rott, R. (1978) On the origin of the human influenza virus subtypes H2N2 and H3N2. *Virology* **87**, 13–20.

Sharp, G.B., Kawaoka, Y., Wright, S.M., Turner, B., Hinshaw, V. & Webster, R.G. (1993) Wild ducks are the reservoir for only a limited number of influenza A subtypes. *Epidemiol Infect* **110**, 161–76.

Slemons, R.D., Johnson, D.C., Osborne, J.S. & Hayes, F. (1974) Type A influenza viruses isolated from wild free-frying ducks in California. *Avian Dis* **18**, 119–24.

Snyder, M.H., Buckler-White, A.J., London, W.T., Tierney, E.L. & Murphy, B.R. (1987) The avian influenza virus nucleoprotein gene and a specific constellation of avian and human virus polymerase genes each specify attenuation of avian–human influenza A/Pintail/79 reassortant viruses for monkeys. *J Virol* **61**, 2857–63.

Stieneke-Grober, A., Vey, M., Angliker, H. *et al.* (1992) Influenza virus hemagglutinin with multibasic cleavage site is activated by furin, a subtilisin-like endoprotease. *EMBO J* **11**, 2407, 2414.

Sutter, G., Wyatt, L.S., Foley, P.L., Bennink, J.R. & Moss, B. (1994) A recombinant vector derived from the host range-restricted and highly attenuated MVA strain of vaccinia virus stimulates protective immunity in mice to influenza virus. *Vaccine* **12**, 1032–40.

Tashiro, M., Reinacher, M. & Rott, R. (1987) Aggravation of pathogenicity of an avian influenza virus by adaptation to quails. *Arch Virol* **93**, 81–95.

Taylor, J., Weinberg, R., Kawaoka, Y., Webster, R.G. & Paoletti, E. (1988) Protective immunity against avian influenza induced by a fowlpox virus recombinant. *Vaccine* **6**, 504–8.

Tripathy, D.N. & Schnitzlein, W.M. (1991) Expression of avian influenza virus hemagglutinin by recombinant fowlpox virus. *Avian Dis* **35**, 186–91.

Uys, C.J & Becker, W.B. (1967) Experimental infection of chickens with influenza A/Tern/South Africa/1961 and Chicken/Scotland/1959 viruses. II. Pathology. *J Comp Pathol* **77**, 167.

Vey, M., Orlich, M., Adler, S., Klenk, H.D., Rott, R. & Garten, W. (1992) Hemagglutinin activation of pathogenic avian influenza viruses of serotype H7 requires the protease recognition motif R-X-K/R-R. *Virology* **188**, 408–13.

Webster, R.G., Hinshaw, V.S., Bean, W.J., van Wyke, K.L., Geraci, J.R. & Petursson, G. (1981) Characterization of an influenza A virus from seals. *Virology* **113**, 712–24.

Webster, R.G. & Kawaoka, Y. (1988) Avian Influenza. In: *The CRC Critical Reviews in Poultry Biology*, Vol. 1, pp. 211–46. CRC Press, Boca Raton, Florida.

Webster, R.G., Kawaoka, Y., Taylor, J., Weinberg, R. & Paoletti, E. (1991) Efficacy of nucleoprotein and haemagglutinin antigens expressed in fowlpox virus as vaccine for influenza in chickens. *Vaccine* **9**, 303–8.

Webster, R.G. & Laver, W.G. (1972) The origin of pandemic influenza. *Bull WHO* **47**, 449–52.

Webster, R.G. & Rott, R. (1987) Influenza virus A pathogenicity: the pivotal role of hemagglutinin. *Cell* **50**, 665–6.

Webster, R.G., Yakhno, M., Hinshaw, V.S., Bean, W.J & Murti, K.G. (1978) Intestinal influenza: replication and characterization of influenza viruses in ducks. *Virology* **84**, 268–78.

Wood, J.M., Kawaoka, Y., Newberry, L.A., Bordwell, E. & Webster, R.G. (1985) Standardization of inactivated H5N2 influenza vaccine and efficacy against lethal A/Chicken/Pennsylvania/1370/83 infection. *Avian Dis* **29**, 867–72.

CHAPTER 13

Influenza in Pigs and their Role as the Intermediate Host

Christoph Scholtissek, Virginia S. Hinshaw and Christopher W. Olsen

Infection of pigs with influenza A viruses is of substantial importance to the swine industry throughout the world and to the epidemiology of human influenza A viruses. Phylogenetic analyses indicate that influenza A viruses have survived in avian reservoirs—especially in waterfowl (Hinshaw & Webster 1982)—for centuries, and from such reservoirs, avian viruses have occasionally crossed species barriers and entered mammals. Thereafter, and as a rare event, such an avian virus can come under strong selection pressure and form a stable lineage in the new host (Gammelin et al. 1990; Gorman et al. 1990; see also Chapter 10). Avian influenza viruses do not spread in the human population and, vice versa, human viruses do not establish themselves in bird populations. Thus, the species barrier between birds and humans is quite tight. However, it is shown in this chapter that pigs can be infected by avian or human influenza A viruses relatively easily (most avian influenza A viruses multiply to reasonable titres in pigs; Hinshaw et al. 1981; Kida et al. 1994) and that the species barriers between pigs and birds or humans are much less stringent. Therefore, pigs may function as intermediate hosts in establishing new influenza virus lineages in humans (Gorman et al. 1991; Scholtissek et al. 1993; Ludwig et al. 1995).

The segmented genome of influenza viruses (see Chapter 4) allows individual avian influenza virus genes to be incorporated into human influenza viruses by reassortment (antigenic shift). Because pigs are susceptible to infection with influenza viruses of both avian and human origin, they have been implicated as the 'mixing vessels' for reassortment (for a review see Scholtissek 1990). The

recent isolation of such reassortants from pigs in Italy demonstrates that this can and does occur in pigs raised under natural conditions (Castrucci et al. 1993).

Finally, pigs can also serve as direct sources for zoonotic transmission of swine influenza viruses to humans, sometimes resulting in death (Rota et al. 1989; Wentworth et al. 1994). However, these viruses did not spread to additional human contacts. Therefore, those influenza viruses that are able to spread in a population and establish long-living stable lineages are likely to have additional, as yet unknown properties.

This chapter describes the role of pigs as intermediate hosts for the introduction of avian influenza viruses (or, by reassortment, individual genes) into the human population and the factors that may be required for these events to occur.

Pigs as a reservoir for influenza A viruses

Classical swine influenza (H1N1) in the USA and in other countries

The first influenza A virus was isolated from diseased pigs in the USA by R.E. Shope (1931). As will be shown below, this H1N1 virus was presumably introduced into the North American pig population at about the beginning of this century and has been enzootic there since that time. Antigenic drift variants of these so-called 'classical' H1N1 swine influenza viruses have also appeared in the USA, although their importance in the epidemiology of disease in pigs remains unclear (Olsen et al. 1992).

In the 1970s, classical H1N1 swine influenza virus was introduced to Asia (Taiwan, Hong Kong, Japan), presumably following the importation of pigs from the USA, and these viruses have now spread to many Asian countries (Kupradinum *et al.* 1991). In Europe, classical swine influenza viruses circulated (mainly in Italy) starting in 1976 (Nardelli *et al.* 1978; Gammelin *et al.* 1989; Donatelli *et al.* 1991). However, these viruses have now been replaced by H1N1 viruses of avian origin (see below), emphasizing the weak species barrier for transmission of avian influenza viruses to pigs.

Swine influenza in Northern Ireland and England

In the late 1930s, there were outbreaks of influenza-like illness among pigs in the British Isles. These H1N1 viruses were antigenically different from the classical swine viruses (Lamont 1938; Blakemore & Gledhill 1941). The haemagglutinin (HA) of two strains studied in detail were antigenically more closely related to early human H1N1 strains than to classical swine viruses of the time (Gompels 1953; Meier-Ewert *et al.* 1970; Neumeier & Meier-Ewert 1992; Kanegae *et al.* 1994). When the other seven gene segments of these British isolates were sequenced, it was clear that they were introduced into the swine population from humans (Neumeier *et al.* 1994). This is remarkable since pigs experimentally infected with early human H1N1 viruses exhibited minimal to no signs of disease (Shope & Frances 1936). These human-like H1N1 viruses disappeared from the British swine population in the early 1940s and did not spread to the European continent.

A new H1N1 lineage of swine influenza virus in Europe

Except for the outbreaks in the UK from 1938 until 1940, and in Italy from 1976 until the early 1980s, Europe was free of swine influenza until 1979. In the winter of 1979–80, influenza outbreaks were reported among pigs in northern Europe. Since then, this virus has spread throughout Europe and has replaced the classical swine virus in Italy. This new H1N1 virus is antigenically and genetically

distinct from classical swine viruses, but is closely related to avian H1N1 influenza A viruses (Ottis *et al.* 1981; Pensaert *et al.* 1981; Witte *et al.* 1981; Scholtissek *et al.* 1983; Hinshaw *et al.* 1984; Schultz *et al.* 1991; Ludwig *et al.* 1994). Thus, at the present time, there are two different H1N1 swine viruses circulating as stable lineages in the world, the classical swine viruses in North America and the European H1N1 swine viruses.

H3N2 influenza A viruses in pigs

Influenza A viruses of the H3N2 subtype were first isolated from pigs during a human epidemic in Taiwan (Kundin 1970). Since that time, infection of pigs with human H3N2 viruses has been documented by serological means and by virus isolation from pigs in several parts of the world (Shortridge *et al.* 1977; Shortridge 1992; Castrucci *et al.* 1993; Bikour *et al.* 1995b; Brown *et al.* 1995b; Nerome *et al.* 1995; Zhou *et al.* 1996). Unlike the H1N1 strains, however, these viruses do not appear to cause significant disease and, as a rule, their circulation is limited. In the USA, H3N2 virus infection in pigs is quite rare, compared to the prevalence of H1N1 viruses (Hinshaw *et al.* 1978; Chambers *et al.* 1991).

Origin of swine influenza viruses and crossing of species barriers

Classical H1N1 swine virus

With the advent of methods to sequence viral RNA genomes and computer programs to establish phylogenetic relationships, the origin of influenza viruses can be quite easily determined. Sequence analyses of the gene for the nucleoprotein (NP), a major determinant of influenza A virus host specificity (Scholtissek *et al.* 1985; Snyder *et al.* 1987), established that avian influenza viruses in birds remain in evolutionary stasis, whereas mammalian viruses are under strong selection pressure to change (Gammelin *et al.* 1990; Gorman *et al.* 1990). From this observation, it was concluded that avian influenza viruses persist almost unchanged in bird populations for centuries and that mammalian influenza viruses have an avian ancestor. By drawing regression lines relating the year of isolation with nucleotide substitutions or amino acid replacements, mutational or evolutionary rates, respectively, can be calculated (Fig. 13.1). Using this approach, the time axis is reached close to the beginning of this century, the classical swine viruses appearing somewhat earlier when compared with the human viruses (Scholtissek *et al.* 1993). This suggests that around 1900, an avian influenza virus passed the species barrier, presumably first to pigs and possibly from there to humans (Scholtissek *et al.* 1993). Similar observations were made by analysing the HA and other viral genes (Sugita *et al.* 1991; Kanegae *et al.* 1994), suggesting that avian influenza viruses can pass the species barrier to mammals *in toto*, without reassortment (Gorman *et al.* 1991; Schultz *et al.* 1991). However, while the

mutational rates (at the level of nucleotide substitutions) of classical swine and human viruses are almost the same (see Fig. 13.1), there are great differences in the evolutionary rates (at the level of amino acid replacements; Gorman *et al.* 1991; Sugita *et al.* 1991; Scholtissek *et al.* 1993). Finally, it should be noted that classical H1N1 swine viruses have also crossed the species barrier back to turkeys (Hinshaw *et al.* 1983).

European H1N1 virus

Unfortunately, H1N1 isolates from pigs or humans around 1900 are not available and, thus, the conclusions on the origin of these viruses reached by extrapolation of regression lines (see Fig. 13.1) cannot be confirmed by virological analysis. However, in 1979, another H1N1 virus (which proved to have originated from an avian reservoir; see above) was isolated from diseased pigs in northern Europe. Sequence analysis of all genes from this virus demonstrated that an avian H1N1 influenza virus passed the species barrier again *in toto*. A more exact phylogenetic analysis (Fig. 13.2) revealed that this avian virus was introduced into the pig population in 1978, forming a stable lineage in the new host. Another interesting observation was that following introduction of this virus into pigs, its evolutionary rate was significantly higher than the rates for classical swine and human viruses (Schultz *et al.* 1991; Ludwig *et al.* 1994, 1995). Finally, these northern European swine viruses have also crossed the species barrier back to turkeys and caused disease in these birds (Andral *et al.* 1985; Ludwig *et al.* 1994; see Fig. 13.2).

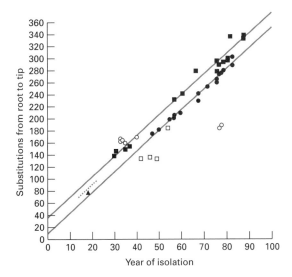

Fig. 13.1 Evolutionary rate determinations for the nucleoprotein genes for human (circles) and classical swine (squares) virus isolates. The evolutionary rates are estimated by regression of the years of isolation (horizontal scale) against the branch distance from the common ancestor node of the nucleotide phylogenetic tree (total nucleotide substitutions vertical scale). Only the closed symbols were used for the calculations of the best fitting lines. The closed triangle is the assumed human–pig divergence point plotted at 1918. (Reprinted from Schotissek *et al.* (1993), 193–201, with kind permission from Elsevier Science – NL, Sara Burgerhartstraat 25, 1055 KV Amsterdam, the Netherlands.)

Occasional introduction of human H3N2 and H1N1 influenza viruses into pigs

As mentioned above, H3N2 influenza viruses have been isolated from pigs worldwide. These viruses are antigenically and genetically similar to viruses that circulated in the human population prior to their isolation from pigs. A phylogenetic analysis revealed that there have been multiple independent introductions of H3 human viruses to pigs in Asia between 1976 and 1982 (Nerome *et al.* 1995).

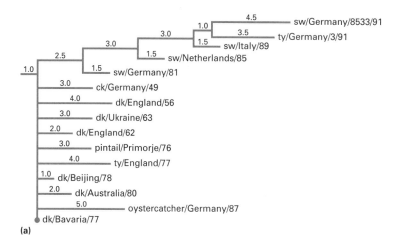

(a)

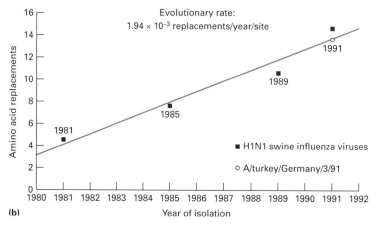

(b)

Fig. 13.2 Phylogenetic tree of the nucleoproteins of influenza A (a), and 'time plot' (b) as constructed from the phylogenetic tree for the north European swine viruses. (From Ludwig *et al.* 1994, with permission from Academic Press.)

Similar observations were made with human H1N1 viruses. In 1992, two H1N1 viruses were isolated from pigs in northern Japan. These isolates contained glycoprotein genes that were closely related to human H1N1 viruses circulating between 1990 and 1992 (Katsuda *et al.* 1995). To date, none of these viruses of human origin have established stable lineages in pigs. However, pigs could form a reservoir where these viruses persist until a new immunologically naive human generation was available (Bikour *et al.* 1995a). These viruses might then have the potential to cause pandemics of disease among children and young adults as happened in 1977 (Nakajima *et al.* 1978; Scholtissek *et al.* 1978a).

Pigs as 'mixing vessels' for the creation of new viruses by reassortment

Antigenic shift

Reassortment of viral RNA segments during dual infection with an avian and a human influenza virus provides a mechanism by which a new virus is created. In this way, a virus can be generated that has surface antigens against which the human population does not have neutralizing antibodies and is not protected (antigenic shift). This new virus could then spread easily, with the potential for causing a worldwide pandemic of disease. This happened in 1957 and 1968. In 1957, the HA, neuraminidase (NA) and polymerase PB1 genes were replaced with segments from an avian virus. In 1968, the HA gene, and probably the PB1 gene, were replaced again with genes of avian origin (Scholtissek *et al.* 1978b; Kawaoka *et al.* 1989).

In order for reassortment and antigenic shift to occur, a host must be dually infected with an avian and a human virus. Since avian influenza viruses do not spread in the human population, it is unlikely that reassortment occurs directly in humans. Pigs, however, are uniquely susceptible to infection with both avian and human viruses and have been implicated as the intermediate hosts for reassortment (Scholtissek *et al.* 1985; Scholtissek 1990). Given this potential, the fact that pigs live in close proximity to their farmers in South-East Asia, sometimes even sharing the same dwellings and water supplies, may explain why the pandemics of recent times originated in this part of the world. In addition, pigs and ducks are often in direct contact in rice fields and the special practice of fish farming in Asia would further enhance interspecies contact and the potential for dual infection of pigs (Shortridge & Stuart-Harris 1982; Scholtissek & Naylor 1988; Scholtissek 1990; Shortridge 1992). In a recent study, Shu *et al.* (1994) found that three of 32 H3N2 virus isolates from pigs in China were reassortants between human and classical swine viruses, in which the surface glycoproteins were of human origin. In contrast, no reassortants were found among 104 H1N1 isolates, all genes being derived from a classical swine virus. More recently, however, Guan *et al.* (1996) isolated avian-like H1N1 influenza viruses from pigs in Hong Kong. Clearly, the possibility of creating a pandemic strain by reassortment in pigs exists in South-East Asia. But as described below, this potential may also exist elsewhere in the world.

H1N2 swine viruses in France and Japan

Since 1981, avian-like H1N1 and human H3N2 strains have circulated in separate outbreaks or concomitantly in pigs. Therefore, it was not too surprising that Gourreau *et al.* (1994) isolated H1N2 reassortants from diseased pigs in northern France in 1987 and 1988. The HA of these viruses was found to be closely related to that of avian-like swine virus, while the NA was derived from human H3N2 strains. Reassortment in the laboratory or during isolation could be excluded, since pig sera contained only antibodies to H1 and N2, and not to H3 and N1. Thus, the recombination event must have occurred in another swine herd or in another species.

Similar H1N2 viruses were isolated in Japan in 1978, 1980 and during the winter of 1989–90. These reassortants contained an HA closely related to classical swine virus, but the NA was again derived from human H3N2 strains. In the latest outbreak, the remaining six viral gene segments of the reassortants were shown, by sequence analysis, to be of classical swine virus origin (Sugimura *et al.* 1980; Yasuhara *et al.* 1983; Nerome *et al.* 1983, 1985; Ouchi *et al.* 1996). So far, there is no indication that these reassortants formed stable lineages in pigs. However, Brown *et al.* (1995a) isolated an H1N2 reassortant on at least three separate farms in the UK and suggest that this virus may be widespread in the British pig population. In addition, an unusual H1N7 reassortant has also been isolated from pigs in the UK. Although this virus was of low pathogenicity for pigs, it was able to spread from pig to pig during experimental infection studies (Brown *et al.* 1994).

Human–avian reassortants in European pigs and children

In 1993, Castrucci *et al.* (1993) isolated reassortant viruses from pigs in Italy that contained the internal viral protein genes from the avian-like swine viruses circulating in Europe and the surface glycoprotein genes from an H3N2 human virus. In fact, although all eight gene segments of H3N2 swine virus isolates from 1977 and 1983 were most closely related to those of human viruses, all of the H3N2 viruses they isolated from swine between 1985 and 1989 were reassortants. It still remains to be determined whether these new reassortants will form a stable lineage. However, these results demonstrate that pigs can function as 'mixing vessels' outside of South-East Asia. In addition, similar reassortants were recently isolated from children in the Netherlands (Claas *et al.* 1994). This observation is very important because it demonstrates that avian-human reassortants can cross the swine-human species barrier. However, there is no evidence to date that these reassortants have spread further in the human population.

Swine-avian reassortants in turkeys

During a survey between 1976 and 1990 in the USA, Wright *et al.* (1992) analysed 73 swine and 11 turkey influenza A isolates genetically. None of the classical swine viruses were found to be reassortants, but 73% of the turkey isolates contained genes from classical swine and avian viruses. In the light of this, it is important to realize that turkeys infected with classical swine influenza viruses can serve as sources for zoonotic transmission to humans (Hinshaw *et al.* 1983).

Possible prerequisites for crossing species barriers

Crossing species barriers *in toto* (without reassortment)

Influenza A viruses cross species barriers relatively easily and often. The establishment of stable lineages and spread over continents are, however, rare events. For the latter event to occur, we have to assume that additional properties are required of such viruses. The early isolates (1979–85) of the avian-like northern European H1N1 swine lineage are genetically extremely unstable, with elevated mutational and evolutionary rates when compared with human viruses. Furthermore, their plaque morphology is heterogeneous over many passages, and the escape rate against specific monoclonal antibodies is extremely high—in contrast to North German isolates from 1991 and later (Ludwig *et al.* 1995). The interpretation of these observations is that the early swine isolates might contain a strong mutator mutation in one of the viral RNA polymerase components. Less significant mutator mutations have been observed previously in a normal influenza virus population (Suàres *et al.* 1992). Ludwig *et al.* (1995) speculated that mutator

mutations in avian viruses might be the prerequisite for crossing the species barrier to pigs and for the establishment of a new stable lineage. A mutator mutation would offer a large number of variants from which pigs could rapidly select the best fitting strains. Consequently, if a virus has passed the species barrier, but does not contain a mutator mutation, it may not have the ability to establish a new stable lineage. Since a mutator mutation may not be an advantage for a virus under normal conditions, it is not surprising that this putative mutation is lost again after a new lineage has been established. However, as long as a mutator mutation is present in a swine virus, it may allow the virus to cross the species barrier a second time, e.g. to humans. This is likely to be what happened just before the Spanish flu pandemic of 1918–19. If this is true, the pandemic of 1918–19 might—as an exception—not have originated in South-East Asia, but in the USA. Correspondingly, could the next pandemic start in Europe, originating from an avian-like European swine viruses still containing a mutator mutation?

Crossing species barriers by reassortment of individual genes

As shown above, pigs can and do become doubly infected by avian and human influenza A viruses. Nevertheless, antigenic shifts and corresponding pandemics occur relatively infrequently. We have to assume therefore that for the introduction of a foreign gene into a new genetic constellation by reassortment, a corresponding adaptation must occur for optimal function of the new gene product within the framework of the existing viral proteins. For instance, during our efforts to rescue temperature-sensitive mutants of fowl plague virus by human viruses, we never found segregation of the matrix (M) and HA genes, but this happened easily when rescue was accomplished with avian strains. Only after strong selection pressure by specific antisera could human–avian reassortants be obtained, and even then these grew only to low titres and formed small fuzzy plaques. Thus, during an antigenic shift, human M-gene product(s) and the avian HA probably have to adapt rapidly. A mutator mutation would again be helpful in this situation. Reassortment amongst components of the polymerase complex—as is known to have occurred in the antigenic shifts of 1957 and 1968—might also create a more error-prone polymerase. However, no one has examined this possibility yet.

Outlook

This chapter has shown that, for influenza viruses, the species barrier to pigs is relatively low when compared with the barrier between birds and humans. Therefore, pigs may function as intermediates and 'mixing vessels' for the creation of new pandemic strains, either by introduction of avian viruses into pigs *in toto* or by reassortment of individual genes during antigenic shifts. It has been suggested that mutator mutations or reassortment among the components of the polymerase complex may also be prerequisites for such events to occur. More research is necessary to clarify this point. However, if pigs are important as intermediates, then influenza virus activity in this species—in addition to the worldwide human influenza surveillance—needs to be monitored. Simple tests for determining the genetic stability of new swine influenza viruses and reassortants should also be established, since only those strains that are genetically unstable are likely to be of concern.

Finally, changes in agricultural practices in South-East Asia could reduce the potential for dual infection of pigs with avian and human viruses. However, clearly the potential for pigs to act as mixing vessels extends beyond South-East Asia and surveillance must be vigilant in other regions of the world. Another potential mechanism to exclude pigs from the chain of transmission of influenza viruses (or their genes) from birds to humans is to create transgenic pigs carrying cDNA copies of the murine Mx1 protein to confer resistance against infections (Müller *et al.* 1992). Although this approach has not yet been successful, further research in this area and in the development of new approaches to vaccination against swine influenza is warranted.

References

Andral, B., Toquin, D., Madec, F. *et al.* (1985) Disease in turkeys associated with H1N1 influenza virus following an outbreak of the disease in pigs. *Vet Rec* **116**, 617–18.

Bikour, M.H., Frost, E.H., Deslandes, S., Talbot, B. & Elazhary, Y. (1995a) Persistence of a 1930 swine influenza A (H1N1) virus in Quebec. *J Gen Virol* **76**, 2539–47.

Bikour, M.H., Frost, E.H., Deslandes, S., Talbot, R., Weber, J.M. & Elazhary, Y. (1995b) Recent H3N2 swine influenza virus with haemagglutinin and nucleoprotein genes similar to 1975 human strains. *J Gen Virol* **76**, 697–703.

Blakemore, F. & Gledhill, A.W. (1941) Some observations on an outbreak of swine influenza in England. *Vet Rec* **53**, 227–30.

Brown, I.H., Alexander, D.J., Chakraverty, P., Harris, P.A. & Manvell, R.J. (1994) Isolation of an influenza A virus of unusual subtype (H1N7) from pigs in England, and the subsequent experimental transmission from pig to pig. *Vet Microbiol* **39**, 125–34.

Brown, I.H., Chakraverty, P., Harris, P.A. & Alexander, D.J. (1995a) Disease outbreaks in pigs in Great Britain due to an influenza A virus of H1N2 subtype. *Vet Rec* **136**, 328–9.

Brown, I.H., Harris, P.A. & Alexander, D.j. (1995b) Serological studies of influenza viruses in pigs in Great Britain. 1991–2. *Epidemiol Infect* **114**, 511–20.

Castrucci, M.R., Donatelli, I., Sidoli, L., Barigazzi, G., Kawaoka, Y. & Webster, R.G. (1993) Genetic reassortment between avian and human influenza A viruses in Italian pigs. *Virology* **193**, 503–6.

Chambers, T.M., Hinshaw, V.S., Kawaoka, Y., Easterday, B.C. & Webster, R.G. (1991) Influenza viral infection of swine in the United States 1988–89. *Arch Virol* **116**, 261–5.

Claas, E.C., Kawaoka, Y., de Jong, J.C., Masurel, N. & Webster, R.G. (1994) Infection of children with avian-human reassortant influenza virus from pigs in Europe. *Virology* **204**, 453–7.

Donatelli, I., Campitelli, L., Castrucci, M.R., Ruggieri, A., Sidoli, L. & Oxford, J.S. (1991) Detection of two antigenic subpopulations of A (H1N1) influenza viruses from pigs: antigenic drift or interspecies transmission? *J Med Virol* **34**, 248–57.

Gammelin, M., Altmüller, A., Reinhardt, U. *et al.* (1990) Phylogenetic analysis of nucleoproteins suggests that human influenza A viruses emerged from a 19th-century avian ancestor. *Molec Biol Evol* **7**, 194–200.

Gammelin, M., Mandler, J. & Scholtissek, C. (1989) Two subtypes of nucleoproteins (NP) of influenza A viruses. *Virology* **170**, 71–80.

Gompels, A.E.H. (1953) Antigenic relationships of swine influenza virus. *J Gen Microbiol* **9**, 140–8.

Gorman, O.T., Bean, W.J., Kawaoka, Y., Donatelli, I., Guo, Y. & Webster, R.G. (1991) Evolution of influenza A virus nucleoprotein genes: implications for the origin of H1N1 human and classical swine viruses. *J Virol* **65**, 3704–14.

Gorman, O.T., Bean, W.J., Kawaoka, Y. & Webster, R.G. (1990) Evolution of the nucleoprotein gene of influenza A virus. *J Virol* **64**, 1487–97.

Gourreau, J.M., Kaiser, C., Valette, M., Douglas, A.R., Labic, J. & Aymard, M. (1994) Isolation of two H1N2 influenza viruses from swine in France. *Arch Virol* **135**, 365–82.

Guan, Y., Shortridge, K.F., Krauss, S., Li, P.H., Kawaoka, Y. & Webster, R.G. (1996) Emergence of avian H1N1 influenza viruses in pigs in China. *J Virol* **70**, 8041–6.

Hinshaw, V.S., Alexander, D.J., Aymard, M. *et al.* (1984) Antigenic comparison of swine influenza-like H1N1 isolates from pigs, birds and humans: an international collaborative study. *Bull WHO* **62**, 871–8.

Hinshaw, V.S., Bean, W.J., Webster, R.G. & Easterday, B.C. (1978) The prevalence of influenza viruses in swine and the antigenic and genetic relatedness of influenza viruses from man and animals. *Virology* **84**, 51–62.

Hinshaw, V.S. & Webster, R.G. (1982) The natural history of influenza viruses. In: Beare, A.S. (ed.) *Basic and Applied Influenza Research*, pp. 79–104. CRC Press, Boca Raton.

Hinshaw, V.S., Webster, R.G., Bean, W.J., Downie, J. & Senne, D.A. (1983) Swine influenza-like viruses in turkeys: potential source of virus for humans? *Science* **220**, 206–8.

Hinshaw, V.S., Webster, R.G., Easterday, B.C. & Bean, W.J. (1981) Replication of avian influenza A viruses in mammals. *Infect Immun* **34**, 354–61.

Kanegae, Y., Sugita, S., Shortridge, K.F., Yoshioka, Y. & Nerome, K. (1994) Origin and evolutionary pathways of the H1 haemagglutinin gene of avian, swine and human influenza viruses: cocirculation of two distinct lineages of swine virus. *Arch Virol* **134**, 17–28.

Katsuda, K., Sato, S., Shirahata, T. *et al.* (1995) Antigenic and genetic characteristics of H1N1 human influenza virus isolated from pigs in Japan. *J Gen Virol* **76**, 1247–9.

Kawaoka, Y., Krauss, S. & Webster, R.G. (1989) Avian-to-human transmission of the PB1 gene of influenza A viruses in the 1957 and 1968 pandemics. *J Virol* **63**, 4603–8.

Kida, H., Ito, T., Yasuda, J. *et al.* (1994) Potential for transmission of avian influenza viruses to pigs. *J Gen Virol* **75**, 2183–8.

Kundin, W.D. (1970) Hong Kong A-2 influenza virus infection among swine during a human epidemic in Taiwan. *Nature* **228**, 857.

Kupradinum, S., Peanpijit, P., Brodhikosoom, C., Yoshioka, Y., Endo, A. & Nerome, K. (1991) The first isolation of swine H1N1 influenza viruses from pigs in Thailand. *Arch Virol* **118**, 289–97.

Lamont, H.G. (1938) The problems of the practitioner in connection with the differential diagnosis and treatment of disease of young pigs. *Vet Rec* **50**, 1377–400.

Ludwig, S., Haustein, A., Kaleta, E.F. & Scholtissek, C. (1994) Recent influenza A (H1N1) infections in pigs and turkeys in northern Europe. *Virology* **202**, 281–6.

Ludwig, S., Stitz, L., Planz, O., Van, H., Fitch, W.M. & Scholtissek, C. (1995) European swine virus as a possible source for the next influenza pandemic? *Virology* **212**, 555–61.

Luoh, S.M., McGregor, M.W. & Hinshaw, V.S. (1992) Hemagglutinin mutations related to antigenic variation in H1 swine influenza viruses. *J Virology* **66**, 1066–73.

Meier-Ewert, H., Gibbs, A.J. & Dimmock, N.J. (1970) Studies on antigenic variations of the haemagglutinin and neuraminidase of swine influenza virus isolates. *J Gen Virol* **6**, 409–19.

Müller, M., Brenig, B., Winnacker, E.L. & Brem, G. (1992) Transgenic pigs carrying cDNA copies encoding the murine Mx1 protein which confers resistance to influenza virus infection. *Gene* **121**, 263–70.

Nakajima, K., Desselberger, U. & Palese, P. (1978) Recent human influenza A viruses are closely related genetically to strains isolated in 1950. *Nature* **274**, 334–9.

Nakajima, K., Nakajima, S., Shortridge, K.F. & Kendal, A.P. (1982) Further genetic evidence for maintenance of early Hong Kong-like influenza A (H3N2) strains in swine until 1976. *Virology* **116**, 562–72.

Nardelli, L., Pascucci, S., Gualandi, G.L. & Loda, P. (1978) Outbreaks of classical wine influenza in Italy in 1976. *Zentralblatt Vet* **B25**, 853–7.

Nerome, K., Kanegae, Y., Shortridge, K.F., Sugita, S. & Ishida, M. (1995) Genetic analysis of porcine H3N2 viruses originating in southern China. *J Gen Virol* **76**, 613–24.

Nerome, K., Sakamoto, S., Yano, N. *et al.* (1983) Antigenic characteristics and genome composition of a naturally occurring recombinant influenza virus isolated from a pig in Japan. *J Gen Virol* **64**, 2611–20.

Nerome, K., Yoshioka, Y., Sakamoto, S., Yasuhara, M. & Oya, A. (1985) Characterization of a 1980-swine recombinant influenza virus possessing H1 haemagglutinin and N2 neuraminidase similar to that of the earliest Hong Kong (H3N2) viruses. *Arch Virol* **86**, 197–211.

Neumeier, E. & Meier-Ewert, H. (1992) Nucleotide sequence analysis of the HA1 coding portion of the haemagglutinin gene of swine H1N1 influenza viruses. *Virus Res* **23**, 107–17.

Neumeier, E., Meier-Ewert, H. & Cox, N.J. (1994) Genetic relatedness between influenza A (H1N1) viruses isolated from humans and pigs. *J Gen Virol* **75**, 2103–7.

Noble, S., McGregor, M.G., Wentworth, D.E. & Hinshaw, V.S. (1993) Antigenic and genetic conservation of the haemagglutinin in H1N1 swine influenza viruses. *J Gen Virol* **74**, 1197–200.

Olsen, C.W., McGregor, M.W., Cooley, A.J., Schantz, B., Hotze, B. & Hinshaw, V.S. (1992) antigenic and genetic analysis of a recently isolated H1N1 swine influenza virus. *Am J Vet Res* **54**, 1630–6.

Ottis, K., Bollwahn, W., Bachmann, P.A. & Henritzi, K. (1981) Ausbruch von Schweineinfluenza in der Bundesrepublik Deutschland: Klinik, Nachweis und Differenzierung. *Tierärztliche Umschau* **36**, 608–12.

Ottis, K., Sidoli, L., Bachmann, P.A. *et al.* (1982) Human influenza A viruses in pigs: isolation of a H3N2 strain antigenically related to A/England/42/72 and evidence for continuous circulation of human viruses in the pig population. *Arch Virol* **73**, 103–8.

Ouchi, A., Nerome, K., Konegae, Y. *et al.* (1996) Large outbreaks of swine influenza in southern Japan caused by reassortant (H1N2) influenza viruses: its epizootic background and characterization of the causative viruses. *J Gen Virol* **77**, 1751–9.

Pensaert, M., Ottis, K., Vandeputte, J., Kaplan, M.M. & Bachmann, P.A. (1981) Evidence of natural transmission of influenza A virus from wild ducks to swine and its potential importance for man. *Bull WHO* **59**, 75–8.

Rota, P.A., Rocha, E.P., Harmon, M.W. *et al.* (1989) Laboratory characterization of a swine influenza virus isolated from a fatal case of human influenza. *J Clin Microbiol* **27**, 1413–16.

Scholtissek, C. (1990) Pigs as 'mixing vessels' for the creation of new pandemic influenza A viruses. *Med Principles Pract* **2**, 65–71.

Scholtissek, C., Bürger, H., Bachmann, P.A. & Hannoun, C. (1983) Genetic relatedness of haemagglutinins of the H1 subtype of influenza A viruses isolated from swine and birds. *Virology* **129**, 521–3.

Scholtissek, C., Bürger, H., Kistner, O. & Shortridge, K.F. (1985) The nucleoprotein as a possible major factor in determining host specificity of influenza H3N2 viruses. *Virology* **147**, 287–94.

Scholtissek, C., Ludwig, S. & Fitch, W.M. (1993) Analysis of influenza A virus nucleoproteins for the assessment of molecular genetic mechanisms leading to new phylogenetic virus lineages. *Arch Virol* **131**, 237–50.

Scholtissek, C. & Naylor, E. (1988) Fish farming and influenza pandemics. *Nature* **331**, 215.

Scholtissek, C., Rohde, W., von Hoyningen, V. & Rott, R. (1978b) On the origin of the human influenza virus subtypes H2N2 and H3N2. *Virology* **87**, 13–20.

Scholtissek, C., Schultz, U., Ludwig, S., & Fitch, W.M. (1993) The role of swine in the origin of pandemic influenza. In: Hannoon, C., Kendal, A.P., Klenk, H.D., & Ruben, F.L. (eds) *Options for the Control of Influenza II.* Excerpta Medica, Amsterdam, 193–201.

Scholtissek, C., von Hoyningen, V. & Rott, R. (1978a) Genetic relatedness between the new 1977 epidemic strain (H1N1) of influenza and human influenza strains isolated between 1947 and 1957 (H1N1). *Virology* **89**, 613–17.

Schultz, U., Fitch, W.M., Ludwig, S., Mandler, J. & Scholtissek, C. (1991) Evolution of pig influenza viruses. *Virology* **183**, 61–73.

Sheerar, M.C., Easterday, B.C. & Hinshaw, V.S. (1989) Antigenic conservation of H1N1 swine influenza viruses. *J Gen Virol* **70**, 3297–303.

Shope, R.E. (1931) Swine influenza. III. Filtration experiments and aetiology. *J Exp Med* **54**, 373–85.

Shope, R.E. & Frances, T. Jr (1936) The susceptibility of swine to the virus of human influenza. *J Exp Med* **64**, 791.

Shortridge, K.F. (1992) Pandemic influenza: a zoonosis? *Sem Resp Infect* **7**, 11–25.

Shortridge, K.F. & Stuart-Harris, C.H. (1982) An influenza epicentre? *Lancet* **ii**, 812–13.

Shortridge, K.F., Webster, R.G. & Butterfield, W.K. (1977) Persistence of Hong Kong influenza virus variants in pigs. *Science* **196**, 1454–5.

Shu, L.L., Lin, Y.P., Wright, S.M., Shortridge, K.F. & Webster, R.G. (1994) Evidence for interspecies transmission and reassortment of influenza A viruses in pigs in southern China. *Virology* **202**, 825–33.

Snyder, M.H., Buckler-White, A.J., London, W.T., Tierney, E.L. & Murphy, B.R. (1987) The avian influenza virus nucleoprotein gene and a specific constellation of avian and human virus polymerase genes each specify attenuation of avian-human influenza A/Pintail/79 reassortant virus for monkeys. *J Virol* **61**, 2857–63.

Suáres, P., Valcácel, J. & Ortin, J. (1992) Heterogeneity of the mutation rates of influenza A viruses: Isolation of mutator mutants. *J Virol* **66**, 2491–4.

Sugimura, T., Yonemochi, H., Ogawa, T., Tanaka, Y. & Kumagai, T. (1980) Isolation of a recombinant influenza virus (Hsw1N2) from swine in Japan. *Arch Virol* **66**, 271–4.

Sugita, S., Yoshioka, Y., Itamura, S. *et al.* (1991) Molecular evolution of haemagglutinin genes of H1N1 swine and human influenza A viruses. *J Molec Evol* **32**, 16–23.

Wentworth, D.E., Thompson, B.L., Xu, X. *et al.* (1994) An influenza A (H1N1) virus, closely related to swine influenza virus, responsible for a fatal case of human influenza. *J Virol* **68**, 2051–8.

Witte, K.H., Nienhoff, H., Ernst, H., Schmidt, U. & Prager, D. (1981) Erstmaliges Auftreten einer durch das Schweineinfluenzavirus verursachten Epizootie in Schweinebeständen der Bundesrepublik Deutschland. *Tierärztliche Umschau* **36**, 591–606.

Wright, S.M., Kawaoka, Y., Sharp, G.B., Senne, D.A. & Webster, R.G. (1992) Interspecies transmission and reassortment of influenza A viruses in pigs and turkeys in the United States. *Am J Epidemiol* **136**, 488–97.

Yasuhara, H., Hirahara, T., Nakai, M. *et al.* (1983) Further isolation of a recombinant virus (H1N2), formerly (Hsw1N2) from a pig in Japan in 1980. *Microbiol Immunol* **27**, 43–50.

Zhou, N., He, S., Zhang, T. *et al.* (1996) Influenza infection in humans and pigs in south-western China. *Arch Virol* **141**, 649–61.

CHAPTER 14

Equine Influenza

Jennifer A. Mumford and Thomas M. Chambers

Introduction

Horses are one of the three common mammalian hosts for influenza A viruses, the others being swine and humans. Equine influenza is caused by two subtypes of influenza A virus, equine-1, an H7N7 virus (Sovinova *et al.* 1958), and equine-2 (Waddell *et al.* 1963), an H3N8 virus. Influenza caused by A/equine-1 virus has not been confirmed since the early 1980s although there is serological evidence for the persistence of this virus in the equine population (Webster 1993). In contrast, influenza A/equine-2 virus is frequently implicated in epidemic and endemic respiratory disease in equids on an almost worldwide basis. Although vaccines containing both subtypes are available in many countries, they are used in only a small proportion of horses. During the 30 years that vaccines have been used to control equine influenza, there have been no reports of vaccine breakdown during A/equine-1 epidemics but their efficacy in controlling infection and disease caused by A/equine-2 viruses is variable and often poor.

The epizootiology and ecology of equine influenza are influenced by the purpose for which domestic equids are used in different countries. In the developing world where equids used for transport and draft power are seldom vaccinated and seldom benefit from veterinary care epidemics may result in severe disease, secondary bacterial complications and even death. In developed countries equids are largely maintained for competition and leisure purposes and may be transported by road and air for long distances, both nationally and internationally, and mixed with other animals from distant geographical origins. Competition horses are often subject to vaccination policies and benefit from good health care. In these animals the disease is usually transient and self-limiting, provided that rest is given when infection occurs.

Equine competitive events and the breeding industry operate globally and horses travel for competitions on temporary import licences, allowing them to move between countries with minimum quarantine restrictions. This movement is based on a system of health certification and compulsory vaccination schemes agreed between exporting and importing countries. Although based on guidelines formulated by the Code Commission of the Office International des Epizooties (OIE), quarantine requirements vary widely between countries (Mumford *et al.* 1998). Thus vaccination policies and the quality of vaccines as well as diagnostic capabilities available to those involved in transport of horses have a major influence on the spread of equine influenza on a global basis. If mild or subclinical disease is unrecognized in vaccinated animals to be transported, equine influenza may be carried rapidly by air travel and introduced, with disastrous consequences, into susceptible indigenous populations far distant from the original source of virus (Kawaoka & Webster 1989; Lai *et al.* 1994).

The disease

Equine influenza infects the ciliated epithelial cells of the upper and lower airways causing deciliation of large areas of the respiratory tract within 4–6 days. As a result the mucociliary clearance mechanism is compromised and tracheal clearance rates may be reduced for up to 32 days following infection (Willoughby *et al.* 1992). Bronchitis and bronchiolitis develop followed by an interstitial pneumonia accompanied by congestion, oedema and neutrophil infiltration. In general, H3N8 viruses produce more severe clinical disease and appear to be more pneumotropic (Blaskovic *et al.* 1966, 1969; Lucam *et al.* 1974).

Clinical signs in previously naive animals are easily recognizable and include short incubation period, high temperature which is usually biphasic, depression, anorexia, dyspnoea and a harsh dry cough, followed by a mucopurulent nasal discharge and on occasions pneumonia, the latter as a consequence of secondary bacterial infection (Gerber 1970). The severity of the disease varies with the dose and strain of a virus and the immune status of the horse (Mumford *et al.* 1988, 1990), but spread of infection through a group is always rapid.

While classical influenza is rarely fatal in previously healthy adult horses, relatively high rates of mortality have been recorded in donkeys, animals in poor condition and foals. If maternal antibody is absent at the time of exposure young foals may develop a viral pneumonia leading rapidly to death (Miller 1965). In the epidemic in India in 1987, mortality rates of around 1% were reported in adult equids (Uppal & Yadav 1988), and in the 1993 epidemic of influenza in China, affecting 2.2 million animals, mortality was similarly about 1% (Shortridge *et al.* 1995). Deaths among adult animals are usually a consequence of secondary bacterial infection leading to pneumonia and purpura haemorrhagica (Rose *et al.* 1970; Uppal *et al.* 1990; Guo *et al.* 1995). An unusually high mortality rate was recorded during the 1989 epidemic in China caused by an H3N8 virus of avian origin. In this outbreak clinical signs included respiratory and enteric disease and resulted in up to 20% mortality in some groups of animals (Guo *et al.* 1990, 1992; Webster *et al.* 1991).

Clinical signs in animals partially immune as a result of vaccination or previous infection are difficult to recognize. Outbreaks have been described in which the infection circulated subclinically for 18 days before inducing recognizable clinical signs (Powell *et al.* 1995), and outbreaks in which little or no coughing or pyrexia were recorded have also been described (Jaeschke & Lange 1993; Newton & Mumford 1995).

Epizootiology

Influenza-like respiratory syndromes have been recognized in horses almost as long as in humans. Equine influenza virus is one of the most common respiratory pathogens of horses. Throughout the world, only Australia, New Zealand and Iceland are known to have remained entirely free from this disease. Equine influenza is now considered enzootic in the USA and the UK (Mumford & Wood 1993), and is probably enzootic in diverse regions including Sweden, China/Mongolia and Argentina based on nearly annual incidence of epizootics in recent years. Several European mainland countries, India, Hong Kong and, on the African continent, Egypt, Nigeria and South Africa have all experienced outbreaks in the decade since 1986.

Unlike influenza in humans, equine influenza does not follow seasonal patterns. Instead, in countries where there is heavy horse traffic, it is likely to occur at sales or race meets for which young horses are brought together from different national or international sources. The large epizootics of equine influenza in Japan (1971), South Africa (1986) and Hong Kong (1992) were all triggered by importation of infected horses into regions where the disease had in recent times been unknown. A detailed epizootiological description of a recent equine influenza outbreak is provided by Powell *et al.* (1995). As with human influenza, the spread of virus is facilitated by the short incubation period, typically 1–3 days (Gerber 1970). Morbidity rates as high as 98% have been reported (Gerber 1970).

Figure 14.1 provides a graphical summary of the history and likely prehistory of known equine influenza viruses, which will be explained in detail in the following section. The first association of influenza virus with equine respiratory disease was demonstrated by Heller *et al.* (1957) in serological studies of a 1955 epizootic. The first strain of equine influenza virus, influenza A/equine/Prague/56, was isolated from an outbreak in Czechoslovakia in

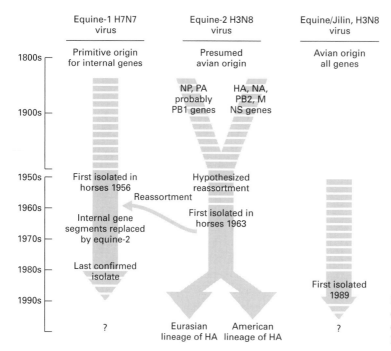

Fig. 14.1 Time lines of known (solid) or unknown (hypothetical/extrapolated) (hatched) genetic histories of equine influenza viruses.

1956 (Sovinova *et al.* 1958). Serological studies suggested this virus subtype, termed equine-1, might have circulated in horses in England as early as 1948 (Beveridge *et al.* 1965) or in the USA by the mid-1950s (Doll 1961).

In 1963 a new equine influenza virus strain of subtype H3N8 appeared and spread internationally. This subtype is termed equine-2, with prototype virus influenza A/equine/Miami/63 (Waddell *et al.* 1963). The appearance of equine-2, subtype H3 influenza virus in 1963, followed by the human pandemic with serologically cross-reacting H3 influenza in 1968, raised the possibility that equine and human H3 influenza viruses might be related. Further, seroarchaeological studies indicated that an H3N8 virus had previously circulated in humans starting with a pandemic in 1890 (e.g. Minuse *et al.* 1965; Schild & Stuart-Harris 1965), and on this basis it was suggested that equine-2 influenza viruses may have been a source of genes for novel or re-emerging human influenza viruses (Kilbourne 1968; Laver & Webster 1973). Against this, sequencing studies show that equine and human H3 HAs emerged independently from avian ancestors (Bean *et al.* 1992). Thus equine-2

influenza virus was not a progenitor of human H3 influenza virus.

Equine-1 and equine-2 virus subtypes cocirculated in horses from 1963 to at least 1980. In some outbreaks viruses of both subtypes were isolated (Tumova *et al.* 1972). The cocirculation of these two major subtypes of influenza A virus in horses had no parallel in human experience of influenza A prior to 1977. Antigenic shift as has occurred in humans, whereby virus of a new HA/NA subtype completely replaces the previous virus in worldwide circulation, has not been demonstrated in horses. It is possible that equine populations have insufficient intermingling to allow a new influenza virus strain to trigger a sudden panzootic, so instead of abrupt shifts we observe gradual changes in the proportions of different equine influenza viruses over time.

Equine-1 influenza viruses have not been isolated in North or South America or western Europe since 1980, and so have been considered either extinct or nearly so. However, equine-1 virus isolations were reported in India in 1987 (Singh 1994, 1995) and in Egypt in 1989 (Ismail *et al.* 1990). These isolations have so far been unconfirmed by the international reference laboratories studying equine influenza.

Additionally, reports since 1990 provide serological evidence for exposure of unvaccinated horses to equine-1 virus (Webster 1993). It is clearly premature to conclude that equine-1 influenza viruses may be extinct.

In 1989 a novel strain of influenza virus appeared in horses. This virus, influenza A/equine/Jilin/89 virus, arose in north-east China where it caused a massive outbreak (Guo *et al.* 1992). This virus has not been reisolated since 1990, although serological evidence from 1993 to 1994 indicated it was still in circulation (Guo *et al.* 1995). Jilin/89 virus is subtype H3N8, but genetic analysis revealed that it was not a member of the equine-2 family. Instead, in all gene segments it was most similar to H3N8 influenza viruses of avian species (Guo *et al.* 1992). Serological studies in mice (Webster & Thomas 1993) and horses (Chambers 1992) demonstrated that while there was partial cross-reaction between Jilin/89 HA and equine-2 HA, it was insufficient for existing equine influenza vaccines to protect against the new virus. Since equine-2 influenza has been active in the same region, the possibility exists that Jilin/89-like virus may have survived by reassortment with conventional equine-2 influenza virus. Unpublished data from our laboratories suggest that a subset of other avian influenza viruses are also replication-competent in the equine trachea, although no disease is associated with them. This makes genetic reassortment between equine and avian influenza viruses theoretically possible in horses, with the potential for generation of a novel, virulent equine influenza virus.

Surveillance and virus characterization

The capacity of equine influenza virus, as with human influenza, for antigenic drift and its ease of spread nationally and internationally by modern modes of fast transport, contribute to both the near-worldwide distribution of equine influenza outbreaks and the relative failure of vaccination to control them. Also, novel influenza viruses infecting equines sometimes occur, e.g. the outbreak of avian-like influenza in horses in Jilin, China in 1989. For these reasons, international surveillance and characterization of the virus strains involved in equine influenza outbreaks have assumed greater importance and these efforts have recently been coordinated under the auspices of the OIE and the World Health Organization (WHO).

Serological studies have sometimes found evidence for antigenic drift of circulating virus strains in comparison with reference viruses, and sometimes not. Such studies mainly use the haemagglutination inhibition test, which appears most sensitive to slight differences among strains. Antigenic analyses of equine-1 influenza viruses showed relatively minor antigenic drift from 1956 to 1977, mostly occurring between 1963 and 1973 isolates (e.g. Appleton & Gagliardo 1992). Similar antigenic analyses of equine-2 isolates have shown that antigenic variation occurs but is not obviously progressive as with human influenza viruses. Cocirculation of antigenic variants has sometimes been observed (e.g. Hinshaw *et al.* 1983; Uppal *et al.* 1989). At least one antigenic epitope on equine-2 HA was conserved from 1963 until at least 1987. Another antigenic determinant present on Miami/63 HA was maintained until about 1976, then disappeared; but thereafter it re-emerged in 1983. New antigenic specificities appeared around 1984 and 1989–1990 (Appleton *et al.* 1987; Kawaoka *et al.* 1989a; Appleton & Gagliardo 1991; Binns *et al.* 1993; Oxburgh *et al.* 1993, 1994). Recent (post-1988) isolates cross-react poorly with the prototype Miami/63 virus (Chambers *et al.* 1994a; Daly *et al.* 1996), and this led to the recommendation of equine influenza experts in 1995 that the Miami/63 strain be dropped from vaccines (Mumford *et al.* 1998). Another commonly used vaccine strain, Fontainebleau/79, has also become poorly cross-reactive with recent isolates (Oxburgh *et al.* 1994). Recently Daly *et al.* (1996) calculated a dendrogram of antigenic resemblance coefficients among isolates from 1963 to 1993 which grouped them into three major antigenic branches. Branch A comprised isolates from the USA plus one isolate from the UK. Branch B comprised isolates from Europe since 1989, whereas Branch C comprised the Hong Kong/92 epizootic virus isolate and a 1991 isolate from Italy. As will be seen below, the antigenic divergence of American/Eurasian isolates reflects diverging evolution of the HA sequences of these viruses (although the antigenicity and sequence-based dendrograms do not precisely match each other) (Daly *et al.* 1996).

Sequencing studies carried out by Gibson *et al.* (1988, 1992) showed that the mutation rate of equine-1 H7 HA was similar to that of equine-2 HA (see below) and much lower than that of human H3 HA. Two groups of isolates were identified: isolates from 1956 to 1963; and from 1964 to 1977. Viruses within groups were more similar (98–99% nucleotide and amino acid homology) than viruses between groups (about 95%).

Most virus characterization efforts have been directed to equine-2 influenza, since this has been the predominant subtype in circulation since 1979. The first sequence of an equine-2 influenza HA, the prototype equine/Miami/63 HA, was described by Daniels *et al.* (1985). Subsequently HA sequences of numerous virus strains have been published. Sequence evidence clearly demonstrates the ongoing accumulation of mutations underlying equine-2 influenza viral antigenic drift, although at a rate only about one third that of human H3 influenza HA: 1.82×10^{-3} nucleotide and 1.41×10^{-3} amino acid substitutions per site per year for equine-2 influenza viruses of 1963–1987, compared to 4.64×10^{-3} nucleotide and 6.00×10^{-3} amino acid substitutions per site per year for human H3 influenza viruses of 1968–1986 (Bean *et al.* 1992; Endo *et al.* 1992). From 1963 to 1987, equine-2 influenza HA was evolving in essentially a single lineage (Kawaoka *et al.* 1989a). However, a recent phylogenetic tree developed by our laboratories (Fig. 14.2; Daly *et al.* 1996) indicates that since 1987 equine-2 influenza strains have evolved in two lines: isolates from Europe, China and Mongolia (the 'Eurasian' family), and isolates from the USA and also Argentina (the 'American' family). The geographical identifications are not absolute: viruses of the 'American' family have been isolated in Europe (Daly *et al.* 1996); whereas one isolate from Canada (influenza A/equine/Saskatoon/90: Bogdan *et al.* 1993) falls within the 'Eurasian' family. In one outbreak viruses from both families were isolated, confirming that antigenic variants of equine-2 influenza could cocirculate even within the same local outbreak.

The relatively small number of HA sequences available from viruses isolated prior to 1989 presently makes it impossible to determine whether the Eurasian/American lineages might have existed previously, and the single-lineage phylogeny of Kawaoka *et al.* (1989a) remains the best overall description for the period 1963–1987. However, a few equine-2 influenza virus isolates from that period are exceptions to the single-lineage conclusion. Kawaoka *et al.* (1989a) themselves noted that two isolates, Tokyo/2/71 and Algiers/72, represented a significant variant branch from the main lineage, which appeared to have died out. Also, Endo *et al.* (1992) identified three other virus isolates, i.e. Tokyo/3/71, Brazil/87 and La Plata (Argentina)/88, that confounded the chronological progression of the main lineage. HAs of these strains resembled the prototype Miami/63 HA far more closely (>99% nucleotide homology in HA1) than any other sequenced strains from Uruguay/63 to the present. One isolate from the 1987 India epizootic (Bhiwani/87) also belongs to that group (Gupta *et al.* 1993). The 'frozen evolution' of these strains suggested that there were hidden reservoirs in which equine-2 influenza virus circulated with extremely low mutation rates. If this were true, it would necessitate retaining old virus strains like Miami/63 as vaccine components despite their lack of effectiveness against the latest strains. Since 1993, however, no new evidence supporting frozen evolution has been presented, and current thinking is that those anachronistic viruses might have been *c.* 1963 isolates that survived in laboratory storage.

The phylogenetic analysis of H3 HA from both human and non-human influenza viruses by Bean *et al.* (1992) yields an estimate of the origin of the equine-2 H3 HA lineage, i.e. the hypothetical common ancestor of all known equine-2 H3 genes, to have existed around 1952, which is well before the first equine-2 virus isolation in 1963. The reason is that the side branch terminating with the Tokyo/2/71 and Algiers/72 HAs ('71–72 branch') appears to have diverged from the main lineage of equine-2 HA before the appearance of Miami/63 virus. The alternative tree (Bean *et al.* 1992; similar to Kawaoka *et al.* 1989a) in which the 71–72 branch shares a common divergence with Miami/63 HA requires

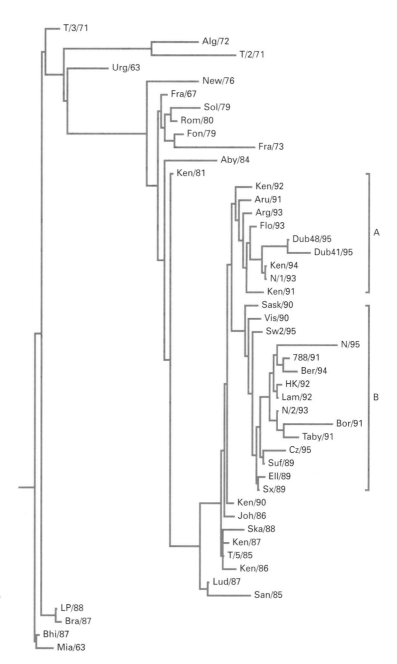

Fig. 14.2 Phylogenetic tree for the amino acid sequence of the HA1 molecules of influenza A/equine-2 (H3N8) viruses. A and B denote the recent 'American' and 'Eurasian' sublineages recently identified (Daly *et al.* 1996). Horizontal lengths of branches are proportional to the sequence differences; vertical lines are for spacing only.

the 71–72 branch's mutation rate to have been much greater than that of the main lineage (4.8 vs. 3.1 nucleotide substitutions per year), although still less than the mutation rate for human H3 HA (7.9 per year). Regardless of the dating of the common ancestral equine-2 HA, this H3 lineage apparently

diverged from other identified avian H3 lineages much earlier, and it is unknown whether H3 influenza viruses might have first entered into horses even before 1952.

Much less attention has been given to equine influenza neuraminidase (NA). For equine-1 virus

NA variation there is no significant information available. Equine-2 viral NA has undergone minor drift based on antigenic and structural analyses (e.g. Hinshaw *et al.* 1983; Berg *et al.* 1990). Complete nucleotide sequences for equine-1 N7 (Cornell/16/74 strain) and equine-2 N8 (Kentucky/81 strain) NAs were first determined by Dale *et al.* (1986). No phylogenetic analysis of equine-1 N7 NA has been done, and the sole analysis of equine-2 N8 NA has been that of Saito *et al.* (1993). Those authors observed similar evolutionary pathways for equine N8 NA to those observed by Bean *et al.* (1992) for equine H3 HA. Again, a side branch represented by NA of Algiers/72 virus appeared to diverge from the main lineage prior to the emergence of Miami/63 NA. The estimated date of origin of the equine N8 NA lineage was estimated as 1951, similar to the 1952 estimate for HA. This suggests that equine-2 HA and NA evolved together and most likely were introduced together into equine influenza viruses, but as with HA, the equine-2 NA lineage had apparently already diverged from identified avian N8 NA lineages long prior to 1951. Observed mutation rates from 1963 to 1991 were 2.9 nucleotide and 0.82 amino acid substitutions per year, also similar to equine H3 HA, suggesting that equine immunological selective pressures are similar on both viral surface antigens.

Phylogenies of the genes encoding the 'internal' proteins (PB1, PB2, PA, NP, M, NS) of equine-1 virus show the uniqueness of the equine-1/Prague/56 strain: it is possibly the most primitive of all known influenza A viruses. Wherever their phylogenic relationship has been determined (which to date includes NP, M, PB2 and NS genes), Prague/56 viral genes are the most divergent from those of all other influenza A viruses, always forming a separate lineage whose branchpoint is closest to the presumptive common ancestor between type A and type B influenza viruses and estimated to have occurred around 1800 (Bean 1984; Kawaoka *et al.* 1989b; Okazaki *et al.* 1989; Gorman *et al.* 1990a, 1990b, 1991; Ito *et al.* 1991).

Equine-2 influenza virus 'internal' genes show different ancestries. For our purposes the 'internal' genes from equine-1 viruses isolated after 1970 will be considered as 'equine-2' because, as first sug-gested by Bean (1984), reassortment between equine-2 viruses and the original, Prague/56-like equine-1 viruses must have occurred sometime between 1964 and 1973, resulting in substitution of equine-1 viral H7 and N7 onto a background of equine-2 viral 'internal' genes. The original Prague/56-like equine-1 viruses probably became extinct, replaced by the reassortant equine-1 virus bearing equine-2 derived genes.

Equine-2 NP and PA genes share similar phylogenies which place their divergence from a presumptive ancestral avian lineage prior to the divergence of human NP and PA genes around 1910 (Okazaki *et al.* 1989; Gammelin *et al.* 1990; Gorman *et al.* 1990a, 1991). Thus equine-2 NP and PA probably diverged from an avian ancestor in the latter 19th century. Equine-2 PB1 appears to have derived from a common ancestor with PB1 of human/swine H1N1 influenza viruses (Kawaoka *et al.* 1989b). As these are also thought to have diverged from an avian lineage around 1910, this implies that equine-2 PB1 gene may have originated after equine-2 NP and PA genes. However, these equine-2 gene phylogenies are based on very limited sequence information, and deductions from their backward extrapolations must be viewed with caution.

Equine-2 PB2, M and NS genes clearly diverged relatively recently from a common ancestor with North American avian lineages (Gorman *et al.* 1990b; Nakajima *et al.* 1990; Ito *et al.* 1991). The origin of the equine lineage is dated around 1952 in the case of NS (Y. Kawaoka, unpublished data), the same estimate as for the common ancestors of equine-2 HA and NA (which however, had already diverged from other avian lineages). Thus the virus family we know as equine-2 probably originated in the latter 19th century, but subsequently acquired new, avian-derived PB2, M and NS genes in the middle of the 20th century. Possibly the equine-2 HA and NA genes were acquired around that same time, but from an unknown source. Could that source have been related to the human H3N8 influenza virus of *c.* 1890?

Due to the paucity of sequences for the 'internal' equine-2 genes, evolutionary rates have been determined only for NP and NS, for the period

1963–1986. Equine-2 NP evolved at rates of 0.78×10^{-3} nucleotide and 0.66×10^{-3} amino acid substitutions per site per year (Gorman *et al.* 1990a), whereas equine-2 NS evolved at rates of 0.84×10^{-3} nucleotide and 0.14 (NS1) or 1.03 (NS2) $\times 10^{-3}$ amino acid substitutions per site per year (Y. Kawaoka, unpublished data). These rates are slower than the analogous rates for human influenza viruses.

Diagnosis

As with other influenza viruses, infections can be diagnosed serologically using the HI test; however, problems of sensitivity arise when measuring antibody to A/equine-2 (H3N8) viruses (Burrows *et al.* 1981; Wood *et al.* 1983a). While whole virus antigen may be used for A/equine-1 viruses, antigen disrupted with Tween 80–ether is required to enhance the sensitivity of HI tests with A/equine-2 viruses (John & Fulginiti 1966). In heavily vaccinated horses, infection may fail to stimulate a four-fold increase on HI antibody required for a definite diagnosis, and if horses are vaccinated in the face of infection, vaccine- and infection-induced antibodies cannot be differentiated by HI. The application of the single radial haemolysis (SRH) test overcomes the problem of sensitivity and enables detection of smaller increases (two-fold) in infection-induced antibody in heavily vaccinated horses (Livesay *et al.* 1993). Differentiation between vaccine- and infection-induced antibodies may be achieved by measurement of antibody responses to the non-structural protein, NS1 (Birch-Machin *et al.* 1997).

More immediate diagnosis may be achieved by the direct detection of viral antigen in nasal secretions by immunofluorescence of infected epithelial cells (Anestad & Maagaard 1990); by detection of viral genome by the polymerase chain reaction (PCR) using primers directed against a conserved segment of the matrix gene (Donofrio *et al.* 1994); or by antigen-capture ELISA using a monoclonal antibody to the nucleoprotein (Cook *et al.* 1988; Chambers *et al.* 1994b; Shortridge *et al.* 1994; Morley *et al.* 1995). However, in heavily vaccinated horses which experience subclinical infections in which only low levels of replication occurs, virus may only be detected after multiple passages in eggs. Eggs are preferable to tissue culture for primary isolation of equine influenza and subsequent antigenic and genetic analysis because egg-grown viruses display less antigenic heterogeneity than virus grown in Madin–Darby canine kidney (MDCK) cells and are more likely to resemble virus in clinical specimens (Ilobi *et al.* 1994; Wood *et al.* 1994).

This panel of tests provides the technology to diagnose infections, even those of a subclinical nature, before animals are moved from one population to another. However, it is only available to veterinarians in relatively few countries, and judgements on the suitability of horses to travel are still largely made on the basis of clinical observation. Much reliance is placed therefore on vaccines and vaccination policies to prevent transmission of infection, particularly when rigorous quarantine procedures are not in place.

Vaccines

Introduction

Inactivated equine influenza vaccines have been in use since the late 1960s and contain A/equine-1 (H7N7) and A/equine-2 (H3N8) viruses (Bryans 1966). Different formulations include whole or split virus vaccines, the latter in the form of micelles or immune stimulating complexes (Mumford *et al.* 1994b; van de Hoven *et al.* 1994). Adjuvants are normally included to enhance the height and duration of the antibody response, particularly to the A/equine-2 component, as in horses the antibody response to HA declines rapidly (Burrows *et al.* 1977). Immune stimulating complexes and the adjuvant Carbopol have been particularly successful in this regard (Morein *et al.* 1984; Mumford *et al.* 1994a, 1994b, 1994c).

Recommended vaccination schedules vary from 6 to 12 months between booster doses, following an initial immunization course of three doses at 0, 1 and 6 months. However, in countries where perceived vaccine efficacy is low, horses may be revaccinated every 1–2 months. Until recently, there was little information on protective levels of antibody and therefore many recommended vaccination schedules were inappropriate for the duration of immunity provided. Recognizing this, the Code Commission of the OIE recommends that an importing country free from equine influenza should require that all horses coming from an endemic area be fully vaccinated and should have received their last booster dose within 2–8 weeks prior to shipment (OIE Code 1997).

This advice assumes that the vaccines are all capable of eliminating not only clinical signs of disease but also virus shedding, if vaccinated animals are exposed to influenza prior to or during shipment. This is clearly not the case and many examples of virus shedding in recently vaccinated and clinically protected horses have been reported (Livesay *et al.* 1993; Powell *et al.* 1995). Many problems with vaccine efficacy arise from the fact that there is no international standardization of vaccine potency. Further, the need to include epidemiologically relevant strains in vaccines, an important aspect of vaccine design and highly relevant to elimination of virus shedding, is only now gaining acceptance (Mumford & Wood 1993).

Vaccine standardization

Measurement of HA content

Historically equine influenza vaccine potency has been standardized on the basis of HA content measured by the chick cell agglutination test (CCA). The inherent unreliability of this measurement was established for human influenza when it was discovered CCA values did not always correlate with vaccine immunogenicity (see Chapter 23). In spite of this, its use for equine vaccines has persisted to the present time and is probably responsible, at least in part, for the wide variation in the efficacy of equine influenza vaccines currently available.

Attempts have been made to introduce the single radial diffusion (SRD) test for standardization of vaccines, as its reproducibility and usefulness were established as early as 1983. Dose-response studies with aqueous whole virus vaccines containing Prague/56 and Miami/63 strains demonstrated a clear correlation between HA content of vaccines measured by SRD and antibody to HA stimulated in the target species, measured by SRH (Wood *et al.* 1983b; Mumford *et al.* 1988). The reluctance to adopt SRD as an *in vitro* potency test results in part from the fact that it cannot be used on the final product, as adjuvant interferes with the test. As a result, SRD can only be used as an 'in process' test prior to final mixing of inactivated antigen and adjuvant. Potency testing of final products has relied on measurement of antibody in small animals (guinea-pigs, mice) and the target species (OIE 1996).

Measurement of antibody responses

Because no challenge model in horses was available when vaccines were first developed, efficacy was assessed for many years on the basis of HI antibody stimulated in small animals or horses. However, difficulties in standardization of the HI test (Burrows *et al.* 1981), variability in the responsiveness of small animal models, and the failure to use unprimed horses for vaccination trials have led to the licensing of vaccines of highly variable and uncertain potency. Attempts to identify HI antibody levels consistent with protection have been confounded by the lack of standardization of the antibody measurement. HI antibody levels ranging from 8 to 128 have been quoted as protective against A/equine-2 infections based on observations during epidemics and experimental infections in horses (Mumford 1992).

Challenge models for equine influenza in horses

Attempts to reproduce influenza in horses were made as early as 1961 (Doll 1961) and while infection could usually be achieved, typical clinical disease was not reproducible particularly for the less pathogenic A/equine-1 viruses (Blaskovic *et al.* 1966, 1969). In the 1980s a series of experiments using different strains, challenge doses and methods of inoculation was performed to establish a reliable challenge model for A/equine-2 viruses. It was found that exposure to nebulized aerosols of virus provided a reproducible method of inducing typical clinical disease, and the severity of disease and levels of virus excretion were dose dependent (Mumford *et al.* 1990). This model provided for the first time a means of evaluating the efficacy of vaccines to prevent infection, virus excretion and clinical signs. It has been possible to establish levels of antibody to HA (measured by SRH) which are consistent with protection and which may be used to predict immunity stimulated by inactivated vaccines. SRH antibody levels of 120–154 mm^2 were shown to be protective against aerosol challenge in studies in which challenge and vaccine viruses were antigenically similar. Correlations between prechallenge SRH antibody and duration of clinical signs and virus excretion have also been demonstrated (Mumford & Wood 1992).

An opportunity to validate conclusions from experimental challenge studies arose when an outbreak of equine influenza caused by an equine-2 virus occurred in South Africa in a previously uninfected and unvaccinated population (Kawaoka & Webster 1989). From this study it was estimated that an SRH value of >160 mm^2 was consistent with a 90% protection rate, based on the proportion of vaccinated horses which seroconverted when exposed to infection (Mumford & Wood 1992). This value was close to that calculated in a vaccination and challenge study in which ponies were exposed by aerosol to a high dose of challenge virus (Mumford *et al.* 1994c) and provided support for the relevance of the challenge model for evaluating vaccine efficacy in the field.

Virus strains

Early vaccines contained the prototype strains A/equine-1/Prague/56 (H7N7) and A/equine-2/Miami/63 (H3N8), or similar viruses isolated at those times. Unlike human influenza vaccines, for many years there was no formal review of vaccine strains and their relevance to epidemic strains, and as a result the original prototype viruses have been used in some vaccines for more than 30 years. Surveillance of antigenic and genetic drift was performed on an *ad hoc* basis, and while drift was demonstrated its significance with respect to vaccine efficacy could only be surmised. The need to update vaccine strains was questioned on the basis that sera from repeatedly vaccinated ponies were cross-reactive and did not recognize large antigenic

differences between recently isolated viruses and the prototype strain (Burrows & Denyer 1982).

However, convincing field evidence for the effect of antigenic drift on vaccine efficacy came from epizootiological studies of the 1989 outbreak of equine influenza in the UK, caused by Suffolk/89 and related virus strains. The disease was first identified in regularly vaccinated horses which had high levels of vaccine-induced antibody at the time of exposure. In spite of this they succumbed to infection and disease, although clinical signs were generally mild compared to those in poorly vaccinated individuals. Thus it appeared that vaccines, while ameliorating clinical disease, failed to suppress virus shedding and spread of infection (Livesay *et al.* 1993). Infected horses in that outbreak had much higher levels of antibody than those expected to provide protection on the basis of previous studies (see 'Challenge models for equine influenza in horses' below). Only horses with antibody levels in excess of 190 mm^2 against Suffolk/89 virus were protected against field infection with the 1989 virus (Mumford & Wood 1992).

These observations raised the possibility that vaccine-induced SRH antibody raised against pre-1989 viruses was ineffective in suppressing replication of the recent Suffolk/89 virus, despite being cross-reactive in SRH and to a lesser extent HI tests. This was tested in a vaccination and challenge study in which groups of 10 ponies each received two doses of monovalent vaccine containing 50 μg HA of H3N8 virus—either Miami/63, Fontainbleau/79, Kentucky/81 or Suffolk/89 strains, and were subsequently challenged by exposure to nebulized aerosol of Sussex/89 (H3N8). Results showed that the ability to reduce virus excretion was directly correlated to the antigenic relatedness of the vaccine strain to the challenge strain, with the Suffolk/89 vaccine being most effective, and the Miami/63 virus being least effective (Fig. 14.3).

These data supported the conclusion that the antigenic drift which has occurred in recent years has rendered vaccine containing A/equine-2 isolates from 1981 or earlier less effective in preventing infection and virus shedding by recent virus strains, and provided an explanation for the 1989 observation that in the field only vaccinated horses

Miami/63 vaccine group							
SRH antibody to Suffolk/89 mm²	Days post infection						
	1	2	3	4	5	6	7
167	–	–	–	–	2.5*	2	–
126	–	2.5	1	2	2	2.5	1.5
179	–	–	–	–	1	–	1
132	–	1	1	1	1.5	2	–
196	–	–	–	–	–	–	–
172	–	–	–	–	>2.5	–	1.5
118	–	4	2.5	3.5	3	1.5	–
68	–	1.5	3.5	–	2.5	1	–
128	–	–	1.5	2	1.5	1	1
151	–	4	3.5	3.5	1.5	2	–

Suffolk/89 vaccine group							
SRH antibody to Suffolk/89 mm²	Days post infection						
	1	2	3	4	5	6	7
–	–	–	1	–	–	1	–
54	–	–	1	1	–	–	–
132	–	–	–	–	–	–	–
–	–	–	–	3.2	–	1.5	–
130	–	–	–	–	1	–	2
194	–	–	–	–	–	–	–
140	–	–	–	–	–	–	–
102	–	–	–	–	–	–	–
–	–	>4.0	>4.0	>4.0	>4.0	1	1

*$\log_{10}$ EID$_{50}$/ml nasal swab extract

Unvaccinated controls						
Days post infection						
1	2	3	4	5	6	7
–	1.5	3	2	3	1.5	–
–	1.5	3	1	3	2.5	3
–	2.5	2.5	2	2	1.5	1.5
–	3.5	1.5	3.5	3.5	2.5	1.5
–	>4.0	3.5	2.5	2.5	1	–
–	1.5	2.5	1	1	1	–
–	1.5	–	2.5	2.5	2	–
–	1	–	–	–	1	–
–	2.5	1.5	–	–	1	1.5
–	3.5	1	2.5	2.5	2.5	–

Fig. 14.3 Virus excretion ($\log_{10}$ EID$_{50}$/ml swab extract) in ponies vaccinated with two doses of aqueous vaccine containing 50 µg haemagglutinin of either Miami/63 (H3N8) or Suffolk/89 (H3N8) and challenged with an aerosol of Sussex/89 (H3N8) 3 weeks after the second dose of vaccine.

with very high levels of antibody were protected against influenza. As a result the OIE now publishes annually the recommendations from an Expert Surveillance Panel, including WHO and OIE reference laboratories, on appropriate strains for inclusion into equine influenza vaccines (Mumford et al. 1997).

Host cell selection

Viruses for equine vaccines are propagated both in eggs and in tissue culture (MDCK and Vero cells), although most isolates from which vaccines are derived have been isolated originally in eggs. Unlike human influenza viruses, equine viruses grow preferentially in eggs, and cell culture (MDCK cells) is more likely to select variant viruses which do not represent the virus most prevalent in clinical specimens (Ilobi et al. 1994; Wood et al. 1994). This is probably related to the receptor specificity of equine-2 HA: whereas human/swine H3 HA binds almost exclusively to sialyloligosaccharides terminating with sialic acid α(2,6)-galactose, equine-2 HA is similar to avian HA in

preferentially binding to sialic acid α(2,3)-galactose linkages (Rogers & Paulson 1983; Rogers et al. 1983). Connor et al. (1994) have shown that this receptor specificity is well correlated with the H3 HA amino acid sequence at residues 226 and also 228: equine and most avian influenza H3 HAs share Glu226 and Gly228 compared to Leu226 and Ser228 in human and some swine H3 HAs. Equine and avian HA receptor specificities are not precisely the same, however (Kawaoka 1991). The phenomenon of host cell selection is significant for the efficacy of equine vaccines because there is a trend for vaccine manufacturers to replace culture in eggs with tissue culture systems. Studies in horses have shown that an egg-grown vaccine prepared from a virus isolated in eggs was equally effective against both egg-grown and cell-grown challenge viruses in suppressing virus excretion; whereas a cell-grown vaccine derived from a virus isolated in tissue culture from the same clinical specimen did not reduce virus excretion effectively following challenge with an egg-grown challenge virus. These results imply that the cell-grown vaccine represented a variant virus subpopulation distinct from the challenge virus grown in eggs and also used for the egg-grown vaccine (Mumford et al. 1994d).

Performance in the field

The presence of vaccinated but still seronegative

horses may be explained on the basis of insensitive serological techniques, vaccines of low potency or inappropriate vaccine schedules, but on occasions individuals or groups of animals are found to have surprisingly low antibody levels in spite of recent vaccination with products of known potency. Non-responsiveness has been observed in young foals at the beginning of their vaccination programme and this has been attributed to delivery of vaccine in the face of maternal antibody (Maanen *et al.* 1992; Oirschot *et al.* 1991). This phenomenon is well known for many viral vaccines, but foals have been reported to fail to respond to equine influenza vaccine even after three doses given between 6 and 10 months of age, beyond the accepted lifetime of equine maternal antibodies (Maanen *et al.* 1992; A. Cullinane, personal communication). The immunological basis for this long-term lack of responsiveness has not been explained. Individual poor responders have also been identified among vaccinated older animals, and are more common among animals receiving split or non-adjuvanted vaccines (Mumford *et al.* 1994a; van de Hoven *et al.* 1994). These poor responders appear to play an important role in the epidemiology of influenza. During the 1989 epizootic, index cases in training yards investigated were invariably animals who had low vaccinal SRH antibody levels ($< 50\,\mathrm{mm}^2$) despite having received similar vaccination regimes to cohorts with high antibody levels (Wood 1991). Equine immunological responses to viral antigens may have a genetic component; however, no specific linkage has been made between HLA type and lack of responsiveness to influenza vaccines (Bodo *et al.* 1994).

Immunological responses to infection and vaccination

Infection with influenza stimulates cellular responses measurable in lymphocyte stimulation (LS) assays and genetically restricted cytotoxic T lymphocyte (CTL) responses, as well as mucosal and humoral neutralizing antibody to the HA (Hannant *et al.* 1988; Hannant & Mumford 1989). Circulating antibody to HA is short lived following infection, declining to low or undetectable levels

within 3–6 months of infection. In spite of this, infection-induced immunity may persist for a year or more, implying that priming of the CTL and mucosal antibody responses is important in natural immunity (Hannant *et al.* 1988).

In contrast, immunization with most inactivated vaccines, although inducing LS response, does not stimulate CTL responses. Where LS responses have been detected following vaccination, they have not correlated with protection (Hannant *et al.* 1994). Although mucosal antibody has been detected in respiratory tract secretions following vaccination with inactivated antigens, the neutralizing capacity of this antibody has not been demonstrated. Therefore, the efficacy of traditional vaccines is probably largely reliant on the stimulation of strong and durable humoral neutralizing antibody responses to HA.

Interestingly, recent studies comparing the equine antibody isotypes stimulated by experimental infection with one brand of commercial adjuvanted inactivated virus vaccine showed that the antibody profiles largely did not overlap: infection stimulated predominantly IgG(a), IgG(b) and IgA; whereas conventional immunization stimulated almost exclusively IgG(T). The significance of IgG(T) antibody in protection from influenza is not well understood, but these results might mean that for optimal immunization, attention needs to be paid to levels of individual antibody isotypes and not merely to overall antibody titres (D.P. Lunn, personal communication).

New approaches

In attempts to broaden the repertoire of equine immunological responses to vaccination a variety of strategies for developing safe live attenuated virus vaccines for equine influenza have been followed. Temperature-sensitive human/equine influenza reassortants have been produced which include either the H7N7 or the H3N8 equine surface antigens (Brundage-Anguish *et al.* 1982). In horses these reassortants provide at least short-term protection against challenge with virulent virus and this protection is not dependent on high levels of circulating antibody to HA (Holmes *et al.* 1988, 1992).

Reassortant viruses derived from avian (Mallard New York/89 (H2N2)) and equine (Newmarket/79 (H3N8)) influenza viruses containing equine HA and NA and avian internal and non-structural proteins have also been evaluated as candidate vaccines (Mumford 1992). Although good protection was demonstrated against virulent virus in hamsters, this strategy was abandoned for horses when an H7N7 equine/avian reassortant was shown to be virulent for chickens (Banbura *et al.* 1991) and an H3N8 virus of avian origin infected horses in China (Guo *et al.* 1992).

The use of vaccinia virus as a vector for equine influenza genes has also been explored. Four recombinants expressing H7 HA, H3 HA, N7 NA and N8 NA have been used to immunize horses. Neutralizing antibody responses were stimulated by the HA and to a lesser extent by the NA recombinants but no information on protective efficacy is available (Dale *et al.* 1988).

The success of immunization with DNA encoding HA of avian and human influenza viruses has been repeated for equine influenza. Mice immunized by gene gun delivery with plasmid DNA encoding the HA gene of Kentucky/81 (H3N8) virus developed neutralizing antibodies and were protected against challenge with homologous virus (Olsen *et al.* 1997). Initial studies in horses have shown similar promise and justify continued effort with this approach (D.P. Lunn, personal communication), the particular advantages being the generation of strong and long-lasting B- and T-cell responses, the ease with which new HA genes can be incorporated into updated vaccines and the potential for more cross-reactive neutralizing antibody generation.

At present there is little information on the role of individual influenza viral proteins in stimulating cellular immune responses in the horse, but construction of recombinants carrying single genes or immunization with DNA vaccines based on individual viral genes will provide opportunities to identify the role of these proteins. The relative importance of stimulating mucosal antibody has been little studied. However, recent results have shown that the common mucosal system functions in the horse and that virus-neutralizing mucosal antibody can be induced by vaccination with inactivated influenza virus coupled to cholera toxin (Hannant *et al.* 1996). Amounts of antibody in nasal washes taken from horses after mucosal vaccination were similar to those stimulated by infection and horses vaccinated by the mucosal route were protected against challenge infection with homologous virus (Easeman 1997).

Antiviral agents in horses

The anti-influenza agents amantadine and rimantadine both inhibit equine-2 influenza virus replication *in vitro* (Rees *et al.* 1997). Rimantadine is generally approximately 10-fold more mass-effective than amantadine. Bryans *et al.* (1966) first demonstrated that amantadine (20 mg/kg b.i.d.) effectively reduced the mean duration of virus shedding by equine-2 influenza-infected horses from 6 days to 1 day. In horses, amantadine and rimantadine have lower bioavailability and shorter half-lives than in humans (25–60% and 2.2–3.4 h, vs. 80% and 16 h in humans). This necessitates frequent administration of large quantities of drug, with a risk of fatal seizures if the intravenous route is used (Rees *et al.* 1997). Nonetheless, in our hands an influenza treatment protocol for horses using rimantadine (30 mg/kg b.i.d. by oral intubation) ameliorated clinical signs of experimental influenza infection compared to controls. It did not reduce the duration of virus shedding, suggesting that rimantadine-resistant virus was generated (W.A. Rees & T.M. Chambers, unpublished data). Thus amantadine/rimantadine control of influenza in horses can be effective but would also be laborious and expensive. Non-specific immune stimulants including interferon are also sometimes used as equine influenza treatments, but so far there is no clear evidence for their effectiveness.

References

Anestad, G. & Maagaard, O. (1990) Rapid diagnosis of equine influenza. *Vet Rec* **126**, 550–1.

Appleton, J. & Gagliardo, L. (1991) Fine specificity of the pony antibody response against the equine influenza virus H3 haemagglutinin analysed *in vitro*.

In: Plowright, W., Rossdale, P. & Wade, J. (eds) *Equine Infectious Diseases VI*, pp. 259–62. R & W Publications, Newmarket.

Appleton, J. & Gagliardo, L. (1992) Diversity of the antibody responses produced in ponies and mice against the equine influenza A virus H7 haemagglutinin. *J Gen Virol* **73**, 1569–73.

Appleton, J., Antczak, D. & Lopes, A. (1987) Characterization of the equine influenza virus H3 with monoclonal antibodies. *Archiv Virol* **94**, 339–46.

Banbura, M., Kawaoka, Y., Thomas, T. & Webster, R. (1991) Reassortants with equine 1 (H7N7) influenza virus haemagglutinin in an avian influenza virus genetic background are pathogenic in chickens. *Virology* **184**, 469–71.

Bean, W. (1984) Correlation of influenza A virus nucleoprotein genes with host species. *Virology* **133**, 438–42.

Bean, W., Schell, M., Katz, J. *et al.* (1992) Evolution of the H3 influenza virus haemagglutinin from human and nonhuman hosts. *J Virol* **66**, 1129–38.

Berg, M., Desselberger, U., Abusugra, I., Klingeborn, B. & Linne, T. (1990) Genetic drift of equine 2 influenza A virus (H3N8), 1963–1988: analysis by oligonucleotide mapping. *Vet Microbiol* **22**, 225–36.

Beveridge, W., Mahaffey, L. & Rose, M. (1965) Influenza in horses. *Vet Rec* **77**, 57–9.

Binns, M., Daly, J., Chirnside, E. *et al.* (1993) Genetic and antigenic analysis of an equine influenza H3 isolate from the 1989 epidemic. *Archiv Virol* **130**, 33–43.

Birch-Machin, I., Rowan, A., Pick, J., Mumford, J. & Binns, M. (1997) Expression of the nonstructural protein NS1 of equine influenza A virus: detection of anti-NS1 antibody in post infection equine sera. *J Virol Meth* **65**, 255–63.

Blaskovic, D., Szanto, J., Kapitancik, B., Lesso, J., Lackovic, V. & Skarda, R. (1966) Experimental pathogenesis of A/equi 1 influenza virus infection in horses. *Acta Virol* **10**, 513–20.

Blaskovic, D., Kapitancik, B., Sabo, A., Styk, B., Vrtiak, O. & Kaplan, M. (1969) Experimental infection of horses with A-equi 2/Miami/63 and human A2/Hong Kong/1/68 influenza viruses. 1. The course of infection and virus recovery. *Acta Virol* **13**, 499–506.

Bodo, G., Marti, E., Gaillard, C. *et al.* (1994) Association of the immune response with the major histocompatibility complex in the horse. In: Nakajima, H. & Plowright, W. (eds) *Equine Infectious Diseases VII: Proceedings of the Seventh International Conference, Tokyo*, pp. 143–51. R & W Publications, Newmarket.

Bogdan, J., Morley, P., Townsend, H. & Haines, D. (1993) Effect of influenza A/equine/H3N8 virus isolate variation on the measurement of equine antibody responses. *Can J Vet Res* **57**, 126–30.

Brundage-Anguish, L.J., Holmes, D.F., Hosier, N.T. *et al.* (1982) Live temperature-sensitive equine influenza virus vaccine: generation of the virus and efficiency in hamsters. *Am J Vet Res* **43**, 869–74.

Bryans, J. (1966) Control of equine influenza. In: Bryans, J.T. (ed.) *Proceedings of the First International Conference on Equine Infectious Diseases*, pp. 157–65. Grayson Foundation, Lexington.

Bryans, J., Zent, W., Grunert, R. & Boughton, D. (1966) 1-Adamantanamine hydrochloride prophylaxis for experimentally induced A/equine 2 influenza virus infection. *Nature* **212**, 1542–4.

Burrows, R. & Denyer, M. (1982) Antigenic properties of some equine influenza viruses. *Archiv Virol* **73**, 15–24.

Burrows, R., Spooner, P.R. & Goodridge, D. (1977) A three-year evaluation of four commercial equine influenza vaccines in ponies maintained in isolation. *International Symposium on Influenza Immunization (II)* **39**, 341–6.

Burrows, R., Denyer, M., Goodridge, D. & Hamilton, F. (1981) Field and laboratory studies of equine influenza viruses isolated in 1979. *Vet Rec* **109**, 353–6.

Chambers, T. (1992) Cross-reactivity of existing equine influenza vaccines with a new strain of equine influenza virus from China. *Vet Rec* **131**, 388–91.

Chambers, T., Lai, A., Franklin, K. & Powell, D. (1994a) Recent evolution of the haemagglutinin of equine-2 influenza virus in the USA. In: Nakajima, H. & Plowright, W. (eds) *Equine Infectious Diseases VII: Proceedings of the Seventh International Conference, Tokyo*, pp. 175–80. R & W Publications, Newmarket.

Chambers, T.M., Shortridge, K.F., Li, P.H., Powell, D.G. & Watkins, K.L. (1994b) Rapid diagnosis of equine influenza by the Directigen FLU-A enzyme immunoassay. *Vet Rec* **135** (12), 275–9.

Connor, R., Kawaoka, Y., Webster, R. & Paulson, J. (1994) Receptor specificity in human, avian, and equine H2 and H3 influenza virus isolates. *Virology* **205**, 17–23.

Cook, R.F., Sinclair, R. & Mumford, J.A. (1988) Detection of influenza nucleoprotein antigen in nasal secretions from horses infected with A/equine influenza (H3N8) viruses. *J Virol Meth* **20**, 1–12.

Dale, B., Brown, R., Miller, J., White, R., Air, G. & Cordell, B. (1986) Nucleotide and deduced amino acid sequence of the influenza neuraminidase genes of two equine serotypes. *Virology* **155**, 460–8.

Dale, B., Brown, R., Kloss, J.M., Cordell, B., Moore, B.O. & Yilma, T. (1988) Generation of vaccinia virus-equine influenza A virus recombinants and their use as immunogens in horses. In: Powell, D.G. (ed.) *Equine Infectious Diseases V*, pp. 80–7. Kentucky University Press, Lexington.

Daly, J., Lai, A., Binns, M., Chambers, T., Barrandeguy, M. & Mumford, J. (1996) Recent worldwide antigenic and genetic evolution of equine H3N8 influenza A viruses. *J Gen Virol* **77**, 661–71.

Daniels, R., Skehel, J. & Wiley, D. (1985) Amino acid sequences of haemagglutinins of influenza viruses of the H3 subtype isolated from horses. *J Gen Virol* **66**, 457–64.

Doll, E. (1961) Influenza of horses. *Am Rev Resp Dis* **83**, 48–50.

Donofrio, J.C., Coonrod, J.D. & Chambers, T.M. (1994) Diagnosis of equine influenza by the polymerase chain reaction. *J Vet Diag Invest* **6 (1)**, 39–43.

Easeman, R.L. (1997) *Induction of mucosal immune responses in the horse.* PhD thesis, Open University, UK.

Endo, A., Pecoraro, R., Sugita, S. & Nerome, K. (1992) Evolutionary pattern of the H3 haemagglutinin of equine influenza viruses: multiple evolutionary lineages and frozen replication. *Archiv Virol* **123**, 73–87.

Gammelin, M., Altmuller, A., Reinhardt, U. *et al.* (1990) Phylogenetic analysis of nucleoproteins suggests that human influenza A viruses emerged from a 19th-century avian ancestor. *Molec Biol Evol* **7**, 194–200.

Gerber, H. (1970) Clinical features, sequelae, and epidemiology of equine influenza. In: Bryans, J.T. & Gerber, H. (eds) *Equine Infectious Diseases II*, pp. 63–80. Karger, Basel.

Gibson, C., Daniels, R., McCauley, J. & Schild, G. (1988) Hemagglutinin gene sequencing studies of equine-1 influenza A viruses. In: Powell, D.G. (ed.) *Equine Infectious Diseases V*, pp. 51–9. University Press of Kentucky, Lexington.

Gibson, C., Daniels, R., Oxford, J. & McCauley, J. (1992) Sequence analysis of the equine H7 influenza virus haemagglutinin gene. *Virus Res* **22**, 93–106.

Gorman, O., Bean, W., Kawaoka, Y. & Webster, R. (1990a) Evolution of the nucleoprotein gene of influenza A virus. *J Virol* **64**, 1487–97.

Gorman, O., Donis, R., Kawaoka, Y. & Webster, R. (1990b) Evolution of influenza A virus PB2 genes: implications for evolution of the ribonucleoprotein complex and origin of human influenza A virus. *J Virol* **64**, 4893–902.

Gorman, O., Bean, W., Kawaoka, Y., Donatelli, I., Guo, Y. & Webster, R. (1991) Evolution of influenza A virus nucleoprotein genes: implications for the origins of H1N1 human and classical swine viruses. *J Virol* **65**, 3704–14.

Guo, Y.J., Wang, M. & Zheng, H.Y. (1990) Equine influenza epidemic again in North-East China. *Virus Information Exchange Newsletter for South-East Asia and the Western Pacific* **7**, 146–7.

Guo, Y., Wang, M., Kawaoka, Y. *et al.* (1992) Characterization of a new avian-like influenza A virus from horses in China. *Virology* **188 (1)**, 245–55.

Guo, Y., Wang, M., Zheng, G., Li, W., Kawaoka, Y. & Webster, R. (1995) Seroepidemiological and molecular evidence for the presence of two H3N8 equine influenza viruses in China in 1993–1994. *J Gen Virol* **76**, 2009–14.

Gupta, A., Yadav, M., Uppal, P., Mumford, J. & Binns, M. (1993) Characterization of equine influenza isolates from the 1987 epizootic in India by nucleotide sequencing of the HA1 gene. *Equine Vet J* **25**, 99–102.

Hannant, D. & Mumford, J.A. (1989) Cell mediated immune responses in ponies following infection with equine influenza virus (H3N8): the influence of induction culture conditions on the properties of cytotoxic effector cells. *Vet Immunol Immunopathol* **21**, 327–37.

Hannant, D., Mumford, J.A. & Jessett, D.M. (1988) Duration of circulating antibody and immunity following infection with equine influenza virus. *Vet Rec* **122**, 125–8.

Hannant, D., Jessett, D.M., O'Neill, T., Livesay, J. & Mumford, J.A. (1994) Cellular immune responses stimulated by inactivated virus vaccines and infection with equine influenza virus (H3N8). In: Nakajima, H. & Plowright, W. (eds) *Equine Infectious Diseases VII: Proceedings of the Seventh International Conference, Tokyo*, pp. 169–74. R & W Publications, Newmarket.

Hannant, D., Easeman, R.L., Evers, E. & Mumford, J.A. (1996) Mucosal vaccination with inactivated equine influenza virus stimulates neutralizing antibody in the nasopharynx of horses. *Vet Immunol Immunopathol* **54**, 205.

Heller, L., Espmark, A. & Viriden, P. (1957) Immunological relationship between the infectious cough in horses and human influenza A. *Archiv Gesamte Virusforschung* **7**, 120–4.

Hinshaw, V., Naeve, C., Webster, R., Douglas, A., Skehel, J. & Bryans, J. (1983) Analysis of antigenic variation in equine 2 influenza A viruses. *Bull WHO* **61**, 153–8.

Holmes, D.F., Lamb, L.M., Anguish, L.M., Coggins, L., Murphy, B.R. & Gillespie, J.H. (1988) Live temperature-sensitive equine-1 influenza A virus vaccine: efficacy in experimental ponies. In: Powell, D.G. (ed.) *Equine Infectious Diseases V*, pp. 88–93. Kentucky University Press, Lexington.

Holmes, D.F., Lamb, L.M., Coggins, L., Murphy, B.R. & Gillespie, J.H. (1992) Live temperature-sensitive equine 2 influenza A virus production and efficacy in experimental ponies. In: Plowright, W., Rossdale, P.D. & Wade, J.F. (eds) *Equine Infectious Diseases VI*, pp. 253–8. R & W Publications, Newmarket.

Ilobi, C., Henfrey, R., Robertson, J., Mumford, J., Erasmus, B. & Wood, J. (1994) Antigenic and molecular characterization of host cell-mediated variants of equine H3N8 influenza viruses. *J Gen Virol* **75**, 669–73.

Ismail, T., Sami, A., Youssef, H. & Abou Zaid, A. (1990) An outbreak of equine influenza type 1 in Egypt in 1989. *Vet Med J Giza* **38**, 195–206.

Ito, T., Gorman, O., Kawaoka, Y., Bean, W. & Webster, R. (1991) Evolutionary analysis of the influenza A virus M gene with comparison of the M1 and M2 proteins. *J Virol* **65**, 5491–8.

Jaeschke, G. & Lange, W. (1993) Equine influenza outbreaks with viral antigenic drift in Berlin 1988–1991. *Berliner und Munchener Tierarztliche Wochenschrift* **106**, 119–23.

John, T.J. & Fulginiti, V.A. (1966) Parainfluenza 2 virus: Increase in haemaglutinin titer on treatment with tween-80 and ether. *Proc Soc Exp Biol Med* **212**, 109–11.

Kawaoka, Y. (1991) Difference in receptor specificity among influenza A viruses from different species of animals. *J Vet Med Sci* **53**, 357–8.

Kawaoka, Y. & Webster, R. (1989) Origin of the hae-magglutinin on A/Equine/Johannesburg/86 (H3N8): the first known equine influenza outbreak in South Africa. *Archiv Virol* **106**, 159–64.

Kawaoka, Y., Bean, W. & Webster, R. (1989a) Evolution of the haemagglutinin of equine H3 influenza viruses. *Virology* **169**, 283–92.

Kawaoka, Y., Krauss, S. & Webster, R. (1989b) Avian-to-human transmission of the PB1 gene of influenza A viruses in the 1957 and 1968 pandemics. *J Virol* **63**, 4603–8.

Kilbourne, E. (1968) Recombination of influenza A viruses of human and animal origin. *Science* **160**, 74–6.

Lai, A., Lin, Y., Powell, D. *et al.* (1994) Genetic and antigenic analysis of the influenza virus responsible for the 1992 Hong Kong equine influenza epizootic. *Virology* **204**, 673–9.

Laver, W. & Webster, R. (1973) Studies on the origin of pandemic influenza. 3. Evidence implicating duck and equine influenza viruses as possible progenitors of the Hong Kong strain of human influenza. *Virology* **51**, 383–91.

Livesay, G.J., O'Neill, T., Hannant, D., Yadav, M.P. & Mumford, J.A. (1993) The outbreak of equine influenza (H3N8) in the United Kingdom in 1989: diagnostic use of an antigen capture ELISA. *Vet Rec* **133**, 515–19.

Lucam, F., Fedida, M., Dannacher, G., Coudert, M. & Peillon, M. (1974) La grippe equine. Charactères de la maladie experimentale et de l'immunité postvaccinale. *Rev Med Vet* **125**, 1273–393.

Maanen, C., van Bruin, G., de Boer-Luijtze, E., Smolders, G. & de Boer, G.F. (1992) Interference of maternal antibodies with the immune response of foals after vaccination against equine influenza. *Vet Quart* **14 (1)**, 13–17.

Miller, W.M.C. (1965) Equine influenza. Further observations on the 'coughing' outbreak 1965. *Vet Rec* **77**, 455–6.

Minuse, E., McQueen, J., Davenport, F. & Francis, T. Jr (1965) Studies of antibodies to 1956 and 1963 influenza viruses in horses and man. *J Immunol* **94**, 563–6.

Morein, B., Sundquist, B., Hoglund, S., Dalsgard, K. & Osterhause, A. (1984) Iscom, a novel structure for antigenic presentation of membrane proteins from enveloped viruses. *Nature* **308**, 457–60.

Morley, P.S., Bogdan, J.R., Townsend, H.G. & Haines, D.M. (1995) Evaluation of Directigen Flu A assay for detection of influenza antigen in nasal secretions of horses. *Equine Vet J* **27 (2)**, 131–4.

Mumford, J.A. (1992) Progress in the control of equine influenza. In: Plowright W., Rossdale P.D. & Wade J.F. (eds) *Equine Infectious Diseases VI*, pp. 207–18. R & W Publications, Newmarket.

Mumford, J.A. & Wood, J. (1992) Establishing an acceptable threshold for equine influenza vaccines. *Dev Biol Stand* **79**, 137–46.

Mumford, J. & Wood, J. (1993) WHO/OIE meeting: consultation on newly emerging strains of equine influenza. 18–19 May, Animal Health Trust, Newmarket, Suffolk, UK. *Vaccine* **11**, 1172–5.

Mumford, J.A., Wood, J.M., Folkers, C. & Schild, G.C. (1988) Protection against experimental infection with influenza virus A/equine/Miami/63 (H3N8) provided by inactivated whole virus vaccines containing homologous virus. *Epidemiol Infect* **100**, 501–10.

Mumford, J.A., Hannant, D. & Jessett, D.M. (1990) Experimental infection of ponies with equine influenza (H3N8) viruses by intranasal inoculation or exposure to aerosols. *Equine Vet J* **22 (2)**, 93–8.

Mumford, J.A., Jessett, D., Dunleavy, U. *et al.* (1994a) Antigenicity and immunogenicity of experimental equine influenza ISCOM vaccines. *Vaccine* **12**, 857–63.

Mumford, J.A., Jessett, D.M., Rollinson, E.A., Hannant, D. & Draper, M.E. (1994b) Duration of protective efficacy of equine influenza immunostimulating complex/tetanus vaccines. *Vet Rec* **134**, 158–62.

Mumford, J.A., Wilson, H., Hannant, D. & Jessett, D.M. (1994c) Antigenicity and immunogenicity of equine influenza vaccines containing a Carbomer adjuvant. *Epidemiol Infect* **112 (2)**, 421–37.

Mumford, J.A., Wood, J., Jessett, D.M. & Cook, R.F. (1994d) Efficacy of H3N8 influenza vaccines prepared from virus cultured in eggs or mammalian cells. In: Nakajima, H. & Plowright, W. (eds) *Equine Infectious Diseases VII: Proceedings of the Seventh International Conference, Tokyo*, pp. 342–3. R & W Publications Limited, Newmarket.

Mumford, J.A., Chambers, T.M. & Wood, J. (1998) Equine influenza: progress in surveillance and application to vaccine strain selection. *Vaccine* (in press).

Nakajima, K., Nobusawa, E. & Nakajima, S. (1990) Evolution of the NS genes of the influenza A viruses. I. Genetic relatedness of the NS1 genes of animal influenza viruses. *Virus Genes* **4**, 15–26.

Newton, R. & Mumford, J.A. (1995) Equine influenza in vaccinated horses. *Vet Rec* **137 (19)**, 495–6.

OIE International Animal Health Code (1997) Chapter 3.4.5. OIE (eds), Paris, France.

OIE Manual of Standards for Diagnostic Tests & Vaccines, 3rd edn (1996), pp. 412–14. OIE (eds), Paris, France.

Oirschot, J.T., van Bruin, G., de Boer-Luytze, E. & Smolders, G. (1991) Maternal antibodies against equine influenza virus in foals and their interference with vaccination. *J Vet Med Series B* **38**, 391–6.

Okazaki, K., Kawaoka, Y. & Webster, R. (1989) Evolutionary pathways of the PA genes of influenza A viruses. *Virology* **172**, 601–8.

Olsen, C.W., McGregor, M.W., Dybdahl-Sissoko, N. *et al.* (1997) Immunogenicity and efficacy of baculovirus-expressed and DNA-based equine influenza virus haemagglutinin vaccines in mice. *Vaccine* **15**, 1149–56.

Oxburgh, L., Berg, M., Klingeborn, B., Emmoth, E. & Linne, T. (1993) Equine influenza virus from the 1991 Swedish epizootic shows major genetic and antigenic divergence from the prototype virus. *Virus Res* **28**, 263–72.

Oxburgh, L., Berg, M., Klingeborn, B., Emmoth, E. & Linne, T. (1994) Evolution of H3N8 equine influenza virus from 1963 to 1991. *Virus Res* **34**, 153–65.

Powell, D., Watkins, K., Li, P. & Shortridge, K. (1995) Outbreak of equine influenza among horses in Hong Kong during 1992. *Vet Rec* **136**, 531–6.

Rees, W., Harkins, J., Woods, W. *et al.* (1997) Amantadine and equine influenza: pharmacology, pharmacokinetics and neurological effects in the horse. *Equine Vet J* **29**, 104–10.

Rogers, G. & Paulson, J. (1983) Receptor determinants of human and animal influenza virus isolates: differences in receptor specificity based on species of origin. *Virology* **127**, 361–73.

Rogers, G., Pritchett, T., Lane, J. & Paulson, J. (1983) Differential sensitivity of human, avian, and equine influenza A viruses to a glycoprotein inhibitor of infection: selection of receptor specific variants. *Virology* **131**, 394–408.

Rose, M., Round, M. & Beveridge, W. (1970) Influenza in horses and donkeys in Britain, 1969. *Vet Rec* **86**, 768–9.

Saito, T., Kawaoka, Y. & Webster, R. (1993) Phylogenetic analysis of the N8 neuraminidase gene of influenza A viruses. *Virology* **193**, 868–76.

Schild, G. & Stuart-Harris, C. (1965) Serological and epidemiological studies with influenza A viruses. *J Hygiene* **63**, 479–90.

Shortridge, K.F., Watkins, K.L. & Powell, D.G. (1994) Steps to prevent entry of equine influenza into Hong Kong: application of Directigen FLU-A enzyme immunoassay. In: Nakajima, H. & Plowright, W. (eds) *Equine Infectious Diseases VII: Proceedings of the Seventh International Conference, Tokyo*, pp. 308–9. R & W Publications, Newmarket.

Shortridge, K., Chan, W. & Guan, Y. (1995) Epidemiology of the equine influenza outbreak in China, 1993–1994. *Vet Rec* **136**, 160–1.

Singh, G. (1994) Characterization of A/eq-1 virus isolated during the equine influenza epidemic in India. *Acta Virol* **38**, 25–6.

Singh, G. (1995) A note on the concurrent isolation, from horses and ponies, of influenza A/EQ-1 and A/EQ-2 viruses from an epidemic of equine influenza in India. *Comp Immunol Microbiol Infect Dis* **18**, 73–4.

Sovinova, O., Tumova, B., Pouska, F. & Nemec, J. (1958) Isolation of a virus causing respiratory diseases in horses. *Acta Virol* **1**, 52–61.

Tumova, B., Easterday, B. & Stumpa, A. (1972) Simultaneous occurrence of A-equi-1 and A-equi-2 influenza viruses in a small group of horses. *Am J Epidemiol* **95**, 80–7.

Uppal, P.K. & Yadav, M.P. (1988) Sero-epidemiological observations on equine influenza in Madhya Pradesh. *Indian J Animal Sci* **3**, 213–20.

Uppal, P., Yadav, M. & van Oberoi, M. (1989) Isolation of A/Equi-2 virus during 1987 equine influenza epidemic in India. *Equine Vet J* **21**, 364–6.

Uppal, P.K., Yadav, M.P. & Manchanda, V.P. (1990) Observations on strangles and purpura haemorrhagica as a sequela to equine influenza infection. *Indian J Animal Sci* **60 (10)**, 1149–53.

van de Hoven, R., Hellander, J. & Minke, J.M. (1994) A comparison of vaccine-induced SRH titres by various commercially available equine influenza vaccines. In: Nakajima, H. & Plowright, W. (eds) *Equine Infectious Diseases VII: Proceedings of the Seventh International Conference, Tokyo*, pp. 343. R & W Publications, Newmarket.

Waddell, G., Teigland, M. & Sigel, M. (1963) A new influenza virus associated with equine respiratory disease. *J Am Vet Med Assoc* **143**, 587–90.

Webster, R. (1993) Are equine 1 influenza viruses still present in horses? *Equine Vet J* **25**, 537–8.

Webster, R. & Thomas, T. (1993) Efficacy of equine influenza vaccines for protection against A/Equine/Jilin/89 (H3N8)—a new equine influenza virus. *Vaccine* **11**, 987–93.

Webster, R., Kawaoka, U. & Guo, Y. (1991) Equine influenza in China. *Foreign Animal Disease Rep* **19**, 1–3.

Willoughby, R., Ecker, G., McKee, S. *et al.* (1992) The effects of equine rhinovirus, influenza virus and herpesvirus infection on tracheal clearance rate in horses. *Can J Vet Res* **56 (2)**, 115–21.

Wood, J.L.N. (1991) *Equine influenza: history and epidemiology and a description of a recent outbreak*. MSc dissertation, London School of Hygiene and Tropical Medicine, University of London.

Wood, J., Mumford, J., Folkers, C., Scott, A. & Schild, G. (1983a) Studies with inactivated equine influenza vaccine. 1. Serological responses of ponies to graded doses of vaccine. *J Hygiene* **90**, 371–84.

Wood, J.M., Schild, G.C., Folkers, C., Mumford, J. & Newman, R.W. (1983b) The standardization of inactivated equine influenza vaccines by single-radial immunodiffusion. *J Biol Standard* **11**, 133–6.

Wood, J.M., Ilobi, C., Mumford, J.A. & Robertson, J.S. (1994) Impact of host cell selection on antigenic and genetic variation of the H3N8 equine influenza virus HA. In: Nakajima, H. & Plowright, W. (eds) *Equine Infectious Diseases VII: Proceedings of the Seventh International Conference, Tokyo*, pp. 159–164. R & W Publications, Newmarket.

CHAPTER 15

Influenza in other Species (Seal, Whale and Mink)

Virginia S. Hinshaw

Influenza viruses infect many different avian and mammalian species in nature; however, some of the more unusual animal populations experiencing influenza epizootics are marine mammals, such as seals and whales, and semiaquatic mammals, such as mink. One feature which is common to the viruses isolated from these mammals is that all appear to be of avian origin. This indicates that avian influenza viruses are quite capable of crossing species barriers and producing disease and death in mammals.

Seals

There is clear evidence, as described below, that harbour seals (*Phoca vitulina*) in North America experience influenza virus infections. Additionally, serological evidence of influenza infection suggests that grey, harp and hooded seals may also be involved at locations in the North Atlantic distant from the New England coast (Geraci *et al.* 1982; Stuen *et al.* 1994). The repeated isolation of influenza viruses from seals, including four different subtypes (H7N7, H4N5, H4N6 and H3N3), indicates that this species is susceptible to infection with influenza viruses, and in each case these viruses appear to originate from an avian reservoir. It is possible that viruses capable of infecting and replicating in seals may be more adapted to mammalian, rather than avian, hosts. So, the potential for transmission to other species, plus the possibility of genetic reassortment, emphasizes the importance of continued surveillance of influenza viruses in seals.

H7N7 viruses

A severe epizootic of pneumonia in harbour seals off the New England coast occurred between December 1979 and October 1980 (Webster *et al.* 1981b; Geraci *et al.* 1982). During this outbreak, approximately 600 seals died and H7N7 influenza viruses were isolated from the lungs and brains of the dead seals. Extensive antigenic and genetic analyses on these isolates showed that all of the genes of the seal viruses were derived from avian viruses. However, 'in vivo' studies (Webster *et al.* 1981b; Murphy *et al.* 1983) indicated that the seal viruses resembled mammalian viruses in that A/Seal/MA/1/80 replicated to high titres in experimentally infected mammals (ferrets, pigs, cats and squirrel monkeys), but replicated poorly, if at all, in avian species (chickens, ducks, turkeys and parakeets). Another marked distinction from avian viruses was that the seal virus was not enterotropic in birds.

The 'mammalian' tropism of this seal virus also extended to humans. During experimental infection studies, a seal infected with A/Seal/MA/1/80 sneezed into the face and eyes of an investigator who then developed severe conjunctivitis (Webster *et al.* 1981a). The seal virus was recovered from the eye of the individual; however, haemagglutination inhibition (HI) assays did not detect any antibodies to the seal virus in postinfection sera and lacrimal secretions from this person. The infected individual recovered completely. It was interesting that a number of field workers had also complained of conjunctivitis after conducting necropsies on the stranded seals. Since such infections appear to be serologically undetectable, it will be particularly difficult to determine the frequency of such events in nature. However, it is clear that avian viruses can reach and infect humans via other hosts in nature, in this case, birds to seals to humans.

This first documentation of an influenza outbreak in seals raised awareness of this infection as a potential explanation for seal strandings (Geraci *et al.* 1982). At the time of this outbreak, environmental and density factors may have contributed to the extent of the epizootic. There were an unusually large number of seals in the area and the weather was unseasonably warm which encouraged seals to spend more time on shore. These factors could well have increased transmission, resulting in widespread disease and the subsequent stranding.

H4N5 viruses

A second milder epizootic of pneumonia in seals occurred from June 1982 to August 1983 and was associated with an H4N5 influenza virus, A/Seal/MA/133/82 (Hinshaw *et al.* 1984). Similar to the earlier findings, these H4N5 isolates were examined antigenically and genetically and shown to be of avian origin. Another common factor was that the weather was unusually warm, so the seals were staying in the area longer than usual. However, there were distinctions between this situation and the earlier one. The viruses were clearly of different subtypes, but a more intriguing difference was that the H4N5 virus replicated quite well in birds and was also enterotropic, similar to avian influenza viruses and in contrast to the seal H7N7 viruses. Thus, the H4N5 isolate was antigenically, genetically and biologically most similar to avian influenza viruses. Whether this made the virus less virulent in seals is not known, but it is interesting that there was also no evidence of human infections among individuals working with the seals in this outbreak.

H4N6 and H3N3 viruses

Continuing surveillance for influenza virus infection in seals along the New England coast has yielded additional influenza isolates (Callan *et al.* 1995). In January 1991, H4N6 viruses were isolated from the lung tissues of two harbour seals which had acute interstitial and/or haemorrhagic pneumonia and subcutaneous emphysema. In January–February 1992, H3N3 viruses were isolated from three harbour seals, also with similar pathological lesions. Although there was not extensive morbidity and mortality reported during 1991–92, there was an increase in the number of strandings during those periods when virus was isolated, as compared to previous years.

The detection of the H3 subtype in seals was interesting because H3 viruses commonly infect other species including humans, pigs, horses and birds. Therefore, antigenic and genetic studies of the haemagglutinin (HA) from these seal H3N3 viruses were performed to evaluate their relationship with H3 subtype influenza viruses isolated from other species. In HI assays using H3-specific antisera and monoclonal antibodies, the reactivity patterns of two of the three seal viruses (A/Seal/MA/3911/92 and A/Seal/MA/4007/92) had patterns similar to the avian virus, A/Duck/Ukraine/1/63, and one virus (A/Seal/MA/3984/92) had a pattern more similar to the human virus, A/Aichi/2/68. This suggested these seal viruses could have originated from different host species. However, the viral HAs were sequenced and their comparison revealed that the two seal virus H3 sequences were virtually identical (99.7% identical at the nucleotide level and 99.3% identical at the amino acid level). The four nucleotide differences between the two sequences each conferred an amino acid change which explained the antigenic differences since both changes in the HA1 were associated with described antigenic sites (A and D) of the HA molecule (Wiley & Wilson 1981). The H3 seal virus HA nucleotide sequences were most similar to that of A/Mallard/New York/6874/78 (94.6% identity), suggesting both viruses were of avian host origin. Phylogenetic analysis of the HA nucleotide sequences supported the previous findings of Bean *et al.* (1992) which indicated that there are three major lineages of H3 viruses, i.e. the equine viruses, viruses predominantly isolated from birds in North America, and the remaining avian, swine and human H3 viruses. In the case of the H3 seal viruses, they were most closely related to H3 influenza viruses isolated from North American birds. This finding, along with the N3 neuraminidase subtype, suggest that these viruses are of avian origin. This is consistent with the conclusions from studies of previous seal influenza virus isolates (Hinshaw *et al.* 1984; Webster *et al.* 1981b). It is likely that close contact between coastal birds and seals is the basis for the interspecies transmission. This does emphasize that this reservoir of H3 viruses in North American birds is capable of adapting to seals, and possibly other mammalian hosts like pigs and humans.

A factor of interest in the host specificity of H3 viruses is the receptor binding site sequence (residues 225–230) (Naeve *et al.* 1984). Mutations at residues 226 and 228 of the receptor binding site are associated with changes in the biological properties and the specificity of sialic acid binding sites of H3 viruses (Rogers & Paulson 1983; Rogers *et al.* 1983; Naeve *et al.* 1984). Residues 226 and 228 of the seal isolates are glutamine and glycine, respectively, which coincide with the consensus for the receptor binding site of most avian and equine H3 viruses. Conversely, most human and swine H3s have leucine and serine for residues 226 and 228, respectively. The H7N7 (A/Seal/MA/1/80) and the H4N5 (A/Seal/MA/133/82) viruses previously isolated from seals also have the same avian receptor binding sequence (Naeve & Webster 1983; Donis *et al.* 1989), suggesting that this binding sequence may be well adapted for seals since mutations altering this sequence have not been observed in seals.

Natural infection of seals with the H4N6 and H3N3 influenza isolates during 1991–92 did not cause a severe epizootic of pneumonia in the seal population as experienced in 1979–80 (A/Seal/MA/1/80, H7N7) and 1982–83 (A/Seal/MA/133/82, H4N5). It may be that these more recent isolates (H4N6 and H3N3) are less pathogenic in seals. Alternatively, environmental conditions and/or secondary pathogens may be additional factors involved in the development of epizootics in the seal population (Geraci *et al.* 1982).

Whales

Whales are also marine mammals from which influenza viruses have been isolated. Lvov *et al.* (1978) described the isolation of H1N3 influenza A viruses from the lungs and liver of striped whales (*Balaenopteridae*) collected during a whaling expedition in the South Pacific from 1976 to 1977. Similar to the viruses in seals, A/whale/Pacific Ocean/76 (H1N3) was closely related antigenically to avian viruses. Whether this virus was responsible for any disease in the whales remains unknown.

In the autumn of 1984, two major pilot whale strandings occurred on the New England coast (Hinshaw *et al.* 1986). One whale was having difficulty swimming and was obviously in very poor condition, so it was removed from the water, euthanized and necropsied. This animal had haemorrhagic lungs, sloughing skin, extreme emaciation, an enlarged hilar node and a small, friable liver. Influenza viruses of the H13N2 subtype were isolated from the lung and both H13N2 and H13N9 subtypes were isolated from the hilar node of this pilot whale. The antigenic, genetic and biological comparisons of both whale viruses suggested that they were most closely related to viruses in gulls. It is possible that, while feeding, whales could have been exposed to the virus via faeces from infected gulls, because gulls and whales do share habitats.

It is interesting that a comparison of the nucleoprotein (NP) genes from A/Whale/PO/19/76 and A/Whale/Maine/328/84 showed that their NP genes were most closely related to avian viruses, but relatively distantly related to each other (Mandler *et al.* 1990). The NPs were closely related to different avian NPs, i.e. A/Whale/Maine/328/84 was most closely related to a gull isolate from the Atlantic coast of North America and A/Whale/PO/19/76, most closely related to a tern isolate from the Caspian Sea. Their analyses suggested that the NP genes in these whale viruses originated from avian species in the same specific geographical region as the whales themselves and that the introductions were relatively recent. It also seems that the appearance of the viruses in whales and seals are independent transmission events from birds, rather than a continual circulation of the viruses among marine mammals.

It remains unknown whether the influenza virus was responsible for the disease or the stranding (or neither) of the pilot whales. Continued surveillance of these stranded animals should indicate whether avian influenza viruses cause significant disease in whales—it seems quite possible in view of the situation in seals.

Mink

Like ferrets, mink belong to the genus *Mustela* and are quite susceptible to experimental infection with influenza virus (Matsuura *et al.* 1979) and serological surveys indicated evidence of influenza infections in mink (Yagyu *et al.* 1982; Okazaki *et al.* 1983). In October 1994, an epizootic of influenza occurred on several mink farms in the south of Sweden (Klingeborn *et al.* 1985). In this case, viruses were isolated from the mink and all were characterized as H10N7, typically a subtype found in birds. The infected mink experienced anorexia, sneezing, coughing and nasal and ocular discharges; necropsies revealed acute interstitial pneumonia. The extent of this outbreak was impressive in that there was 100% morbidity and 3000 deaths in the 100 000 mink on the 33 farms involved. It is unclear as to how the virus started and then spread in the mink; however, the farms were close to the sea and the mink were housed in outside cages. It is possible that seabirds, particularly gulls, may have spread their influenza viruses to the mink when the gulls tried to eat the food in the mink cages.

Acknowledgements

The author acknowledges support by Public Health Service research grant AI 24902 from the National Institute of Allergy and Infectious Disease and by grants 3101 and 3414 from the US Department of Agriculture. The author thanks all of the people who work on marine mammal strandings, especially the New England Aquarium, for their dedication and help.

References

Bean, W.J., Schell, M., Katz, J. *et al.* (1992) Evolution of the H3 influenza virus haemagglutinin from human and non-human hosts. *J Virol* **66**, 1129–38.

Callan, R.J., Early, G., Kida, H. & Hinshaw, V.S. (1995) The appearance of H3 influenza viruses in seals. *J Gen Virol* **76**, 199–203.

Donis, R.O., Bean, W.J., Kawaoka, Y. & Webster, R.G. (1989) Distinct lineages of influenza virus H4 haemagglutinin genes in different regions of the world. *Virology* **169**, 408–17.

Geraci, J.R., St Aubin, D.J., Barker, I.K. *et al.* (1982) Mass mortality of harbor seals: pneumonia associated with influenza A virus. *Science* **215**, 1129–31.

Hinshaw, V.S., Bean, W.J., Geraci, J., Fiorelli, P., Early, G. & Webster, R.G. (1986) Characterization of two influenza A viruses from a pilot whale. *J Virol* **58**, 655–6.

Hinshaw, V.S., Bean, W.J., Webster, R.G. *et al.* (1984) Are seals frequently infected with avian influenza viruses? *J Virol* **51**, 863–5.

Klingeborn, B., Englund, L., Rott, R., Juntti, N. & Rockborn, G. (1985) An avian influenza A virus killing a mammalian species—the mink. *Arch Virol* **86**, 347–51.

Lvov, D.K., Zdanov, V.M., Sazonov, A.A. *et al.* (1978) Comparison of influenza viruses isolated from man and from whales. *Bull WHO* **56**, 923–30.

Mandler, J., Gorman, O.T., Ludwig, S. *et al.* (1990) Derivation of the nucleoproteins (NP) of influenza A viruses isolated from marine mammals. *Virology* **176**, 255–61.

Matsuura, Y., Yanagawa, R. & Noda, H. (1979) Experimental infection of mink with influenza A viruses. *Arch Virology* **62**, 71–6.

Murphy, B.R., Harper, J., Sly, D.L., London, W.T., Miller, N.T. & Webster, R.G. (1983) Evaluation of the A/Seal/ Mass/1/80 virus in squirrel monkeys. *Infect Immun* **42**, 424–6.

Naeve, C.W., Hinshaw, V.S. & Webster, R.G. (1984) Mutations in the haemagglutinin receptor-binding site can change the biological properties of an influenza virus. *J Virol* **51**, 567–9.

Naeve, C.W. & Webster, R.G. (1983) Sequence of the haemagglutinin gene from influenza virus A/Seal/ Mass/1/80. *Virology* **129**, 298–308.

Okazaki, K. & Yanagawa, R. & Kida, H. (1983) Human influenza virus infection in mink: serological evidence of infection in summer and autumn. *Vet Microbiol* **8**, 251–7.

Rogers, G.N. & Paulson, J.C. (1983) Receptor determinants of human and animal influenza virus isolates: differences in receptor specificity of the H3 haemagglutinin based on species of origin. *Virology* **127**, 361–73.

Rogers, G.N., Paulson, J.C., Daniels, R.S., Skehel, J.J., Wilson, I.A. & Wiley, D.C. (1983) Single amino acid substitutions in influenza haemagglutinin change receptor binding specificity. *Nature* **304**, 76–8.

Stuen, S., Have, P., Osterhaus, A.D.M.E., Arnemo, J.M. & Moustgaard. (1994) Serological investigation of virus infections in harp seals (*Phoca groenlandica*) and hooded seals (*Cystophora cristata*). *Vet Rec* **7**, 502–3.

Webster, R.G., Geraci, J., Petursson, G. & Skirnisson, K. (1981a) Conjunctivitis in human beings caused by influenza A virus of seals. *N Engl J Med* **304**, 911.

Webster, R.G., Hinshaw, V.S., Bean, W.J. *et al.* (1981b) Characterization of an influenza A virus from seals. *Virology* **113**, 712–24.

Wiley, D.C. & Wilson, I.A. (1981) Structural identification of the antibody-binding sites of Hong Kong influenza haemagglutinin and their involvement in antigenic variation. *Nature* **289**, 373–8.

Yagyu, K., Yanagawa, R., Matsuura, Y., Fukushi, H., Kida, H. & Noda, H. (1982) Serological survey of influenza A virus infection in mink. *Jpn J Vet Sci* **44**, 691–3.

CHAPTER 16

Cocirculation and Divergence of Human Influenza Viruses

Janet M. Daly, John M. Wood and James S. Robertson

The three types of influenza viruses (A, B and C) vary greatly in their epidemiological significance. The epidemiology of influenza A viruses has been well studied in relation to the occurrence of epidemics and pandemic episodes of disease in humans. Influenza B viruses also cause epidemics of influenza in people whereas influenza C viruses cause only mild respiratory infections affecting mainly the immunologically naive (children) or the elderly. The continuing occurrence of influenza epidemics is caused by rapid evolution of the viral genome. This can be monitored by antigenic analyses and by sequence analysis of genes, particularly the haemagglutinin (HA) gene, of influenza virus field strains.

Antigenic shift and antigenic drift in influenza A viruses

The ability of human influenza A viruses to cause recurrent epidemics and repeated infections during the lifetime of an individual is due to the remarkable variability of the virus. Antigenic variation of influenza A viruses involves several different mechanisms. Antigenic shift involves the sudden appearance of a different HA subtype, which may or may not be accompanied by a change in neuraminidase (NA) subtype (WHO 1979). This gives rise to pandemic disease because the new virus is not recognized and neutralized by the human immune system. There is good evidence that the main mechanism for antigenic shift is reassortment of the genes coding for the surface glycoproteins. Direct interspecies transmission and re-emergence of previously circulating strains have also been pro-posed as causes of the sudden appearance of new influenza subtypes.

Antigenic drift occurs by the accumulation of point mutations resulting in amino acid changes in the surface glycoproteins, particularly the HA, which allows new variants to escape immunity induced by prior influenza infection or vaccination (reviewed by Wiley et al. 1981; Webster et al. 1982). Gene sequence analyses of viruses of the H3 subtype have indicated that the amino acid substitutions resulting in antigenic drift accumulate primarily in five antigenic regions, A–E, located on the surface of the HA1 domain of the H3 HA molecule (Wiley et al. 1981; Both et al. 1983; Wiley & Skehel 1987). Studies of H1 subtype viruses also revealed antigenically significant regions of the H1 HA similar to those described for the H3 HA molecule (Caton et al. 1982). Similarly, comparison of NA genes of field isolates and information collected from monoclonal antibody-selected variants (Laver et al. 1982; Webster et al. 1982) has demonstrated that antigenic drift also occurs in the NA by a similar mechanism as for HA.

Antigenic drift between epidemic influenza virus strains is associated with amino acid changes in one or more antigenic sites of the HA molecule (Both et al. 1983; Raymond et al. 1986; Nakajima et al. 1988; Cox et al. 1989, 1993). In vitro, the frequency of selection of escape mutants with an amino acid change in a single site using monoclonal antibodies is 10^{-4}-10^{-5} (Yewdell et al. 1979). Since a single antibody recognizing any one of the five antigenic regions may be sufficient for neutralization, the calculated probability of a mutant arising with changes in several antigenic sites is so low that the production of a new epidemic strain in the presence of host antibodies recognizing several different epitopes is unlikely to occur. However, most people, especially children, mount a limited antibody response to influenza which, in the case of HA, is restricted to one or two antigenic sites (Wang *et al.* 1986). Furthermore, the spectrum of antibodies produced differs between individuals. It is therefore more likely that epidemic viruses evolve in a stepwise manner through successive infections of individuals possessing different and limited antibody repertoires.

In 1957, H1N1 viruses that had been circulating in the human population since at least 1933 when the virus was first isolated were replaced by viruses of the H2N2 subtype. The H2 HA and N2 NA underwent antigenic drift between 1957 and 1968 until the HA was replaced in 1968 by the emergence of the H3N2 influenza subtype, after which the N2 NA continued to drift along with the H3 HA.

Evolution of influenza A viruses

H3 haemagglutinin

Viruses of the H3N2 subtype emerged in humans during the 1968 pandemic and have circulated continuously since, causing morbidity and mortality in successive epidemics.

Sequencing studies of human influenza A viruses have suggested that they evolve along a single lineage (Yamashita *et al.* 1988). However, separate sublineages of influenza A (H3N2) subtypes can cocirculate in humans for short periods. Two distinct groups of antigenic variants of the influenza A (H3N2) subtype were recognized in HI tests with postinfection ferret sera between 1989 and 1990 (CDC 1991). They were represented by the strains A/Beijing/353/89 or A/Shanghai/24/90 and related viruses cocirculated between 1990 and 1992. In 1992, strains similar to a new variant (A/Beijing/32/92), which were antigenically and genetically related to the A/Shanghai/24/90 reference strain, began to circulate worldwide and became the major epidemic strains (CDC 1993). Figure 16.1 shows an evolutionary tree derived from the number of nucleotide differences in the HA1 domains of the

HAs of 30 H3N2 field strains. This figure shows that the A/Beijing/353/89 and A/Beijing/32/92 viruses are located on different branches of the evolutionary tree and that the A/Beijing/353/89-like strains appear to have been superseded by A/Beijing/32/92-like viruses and their descendants.

As H3N2 viruses are frequently associated with excess mortality in the elderly population and others who are at high risk of complications due to influenza, it is especially important to match this vaccine component to the circulating strains. In the 10-year period spanning 1986–96, nine different strains of H3N2 virus have been used as vaccine components.

Although considerable sequence variation exists between epidemic variants, the degree of sequence homogeneity within an epidemic can be surprising. Soon after the emergence of a novel epidemic variant there may be little sequence variation at the amino acid level. For example, geographically distinct H3N2 strains isolated over a 9-month period during 1987 showed few amino acid changes in their HA molecules (Cox *et al.* 1993). The slight genetic and corresponding antigenic variation that was observed among these strains (CDC 1988) is more likely to be a result of host-cell selection during isolation and passage of the viruses in the laboratory. Human influenza virus isolates are routinely adapted to growth in embryonated hens' eggs prior to antigenic characterization for epidemiological purposes, and such procedures result in the selection of variants (Robertson *et al.* 1985, 1987). These variants have single amino acid substitutions in the HA in the vicinity of the receptor binding site (reviewed by Robertson 1993), which can have considerable effects on the antigenicity of the virus (Katz *et al.* 1987). It is important, therefore, to monitor HA sequences for such laboratory-derived changes to distinguish them from those occurring in the wild.

H1 haemagglutinin

Influenza A viruses of the H1N1 subtype have circulated over two distinct periods this century, the first being between approximately 1918 and 1957, and the second being from 1977 to the present time.

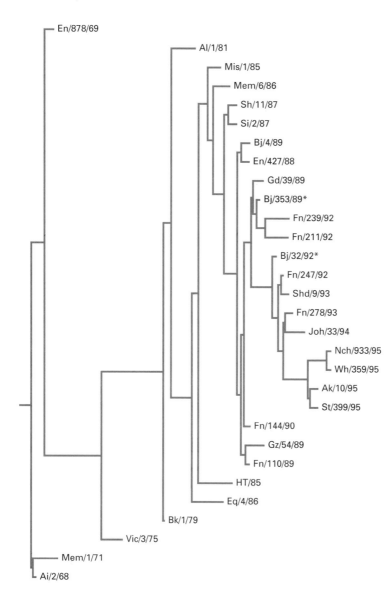

Fig. 16.1 Evolutionary tree of the HA1 domain of influenza A (H3N2) viruses isolated at different times and in different regions. The sequence data were obtained from GenBank, with additional recent sequences kindly provided by Dr N.J. Cox, Centers for Disease Control and Prevention. The maximum likelihood method (DNAML) of the Phylogeny Inference Package (Phylip), version 3.5, was used to estimate phylogenies from nucleotide sequences. Horizontal lines are proportional to the number of nucleotide changes; vertical lines are for spacing only.

During the second period of circulation, disease mainly occurred in children and young adults, whereas older people who were exposed to similar viruses prevalent prior to 1957 were protected against disease. In a sequence analysis of H1N1 field strains there was remarkable genetic similarity between the HA of a 1950 virus, A/Fort Warren/50, and the re-emergent 1977 strain, A/USSR/77 (Raymond *et al.* 1986). The re-emergent viruses appear to be evolving at the same rate as those circulating in the 1950s. On the basis of the calculated rate of 1.7 nucleotide substitutions per year in the non-structural (NS) gene, if evolution had continued during the intervening 'latent' period, 46 substitutions would be predicted to have occurred in the NS gene between A/Fort Warren/50 and A/USSR/77. However, only five substitutions have occurred.

Monitoring of sequence changes occurring in the HA1 coding region since the re-emergence of H1N1 strains in 1977, suggests that evolution is occurring along a single pathway with short side branches (Raymond *et al.* 1986; Cox *et al.* 1989; Nakajima *et al.* 1991; Xu *et al.* 1993; Pyhälä *et al.* 1995) (Fig. 16.2). However, it has been demonstrated that, as with H3N2 viruses, separate lineages of H1N1 viruses can cocirculate (Cox *et al.* 1993), which is an added complication to the process of vaccine strain selection.

In April 1986, H1N1 viruses were isolated that were antigenically distinguishable from all reference strains current at that time, including A/Chile/83, which had recently been recommended by the World Health Organization (WHO) as the H1N1 vaccine component for the forthcoming influenza season. Spread of these variant viruses prompted a second WHO recommendation, close to the time of vaccine administration in the Northern Hemisphere, for an additional vaccine containing an A/Singapore/6/86-like strain (WHO

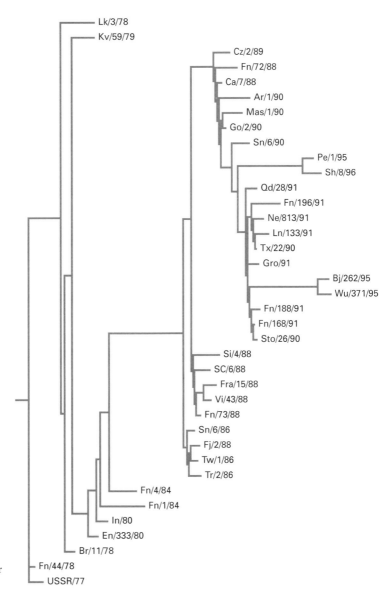

Fig. 16.2 Evolutionary tree of the HA1 domain of influenza A (H1N1) viruses prepared as described for Fig. 16.1. The sequence data were obtained from GenBank, with additional recent sequences kindly provided by Dr N.J. Cox, Centers for Disease Control and Prevention.

1986). Sequence analysis demonstrated that the A/Singapore/6/86-like strains did not evolve directly from viruses related to the preceding epidemic strains, represented by A/Chile/83, but from viruses isolated in the Hong Kong region in 1982 and 1983, A/Hong Kong/2/82 and A/Hong Kong/32/83 (Robertson 1987). Following the emergence of the A/Singapore/6/86-like variants, little antigenic variation has been detected among H1N1 viruses circulating worldwide and the H1N1 component of the vaccine has remained the same for 10 years. The variation that has been observed generally has followed a linear pathway. However, in the winter of 1996–97, an increasing number of H1 variants was detected, which prompted the recommendation of a new H1N1 vaccine component, A/Bayern/7/95-like strains, for the 1997/98 winter season.

Neuraminidase

Although anti-NA antibodies do not neutralize viral infectivity, they do appear to modify disease (Deroo *et al.* 1996) and as such the immune response to NA also has a role in the epidemiology of influenza.

Comparison of five N1 genes from viruses isolated between 1933 and 1983 show a high degree of sequential nucleotide and amino acid mutation occurring over time. In addition, phylogenetic analysis of the nucleotide sequence of N2 genes from 33 influenza A (H3N2) epidemic strains isolated between 1968 and 1995 demonstrated that the NA genes like the H3 HA genes, have evolved as two distinct lineages represented by the strains A/Beijing/353/89 and A/Beijing/32/92 or A/Shanghai/24/90 (Xu *et al.* 1996). Furthermore, genetic reassortment of N2 genes between the two lineages occurred during their cocirculation. Genetic reassortants that bear an A/Beijing/32/92-like HA and an A/Beijing/353/89-like NA have circulated worldwide. However, these reassortants would not be expected to have an increased epidemic potential compared with their parents because a significant part of the population had already developed immunity to these antigens from previous infection or immunization.

Evolution of influenza C viruses

Influenza C viruses usually cause only mild respiratory infections in humans (Katagiri *et al.* 1983). For this reason, influenza C viruses are not included in influenza vaccines and their epidemiology is less well studied than that of influenza types A and B. Early evidence from studies with polyclonal immune sera (Chakraverty 1978) suggests that influenza C viruses are antigenically more stable than influenza A viruses.

Sequence analysis of influenza C virus genes reveal an evolutionary pattern very different from that of influenza A viruses. From a comparison of the HA esterase (HE) sequence of eight human influenza C viruses isolated between 1947 and 1983, the appearance of nucleotide substitutions in the HE genes could not be correlated with the year of their isolation (Buonagurio *et al.* 1985). Dramatic conservation of sequence in the HE gene of influenza C viruses has been observed. For example, two strains isolated 31 years apart (C/Ann Arbor/50 and C/Yamagata/81) had almost identical HE gene sequence, indicating that influenza C virus genes can exist unchanged for decades (Fig. 16.3). In contrast, C/Yamagata/81 had many changes compared with a strain isolated only 1 year before (C/Mississippi/80). These findings were also reflected in a study of the NS genes of the same eight strains (Buonagurio *et al.* 1986a), in which there was no correlation between the number of amino acid changes observed between strains and the year of their isolation. In addition phylogenetic trees constructed from the NS gene sequences were distinct from those constructed for the corresponding HE genes, a finding that could be explained by the occurrence of reassortment between different viral lineages (Buonagurio *et al.* 1986a). It appears that the epidemiology of influenza C viruses is characterized by the presence of multiple evolutionary lineages of the virus, rather than a single dominant lineage as occurs with influenza A viruses.

Evolution of influenza B viruses

Although disease caused by influenza B viruses is less severe than that due to influenza A viruses,

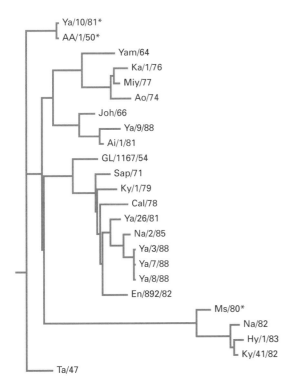

Fig. 16.3 Evolutionary tree of the HE influenza C viruses prepared as described for Fig. 16.1. The sequence data were obtained from GenBank.

small number of viruses, it was originally proposed that the evolution of influenza B virus is similar to that of influenza A virus (Krystal *et al.* 1983; Verhoeyen *et al.* 1983). However, several other studies involving genetic and antigenic analysis suggest that the evolutionary pattern of influenza B viruses is more complex. Multiple genetic variants of influenza B viruses have been shown to cocirculate during a single epidemic (Lu *et al.* 1983) and two distinct lineages of influenza B viruses, represented by the strains B/Yamagata/16/88 and B/Victoria/2/87, have been maintained for at least 4 years (Rota *et al.* 1990) (Fig. 16.4). In a comparison of the NS sequences of 14 isolates and the HA sequences of 10 isolates, Yamashita *et al.* (1988) described a pattern of evolution resembling that of influenza C, with multiple evolutionary lineages that can coexist for considerable periods of time. However, there was also evidence of linear evolution within subsets of strains leading to the conclusion that influenza B virus evolution is intermediary to that of influenza A and C viruses. This complexity of the evolutionary pattern of influenza type B makes the choice of strain for the type B component of influenza vaccines quite difficult.

Comparison of evolutionary patterns of influenza A, B and C viruses

Comparison of the sequence divergence among genes of type A, B and C viruses suggests that in humans influenza B and C viruses evolve more slowly than A viruses. The evolutionary rates obtained in different laboratories for the same type or subtype of genes vary. Despite this, evolutionary rates calculated for influenza B are approximately two-fold slower than for influenza A viruses, i.e. $1.1–1.96 \times 10^{-3}$ nucleotide substitutions per site per year (Yamashita *et al.* 1988; Cox *et al.* 1993) for B HA as opposed to 4.0×10^{-3} nucleotide substitutions per site per year for HA of influenza A H3N2 viruses (Cox *et al.* 1993) and 4.4×10^{-3} nucleotide substitutions per site per year for H1N1 viruses (Raymond *et al.* 1986). In a recent study of influenza C strains isolated in Japan between 1964 and 1988 (Muraki *et al.* 1996), viruses in one lineage

influenza B virus epidemics occur regularly and an influenza B virus is included in the vaccine. There is no evidence of antigenic shift in influenza B viruses, possibly due to the absence of an animal reservoir of influenza B viruses (Pereira 1969). Also, there are no subdivisions of the surface antigens of influenza B as exists with influenza A viruses, and reassortment occurs within but not between types of influenza viruses.

Less information is available concerning the physical and antigenic structure of the HA of influenza B virus than of influenza A HA. Despite recognized similarities between the HA sequence of influenza A and B viruses, which suggests a similarity in the basic structure of the two molecules (Krystal *et al.* 1982), information on the number and organization of immunodominant sites on the influenza B HA is less detailed than for influenza A HA.

On the basis of studies of the HA sequence of a

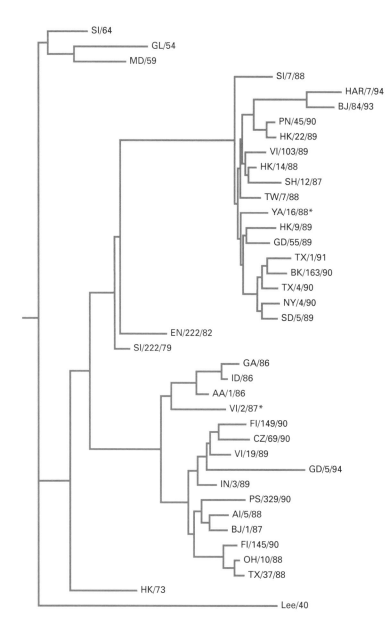

Fig. 16.4 Evolutionary tree of the HA1 domain of influenza B viruses prepared as described for Fig. 16.1. The sequence data were obtained from GenBank, with additional recent sequences kindly provided by Dr N.J. Cox, Centers for Disease Control and Prevention.

demonstrated sequential evolution, permitting the evolutionary rate for the HE gene to be estimated at 0.49×10^{-3} nucleotide substitutions per site per year, almost one-tenth of the value of the rates calculated for human influenza A HA genes.

Why do influenza A viruses have a faster rate of evolutionary change? The rate of evolution of an RNA genome is dependent on several factors including the intrinsic error frequency of the RNA-replicating enzymes, selection for variants by the immune system of a partially immune population and selection against variants imposed by structural and functional constraints of viral proteins.

There has been controversy as to whether influenza evolution is a result of positive selection or random neutral change. Most protein sequences are more strongly conserved than nucleotide sequences. Random mutations among the 61 codons specifying amino acids will result in a coding change in 24% of the codons. In influenza A, about 50% of nucleotide changes in HA and NA sequences result in amino acid changes (Air *et al.* 1990). This can be taken as an indication of positive selection to change the protein sequence, with the most likely selection pressure being the immune system of the host. In influenza B viruses, there is less apparent direct selection to change the protein, with approximately 30% of nucleotide changes giving rise to amino acid substitutions in the surface glycoprotein molecules (Air *et al.* 1990).

Though the reason for the characteristically high frequency of antigenic change of influenza A viruses remains unclear, it seems likely that the existence of virus reservoirs in other species and their transmission to humans at infrequent intervals (antigenic shift) are major factors in disturbing the equilibrium that similar but less variable viruses such as influenza B and C viruses appear to have achieved.

Variation in genes for internal proteins

Continuing evolution is most prominent in the surface glycoproteins, but also occurs in each of the other six gene segments of influenza A and B viruses. Where evolutionary rates have been determined for internal protein genes (Altmüller *et al.* 1991; Kawaoka *et al.* 1989; Okazaki *et al.* 1989; Gorman *et al.* 1990, 1991), they are much lower than those of the surface glycoproteins. Also, the proportion of non-coding (silent) to total nucleotide changes is much higher in the internal protein genes (PB2, NP and M1) than for H3 HA (81–96% as opposed to 57%), which reveals differences in their respective modes of evolution. In addition, within the M segment, which contains two overlapping reading frames, the M1 and M2 genes are evolving very differently from one another. The gene coding for M2, an ion channel protein, is evolving more rapidly and with a higher proportion of non-silent nucleotide changes than the M1 gene, which showed almost no accumulation of coding changes over a 55-year period (Ito *et al.* 1991).

Conclusion

In addition to intensive international strain surveillance, a better understanding of variation and evolution of influenza viruses is of enormous practical use in ensuring that viruses chosen for use in influenza vaccines are closely related to viruses in circulation. Although serological assays, such as HI, are essential to monitor rapidly antigenic changes in the HA of new influenza strains, the data can be misleading if used to assign evolutionary relationships between viruses. As an example, viruses that are evolving on separate evolutionary lineages may appear to be antigenically related because they share a key antigenic site. This is the reason antigenic analysis should be performed in tandem with sequencing of the HA1 domain of the HA gene, the main gene of antigenic drift. Thus the amino acid residues associated with antigenic drift can be identified and help establish a more precise evolutionary relationship between viruses.

Acknowledgements

The authors are grateful to Dr Nancy Cox of the Centers for Disease Control and Prevention, Atlanta, USA for supplying additional unpublished HA1 sequences of influenza A (H3N2) and (H1N1) and influenza B viruses.

References

Air, G., Gibbs, A., Laver, W. & Webster, R. (1990) Evolutionary changes in influenza B viruses are not primarily governed by antibody selection. *Proc Natl Acad Sci (USA)* **87**, 3882–8.

Altmüller, A., Kunerl, M., Müller, K., Hinshaw, V., Fitch, W. & Scholtissek, C. (1991) Genetic relatedness of the nucleoprotein (NP) of recent swine, turkey, and human influenza A virus (H1N1) isolates. *Virus Res* **22**, 79–87.

Both, G., Sleigh, M., Cox, N. & Kendal, A. (1983) Antigenic drift in influenza virus H3 haemagglutinin from 1968 to 1980: multiple evolutionary pathways and sequential amino acid changes at key antigenic sites. *J Virol* **48**, 52–60.

Buonagurio, D., Nakada, S., Desselberger, U., Krystal, M. & Palese, P. (1985) Non-cumulative sequence changes in the haemagglutinin genes of influenza C virus isolates. *Virology* **153**, 221–32.

Buonagurio, D., Nakada., S., Fitch, W. & Palese, P. (1986a) Epidemiology of influenza C virus in man: multiple evolutionary lineages and low rate of change. *Virology* **153**, 12–21.

Buonagurio, D., Nakada, S., Parvin, J., Krystal, M., Palese, P. & Fitch, W. (1986b) Evolution of human influenza A viruses over 50 years: rapid uniform rate of change in NS gene. *Science* **232**, 980–2.

Caton, A., Brownlee, G., Yewdell, J. & Gerhard, W. (1982) The antigenic structure of the influenza virus A/PR/8/34 haemagglutinin (H1 subtype). *Cell* **31**, 417–27.

CDC (Centers for Disease Control and Prevention) (1988) Update: influenza activity—worldwide, and influenza vaccine availability—United States. *MMWR* **37**, 599–601.

CDC (Centers for Disease Control and Prevention) (1991) Update: influenza activity—United States and worldwide, and the composition of the 1991-92 influenza vaccine. *MMWR* **40**, 231–9.

CDC (Centers for Disease Control and Prevention) (1993) Update: influenza activity—United States and worldwide, and composition of the 1993-94 influenza vaccine. *MMWR* **42**, 177–80.

Chakraverty, P. (1978) Antigenic relationship between influenza C viruses. *Arch Virol* **58**, 341–8.

Cox, N., Black, R. & Kendal, A. (1989) Pathways of evolution of influenza A (H1N1) viruses from 1977 to 1986 as determined by oligonucleotide mapping and sequencing studies. *J Gen Virol* **70**, 299–313.

Cox, N., Xu, X., Bender, C. *et al.* (1993) Evolution of haemagglutinin in epidemic variants and selection of vaccine viruses. In: Hannoun, C. *et al.* (eds) *Options for the Control of Influenza II*, pp. 223–30. Elsevier, North Holland.

Deroo, T., Min Jou, W. & Fiers, W. (1996) Recombinant neuramindase vaccine protects against lethal influenza. *Vaccine* **14**, 561–9.

Gorman, O., Bean, W., Kawaoka, Y., Donatelli, I., Guo, Y. & Webster, R. (1991) Evolution of influenza A virus nucleoprotein genes: implications for the origin of H1N1 human and classical swine viruses. *J Virol* **65**, 3704–14.

Gorman, O., Donis, R., Kawaoka, Y. & Webster, R. (1990) Evolution of influenza A virus PB2 genes implications for the evolution of the nucleoprotein complex and origin of human influenza A virus. *J Virol* **64**, 4893–902.

Ito, T., Gorman, O., Bean, W. & Webster, R. (1991) Evolutionary analysis of the influenza A virus M gene with comparison of the M1 and M2 proteins. *J Virol* **65**, 5491–8.

Katagiri, S., Ohizumi, A. & Homma, M. (1983) An outbreak of type C influenza in a children's home. *J Infect Dis* **148**, 51–6.

Katz, J., Naeve, C. & Webster, R. (1987) Host cell-mediated variation in H3N2 influenza viruses. *Virology* **156**, 386–95.

Kawaoka, Y., Krauss, S. & Webster, R.G. (1989) Avian-to-human transmission of the PB1 gene of influenza A viruses in the 1957 and 1968 pandemics. *J Virol* **53**, 4603–8.

Krystal, M., Elliott, R., Benz, E., Young, J. & Palese, P. (1982) Evolution of influenza A and B viruses: conservation of structural features in the haemagglutinin genes. *Proc Natl Acad Sci (USA)* **79**, 4800–4.

Krystal, M., Young, J., Palese, P., Wilson, I., Skehel, J. & Wiley, D. (1983) Sequential mutations in haemagglutinins of influenza B virus isolates: definition of antigenic domains. *Proc Natl Acad Sci (USA)* **80**, 4527–31.

Laver, W., Air, G., Webster, R. & Markoff, L. (1982) Amino acid sequence changes in antigenic variants of type A influenza virus N2 neuraminidase. *Virology* **122**, 450–60.

Lu, B.-L., Webster, R., Brown, L. & Nerome, K. (1983) Heterogeneity of influenza B viruses. *Bull WHO* **61**, 681–7.

Muraki, Y., Hongo, S., Bugawara, K., Kitame, F. & Nakamura, K. (1996) Evolution of the haemagglutinin-esterase gene of influenza C virus. *J Gen Virol* **77**, 673–9.

Nakajima, R., Nakamura, K., Nishikawa, F., Nakamura, K. & Nakajima, K. (1991) Genetic relationship between the HA genes of type A influenza viruses isolated in off-seasons and epidemic seasons. *Epidemiol Infect* **106**, 383–95.

Nakajima, S., Takeuchi, Y. & Nakajima, K. (1988) Location on the evolutionary tree of influenza H3 haemagglutinin genes of Japanese strains isolated during 1985–86 season. *Epidemiol Infect* **100**, 301–10.

Okazaki, K., Kawaoka, Y. & Webster, R. (1989) Evolutionary pathways of the PA genes of influenza A viruses. *Virology* **172**, 601–8.

Pereira, H. (1969) Influenza: antigenic spectrums. *Progr Med Virol* **11**, 46–69.

Pyhälä, R., Ikonen, N., Forsten, T., Alanko, S. & Kinnunen, L. (1995) Evolution of the HA1 domain of human influenza A (H1N1) virus: loss of glycosylation sites and occurrence of herald and conserved strains. *J Gen Virol* **76**, 205–10.

Raymond, F., Caton, A., Cox, N., Kendal, A. & Brownlee, G. (1986) The antigenicity and evolution of influenza H1 haemagglutinin from 1950 to 1957 and 1977–83; two pathways from one gene. *Virology* **148**, 275–87.

Robertson, J. (1987) Sequence analysis of the haemagglutinin of A/Taiwan/1/86, a new variant of human influenza A (H1N1). *J Gen Virol* **70**, 299–313.

Robertson, J. (1993) Clinical influenza virus and the embryonated hens' eggs. *Rev Med Virol* **3**, 97–106.

Robertson, J., Bootman, J., Newman, R. *et al.* (1987) Structural changes in the haemagglutinin which accompany egg adaptation of an influenza A (H1N1) virus. *Virology* **160**, 31–7.

Robertson, J., Naeve, C., Webster, R., Bootman, J., Newman, R. & Schild, G. (1985) Alterations in the haemagglutinin associated with adaptation of influenza B virus to growth in eggs. *Virology* **143**, 166–74.

Rota, P., Wallis, T., Harmon, M., Rota, J., Kendal, A. & Nerome, K. (1990) Cocirculation of two distinct evolutionary lineages of influenza type B virus since 1983. *Virology* **175**, 59–68.

Verhoeyen, M., Rompuy, L., Jou, W., Huylebroeck, D. & Fiers, W. (1983) Complete nucleotide sequence of the influenza B/Singapore/222/79 virus haemagglutinin gene and comparison with the B/Lee/40 haemagglutinin. *Nucl Acids Res* **11**, 4703–12.

Wang, M.-L., Skehel, J. & Wiley, D. (1986) Comparative analyses of the specificities of anti-influenza haemagglutinin antibodies in human sera. *J Virol* **57**, 124–8.

Webster, R., Laver, W., Air, G. & Schild, G. (1982) Molecular mechanisms of variation in influenza viruses. *Nature* **296**, 115–21.

WHO (1979) A reconsideration of influenza A virus nomenclature: a WHO memorandum. *Bull WHO* **57**, 227–33.

WHO (1986) Composition of influenza virus vaccines for use in the 1986–87 season: an update. *WHO Weekly Epidemiol Rec* **31**, 237–8.

Wiley, D. & Skehel, J. (1987) The stucture and function of the haemagglutinin membrane glycoprotein of influenza virus. *Ann Rev Biochem* **56**, 365–94.

Wiley, D., Wilson, I. & Skehel, J. (1981) Structural identification of the antibody-binding sites of Hong Kong influenza haemagglutinin and their involvement in antigenic variation. *Nature* **289**, 373–8.

Xu, X., Cox, N., Bender, C., Regnery, H. & Shaw, M. (1996) Genetic variation in neuraminidase genes of influenza A (H3N2) viruses. *Virology* **224**, 175–83.

Xu, X., Rocha, E., Regenery, H., Kendal, A. & Cox, N. (1993) Genetic and antigenic analyses of influenza A (H1N1) viruses, 1986–91. *Virus Res* **28**, 37–55.

Yamashita, M., Krystal, M., Fitch, W. & Palese, P. (1988) Influenza B virus evolution: cocirculating lineages and comparison of evolutionary pattern with those of influenza A and C viruses. *Virology* **163**, 112–22.

Yewdell, J., Webster, R. & Gerhard, W. (1979) Antigenic variation in three distinct determinants of an influenza type A haemagglutinin molecule. *Nature* **219**, 246–8.

Section 4
Epidemiology and Surveillance
of Human Influenza

CHAPTER 17

Epidemiology of Influenza

Jonathan S. Nguyen-Van-Tam

The origins of influenza epidemiology lie in an era of relative uncertainty in terms of both clinical diagnoses and population statistics. Epidemic fevers have been described in the medical literature since the time of Hippocrates (*c.* 460–357 BC) but influenza was not reliably described until the middle of the 16th century (Creighton 1965). Even so, the epidemiological study of influenza predates both the introduction of statutory death registration in 1874 (Ashley *et al.* 1991a), and discovery of the virus itself almost 60 years later in 1933 (Smith *et al.* 1933). From an epidemiological perspective the disease remains constantly challenging, because of the changeable nature of the virus—a moving target, the unpredictability of its activity, and the frailty of routinely collected data sources in establishing the true burden of disease. This chapter discusses the main epidemiological features of influenza by drawing on examples taken from the many human influenza epidemics and rather fewer pandemic periods which have been well documented. Greatest emphasis is given to influenza types A and B because these are responsible for the vast majority of influenza-related morbidity and mortality, and have been far more widely studied than influenza type C.

Excess mortality

In Britain epidemiological descriptions of influenza epidemics first appeared with reasonable certainty in about 1557; in virtually all of these early reports, high mortality was mentioned as a characteristic feature and often formed the basis upon which influenza was distinguished from other epidemic 'grippes, catarrhs and colds' (Creighton 1965). The now familiar concept of excess mortality was first formally described during an influenza epidemic in London in 1847 by Dr William Farr, the first Registrar General of England; it was noted that the total number of deaths from all causes recorded during the epidemic was substantially higher than would normally have been expected at that time of year (Farr 1885). Studies of excess burials in British churchyards by Hope-Simpson (1983, 1986) now suggest that, although first described in 1847, this phenomenon occurred in association with influenza epidemics from as early as 1558. This concept of excess mortality is now established as one of the cornerstones of influenza epidemiology and it is well recognized that estimates of influenza-related mortality during epidemics must include excess deaths certified to causes other than influenza itself.

Towards the end of the 19th century, the 1889–94 influenza pandemic marked the first period of influenza activity for which it proved possible to obtain retrospective serological evidence of the influenza A virus (Masurel & Marine 1973; Davenport 1977; Rekart *et al.* 1982; Masurel & Heijtink 1983). This was also the first period of substantial influenza activity for which reliable mortality data were available because ascertainment of cause of death by a registered medical practitioner was not made compulsory in Britain until 1874 (Ashley *et al.* 1991a). In London, during each of the four epidemic periods between 1889 and 1894 weekly numbers of deaths from certified influenza rose from 10–20 per week to several hundred, with similar increases in deaths from bronchitis and pneumonia. In addition death rates from all causes (typically 20/1000 population per annum) rose to 30–50/1000 during each epidemic period (Creighton 1965).

The 1918–19 influenza pandemic which began during the final months of the Great War in Europe, demonstrated the ability of influenza to inflict massive worldwide mortality, when it is estimated that some 20 million deaths occurred. In Britain calculations of excess deaths were complicated by the fact that, in 1918 reliable mortality data for males were only available for civilians — a population already dramatically modified in terms of health status and age by the enlistment of able-bodied men into the armed services between 1913 and 1917. Nevertheless it was estimated that 198 000 excess civilian deaths occurred during the three waves of the pandemic (HMSO 1920). In the USA a study of the mortality records of 40 large cities showed that mortality rates rose by an average factor of 4.75 above baseline in a 25-week period ending on 1 March 1919 (Pearl 1919). In San Francisco and New York City between 1910 and 1917, death rates from pneumonia and influenza peaked each winter at about 400/100 000 population per annum; however, in autumn 1918 these rose eight-fold to above 3500/100 000 in both cities (Frost 1919). In the USA a total of 500 000 excess deaths were attributed to the 1918–19 pandemic (Kilbourne 1987; Crosby 1989).

In the 1930s, Collins refined the study of excess mortality during influenza epidemics by adjusting for normal seasonal variation and long-term trends in death rates when establishing a baseline for expected deaths (Collins 1930; Collins *et al.* 1930; Collins & Lehmann 1951). Of possibly greater significance was the quantification of excess deaths during epidemics ascribed to other chronic diseases including heart disease, tuberculosis, 'intracranial vascular lesions', nephritis, diabetes mellitus, and puerperal disorders; these calculations revealed that deaths attributable to influenza occurred under a wide variety of other diagnoses (Collins 1932; Collins & Lehmann 1953; Eickhoff *et al.* 1961). More recently Sprenger *et al.* (1989) examined Dutch mortality data between 1967 and 1982, concluding that for each recorded influenza death 1–1.5 further deaths (attributable to influenza) were recorded due

to heart disease, pneumonia and other chronic lung diseases. Tillet *et al.* (1983) reported 120 000 excess deaths in England and Wales due to influenza between 1968–69 and 1977–80 (Fig. 17.1) of which 67% were certified to respiratory causes, but another 31% to circulatory causes, mainly ischaemic heart disease and cerebrovascular disease. During the 1989–90 epidemic, Ashley *et al.* (1991b) demonstrated that only 10% of excess deaths which occurred in Britain were certified due to influenza the remainder being ascribed to other causes.

In the 1960s Serfling proposed modifications to the method by which excess deaths were calculated, and these still form the basis for the techniques currently used by the Communicable Disease Center in Atlanta, USA (Serfling 1963; Assad *et al.* 1973). In Britain this method was refined by employing a regression model to relate total mortality to other clinical indices of influenza, in an attempt to produce a more accurate estimation of the number of deaths expected in the absence of an influenza epidemic (Clifford *et al.* 1977). In the USA autoregressive integrated moving average (ARIMA) modelling has also been employed, based on Box and Jenkins' methodology, and is claimed to be more accurate in making predictions than Serfling's technique (Choi & Thacker 1981). Figure 17.2 shows excess annual death rates in Massachusetts and other American cities between 1887 and 1957. It should be noted that excess mortality did not occur

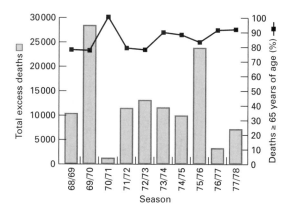

Fig. 17.1 Estimated excess deaths among adults attributable to influenza and percentage occurring in elderly subjects: England and Wales, 1968/69–1977/78. (From Tillet *et al.* 1983.)

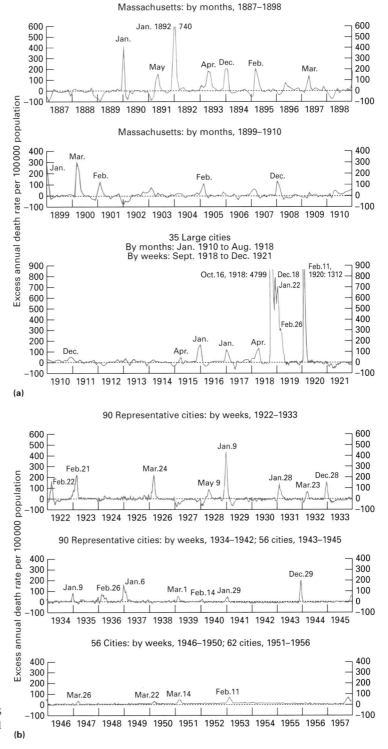

Fig. 17.2 Excess annual death rates for Massachusetts (a) and for representative cities in the USA (b) from 1887 to 1957. (Redrawn from US Department of Health Education and Welfare 1957.)

on an annual basis, and many (but not all) of the peaks in mortality were followed by small troughs lasting perhaps 1–2 months. A deficit of deaths observed immediately after an influenza epidemic was also described by Ashley *et al.* (1991b) for the 1989–90 influenza epidemic in Britain. The implication of this finding is that influenza epidemics hasten the deaths of certain frail individuals whose deaths were already imminent. On this basis the initial estimate of 29 000 excess deaths in Britain during the 1989–90 epidemic was later modified to 17 000 (Ashley *et al.* 1991b).

In studies based on regression modelling, excess deaths from all causes, and those specifically from pneumonia and influenza have been shown to correlate closely with other indices of influenza activity such as 'sentinel practice' primary care consultation data in Britain, and laboratory virus isolates in the USA (Clifford *et al.* 1977; Alling *et al.* 1981; Tillett *et al.* 1983). Some researchers assert that much of the excess mortality assigned to non-respiratory causes is caused by influenza-related pneumonia which is masked by the rules governing the interpretation of death certificates whereby only one underlying cause may be recorded in official statistics (Barker & Mullooly 1981; Barker & Mullooly 1982a).

Possible 'interference' between influenza and other respiratory viruses, especially parainfluenza viruses and respiratory syncytial virus (RSV), has been described by Glezen *et al.* (1980b) and Anestad (1982, 1987). High levels of activity from one epidemic respiratory infection temporarily suppress transmission of the remainder, possibly through the action of interferon. However, the evidence to support this theory is not overwhelming; other studies document concurrent RSV and influenza A activity, and dual infection has also been recognized (Mathur *et al.* 1980; Nicholson *et al.* 1990; Falsey *et al.* 1995). Two recent studies have explored the relationship between RSV and excess winter mortality, concluding that this may be as important a cause of excess deaths as influenza itself, and possibly more so (Fleming & Cross 1993; Nicholson 1996). These data suggest that the excess mortality in Britain ascribed to influenza during the 1975–76 and 1989–90 epidemics may have been over-

estimated because of the simultaneous occurrence of high levels of RSV infection.

Substantial variation has been observed in both the number of excess deaths reported during epidemics and their age distribution. Excess mortality is not detected each year, even though influenza viruses continue to circulate annually (Pereira & Chakraverty 1977; Sabin 1977; Chakraverty *et al.* 1986). Much of this variation undoubtedly relates to factors such as the introduction of new antigenic subtypes (antigenic shift) or strains (antigenic drift), variations in herd immunity, demographic patterns and subsequent alterations in the attack rate and virulence of influenza.

Excess morbidity

In addition to excess mortality, influenza epidemics also cause considerable social and commercial disruption and exert considerable pressure on healthcare services. However, in contrast with excess mortality, fewer studies have attempted to quantify excess morbidity using population-based data. Few precise morbidity measures exist and greater reliance must be placed on indirect measures which are more difficult to interpret. Suitable sources of information include new claims for sickness benefit, emergency room visits, hospitalizations for acute respiratory disease, and school or workplace absenteeism (Goldstein & Block 1976; Glass *et al.* 1978; Campbell *et al.* 1988).

Consultation rates

Primary care data from British general practitioners have been available since 1939, becoming formally established as the Royal College of General Practitioners Weekly Returns Service in 1967 (Fleming *et al.* 1991). Consultation rates for influenza and influenza-like illness are therefore available for all recent periods of influenza activity in England and Wales. Data from the 9-year period 1986–95 show typical winter weekly consultation rates of 30–70 consultations per 100 000 population for influenza and influenza-like illness combined. However, during epidemic years they have risen and fallen dramatically over a 5–6-week period, peaking at

800/100 000 in 1975–76 and 600/100 000 in 1989–90 (Birmingham Research Unit of the Royal College of General Practitioners 1977; Fleming 1996). From these data it has been estimated that 4.9% of the population of England and Wales (2.4 million people) consulted a general practitioner with influenza during the epidemic in 1976 (Birmingham Research Unit of the Royal College of General Practitioners 1977); more recent calculations suggest that during the 1989–90, 1993–94, and 1994–95 seasons the number of people in England and Wales who consulted a general practitioner with 'influenza' in each of the 4–6-week epidemic periods was 755 000 (1.5%), 469 000 (0.9%) and 172 000 (0.3%), respectively (Fleming 1996). Similarly, Barker and Mullooly (1980) reported a 30–50% excess in ambulatory care (primary care) visits compared with baseline in an adult population in Portland, Oregon, USA during two epidemics in 1968–69 and 1972–73. In Michigan, Monto (1987) demonstrated that influenza accounted for 29% of all respiratory viruses isolated during community surveillance, but 66% of those isolated by doctors during consultations; this demonstrates the greater severity of influenza and the increased likelihood of doctor involvement compared with other respiratory viruses. About 50% of patients in whom influenza A/H3N2 had been isolated consulted a doctor, compared with 40% for influenza B and 0–25% for A/H1N1; among adults the median duration of these illnesses was 15, 13 and 10 days, respectively, and 3 days shorter in children and teenagers.

Claims for sickness benefit

In Britain statutory sickness benefit claims among working-age adults provide a means of estimating absenteeism of greater than 3 days and its cause, including influenza. These data should be interpreted with caution because the take-up of benefit is not universal and claims up to 7 days are based on self-certification; nonetheless they give some indication of the burden of excess morbidity. At the height of the Asian influenza pandemic in September–October 1957 an extra 4% of the British national workforce (some 500 000 adults) claimed sickness benefit compared with the 1953–54 season

(McDonald 1958). Multiple regression models have been used to estimate excess new claims attributable to influenza over 12 winter seasons between 1967–68 and 1978–79 (Clifford *et al.* 1977; Tillett *et al.* 1980). During the epidemic in 1975–76 there were 908 000 excess new claims among working-age adults attributable to influenza; in contrast there were between 237 000 and 364 000 excess new claims in each of the following three winters when levels of influenza activity were somewhat lower.

School absenteeism

Among children school absenteeism due to influenza is a useful indirect measure of morbidity (see Fig. 33.1, p. 437). In 1977, during an epidemic of influenza B in two rural parishes in Louisiana, USA, total school absenteeism and absenteeism specifically due to influenza-like illness were shown to correspond closely with the epidemic curve (Retailliau *et al.* 1979). Data obtained in Glasgow, UK during the 1976 influenza epidemic show an equally clear relationship (Campbell *et al.* 1988). Similar observations were made in Houston, USA during the 1976 A/H3N2 epidemic and the influenza B epidemic in 1977; however, such obvious increases were less apparent during the A/Port Chalmers/H3N2 epidemic in 1975, an influenza B epidemic in 1980, and in two consecutive outbreaks in New Jersey, USA (Glass *et al.* 1978; Glezen & Couch 1978; Glezen *et al.* 1980a; Frank *et al.* 1983a). In both 1976 and 1977 rates of school absenteeism in Houston rose from a baseline of 8–9% over a 5-week period, peaking at about 12%; an estimated 37% of all enrolled schoolchildren suffered absence due to influenza (Glezen & Couch 1978; Glezen et al. 1980a). Industrial absenteeism among adults due to respiratory complaints followed a similar pattern in both years; however, these curves lagged behind school absenteeism by 2–3 weeks, and peaked higher at about 40% (Glezen & Couch 1978; Glezen *et al.* 1980a).

Hospital services

Influenza epidemics also place secondary care (hospital) services under considerable pressure.

Studies in Houston during an influenza A/H3N2 epidemic in 1976 revealed increases in both the number of emergency room attendances and the proportion of those presenting with respiratory symptoms (Glezen & Couch 1978). Similar increases in hospital attendance were observed by Glass *et al.* (1978) in New Jersey during two separate influenza epidemics in 1977–78 (A/H3N2 followed by A/H1N1), and by Goldstein and Block (1976) in New York City during 1969–71; however, this trend was not apparent during an influenza B epidemic in 1977 (Glezen *et al.* 1980a).

In economic terms the impact of influenza is of greatest significance in relation to acute hospital admissions rather than emergency room attendances (Retailliau *et al.* 1979). Increases in admissions due to acute respiratory disorders including influenza, pneumonia and lower respiratory tract infections have been well described during influenza epidemics among both adults and children (Glass *et al.* 1978; Glezen & Couch 1978; Glezen *et al.* 1980a). Perrotta *et al.* (1985) studied hospital discharge data from 11 hospitals in Harris County, Texas, USA between July 1978 and June 1981. Admissions for acute respiratory disease (ICD-9: 460–487) showed a close correlation with both the number of febrile respiratory illnesses reported at sentinel primary care sites, and the number of positive cultures for influenza virus. Whilst 54% of discharge diagnoses related to pneumonia, only 4% were assigned to influenza itself.

Barker and Mullooly (1980) studied excess hospital admissions during two epidemics of influenza A in Portland, Oregon in 1968–69 and 1972–73, using data from 1970 to 1971 as a baseline for comparison. Overall, annual hospitalization rates for pneumonia and influenza increased by about 80/100 000 population; the rate of excess (140–150% overall) was strongly associated with both increasing age and the presence of underlying high-risk diseases. In a later study Barker (1986) analysed American National Hospital Discharge data from 1970 to 1978 to calculate excess rates of hospitalization during epidemic periods from pneumonia and influenza, 'other' respiratory conditions and acute cardiac conditions. Between January and March during epidemic years excess annual hospitalization rates for pneumonia and influenza were 25/100 000 among children, 93/100 000 among adults aged 45–64 years, and 370/100 000 among the elderly (≥ 65 years). For 'other' respiratory conditions a similar age-related trend was observed although these excess rates were substantially lower than for pneumonia and influenza overall (maximum 40/100 000). Finally, for acute cardiac conditions a very small excess was observed among the elderly population. In contrast to observations of excess mortality there did not appear to be any compensatory deficit in admissions during the months immediately after the epidemic, suggesting that true excess morbidity had been detected.

Patterns of transmission in communities and households

In common with many aspects of influenza epidemiology, transmission studies are fraught with methodological problems. Transmissibility of any infectious agent is usually judged by measuring secondary attack rates among contacts. In the case of influenza these measurements can be problematic due to difficulties in establishing the diagnosis and the presence of other respiratory viral infections clinically indistinguishable from influenza (Longini *et al.* 1982). Fox *et al.* (1982b) failed to isolate influenza viruses from at least 73% of subjects with serologically proven infection; and in Michigan, USA between 1966 and 1971, the overall viral isolation rates for influenza among individuals with symptomatic respiratory disease were 1.4% for influenza A and 1.5% for type B compared with serological attack rates of 17% and 8%, respectively (Monto & Kioumehr 1975). While virus isolation rates have clearly underestimated morbidity, serologically confirmed infections do not always reflect symptomatic infection. In 1968–69 a serological study of high school students in Kansas, USA during the A/Hong Kong/68 epidemic showed that only 58% of serological infections were accompanied by clinical illness (Davis *et al.* 1970). Fox *et al.* (1982a) showed that among children and teenagers with $\geq$ four-fold rises in antibody 69–83%

suffered clinical illness, and in adults the percentage was 40–81%. More recently Elder *et al.* (1996) discovered that only 41% of hospital workers in Glasgow, UK with serological evidence of recent influenza infection could recall a flu-like illness.

Population (community) attack rates

The most reliable epidemiological data originate from studies combining clinical surveillance with serology and virus isolation techniques. A longitudinal study of respiratory illness among families in Tecumseh, Michigan, USA (population ~10 000) commenced in November 1965. Participating families comprised at least one child of school age or younger with parents who were aged under 45 years. Self-reported details of respiratory illnesses were combined with nasal and throat swabs and interval serological data (Monto *et al.* 1971). The number of families on report at any given time varied between 100 and 300 with a mean weekly surveillance population of 922 people (Monto & Cavallaro 1971). During the 6 full years of surveillance between 1966 and 1971, influenza A viruses were isolated annually; these were initially H2N2 strains until superseded by H3N2 strains from 1968 to 1969 onwards. Influenza B was detected in 1966, 1969 and 1971 (Monto & Kioumehr 1975). A similar study took place between 1965 and 1969 and 1975–79, in Seattle, Washington, USA. Over 215 families with young children were studied for influenza infections by illness reporting, virus isolation and interval serological sampling (Hall *et al.* 1973; Fox et al. 1982b). The first study period coincided with two winter epidemics of influenza A/H2N2 and a third of the emergent H3N2 subtype in the final season. The second period covered a type B epidemic in 1975–76, A/H3N2 epidemics in 1975–76 and 1977–78, and A/H1N1 in 1978–79.

In Michigan between 1966 and 1971 estimates of annual attack rate based on serology, with or without symptoms, were 17 and 8% for types A and B, respectively (Monto & Kioumehr 1975). In Seattle between 1965 and 1969 serologically confirmed influenza infection, with or without symptoms, occurred at a rate of 19% for type A viruses and 20% for type B (Hall *et al.* 1973). In the epidemic seasons of 1975–76 and 1977–78 influenza A/H3N2 infection rates as defined by virus isolation or serology, with or without symptoms, were 18 and 24%, respectively; in non-epidemic seasons these rates ranged between 0.4 and 6%. In 1975–76 influenza B produced an attack rate of 17%, but only 2–3% in subsequent non-epidemic seasons. Finally the influenza A/H1N1 epidemic in 1978–79 produced an attack rate of 31%, almost exclusively confined to children (Fox *et al.* 1982b). These data serve to illustrate the great variability in population attack rates which is seen in consecutive seasons; such fluctuations and their relative unpredictability have profound implications for the cost-effectiveness of influenza vaccine and other control measures (Patriarca & Strikas 1995). As judged by haemagglutination inhibition (HI) antibody seroconversion, typical annual (seasonal) community attack rates range from 5 to 15% during epidemic seasons (Patriarca & Strikas 1995).

Many studies worldwide have identified that the highest attack rates for influenza occur in children (Philip *et al.* 1961; Chin *et al.* 1963; Hall *et al.* 1973; Monto & Kioumehr 1975; Jennings & Miles 1978; Fox *et al.* 1982a, 1982b; Hope-Simpson 1984). Studies from the 1950s and early 1960s suggested that schoolchildren are most important for causing spread within communities (Philip *et al.* 1961; Chin *et al.* 1963). However, in Michigan annual attack rates for influenza A were highest in infants less than one year old (23%) but remained relatively high at all ages up to 39 years (typically 15–20%) before falling off to 12% in subjects aged 40 years and over; in contrast attack rates for influenza B were far higher among children aged 5–9 years (13%) and teenagers (14%) compared with adults of any age (3–9%) (Monto & Kioumehr 1975). In Seattle between 1965 and 1969 attack rates for both type A and B infections were also highest in preschool age children (24 and 26%, respectively) compared with adults (14 and 17%, respectively) (Hall *et al.* 1973). Both studies suggest that preschool age children are most important in producing community spread of influenza virus, presumably through casual and organized play activity. Further studies in Seattle between 1975 and 1979 studied only families with at least one school-age child. In all four seasons infection rates were highest among primary schoolchildren (5–9 years) but only marginally lower among preschool children (< 5 years) and older children and teenagers (10–19 years). For influenza A/H3N2, annual attack rates varied from 1 to 35% among primary schoolchildren compared with 0.5 to 12.7% among adults. Influenza B attack rates varied from ~1 to ~34% among older children and teenagers compared with 1 to 6% among adults (Fox *et al.* 1982b). Similar observations were made during two influenza B epidemics in Houston in 1976–77 and 1979–80 (Frank *et al.* 1983a). Data from the three major community studies are summarized in Table 17.1.

Glezen and Couch (1978) demonstrated a shift in the age distribution of virus-positive patients over the course of two influenza A epidemics in Houston; highest attack rates were initially seen in children and teenagers (5–19 years), switching to young adults (20–44 years) as the epidemic progressed in time. Similar observations were made during a period of influenza B activity in 1976–77 (Glezen *et al.* 1980a), suggesting that children and teenagers may initiate community outbreaks of influenza.

Fox *et al.* (1982a) studied how influenza was introduced into individual households; these researchers calculated introduction rates to express the relative importance of different age groups in introducing infection into households. During all seasons by far the highest introduction rates were produced by children and teenagers. Taber *et al.*

(1981) demonstrated that individuals from families with school-age children were twice as likely as other people to become infected. Whilst these findings are not without exception (Hope-Simpson 1970), little doubt remains that children and teenagers suffer the highest influenza attack rates and are therefore of great importance for the transmission of influenza within communities.

Household attack rates

Besides population attack rates, household attack rates (proportion of households affected) are also relevant to the epidemiology of community-based influenza epidemics. During influenza A/H3N2 epidemics in Seattle in 1975–76 and 1977–78 household attack rates of 41 and 53% were reported, as defined by virus isolation or serology, with or without symptoms. The influenza A/H1N1 season in 1978–79 produced a household attack rate of 73%, and in 1975–76 influenza B affected 38% of households (Fox *et al.* 1982b).

Secondary attack rates within households

In Seattle, after the introduction of infection into individual households, secondary attack rates among family members averaged 28% for A/H2N2 infections, 24% for A/H3N2 infections and 32% for influenza B (Hall *et al.* 1973). Later, the importance of misclassification bias in determining secondary infections was recognized; after allowing for

Table 17.1 Age-specific influenza type A attack rates estimated from community studies in Seattle (1975–79), Houston (1976–84) and Tecumseh (1966–71) USA. (Adapted with permission from Monto and Kioumehr 1975; Glezen *et al.* 1996.)

Tecumseh		Seattle		Houston	
Age group (years)	Attack rate (%)	Age group (years)	Attack rate (%)	Age group (years)	Attack rate(%)
< 1	23.5	< 5	25	< 2	35.5
1–2	18.3			2–5	44.5
3–4	15.3			6–10	47.7
5–9	16.8	5–9	33		
10–14	21.1			11–17	40.3
15–19	17.1	10–19	39	18–24	23
20–29	16.1				
30–39	17.5			25–34	21.5
40+	12.2	≥ 20	12	≥ 35	21
Overall	16.7	Overall	24	Overall	32.8

concurrent community acquired infections and third- and fourth-generation infections adjusted secondary attack rates were estimated at 31% for influenza A/H1N1 in 1978–79 (Seattle), 21% (Seattle) to 15% (Michigan) for A/H3N2 in 1977–78, and 13% for influenza B in 1975-76 (Longini *et al.* 1982). In Port Chalmers, New Zealand during an A/H3N2 epidemic in 1973 the secondary attack rate was estimated at 58% (Jennings & Miles 1978), contrasting sharply with secondary attack rates of 17 and 14% in Cirencester, UK during A/H3N2 epidemics in 1968–69 and 1969–70, respectively (Hope-Simpson 1979). Furthermore a 5-year study of influenza in British families between 1973 and 1978 demonstrated very little evidence of transmission within households; although secondary attack rates were not formally calculated, 199 infections in 44 households produced secondary infections in only 12 homes (Mann *et al.* 1981). Other studies reveal secondary attack rates of 20–30% although considerable variation is possible (Jordan *et al.* 1958a, 1958b; Philip *et al.* 1961; Foy *et al.* 1976). Secondary attack rates are higher among children than in adults (Chin *et al.* 1963; Davis *et al.* 1970; Longini *et al.* 1982); they are also related to household size (Davis *et al.* 1970; Retailliau *et al.* 1979; Taber *et al.* 1981; Hirota *et al.* 1992) and to the number of susceptible individuals in each household rather than the total number of occupants (Longini *et al.* 1982).

Reinfections

Reinfections with both influenza A subtypes and influenza B are described, and individuals may be infected with two subtypes of influenza A virus in the same season (Frank *et al.* 1983b). In Seattle between 1965 and 1979 annual reinfection rates were highest among young children for both influenza B (5%) and influenza A/H3N2 (4.7%) (Fox *et al.* 1982b), and reinfection with influenza B appeared to be more common than with influenza A (Hall *et al.* 1973). In Houston, influenza B reinfection during 1976–84 averaged 25% among children but only 2% among adults (Frank *et al.* 1987). Frank *et al.* (1979) studied 57 young children and their families during two influenza A/H3N2 epidemics in the period 1976–78. Over the study period the reinfection rates

were 58% in these young children, 26% in their older siblings, but only 6% among parents.

Influenza in 'closed' populations

Influenza outbreaks in institutions and other 'closed' populations have also been extensively studied. Famous among these observations is the harrowing account of pandemic influenza on board the troopship USS Leviathan which set sail from the USA on 29 September 1918 for northern France. The vessel contained 2000 crew and 10 000 soldiers in cramped conditions; within 24 h 700 troops were reported to be sick, rising to 2000 by the end of the voyage. With no proper medical facilities available 76 soldiers and three crewmen died at sea, and a further 31 soldiers died on 7 October as the ship docked in Brest (Crosby 1989). Reports such as these were widespread among the military units of all nations fighting in Europe towards the end of the Great War. The explosive onset and rapidity of spread of influenza in other close confines have also been noted on board airliners, in nursing homes and on college campuses (Moser *et al.* 1979; Pons *et al.* 1980; Goodman *et al.* 1982; Sobal & Loveland 1982) with epidemic periods typically of brief duration (Penny 1978; Moser *et al.* 1979; Mitchell *et al.* 1991).

In troopships, military bases and remote island communities, attack rates of 30 to 87% have been described (Philip *et al.* 1959; Jordan 1961; Clark *et al.* 1970). These are comparable to attack rates of 20–90% seen in boarding schools (Davies *et al.* 1982, 1984; Stuart-Harris *et al.* 1985). Review of 41 outbreaks in nursing homes revealed an estimated average attack rate of 43% (Patriarca *et al.* 1987), and attack rates up to 60% have been reported (Arden *et al.* 1986). Surveillance of 45 nursing homes in Michigan, USA revealed that 38% of institutions reported an influenza outbreak during the 1989–90 winter season (Arden *et al.* 1995). The likelihood of an influenza outbreak within nursing homes is inversely related to the influenza vaccination rate among residents (Arden *et al.* 1993), and together with other findings suggests that the rate of progress of influenza epidemics in closed communities is affected by levels of herd immunity (Salk & Salk

1977; Patriarca *et al.* 1986; Gross *et al.* 1988). Risk factors for outbreaks of influenza in nursing homes include the number of residents and part-time carers who are also employed in other homes and hospitals (Patriarca *et al.* 1986; Arden *et al.* 1993, 1995; Mukerjee 1994). During epidemics, elderly residential institutions appear to pose significantly increased risks for both influenza death and acute respiratory hospitalization, even after adjusting for age and chronic illnesses (Nguyen-Van-Tam & Nicholson 1992; Ahmed *et al.* 1995, 1997).

Epidemiological differences between influenza types A and B

The epidemiological characteristics of influenza A and B appear similar; both may cause excess mortality and morbidity (Barker & Mullooly 1980; Nolan *et al.* 1980) although influenza B does not produce pandemic influenza because of its inherent antigenic stability. Household and community transmission were comprehensively examined by Longini *et al.* (1982) using data from Michigan and Seattle (Monto & Kioumehr 1975; Fox & Hall 1980). In terms of ease of spread within individual households and the community at large influenza A/H1N1 was estimated to be most readily transmissible, followed by A/H3N2 strains, then influenza B. Community-wide epidemics of influenza B produce overall attack rates which are generally lower than for influenza A; in contrast outbreaks of influenza B in closed populations have tended to produce higher adult attack rates (up to 80%) which are comparable with those produced by influenza A (Clark *et al.* 1970; Hall *et al.* 1981; Arden *et al.* 1986). Influenza B also produces attack rates which are notably higher among children compared with adults (Monto & Kioumehr 1975; Retailliau *et al.* 1979; LaMontagne 1980; Wright *et al.* 1980; Fox *et al.* 1982a,b).

Nosocomial infection

Hospitals are complex and dynamic micro-environments in which staff or patients may contract influenza from a variety of possible sources including the community, newly admitted patients with community-acquired infection, other patients with established nosocomial influenza, staff, and visitors (Hoffman & Dixon 1977); these must be carefully disentangled in order to identify the true burden of nosocomial disease. Moreover studies which concentrate on patients and staff with respiratory symptoms may considerably underestimate the true extent of influenza in hospitals, especially among staff.

Weightman *et al.* (1974) showed that influenza A transmission was three to four times more frequent than RSV on both open wards and those with mainly cubicles. Both influenza types A and B have been implicated in nosocomial outbreaks among children (Brocklebank *et al.* 1972; Bauer *et al.* 1973; Gardner *et al.* 1973; Hall & Douglas 1975; Meibalane *et al.* 1977; Hall 1981), adults with underlying chronic illness (Blumenfeld *et al.* 1959; Kapila *et al.* 1977; Weingarten *et al.* 1988; Serwint *et al.* 1991), and elderly people (Van Voris *et al.* 1982). The reported incidence of hospital-acquired influenza is highly variable. In the 1986–87 season, a prospective surveillance programme in an acute care hospital in Los Angeles, USA detected 43 cases of influenza of which 17 (40%) were among hospital employees; two patients acquired infection nosocomially, giving a rate of 0.3 cases per 100 admissions, and representing 17% of all influenza isolates among inpatients (Weingarten *et al.* 1988). Pachucki *et al.* (1989) observed an attack rate of about 2.5% among patients of a veterans' hospital in Illinois, USA; but in contrast Van Voris *et al.* (1982) noted an attack rate of 20% confined to one hospital ward; O'Donoghue *et al.* (1973) described an attack rate of about 20% among unprotected patients during a trial of amantadine, whilst Yassi *et al.* (1993) described a localized outbreak involving 37% of health-care workers and 47% of patients.

Few studies have focused on nosocomial influenza among hospital workers and even fewer have convincingly demonstrated its occurrence. However, Yassi *et al.* (1991) observed a 35% increase in sickness absence among 'high-risk' hospital workers during an influenza epidemic in 1987–88, but no increase in a comparison non-epidemic season. Elder *et al.* (1996) studied 518 health-care workers at four acute care hospitals in Glasgow, UK during the

1993–94 influenza A epidemic. Only 30% of workers reporting symptoms of influenza showed evidence of seroconversion, indicating that self misdiagnosis was high; furthermore, 59% of seropositive workers could not recall an influenza-like illness, and 28% could not recall any respiratory illness during the season, indicating high levels of subclinical infection. Of possibly greater concern was the fact that 52% of seropositive workers had not taken sick leave for respiratory infections suggesting that there were many opportunities for cross-infecting patients and other staff. An overall serological attack rate of 23% was substantially higher than the community attack rate of 0.15–2.0% estimated from other studies. Whilst it seems reasonable to suppose that transmission of influenza from staff to patients is highly likely, direct evidence in support of this assertion is scanty (Fralick 1985). However, influenza vaccination of health-care workers in long-stay hospitals has recently been shown to reduce mortality among residents, suggesting that such a causal link does exist (Potter *et al.* 1997).

Host factors

Preseason immunity

Infection and illness rates are both inversely related to the presence of circulating HI antibody. In Seattle between 1975 and 1979 infection and reinfection rates (whether serologically proven or virus-positive) were consistently higher among individuals with low HI antibody titres before infection (Fox *et al.* 1982a, 1982b). Overall 70–80% of infections produced symptomatic illnesses; furthermore, illness rates and illness severity were both highest among individuals with low titres of HI antibody prior to infection (Foy *et al.* 1976; Fox *et al.* 1982a). Similarly in Michigan during the 1977–78 A/H3N2 season infection rates were estimated to be about 20% among individuals with the lowest preseason HI antibody titres, decreasing to about 7% among those with highest titres (Longini *et al.* 1982). Similar observations were made in Houston during the influenza A/H3N2 epidemic in 1976–77 and epidemics influenza B in

1976–77 and 1979–80 (Taber *et al.* 1981; Frank *et al.* 1983a).

Chronic illnesses

In his report William Farr (1885) commented on the characteristics of people who died in London during the 1847 influenza epidemic: 'a disease much more deadly in the old than in middle-aged and young people... Influenza attacked those labouring under all sorts of diseases, as well as the healthy. The vital force was extinguished in old age and chronic diseases'. Dr Farr also described influenza as 'fatal to the asthmatic', and showed an excess of deaths among sufferers. Impressively, these basic observations have remained unchallenged for 150 years and old age and chronic illnesses still form the basis of determining the principle risk factors for influenza morbidity and mortality.

There is now widespread agreement about the existence and identity of high-risk patient groups, defined on the basis of those chronic illnesses which are associated with increased likelihood of death or hospitalization during influenza epidemics or pandemics—as illustrated in Fig. 17.3. These include patients with chronic pulmonary diseases including asthma, bronchitis, emphysema and tuberculosis (Farr 1885; Collins 1932; Stocks 1934; Collins & Lehmann 1953; Martin *et al.* 1959; Petersdorf *et al.* 1959; Eickhoff *et al.* 1961; Housworth & Langmuir 1974; Barker & Mullooly 1982b; Blackwelder *et al.* 1982; Glezen *et al.* 1987; Sprenger *et al.* 1989; Ashley *et al.* 1991b; Nguyen-Van-Tam & Nicholson 1992; McBean *et al.* 1993; Strikas *et al.* 1993; Ahmed *et al.* 1995, 1997); rheumatic and ischaemic heart disease (Collins 1932; Stocks 1934; Collins & Lehmann 1953; Martin *et al.* 1959; Petersdorf *et al.* 1959; Eickhoff *et al.* 1961; Housworth & Langmuir 1974; Barker & Mullooly 1982b; Glezen *et al.* 1987; Sprenger *et al.* 1989; Ashley *et al.* 1991b; Nguyen-Van-Tam & Nicholson 1992; McBean *et al.* 1993; Monto *et al.* 1993; Strikas *et al.* 1993; Ahmed *et al.* 1995); diabetes mellitus (Collins 1932; Stocks 1934; Collins & Lehmann 1953; Martin *et al.* 1959; Petersdorf *et al.* 1959; Eickhoff *et al.* 1961; Watkins *et al.* 1970; Housworth & Langmuir 1974;

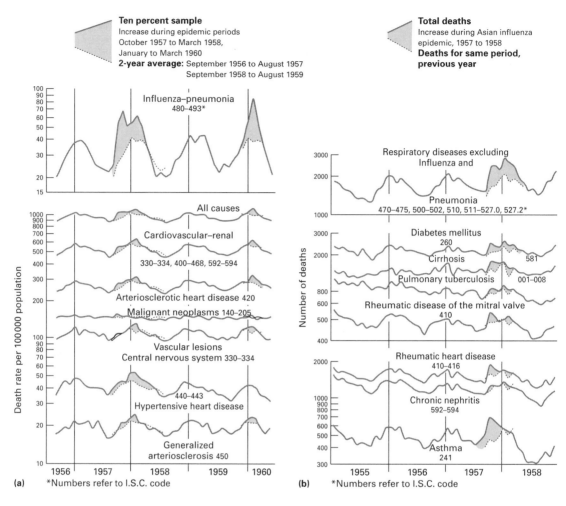

Fig. 17.3 Death rates per month from specified diseases 1956–60 (a) and total deaths per month for specified diseases 1955–58 (b), showing increases during the Asian influenza epidemic 1957–58. (Redrawn from Eickhoff *et al.* 1961.)

Barker & Mullooly 1982b; Diepersloot *et al.* 1990; McBean *et al.* 1993); renal disease including chronic nephritis (Collins 1932; Stocks 1934; Collins & Lehmann 1953; Eickhoff *et al.* 1961; Barker & Mullooly 1982b; Monto *et al.* 1993); neurological diseases including cerebrovascular accident, Parkinson's disease and multiple sclerosis (Collins 1932; Stocks 1934; Collins & Lehmann 1953; Petersdorf *et al.* 1959; Eickhoff *et al.* 1961; Sprenger *et al.* 1989; Nguyen-Van-Tam & Nicholson 1992;

McBean *et al.* 1993; Ahmed *et al.* 1995); cirrhosis (Martin *et al.* 1959; Petersdorf *et al.* 1959; Eickhoff *et al.* 1961); malignancy (Eickhoff *et al.* 1961; Housworth & Langmuir 1974; Barker & Mullooly 1982b; McBean *et al.* 1993); anaemia (Monto *et al.* 1993); and pregnancy (Collins 1932; Collins & Lehmann 1953; Greenberg *et al.* 1958; Martin *et al.* 1959; Petersdorf *et al.* 1959; Hardy *et al.* 1961; Mullooly *et al.* 1986; Ashley *et al.* 1991b). Data from studies of influenza deaths in Britain and the USA show that influenza-related mortality increases with an increasing number of chronic illnesses suffered. Barker and Mullooly (1982b) examined the medical records of individuals whose deaths during two epidemics were ascribed to either pneumonia or influenza; it was discovered that 95% had suffered with one or more chronic diseases at the time of death. Similarly during the influenza A/H3N2 epidemic in Leicestershire, UK Nguyen-Van-Tam and Nicholson (1992) showed that 93% of those with influenza as the certified cause of death also had one or more chronic illnesses.

Age

Although influenza attack rates are known to be highest among children and teenagers, mortality is greatest among the elderly population (Dauer & Serfling 1961; Alling *et al.* 1981; Barker & Mullooly 1982b; Glezen *et al.* 1982b, 1987; Tillett *et al.* 1983; Lui & Kendal 1987; Ashley *et al.* 1991b; Nguyen-Van-Tam & Nicholson 1992; Simonsen *et al.* 1996). It is questionable, however, whether age is an independent risk factor since the majority of deaths occur in those with chronic medical conditions. The situation is even less clearly defined with respect to hospital admissions where conflicting data exist. Perrotta *et al.* (1985) showed that during influenza epidemics elderly people accounted for about 23% of all emergency respiratory admissions; whilst a substantial proportion, this figure nonetheless suggests that old age is not as important a risk factor for hospital admission during influenza epidemics as it may be for death, and that influenza morbidity is more evenly distributed than mortality across age groups. In contrast, other researchers have shown the rate of excess hospitalization for pneumonia and influenza during epidemics to be strongly associated with both increasing age and the presence of underlying high-risk diseases (Barker & Mullooly 1980; Barker 1986).

Cigarette smoking

Cigarette smoking has also been identified as a risk factor for influenza. A study of Israeli military personnel revealed that smokers suffered higher attack rates of influenza A/H1N1 during an epidemic compared with non-smokers in the same unit (68 versus 47%); moreover, illness severity and sickness absence due to influenza are both increased among smokers (Finklea *et al.* 1969; Waldman *et al.* 1969; MacKenzie *et al.* 1976; Kark &

Lebiush 1981; Kark *et al.* 1982; Monto *et al.* 1993; Strikas *et al.* 1993).

Seasonality and herald waves

The conventional understanding of influenza as a disease which is spread person to person by virus-laden respiratory secretions, and whose survival depends upon serial transmission between infected hosts and non-immune contacts, fails to explain fully a number of unique epidemiological behaviours attributed to the virus since its discovery in 1933. These distinguishing features were described by Hope-Simpson (1979); some of these are shown in Table 17.2.

Seasonality

In the temperate zones of both Northern and Southern Hemispheres influenza tends to be seasonal, occurring during the coldest months of the year (Hope-Simpson 1981; Thacker 1986; Kilbourne 1987). In tropical zones evidence of seasonality is more difficult to elicit although activity is more likely during monsoon and wet seasons (Hope-Simpson 1979, 1981; Kilbourne 1987). Even to this day the precise reasons for seasonal variation remain unknown. Several environmental factors are thought to favour the seasonal transmission of influenza. Indoor crowding (including school attendance) under conditions of reduced ventila-

Table 17.2 Some important epidemiological features of type A influenza. (Adapted with permission from Hope-Simpson, R.E. Epidemic mechanisms of type A influenza, 1979, *Journal of Hygiene*, Cambridge, Cambridge University Press.)

- Antigenic drift
- Antigenic shift
- Seasonal occurrence
- Worldwide conformity in appearance of new strains/sub-types and disappearance of old ones
- Low transmission rates out-of-season
- Explosive onset of epidemics
- Rapid termination of epidemics despite continued abundance of susceptible persons
- Worldwide distribution throughout recorded history, at all inhabited latitudes and longitudes, in all climates

tion is most likely to occur in winter and during tropical wet seasons and monsoons and has been proposed to explain the seasonality of influenza outbreaks (Jordan 1961; Fine & Clarkson 1982; Thacker 1986). It has also been noted that influenza viruses survive more readily in aerosols under the conditions of low temperature and low humidity that are found in temperate zones during the winter months (Hemmes *et al.* 1960; Schaffer *et al.* 1976). There has been much speculation on the methods by which interhemispheric spread might occur (Andrewes 1942; Webster *et al.* 1980; Hope-Simpson 1981, 1983, 1986; Hammond *et al.* 1989). Suggested vehicles include migratory birds and the transport of aerosolized virus within the upper atmosphere. However, descriptions of seasonality belie the fact that in many communities influenza viruses have been isolated throughout the year (Jordan *et al.* 1958b; Philip *et al.* 1961; Hall *et al.* 1973; Dowdle *et al.* 1974; Monto & Kioumehr 1975; Pereira & Chakraverty 1977; Fox *et al.* 1982b), although in the Northern Hemisphere summertime outbreaks of influenza, resulting in appreciable morbidity and mortality, are hardly ever reported (Dowdle *et al.* 1974; Kohn *et al.* 1995). Interestingly influenza A/H2N2 (Asian) in 1957 and A/H3N2 (Hong Kong) in 1968 failed to produce epidemic activity in the USA during the summer months, despite widespread population susceptibility, but caused greater morbidity and mortality several months later (Trotter *et al.* 1959; Langmuir 1961; Cockburn *et al.* 1969; Sharrar 1969). In Britain the appearance of influenza A/H3N2 in winter 1968–69 failed to produce a severe epidemic in spite of the novelty of the virus; yet in winter 1969–70 the same virus caused widespread disruption (Hope-Simpson 1979; Tillett *et al.* 1983).

Herald waves

During 3 successive years (1976–79), the community surveillance system of the Houston Influenza Research Center identified a 'wave' of influenza virus activity, which occurred during the latter part of one season and heralded the epidemic virus for the next season (Glezen *et al.* 1980a, 1982a). These isolations provide the benefit of obtaining infor-

mation on the virus most likely to cause outbreaks during the next season. However, the influenza B herald viruses identified in spring 1976 in Houston, represented only 3% of all influenza isolates and 1% of persons consulting a doctor with respiratory illness. In subsequent herald waves the percentage of novel isolates varied between 0.4 and 2.0%, suggesting that herald waves are difficult to identify without continuous, large-scale virological surveillance (Glezen *et al.* 1982a). Glezen *et al.* (1980a, 1982a) and Fox *et al.* (1982b) were unable to isolate herald viruses in the period between the herald waves and their apparent re-emergence some 6–9 months later.

It is plausible that herald viruses are maintained within the population at very low levels until the next respiratory season when environmental factors favour more widespread transmission. An alternative theory is that herald viruses migrate to the Southern Hemisphere during spring and summer, before reverse migration and reintroduction the next winter. This theory is supported by evidence showing that the A/H1N1 viruses identified in Houston, USA during the winter season of 1978–79 contained recombinant genetic material from viruses which were not active in Houston previously (Glezen *et al.* 1982a). Data from the Public Health Laboratory Service in Britain support this theory. During the winter of 1971–72 an isolate of influenza A/England/42/72 was detected which differed antigenically from the widely prevalent A/Hong Kong/68 virus; in retrospect it could be argued that with more intensive community surveillance this might have been recognized as a herald wave. The new strain was then isolated frequently during outbreaks in the Southern Hemisphere during the summer of 1972, before viruses identical to A/England/42/72 re-emerged in Britain from November onwards (Pereira & Chakraverty 1977). Herald waves do not appear to be a consistent annual phenomenon. Monto *et al.* (1985) failed to identify a herald wave prior to two type B influenza outbreaks, two due to A/H3N2 viruses, and three due to A/H1N1 in Michigan, USA between 1976/77 and 1980/81. Community virological surveillance was less intense than in Houston but was probably sufficient to detect herald waves had they existed.

With the development of more rapid methods of vaccine production the practical value of the herald wave phenomenon could be immense.

Pandemic influenza

Pandemics, defined as worldwide epidemics of influenza with high morbidity and mortality, have resulted from antigenic shift—the incorporation of a novel haemagglutinin (with or without a change in neuraminidase) against which there is no existing population immunity (Kilbourne 1973). Precise data on the epidemiology of influenza A in general, and antigenic shifts in particular, only became available after discovery of the virus in 1933 (Smith *et al.* 1933), and seroarchaeological studies provide additional but less certain data from the mid-19th century onwards. On the basis of these data only three haemagglutinins (H1 to H3) and neuraminidases (N1, N2, N8) have been implicated in extensive human outbreaks.

Pandemics and the process of antigenic shift are both unpredictable and infrequent. There have been at least three such events this century, in 1918 (swine-like virus: A/H$_{SW}$1N1, later reclassified A/H1N1), 1957 (Asian influenza: A/H2N2) and 1968 (Hong Kong influenza: A/H3N2). Extensive mutation from previously circulating H1 strains occurred in 1946–47 resulting in worldwide spread of a novel ('A-prime') influenza A/FM/1/47 (H1N1) virus, yet with remarkably low mortality (Sartwell & Long 1948); it is still debated whether this was a true pandemic. In 1976 a novel A/H$_{SW}$1N1 swine virus caused human influenza at Fort Dix, New Jersey, USA but a widely anticipated pandemic did not follow (Goldfield *et al.* 1977; Top & Russell 1977). The following year influenza A/H1N1 of a type nearly identical to virus strains circulating from 1947 to 1957 re-emerged. Although it spread rapidly around the globe it did not cause significant mortality and set a precedent by continuing to circulate with A/H3N2 viruses without establishing dominance (Gregg *et al.* 1978; Nakajima *et al.* 1978). The reasons why A/USSR/90/77 (H1N1) and its subsequent antigenic variants failed to displace the predominant A/H3N2 strains, but instead began cocirculation are unknown. This may

have happened once before in ~1908–18 but the evidence from that era is less certain (Masurel & Heijtink 1983). One theory is that until 1977 the world population was not large enough to support more than one subtype in continuous transmission (Fine 1982).

The reasons for the decline of dominant viral subtypes and the emergence of new pandemic strains remain speculative. The emergence of new pandemic strains in 1957 and 1968 were both associated with the rapid disappearance of the previous subtype. This disappearance is possibly apparent rather than real, since Napiorkowski and Black (1974) showed evidence of influenza A/H2N2 infections in Amazonian tribesmen 2 years after the disappearance of this subtype elsewhere and its replacement with A/H3N2. Certainly disappearance does not equate with extinction as old 'human' influenza viruses have been identified in animals (Webster *et al.* 1980), and have the potential to re-emerge as in 1977 (A/H1N1) (Kilbourne 1987). Kilbourne (1987) proposed a model whereby population immunity to an existing influenza subtype broadens during a sustained period of dominance (interpandemic period); a point is then reached when the virus loses its capacity for further antigenic mutation capable of eluding host defences, and virus survival is threatened. At this point the necessary conditions are in place to allow for the entry or re-emergence of a different (pandemic) subtype. The logical successor is a virus with human pathogenic potential and an antigenic composition of sufficient novelty to render current protective antibodies ineffective (Fig. 17.4). The model is supported by antibody studies in schoolchildren and families showing increasing levels of herd immunity over time (Hayslett *et al.* 1962; Jennings & Miles 1978; Davies *et al.* 1982, 1984). However, other data from Sheffield, UK show population HI antibodies against influenza A/Victoria/75 between 1975 and 1981, and A/Texas/77 between 1978 and 1980 were acquired rapidly but waned over several years (Stuart-Harris *et al.* 1985). Furthermore, the persistence of both influenza B and C in humans is not adequately explained by this model as neither have produced new subtypes.

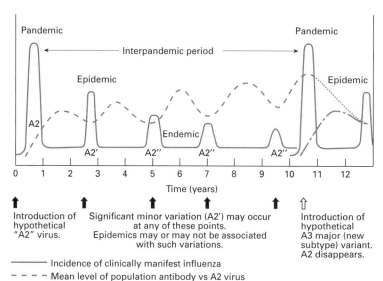

Fig. 17.4 Schematic diagram showing the effects of major (pandemic) and minor (interpandemic) influenza virus antigenic variation (global trends). (Redrawn with permission from Kilbourne 1975.)

Pandemic patterns of mortality and morbidity

Between 1890 and 1917 deaths from certified influenza among girls (0–15 years) and young women (15–35) in England represented 7–11% of all female influenza deaths. However, during the 1918–19 pandemic these percentages suddenly increased to 25% for girls and 45% for young women; in contrast, the proportion of total deaths occurring in older women aged 55 years and over decreased in reciprocal fashion from 60–70 to 12% (HMSO 1920); the same phenomenon was also observed in the USA (Stuart-Harris *et al.* 1985; Crosby 1989) The near complete reversal of patterns of influenza mortality by age during the 1918–19 pandemic is still without precedent. The changes in age-specific death rate among females in England and Wales between the first and fourth quarters of 1918 are illustrated in Fig. 17.5.

The emergence of subsequent pandemic influenza subtypes in 1946–47 (H1N1), 1957 (H2N2) and 1968 (H3N2) have also been associated with transient shifts in the age distribution of mortality towards the young, compared with immediately preceding seasons. In relative terms excess deaths increased most among young adults, even though the majority of excess deaths still occurred among elderly people (Dauer & Serfling 1961; Alling *et al.*

1981; Simonsen *et al.* 1996). These increases have become progressively smaller and smaller with each new pandemic. This may partly be due to the development of effective antibiotics for the treatment of bacterial pneumonias which may complicate influenza infection (Dowdle *et al.* 1974; Simonsen *et al.* 1996). However, the occurrence of antigenic recycling, which can provide a degree of residual cross-protection against antigenically similar viruses among older subgroups of the population may well be of crucial importance. Sera from individuals born as long ago as 1857, but

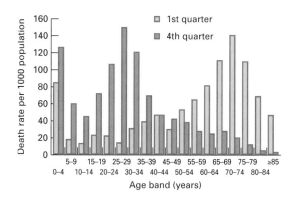

Fig. 17.5 Age-specific influenza death rates among females in England and Wales during first and fourth quarters of 1918. (From HMSO 1920.)

collected from 1957 onwards, prior to the emergence of new pandemic strains, reveal compelling evidence of previous eras of circulation of influenza A/H3N8 (~1900–18), A/H2N2 (~1889–1901) and A/H1N1 (~1908 onwards) (Masurel & Marine 1973; Davenport 1977; Rekart *et al.* 1982; Masurel & Heijtink 1983). During 1977–78, 97% of influenza A/H1N1 isolates in the USA were recovered from individuals less than 26 years of age supporting the fact that partial immunity from a previous era had persisted among older people (Kendal *et al.* 1979). Similarly at the beginning of the A/Hong Kong/68 (H3N2) pandemic the attack rate among individuals born before 1890 was about one-third of the rate among people born after 1899, suggesting prior exposure to H3N2 antigens among the very elderly population (Schoenbaum *et al.* 1976). Collectively these unique data suggest that antigens present during the latter part of the 20th century were recycled.

An important and interesting feature of pandemic influenza is the apparent existence of several epidemic waves with differing patterns of morbidity and mortality. The initial wave of 'swine influenza' in spring 1918 produced substantial attack rates but mortality was not unusually raised. A second wave of influenza began in August 1918. Reports of devastating mortality emerged almost simultaneously in Freetown, Sierra Leone, in Brest, north-west France, and Boston, Massachusetts (Crosby 1989). Historical records suggest that large-scale mobilization and troop movements, often in overcrowded conditions, contributed to the rapid spread of influenza which seemed to focus early on the military population. However, it should be remembered that in 1918 the availability of written records in the military was probably far greater than in the surrounding civilian community, and most other parts of the world, leading to reporting bias. The most detailed historical records of these events can be found in American naval logs because large numbers of soldiers were still crossing the Atlantic Ocean bound for service in France. Mortality from influenza in the American navy peaked during the first week in October (651 deaths) and in the American army 1 week later (6170 deaths) (Crosby 1989). Among the American

civilian population the second wave began in mid–late September along the eastern seaboard, spreading westwards to affect all states by the first week in October, at the same time as western Europe was affected (HMSO 1920; Crosby 1989). A third wave of influenza was recorded worldwide in February–March 1919. In terms of mortality this was less devastating than the second wave, but nonetheless considerable excess mortality was recorded (HMSO 1920). Differences in the level of mortality between the first and second waves suggest that the pandemic virus underwent a process of adaptation to its human host. The evidence for secondary and tertiary waves in subsequent pandemic periods is less clear-cut. However, in 1957 Japan experienced a wave of Asian influenza between June and July as the disease spread outwards from China; it then disappeared in August before a second wave occurred in September–October (Dunn 1958). Similar recrudescences were observed in Britain and the USA in January–February 1958 (McDonald 1958; Langmuir 1961).

Collins and Lehmann (1953) demonstrated a decline in annual excess death rates during influenza epidemics from 1918 to 1951; similarly Fleming *et al.* (1990) demonstrated a decline in mean weekly consultation rates during winter seasons between 1969/70 and 1989/90. Whilst neither of these trends is absolutely consistent, they nonetheless suggest that morbidity and mortality both decrease with increasing interval from the emergence of a pandemic virus. This phenomenon could be partially explained by gradually increasing levels of population immunity, although changes in viral virulence may also be important.

Global spread of pandemic influenza

The origin of the 1918 influenza pandemic (A/H1N1) is not known but outbreaks were reported in American military establishments, at the Ford Motor Company in Detroit and in San Quentin prison, California in March 1918. The first reports in Europe came shortly afterwards in April from French Atlantic ports where elements of the US Expeditionary Force were off-loading from troopships (Collier 1974; Crosby 1989). In the months that followed all of the armies fighting in Europe witnessed the rapid spread of influenza through their ranks. Outbreaks were known by various names such as '3-day fever', 'Blitzkattarh' and 'Flanders fever' (Crosby 1989). These reports strongly suggest that the 1918 pandemic originated in north America, and are consistent with what is known about the occurrence of swine influenza in the American Midwest and its close similarity to the human pandemic strain (Andrewes *et al.* 1935; Francis & Shope 1936). However, Vaughan (1921) reported epidemic influenza in mainland China at about the same time, and the possibility that it was introduced into the USA by labourers migrating from China cannot be discounted.

Evidence for a single point of origin of the Asian influenza pandemic in 1957 (A/H2N2) is clearer. This began in late February in Kweichow province, China, before spreading rapidly to the remainder of South-East Asia and Australia by June; thereafter it spread to the Middle-East, most of Africa, parts of southern Europe, Oceania and South America in July–September. Finally northern Europe (including the USSR) and north America were affected and it is estimated that by December 1957 every continent including Antarctica had experienced the pandemic (Dunn 1958). Morbidity and mortality were universally severe. Langmuir described the spread of Asian influenza in the USA in greater detail where it was apparent that the virus had seeded in the population from May–June 1957 onwards, causing localized outbreaks. There is some evidence that introduction occurred separately on both eastern and western seaboards, possibly reflecting simultaneous spread from both Europe and Oceania (Langmuir 1961).

Similarly, a great deal is known about the global spread of pandemic influenza in 1968 (A/H3N2). This also began in China, in July, spreading rapidly to Hong Kong where formal identification took place (Chang 1969). As in 1957, further spread occurred rapidly throughout most of South-East Asia; however, in Japan some delay was apparent between the introduction of infection in August and the onset of widespread activity in January 1969 (Cockburn *et al.* 1969). In Britain and most of Europe a slow indolent period of activity occurred between January and April 1969 without substantial excess mortality; the latter occurred 1 year later in the 1969–70 season (Cockburn *et al.* 1969; Assad *et al.* 1973; Hope-Simpson 1979; Tillett *et al.* 1983). In contrast, the Hong Kong virus was introduced to the USA in September 1968 via American marines returning from Vietnam; the first community outbreaks occurred in early October and by the end of 1968 influenza was epidemic across all American states. Unlike in Europe morbidity and mortality were considerable (Sharrar 1969). More recently it has been possible to combine surveillance data from sentinel practices with epidemiological mapping techniques to demonstrate with greater precision patterns of spread of influenza within land masses (Carrat & Valleron 1992).

Infection of humans with animal strains of influenza

Animal influenza viruses are of immense potential epidemiological importance for human disease. A wide range of haemagglutinin–neuraminidase combinations occur in influenza viruses which infect lower animals but the extent to which these hold potential for human disease is not fully known. Both avian and porcine influenzas have produced symptomatic disease in humans by direct transmission (Kurtz *et al.* 1996; Wentworth *et al.* 1997). Furthermore, a population-based serological study in central China revealed evidence for infection of farmers with avian H7 influenza viruses, suggesting that direct transmission from ducks to humans may occur (Zhou *et al.* 1996). Most instances of human infection with animal influenza appear sporadic, without resulting in further transmission between humans. However, in 1976 at Fort Dix, USA limited transmission of a swine influenza virus ($H_{SW}1N1$) occurred within a closed military camp, but widely predicted spread into the general population did not follow (Top & Russell 1977).

The haemagglutinins and neuraminidases associated with human influenza infection also cause disease in lower animals, giving rise to the suggestion that interspecies transmission occurs through a process of genetic reassortment, first postulated by Hirst (1962). Isolates of human and swine influenzas (A/H1N1) in the 1930s showed considerable antigenic similarity (Andrewes *et al.* 1935; Francis & Shope 1936), suggesting that the 1918 pandemic virus may have resulted from a swine influenza virus. Genes from human H2N2 and H3N2 viruses have also been identified in avian, equine and porcine influenzas (Tumova & Easterday 1969; Kundin 1970; Kendal *et al.* 1973; Fang *et al.* 1981; Kendal 1987; Kawaoka *et al.* 1989), illustrating the potential for interspecies transfer of genetic material. Phylogenetic studies have confirmed the existence of human–avian reassortant viruses in pigs in Italy (Castrucci *et al.* 1993), and symptomatic children in The Netherlands (Claas *et al.* 1994); these studies illustrate the pathogenic potential of human–animal reassortant viruses and suggest that pigs play a pivotal role in interspecies transmission (Kawaoka *et al.* 1993; Scholtissek *et al.* 1993; Webster *et al.* 1995). One of the most popular theories advanced to explain the mechanism of genetic reassortment between human and animal influenza viruses relates to social and agricultural practices in China (and South-East Asia). Many researchers have identified this part of the world as the site of emergence of most recent pandemic viruses and many other smaller virus mutations (antigenic drift) (Chang 1969; Cockburn *et al.* 1969; Shortridge & Stuart-Harris 1982). It has been suggested that the presence of large numbers of peasant farmers in the region living in close proximity to both ducks and pigs creates opportunities for genetic reassortment between human and avian influenza viruses, and that pigs, being susceptible to both human and avian influenzas, provide a biological medium—a 'mixing bowl'—for this interchange (Shortridge & Stuart-Harris 1982; Scholtissek & Naylor 1988; Scholtissek *et al.* 1993; Webster *et al.* 1995).

Interpandemic influenza

Although morbidity and mortality from influenza may decline during interpandemic periods, the cumulative effects of regular seasonal activity far exceed those observed during the first waves of pandemic influenza. Since 1977, both influenza A

H1N1 and H3N2 and influenza B have cocirculated. One type usually predominates in each season but concurrent outbreaks of an influenza A subtype and influenza B have been recorded, as have mixed outbreaks of two influenza A subtypes (Frank *et al.* 1983b; Spelman & McHardy 1985).

Just as it remains unclear why influenza shows seasonal activity, it is also unclear why, during epidemic periods, the upsurge in activity lasts only 5–6 weeks before declining sharply, even though many susceptible individuals remain in the population (Gregg 1980; Kendal 1987; Glezen 1996). Thacker (1986) suggests that since host populations are heterogeneous and do not mix at random it is possible that influenza could affect a sufficiently large number of individuals in one locality in a short space of time so as to cause its disappearance until a pool of susceptible individuals reforms. This hypothesis seems plausible considering many infections are subclinical (Jordan 1961; Davis *et al.* 1970; Monto & Kioumehr 1975; Foy *et al.* 1976; Taber *et al.* 1981; Fox *et al.* 1982a), and frequent antigenic drift helps maintain population susceptibility.

References

Ahmed, A.H., Nicholson, K.G. & Nguyen-Van-Tam, J.S. (1995) Reduction in mortality associated with influenza vaccine during 1989–90 epidemic. *Lancet* **346**, 591–5.

Ahmed, A.H., Nicholson, K.G., Nguyen-Van-Tam, J.S. & Pearson, J.C.G. (1997) Effectiveness of influenza vaccine in reducing hospital admissions during the 1989–90 epidemic. *Epidemiol Infect* **118**, 27–33.

Alling, D.W., Blackwelder, W.C. & Stuart-Harris, C.H. (1981) A study of excess mortality during influenza epidemics in the United States, 1968–76. *Am J Epidemiol* **113**, 30–8.

Andrewes, C.H. (1942) Thoughts on the origin of influenza epidemics. *Proc Roy Soc Med* **36**, 1–10.

Andrewes, C.H., Laidlaw, P.P. & Smith, W. (1935) Influenza: observations on the recovery of virus from man and on the antibody content of human sera. *Br J Exp Pathol* **16**, 566–81.

Anestad, G. (1982) Interference between outbreaks of respiratory syncytial virus and influenza virus infection. *Lancet* **i**, 502.

Anestad, G. (1987) Surveillance of respiratory viral infections by rapid immunofluorescence diagnosis, with emphasis on virus interference. *Epidemiol Infect* **99**, 523–31.

Arden, N., Bidol, S., Ohmit, S.E. & Monto, A.S. (1993) Effect of nursing home size and influenza vaccination rates on the risk of institutional outbreaks during an influenza A (H3N2) epidemic. In: Hannoun, C., Kendal, A.P., Klenk, H.D. & Ruben, F.L. (eds) *Options for the Control of Influenza II*, pp. 161–5. Elsevier, Amsterdam.

Arden, N., Monto, A.S. & Ohmit, S.E. (1995) Vaccine use and the risk of outbreaks in a sample of nursing homes during an influenza epidemic. *Am J Public Health* **85**, 399–401.

Arden, N.H., Patriarca, P.A. & Kendal, A.P. (1986) Experiences in the use and efficacy of inactivated influenza vaccine in nursing homes. In: Kendal, A.P. & Patriarca, P.A. (eds) *Options for the Control of Influenza*, pp. 155–68. Liss, New York.

Ashley, J.S.A., Cole, S.K. & Kilbane, M.P.J. (1991a) Health information resources: UK health and social factors. In: Holland, W.W., Detels, R. & Knox, G. (eds) *Oxford Textbook of Public Health, Vol. II. Methods of Public Health*, 2nd edn, pp. 29–53. Oxford Medical Publications, Oxford.

Ashley, J., Smith, T. & Dunnell, K. (1991b) Deaths in Great Britain associated with the influenza epidemic of 1989/90. *Population Trends* **65**, 16–20.

Assad, F., Cockburn, W.C. & Sundaresan, T.K. (1973) Use of excess mortality from respiratory diseases in the study of influenza. *Bull WHO* **49**, 219–33.

Barker, W.H. (1986) Excess pneumonia and influenza associated hospitalization during influenza epidemics in the United States, 1970–78. *Am J Public Health* **76**, 761–5.

Barker, W.H. & Mullooly, J.P. (1980) Impact of epidemic type A influenza in a defined adult population. *Am J Epidemiol* **112**, 798–811.

Barker, W.H. & Mullooly, J.P. (1981) Underestimation of the role of pneumonia and influenza in causing excess mortality. *Am J Public Health* **71**, 643–5.

Barker, W.H. & Mullooly, J.P. (1982a) A study of excess mortality during influenza epidemics in the United States, 1968–76. *Am J Epidemiol* **115**, 479–80.

Barker, W.H. & Mullooly, J.P. (1982b) Pneumonia and influenza deaths during epidemics: implications for prevention. *Arch Int Med* **142**, 85–9.

Bauer, C.R., Elie, K., Spence, L. & Stern, L. (1973) Hong Kong influenza in a neonatal unit. *J Am Med Assoc* **223**, 1233–5.

Birmingham Research Unit of the Royal College of General Practitioners (1977) Influenza (Collective Research in General Practice). *J Roy Coll Gen Pract* **27**, 544–51.

Blackwelder, W.C., Alling, D.W. & Stuart-Harris, C.H. (1982) Association of excess mortality from chronic nonspecific lung disease with epidemics of influenza. *Am Rev Resp Dis* **125**, 511–16.

Blumenfeld, H.I., Kilbourne, E.D., Louria, D.B. & Rogers, D.E. (1959) Studies on influenza in the pandemic of 1957–58: I. An epidemiologic, clinical and serologic investigation of an intrahospital epidemic, with a note on vaccination efficacy. *J Clin Invest* **38**, 199–212.

Brocklebank, J.T., Court, S.D.M., McQuillin, J. & Gardner, P.S. (1972) Influenza A infection in children. *Lancet* **ii**, 497–500.

Campbell, D.M., Paixao, M.T. & Reid, D. (1988) Influenza and the 'spotter' general practitioner. *J Roy Coll Gen Pract* **38**, 418–21.

Carrat, F. & Valleron, A. (1992) Epidemiologic mapping using the 'Kriging' method: application to an influenza-like illness epidemic in France. *Am J Epidemiol* **135**, 1293–300.

Castrucci, M.R., Donatelli, I., Sidoli, L., Barigazzi, G., Kawaoka, Y. & Webster, R.G. (1993) Genetic reassortant between avian and human influenza A viruses in Italian pigs. *Virology* **193**, 503–6.

Chakraverty, P., Cunningham, P., Shen, G.Z. & Pereira, M.S. (1986) Influenza in the UK 1982–85. *J Hygiene, Cambridge* **97**, 347–58.

Chang, W.K. (1969) National influenza experience in Hong Kong, 1968. *Bull WHO* **41**, 349–51.

Chin, D.Y., Mosley, W.H., Poland, J.D., Rush, D. & Johnson, O. (1963) Epidemiologic studies of type B influenza in 1961-62. *Am J Public Health* **53**, 1068–74.

Choi, K. & Thacker, S.B. (1981) An evaluation of influenza mortality surveillance, 1962–79. I. Time series forecasts of expected pneumonia and influenza deaths. *Am J Epidemiol* **113**, 215–26.

Claas, E.C.J., Kawaoka, Y., de Jong, J.C. & Webster, R.G. (1994) Infection of children with avian–human reassortant influenza virus from pigs in Europe. *Virology* **204**, 453–7.

Clark, P.S., Feltz, E.T., List-Young, B., Ritter, D.G. & Noble, G.R. (1970) An influenza B epidemic within a remote Alaska community: serologic, epidemiologic, and clinical observations. *J Am Med Assoc* **214**, 507–12.

Clifford, R.E., Smith, J.W.G., Tillett, H.E. & Wherry, P.J. (1977) Excess mortality associated with influenza in England and Wales. *Int J Epidemiol* **6**, 115–28.

Cockburn, W.C., Delon, P.J. & Ferreira, W. (1969) Origin and progress of the 1968-69 Hong Kong influenza epidemic. *Bull WHO* **41**, 345–8.

Collier, R. (1974) *The Plague of the Spanish Lady: the Influenza Pandemic of 1918–19*. Macmillan, London.

Collins, S.D. (1930) Influenza–pneumonia mortality in a group of about 95 cities in the United States, 1920–29. *Public Health Rep* **45**, 361–406.

Collins, S.D. (1932) Excess mortality from causes other than influenza and pneumonia during influenza epidemics. *Public Health Rep* **47**, 2159–89.

Collins, S.D., Frost, W.H., Gover, M. & Sydenstricker, E. (1930) Mortality from influenza and pneumonia in 50 large cities of the United States, 1910–29. *Public Health Rep* **45**, 2277–329.

Collins, S.D. & Lehmann, J. (1951) Trends and epidemics of influenza and pneumonia, 1918–51. *Public Health Rep* **66**, 1487–516.

Collins, S.D. & Lehmann, J. (1953) *Excess Deaths from Influenza and Pneumonia and from Important Chronic Diseases during Epidemic Periods, 1918–51* (ed. Public Health Service). Monograph No. 10, pp. 1–22. Public Health Service, Washington DC.

Creighton, C. (1965) Influenzas and epidemic agues. In: Creighton, C. (ed.) *A History of Epidemics in Britain*, 2nd edn, pp. 300–433. Frank Cass, London.

Crosby, A.W. (1989) *America's Forgotten Pandemic: The Influenza of 1918*, 2nd edn. Cambridge University Press, Cambridge.

Dauer, C.C. & Serfling, R.E. (1961) Mortality from influenza 1957–58 and 1959–60. *Am Rev Resp Dis* **83**, 15–28.

Davenport, F.M. (1977) Reflections on the epidemiology of myxovirus infections. *Med Microbiol Immunol* **164**, 69–76.

Davies, J.R., Grilli, E.A. & Smith, A.J. (1984) Influenza A: infection and reinfection. *J Hygiene, Cambridge* **92**, 125–7.

Davies, J.R., Smith, A.J., Grilli, E.A. & Hoskins, T.W. (1982) Christ's Hospital 1978–79: an account of two outbreaks of influenza A H1N1. *J Infect* **5**, 151–6.

Davis, L.E., Caldwell, G.G., Lynch, R.E., Bailey, R.E. & Chin, D.Y. (1970) Hong Kong influenza: the epidemiologic features of a high school family study analysed and compared with a similar study during the 1957 Asian influenza epidemic. *Am J Epidemiol* **92**, 240–7.

Diepersloot, R.J.A., Bouter, K.P. & Hoekstra, J. (1990) Influenza infection and diabetes mellitus. *Diabetes Care* **13**, 876–82.

Dowdle, W.R., Coleman, M.T. & Gregg, M.B. (1974) Natural history of influenza A in the United States, 1957–72. *Prog Med Virol* **17**, 91–135.

Dunn, F.L. (1958) Pandemic influenza in 1957: review of international spread of new Asian strain. *J Am Med Assoc* **166**, 1140–8.

Eickhoff, T.C., Sherman, I.L. & Serfling, R.E. (1961) Observations on excess mortality associated with epidemic influenza. *J Am Med Assoc* **176**, 776–82.

Elder, A.G., O'Donnell, B., McCruden, E.A.B., Symington, I.S. & Carman, W.F. (1996) Incidence and recall of influenza in a cohort of Glasgow healthcare workers during the 1993–4 epidemic: results of serum testing and questionnaire. *Br Med J* **313**, 1241–2.

Falsey, A.R., Cunningham, C.K., Barker, W.H. *et al.* (1995) Respiratory syncytial virus and influenza A infections in the hospitalized elderly. *J Infect Dis* **172**, 389–94.

Fang, F., Jou, W.M., Huylebroeck, D., Devos, R. & Fiers, W. (1981) Complete structure of A/Duck/Ukraine/63 influenza haemagglutinin gene: animal virus as progenitor of human H3 Hong Kong 1968 influenza haemagglutinin. *Cell* **25**, 315–23.

Farr, W. (1885) Untitled. In: Humphreys, N.A. (ed.) *Vital Statistics: a memorial volume of selections from the reports and writings of William Farr*, pp. 330. Office of the Sanitary Institute, London.

Fine, P.E.M. (1982) Herd immunity (1). In: Selby, P. (ed.) *Influenza Models: Prospects for Development and Use*, pp. 189–94. MTP Press, Lancaster.

Fine, P.E.M. & Clarkson, J.A. (1982) Measles in England and Wales. I. An analysis of factors underlying seasonal patterns. *Int J Epidemiol* **11**, 5–14.

Finklea, J.F., Sandifer, S.H. & Smith, D.D. (1969) Cigarette smoking and epidemic influenza. *Am J Epidemiol* **90**, 390–9.

Fleming, D.M. (1996) The impact of three influenza epidemics on primary care in England and Wales. *PharmacoEcon Suppl* **9**, 38–45.

Fleming, D.M., Crombie, D.L. & Norbury, C.A. & Cross, K.W. (1990) Observations on the influenza epidemic of November/December 1989. *Br J Gen Pract* **40**, 495–7.

Fleming, D.M. & Cross, K.W. (1993) Respiratory syncytial virus or influenza? *Lancet* **342**, 1507–10.

Fleming, D.M., Norbury, C.A. & Crombie, D.L. (1991) *Annual and Seasonal Variation in the Incidence of Common Diseases*. Occasional paper 53. Royal College of General Practitioners, London.

Fox, J.P., Cooney, M.K., Hall, C.E. & Foy, M.F. (1982a) Influenza virus infections in Seattle families, 1975–79. II. Pattern of infection in invaded households and relation of age and prior antibody to occurrence of infection and related illness. *Am J Epidemiol* **116**, 228–42.

Fox, J.P. & Hall, C.E. (1980) *Viruses in Families*. PSG, Littleton, MA.

Fox, J.P., Hall, C.E., Cooney, M.K. & Foy, M.F. (1982b) Influenza virus infections in Seattle families, 1975–79. I. Study design, methods and the occurrence of infections by time and age. *Am J Epidemiol* **116**, 212–27.

Foy, M.F., Cooney, M.K. & Allan, I. (1976) Longitudinal studies of types A and B influenza among Seattle schoolchildren and families, 1968–74. *J Infect Dis* **134**, 362–9.

Fralick, R.A. (1985) Absenteeism among hospital staff during influenza epidemic (letter). *Canad Med Assoc J* **133**, 641–2.

Francis, T., Jr. & Shope, R.E. (1936) Neutralization tests with sera of convalescent or immunized animals and the viruses of swine and human influenza. *J Exp Med* **63**, 645–53.

Frank, A.L., Taber, L.H., Glezen, W.P., Geyer, E.A., McIlwain, S. & Paredes, A. (1983a) Influenza B virus infections in the community and the family: the epidemics of 1976–77 and 1979–80 in Houston, Texas. *Am J Epidemiol* **118**, 313–25.

Frank, A.L., Taber, L.H., Glezen, W.P., Paredes, A. & Couch, R.B. (1979) Reinfection with influenza A (H3N2) virus in young children and their families. *J Infect Dis* **140**, 829–36.

Frank, A.L., Taber, L.H. & Porter, C.M. (1987) Influenza B virus reinfection. *Am J Epidemiol* **125**, 576–86.

Frank, A.L., Taber, L.H. & Wells, J.M. (1983b) Individuals infected with two subtypes of influenza A virus in the same season. *J Infect Dis* **147**, 120–4.

Frost, W.H. (1919) The epidemiology of influenza. *Public Health Rep* **34**, 1823–7.

Gardner, P.S., Court, S.D.M., Brocklebank, J.T., Downham, M.A.P.S. & Weightman, D. (1973) Virus cross-infection in paediatric wards. *Br Med J* **2**, 571–5.

Glass, R.I.M., Brann, E.A., Slade, J.D. *et al.* (1978) Community-wide surveillance of influenza after outbreaks due to H3N2 (A/Victoria/75 and A/Texas/77) and H1N1 (A/USSR/77) influenza viruses, Mercer County, New Jersey, 1978. *J Infect Dis* **138**, 703–6.

Glezen, W.P. (1996) Emerging infections: pandemic influenza. *Epidemiol Rev* **18**, 64–76.

Glezen, W.P. & Couch, R.B. (1978) Interpandemic influenza in the Houston area, 1974–76. *N Engl J Med* **298**, 587–92.

Glezen, W.P., Couch, R.B., Taber, L.H. *et al.* (1980a) Epidemiologic observations of influenza B virus infections in Houston, Texas, 1976–77. *Am J Epidemiol* **111**, 13–22.

Glezen, W.P., Couch, R.B. & Six, H.R. (1982a) The influenza herald wave. *Am J Epidemiol* **116**, 589–98.

Glezen, W.P., Decker, M. & Perrotta, D.M. (1987) Survey of underlying conditions of persons hospitalized with acute respiratory disease during influenza epidemics in Houston, 1978–81. *Am Rev Resp Dis* **136**, 550–5.

Glezen, W.P., Paredes, A. & Taber, L.H. (1980b) Influenza in children. Relationship to other respiratory agents. *J Am Med Assoc* **243**, 1345–9.

Glezen, W.P., Payne, A.A., Snyder, D.N. & Downs, T.D. (1982b) Mortality and influenza. *J Infect Dis* **146**, 313–20.

Goldfield, M., Bartley, J.D., Pizzuti, W., Black, H.C., Altman, R. & Halperin, W.E. (1977) Influenza in New Jersey in 1976: isolations of influenza A/New Jersey/76 virus at Fort Dix. *J Infect Dis* **136** (suppl), S347–55.

Goldstein, I.F. & Block, G. (1976) A method for surveillance of influenza epidemics. *Am J Public Health* **66**, 992–3.

Goodman, R.A., Orenstein, W.A., Munro, T.F., Smith, S.C. & Sikes, R.K. (1982) Impact of Influenza A in a nursing home. *J Am Med Assoc* **247**, 1451–3.

Greenberg, M., Jacobziner, H., Pakter, J. & Weisl, B.A.G. (1958) Maternal mortality in the epidemic of Asian influenza, New York City, 1957. *Am J Obstet Gynaecol* **76**, 897–902.

Gregg, M.B. (1980) The epidemiology of influenza in humans. *Ann NY Acad Sci* **353**, 45–53.

Gregg, M.B., Hinman, A.R. & Craven, R.B. (1978) The Russian flu: its history and implications for this year's influenza season. *J Am Med Assoc* **240**, 2260–3.

Gross, P.A., Rodstein, M., LaMontagne, J.R. *et al.* (1988) Epidemiology of acute respiratory illness during an influenza outbreak in a nursing home: a prospective study. *Arch Int Med* **148**, 559–61.

Hall, C.B. (1981) Nosocomial viral respiratory infections: perennial weeds on pediatric wards. *Am J Med* **70**, 670–6.

Hall, C.E., Cooney, M.K. & Fox, J.P. (1973) The Seattle Virus Watch: IV. Comparative epidemiologic observations of infections with influenza A and B viruses, 1965–69, in families with young children. *Am J Epidemiol* **98**, 365–80.

Hall, C.B. & Douglas, R.G. Jr (1975) Nosocomial influenza infection as a cause of intercurrent fevers in infants. *Pediatrics* **55**, 673–7.

Hall, W.N., Goodman, R.A., Noble, G.R., Kendal, A.P. & Steece, R.S. (1981) An outbreak of influenza B in an elderly population. *J Infect Dis* **144**, 297–302.

Hammond, G.W., Raddatz, R.L. & Gelskey, D.E. (1989) Impact of atmospheric dispersion and transport of viral aerosols on the epidemiology of influenza. *Rev Infect Dis* **2**, 494–7.

Hardy, J.M.B., Azarowicz, E.N., Mannini, A., Medearis, D.N. & Cooke, R.E. (1961) The effect of Asian influenza on the outcome of pregnancy, Baltimore, 1957–58. *Am J Public Health* **51**, 1182–8.

Hayslett, J., McCarroll, J., Brady, E., Deuschle, K., McDermott, W. & Kilbourne, E.D. (1962) Endemic influenza: I. Serologic evidence of continuing and subclinical infection in disparate populations in the postpandemic period. *Am Rev Resp Dis* **85**, 1–8.

Hemmes, J.H., Winkler, K.C. & Kool, S.M. (1960) Virus survival as a seasonal factor in influenza and poliomyelitis. *Nature* **188**, 430–1.

Hirota, Y., Takeshita, S., Ide, S. *et al.* (1992) Various factors associated with the manifestation of influenza-like illness. *Int J Epidemiol* **21**, 574–82.

Hirst, G.K. (1962) Genetic recombination with Newcastle disease virus, polioviruses, and influenza. *Cold Spring Harbor Symp Quant Biol* **27**, 303–9.

HMSO (1920) *Supplement to the 81st Annual Report of the Registrar General: report on the mortality from influenza in England and Wales during the epidemic of 1918–19*, pp. 1–47. HMSO, London.

Hoffman, P.C. & Dixon, R.E. (1977) Control of influenza in the hospital. *Ann Int Med* **87**, 725–8.

Hope-Simpson, R.E. (1970) First outbreak of Hong Kong influenza in a general practice population in Great Britain. A field and laboratory study. *Br Med J* **iii**, 74–7.

Hope-Simpson, R.E. (1979) Epidemic mechanisms of type A influenza. *J Hygiene, Cambridge* **83**, 11–26.

Hope-Simpson, R.E. (1981) The role of season in the epidemiology of influenza. *J Hygiene, Cambridge* **86**, 35–47.

Hope-Simpson, R.E. (1983) Recognition of historic influenza epidemics from parish burial records: a test of prediction from a new hypothesis of influenzal epidemiology. *J Hygiene, Cambridge* **91**, 293–308.

Hope-Simpson, R.E. (1984) Age and secular distributions of virus-proven influenza patients in successive epidemics 1961–76 in Cirencester: Epidemiological significance discussed. *J Hygiene, Cambridge* **92**, 303–36.

Hope-Simpson, R.E. (1986) The method of transmission of epidemic influenza: further evidence from archival mortality data. *J Hygiene, Cambridge* **96**, 353–75.

Housworth, J. & Langmuir, A.D. (1974) Excess mortality from epidemic influenza, 1957–66. *Am J Epidemiol* **100**, 40–8.

Jennings, L.C. & Miles, J.A.R. (1978) A study of acute respiratory disease in the community of Port Chalmers. II. Influenza A/Port Chalmers/1/73: intrafamilial spread and the effect of antibodies to the surface antigens. *J Hygiene, Cambridge* **81**, 67–75.

Jordan, W.S. Jr (1961) The mechanism of spread of Asian influenza. *Am Rev Resp Dis* **2**, 29–40.

Jordan, W.S. Jr, Badger, G.F. & Dingle, J.H. (1958a) A study of illness in a group of Cleveland families. XVI. The epidemiology of influenza, 1948–53. *Am J Hygiene* **68**, 169–89.

Jordan, W.S. Jr, Denny, F.W. Jr, Badger, G.F. *et al.* (1958b) A study of illness in a group of Cleveland families. XVII. The occurrence of Asian influenza. *Am J Hygiene* **68**, 190–212.

Kapila, R., Lintz, D.I., Tecson, F.T., Ziskin, L. & Louria, D.B. (1977) A nosocomial outbreak of influenza A. *Chest* **71**, 576–9.

Kark, J.D. & Lebiush, M. (1981) Smoking and epidemic influenza-like illness in female military recruits: a brief survey. *Am J Public Health* **71**, 530–2.

Kark, J.D., Lebiush, M. & Rannon, L. (1982) Cigarette smoking as a risk factor for epidemic A (H1N1) influenza in young men. *N Engl J Med* **307**, 1042–6.

Kawaoka, Y., Bean, W.J., Gorman, O.T. *et al.* (1993) The roles of birds and pigs in the generation of pandemic strains of human influenza. In: Hannoun, C., Kendal, A.P., Klenk, H.D. & Ruben, F.L. (eds) *Options for the Control of Influenza II*, pp. 187–91. Elsevier Science, Amsterdam.

Kawaoka, Y., Krauss, S. & Webster, R.G. (1989) Avian-to-human transmission of the PB1 gene of influenza A virus in the 1957 and 1968 pandemics. *J Virol* **63**, 4603–8.

Kendal, A.P. (1987) Epidemiologic implications of changes in the influenza virus genome. *Am J Med* **82** (suppl 6A), 4–14.

Kendal, A.P., Joseph, J.M., Kobayashi, G. *et al.* (1979) Laboratory-based surveillance of influenza virus in the United States during the Winter of 1977–78. *Am J Epidemiol* **110**, 449–61.

Kendal, A.P., Minuse, E., Maassab, H.F., Hennessy, A.V. & Davenport, F.M. (1973) Influenza neuraminidase antibody patterns of man. *Am J Epidemiol* **98**, 96–103.

Kilbourne, E.D. (1973) The molecular epidemiology of influenza. *J Infect Dis* **127**, 478–87.

Kilbourne, E.D. (1975) *The Influenza Viruses and Influenza.* Academic Press, Orlando.

Kilbourne, E.D. (1987) *Influenza.* Plenum, New York.

Kohn, M.A., Farley, T.A., Sundin, D., Tapia, R., McFarland, L.M. & Arden, N.H. (1995) Three summertime outbreaks of influenza type A. *J Infect Dis* **172**, 246–9.

Kundin, W.D. (1970) Hong Kong A2 influenza virus infection among swine during a human epidemic in Taiwan. *Nature* **228**, 857.

Kurtz, J., Manvell, R.J. & Banks, J. (1996) Avian influenza virus isolated from a woman with conjunctivitis. *Lancet* **348**, 901–2.

LaMontagne, J.R. (1980) Summary of a workshop on influenza B viruses and Reye's syndrome. *J Infect Dis* **142**, 452–65.

Langmuir, A.D. (1961) Global epidemiology: epidemiology of Asian influenza. *Am Rev Resp Dis* **83**, 2–14.

Longini, I.M., Jr, Koopman, J.S., Monto, A.S. & Fox, J.P. (1982) Estimating household and community transmission parameters for influenza. *Am J Epidemiol* **115**, 736–51.

Lui, K. & Kendal, A.P. (1987) Impact of influenza epidemics on mortality in the United States from October 1972 to May 1985. *Am J Public Health* **77**, 712–16.

McBean, A.M., Babish, J.D., Warren, J.L. & Melson, E.A. (1993) The effect of influenza epidemics on the hospitalization of persons 65 years and older. In: Hannoun, C., Kendal, A.P., Klenk, H.D. & Ruben, F.L. (eds) *Options for the Control of Influenza II*, pp. 25–37. Elsevier Science, Amsterdam.

McDonald, J.C. (1958) Asian influenza in Great Britain 1957–58. *Proc Roy Soc Med* **51**, 36–8.

MacKenzie, J.S., MacKenzie, I.H. & Holt, P.G. (1976) The effect of cigarette smoking on susceptibility to epidemic influenza and on serological responses to live attenuated and killed subunit influenza vaccines. *J Hygiene, Cambridge* **77**, 409–17.

Mann, P.G., Pereira, M.S., Smith, J.W.G., Hart, R.J.C. & Williams, W.O. (1981) A 5-year study of influenza in families. *J Hygiene, Cambridge* **87**, 191–200.

Martin, C.M., Kunin, C.M., Gottlieb, L.S., Barnes, M.W., Liu, C. & Finland, M. (1959) Asian influenza A in Boston, 1957–58. *Arch Int Med* **103**, 515–31.

Masurel, N. & Heijtink, R.A. (1983) Recycling of H1N1 influenza A virus in man—a haemagglutinin antibody study. *J Hygiene* **90**, 397–402.

Masurel, N. & Marine, W.M. (1973) Recycling of Asian and Hong Kong influenza A virus haemagglutinins in man. *Am J Epidemiol* **97**, 44–9.

Mathur, U., Bentley, D.W. & Hall, C.B. (1980) Concurrent respiratory syncytial virus and influenza A infections in the institutionalized elderly and chronically ill. *Ann Int Med* **93**, 49–52.

Meibalane, R., Sedmak, G.V., Sasidharan, P., Garg, P. & Grausz, J.P. (1977) Outbreak of influenza in a neonatal intensive care unit. *J Pediatr* **91**, 974–6.

Mitchell, E., Sethi, S., Rowland, M.G.M. *et al.* (1991) An unusual community outbreak of influenza A. *J Public Health Med* **13**, 214–18.

Monto, A.S. (1987) Influenza: quantifying morbidity and mortality. *Am J Med* **82**, 20–5.

Monto, A.S. & Cavallaro, J.J. (1971) The Tecumseh Study of Respiratory Illness. II. Patterns of occurrence of infection with respiratory pathogens, 1965–69. *Am J Epidemiol* **94**, 280–9.

Monto, A.S. & Kioumehr, F. (1975) The Tecumseh Study of Respiratory Illness. IX. Occurrence of influenza in the community, 1966–71. *Am J Epidemiol* **102**, 553–63.

Monto, A.S., Koopman, J.S. & Longini, I.M. & Jr. (1985) Tecumseh Study of Illness XII. Influenza infection and disease, 1976–81. *Am J Epidemiol* **121**, 811–22.

Monto, A.S., Napier, J.A. & Metzner, H.L. (1971) The Tecumseh Study of Respiratory Illness. I. Plan of study and observations on syndromes of acute respiratory disease. *Am J Epidemiol* **94**, 269–79.

Monto, A.S., Ohmit, S.E., Foster, D.A., Furumoto-Dawson, A. & Arden, N. (1993) Case–control study in Michigan on prevention of hospitalization by vaccination, 1989–91. In: Hannoun, C., Kendal, A.P., Klenk, H.D. & Ruben, F.L. (eds) *Options for the Control of Influenza II*, pp. 135–41. Elsevier Science, Amsterdam.

Moser, M.R., Bender, T.R., Margolis, H.S., Noble, G.R., Kendal, A.P. & Ritter, D.G. (1979) An outbreak of influenza aboard a commercial airliner. *Am J Hygiene* **110**, 1–6.

Mukerjee, A. (1994) Spread of influenza: a study of risk factors in homes for the elderly in Wales. *J Epidemiol Commun Health* **48**, 602–3.

Mullooly, J.P., Barker, W.H. & Nolan, T.F. Jr (1986) Risk of acute respiratory disease among pregnant women during influenza A epidemics. *Public Health Rep* **101**, 205–11.

Nakajima, K., Desselberger, U. & Palese, P. (1978) Recent human influenza A (H1N1) viruses are closely related genetically to strains isolated in 1950. *Nature* **274**, 334–9.

Napiorkowski, P.A. & Black, F.L. (1974) Influenza A in an isolated population in the Amazon. *Lancet* **ii**, 1390–1.

Nguyen-Van-Tam, J.S. & Nicholson, K.G. (1992) Influenza deaths in Leicestershire during the 1989–90 epidemic: implications for prevention. *Epidemiol Infect* **108**, 537–45.

Nicholson, K.G. (1996) Impact of influenza and respiratory syncytial virus on mortality in England and Wales from January 1975 to December 1990. *Epidemiol Infect* **116**, 51–63.

Nicholson, K.G., Baker, D.J., Farquhar, A., Hurd, D., Kent, J. & Smith, S.H. (1990) Acute upper respiratory tract viral illness and influenza immunization in homes for the elderly. *Epidemiol Infect* **105**, 609–18.

Nolan, T.F. Jr, Goodman, R.A., Hinman, A.R., Noble, G.R., Kendal, A.P. & Thacker, S.B. (1980) Morbidity and mortality associated with influenza B in the United States, 1979–80: A report from the Centre for Disease Control. *J Infect Dis* **142**, 360–2.

O'Donoghue, J.M., Ray, C.G., Terry, D.W. Jr & Beaty, H.N. (1973) Prevention of nosocomial influenza infection with amantadine. *Am J Epidemiol* **97**, 276–83.

Pachucki, C.T., Pappas, S.A.W., Fuller, G.F., Krause, S.L., Lentino, J.R. & Schaaff, D.M. (1989) Influenza A among hospital personnel and patients: implications for recognition, prevention, and control. *Arch Int Med* **149**, 77–80.

Patriarca, P.A., Arden, N., Koplan, J.P. & Goodman, R.A. (1987) Prevention and control of type A influenza infections in nursing homes: benefits and costs of four approaches using vaccination and amantadine. *Ann Int Med* **107**, 732–40.

Patriarca, P.A. & Strikas, R.A. (1995) Influenza vaccine for healthy adults? *N Engl J Med* **333**, 933–4.

Patriarca, P.A., Weber, J.A., Parker, R.A. *et al.* (1986) Risk factors for outbreaks of influenza in nursing homes: a case-control study. *Am J Epidemiol* **124**, 114–19.

Pearl, R. (1919) Influenza studies: 1. On certain general statistical aspects of the 1918 epidemic in American cities. *Public Health Rep* **34**, 1743–61.

Penny, P.T. (1978) Epidemic influenza in schools. *Br Med J* **1**, 298–9.

Pereira, M.S. & Chakraverty, P. (1977) The laboratory surveillance of influenza epidemics in the United Kingdom 1968–76. *J Hygiene, Cambridge* **79**, 77–87.

Perrotta, D.M., Decker, M. & Glezen, W.P. (1985) Acute respiratory disease hospitalizations as a measure of impact of epidemic influenza. *Am J Epidemiol* **122**, 468–76.

Petersdorf, R.G., Fusco, J.J., Harter, D.H. & Albrink, W.S. (1959) Pulmonary infections complicating Asian influenza. *Arch Int Med* **103**, 262–72.

Philip, R.N., Bell, J.A., Davis, D.J. *et al.* (1961) Epidemiologic studies on influenza in familial and general population groups, 1951–56. II. Characteristics of occurrence. *Am J Hygiene* **73**, 123–37.

Philip, R.N., Weeks, W.T., Reinhard, K.R., Lackman, D.B. & French, R.N. (1959) Observations on Asian influenza on two Alaskan islands. *Public Health Rep* **74**, 737–45.

Pons, V.G., Canter, J. & Dolin, R. (1980) Influenza A/USSR/77 (H1N1) on a university campus. *Am J Epidemiol* **111**, 23–30.

Potter, J., Stott, D.J., Roberts, M.A. *et al.* (1997) Influenza vaccination of health care workers in long-term care hospitals reduces the mortality of elderly patients. *J Infect Dis* **175**, 1–6.

Rekart, M., Rupnik, K., Cesario, T.C. & Tilles, J.G. (1982) Prevalence of haemagglutination inhibition antibody to current strains of the H3N2 and H1N1 subtypes of influenza: a virus in sera collected from the elderly in 1976. *Am J Epidemiol* **115**, 587–97.

Retailliau, H.F., Storch, G.A., Curtis, A.C., Horne, T.J., Scally, M.J. & Hattwick, M.A.W. (1979) The epidemiology of influenza B in a rural setting in 1977. *Am J Epidemiol* **109**, 639–49.

Sabin, A. (1977) Mortality from pneumonia and risk conditions during influenza epidemics: high influenza morbidity during nonepidemic years. *J Am Med Assoc* **237**, 2823–8.

Salk, J. & Salk, D. (1977) Control of influenza and poliomyelitis with killed virus vaccines. *Science* **195**, 834–47.

Sartwell, P.E. & Long, A.P. (1948) The army experience with influenza, 1946–47. I. Epidemiological aspects. *Am J Hygiene* **47**, 135–41.

Schaffer, F.L., Soergel, M.E. & Straube, D.C. (1976) Survival of airborne influenza virus: effects of propagating host, relative humidity, and composition of spray fluids. *Arch Virol* **51**, 263–73.

Schoenbaum, S.C., Coleman, M.T., Dowdle, W.R. & Mostow, S.R. (1976) Epidemiology of influenza in the elderly: evidence of virus recycling. *Am J Epidemiol* **103**, 166–7.

Scholtissek, C. & Naylor, E. (1988) Fish farming and influenza pandemics. *Nature* **331**, 215.

Scholtissek, C., Schultz, U., Ludwig, S. & Fitch, W.M. (1993) The role of swine in the origin of pandemic influenza. In: Hannoun, C., Kendall, A.P., Klenk, H.D. & Ruben, F.L. (eds) *Options for the Control of Influenza II*, pp. 193–201. Elsevier Science, Amsterdam.

Serfling, R.E. (1963) Methods for current statistical analysis of excess pneumonia–influenza deaths. *Public Health Rep* **78**, 494–506.

Serwint, J.R., Miller, R.M. & Korsch, B.M. (1991) Influenza type A and B infections in hospitalized pediatric patients: who should be immunized? *Am J Dis Child* **145**, 623–6.

Sharrar, R.G. (1969) National influenza experience in the USA, 1968–69. *Bull WHO* **41**, 361–6.

Shortridge, K.F. & Stuart-Harris, C.H. (1982) An influenza epicentre? *Lancet* **ii**, 812–13.

Simonsen, L., Schonberger, L.B., Stroup, D.F., Arden, N.H. & Cox, N.J. (1996) The impact of influenza on mortality in the USA. In: Brown, L.E., Hampson, A.W. &Webster, R.G. (eds) *Options for the Control of Influenza III*, pp. 26–33. Elsevier Science, Amsterdam.

Smith, W., Andrewes, C.H. & Laidlaw, P.P. (1933) A virus obtained from influenza patients. *Lancet* **ii**, 66–8.

Sobal, J. & Loveland, F.C. (1982) Infectious disease in a total institution: a study of the influenza epidemic of 1978 on a college campus. *Public Health Rep* **97**, 66–72.

Spelman, D.W. & McHardy, C.J. (1985) Concurrent outbreaks of influenza A and influenza B. *J Hygiene, Cambridge* **94**, 331–9.

Sprenger, M.J.W., Van Naelten, M.A.M.G., Mulder, P.G.H. & Masurel, N. (1989) Influenza mortality and excess deaths in the elderly, 1967–82. *Epidemiol Infect* **103**, 633–41.

Stocks, P. (1934) The effect of influenza epidemics on the certified causes of death. *Lancet* **ii**, 386–95.

Strikas, R.A., Cook, P., Kuller, L. *et al.* (1993) Case–control study in Ohio and Pennyslvania on prevention of hospitalization by influenza vaccination. In: Hannoun, C.,

Kendal, A.P., Klenk, H.D. & Ruben, F.L. (eds) *Options for the Control of Influenza II*, pp. 153–60. Elsevier Science, Amsterdam.

Stuart-Harris, S.C.H., Schild, G.C. & Oxford, J.S. (1985) *Influenza: The Viruses and the Disease*, 2nd edn. Edward Arnold, London.

Taber, L.H., Paredes, A., Glezen, W.P. & Couch, R.B. (1981) Infection with influenza A/Victoria virus in Houston families, 1976. *J Hygiene, Cambridge* **86**, 303–13.

Thacker, S.B. (1986) The persistence of influenza A in human populations. *Epidemiol Rev* **8**, 129–41.

Tillett, H.E., Smith, J.W.G. & Clifford, R.E. (1980) Excess morbidity and mortality associated with influenza in England and Wales. *Lancet* **i**, 793–5.

Tillett, H.E., Smith, J.W.G. & Gooch, C.D. (1983) Excess deaths attributable to influenza in England and Wales: age at death and certified cause. *Int J Epidemiol* **12**, 344–52.

Top, F.H. Jr & Russell, P.K. (1977) Swine influenza A at Fort Dix, New Jersey (January–February 1976): IV. Summary and speculation. *J Infect Dis* **136** (suppl), S376–80.

Trotter, Y. Jr, Dunn, F.L., Drachman, R.H., Henderson, D.A., Pizzi, M. & Langmuir, A.D. (1959) Asian influenza in the United States, 1957–58. *Am J Hygiene* **70**, 34–50.

Tumova, B. & Easterday, B.C. (1969) Relationship of envelope antigens of animal influenza viruses to human A2 influenza strains isolated in the years 1957–68. *Bull WHO* **41**, 429–35.

US Department of Health, Education and Welfare (1957) Trend and age variation of mortality and morbidity from influenza and pneumonia. In: Public Health Service (ed.) *Long-Time Trends in Illness and Medical Care.* Monograph no. 48, pp. 51–67. Public Health Service, Washington DC.

Van Voris, L.P., Belshe, R.B. & Shaffer, J.L. (1982) Nosocomial influenza B virus infection in the elderly. *Ann Int Med* **96**, 153–8.

Vaughan, W.T. (1921) *Influenza: An Epidemiologic Study Monographic Series No. 1*, pp. 1–116. American Journal of Hygiene, Baltimore, MD.

Waldman, R.H., Bond, J.O., Levitt, L.P. *et al.* (1969) An evaluation of influenza immunization: influence of route of administration and vaccine strain. *Bull WHO* **41**, 543–8.

Watkins, P.J., Soler, N.G., Fitzgerald, M.G. & Malins, J.M. (1970) Diabetic ketoacidosis during the influenza epidemic. *Br Med J* **4**, 89–91.

Webster, R.G., Hinshaw, V.S., Bean, W.J. Jr & Sriram, G. (1980) Influenza viruses: transmission between species. *Phil Trans Roy Soc London* **288**, 439–47.

Webster, R.G., Sharp, G.B. & Claas, E.C. (1995) Interspecies transmission of influenza viruses. *Am J Respir Crit Care Med* **152** (4 part 2), S25–30.

Weightman, D., Downham, M.A.P.S. & Gardner, P.S. (1974) Introduction of a cross-infection rate in children's wards and its application to respiratory virus infections. *J Hygiene, Cambridge* **73**, 53–60.

Weingarten, S., Friedlander, M., Rascon, D., Ault, M., Morgan, M. & Meyer, R.D. (1988) Influenza surveillance in an acute care hospital. *Arch Int Med* **148**, 113–16.

Wentworth, D.E., McGregor, M.W., Macklin, M.D., Neumann, V. & Hinshaw, V.S. (1997) Transmission of swine influenza virus to humans after exposure to experimentally affected pigs. *J Infect Dis* **175**, 7–15.

Wright, P.F., Bryant, J.D. & Karzon, D.T. (1980) Comparison of influenza B/Hong Kong virus infections among infants, children, and young adults. *J Infect Dis* **141**, 430–5.

Yassi, A., Kettner, J., Hammond, G., Cheang, M. & McGill, M. (1991) Effectiveness and cost-benefit of an influenza vaccination program for health care workers. *Canad J Infect Dis* **2**, 101–8.

Yassi, A., McGill, M., Holton, D. & Nicolle, L. (1993) Morbidity, cost and role of health care worker transmission in an influenza outbreak in a tertiary care hospital. *Canad J Infect Dis* **4**, 52–6.

Zhou, N., He, S., Zhang, T. *et al.* (1996) Influenza infection in humans and pigs in south-eastern China. *Arch Virol* **141**, 649–61.

CHAPTER 18

Surveillance of Influenza

John M. Watson

Although influenza viruses were not isolated and identified until 1933, the disease has been recognized and its occurrence monitored for many centuries on the basis of its clinical and epidemiological characteristics. The combination of virological identification and clinical/epidemiological monitoring forms the mainstay of surveillance for influenza today.

Epidemics of influenza occur in most temperate countries every 1–3 years. There are clear descriptions of epidemics in Britain from at least the 16th century (Thompson 1852). Worldwide epidemics, or pandemics, of influenza have occurred at less frequent and irregular intervals, but there may have been more than 30 since the 16th century (Betts 1995). The 'Spanish' influenza pandemic of 1918–19 was probably the largest and is estimated to have been responsible for at least 20 million deaths and probably considerably more (Kilbourne 1987; Van Hartesveldt 1992). This pandemic occurred, in most places, in three waves with the greatest morbidity and mortality occurring during the second wave. The first wave began in the summer of 1918, outside the traditional influenza season in the Northern Hemisphere, but was relatively mild or even unnoticed in some localities (Hope-Simpson 1992). The 1918–19 pandemic was notable for the relatively high proportion of young adults affected, and the proportion of cases developing pneumonia, presumed in many to be primary viral pneumonia. This pandemic was subsequently shown to be due to influenza A, subtype H1N1, which continued to circulate until 1957 when it disappeared to be replaced by the H2N2 subtype in the 'Asian' influenza pandemic. In 1968 this subtype was in turn replaced by 'Hong Kong' influenza, due to the H3N2 subtype, which was responsible for the pandemic of 1968/69. The morbidity and mortality associated with both these new subtypes of influenza A was substantial, although not as great as that seen in 1918–19. In 1977, the H1N1 subtype reappeared but failed either to cause a major pandemic or to oust the circulation of the H3N2 subtype. This may have been due, at least in part, to the previous exposure of those aged over 20 years to related strains of H1N1 subtype in the 1918–57 era (Betts 1995). Both the H1N1 and the H3N2 subtypes have cocirculated since 1977.

Despite the substantial impact of pandemics, epidemics of influenza cause the greater overall burden of morbidity and mortality. In epidemic years, 10–20% of the general population may be affected and an appreciable excess mortality due to influenza is measurable in most years (Tillett et al. 1980). In England and Wales (population 51.8 million in 1995) most influenza seasons are associated with an excess of 3000–5000 deaths and larger epidemics, such as that seen in 1989/90, with up to 30 000 excess deaths (Curwen et al. 1990).

The period during which influenza viruses circulate in the population appears to be limited, although different types, subtypes or strains may cocirculate or circulate at different times in the same influenza season. In general, after the detection of an influenza virus in a community, often initially in children, the frequency with which the virus is isolated increases rapidly over a 3–6-week period and then diminishes equally rapidly. Despite continued routine surveillance of respiratory viruses, or detailed local studies, influenza viruses are rarely isolated in the Northern Hemisphere outside the recognized period of circulation.

The epidemic potential of influenza virus, with its ability to cause substantial morbidity and mortality in a short space of time, is unique among the respiratory viruses. Nevertheless other viruses, such as respiratory syncytial virus (RSV), do causes widespread illness, particularly in certain subgroups of the population and may be responsible for an overall burden of disease that is comparable to influenza virus (Fleming & Cross 1993). RSV is well recognized as a cause of acute respiratory illness, particularly bronchiolitis, in neonates and infants, but its role in acute respiratory illness in adults and especially in elderly people is increasingly being recognized (Nicholson 1996). Other respiratory viruses, such as parainfluenza virus, adenovirus, coronavirus and rhinovirus probably also contribute to the range of acute respiratory illnesses that occur with greater frequency in the colder months, but do not generally cause substantial outbreaks (Monto & Sullivan 1993).

The association of influenza activity with the colder months of the year, in the temperate parts of the world is well recognized, although poorly understood. Thus the influenza season stretching from October to April in the Northern Hemisphere is matched by a similar season from April to October in the Southern Hemisphere. The virus strains seen during an influenza season in one hemisphere are often detected again in the subsequent season in the other hemisphere. In tropical areas influenza activity may be detectable at any time of year but is sometimes more evident after periods of cold or wet weather (Kilbourne 1987).

Aims of influenza surveillance and its limitations

Influenza surveillance must achieve a public health goal if it is to be justified as an activity outside the setting of research. The purpose of influenza surveillance is to collect, collate, analyse and disseminate information on influenza activity that will assist in the assessment, prevention and control of the morbidity and mortality associated with the infection and its complications. The surveillance must provide sufficiently accurate and current information to guide the effective application of control measures (Langmuir & Housworth 1969). Specifically surveillance is designed to fulfil the following:

• to identify the onset of influenza activity in a population at the earliest opportunity and to obtain virus isolates for characterization throughout the period of activity. This is essential for providing the data that contribute to the decision on the composition of the influenza vaccines to be used in the subsequent season

• to assess the extent of morbidity and mortality due to influenza-like illness in the community and the contribution of influenza virus and other respiratory pathogens to this illness burden

• to predict the likely types of influenza, and extent of activity, in a population over the subsequent weeks, months or years. In practice the extent to which any reliable prediction of influenza activity is possible is very limited.

Some influenza surveillance activities are carried out to provide the most up-to-date information about current levels of influenza activity to be used for control and prevention decisions while influenza activity is continuing. These include surveillance activities which identify the virus and its relatedness to recently circulating strains and the components of the current vaccine. It also includes estimates of the extent of current clinical activity, its severity and its relative impact in different groups within the population, especially those in different age groups. Other influenza surveillance activities are used to assess the impact of influenza epidemics and are generally employed retrospectively when all the relevant information is available. The impact of influenza on mortality is usually assessed retrospectively, although rapid collation of death registration data may permit timely assessment of mortality associated with current influenza activity (CDC 1997).

One of the major difficulties in the surveillance of influenza activity is the non-specific nature of the illness. Many viruses, and some other pathogenic organisms, may cause influenza-like illnesses although they rarely cause large outbreaks on the scale seen with influenza. Conversely, influenza virus infection may be asymptomatic, or may cause a range of clinical syndromes from rhinitis through 'typical' influenza-like illness to fulminant pneumonia. The clinical features associated with influenza infections, such as fever and cough, may not be apparent in certain groups such as the elderly, the very young and the immunosuppressed.

Surveillance of influenza virus activity is further complicated by the fact that most patients developing an illness due to influenza infection do not present for medical attention but, very sensibly, care for themselves with self-medication at home. If they do present to their family doctor, samples are rarely taken for microbiological diagnosis. More often those who present for medical attention are those in whom the illness has been present, without improvement, for some days or in whom the original viral illness has been followed by a bacterial superinfection. Whilst serological examination may provide retrospective indication of recent influenza virus infection, the results may be difficult to interpret and other tests to detect the influenza virus directly (such as isolation, antigen detection and polymerase chain reaction methods) may be negative at this stage.

Consequently, neither epidemiological nor virological surveillance alone is adequate to monitor influenza activity in a population and it is usual to combine information from a variety of sources to obtain a representative picture.

Virological surveillance

An international network for the surveillance of influenza viruses was established by the World Health Organization in 1947 (Hampson & Cox 1996). The network consists of three collaborating centres for influenza reference and research in London, Atlanta and Melbourne (the WHO Collaborating Centre for Influenza Epidemiology in Tokyo also contributes to this WHO network) and 110 designated national influenza centres in 80 countries. The objectives of the collaborating centres are to provide information about the types of influenza viruses circulating around the world, advise on the appropriate strains for inclusion in the next influenza vaccine, examine and store strains of interest and make them available to other laboratories, and provide teaching on relevant virological techniques (Anonymous 1979). The extent to which updated vaccines will provide protection against currently circulating influenza virus strains is also assessed by the collaborating centres using serology.

The national influenza centres submit viral isolates to the collaborating centres for further antigenic and genetic analysis. These national centres receive most of the strains that they isolate from sources within their own countries, but the methods used to obtain these samples vary considerably. In some countries the national influenza centres receive clinical samples from patients with influenza-like or related illnesses, and carry out the primary isolation of the influenza viruses. As little influenza virus isolation work is performed outside these centres, they examine most of the isolates that are available for that country. In some other countries, a wider range of hospital microbiology laboratories (often academic centres or public health laboratories) carry out the primary isolation and submit isolates to the national influenza centres, which confirm the type or subtype of virus, determine the strain and may carry out further antigenic or genetic analysis. Many of the national influenza centres carry out both primary isolation and secondary reference functions (Hannoun *et al.* 1989; Hutchinson *et al.* 1996).

The adequacy of virological surveillance will depend upon the specific objectives for the influenza surveillance in a geographical region. These objectives may include:

- identification, as early as possible, of the circulating strains of influenza virus
- quantification of the extent of influenza virus circulation in the community in comparison to previous period of influenza activity
- assessment of the relative contribution of different types, subtypes or strains of influenza virus to the occurrence of illness, including influenza-like illness, in the community
- assessment of the contribution of influenza viruses to illness in different groups within the population, particularly by geographical region, age group and whether seen in hospital or in community-based patients.

In practice, virological surveillance in many countries contributes information on all of these objectives but the methods used in the surveillance process can influence the representativeness of the information collected. Early identification of newly circulating strains of influenza virus, for example, can be facilitated by collaborative schemes between family practitioners and laboratories, so that small increases in the number of patients with influenza-like illness syndromes may be identified early and samples taken for rapid analysis (Fleming *et al.* 1995). The selection of patients with classical influenza symptoms and signs by an experienced doctor can increase the diagnostic yield (proportion of patients found to have true influenza virus infection) and the selection of specimens from children may also contribute to a high yield, as they are often the first in the community to become infected with a newly circulating strain.

The number of influenza viruses isolated during a period of influenza activity is dependent on a wide range of factors including:
• the severity of the illness caused: patients with milder illness are less likely to present for medical examination
• methods used for taking specimens: combined nose and throat swabs, or nasal pharyngeal washings, may be more sensitive than simple throat swabbing (Westmoreland *et al.* 1989; Fleming *et al.* 1995)
• characteristics of the virus in relation to laboratory isolation: the ease with which influenza viruses can be cultured appears to vary with different strains, laboratory methods and reagents
• the number of patients examined, the clinical criteria triggering examination, the ages of the patients and the stages of illness when sampled all influence the number of isolates ultimately identified.

Consequently, care should be exercised when assessing the relative size and severity of periods of influenza activity on the basis of virological information only.

The assessment of the relative contribution of influenza viruses to the occurrence of illness, including influenza-like illness, in the community and distinction from illness caused by other pathogens, may be influenced by all the factors affecting the estimation of the extent of virus circulation above. The adoption of standard epidemiological methods, employing a case definition, as well as standard virological methods and identification of other respiratory pathogens, may help to provide a more accurate assessment of the relative role of different aetiological agents in the cause of influenza-like illness and other acute respiratory illnesses in the community.

Influenza activity may vary in different regions of a country, and even between small areas within the same region of a country. The representativeness of the isolates examined will be improved if samples are obtained from all parts of the area under surveillance, and from all age groups. In addition, the picture of the relative activity of different influenza viruses in an area may be influenced by the severity of the associated illness: a greater proportion of patients with infection due to a virus causing more severe illness are likely to be examined in hospital. Surveillance dependent primarily on samples originating in hospitalized patients may over-represent the occurrence of the virus causing more severe illness and under-represent a more common virus causing milder illness in the community (Claas *et al.* 1995). In general surveillance based predominantly on samples that derive from family practitioners is likely to give a more representative picture of the circulating viruses in the community, although the picture from hospitalized patients may give a better indication of those viruses causing more severe morbidity (de Jong *et al.* 1995; Watson *et al.* 1995).

'Direct virological surveillance' schemes have been employed in some countries to link the occurrence of clinical cases in epidemiological surveillance schemes to virological surveillance (Fleming *et al.* 1995). These schemes generally involve networks of family doctors who take samples for virus isolation from patients conforming to a surveillance case definition. Such schemes have proved valuable in assuring an early and continuous flow of specimens for viral isolation, but need to be large (and therefore expensive) if they are to produce results that can be considered to be representative of influenza activity in the whole population.

Despite these reservations, virological surveillance in many countries achieves its main objectives of providing isolates for examination at an early stage in and throughout the period of influenza activity, and provides an approximate indication of the relative size of influenza epidemics and their impact in different subgroups of the population. The value of this information is enhanced when combined with epidemiological surveillance.

Epidemiological surveillance

A wide range of indices has been used to monitor clinical influenza activity. Rates of consultations with general practitioners for illness that might be caused by influenza virus infection are monitored in many areas, and variations in weekly death rates, and associated causes, have been monitored for a century or more in some countries. Other non-specific indices of clinical influenza activity are employed in some countries including assessment of overall influenza activity in regions within a country by public health doctors, sickness absence among employed persons, illness rates among schoolchildren, rates of purchasing from pharmacies of remedies for colds and influenza symptoms, and indices of demand for hospital beds for acutely ill patients (Hutchinson *et al.* 1996; CDC 1997). Figures 18.1–18.3 show three indices of influenza activity (consultation rates for influenza-like illness, laboratory reports of influenza A infections, and deaths from all causes) for three contrasting

influenza seasons in England and Wales during which influenza A subtype H3N2 was the predominant virus: 1989/90, during which a major epidemic of influenza occurred associated with substantial mortality; 1993/94, during which a moderate epidemic occurred with only a limited impact on mortality; and 1995/96, during which influenza activity appeared more limited on the basis of general practitioner consultations, but was associated with substantial mortality and large numbers of laboratory identified infections.

Sentinel practitioner surveillance schemes

Many patients with illnesses that may be caused by influenza virus infection seek advice and treatment from general practitioners (family doctors), and schemes have been developed for monitoring the consultation rates with representative samples of practitioners in an area. Although simple in concept and sharing the same general aim, these schemes vary widely in the methods employed to monitor consultation rates (Hannoun *et al.* 1989; Palmer & Smith 1991; Szecsenyi *et al.* 1995; Boussard *et al.* 1996; Hutchinson *et al.* 1996). These variations, discussed below, mean that comparisons between the rates recorded by such schemes should be made with care although comparison from week to week, or year to year, within the same scheme is usually safe. The consultation rates for influenza-like illness in the 1995/96 influenza season in England (Royal College of General Practitioners), Wales and

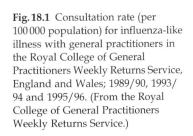

Fig. 18.1 Consultation rate (per 100 000 population) for influenza-like illness with general practitioners in the Royal College of General Practitioners Weekly Returns Service, England and Wales; 1989/90, 1993/94 and 1995/96. (From the Royal College of General Practitioners Weekly Returns Service.)

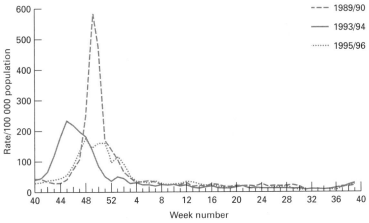

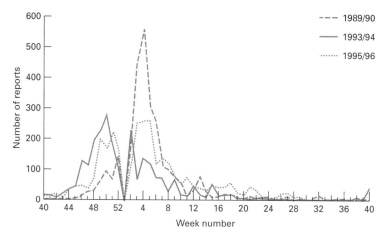

Fig. 18.2 Laboratory reports of influenza A infections in England and Wales, received by the PHLS Communicable Disease Surveillance Centre; 1989/90, 1993/94 and 1995/96 (includes diagnoses based on isolation, direct antigen detection and serology). (From PHLS data.)

Scotland are shown in Fig. 18.4. Although the severity of the epidemic was considered to be reasonably similar on the basis of comparison of local reports, the reported consultation rates in the sentinel practitioner schemes varied substantially.

Definitions

Some schemes invite participating practitioners to report cases of influenza relying on individual clinical judgement to determine what constitutes a case of influenza. Others offer diagnostic guidelines or written case definitions. In an ideal surveillance system, a consistent definition of a case for reporting should be used but influenza poses special problems in this regard because of the non-specific nature of the symptoms, particularly in certain

groups such as the very young or very old. No single definition is both sufficiently sensitive and specific for all surveillance purposes.

Denominators

The type of denominator used to produce consultation rates varies according to the organization of the local health service. In some countries the size of the population covered by each sentinel practitioner is known, and rates can be calculated per 100 000 population. In other schemes, where medical practitioners do not provide care for a defined population, consultation rates for influenza-like illness are estimated as a proportion of consultations for all causes, or as consultation rates per participating sentinel practitioner.

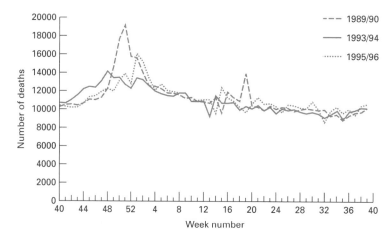

Fig. 18.3 Weekly number of deaths from all causes, England and Wales; 1989/90, 1993/94 and 1995/96. (From the Office for National Statistics, London.)

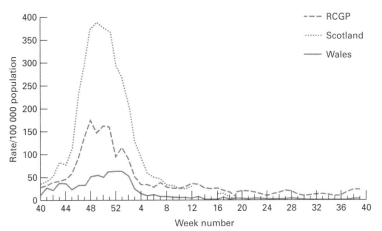

Fig. 18.4 Consultation rate (per 100 000 population) for influenza-like illness with general practitioners in England, Wales and Scotland in 1995/96. (From the Royal College of General Practitioners Weekly Returns Service, Communicable Disease Surveillance Centre Welsh Unit and Scottish Centre for Infection and Environmental Health.)

Reporting method

In some schemes, all patients consulting a doctor are recorded with a diagnostic label and consequently 'influenza-like illness' may be only one of a range of diagnoses which may also include other acute respiratory illnesses. In other schemes, influenza is the sole focus of the surveillance and only consultations by patients considered to have an influenza-like illness prompt a report. In the former type of scheme, a steady trickle of patients with influenza-like illness may be reported throughout the year with a clearly evident increase during periods of established influenza virus activity. In the latter type of scheme, influenza-like illness may be reported only rarely during most of the year, with a very large increase in reporting during periods when influenza virus is known to be active. If the reporting scheme involves an additional albeit small workload, 'reporting fatigue' may be apparent during periods when excessive influenza case loads reduces the time available for reporting.

Representativeness

The number of sentinel practitioners in a reporting scheme (in relation to the size of the population covered), their geographical distribution, the demography of the population from which they draw patients (e.g. age distribution, presence of conditions predisposing to the complications of influenza infection) and the local influenza vaccine coverage rates, may all influence the representativeness of the results of influenza surveillance from a sentinel scheme and its applicability to the population as a whole. Most sentinel practitioner schemes appear to give a sufficiently robust indication for most purposes of overall levels of influenza-like illness in the population covered, but care needs to be taken when extrapolating from results in subgroups by, for example, geographical region or age group.

The data from sentinel schemes are particularly valuable for monitoring trends in activity, particularly when linked with virological data from the same population and other indicators of clinical activity. Further benefit, including the possibility of early warning of epidemics, is derived from the pooling of information derived from clinical and virological surveillance between countries as in the collaborative project between a growing number of European countries (Snacken *et al.* 1995; Fleming & Cohen 1996).

Mortality surveillance

Influenza virus infection may lead to death as a result of the primary infection, bacterial superinfection, or exacerbation of an underlying chronic condition. The most readily identifiable deaths attributable to influenza are those in which influenza is indicated as a contributory cause on the death certificate but, even during periods of known influenza virus activity, this cause of death is relatively infrequently cited not least because virological investigation confirming influenza infection is rarely carried out. Deaths from respiratory causes increase sharply during periods of influenza activity and are consistent with the well-recognized occurrence of bacterial super-infection (Langmuir & Housworth 1969). However, even assessment of the number of excess respiratory deaths at times of influenza virus activity will underestimate the true burden due to the infection as half or more of the excess deaths are attributed to other causes including a range of cardiac conditions (e.g. acute myocardial infarction, heart failure) cerebrovascular conditions (e.g. cerebrovascular accidents) and other conditions (e.g. diabetic ketoacidosis) (Curwen *et al.* 1990).

In countries where information on total mortality, or mortality by cause, is available for the whole population (or a representative sample) of the population on a weekly basis within a few weeks of the week in question, monitoring mortality may provide timely data on the impact of the current epidemic in a population (CDC 1997). More often, however, this impact is determined retrospectively (Clifford *et al.* 1977).

Excess mortality due to influenza is calculated by estimating a baseline representing the number of deaths that would be expected in the absence of influenza virus activity, and the number of deaths actually observed. The estimates of excess deaths obtained depend heavily on the methods used to estimate the number of expected deaths and the period over which the excess is estimated (Tillett *et al.* 1991). In addition, the occurrence of other factors, such as low or changing ambient atmospheric temperature and the presence of non-influenza respiratory virus activity should be taken into account. Comparison of excess deaths between different influenza seasons or different countries should be made, where possible, using the same methods.

Other non-specific indicators of influenza activity

The dramatic nature of influenza epidemics and their effect on the functioning of a significant pro-

portion of a population at any one time means that some non-specific indicators reflect, surprisingly well, the level of influenza activity in a community (Dedman *et al.* 1994). Sickness absence records are monitored in some countries, or subgroups within a country, and while a proportion of employees would be expected to be off sick at any one time, the proportion absent rises sharply during influenza epidemics. This indicator, however, reflects exclusively the occurrence of illness among the working age population and provides no indication of the impact in children and the elderly people.

Collaborative schemes with schools, monitoring either school absence generally, or sickness absence due to influenza-like illness specifically, may give a clear indication of the occurrence of influenza in children, and may also provide especially timely warning in the occurrence in the population generally as infection in children may precede that in their families and other adult contacts.

Demand for hospital beds for acutely ill patients is monitored in London by the Emergency Bed Service. Although there is a constant demand for beds for ill patients which rises during the winter, rapid rises at periods of especially heavy demand are seen during influenza epidemics.

Timeliness of influenza surveillance information

The process of collection and collation of information on influenza activity inevitably leads to a delay between the onset of influenza illness and the availability of data demonstrating an increase. Sentinel practitioner schemes generally provide the most timely data: consultations for influenza-like illnesses during a particular week may be reported at the end of the same week, aggregated over the next few days and the information disseminated by the end of the subsequent week. Information from virological surveillance may be more delayed as, following the consultation of the patient and specimen collection, the specimen needs to be processed and the results reported. Isolation of influenza viruses from clinical specimens generally takes a few days and may take a week or more. Information on mortality may be the most delayed:

a patient becoming ill with influenza may develop a secondary infection after a number of days or weeks, and may die some days or weeks after that; following death, registration of the cause of death may take a few days, and the collation of information on death registration may involve a further delay. Hence increased mortality in a community as a result of influenza may not be apparent in mortality statistics for a month or more after the increase in influenza activity.

Despite these delays in 'official' statistics, individual communities and the news media that serve them, are often aware at an early stage of increasing influenza illness and can provide a useful early warning of increasing influenza virus activity in the population generally (Hunt 1995).

Epidemic definitions and thresholds

Epidemics exist when the number of cases of a disease exceeds the number expected (Last 1988). On this basis influenza epidemics can be said to occur at some point every year in countries with temperate climates as some influenza virus activity is invariably detected but its timing cannot be predicted. However, in some years the level of influenza activity is low by comparison to the years when well-recognized epidemics have occurred. Consequently, the formal definition of influenza has little practical relevance for describing current, or past, influenza activity for the purposes of public health action or public/press information. Nevertheless there is a need for terms to describe levels of influenza activity that can be used to trigger public health action as well as inform a wider audience. The term epidemic is used widely in this context but needs to be clearly defined if it is to be useful and used consistently.

Various approaches to defining 'epidemic' influenza have been adopted. In the USA, an epidemic threshold for mortality is based on estimates of the expected number of deaths in a given week along with 95% confidence limits around this estimate (CDC 1997). Epidemic activity is reported to be occurring when the upper 95% confidence limit is exceeded. In Britain a simpler approach has been adopted based on retrospective assessment of the impact of previous epidemics: using indices based on sentinel practitioner consultation rates, thresholds have been used to indicate 'baseline activity', 'normal seasonal activity', 'higher than expected seasonal activity' and 'epidemic activity' (Anonymous 1997). In this British example the term epidemic has been reserved for relatively high levels of influenza activity. Although the thresholds selected reflect levels at which health authorities and other providers of health care may usefully be warned of current influenza activity and the need to take preparatory action, the selection of these thresholds is essentially arbitrary.

References

Anonymous (1979) Influenza: the WHO programme. *WHO Chronicle* **33**, 7–8.

Anonymous (1997) News media are the first to catch influenza. *Communicable Dis Rep* **7**, 1–4.

Betts, R.F. (1995) Influenza virus. In: Mandell, G.L., Bennett, J.E. & Dolin, R (eds) *Mandell, Douglas and Bennett's Principles and Practice of Infectious Diseases*, 4th edn, pp. 1546–67. Churchill Livingstone, New York.

Boussard, E., Flahault, A., Vibert, J. & Valleron, A. (1996) Sentiweb: French communicable disease surveillance on the world wide web. *Br Med J* **313**, 1381–2.

CDC (1997) Update: influenza activity—United States and worldwide, 1996–97 season, and composition of the 1997–98 influenza vaccine. *MMWR* **46**, 325–30.

Claas, E.J., de Jong, J.C., Bartelds, A.I.M. *et al.* (1995) Influenza types and patient population. *Lancet* **346**, 180.

Clifford, R.E., Smith, J.W.G., Tillett, H.E. & Wherry, P.J. (1977) Excess mortality associated with influenza in England and Wales. *Int J Epidemiol* **6**, 115–28.

Curwen, M., Dunnell, K. & Ashley, J. (1990) Hidden influenza deaths: 1989–90. *Pop Trends* **Autumn**, 31–3.

de Jong, J.C., Claas, E.C.J. & Osterhaus, A.D.M.E. (1995) Influenza types and patient population. *Lancet* **346**, 1713–14.

Dedman, D.J., Joseph, C.A., Chakraverty, P., Fleming, D.M. & Watson, J.M. (1994) Influenza surveillance, England and Wales: October 1993 to June 1994. *Communicable Dis Rep* **4**, R164–8.

Fleming, D.M., Chakraverty, P., Sadler, C. & Litton, P. (1995) Combined clinical and virological surveillance of influenza in winters of 1992 and 1993–4. *Br Med J* **311**, 290–1.

Fleming, D.M. & Cohen, J.M. (1996) Experience of European collaboration in influenza surveillance in the winter of 1993–94. *J Public Health Med* **18**, 133–42.

Fleming, D.M. & Cross, K.W. (1993) Respiratory syncytial virus or influenza? *Lancet* **342**, 1507–10.

Hampson, A.W. & Cox, N.J. (1996) Global surveillance for pandemic influenza: are we prepared? In: Brown, L.E., Hampson, A.W. & Webster, R.G. (eds) *Options for the Control of Influenza*, Vol. 3. Elsevier, Amsterdam.

Hannoun, C., Dab, W. & Cohen, J.M. (1989) A new influenza surveillance system in France: the Ile-de-France 'Grog'. 1. Principles and methodology. *Eur J Epidemiol* **5**, 285–93.

Hope-Simpson, R.E. (1992) *The Transmission of Epidemic Influenza*. Plenum Press, New York.

Hunt, L. (1995) Epidemic fear as flu outbreak gains momentum. *Independent* (1 Dec).

Hutchinson, E.J., Joseph, C.A., Zambon, M., Fleming, D.M. & Watson, J.M. (1996) Influenza surveillance in England and Wales: October 1995 to June 1996. *Communicable Dis Rep* **6**, R163–9.

Kilbourne, E.D. (1987) *Influenza*. Plenum, New York.

Langmuir, A.D. & Housworth, J. (1969) A critical evaluation of influenza surveillance. *Bull WHO* **41**, 393–8.

Last, J.M. (1988) *A Dictionary of Epidemiology*. Oxford University Press, Oxford.

Monto, A.S. & Sullivan, K.M. (1993) Acute respiratory illness in the community. Frequency of illness and the agents involved. *Epidemiol Infect* **110**, 145–60.

Nicholson, K.G. (1996) Impact of influenza and respiratory syncytial virus on mortality in England and Wales from January 1975 to December 1990. *Epidemiol Infect* **116**, 51–63.

Palmer, S.R. & Smith, R.M.M. (1991) GP surveillance of infections in Wales. *Communicable Dis Rep* **1**, R25–8.

Snacken, R., Bensadon, M. & Strauss, A. (1995) The CARE Telematics Network for the surveillance of influenza in Europe. *Meth Inform Med* **34**, 1–5.

Szecsenyi, J., Uphoff, H., Ley, S. & Brede, H. (1995) Influenza surveillance: experiences from establishing a sentinel surveillance system in Germany. *J Epidemiol Commun Health* **49**, 9–13.

Thompson, T. (1852) *Anonymous Annals of Influenza in Great Britain 1510–1837*. Sydenham Society, London.

Tillett, H.E., Nicholas, S. & Watson, J.M. (1991) Unusual pattern of influenza mortality in 1989/90 (letter). *Lancet* **338**, 1590–1.

Tillett, H.E., Smith, J.W.G. & Clifford, R.E. (1980) Excess morbidity and mortality associated with influenza in England and Wales. *Lancet* **i**, 793–5.

Van Hartesveldt, F.R. (1992) *The 1918–19 Pandemic of Influenza: The Urban Impact in the Western World*. Edwin Mellen Press, Lewiston.

Watson, J.M., Dedman, D., Joseph, C., Zambon, M. & Timbury, M.C. (1995) Influenza types and patient population (letter). *Lancet* **346**, 515–16.

Westmoreland, D., Player, V. & Weymont, G. (1989) Simple samples for diagnosing influenza (letter). *J Infect* **18**, 196–8.

Section 5
Human Influenza

CHAPTER 19

Human Influenza

Karl G. Nicholson

Introduction

Influenza is the name given to an acute, febrile respiratory illness of global importance caused by A, B and C serotypes of influenza viruses. The origin of the name 'influenza' is uncertain, although the chronicles of a Florentine family used it in reference to the possible influence of the planets at times of respiratory epidemics (Stuart-Harris & Schild 1976). The term 'influenza' was used in England during the outbreak of 1743 (Francis 1953), and earlier references to influenzal illness include 'newe acquayantance', the gentle correction, epidemic catarrh, or catarrhal fever (Francis 1953; Creighton 1965). Influenza has no pathognomonic features so a precise picture of its impact was impossible before the first isolations of influenza A in 1933 (Smith *et al.* 1933), influenza B in 1940 (Francis 1940; Magill 1940) and influenza C in 1947 (Taylor 1949). Further knowledge of the illness came with the discovery of the haemagglutinating properties of influenza virus in 1941 (Hirst 1941) and development of diagnostic methods based on haemagglutination inhibition. However, in the absence of these tools, a combination of the explosive nature of influenza, its respiratory and systemic features, its tendency for seasonality, and its high attack rates and associated mortality in people of advanced age provides an insight into influenza since ancient times.

Influenza in man occurs in two epidemiological forms (Table 19.1). The first is pandemic influenza which results from the emergence of a new influenza A virus—termed antigenic shift—to which the population possesses little or no immunity. It therefore normally spreads with high attack rates throughout all parts of the world. The second is interpandemic influenza, occurring as sporadic infections, a localized outbreak or epidemic, the latter representing an outbreak in a given community which usually occurs abruptly, peaks within 2–3 weeks, lasts 5–6 weeks, and is associated with significant 'drift' of the surface antigens. Epidemics occur virtually every year almost exclusively in the 'winter' months in the northern hemisphere (October to April), and in May to September in the southern hemisphere. Virological, sero-archaeological and molecular studies have revealed that although all 15 haemagglutinin and nine neuraminidase subtypes of influenza A have been isolated from birds in most probable combinations, only a limited number (see Chapter 11) have caused outbreaks in man. This chapter describes the transmission of human influenza, and its clinical features, complications, risk factors and pathology.

Transmission

Influenza is spread by virus-laden respiratory secretions from an infected to a susceptible person. Most influenza infections appear to be transmitted by droplets several microns in diameter that are expelled during coughing and sneezing, rather than by fine-droplet nuclei (Alford *et al.* 1966; Moser *et al.* 1979). Emphasis has also been given to large-particle droplets ($>5\,\mu m$) as an important mode of transmission, and direct or indirect contact is another mode of transmission (Tablan *et al.* 1994). Influenza virus may survive drying at room

Table 19.1 Comparison of pandemic and interpandemic influenza.

Type of influenza	Cause	Immune status of population	Outcome
Pandemic	Antigenic 'shift' resulting in emergence of a new or recycled subtype of influenza A virus	Partial immunity of the elderly if 'recycling' has occurred, otherwise little or no immunity	Usually high attack rates, with high morbidity and mortality in all parts of the world, especially during first to third waves of infection
Interpandemic	Antigenic 'drift' of existing strains of influenza A or B	Crossreacting antibody in much of the population induced by recent antigenic variants; little or no immunity in infants	Variable attack rates, resulting in sporadic infections, outbreaks or epidemics with variable morbidity and mortality. Young children are especially vulnerable

temperature for some days and has been demonstrated to survive in dust for up to a fortnight (Edward 1941). The human infectious dose 50 (HID_{50}) of influenza A virus was 127–320 tissue culture infectious dose 50s ($TCID_{50}$) for virus administered by nosedrops (Couch *et al.* 1971, 1974), but significantly less, 0.6–3.0 $TCID_{50}$, for virus delivered by aerosol (Alford *et al.* 1966). These studies were carried out in different laboratories with different strains of influenza virus and it is questionable whether infectivity is greater in the lung than in the nasopharynx. More recent studies in adults with haemagglutination inhibition titres of $\leq 1:8$ found that intranasal inoculation of $\sim 10^3$, 10^5, and 10^7 $TCID_{50}$ of A/Texas/91 (H1N1) caused infections in 50%, 75% and 80%, respectively (Hayden *et al.* 1996), and $\sim 10^7$ $TCID_{50}$ of A/Kawasaki (H1N1) infected 100% (Skoner *et al.* 1996). Pathological evidence suggests initial or early involvement of pulmonary alveolar cells, a site only accessible to droplets up to 5 μ in diameter.

Replication and shedding

It is considered that infection begins in the tracheobronchial epithelium and then spreads. Lesions have been identified in the tracheo-bronchial mucosa in bronchoscopic biopsies from young adults with uncomplicated Asian influenza (Walsh *et al.* 1961) which correspond with, but are not so severe as, those found in the trachea and bronchi of fatal cases (Hers 1966). Histological studies of fatal cases, nasal exudate cells and tracheal biopsies indicate that virus replication may occur throughout the entire respiratory tract (Liu 1956; Hers *et al.* 1957; Louria *et al.* 1959; Lindsay *et al.* 1970), the principal site of infection occurring in ciliated columnar epithelial cells (Hers 1966; Walsh *et al.* 1961).

In vitro studies suggest that the cycle of replication takes about 4 hours. Thereafter virus is released for several hours before cell death and progeny virions initiate infection in adjacent cells, so that within a short period many cells in the respiratory tract are either infected, releasing virus or dying. The pattern of virus replication in relation to clinical symptoms and immune responses has been studied by several investigators. Virus can be detected shortly before the onset of illness, usually within 24 hours, rises to a peak of 10^3–10^7 $TCID_{50}$/ml of nasopharyngeal wash, remains elevated for 24–72 hours, and falls to low levels by the fifth day (Murphy *et al.* 1973). In young children virus shedding at high titres is generally more prolonged and virus can be recovered up to 6 days before and 21 days after the onset of symptoms (Hall & Douglas 1975; Frank *et al.* 1981; Hall *et al.* 1979). In adults the amount of virus shedding is related to the severity of illness and temperature elevation and is also affected by immunosuppression.

Attempts to demonstrate viraemia have been inconclusive—a few investigators have demonstrated viraemia, even before the onset of symptoms (Naficy 1963; Stanley & Jackson 1966; Khakpour *et al.* 1969), but others have been unsuccessful (Kilbourne 1959; Minuse *et al.* 1962; Morris *et al.* 1966). Nonetheless influenza virus has occasionally been identified in the heart and brain, and it can cross the placenta.

The incubation period of influenza ranges from 1 to 7 days but is commonly 2–3. This short period coupled with the relatively high titres in nasopharyngeal secretions, the fairly lengthy periods of virus shedding (especially in children), and the relatively small amounts necessary to initiate infection in susceptible individuals explains the explosive nature of influenza outbreaks.

Clinical features

The spectrum of influenza is extremely broad ranging from asymptomatic infection; through respiratory illness with systemic features; multisystem complications affecting the lung, heart, brain, liver, kidneys and muscle; to death, most commonly due to primary viral or secondary bacterial pneumonia. The clinical outcome may be influenced by a number of potentially confounding factors including the age of the patient, prior infection with an antigenically related strain, intrinsic properties of the virus (e.g. whether influenza A H1N1 or H3N2 or influenza B, and possibly the adaptation of newly emerged pandemic strains to man), the presence of chronic medical conditions such as heart or lung disease, renal failure and disorders of immunity, and also pregnancy and smoking. Thus the incidence of clinical features and complications may vary from one cohort to another.

Review of previous descriptions of 'influenza' reveals many instances of selection bias with writers focusing mostly on febrile patients with a typical 'influenzal' illness during a known outbreak, or on seriously ill cases in hospital. Reports that lack virological confirmation of the diagnosis (e.g. cases during the 1918/19 pandemic) will also include patients with other respiratory viral infections or bacterial pneumonia. Nonetheless it is remarkable how little the clinical descriptions of 'influenza'

have varied over decades of observation. Indeed, it has been said: 'Epidemics come and epidemics go, but the clinical picture of influenza remains remarkably unchanged' (Stuart-Harris 1961); and 'Influenza ... is an unvarying disease ... caused by a varying virus' (Kilbourne 1973). While reviews of the older literature generally support this view it is now accepted that influenza is quite protean in its manifestations. Influenza cannot be distinguished readily on clinical grounds from other acute respiratory infections, and during virologically confirmed outbreaks of influenza the proportion of influenzal illnesses confirmed by laboratory tests as being influenza is currently about half.

Adults

Influenza A

The symptoms recorded during 10 studies of adults with uncomplicated virologically confirmed influenza A during the period 1937–1992 are shown in Fig. 19.1 (Jordan *et al.* 1958; Burch *et al.* 1959; Stuart-Harris 1961; Lindsay *et al.* 1970; Gaydos *et al.* 1977; Ksiazek *et al.* 1980; Mathur *et al.* 1980; Wright *et al.* 1980; Weingarten *et al.* 1988; Wald *et al.* 1995). Descriptions of uncomplicated 'influenza' during the pandemics in 1889/90 and 1918 also reveal clinical pictures similar to those in Fig. 19.1 with wide variations in the reported frequency of symptoms (Bristowe 1890; Preston 1890; Robertson & Elkins 1890; Influenza Committee of the Advisory Board to the D.G.M.S., France 1918; Martin 1918; Wirgman 1918). Review of the syndromes due to H1N1, Hsw1N1, H2N2, and H3N2 strains of influenza reveals no important differences, but the frequency of symptoms in Fig. 19.1 can be seen to vary considerably from report to report. Comparative studies carried out during the late 1970s and early 1980s suggest that H3N2 infections produce more severe illness than H1N1 (Wright *et al.* 1980; Frank *et al.* 1985; Monto *et al.* 1985) and that influenza B is intermediate in severity between H3N2 and H1N1 (Monto *et al.* 1985).

The onset of illness due to influenza A is typically abrupt after an incubation period of several days. Systemic features are often evident at the onset and

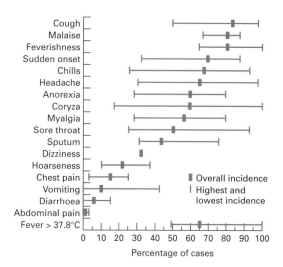

Fig. 19.1 Overall incidence and the highest and lowest incidence of symptoms recorded during 10 studies of 520 adults with virologically confirmed uncomplicated influenza A during the period 1937–1992. Data from: Jordan *et al.* 1958; Burch *et al.* 1959; Stuart-Harris 1961; Lindsay *et al.* 1970; Gaydos *et al.* 1977; Ksiazek *et al.* 1980; Mathur *et al.* 1980; Wright *et al.* 1980; Weingarten *et al.* 1988; Wald *et al.* 1995).

include malaise and feverishness, chills, headache, anorexia, myalgia affecting the back and limbs, and dizziness (Fig. 19.1). The early systemic features are usually accompanied by a non-productive cough, nasal discharge or obstruction and sneezing, and less frequently by productive cough, hoarseness and substernal soreness. Photophobia and other ocular symptoms including lacrimation, burning and pain on moving the eyes occur in up to a fifth of cases. Vomiting is reported in 10% of virologically confirmed cases, diarrhoea is a feature in ~6% and abdominal pain is seldom reported. During the 'Asian' influenza pandemic, headache and sore throat were the most frequent initial symptoms, and headache, myalgia and cough were usually the most troublesome (Woodall *et al.* 1958).

Fever is the most prominent sign of infection and although it was as high as 41 °C in about a quarter of cases during the pandemic in 1957 it is more commonly 38–40 °C (Jordan *et al.* 1958). The pyrexia peaks at the height of systemic features and is typically of 3 days' duration but may last for 1–5 days. Clinical examination often reveals a toxic

appearance early in the course of the illness: the skin is often hot and moist, the face appears flushed, the eyes may have a glistening, injected, sometimes weepy appearance, the mucous membranes of the nose and pharynx are hyperaemic and devoid of an exudate, and breathing may appear labored with a clear nasal discharge or blocked nose. Small, tender, cervical lymph nodes are palpable in about 10–15% of cases and crackles and/or wheezing are heard in ~10% (Jordan *et al.* 1958; Burch *et al.* 1959; Lindsay *et al.* 1970). This constellation of symptoms and signs typically persists for 3–4 days, but cough, lassitude and malaise may persist for 1–2 weeks after the fever has settled. These features relate to a typical case, but infection is often subclinical. Alternatively it may present as a common cold, pharyngitis or tracheobronchitis, or as a systemic illness without respiratory features or with one or more complications.

Influenza B and C

Because of the greater antigenic stability of the surface glycoproteins of influenza B in comparison with influenza A, illness due to influenza B tends to occur mostly in younger age groups, particularly school-age children (Chin *et al.* 1963; Clark *et al.* 1970; Monto & Kioumehr 1975; Retailliau *et al.* 1979). It is clinically indistinguishable from influenza A (Jackson 1946; Burnet *et al.* 1946; Finland *et al.* 1948; Clark *et al.* 1970).

Comparatively little is known of the manifestations of influenza C. Antibody to the virus is widespread among adults (Davenport *et al.* 1953; Hilleman *et al.* 1953; Broun *et al.* 1960; Jennings 1968), but evidence of influenza C among subjects with typical influenzal symptoms has seldom been reported (Andrews & McDonald 1955; Dykes *et al.* 1980; Katagiri *et al.* 1983). Influenza C is a cause of the 'common cold' (Dykes *et al.* 1980); occasionally it is associated with bronchitis and pneumonia in both adults and children (Grist 1955; Moriuchi *et al.* 1991).

Infants and children

Most studies of the symptoms of influenza have focused on hospitalized children and thus emphasize the more severe aspects of infection. Although the manifestations of influenza A in infants and children are similar to those in adults—the onset usually being sudden with fever, headache, cough and sore throat as the most common complaints (Podosin & Felton 1958; Woodall *et al.* 1958)—some differences are apparent. Maximal temperatures tend to be higher among children (Jordan *et al.* 1958; Monto *et al.* 1985) though not in young infants (Paisley *et al.* 1978); and among hospital admissions of children less than 5 years of age febrile convulsions are especially prominent, occurring in more than 20% of all children hospitalized with influenza in seven studies (Taylor *et al.* 1967; Brocklebank *et al.* 1972; Kerr *et al.* 1975; Price *et al.* 1976; Paisley *et al.* 1978; Olsen *et al.* 1992; Sugaya *et al.* 1992). Among hospital admissions there is a relative prominence of otitis media and gastrointestinal manifestations, notably abdominal pain, diarrhoea and vomiting, especially in children aged 6 months or less (Jordan *et al.* 1958; Woodall *et al.* 1958; Brocklebank *et al.* 1972; Kerr *et al.* 1975; Price *et al.* 1976; Heikkinen *et al.* 1991).

Infection in hospitalized neonates often presents non-specifically with lethargy, poor feeding and apnoea (Meibalane *et al.* 1977), unexplained fever or pneumonia (Glezen *et al.* 1980), while in hospitalized infants influenza can present as croup or bronchiolitis (Brocklebank *et al.* 1972; Kim *et al.* 1979). Kim *et al.* (1979) associated influenza virus infection with more than 5% of admissions to a children's hospital for acute respiratory tract illness and showed that 14.3% of 860 patients with croup had influenza. In the community, the incidence of drowsiness associated with influenza decreases with increasing age from about 50% in children less than 4 years of age to about 10% in children 5–14 years of age, and is uncommon in adults (Woodall *et al.* 1958). In contrast, myalgia, sweats, sputum production and other lower respiratory symptoms are more common in adults than in children (Jordan *et al.* 1958; Monto *et al.* 1985).

Infants beyond the age when passively acquired antibody provides protection and those with congenital abnormalities are at particular risk from the complications of influenza (Brocklebank *et al.* 1972; Bauer *et al.* 1973; Hall & Douglas 1975). A review of

15 fatalities occurring among children hospitalized with influenza reveals that 10 of the children had congenital abnormalities, nine out of 14 (whose age was reported) were ≤ 3 years of age, and only three fatalities occurred in previously well children ≥ 4 years of age (Taylor *et al.* 1967; Brocklebank *et al.* 1972; Kerr *et al.* 1975; Price *et al.* 1976; Paisley *et al.* 1978; Glezen *et al.* 1980; Armstrong *et al.* 1991). The overall fatality rate among children hospitalized with proven influenza in the above reports and those described by Sugaya *et al.* (1992) was 3.8% (15 out of 392).

The incidence and nature of complications and the risk of hospital admission have been studied in the community. X-ray evidence of pneumonia was found in 26 out of 504 (5.1%) symptomatic children with 'Asian' influenza (Podosin & Felton 1958), and five (8%) of 121 young seronegative children developed clinical and X-ray evidence of pneumonia during an outbreak of H3N2 influenza in 1974 (Wright *et al.* 1977). Otitis media occurred during 4.2% of 616 symptomatic infections with 'Asian' influenza and exacerbations of asthma occurred during 4.1% (Podosin & Felton 1958). The risk of hospital admission for children less than 5 years of age in Harris County, Texas, was estimated to be 6.9 per 1000 during the A/Victoria/75 outbreak, 1976 (Glezen 1982). Review of three later epidemics (H1N1, H3N2 and influenza B) in Harris County identified hospitalization rates of at least 5 per 1000 regardless of the type of influenza virus (Perrotta *et al.* 1985). Given the overall mortality rate of about 4% for paediatric admissions with influenza, these hospitalization rates suggest that epidemics of influenza A and B result in the death of ~1 in 5000 infants in the community.

Influenza in risk groups

Certain complications of influenza are unique to particular risk groups (e.g. diabetic ketoacidosis in patients with diabetes, asthma exacerbations in asthmatics) whereas other groups are at a generally increased risk of symptomatic illness and serious morbidity and mortality from influenza (e.g. smokers and those with chronic heart and lung disease). Because of the increase in morbidity and mortality from influenza associated with the following 'risk factors', most are incorporated in national recommendations to receive annual vaccination against influenza.

Vascular disease

Studies of influenza pandemics and epidemics indicate that they are accompanied by considerable increases in mortality from certain chronic disorders. During the 1889–1890 influenza pandemic in Paris, for example, certified deaths from 'paralysis' increased 2.5-fold in comparison with the average number in the same period during the 3 previous years (Parsons 1891). Cardiac deaths increased 1.8-fold. During the period 1921–1933 Stocks (1935) identified a slight increase in central nervous system deaths during epidemics, especially those due to 'cerebral haemorrhage'. In addition, study of excess mortality in the USA from 1957 to 1966 revealed significant excesses of deaths from arteriosclerotic heart disease during all eight epidemic periods (Housworth & Langmuir 1974).

An insight into the role of influenza in causing cardiac events was recently provided by a large cohort study of the effectiveness of influenza vaccine (Nichol *et al.* 1996). Among elderly people 65 years of age or older, influenza vaccine resulted in a mean reduction of 28.6% in congestive heart failure hospitalizations during the three seasons 1990–91 to 1992–93. Prompted by observations that within the first few days of influenza being recognized in the community the number of admissions for acute myocardial infarction began to increase, Bainton *et al.* (1978) studied the number of deaths from ischaemic heart disease at the time of influenza, during the period 1953–1973, and allowed for changes in temperature. Deaths from ischaemic heart disease were found to be increased at all ages during influenza outbreaks. Vullers *et al.* (1980) related influenza to heart attacks in five men aged 53–75 years and considered influenza to be an important risk factor for myocardial infarction. A study by Bondarenko and Tumanov (1992) suggests that one in two patients with influenza pneumonia who have a prior history of myocardial infarction may develop further cardiac complications.

Respiratory conditions

Asthma

In normal individuals with uncomplicated influenza, pulmonary function tests have revealed frequent airway hyperreactivity, peripheral airway dysfunction and abnormalities in gas exchange that can persist for some weeks after clinical recovery (Johanson *et al.* 1969; Horner & Gray 1973; Hall *et al.* 1976). However, no changes in bronchial reactivity to inhaled methacholine occurred in healthy subjects with and without allergic rhinitis who were inoculated intranasally with influenza A/Kawasaki (H1N1) virus (Skoner *et al.* 1996).

Bendkowski (1958), a general practitioner, compared the incidence of respiratory complications in 124 patients with allergies (of whom 55 had asthma), 59 non-allergic individuals—but who came from allergic families, and 161 non-allergic cases. Bendkowski noted that bronchitis with asthma complicated 47 (38%) of the 124 'influenzal' infections in the allergic group and clinical improvement was slow; only one of the 230 infections in the 'non-allergic' group resulted in an episode of asthma. Bendkowski's data show that the incidence of pneumonia in the allergic group (14/124, 11%) was higher than in those without a history of allergy (9/230, 4%; $p < 0.02$), suggesting that influenzal pneumonia may be more common in people with allergy. Interestingly Podosin and Felton (1958) showed that among boy scouts with Asian influenza the incidence of pulmonary infiltrates or bronchial markings was higher ($p < 0.001$) in asthmatics (8/27) than in non-asthmatics (38/504).

Influenza virus infections have consistently precipitated attacks of wheezing in asthmatic children and adults—for example, a study by Minor *et al.* (1976), which involved 41 children aged 3–17 years and eight adults with a history of 'infectious' asthma, showed that 55% of all respiratory infections precipitated asthma. Five patients had influenza A infections and four of these (80%) were associated with asthma. Kondo and Abe (1991) studied the time course of influenza-induced asthma in a residential asthma clinic from 5 days before to 10 days after onset of influenza A and B infection in 20 asthmatic children in Japan from 1978 to 1985. Fifteen (75%) children had a decrease in forced expiratory volume in one second (FEV_1) of more than 20% from baseline during the acute stage. The FEV_1 continuously dropped on the second day, when the mean decrease in FEV_1 was maximal at –30.3%, and returned to within 10% difference on the seventh to tenth day. Exacerbations associated with influenza A and B were comparable, and the time course of decline in FEV_1 was similar to that reported by Roldaan and Masural (1982) who observed declines in FEV_1 ranging from 55 to 75% in three children with influenza A.

Such exacerbations are not uncommon. During a 16-month study of the role of microbial agents in acute exacerbations of asthma, Gbadero *et al.* (1995) reviewed young children in hospital in an urban tropical setting in Nigeria and found influenza type A infection in 12 out of 74 (16%) exacerbations. Rhinovirus studies were not undertaken, but other respiratory viruses were identified in 53% of exacerbations. These findings underscore the importance of viral upper respiratory infections, including influenza, in asthma exacerbations in the tropical setting. In adults, almost 50% of upper respiratory tract viral infections in asthmatics are associated with exacerbations, and a similar percentage of asthmatic episodes are associated with a virus, chiefly rhinoviruses and coronaviruses, but also influenza (Nicholson *et al.* 1993).

Severe epidemics of influenza result in a small but significant excess mortality attributed to asthma. Housworth & Langmuir (1974) studied asthma excess mortality during seven periods of influenza activity between 1957 and 1966. Asthma deaths increased by 19–46% during influenza A outbreaks in 1957, 1958, 1960 and 1963, but were either insignificant or barely significant during the milder epidemics with some influenza B activity. During the worst period, excess mortality from asthma increased by an estimated 3.8 per million population.

Chronic obstructive airways disease

Between a quarter and two-thirds of exacerbations of chronic obstructive airways disease are asso-

ciated with viruses, and data collated from several studies has revealed serological evidence of influenza A and B infection in up to 28% of exacerbations (Carilli *et al.* 1964; Eadie *et al.* 1966; Grist 1967; Lamy *et al.* 1973; Buscho *et al.* 1978). The association between influenza and deaths from chronic bronchitis was recognized during the 19th century and was highlighted by Stocks (1935) who showed that deaths from chronic bronchitis increased by up to 52% during epidemics from 1921 to 1933. Smith *et al.* (1980) examined the hypothesis that respiratory viral infections may contribute to the progressive deterioration of airways function in chronic bronchitis. They studied 100 separate respiratory viral infections in 84 patients over an 8-year period. A transient decline in pulmonary function followed some viral infections and the greatest deterioration followed infection with influenza.

Cystic fibrosis

Recent studies have highlighted the role of respiratory viral infections in deterioration of pulmonary function, bacterial colonization and disease progression in patients with cystic fibrosis (Wang *et al.* 1984; Hordvik *et al.* 1989; Smyth *et al.* 1995; Collinson *et al.* 1996). Respiratory viral infections including influenza precede 18–38% of pulmonary exacerbations (Wright *et al.* 1976; Ong *et al.* 1989; Pribble *et al.* 1990). During a 2-month period, January–February, Wright *et al.* (1976) identified influenza A in association with three out of 18 (17%) 'major' exacerbations. During an 8-month period, October–May 1978, Petersen *et al.* (1981) found that about one in 25 (4%) exacerbations were caused by influenza A or B, but these investigators relied upon the relatively insensitive complement fixation test. Pribble *et al.* (1990) examined the role of viruses in 71 exacerbations between September 1986 and April 1987, but paired serological specimens were available for only 40 exacerbations. Influenza A and B were identified in nine, indicating that influenza was implicated in at least 13% of exacerbations. Hordvik *et al.* (1989) showed that the magnitude of the abnormalities of peak expiratory flow during influenza A and B was 33%. During the winter of 1989–1990, Conway *et al.* (1992) admitted three patients with acute severe deterioration who were infected with influenza A. They were hospitalized for periods of 2–3 weeks and in the light of the available data the authors suggested that all patients with cystic fibrosis should be offered immunization at the beginning of each influenza season.

Age

Deaths above the normal winter increase are recorded regularly in association with influenza epidemics and about 90% of these excess deaths are among people aged 65 and over (Tillett *et al.* 1980; Lui & Kendal 1987; Ashley *et al.* 1991; Sprenger *et al.* 1993). Serfling *et al.* (1967) estimated excess pneumonia–influenza deaths during three major influenza epidemics in the USA in late 1957 to early 1958, 1960 and 1963. Mortality among infants aged less than 12 months ranged from 3.7 to 11.6 per 100 000 (mean 7.3 per 100 000). It fell to 0.8–3.1 per 100 000 (mean 1.8) among those aged 1–4 years, and to 0.1–1.4 per 100 000 (mean 0.5 per 100 000) among 5–14-year-olds. It then increased to 0.2–2.5 per 100 000 (mean 0.95 per 100 000) among 15–19-year-olds, 0.9–2.7 per 100 000 (mean 1.6 per 100 000) among 20–44-year-olds, 5–8.9 per 100 000 (mean 7 per 100 000) among 45–64-year-olds, 16.7–33.1 per 100 000 (mean 25 per 100 000) among 65–74-year-olds, to 51.3–101.6 per 100 000 (mean 73.1 per 100 000) in those aged ≥ 75 years. Comparable rates for deaths certified as due to influenza were seen in England and Wales during the 15 years 1974–1988. The lowest mortality (0.04 per 100 000) was again noted in 5–14 year olds; mortality increased in successive 10-year age bands three-fold, four-fold, six-fold, 11-fold, 32.5-fold, 100-fold, and 765-fold to a mean of 30.6 per 100 000 (range 3.4–190.2) in those aged 75 years and over. Examination of 1989–1990 mortality data for England and Wales (Curwen *et al.* 1990) showed that certified influenza deaths represented fewer than 10% of the excess mortality associated with influenza, so it is possible that mortality from influenza in the over 75s could be nearer 2% during the most severe epidemics.

Although these data indicate increasing mortality with increasing age, about half of the population aged 65 years and older have one or more chronic medical conditions (Nicholson 1993). This raises the question whether age or underlying chronic ill-health is the principal risk factor. Barker and Mullooly (1982) examined the risks of death from pneumonia and influenza among 230 000 people in a health maintenance organization during epidemics in 1968–1969 and 1972–1973. The death rate was 9 per 100 000 for the over 65s without high-risk conditions, but was 20-fold greater in the over 65s with one 'high-risk' medical condition and 30-fold greater in those with two or more. As part of a vaccine effectiveness study, Ahmed and colleagues (1995) reviewed the medical records of people whose primary or contributory cause of death was certified as influenza. They found that more than 80% had one or more 'high-risk' medical conditions. Similarly 70–90% of the people 65 years of age and older who are hospitalized with pneumonia- and influenza-related diagnoses have chronic medical conditions (Foster *et al.* 1992; Ohmit & Monto 1995). Thus, although mortality increases with age, the presence of underlying ill-health represents the principal risk.

Residential status

There have been numerous reports of influenza in homes for the elderly with high attack rates and case fatality. As examples mortality rates attributable to influenza were 4–8% during a 3-year period in Cardiff (Howells *et al.* 1975). Similarly mortality rates of 3.7% and 0.2% were seen during A/Victoria/75 (H3N2) and B/Hong Kong/73 outbreaks in Paris (Serie *et al.* 1977); a rate of 4.5% was seen in seven nursing homes in Michigan when A/Bangkok/1/79 (H3N2) was circulating (Patriarca *et al.* 1985); and the mortality was 17.7% in an unvaccinated population during an influenza A/Arizona/ 80 (H3N2) outbreak in a New York home for the elderly (Gross *et al.* 1988).

Nguyen-Van-Tam and Nicholson (1992) examined certified influenza deaths among a population of 892 000 in Leicestershire during the 1989–1990 epidemic. Influenza was reported as the cause of death for 18 men and 29 women aged 67–97 (mean age 84); 41 (87%) were aged ≥ 75 years. There were no deaths in younger subjects with chronic medical conditions, and the estimated mortality for the fit elderly was ~7 per 100 000, i.e. similar to the rate observed by Barker and Mullooly (1982). Among non-residential subjects the rate for influenza-certified deaths was 11.6 and 23.1 per 100 000 for those with lung and heart disease, respectively. The major impact of influenza was seen in the residential care facilities where the rates were 343, 499 and 2703 per 100 000, respectively, for people with one, two and three or more medical conditions.

Case-control studies of vaccine effectiveness carried out by the same investigators during the 1989–1990 epidemic examined the residential status of (i) people with influenza as a certified cause of death in five health regions in England; and (ii) patients admitted to Leicestershire hospitals with pneumonia- and influenza-related conditions (Ahmed *et al.* 1995, 1997). More than half of those who died lived in residential care (odds ratio 2.08, 95% CI 1.48–2.9), as did over 15% of the admissions for pneumonia and influenza in Leicester (odds ratio 2.96, 95% CI 1.35–6.53). Since only about 5% of the elderly population in England live in residential care, it is evident that this group are at the greatest risk of serious morbidity and mortality.

Diabetes mellitus

People with late-onset diabetes are 1.7 times more likely to die from pneumonia and influenza than the general population and one in 33 die from these conditions overall (Moss *et al.* 1991). A similar but non-significant trend towards increased pneumonia and influenza deaths has also been observed among younger, insulin-dependent diabetics (Moss *et al.* 1991). People with diabetes are at significantly increased risk from death during epidemics of influenza than during non-epidemic periods. During the 1889–1890 influenza pandemic in Paris, for example, it was noted that there were twice as many 'diabetes' deaths during the outbreak as compared with the average number during the same period during the 3 previous years (Parsons 1891). Since these early observations—when diagnosis and treatments were both rudimentary—there have been several further reports of increases

in diabetic deaths during pandemic and interpandemic outbreaks.

The first wave of the 'Asian' influenza pandemic in Holland in 1957 saw an increase in diabetic deaths of 25% in comparison to the pre-epidemic years of 1954–1956 (Polak 1959). Housworth and Langmuir (1974) studied excess mortality from epidemic influenza in the USA from 1957 to 1966. They identified seven epidemic periods associated with influenza A or B or both. Excess deaths from diabetes were significant in six of the seven epidemics. The first wave of the epidemic during October–December 1957 saw diabetic deaths increase by 3.62 per million population (by 9.2%), and by 3.25 per million (by 7.9%) during the second wave during January–March 1958. During the epidemics of 1960–1966, deaths from diabetes increased by 5–12%. Increases in diabetic deaths of 5–15% were seen in the years during the period 1921–1932 with the highest influenza death rates (Stocks 1935). Endocrine deaths (mostly diabetic) increased by about 1350 (i.e. by 30%) in England and Wales during the period 25 November 1989 to 8 January 1990 compared with the comparable days in 1985–1986.

The risk of death in a health maintenance organization with more than 230 000 members was examined by Barker and Mullooly (1982) during epidemics in 1968–1969 and 1972–1973. The pneumonia and influenza death rates among people with underlying cardiovascular disease was estimated at 104 per 100 000 during influenza A epidemics, but increased more than four-fold to 481 per 100 000 (i.e. 1 in 208) in those with both cardiovascular disease and diabetes.

The effect of influenza on ketoacidosis, pneumonia and deaths in people with diabetes mellitus was examined using a hospital register survey in Holland during 1976–1979 (Bouter *et al.* 1991). Influenza epidemics occurred during 1976 and 1978, whereas 1977 and 1979 were considered, on the basis of consultation rates in sentinel practices, to be non-epidemic years. Patients with duodenal ulcer served as controls. Compared to controls, the estimated relative risk for hospitalization for 'influenza' was estimated to be 5.7 in 1977 and 6.2 in 1979, but only 1.1 and 1.0

during non-epidemic years. An increased relative risk was also noted for pneumonia, being 25.6 for both epidemic years. The highest consultation rates in sentinel practices occurred during 1978. During this year the number of admissions for ketoacidosis increased by 50% in comparison with the other 3 years. During the 1978 epidemic it was estimated that one out of every 1300 patients with diabetes mellitus was hospitalized for pneumonia, and one out of every 260 with insulin-dependent diabetes was hospitalized for diabetic ketoacidosis. The combination of pneumonia and diabetes appears especially serious; in one study six out of nine diabetics with influenzal pneumonia died, four of whom were admitted in coma (Oswald *et al.* 1958).

Given that influenza vaccine is effective in preventing deaths and hospital admissions for pneumonia and influenza, its effectiveness in preventing admissions among people with diabetes can be used as a surrogate to assess the impact of influenza. The estimated effectiveness of influenza vaccine in reducing hospital admissions was 79% (95% CI 19–95%) during epidemics in 1989–1990 and 1993 (Nicholson *et al.* 1996). Interestingly, of the 37 cases who were admitted, 32 (86%) were admitted for reasons of diabetic control rather than because of acute respiratory conditions. Thus even during an era of improved diabetic control, influenza is still responsible for appreciable morbidity among people with diabetes.

Disorders of the central nervous system

Although dementia, seizure disorders, cerebrovascular disease, difficulty with oropharyngeal secretions and 'neuromuscular disease' have all been identified as risk factors for the development of nosocomial pneumonia and pneumococcal infection (Lipsky *et al.* 1986; Marrie *et al.* 1986; Harkness *et al.* 1990; Hanson *et al.* 1992), the evidence that chronic disorders of the central nervous system increase the risk for serious morbidity and mortality from influenza is not strong. During the 1989–1990 influenza A epidemic in England, chronic neurological disease (including dementia, Parkinson's disease and cerebrovascular disease)

was found to be a risk factor (odds ratio 1.65; 95% CI 1.19–2.28) for certified influenzal death (as either a primary or contributory cause) (Ahmed *et al.* 1995), but was not identified as a risk factor for hospitalization for 'pneumonia and influenza' (Ahmed *et al.* 1997). Gorell *et al.* (1994) compared the underlying cause of death for patients with and without Parkinson's disease. Persons with Parkinson's disease were three to four times more likely to die from pneumonia and influenza than the general population, presumably because of their relative immobility towards the end of life.

Immunosuppression

Transplant recipients and persons with malignancy

A number of reports have focused on the increase in susceptibility to influenza and in serious pulmonary complications of influenza and death in transplant recipients and persons with malignancy. Kempe *et al.* (1989) prospectively followed a group of unimmunized immunosuppressed children with cancer and found that the incidence of influenza (23/73, 32%) was higher than in community controls (10/70, 14%). Moreover although a preseason haemagglutination inhibition titre of $\geq 1{:}32$ was protective for all children in the control group, it was not protective in some patients with cancer.

The occurrence of pneumonia and death associated with documented infection with influenza among adult and paediatric transplant recipients and patients with haematological malignancy is shown in Table 19.2. Pneumonia occurred in 65% of adults and 36% of children with influenza and 20% of both adults and children died from the infection. These rates are much higher than in immunocompetent subjects and reveal the immunocompromised to be at an especially high risk of serious morbidity and mortality. Most fatal pneumonias complicating influenza in the immunocompromised are viral rather than secondary bacterial in aetiology (Couch *et al.* 1997; Yousuf *et al.* 1997). Three risk factors found to be associated with death from parainfluenza virus or influenza are: young age; the onset of infections soon after transplantation; and augmentation of immunosuppression with steroid boluses or murine

Table 19.2 Incidence of pneumonia and death during influenza infection of adults and children who have received transplants or have haematological malignancy.

	Pneumonia (numerator/denominator (%))		Deaths (numerator/denominator (%))	
	Adults	Children	Adults	Children
Bone marrow transplant	18/26	1/4	8/44	1/4
Solid organ transplant	14/25	7/18	2/25	3/18
Haematological malignancy	24/35	1/3	11/35	1/3
Total	56/86 (65%)	9/25 (36%)	21/104 (20%)	5/25 (20%)

Data from Connolly *et al.* 1984; Beyer *et al.* 1987; Bell *et al.* 1988; Potter *et al.* 1991; Hirschorn *et al.* 1992; Ljungman *et al.* 1993; Mauch *et al.* 1994; Apalsch *et al.* 1995; Embrey & Geist 1995; Klimov *et al.* 1995; Ljungman 1997; Whimbey *et al.* 1997.

monoclonal anti-CD3 antibody (OKT3) (Apalsch *et al.* 1995). Yousuf *et al.* (1997) showed a non-significant trend towards a higher frequency of pulmonary complications and death from influenza among patients who had recently received chemotherapy and who had more chemotherapy-induced immunosuppression. The patients who died also tended to be the most neutropenic.

Graft rejection, possibly arising from the temporary suspension of immunosuppression, is potentially a complication of influenza infection in transplant recipients (Feldman *et al.* 1977; Kempe *et al.* 1989). Three out of 12 paediatric solid organ transplant recipients with influenza B had concurrent allograft rejection in the series reported by Mauch *et al.* (1994), and influenza A/Victoria may also have triggered acute renal allograft rejection (Keane *et al.* 1978). However, Apalsch *et al.* (1995) showed that the rate of rejection among liver transplant recipients with parainfluenza or influenza virus infections was not increased.

Human immunodeficiency virus (HIV)

In contrast to patients with organ transplants or haematological malignancy, there are few data pointing to an increase in morbidity or mortality from influenza in patients infected with HIV. In cities with a high incidence of HIV infection, an increase in the pneumonia deaths among persons aged 25–44 during the peak influenza months provides the only evidence supporting an increase in severity of influenza in adults with HIV (Morbidity

and Mortality Weekly Report 1988). During a retrospective study in Cincinnati, Connolly *et al.* (1994) obtained 1199 specimens of bronchoalveolar lavage (BAL) fluid from 895 patients, most of whom had immunosuppression due to AIDS, transplantation, malignancy or immunosuppressive therapy. Influenza virus was isolated on only 11 occasions during 6 years, but not from any of the 757 BAL fluids from patients with AIDS. Similarly, during the winter of 1994–1995, Miller *et al.* (1996) examined BAL fluid from 44 consecutive HIV-1 antibody-positive patients who underwent 47 diagnostic bronchoscopies for lower respiratory disease; influenza virus was detected in none. Safrin *et al.* (1990) reported influenza infection in six HIV-infected patients at San Francisco General Hospital. One of the six developed pneumonia, but the overall course of the illness in this cohort suggested that it was not worsened in comparison with immunocompetent subjects. However, all subjects had CD4+ lymphocyte counts of > 300 per cu mm, and the mean count was in excess of 500 per cu mm, i.e. at a level where opportunistic infections are unusual.

Virus shedding in the immunocompromised and the risk of nosocomial infection

Almost 70% of influenza A or B infections in immunocompromised patients are nosocomial (Aschan *et al.* 1989; Mauch *et al.* 1994; Whimbey *et al.* 1994). Immunosuppressed patients with influenza shed influenza virus for much longer periods than the immunocompetent. Whereas healthy children may shed influenza virus for up to 14 days after onset of illness (Frank *et al.* 1981), and infants with nosocomially acquired infection for up to 21 days (Hall & Douglas 1975), an HIV-infected child with an extremely low CD4+ lymphocyte count shed influenza A virus for a period of 9 weeks (Evans & Kline 1995). Klimov *et al.* (1995) demonstrated continuous shedding of influenza A virus from a child with severe combined immunodeficiency for a period of approximately 5 months. These investigators also detected amantadine-resistant mutants from two immunodeficient patients undergoing treatment with amantadine (Klimov *et al.* 1995). These observations, together with the rapid development of resistance in other immuno-compromised patients (Whimbey *et al.* 1997) and the immunocompetent (see Chapter 35), indicate that treatment with amantadine or rimantadine alone may prove little benefit to immunocompromised patients with influenza A.

Influenza during pregnancy

Maternal death

Women who are pregnant appear to be at increased risk of hospital admission, severe pulmonary complications of influenza and death during the second and third trimesters, but the overall risk appears to be small, particularly during inter-pandemic years. Mullooly *et al.* (1986) examined the use of medical services for approximately 1000 pregnant women and 3000 non-pregnant women during four epidemics, and a non-epidemic period. Pregnant women sought medical attention more often than non-pregnant women, but hospitalization rates for acute respiratory disease were low among pregnant women (2 per 1000), and there were no maternal deaths. Ashley *et al.* (1991) compared cause of death among a one in 15 random sample of deaths that occurred between 25 November 1989 and 8 January 1990 with deaths occurring during the same period in 1985/6. Analysis revealed a four-fold increase in maternal deaths during the 1989/90 epidemic and suggested that the epidemic in Great Britain accounted for about 90 excess deaths during pregnancy.

The Public Health Laboratory Service (1958) report on the Asian influenza pandemic in England and Wales during 1957–1958 commented that 12 out of 103 fatal cases in females aged 15–44 years of age were in pregnant women, which is about double the expected proportion for this age group. During the first wave of Asian influenza in the Netherlands a total of 1230 influenzal deaths occurred among a population of 11 million inhabitants, and 11 deaths occurred during pregnancy (Polak 1959). In the group 20–39 years of age the mortality of pregnant women was twice that of non-pregnant females. Similarly, about three to four times the expected number of pregnant women (10 out of 24 females aged 16–40 years were pregnant) were seen among an American series of 91 patients with pneumonia complicating Asian influenza (Petersdorf *et al.* 1959). All but one were in the last trimester or at term.

During the Asian influenza epidemic in New Orleans, Burch *et al.* (1959) admitted 34 women with proven influenza of whom 13 were pregnant—three in the second trimester and 10 in the third. Three terminated in the death of the infant—one, a full-term infant, died on the ninth day of life with pulmonary haemorrhages believed to be influenzal; two others were stillborn during the sixth and seventh months of pregnancy. Here again the proportion of admissions who were pregnant was several times higher than expected.

Most of the above reports do not make it clear whether the severe outcome during pregnancy was associated with underlying chronic medical conditions. Of 379 patients with influenzal pneumonia reported by Oswald *et al.* (1958), seven were in the 'later' stages of pregnancy, two of the seven died, and one of these had mitral stenosis. In the series reported by Petersdorf *et al.* (1959) one of the 10 pregnant women with influenza went into premature labour, delivered a dead fetus, and died 15 hours later. Neither she nor the other nine pregnant women had any other risk factor. Soto *et al.* (1959) reported nine deaths due to Asian influenza. Four of the five women who died were in the second or third trimester of pregnancy; two of the four had underlying mitral stenosis. Two of 15 women with Asian influenzal pneumonia reported by Louria *et al.* (1959) were pregnant, one had rheumatic heart disease with mitral stenosis, but both recovered. During the same epidemic, Martin *et al.* (1959a) reported 10 fatal cases among women aged 15–44, of whom four were pregnant. As noted above, the proportion of admissions who were pregnant was several times higher than expected and only one of the four pregnant women had a chronic medical condition, myasthenia gravis. Giles and Shuttleworth (1957) reported the death of a 17-year-old pregnant girl among 14 women who died from Asian influenza in Stoke on Trent. Postmortem examination revealed cardiac hypertrophy, but the girl was not known previously to have had cardiac disease. Ramphal *et al.* (1980) describe a fatal A/Texas/77 infection in a woman with ventricular septal defect. Fetal heart sounds stopped suddenly 48 hours after admission and the patient died 12 hours later with a pneumococcal septicaemia. These cases indicate that few pregnant women hospitalized for complications of influenza have chronic medical conditions (2/19, 11%).

Influenza complicating mitral valve disease in pregnancy appears especially serious. Govan and Macdonald (1957) identified nine such patients of whom four died. Three out of five patients who went into labour during the acute stage of the illness died.

Transplacental passage of virus

Few attempts have been made to demonstrate transplacental passage of influenza virus to the fetus. Martin *et al.* (1959a) and Ramphal *et al.* (1980) failed to identify the presence of influenza antigen in fetuses from four mothers with fatal influenza. Yawn *et al.* (1971), however, recovered the virus from extrapulmonary tissues of a mother who died in the third trimester and from the amnion and myocardium of the fetus, but there were no abnormalities in the tissues from which the virus was isolated. Influenza A/Bangkok (H3N2) was isolated from the amniotic fluid obtained by amniocentesis within 1 day of the onset of influenza from a mother with suspected bacterial amnionitis at 36 weeks of gestation. The infant, who was born at 39 weeks, had evidence of infection but remained well (McGregor *et al.* 1984).

Congenital malformations

Conover and Roessman (1990) recently described an infant with complex malformations of the central nervous system in the brain of whom influenza antigens were demonstrated at postmortem. There have been reports of an increase in various congenital abnormalities following influenzal illness during pregnancy (Coffey & Jessop 1959; Hardy *et al.* 1961; Hakosalo & Saxen 1971; Griffiths *et al.* 1980; Aro 1983; Lynberg *et al.* 1994), but there is no consistent association between specific defects and illness, and the virus has not been conclusively implicated.

During the period 1 October 1957–1 June 1958, Coffey & Jessop (1959) asked women who attended antenatal clinics whether they had clinical influenza during pregnancy. Influenza infection was not confirmed in any of the 663 'cases' nor was subclinical infection excluded in any of the controls. Moreover no data were provided on the stage of pregnancy when illness occurred. The overall incidence of abnormalities in the 'infected' group was 3.6% and in the controls 1.5%. Here most abnormalities affected the central nervous system (CNS) and the difference in the incidence achieved statistical significance.

Hardy *et al.* (1961) noted major congenital abnormalities in 5.3% of 80 women whose influenza infections occurred during the first trimester compared with 2.1% of 183 women infected during the second trimester and 1.1% infected during the third. Hakosalo and Saxen (1971) studied a cohort of children for evidence of congenital abnormalities. The children were divided into three groups—those whose mothers were in the 5th to 11th weeks of gestation during the epidemic of Asian influenza, those who were beyond this stage, and finally those who were conceived after the epidemic. Comparison of the incidence of CNS abnormalities in the three groups again revealed a significant difference, with rates of 0.81% in the group whose mothers were in the 5th to 11th weeks of gestation, and 0.3% and 0.32% in the two 'control' groups. Griffiths *et al.* (1980) compared the offspring of 77 women with serological evidence of infection with those of uninfected controls. Here there was a slight increase in cardiac and minor orthopaedic abnormalities in the offspring of infected women. Aro (1983) identified independent associations between reduction limb defects and maternal 'influenza', smoking and alcohol. He questioned whether an infection, fever or medication could account for the apparent association with influenza.

To address this issue further Lynberg *et al.* (1994) undertook a case–control study to assess the magnitude of the risk of giving birth to a child with a neural tube defect associated with 'flu' (an ill-defined entity incorporating any influenza-like illness), fever and medications taken for illness. Of 385 mothers of case infants, 31 reported having a febrile 'flu-like illness during the period from 1 month before to 3 months after conception (odds ratio: 3.0, 95% CI 1.9–4.7); infants of mothers who took medication had a higher risk (odds ratio: 4.3, 95% CI 2.6–7.1). There was no increased risk of neural tube defects among the infants of mothers who reported fever from causes other than 'flu. The authors were unable to disentangle the individual contributions of 'flu or medication, and the imprecision of the clinical diagnosis further questions an association.

In contrast to the above, Wilson and Stein (1969) noted no increase in congenital abnormalities among infants who were conceived during the 3-month period when Asian influenza was epidemic and whose mothers had serological evidence of infection. Warrell *et al.* (1981) collected early antenatal blood samples from 25 women who subsequently gave birth to infants with anencephaly or spina bifida. None demonstrated recent influenza infection, indicating that during 1972–1976 influenza in pregnancy was not an important cause of neural tube defects in Oxford. To explore the potential teratogenic effect of influenza on the CNS further, Saxen *et al.* (1990) grouped mothers of 248 anencephalic infants into those whose first trimester had occurred during an epidemic period and those whose pregnancy had commenced during a non-epidemic period. No significant differences in the prevalence of anencephaly were noted.

Prematurity and neonatal mortality

Review of influenza deaths in England during the period 1921–1932 revealed a slight increase in mortality from premature births in association with influenza (Stocks 1935). Wynne-Griffith *et al.* (1972) showed that early neonatal mortality in England and Wales in the second quarter of 1970 after a major influenza epidemic was slightly but significantly higher (from 9.88 per 1 000 live births in 1969 to 10.77 in 1970) than in the corresponding quarter of the previous year. Analysis of infant mortality over the previous quarter century indicated that similar increases occurred in relation to four out of the other five major influenza epidemics during the period, notably in 1951, 1953, 1959 and 1961; the exception was the Asian 'flu epidemic of the autumn of 1957. Hardy *et al.* (1961) reported that the incidence of stillbirths in Baltimore was higher in 332 symptomatic pregnant women with serologically confirmed influenza than in 206 asymptomatic women with serologically confirmed influenza or in 73 uninfected women. A small cluster of early and late fetal deaths in early 1986 prompted a case-control study which revealed that case pregnancies were distinguished by having a significant excess of recent 'flu-like illness, and were significantly more likely than controls to have serological evidence of influenza A infection to an influenza A Christchurch/4/85 (H3N2)-like strain (Stanwell-Smith *et al.* 1994). Ashley *et al.* (1991) showed that perinatal deaths increased 1.6-fold during the 1989–1990 epidemic, by 255 from ~465 to ~720, as compared with a similar period in 1985/6.

Development of illness in offspring later in life

Childhood malignancy. Studies in the USA and the UK indicate a possible relationship between maternal influenza and childhood leukaemia (Fedrick & Alberman 1972; Bithell *et al.* 1973; Hakulinen *et al.* 1973; Austin *et al.* 1975). The relationship, if real, is not a constant finding (Leck & Stewart 1972; Hakulinen *et al.* 1973) and the effect is considered to be very small.

Schizophrenia. It has been shown recently that individuals who later develop schizophrenia are more likely to be born in the late winter and during spring than at other times of the year (O'Callaghan *et al.* 1991; Pallast *et al.* 1994). Against a background of data suggesting that structural abnormalities found in the brains of many schizophrenic patients occurred *in utero*, Mednick *et al.* (1988) claimed that a Finnish birth cohort which had been in the second trimester of pregnancy at the time of the 1957 pandemic of Asian influenza had an increased hospital admission rate for schizophrenia. Since then studies from Japan and several countries in Europe have confirmed that prenatal exposure to influenza is associated with an increased risk of adult schizophrenia (Barr *et al.* 1990; O'Callaghan *et al.* 1991; Kunugi *et al.* 1992; Sham *et al.* 1992; Adams *et al.* 1993). In contrast two American studies have shown only a trend towards an association (Watson *et al.* 1984; Torrey *et al.* 1988); conflicting data were obtained in Scotland (Kendell & Kemp 1989; Mednick *et al.* 1990); and no association at all was found in studies from the UK, Croatia and Holland (Crow *et al.* 1992; Torrey *et al.* 1992; Erlenmeyer-Kimling *et al.* 1994; Susser *et al.* 1994).

The positive findings have implicated exposure during the second trimester (Mednick *et al.* 1988; O'Callaghan *et al.* 1991) and an effect in females but not in males (Mednick *et al.* 1990; Takei *et al.* 1994; O'Callaghan *et al.* 1991). Even if there is real association between prenatal exposure to influenza and development of schizophrenia, the relationship is not necessarily causal, since influenza may lead to drug therapy for relief of symptoms, and obstetric complications (Wright *et al.* 1995). Interestingly other studies — that are not concerned with influenza — have reported an association between obstetric complications and the later development of schizophrenia.

Cigarette smoking

A few studies have examined the relationship between smoking and influenza. These have shown that current smokers have higher rates of both asymptomatic and symptomatic influenza than non-smokers (Finklea *et al.* 1969; Kark & Lebiush 1981; Kark *et al.* 1982; K. G. Nicholson, in preparation). The odds ratio for clinical influenza among young male smokers during an outbreak in a military unit was 2.42 (95% CI 1.53–3.83) (Kark *et al.* 1982) and the risk ratio among female military

recruits who smoked was 1.44 (95% CI 1.03–2.01) in comparison to non-smokers (Kark & Lebiush 1981). The proportion of clinical influenza attributable to smoking was estimated at 13% in the female recruits and 31% in male recruits, and was 72% in a study in the elderly. In the latter study the unadjusted odds ratio for influenza A in current smokers was 4.39 (95% CI 1.6–11.9) in comparison to non-smokers (K. G. Nicholson, in preparation).

Complications of influenza

The complications of influenza are predominantly respiratory. These include acute bronchitis, laryngotracheobronchitis (croup), bronchiolitis, pneumonia, lung abscess, empyema, exacerbations of chronic bronchitis, asthma and cystic fibrosis, together with pneumothorax and surgical emphysema. However, many other complications affecting other body systems are reported (see Table 19.3 for a summary). Some were discussed in the preceding section and the remainder are discussed below.

Respiratory complications

Acute bronchitis

Acute bronchitis is the most common lower respiratory tract complication of influenza. However, the reported incidence in general practice is very variable. Bendkowski (1958) noted acute bronchitis in 48 (30%) out of 161 cases of Asian 'influenza' of all ages in general practice. However, Fry (1958) identified only 10 (1%) cases among 930 cases of Asian 'influenza'. During the H3N2 outbreak in 1989–1990, Connolly *et al.* (1993) found that the incidence of acute bronchitis in general practice in patients with 'influenza' was 19%. These investigators found that the risk of bronchitis complicating influenza was higher in elderly patients and in those with underlying chronic medical conditions. In the hospital setting, Guthrie *et al.* (1957) diagnosed bronchitis in 77 (22%) out of 350 admissions with Asian influenza in Kuwait. Brocklebank *et al.* (1972) found bronchitis in 9 (12%) out of 76 children in hospital with virologically

Table 19.3 Complications of symptomatic influenza.

Complication	Association with influenza*	Estimated incidence during symptomatic illness
Respiratory		
• Acute bronchitis	+++	+++
• Croup	+++	?++ (infants)
• Bronchiolitis	+++	?++ (infants)
• Acute otitis media	+++	++++ (young children)
• Primary viral pneumonia	+++	++ to ++++
• Secondary bacterial pneumonia	+++	++
• Lung abscess	+++	+
• Empyema	+++	+
• Aspergillosis	+++	+
• Exacerbation of asthma	+++	++++ (asthmatics)
• Exacerbation of chronic obstructive airways disease	+++	++++ (people with chronic obstructive airways disease)
• Exacerbation of cystic fibrosis	+++	++++ (children with cystic fibrosis)
• Pneumothorax	+++	+
• Surgical emphysema	+++	+
• Pulmonary fibrosis and obliterative bronchiolitis	+	+
• Respiratory death	+++	+ to ++ (depending on age and risk factors)
Cardiovascular		
• ECG abnormalities	+++	++++
• Heart failure	+++	?+ to ++ (in patients with underlying cardiac disease)
• Myocarditis	+++	+++
• Pericarditis	+++	?+
• Myocardial infarction	+++	?+ to ++ (in patients with underlying vascular disease)
• Death	+++	+ to ++ (depending on age and risk factors)
• Toxic shock syndrome	+++	+
Central nervous system		
• Cerebrovascular disease	++	+
• Febrile convulsions	+++	++ (children < five years of age)
• Encephalitis and immune-mediated parainfectious encephalitis	+++	+
• 'Encephalopathy'	+++	+ to +++
• Guillain–Barré syndrome	++	+
• Transverse myelitis	++	+
• Reye's syndrome	+++	+
• Bacterial meningitis	++	+
• Cerebral abscess	++	+
• Acute psychoses	++	+
• Impaired reaction times	+++	++++
Gastrointestinal		
• Haemorrhagic gastritis, duodenitis and haematemesis	+++	?++
• Reye's syndrome	+++	+
• Parotitis	+++	+
• Ulceration of bowel	+++	?+

Continued

Table 19.3 *Continued*

Complication	Association with influenza	Estimated incidence during symptomatic illness
Musculoskeletal		
• Rupture of rectus abdominis	++	?++ (only reported during 1918–19 pandemic)
• Myositis	+++	++ (mostly children with influenza B)
• Rhabdomyolysis and myoglobinuria	++	+
Renal		
• Myoglobinuric renal failure	+++	+
• Renal failure with disseminated intravascular coagulation	+++	+
• Exacerbation of nephrotic syndrome	+++	?
• Nephritis	+	?
Endocrine		
• Poor diabetic control	+++	++ to +++
• Diabetic deaths	+++	+
• Adrenal haemorrhage	+++	?
Haematological		
• Disseminated intravascular coagulation	+++	+
• Haemophagocytic syndrome	+++	+
• Aplastic anaemia	+	+
Maternofetal		
• Maternal death	+++	+
• Perinatal death	+++	+
Congenital		
• Central nervous system abnormalities	++	++
• Schizophrenia	+	?
• Childhood leukaemia	+	+
Ophthalmic		
• Choroiditis	+	+
• Retinitis	+	+
Immunocompromised		
• Transplant rejection	+	?
• Death in patients with haematological malignancy and transplant recipients in those with documented influenza	+++	++++

* Association with influenza: +++, definite; ++, probable; +, possible. Incidence during symptomatic illness: ++++, $\geq 10\%$; +++, $\geq 1\%$; ++, $\geq 0.1\%$; +, $< 0.1\%$.

confirmed influenza A/Hong Kong. Stocks (1935) showed an increase in death certifications from both acute and chronic bronchitis during influenza epidemics of 1921–1933. During the worst periods deaths from acute bronchitis increased by 93%, and from chronic bronchitis by 52%.

Croup

Influenza viruses are among the aetiological agents associated with acute laryngotracheobronchitis (croup), and croup is a not uncommon finding (5–15%) among children hospitalized with influenza

(Brocklebank *et al.* 1972; Price *et al.* 1976; Paisley *et al.* 1978; Sugaya *et al.* 1992). Croup associated with influenza A virus appears to be more severe, resulting in more frequent hospitalizations and tracheostomies (Howard *et al.* 1972), but occurs less frequently than croup associated with parainfluenza viruses or respiratory syncytial virus infections. Kim *et al.* (1979) showed that whereas influenza viruses (particularly influenza A) ranked second overall after the parainfluenza viruses as a cause of croup, influenza A infection was detected in proportionately more croup patients than the most important croup-producing virus, parainfluenza type 1 when the peak months of influenza A and parainfluenza virus activity were compared. H3N2 viruses appear to have a greater predeliction to producing croup than the H2N2 viruses. During the years 1957–1976, influenza A virus infection was detected in approximately 8% of hospitalized children with croup during the H2N2 era and 24% of such patients during the H3N2 era (Kim *et al.* 1979). During the peak month of a composite of 13 consecutive influenza A virus outbreaks, influenza A virus infection was demonstrated in 67.6% of croup patients and in 35.6% of all hospitalized respiratory patients including croup patients. During the peak month of a composite of six consecutive influenza B outbreaks, influenza B virus infection was demonstrated in 36% of croup patients and in 10.8% of all hospitalized respiratory disease patients including croup patients. These data suggest that influenza A does indeed cause more lower respiratory morbidity in children than influenza B, though the observed differences could be due to lower overall attack rates of influenza B in vulnerable children.

Acute otitis media

Acute otitis media is preceded in many instances by a respiratory viral infection and a simultaneous viral infection has been documented in a quarter to a half of patients with acute otitis media. Acute otitis media and more subtle otological abnormalities are common findings in influenza (see Chapter 39). In a Finnish study 35% of children hospitalized with influenza A appeared to have acute otitis

media (Ruuskanen *et al.* 1989). Subsequently these investigators conducted a prospective study of influenza vaccine in the prevention of otitis media in otitis-prone children aged 1–3 years of age during an outbreak of influenza A (Heikkinen *et al.* 1991). The diagnosis of otitis media was based on signs and symptoms of acute infection and presence of middle-ear fluid detected by pneumatic otoscopy. This was not a double-blind, placebo-controlled study, and the occurrence of otitis media in 18 out of 27 (67%) children with influenza A was higher than in their previous study, which involved older children who were not otitis prone.

Pneumonia

Two main types of pneumonia are recognized—a primary viral pneumonia and secondary bacterial pneumonia. The latter may occur either with viral pneumonia or as a 'late' complication of influenza. The interval between the onset of symptoms and signs of pneumonia is variable. During the 'Spanish' influenza pandemic, pneumonia frequently occurred without an 'influenza' period at all; more often the patient was ill with influenzal symptoms for a day or two before pulmonary complications occurred; in others the influenza had run its course and the temperature had returned to normal, or nearly so, before the onset of pneumonia (Abrahams *et al.* 1919).

During the second wave of the pandemic in 1918, Fildes *et al.* (1918) drew attention to differences between the postmortem findings of rapidly fatal cases and those of longer standing. Rapidly fatal cases were characterized by an absence of pus and by dark red airless lungs. The lungs were full of thin haemorrhagic exudate which flowed from the cut surface; the bronchial tree throughout the lungs was intensely injected and contained bloody fluid which poured into the trachea; and the nasopharynx, pharynx, larynx and trachea were affected similarly. In cases of longer standing, there was a marked bronchopneumonia with pus in addition to the haemorrhagic features. In contrast, other postmortem reports describe the almost universal finding of bronchopneumonia, often found in association with haemorrhagic manifestations

(Influenza Committee of the Advisory Board to the D.G.M.S., France 1918; Abrahams *et al.* 1919; Muir & Wilson 1919; Wilson & Steer 1919). Scadding's search of the literature (1937) revealed records of only two cases (described by Goodpasture 1919) in which bacteria were neither seen in sections nor cultured from the lungs; however, neither case was notably acute or rapid in its course.

Despite differences in clinical presentation, Goodpasture's observations (1919) and those of Fildes (1918) provide the earliest evidence that occasional patients with 'influenza' died of a fulminating illness that was unassociated with known bacterial pathogens. The pneumotropism of influenza virus was revealed shortly after the discovery of influenza A when lung from a patient with fulminating pneumonia yielded both *Staphylococcus aureus* and influenza virus (Scadding 1937).

Incidence of pneumonia. The incidence of pneumonia and the case fatality rate varies considerably from one report to another. A number of factors may be responsible, including intrinsic properties of the virus, the age, immune status and number and type of chronic medical conditions of the host, and whether or not virological tests and X-rays are carried out. It is unusual for virology and radiology to be carried out in primary care, whereas in the hospital setting the investigation of patients with more serious illness represents a source of bias.

During the pre-antibiotic era pneumonia was 'very rare' during the 1889 pandemic in Russia (Clemow 1890). Only 534 (1%) episodes of pneumonia were recognized among 55 263 cases of 'influenza' during the 1889 pandemic in the Prussian army (Rolleston 1919). Similarly, only three (1.7%) cases of pneumonia were observed among 177 schoolgirls with 'Russian' influenza (Bristowe 1890); one (1.2%) case occurred among 85 young men with 'Russian' influenza on a training ship (Preston 1890); and six cases (~3%) of pneumonia were identified among 200 cases of 'Russian' influenza in the family setting (Murphy 1891). In contrast, pneumonia complicated 14 (10%) out of 140 cases of 'Russian' influenza at the Royal Asylum in Edinburgh (Robertson & Elkins 1890).

This exceptionally high rate possibly reflects the harsh conditions and general debility of the insane in asylums during the Victorian era.

Despite improvements in public health during the following 25 years, the pandemic of 'Spanish' influenza during 1918–1919 saw a far greater incidence of pneumonia, particularly during the second wave when the overall influenza case fatality rate was ~4% (Cole 1918; Abrahams *et al.* 1919). Whereas 3% of 1810 patients with influenza developed pneumonia during the first wave (Gotch & Whittingham 1918; Influenza Committee of the Advisory Board to the D.G.M.S., France 1918; Taylor 1919), 18% of 1315 cases developed pneumonia during the second wave (Abrahams *et al.* 1919; Taylor 1919; Watson 1919). Figure 19.2 shows a W-shaped pattern for the age-related complications of pneumonia and death during the 1918–1919 pandemic. Although 5–14-year-olds had the highest incidence of 'influenza', they had the lowest incidence of pneumonia and case fatality rate. Unexplicably the 25–40-year-olds had an intermediate incidence of influenza but the highest incidence of pneumonia and greatest case fatality rate. In contrast, during the epidemic in 1928–1929, both the incidence of pneumonia and the case fatality rate were lowest in young adults (Fig. 19.3).

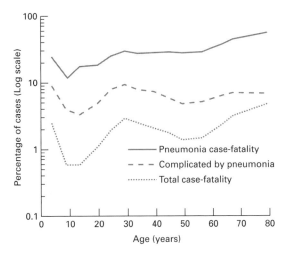

Fig. 19.2 Age-related complications of pneumonia and death, and the pneumonia case fatality rate during the 1918–1919 pandemic.

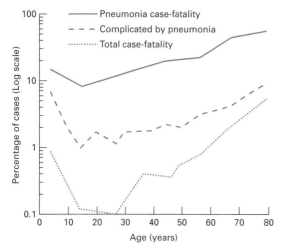

Fig. 19.3 Age-related complications of pneumonia and death, and the pneumonia case fatality rate during the 1928–1929 epidemic.

During the 'Asian' influenza pandemic in 1957 the incidence of influenza-related pneumonia diagnosed clinically in general practice was ~2% (91 of 4033) (Guthrie *et al.* 1957; Holland 1957; Bendkowski 1958; Fry 1958; Rowland 1958; Woodall *et al.* 1958). It was similar for adults and children (Gilroy 1957; Podosin & Felton 1958).

However, other studies in primary care which included diagnostic radiology revealed that more than 5% of cases of 'Asian' influenza developed pneumonia (Gilroy 1957; Podosin & Felton 1958). These studies suggest that the incidence of pneumonia in primary care may be several-fold greater than is generally recognized. Thus the pneumonia rate of 2.9% reported during the H3N2 influenza epidemic in 1989–1990 (Connolly *et al.* 1993) is probably an underestimate. More reliable are the data from studies incorporating both virology and radiology. Using these investigations pneumonia was found in 38% of 13 soldiers with A/New Jersey/76 (Hsw1N1) infections (Gaydos *et al.* 1977); 21% of 24 institutionalized elderly patients with A/Texas/77 (H3N2) infections (Mathur *et al.* 1980); and 5.5% of 36 A/USSR/77 (H1N1) infections aboard a US navy ship (Ksiazek *et al.* 1980).

The incidence of influenza B in the community is less well described. Jackson (1946) observed pneumonia in 9.6% of 219 Bahamian troops with influenza B. In contrast no cases of pneumonia were described among 37 people with influenza B (Foy *et al.* 1987), nor among 43 children with proven influenza B in a paediatric group practice (Hall *et al.* 1979). However, pneumonia requiring hospitalization occurred in 5 (~4%) out of 129 residents of a nursing home who developed symptoms during an influenza B outbreak.

Clinical features. Influenza complicated by pneumonia generally presents with influenzal symptoms and, although there are no clear distinguishing features, cough and chest pain occur more frequently than in uncomplicated influenza—54% vs. 79%, and 31% vs. 51%, respectively, in the series reported by Jamieson *et al.* (1958). The chest pain is of two types—substernal, which presumably reflects the tracheitis commonly seen at postmortem, and pleuritic. During the Asian influenza outbreak the onset of illness in fatal cases was typically abrupt and within 24 hours of onset of symptoms pneumonic or other serious symptoms were observed in one-third of patients (Public Health Laboratory Service 1958). Deterioration was much more rapid in the young than in the elderly with 56% of patients under 5 years of age gravely ill within the day of onset compared with 16% of those >64 years of age (Public Health Laboratory Service 1958). In fatal cases deterioration was particularly rapid; in the Public Health Laboratory Service series of 477 deaths no fewer than 86 occurred before admission to hospital and two-thirds died within 48 hours of admission (Public Health Laboratory Service 1958).

Rapid deterioration was also seen in England during the influenza epidemic of 1989–1990. Figure 19.4 shows the interval between onset of illness and death of 275 cases with 'influenza' registered anywhere on the death certificate. The median interval between onset of illness and death was 6 days. Figure 19.5 shows the interval between admission to hospitals in Leicester for pneumonia and influenza and death. Overall 78 out of 156 (50%) cases died during the admission. More than a third of those who died succumbed within 2 days of hospitalization and less than a third survived for longer than 8 days. Clearly hospital clinicians have

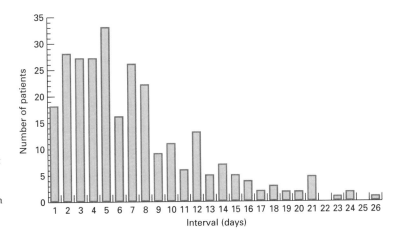

Fig. 19.4 Interval between the onset of illness and death in 275 patients who died during the 1989–1990 influenza epidemic in England with influenza registered on the death certificate.

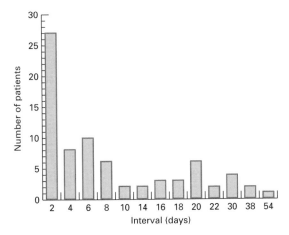

Fig. 19.5 Interval between admission to hospitals in Leicestershire for pneumonia and influenza and death.

little opportunity to modify the outcome in fatal cases. Despite many improvements in health care, including drug development, the mortality from influenzal pneumonia is no less than that observed 60 years ago (Scadding 1937).

Primary viral pneumonia. Prior to the Asian influenza pandemic there were only isolated cases in which no bacterial component of pneumonia could be identified by careful bacteriological studies during life or at autopsy, and influenza virus was grown readily from the lungs (Parker *et al.* 1946). Hers *et al.* (1958) isolated influenza virus from the lungs of 106

(72%) out of 148 virologically confirmed fatal cases of Asian influenza. Overall 30 (20%) were identified as having influenza virus pneumonia without secondary bacterial infection. Bacteria, mostly *Staphylococcus aureus*, were recovered from the lungs of 90 of the 148 cases. These observations indicate: (i) that primary viral pneumonia is both common and life-threatening without secondary bacterial infection; and (ii) that the lungs of most patients with secondary bacterial pneumonia are coinfected with influenza.

Although most reports of primary influenza virus pneumonia concern influenza A, fatal influenza B pneumonia without a secondary bacterial component has also been reported (Troendle *et al.* 1992). Martin *et al.* (1959a) and Louria *et al.* (1959) provide detailed accounts of primary influenza virus pneumonia. Of 32 fatal cases of influenzal pneumonia admitted to Boston hospitals, Martin *et al.* (1959a) found 15 without secondary bacterial infection. Similarly, Louria *et al.* (1959) found six cases of primary virus pneumonia (of whom five died) among 33 patients admitted with pneumonia to the New York Hospital. Pneumonia developed 1–5 days (mean 2.6 days) after onset of influenza in Boston, but onset of pneumonia was inseparable from the initial influenza symptoms in New York and was established within 36 hours of illness onset. Death occurred 12–36 hours following the recognition of complications (Martin et al. 1959a), i.e. within 4–5 days of the onset of influenza (Louria *et al.*

1959; Martin *et al.* 1959a). Auscultation revealed crackles and wheezes, but no signs of consolidation. The X-ray appearance usually showed bilateral abnormalities, and except when cavitation was demonstrable, pure viral pneumonia was generally indistinguishable from those with secondary bacterial involvement (Louria *et al.* 1959; Martin *et al.* 1959a). The total leukocyte counts were elevated throughout the illness and some revealed a polymorph predominance (Louria *et al.* 1959) despite the absence of concurrent bacterial infection.

Kaye *et al.* (1962) described three further examples of severe influenza virus pneumonia and also three cases of segmental pneumonia apparently due to influenza who survived. The prognosis of primary viral pneumonia in hospitalized patients generally appears to be poor. During the pandemic of 1968–1969, four patients with severe influenza pneumonia were recognized at Vanderbilt University Hospital and two died (Burk *et al.* 1971). Winterbawer *et al.* (1977) reported 11 patients with primary viral pneumonia of whom only five survived after prolonged ventilation and oxygen therapy. Poor outcome is heralded by dyspnoea, tachypnoea, cyanosis and haemoptysis, and terminally by shock and signs of pulmonary oedema.

Pathology of viral pneumonia. Postmortem examination of lung reveals no consolidation and bloody fluid can be expressed from the cut surface (Parker *et al.* 1946; Louria *et al.* 1959). The trachea and bronchi often contain serosanguinous fluid and the mucosa is strikingly hyperaemic (Parker *et al.* 1946; Louria *et al.* 1959). Histology of the airways reveals tracheitis, bronchitis, bronchiolitis with haemorrhagic areas and loss of ciliated epithelium (Louria *et al.* 1959; Noble *et al.* 1973). The lungs frequently contain irregular haemorrhagic areas up to several cm in diameter, and the alveoli contain neutrophils, mononuclear cells, fibrin and oedema. Intraalveolar haemorrhage is common, particularly in the lower lobes (Louria *et al.* 1959). Hyaline membranes line many of the alveolar ducts and alveoli, often in areas where there is no cellular exudate (Parker *et al.* 1946; Louria *et al.* 1959), and the septa are infiltrated with large mononuclear cells, lymphocytes and plasma cells.

Walsh *et al.* (1961) examined the potential for influenza to affect the lower airways by biopsy of the trachea and main stem bronchus from six patients with pandemic Asian influenza. The tissue response to infection became more prominent distally. At one extreme, columnar cells persisted, exhibiting vacuolization, oedema and loss of cilia. At the other there was extensive desquamation to the basement membrane. These abnormalities and the frequent abnormalities of pulmonary function during influenza suggest lower airway involvement in most, if not all, cases.

Since autopsy specimens are biased towards the most severe cases, Yeldani & Colby (1994) examined lung biopsies obtained during life from six sporadic cases of influenzal pneumonia, four influenza A, one influenza B, and one influenza A and B, that occurred during the period 1976–1991. Follow-up information was available in five cases: two recovered without specific therapy, two whose biopsies revealed bronchiolitis obliterans with organizing pneumonia (BOOP) recovered promptly with steroids, and one died. The histological changes were non-specific and were less severe in the survivors than in the fatal case, previously reported by Noble *et al.* (1973). They varied from patchy alveolar exudates and hyaline membranes with oedema to severe diffuse alveolar damage with necrosis of bronchiolar mucosa. Reparative changes were seen as proliferation of type II cells and mild interstitial chronic inflammatory infiltrates.

Long-term complications. There have been a few reports of pulmonary fibrosis and obliterative bronchiolitis as long-term complications of influenza (Klimek *et al.* 1976; Laraya-Cuasay *et al.* 1977; Pinsker *et al.* 1981), but it is unclear whether the relationship is causal. Laraya-Cuasay *et al.* (1977) followed three patients who developed influenza A at 5, 24 and 42 months of age. Biopsies taken at 50, 166 and 51 days after the onset of the influenza pneumonia revealed varying degrees of interstitial fibrosis, bronchial and bronchiolar erosions and metaplasia, obliterative bronchiolitis, and interstitial chronic inflammatory infiltrates. Interestingly, influenza A/Hong Kong/68 was isolated from the lung tissue of one patient 8 weeks after the onset of illness. Finckh and Bader (1974) also recovered influenza A/Hong Kong/68 virus from the postmortem lung of nine patients between 4 and 21 days after onset of symptoms. Epithelial cell loss was still prominent in patients whose illness lasted more than 3 weeks, while in the pulmonary parenchyma, there was a continuing exudate within alveolar ducts and alveoli with a web of fibrin in some alveoli and hyaline membrane in others. The diagnosis of influenza A/Hong Kong/ 68 pneumonia was also established serologically in another patient whose history was of 4.5 weeks duration at death. In the bronchial tree there was continuing cellular shedding, regeneration and metaplasia with metaplastic squamous epithelium extending into adjoining fibrotic lung. There was also prominence of hyaline membrane and interstitial organization that had proceeded to advanced fibrosis.

Pinsker *et al.* (1981) described two patients with usual interstitial pneumonia (UIP) following A/Texas influenza. The first had an acute fulminating pneumonia resulting in respiratory failure on the third day of hospitalization. Open lung biopsy performed on day 16 revealed extensive fibrosis and subacute interstitial inflammation; the patient was left with restrictive pulmonary function abnormalities which improved gradually. The second patient had a more chronic course with interstitial fibrosis and focal interstitial inflammatory infiltrates 4 months after the initial presentation. She also suffered a marked deterioration in diffusing capacity for carbon monoxide when retested 9 months later. A similar prolonged reduction in transfer factor, a state compatible with residual pulmonary fibrosis, has also been reported following influenza B complicated by pneumonia (Luksza & Jones 1984).

Secondary bacterial pneumonia. The high incidence of bronchopneumonia during the 1918–1919 pandemic was described above. The literature from this period indicates that one or more pathogens, including pneumococci, haemolytic streptococci, *Haemophilus influenzae*, staphylococci and *Branhamella catarrhalis* were recovered from the airways, lungs and blood. *H. influenzae* was most commonly associated with lower respiratory complications in the British armies in France (Influenza Committee of the Advisory Board to the D.G.M.S., France 1918; Wilson & Steer 1919); streptococci and *H. influenzae* were equally common at a military base hospital in Italy (Barratt 1919); but among American troops in Glasgow *H. influenzae* and pneumococci were recovered in comparable numbers, often together (Muir & Wilson 1919).

During recent pandemics, studies supported by diagnostic virology and bacteriology (Parker *et al.* 1946; Hers *et al.* 1958; Louria *et al.* 1959; Soto *et al.* 1959) or bacteriology only (Giles & Shuttleworth 1957; Jamieson *et al.* 1958; Public Health Laboratory Service 1958; Petersdorf *et al.* 1959; Lindsay *et al.* 1970) revealed that almost three-quarters of patients with fatal or life-threatening influenzal pneumonia had secondary bacterial infection. *S. aureus*, either as sole pathogen or together with other micro-organisms, was identified in the overwhelming majority of bacterial pneumonias that occurred as a complication of virologically confirmed Asian influenza (Table 19.4). *S. aureus* was also prominent in bacterial pneumonias complicating proven infections with H1N1 and H3N2 strains of influenza A, and influenza B (Table 19.4) and during both the Asian and Hong Kong pandemics it was recovered frequently from patients hospitalized with pneumonia (Angeloni & Scott 1958; Robertson *et al.* 1958; Schwarzman *et al.* 1971).

Interval between onset of influenza and secondary bacterial pneumonia. Scadding (1937) was the first to comment on the time of onset of pneumonia associated with influenza. Of 18 cases of consolidation, five had an insidious onset, being continuous with the influenzal symptoms. In 10 the history was that on about the fourth or fifth day of the influenzal attack the patient was feeling somewhat better, when pleuritic pain heralded the onset of pneumonia. In the remaining three cases the onset was much later, occurring on the eleventh to fourteenth days.

Louria *et al.* (1959) likewise classified bacterial pneumonias complicating influenza into those in which there was concomitant viral and bacterial pneumonia and those in which influenza was 'fol-

Table 19.4 Bacteriological findings in fatal cases of influenza A and B in which influenza virus was recovered from the lungs, or influenza was diagnosed serologically.

	'Asian' influenza number of cases (%)	Influenza H1N1, H3N2 and influenza B number of cases (%)
Staphylococcus aureus	369 (69)	10 (45)
'Mixed' infections	95 (18)	5 (23)
Streptococcus pneumoniae	50 (9)	1 (5)
Haemophilus influenzae	11 (2)	–
Streptococci groups A and B	6 (1)	3 (14)
Proteus spp.	2 (< 1)	–
Diphtheroids	1 (< 1)	–
Klebsiella pneumoniae	1 (< 1)	–
Pseudomonas spp.	1 (< 1)	2 (9)
Escherichia coli	–	1 (5)
Total	536	22

Data from: Burnet *et al.* 1946; Parker *et al.* 1946; Giles & Shuttleworth 1957; Hers *et al.* 1958; Jamieson *et al.* 1958; Public Health Laboratory Service 1958; Louria *et al.* 1959; Martin *et al.* 1959a; Petersdorf *et al.* 1959; Soto *et al.* 1959; Lindsay *et al.* 1970; Barber & Stanbridge 1977; Gerber *et al.* 1978; Baine *et al.* 1980; Troendle *et al.* 1992.

lowed' by a secondary bacterial pneumonia. Of the 15 patients in the latter group 10 indicated that there was only a brief improvement in influenzal symptoms before the appearance of symptoms suggesting pulmonary infection; in five the pulmonary symptoms blended with the initial influenza symptoms. Radiology of those with secondary bacterial pneumonia revealed lobar or lobular involvement, they appeared acutely unwell on admission but only one of 15 died (7% mortality). Radiology of those with concomitant viral and bacterial pneumonia revealed both lobar and perihilar infiltrates, they had severe respiratory distress and four out of nine (44%) died.

Antibiotic use and mortality. The introduction of antibiotics into clinical practice has not resulted in an obvious reduction in mortality from secondary bacterial pneumonia. Scadding (1937) reported seven deaths (37% mortality) among 19 patients with consolidation during the winter of 1936–1937. During the 'Asian' influenza pandemic Louria *et al.* (1959) reported 21% mortality from secondary bacterial pneumonia with no difference between those with and without risk factors. During the Hong Kong pandemic, Lindsay *et al.* (1970) reported the deaths of six (46%) out of 13 patients with virologically confirmed influenza complicated by

bacterial pneumonia. These studies and others without laboratory confirmation of influenza show that the mortality from bacterial pneumonia complicating influenza is still comparable to the pneumonia case fatality observed during the 1918–1919 and 1928–1929 outbreaks (Figs 19.2 and 19.3).

Risk factors for fatal bacterial pneumonia complicating 'influenza'. Several factors including age (see Figs 19.2 and 19.3), pre-existing disease and the identity of the invading microbe can affect the outcome of secondary bacterial pneumonia. Angeloni & Scott (1958) reported nine deaths (22% mortality) among 41 adults who developed pneumonia from 1 to 14 days after onset of influenza. Further analysis revealed that the mortality was higher in patients with chronic chest disease than in the previously fit (6/13, 46% vs. 3/28, 11%).

Staphylococcus aureus was frequently isolated from patients with fulminant pneumonia and from postmortem lung during the 1957 pandemic (Oswald *et al.* 1958; Robertson *et al.* 1958). Robertson *et al.* (1958) reported 38 cases of staphylococcal pneumonia with 18 deaths (47% mortality) whereas in non-staphylococcal pneumonia there were 16 deaths among 102 cases (16% mortality, $p \leq 0.001$; overall mortality 24%). In patients with staphylococcal pneumonia the mortality was high in those both with and without underlying high-risk conditions (10/19, 53% vs. 8/19, 42%). In contrast with other microbial pathogens the mortality was higher in patients with chronic medical conditions than in the previously healthy (14/67, 21% vs. 2/35, 6%). In a similar study 71 (46%) of 155 patients with staphylococcal pneumonia were 'severely ill', compared with 34 (23%) of the 145 with non-staphylococcal pneumonia ($p \leq 0.001$) (Oswald *et al.* 1958). The overall mortality of 28% (44/155) for staphylococcal pneumonia was more than twice as high as for non-staphylococcal pneumonia (12%; 18/145; $p \leq 0.001$). Moreover the mortality in the staphylococcal group was similar at all ages, whereas in the non-staphylococcal group mortality was concentrated in those aged $\geq$55 years.

Hospital-acquired staphylococcal pneumonia. Two large studies of hospitalized patients in Dundee (Jamieson *et al.* 1958) and London (Oswald *et al.* 1958) illustrate that many of the staphylococcal infections during the Asian influenza pandemic were nosocomial. The acquisition of staphylococci in hospitals was also shown by the Public Health Laboratory Service (1958) study which related the bacterial flora of the lung or sputum to the interval between hospital admission and death. The percentages of elderly patients who yielded staphylococci were: 13% of those who died on the day of or day after admission; 20% of those who died after 2 or 3 days, 45% after 5–7 days, and 80% after 8 days or more. Moreover, patients who died within 48 hours of admission to hospital, like those who were never admitted, had antibiotic-sensitive staphylococci in about 65% of cases. Patients who died later had drug-resistant strains much more frequently, and none of the patients who died after more than 7 days in hospital had a penicillin-sensitive strain. Rather than benefitting patients, it seems that indiscriminate 'prophylactic' use of broad-spectrum antibiotics or a combination of antibiotics may actually predispose patients with otherwise uncomplicated pneumonia to a more serious staphylococcal pneumonia (Martin *et al.* 1959b).

Immunopathogenesis of staphylococcal pneumonia. During the early 1950s it was considered that there was a special relationship between *Staphylococcus aureus* and influenza, as evidenced by the rapidity with which staphylococcal pneumonia developed and the ease with which the virus could be recovered from the lungs of fatal cases (Annotations 1951). While it is likely that virus-mediated damage to mucosal barriers may predispose to bacterial infections, there is evidence that other factors, notably defects in phagocyte function, play an important role.

Studies of polymorphonuclear leukocytes (polymorphs) from patients infected with influenza virus, or of exposure of polymorphs to influenza virus, have identified a variety of alterations in cellular intermediary activation steps (e.g. lysosome–phagosome fusion, altered actin polymerization, protein phosphorylation) and depression of end-stage functions (i.e. chemotactic, oxidative and secretory) (Larson & Blades 1976; Larson *et al.* 1977, 1980; Ruutu *et al.* 1977; Busse & Sosman 1981; Verhoef *et al.* 1982; Abramson *et al.* 1982, 1985, 1991). This dysfunction appears to be mediated through the sialophorin (CD43) receptor on polymorphs which acts as a receptor for influenza A (Abramson & Hudnor 1995). Several innate immune responses, notably GM-CSF and collectins (serum and surfactant proteins that have Ca^{2+}-dependent lectin activity) seem able to protect neutrophils against the depressing effects of virus on respiratory burst activity (Abramson *et al.* 1991; Little *et al.* 1994; Hartshorn 1996). However, since treatment with GM-CSF failed to protect chinchillas infected with influenza A virus against pneumococcal superinfection (Abramson & Hudnor 1994), this approach appears to be unrewarding.

The production of proteases by bacteria that are capable of activating the haemagglutinin of influenza by proteolytic cleavage may represent another important factor in the pathogenesis of influenzal pneumonia. An interaction between influenza virus and bacteria has been shown for *Staphylococcus aureus* (Tashiro *et al.* 1987a,b) and *Aerococcus viridans*, but other bacterial enzymes have not been found to activate influenza virus infectivity directly (Scheiblauer *et al.* 1992). However, there is some evidence that they may modify or increase host proteases, which in turn activate influenza virus (Scheiblauer *et al.* 1992; reviewed by Rott *et al.* 1995). Jakeman *et al.* (1991) examined the interaction between staphylococcal alpha and gamma toxin and endotoxin with influenza A virus in ferrets. Lethality was enhanced three-fold for staphylococcal gamma toxin, 14-fold for staphylococcal alpha toxin and 84-fold for endotoxin. No increased viral replication occurred; thus the effect of the toxins was exacerbated by the virus infection, not vice versa.

Lung abscess and empyema. Radiology is not considered to reflect the true incidence of abscess formation during the acute stages of bacterial pneumonia, because the ring shadows are often obliterated by surrounding pneumonia and oedema. This was frequently seen by Oswald *et al.* (1958) during their comparison of chest radiographs and necropsy specimens, and applied particularly to the smaller abscesses which occurred commonly during acute staphylococcal pneumonia. Radiological cavitation was observed in 14% of secondary staphylococcal pneumonias, and in 2% of the remainder. Many of the larger abscesses are diagnosed 2 weeks or more after the onset of influenza in patients who have more or less recovered from their 'influenza', but are troubled by excess sputum production. Lung abscess was diagnosed radiologically in eight (29%) out of 28 previously fit adults who developed symptoms of pneumonia between 1 and 14 days after the onset of 'influenza', and empyema occurred in one (Angeloni & Scott 1958). The abscesses varied from a single lesion to multiple cavities throughout both lungs. The physical signs were often inconspicuous. Frank abscess formation was found at postmortem in eight out of 24 influenza deaths studied by Jamieson *et al.* (1958), and in four out of 46 patients studied by Giles and Shuttleworth (1957).

Pleural exudates were found frequently at postmortem during the pre-antibiotic era of the Spanish influenza pandemic in 1918–1919, but death occurred generally before this changed to frank pus. Cole (1918) reported the occurrence of empyema in about 10% of 163 fatal cases, which was usually streptococcal rather than pneumococcal. Barratt (1919) observed empyema in almost one-fifth of fatal cases. More recently it was found

in only four of 379 cases of pneumonia seen at the height of the Asian influenza pandemic (Oswald *et al.* 1958).

Aspergillosis. There have been at least eight case reports of invasive pulmonary aspergillosis as a complication of influenza A in immunocompetent subjects (Horn *et al.* 1983; Lewis *et al.* 1985; Urban *et al.* 1985; Shapiro & Ferris 1986; Kobayashi *et al.* 1992). This is considered to be facilitated by the lymphocytopenia and loss of ciliary function in the trachea and bronchioles that accompany influenza, and by broad-spectrum antibiotics, corticosteroids and diabetes (Horn *et al.* 1983; Lewis *et al.* 1985). Sputum microscopy may be positive for hyphae and mycelia of *Aspergillus*, X-rays may reveal nodular shadowing with subsequent cavitation, and bronchial walls may be lined with an adherent plaque of *Aspergillus*. Only one of the eight cases survived.

Pneumothorax and surgical emphysema. The literature of the 1918–1919 pandemic describes occasional cases of pneumothorax and surgical emphysema complicating influenza (Garrett 1918; Nash 1919; Weber 1919). Abrahams *et al.* (1919) described the occurrence of surgical emphysema in about 7% (15 out of 200) of 'pneumonic' cases of influenza. Surgical emphysema heralded death in almost all cases.

Cardiovascular complications

The possibility that influenza might affect the cardiovascular system was suggested by the near doubling of deaths from heart disease in Paris during the pandemic of 1889–1890 (Parsons 1891). Similarly in Dublin during the 1889–1890 pandemic there was a 2.5-fold increase in mortality from 'diseases of the organs of circulation' (Watson 1900). During the 1918–1919 pandemic reference was made to various cardiovascular complications including hypotension (Cole 1918), relative bradycardia (Gotch & Whittingham 1918), heart failure (Cole 1918), pericarditis (Influenza Committee of the Advisory Board to the D.G.M.S., France 1918), pericardial effusions (Wilson & Steer 1919), pericardial, subpericardial, epicardial and subendocardial haemorrhages (Whittingham & Sims

1918; Influenza Committee of the Advisory Board to the D.G.M.S., France 1918; Wilson & Steer 1919), cardiac dilatation (Whittingham & Sims 1918; Influenza Committee of the Advisory Board to the D.G.M.S., France 1918; Armitage 1919), and friability of the heart muscle (Barratt 1919). Clearly the absence of diagnostic tests for influenza during this era together with the frequent occurrence of secondary bacterial pneumonia and the absence, or rudimentary nature, of electrocardiographic examination made it impossible to draw firm conclusions about the occurrence of cardiac events during influenza and the role of the virus.

Possibly the most convincing evidence of cardiac involvement during the pandemic of 1918–1919 was produced by Cockayne (1918–1919) who commented on the frequent occurrence of bradycardia (with pulse rates of less than 50) and described cases of heart block and extrasystoles; most cases recovered promptly. His clinical observations were supported by the pathological features of myocarditis in patients with 'influenza' first described by Lucke *et al.* (1919). Hyman (1927) also reported bradycardia and heart block during or following influenzal illness.

Myocarditis and pericarditis

In 1945 Finland *et al.* reviewed the literature on the occurrence of myocarditis associated with influenza and identified two cases in which influenza A was confirmed at postmortem. One patient had complete heart block and lymphocytic infiltration of myocardium surrounding necrotic muscle fibres. Similar cases were reported soon thereafter by Parker *et al.* (1946) and Borden (1950). Between 1950 and 1956 Silber (1958) saw 21 patients with myocarditis and two with pericarditis and the diagnosis of influenza was established serologically in six. Silber noted that almost all previous writers on the topic had pointed out: (i) the lack of correlation between the severity of influenza and cardiac disease; and (ii) the infrequency of cardiac complications during the acute respiratory disease. Indeed Silber commented that most cardiac complications had been reported as occurring during convalescence.

More extensive studies of the cardiac complications of influenza were possible during the 'Asian' influenza pandemic in 1957. Adams (1959) saw a total of 13 cases of myopericarditis with laboratory evidence of influenza A or B. He noted an interval of one or more weeks between influenza and the cardiac disorder and found that recovery was generally prompt. Postmortems carried out during the pandemic frequently revealed cardiomegaly, myocardial oedema, necrosis of muscle fibres and lymphocytic infiltration (Giles & Shuttleworth 1957; Martin *et al.* 1959a). Oswald *et al.* (1958) provided details of two cases of fatal staphylococcal pneumonia occurring as complications of 'clinical influenza' during the pandemic in 1957. In one the postmortem findings revealed a dilated heart, pericardial effusion, subpericardial petechiae, and a pale and friable myocardium; and in the other a dilated heart, pale friable myocardium, purulent pericarditis and an abscess in the wall of the ventricle. As in cases described during the 1918–1919 pandemic, the relative contribution of the influenza virus in cases with secondary bacterial infection is unclear.

Electrocardiographic (ECG) abnormalities have been found in up to 81% of patients with influenza in hospital (Gibson *et al.* 1959; Walsh *et al.* 1958; Karjalainen *et al.* 1980) and in 43% of cases in the community (Verel *et al.* 1976), mostly in people without cardiac symptoms. They include T wave abnormalities, described as either inverted, diphasic, significantly lowered or isoelectric; ST segment elevation; sinus bradycardia or tachycardia; nodal rhythm, atrial fibrillation, ventricular extrasystoles, and ventricular fibrillation. They may be transient, lasting no longer than 24 hours (Karjalainen *et al.* 1980), or may occasionally persist for months or years (Lewes *et al.* 1974; Verel *et al.* 1976), and there is evidence that the underlying abnormalities may cause fatal arrhythmia or restrictive cardiomyopathy long after recovery from influenza (Morgan & Chappell 1977; Schmaltz *et al.* 1986). Of 41 serologically confirmed cases of influenza A, multidirectional echocardiography revealed regional myocardial dysfunction in six patients with ECG evidence of myocarditis, of whom only one had cardiac symptoms (Karjalainen et al. 1980).

Elevated levels of the cardiospecific MB–CK iso-enzyme were found in three of the six cases. The ECG findings, echocardiography and enzyme studies indicate that myocarditis is common in influenza, but is mostly asymptomatic.

There have been comparatively few reports of influenzal pericarditis since the influenza pandemic of 1918–1919. More recently, Proby *et al.* (1986) described a case in which acute influenza A infection was associated with elevated MB–CK levels, pericardial effusion and tamponade requiring pericardiocentesis. Franzen *et al.* (1991) describe a 48-year-old man admitted with suspected acute myocardial infarction because of severe precordial pain and ST elevations in the ECG. He subsequently developed a pericardial effusion and a significant rise in antibodies to influenza A. Reichman *et al.* (1997) described a case of acute effusive-constrictive pericarditis due to influenza A infection, which required extensive pericardiectomy.

The pathogenesis of cardiac complications remains unclear. Viral infection of the heart has been established in a few cases only. Martin *et al.* (1959a) studied tissues from 32 fatal cases of influenza. These investigators identified influenza antigen in one heart without myocarditis, but failed to find virus in multiple sections of heart with severe diffuse myocarditis. Oseasohn *et al.* (1959) recovered Asian influenza virus from cardiac muscle at postmortem and Engblom *et al.* (1983) and Ray *et al.* (1989) recovered virus from two patients with fulminant myocarditis.

Microscopic examination of the heart in such cases reveals fragmentation of myocardial fibrils, interstitial haemorrhage and oedema, and lymphocytic infiltration (Verel *et al.* 1976; Engblom *et al.* 1983; Ray *et al.* 1989).

Neurological complications

Viral infection of the central nervous system is normally established by virus isolation, viral antigen detection, serological testing of serum and cerebrospinal fluid, and microscopic and ultrastructural examination of neurological tissue. The diagnosis of viral encephalitis is supported by the finding of abnormal cerebrospinal fluid (CSF), but

abnormalities also occur in immune-mediated parainfectious encephalomyelitis and occasionally in influenza without specific neurological abnormalities (Paisley *et al.* 1978). The literature on influenza at the beginning of the 20th century refers to various neurological complications, including functional disturbances, encephalitis, paralyses, convulsions, bacterial meningitis, transverse myelitis, acute ascending paralysis, peripheral neuropathy and psychoses (Bury 1900; Watson 1900), but their relation to influenza is questionable in view of the lack of diagnostic virology during this period.

Prior to the 'Asian' influenza pandemic there were only a few instances in which virological tests linked influenza to encephalitis or encephalopathy (see Flewett & Hoult 1958; Mellman 1958). The pandemic in 1957 provided sufficient cases to allow the appreciation of the spectrum of neurological complications that occur in association with influenza.

Spectrum of neurological complications linked virologically to influenza

Review of a representative selection of the literature on influenza (Dubowitz 1958; Dunbar *et al.* 1958; Flewett & Hoult 1958; Horner 1958; McConkey & Daws 1958; Mellman 1958; Louria *et al.* 1959; Petersdorf *et al.* 1959; Taylor *et al.* 1967; Wells 1971; Stevens *et al.* 1974; Delorme & Middleton 1979; Baine *et al.* 1980; Glezen *et al.* 1980; Sulkava *et al.* 1981; Hawkins *et al.* 1987; Protheroe & Mellor 1991), which describes patients with neurological complications of infection with influenza A H1N1, A H3N2 and influenza B, provides a number of cases that fall into the following groups.

Group 1 Convulsions, occurring mostly in young children during the acute febrile stage of the illness, and not accompanied by pareses, stupor or coma. This is the most common complication affecting the nervous system, and approximately one-fifth of young children hospitalized with influenza are admitted for this reason.

Group 2 Patients with stupor, coma or paresis, with or without convulsions, with a normal CSF. Some patients may have encephalitis, immune-mediated parainfectious encephalomyelitis or Guillain–Barré syndrome, but these are likely to be found mostly in Group 3.

Group 3 Patients with the above clinical presentation or cerebellar features, but with an increase in the number of cells in the CSF and/or an increase in CSF protein. Most patients will have encephalitis, immune-mediated parainfectious encephalomyelitis or Guillain–Barré syndrome.

Reports of influenza during the 1957 pandemic suggest that neurological complications, excluding febrile convulsions in children, are not uncommon. Figure 19.6 shows the interval between onset of influenzal symptoms and stupor, coma or paresis. The median interval is 5 days (range 0–21) and is somewhat shorter for patients in Group 2, i.e. those without an increase in cells or protein in the CSF, than in Group 3 (median 4.5 vs. 7). The patients in Group 2 are younger than in Group 3 (median 10 vs. 36) and the mortality in Group 2 is greater (6/24 vs. 0/20). The review does not suggest a special neurotropic effect of a particular type of virus; 21 cases were associated with influenza A H2N2, 14 with influenza A H3N2 and 10 with influenza B, and four occurred in association with an unspecified type of influenza A. Strains of influenza A H1N1 are also capable of causing neurological complications (see Mellman 1958 and Flewett & Hoult 1958 for examples).

Clinical presentations include one or more of the following: confusion, stupor, coma, convulsions, hallucinations, aphasia, inability to respond to commands, extensor plantar responses, myoclonus, athetoid movements, nystagmus, cerebellar ataxia, decorticate posturing, opisthotonus, Cheyne-Stokes respiration, papilloedema, cranial nerve palsies, vertical gaze palsy, transverse myelitis and Guillain–Barré syndrome. Review of adequately documented cases reveals six deaths (~13% mortality) among 47 patients. Three-quarters of the cases recovered fully, often shortly after the onset of influenza. The pathogenesis of most complications remains unclear but it is possible that the pyrexia, hypoxia, and pH abnormalities that accompany influenza are responsible for a toxic encephalopathy in some cases, while in others a viral encephalitis or an immune-mediated parainfectious encephalomyelitis are responsible. In addition the literature suggests that a number of cases may be due to Reye's syndrome (Davis & Kornfeld 1980).

CT scan appearance. Hawkins *et al.* (1987) found no abnormalities on computed tomography (CT) or isotope brain scans during investigations of a case of influenza B encephalitis with a cellular CSF. Similarly the CT scans were described as normal in three patients with influenza A (H3N2) infection who developed a 'post-influenzal encephalitis' with a lymphocyte response in the CSF (Sulkava *et al.* 1981).

In contrast, cerebellar oedema was found on CT scanning of a young patient with influenza A-associated encephalopathy who did not have a lumbar puncture (Delorme & Middleton 1979). Protheroe and Mellor (1991) identified bilateral low

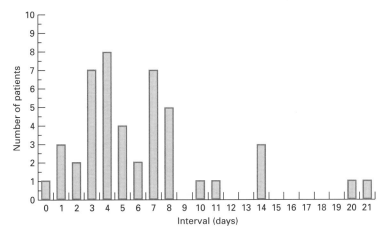

Fig. 19.6 Interval between the onset of influenza and the development of neurological complications of stupor or coma, and paresis or paralysis. Data abstracted from Dubowitz 1958; Dunbar *et al.* 1958; Flewett & Hoult 1958; Horner 1958; McConkey & Daws 1958; Mellman 1958; Louria *et al.* 1959; Petersdorf *et al.* 1959; Taylor *et al.* 1967; Wells 1971; Stevens *et al.* 1974; Delorme & Middleton 1979; Baine *et al.* 1980; Glezen *et al.* 1980; Sulkava *et al.* 1981; Hawkins *et al.* 1987; Protheroe & Mellor 1991.

attenuation changes in the thalami of two patients with influenza A encephalitis, neither of whom had increases in the CSF lymphocyte count. Additional changes included swelling of the midbrain and brainstem and low attenuation in the pons. These investigators suggested that in influenza encephalitis there may be a typical appearance on computed tomography as similar localized hypodense areas had been described in Japan (Okuno *et al.* 1982; Hattori *et al.* 1983).

Nagai *et al.* (1993) compared the CT scans of two children with Reye's syndrome associated with influenza A and two other children with non-Reye influenza 'encephalopathy'. All had symmetrical low-density lesions of the thalamus and brainstem. These lesions were present in the acute stage and decreased in size within a few weeks in all, but were still seen 2 years later in three surviving patients. Liver biopsy showed diffuse lipid droplet infiltration in two, focal infiltration in one, and normal morphology in one. Myelin basic protein was increased in the CSF of two of the three subjects studied — an observation consistent with a diagnosis of immune-mediated parainfectious encephalomyelitis. Nagai *et al.* (1993) suggested that there may be a continuum of Reye's syndrome and virus-associated encephalopathy with significant overlap.

Histology. Gross (and microscopic: Louria *et al.* 1959; Pertersdorf *et al.* 1959) histological abnormalities are often absent in patients with neurological complications who die (Horner 1958; Louria *et al.* 1959; Petersdorf *et al.* 1959; Hoult & Flewett 1960), even in those with abnormal CSF (Oswald *et al.* 1958). Hoult and Flewett (1960) had difficulties in identifying abnormalities. Those that were found consisted mostly of scanty and patchy lymphocytic infiltration of the meninges and perivascular spaces. Subdural empyema, cerebral abscess formation and bacterial meningitis are found occasionally (Oswald *et al.* 1958; Wells 1971). In some cases the findings of perivascular demyelination (Flewett & Hoult 1958; Horner 1958) are typical of an immune-mediated parainfectious encephalomyelitis, while in others (and suspected cases: Dunbar *et al.* 1958) the findings

are those of an acute haemorrhagic leukoencephalitis (Hoult & Flewett 1960) and are essentially identical to those of hyperacute experimental allergic encephalitis produced in rats and monkeys. Attempts to recover influenza virus from the brain postmortem (Flewett & Hoult 1958; Horner 1958) or the CSF antemortem (Louria *et al.* 1959; Hawkins *et al.* 1987) are usually unsuccessful, but few fatal cases have been studied. Occasionally influenza virus is recovered from the brain of patients with neurological complications (Flewett & Hoult 1958; Kapila *et al.* 1958).

Bacterial meningitis

There have been anecdotal reports of an association between outbreaks of influenza A and meningococcal disease. The increase in the number of cases of meningococcal infection 2 weeks after an influenza outbreak in England and Wales during 1989 led Cartwright *et al.* (1991) to investigate the relationship between the two conditions in a case–control study. Patients with meningococcal disease in December 1989 were more likely than age-matched controls to show serological evidence of recent influenza A infection (odds ratio 3.9, 95% CI 1.2–13.9). Hubert *et al.* (1992) assessed the temporal and spatial association between meningococcal disease and 'influenza-like illness' in France over the 6-year period 1985–1990. Although links were demonstrated, the proportion of cases of meningococcal disease that are causally linked to influenza is considered to be small.

Cerebrovascular disease

The possible association between influenza outbreaks and respiratory infections with vascular events has been referred to in a preceding section. The observation of a seasonal variation in the numbers of referrals for treatment of subarachnoid haemorrhage prompted Bowen-Jones (1979) to examine the link between the occurrence of subarachnoid haemorrhage and influenza. Between March and July 1978, the sera of all 25 patients with subarachnoid haemorrhage, 17 patients with various suspected CNS viral disorders, and 25 age-

and sex-matched patients whose blood were sent to the PHLS laboratory for virological screening were assayed for evidence of infection with 14 different viruses. The proportion of those with complement fixation titres >1/16 to influenza A virus was greater in those with subarachnoid haemorrhage (20/25, 80%), than in the neurology control group (3/17, 17%) and the 'matched' control group (3/25, 12%). The observed association is not evidence of causation; rather it could be argued that influenza is more likely to occur in people with a predisposition to subarachnoid haemorrhage.

Encephalitis lethargica

It has been reasoned that the global pandemic of encephalitis lethargica followed by post-encephalitic Parkinson's disease was associated with the 1918 influenza pandemic (Ravenholt & Foege 1982). Others have examined the possible association (Gamboa *et al.* 1974; Weinstein, 1976; Moore 1977; Anonymous 1981), but an association between the two events remains unproven.

Acute psychosis

Acute psychosis that develops 2–10 days after the onset of influenza possibly represents a manifestation of encephalitis or immune-mediated para-infectious encephalitis. Electroencephalograms in three patients with psychoses were diffusely abnormal and improved slowly over a period of weeks (Bental 1958). One report of 19 patients describes the development of acute psychosis with auditory and visual hallucinations during or after presumed 'Asian' influenza (Lloyd-Still 1958). All recovered quickly.

Subtle changes in brain function

Influenza B virus was one of several viruses studied at the MRC Common Cold Unit in Salisbury for its ability to affect simple measures of performance (Smith *et al.* 1989). Volunteers infected with influenza B had significant impairments in reaction times and their ability to perform a visual search task involving five possible target letters was also significantly impaired. Various tests were applied but there was impairment in only the attention tasks. Similar tasks were assessed in students infected naturally with influenza B. Comparison of baseline and symptomatic periods revealed a 37.5% increase in the variable foreperiod simple reaction time, a 13% reduction in response time to a repeated numbers detection task, and a significant reduction in a categoric search task (Smith *et al.* 1993). These effects were comparable to deteriorations seen with alcohol consumption, or working at night. Memory, logical reasoning, and hand–eye coordination were all unimpaired.

Reye's syndrome

Reye's syndrome, a multisystem disorder characterized by encephalopathy and fatty liver degeneration, was first described in 1963. Sixty to 87% of cases have been associated with upper respiratory infections, particularly influenza A and B (Corey *et al.* 1976a; Hurwitz *et al.* 1982). Reye's syndrome occurs primarily in children, with a peak onset between 5 and 14 years of age, but histologically confirmed cases have also occurred in adults (Davis & Kornfeld 1980). During the 1970s Reye's syndrome occurred with an estimated rate of 31–58 cases per 100 000 influenza B infections (Corey *et al.* 1976b; 1977) and from 2.5 to 4.3 cases per 100 000 influenza A infections (Halsey *et al.* 1980). The years with the highest incidence of Reye's syndrome in the USA correlated best with years in which influenza B was most prevalent (Rowley 1985). An increasing body of data has revealed a strong association between the use of salicylates and Reye's syndrome and, possibly because of reduced salicylate usage, recent trends in the USA and UK indicate a decreased incidence of cases (Barrett *et al.* 1986; Hurwitz 1989). In the British Isles recent active surveillance of Reye's syndrome has revealed an annual incidence of about one case per million population aged < 16 years (Newton & Hall 1993).

The clinical manifestations of Reye's syndrome have been divided into five or six stages: an abrupt onset of repetitive vomiting is a cardinal feature and lasts for hours to several days; in stage I, the patient is confused and lethargic but obeys commands; thereafter the patient may progress through stages characterized by delirium (stage II); coma and decorticate posturing (stage III); decerebrate posturing (stage IV); and flaccid coma (stage V). Typically, a previously normal child (or one with a history of Reye's syndrome) develops nausea, vomiting and an altered level of consciousness during convalescence from a respiratory viral illness, usually 4–6 days after the onset. The child is typically afebrile, and has an enlarged liver and normal CSF. The laboratory features include elevated serum transaminases (Monto *et al.* 1981) but bilirubin levels are normal or only slightly elevated. Arterial ammonia levels are elevated, particularly in the early course of the disease, and hypoglycaemia and clotting abnormalities may occur. The CT scan appearance may be normal or reveal cerebral oedema with low-density areas in the deep white matter (Russell *et al.* 1979). The mortality rate is high at approximately 25–40%.

The pathogenesis of Reye's syndrome remains unclear. Although influenza virus has been recovered from the liver, muscle biopsy specimens, CSF and nasotracheal specimens from a patient with Reye's syndrome (Partin *et al.* 1976), virus is rarely recovered from the brain or liver (Lamontagne 1980). Electron microscopy reveals mitochondrial abnormalities within hepatocytes and the majority of the enzymatic abnormalities involve mitochondria. An influenza B model of Reye's syndrome in mice supports the mitochondrial theory of Reye's syndrome (Davis *et al.* 1990), and suggests that a non-permissive viral infection of liver and brain may be responsible for the mitochondrial abnormalities.

Haematological abnormalities

Haemorrhage and disseminated intravascular coagulation

A haemorrhagic tracheobronchitis is generally seen at postmortem in patients dying with influenza. During the 1918–1919 pandemic haemoptysis and epistaxis were observed frequently (Abrahams *et al.* 1919); haematemesis

was much less common and tended to occur in cases in which vomiting occurred (McConnochie 1918); haemorrhage affecting the recti abdominis was not uncommon (Wilson & Steer 1919), but haematuria, purpura, other forms of haemorrhage into the skin and uterine bleeding occurred rarely (Abrahams *et al.* 1919). Haemorrhage into the adrenal glands and elsewhere was seen at necropsy in four out of 89 (4%) patients yielding Asian influenza virus (Jamieson *et al.* 1958), and epistaxis was also noted in patients with Asian 'influenza' in general practice (Fry 1957). Thrombocytopenic purpura was seen in one of 88 virologically confirmed cases during concurrent epidemics of influenza A and B in Scotland (Taylor *et al.* 1967); bilateral submacular haemorrhages were visualized in a 21-year-old nurse, possibly caused by a focal choroiditis (Weinberg & Nerney 1983); and during the influenza A (H1N1) epidemic in Brisbane during 1988 seven children with laboratory evidence of infection developed haematemesis and an erosive gastritis was visualized in three of the seven cases (Armstrong *et al.* 1991).

Bleeding disorders in influenza may be due in part to disseminated intravascular coagulation (DIC) which has been associated with both influenza A and B (Talley & Assumpcao 1971; Davison *et al.* 1973; Whitaker *et al.* 1974; Luksza & Jones 1984). Patients with DIC as a complication of influenza have presented with haematuria, haemoptysis, melaena, vaginal bleeding, purpura, haematemesis, renal failure and jaundice (Davison *et al.* 1973; Whitaker *et al.* 1974).

Virus-associated haemophagocytic syndrome

The virus-associated haemophagocytic syndrome was first described by Risdall *et al.* (1979) in a series of 19 patients with peripheral blood cytopenias associated with marrow histiocytosis and haemophagocytosis. It has been described mostly in association with cytomegalovirus and Epstein–Barr virus, but has also been linked to herpes simplex and zoster, adenovirus, parvovirus and human immunodeficiency virus. Clinical findings include fever, lymphadenopathy and hepatosplenomegaly.

It is possibly caused by the release of virally induced cytokines, and tends to resolve within several months. A proliferative histiocytosis has also been linked to leukaemias and lymphomas in the absence of infection. In most cases the histiocytosis has progressed rapidly and been fatal. At the height of the influenza A epidemic in 1989–1990, Potter *et al.* (1991) identified a cluster of three cases of haemophagocytic syndrome in children with acute leukaemia; influenza was confirmed by virus isolation or immunofluorescence in all cases. In the three cases the clinical and histological findings were compatible with a benign reactive process, and initial recovery in two cases also suggests that it was not a malignant condition. More recently Shirono *et al.* (1996) diagnosed virus-associated haemophagocytic syndrome in a 59-year-old man with influenza and pernicious anaemia. Aplastic anaemia has also been linked to influenza A (Curzon *et al.* 1983), but it is unclear whether this was associated with virus-associated haemophagocytic syndrome.

Toxic shock syndrome

There have been several reports of influenza or an influenza-like illness followed by *Staphylococcus aureus* respiratory tract infection complicated by toxic shock syndrome (TSS) (Wilkins *et al.* 1985; MacDonald *et al.* 1987; Sperber & Francis 1987; Prechter & Gerhard 1989; Conway *et al.* 1991). TSS is an illness characterized by major diagnostic criteria of fever, hypotension and erythroderma followed by desquamation and is found in association with TSST-1- or enterotoxin-producing *S. aureus* infection. In addition to these major criteria, involvement of three or more of the following organ systems are required: mucous membrane inflammation, and abnormalities of liver function, haematology, gastrointestinal tract, kidneys, or of the muscular, cardiopulmonary, or central nervous systems. By 1993 a total of 15 cases had been described, 12 as a complication of influenza B (Tolan 1993); the overall mortality was 40%. Cases without a rash, that might otherwise meet a definition of probable TSS, have also been described in association with influenza B (Jaimovich *et al.* 1992). Langmuir and colleagues

(1985) proposed that the 'Plague of Athens' in 430 BC was due to influenza and that certain inconsistent features could be explained by TSS. They suggested that its name should be changed to 'the Thucydides Syndrome' to honour the Athenian general who described it. However, using a combined epidemiological, historical and clinical approach Morens & Littman (1994) considered that the ancient descriptions of the disease best fitted a zoonosis or vector-borne disease.

Rupture of rectus abdominis muscles

The literature on the pandemic of 'Spanish' influenza refers to degeneration and rupture of the rectus abdominis muscles (Cole 1918; Abrahams *et al.* 1919; Wilson & Steer 1919). Wilson and Steer (1919) noted varying degenerative changes of the fibres of the rectus abdominis muscles in 23 out of 92 (25%) postmortem examinations. Abrahams *et al.* (1919) referred to the finding of ruptured rectus abdominis muscles in more than 20 cases. They likened the postmortem appearance of the muscle to that of 'a badly shot pheasant ... the muscle was dark crimson, of bruised appearance, full of diffusely extravastated dark blood, friable, readily torn by the fingers, and it may be squeezed into a pulpy mass without much force.'

Myositis, rhabdomyolysis, myoglobinuria and renal failure

Myalgia affecting the legs and back is a well-recognized feature of influenza and occurs early during the course of the illness. In contrast, myositis (and myoglobinuria with or without renal failure) is considered an infrequent complication and generally occurs in the recovery phase from a typical influenzal illness. The literature contains a number of reports of myositis complicating both influenza A and influenza B (Simon *et al.* 1970; Morgensen 1974; Dietzman *et al.* 1976; Zamkoff & Rosen 1979; Ruff & Secrist 1982; Bove *et al.* 1983; Kessler *et al.* 1983; Berry & Braude 1991; Holt & Kibblewhite 1995; Karpathios *et al.* 1995).

Middleton *et al.* (1970) reported 26 children who developed bilateral lower-limb myositis, characteristically after a period of rest and at a time when the respiratory symptoms and signs were beginning to subside. Influenza B virus infection was proved in 20 cases and type A infection in one. A further series of paediatric cases is described with evidence of influenza B infection in 11 out of 17 cases (Dietzman *et al.* 1976). In Middleton's series, leg pains and muscle tenderness lasted 1–5 days and no true muscle weakness was apparent, though the children often refused to walk, or did so with a bizarre gait. Muscle enzymes were elevated in two-thirds of the cases and attempts to isolate influenza virus from blood were unsuccessful. In adults the myositis tends to be more diffuse. Microscopy reveals focal muscle cell necrosis with or without cellular infiltrates (Gamboa *et al.* 1979; Kessler *et al.* 1983) while ultrastructural studies show myo-fibrillar disarray with disruption or loss of the sarcoplasmic reticulum, glycogen depletion accompanied by mitochondriopathy, and sub-sarcolemmal mitochondrial aggregates (Bove *et al.* 1983).

It is unclear whether virus infection of muscle is involved in the pathogenesis of this condition. The isolation of influenza virus from the muscle of a patient with Reye's syndrome demonstrates the potential for this to occur (Partin *et al.* 1976). Using electron microscopy Greco *et al.* (1977) found myxovirus-like particles in muscle cells from a patient with a 'postinfluenzal myositis', and Gamboa *et al.* (1979) isolated influenza virus, and obtained immunofluorescent and electron micro-scopic evidence of viral infection of skeletal muscle in a patient with myoglobinuria.

Influenza B-associated cases tend usually to be benign and of short duration, but rhabdomyolysis with myoglobinemia, myoglobinuria and acute renal failure has been described in association with influenza A (Simon *et al.* 1970; Minow *et al.* 1974; Morgensen 1974; Zamkoff & Rosen 1979; Foulkes *et al.* 1990; Berry & Braude 1991; Waka-bayashi *et al.* 1994; Holt & Kibblewhite 1995). During outbreaks influenza A is probably the leading cause of acute myoglobinuric renal failure. Histological examination reveals normal glomeruli with focal tubular necrosis and pigmented casts in some tubules.

Renal complications

Myoglobinuric renal failure, Goodpasture's syn-drome (Wilson & Smith 1972) and renal failure triggered by disseminated intravascular coagula-tion (Talley & Assumpcao 1971; Davison *et al.* 1973; Whitaker *et al.* 1974; Shenouda & Hatch 1976; Luksza & Jones 1984) have all been docu-mented in patients with influenza. MacDonald *et al.* (1986) showed that exacerbations of nephrotic syndrome in children (including children with minimal-change nephrotic syndrome, membrano-proliferative glomerulonephritis and membranous glomerulonephritis) were temporally related to upper respiratory tract infections, including influenza.

Beswick and Finlayson (1959) describe the his-tological appearance of the kidneys of seven cases of influenza who died from viral pneumonia or combined viral and bacterial pneumonia. These subjects had a terminal phase lasting from 1 to 3 days characterized by severe toxaemia and per-ipheral circulatory failure. Tubular lesions were found in the medullae, principally affecting the collecting tubules and to a less severe degree the loops of Henle. Jamieson *et al.* (1958) also noted the occurrence of necrosis of the proximal tubules of three out of 24 fatal cases of influenza. The older literature also refers to the occurrence of an acute nephritis at postmortem (Abrahams *et al.* 1919). However, judging by the absence of clinically important renal complications in series of patients with proven influenza and the dearth of patholo-gical abnormalities in renal tissue, it is evident that influenza rarely affects the kidneys.

Gastrointestinal complications

Ulceration and haemorrhage

Apart from the anorexia, nausea, vomiting and abdominal pain that are reported to varying degrees during epidemics, most observers agree that there is a very low incidence of gastrointestinal complications from influenza. However, the litera-ture relating to the 1889–1890 and 1918–1919 pan-demics describes the occurrence of haematemesis in about 1% of cases (Abrahams *et al.* 1919), melaena and bloody diarrhoea (Tibbles 1890; Cole 1918; Abrahams *et al.* 1919; Armitage 1919), and ulceration of the bowel (Barratt 1919). Autopsy findings during the 1918–1919 pandemic revealed that fulminant 'influenza' was not infrequently associated with a haemorrhagic gastritis, submucosal haemorrhages in the wall of the stomach and intestines, and peritoneal petechiae (Whittingham & Sims 1918; Wilson & Steer 1919). However, the frequent occurrence of secondary bacterial pneumonia and septicaemia during the pandemic together with the lack of a diagnostic test for influenza questioned a causal role of influenza.

During the pandemic of Asian influenza in 1957 petechiae were found at postmortem in the fundus of the stomach in 10 out of 24 cases, sometimes associated with coffee-ground material (Jamieson *et al.* 1958). In two cases acute gastric erosions were observed and in a third, mucosal haemorrhages 1 cm in diameter. More recently, Armstrong *et al.* (1991) reported seven young children with haematemesis among 19 who were hospitalized for virologically confirmed influenza A H1N1; two children died. Postmortem or endoscopy findings included haemorrhagic gastritis with multiple ulcerations and inflammatory infiltrate, and duodenitis. Attempts to identify the antigen or culture it from postmortem specimens failed. Thus the pathogenesis of the haemorrhage, ulceration, nausea, vomiting and diarrhoea still remain obscure.

Parotitis

Parotitis appears to be a rare complication of influenza. During the Spanish influenza pandemic of 1918–1919, Cole (1918) observed over 30 cases of painless parotid swelling as a complication of influenza. Occasionally the swelling was bilateral and fewer than one-fifth of cases were associated with testicular swelling. The ducts were normal, and in only one case was there any suppuration. During the same pandemic, Abrahams and colleagues (1919) described about a dozen cases of painless parotitis complicating influenza. The swellings were either unilateral or bilateral and there was no associated orchitis or suppuration. More than 50

years later, at the height of the 1975–1976 influenza epidemic in Massachusetts, Brill & Gilfillan (1977) reported 12 patients with parotitis in whom evidence of influenza A infection was found in the absence of serological responses to other known causes of parotitis. More recently Krilov and Swenson (1985) isolated influenza A (H3N2) from nasopharyngeal aspirates from a child who developed a painless unilateral swelling occurring 7 days after the onset of an acute respiratory infection.

Ophthalmic complications

Ophthalmic complications of influenza have been described only rarely. As noted above, bilateral submacular haemorrhages were visualized in a 21-year-old nurse, possibly caused by a focal choroiditis (Weinberg & Nerney 1983). Kovacs (1985) reported a case of 'influenza retinitis' with leakage from retinal vessels demonstrated by fluoroangiography. H7N7 virus of avian origin has been recovered from the eyes of two patients with conjunctivitis (Webster *et al.* 1981; Kurtz *et al.* 1996).

References

Abrahams, A., Hallows, N. & French, H. (1919) A further investigation into influenzo-pneumococcal and influenzo-streptococcal septicaemia. *Lancet* 1–11.

Abramson, J. & Hudnor, H. (1994) Effect of priming polymorphonuclear leukocytes with cytokines (GM-CSF and G-CSF) on the host resistance to *Streptococcus pneumoniae* in chinchillas infected with influenza A virus. *Blood* **83**, 1929–34.

Abramson, J.S. & Hudnor, H.R. (1995) Role of the sialophorin (CD 43) receptor in mediating influenza A virus-induced polymorphonuclear leukocyte dysfunction. *Blood* **85**, 1615–19.

Abramson, J.S., Mills, E.L., Giebank, G.S. & Quie, P.G. (1982) Depression of monocyte and polymorphonuclear leukocyte oxidative metabolism and bactericidal capacity by influenza A virus. *Infect Immun* **35**, 350–55.

Abramson, J.S., Wiegand, G.L. & Lyles, G.L. (1985) Neuraminidase activity is not the cause of influenza virus-induced neutrophil dysfunction. *J Clin Microbiol* **22**, 129–31.

Abramson, J.S., Wagner, M.P., Ralston, E.P., Wei, Y. & Wheeler, J.G. (1991) The ability of polymorphonuclear leukocyte priming agents to overcome influenza A virus-induced cell dysfunction. *J Leukocyte Biol* **50**, 160–6.

Adams, C.W. (1959) Postviral myopericarditis associated with the influenza virus. *Am J Cardiol* **4**, 56–67.

Adams, W., Kendell, R.E., Hare, E.H. & Munk-Jørgensen, P. (1993) Epidemiological evidence that maternal influenza contributes to the aetiology of schizophrenia. *Br J Psych* **163**, 522–34.

Ahmed, A.H., Nicholson, K.G. & Nguyen-Van-Tam, J.S. (1995) Reduction in mortality associated with influenza vaccine during 1989–1990 epidemic. *Lancet* **346**, 591–5.

Ahmed, A.H., Nicholson, K.G., Nguyen-Van-Tam, J.S. & Pearson, J.C.G. (1997) Effectiveness of influenza vaccine in reducing hospital admissions during the 1989–1990 epidemic. *Epidemiol Infect* **18**, 27–33.

Alford, R.M., Kasel, J.A., Gerone, P.J. & Knight, V. (1966) Human influenza resulting from aerosol inhalation. *Proc Soc Exp Biol Med* **122**, 800–4.

Andrews, B.E. & McDonald, J.C. (1955) Influenza virus C infection in England. *Br Med J* **2**, 992–4.

Angeloni, J.M. & Scott, G.W. (1958) Lung abscess and pneumonia complicating influenza. *Lancet* **i**, 1255–6.

Annotations (1951) Influenzal pneumonia. *Lancet* **i**, 335.

Anonymous (1981) Encephalitis lethargica *Lancet* **i**, 1396–7.

Apalsch, A.M., Green, M., Ledesma-Medina, J., Nour, B. & Wald, E.R. (1995) Parainfluenza and influenza virus infections in pediatric organ transplant recipients. *Clin Infect Dis* **20**, 394–9.

Armitage, F.L. (1919) Note on influenza and pneumonia. *Br Med J* 272–4.

Armstrong, K.L., Fraser, D.K.B. & Faoagali, J.L. (1991) Gastrointestinal bleeding with influenza virus. *Med J Austral* **154**, 180–2.

Aro, T. (1983) Maternal diseases, alcohol consumption and smoking during pregnancy associated with limb defects. *Early Human Dev* **9**, 49–57.

Aschan, J., Ringdien, O, Ljungman, P., Andersson, J., Lewensohn-Fuchs, I. & Forsgren, M. (1989) Influenza B in transplant patients. *Scand J Infect Dis* **21**, 349–50.

Ashley, J., Smith, T. & Dunell, K. (1991) Deaths in Great Britain associated with the influenza epidemic of 1989/90. *Pop Trends* **65**, 16–20.

Austin, D.F., Karp, S., Dworsky, R. & Henderson, B.E. (1975) Excess leukaemia in cohorts of children born following influenza epidemics. *Am J Epidemiol* **101**, 77–83.

Baine, W.B., Luby, J.P. & Martin, S.M. (1980) Severe illness with influenza B. *Am J Med* **68**, 181–9.

Bainton, D., Jones, G.R. & Hole, D. (1978) Influenza and ischaemic heart disease—a possible trigger for acute myocardial infarction? *Internat J Epidemiol* **7**, 231–9.

Barber, P.V. & Stanbridge, T.N. (1977) Bacterial septicaemia with multiple organisms complicating influenza pneumonia. *Br Med J* **1**, 1511–12.

Barker, W.H. & Mullooly, J.P. (1982) Pneumonia and influenza deaths during epidemics. *Archiv Intern Med* **142**, 85–9.

Barr, C.E., Mednick, S.A. & Munk-Jorgensen, P. (1990) Exposure to influenza epidemics during gestation and adult schizophrenia. *Archiv Gen Psych* **47**, 869–74.

Barratt, J.O.W. (1919) Notes on cases of influenza in a base hospital in Italy. *Br Med J* **i**, 705–6.

Barrett, J.M., Hurwitz, E.S. & Schonberger, L.B. (1986) Changing epidemiology of Reye's syndrome in the United States. *Pediatrics* **77**, 598–602.

Bauer, C.R., Elie, K., Spence, L. & Stern, L. (1973) Hong Kong influenza in a neonatal unit. *J Am Med Assoc* **223**, 1233–5.

Bell, M., Hunter, J.M. & Mostafa, S.M. (1988) Nebulised ribavirin for influenza B viral pneumonia in a ventilated immunocompromised adult. *Lancet* **ii**, 1084–5.

Bendkowski, B. (1958) Asian influenza (1957) in allergic patients. *Br Med J* **2**, 1314–15.

Bental, E. (1958) Acute psychoses due to encephalitis following Asian influenza. *Lancet* **ii**, 18–20.

Berry, L. & Braude, S. (1991) Influenza A infection with rhabdomyolysis and acute renal failure—a potentially fatal complication. *Postgrad Med J* **67**, 389–90.

Beswick, I.P. & Finlayson, R. (1959) A renal lesion in association with influenza. *J Clin Pathol* **12**, 280–5.

Beyer, W.E.P., Diepersloot, R.J.A., Masurel, N., Simoons, M.L. & Weimar, W. (1987) Double failure of influenza vaccination in a heart transplant patient. *Transplantation* **43**, 319.

Bithell, J.F., Draper, G.J. & Gorbach, P.D. (1973) Association between malignant disease in children and maternal virus infections. *Br Med J* **1**, 706–8.

Bondarenko, S.S. & Tumanov, F.A. (1992) The effect of influenza and parainfluenza on the course of ischemic heart disease. *Terapevticheskii Arkiv* **64**, 81–3.

Borden, C. (1950) Acute myocarditis; report of a case with observations on the etiologic factor. *Am Heart J* **39**, 131–5.

Bouter, A.M., Diepersloot, R.J.A., van Romunde, L.K.J. *et al.* (1991) Effect of epidemic influenza on ketoacidosis, pneumonia and death in diabetes mellitus: a hospital register survey of 1976–1979 in the Netherlands. *Diabetes Res Clin Pract* **12**, 61–8.

Bove, K.E., Hilton, P.K., Partin, J. & Farrell, M.K. (1983) Morphology of acute myopathy associated with influenza B. *Ped Pathol* **1**, 51–66.

Brill, S.J. & Gilfillan, R.F. (1977) Acute parotitis associated with influenza type A. *New Engl J Med* **296**, 1391–2.

Bristowe, H.C. (1890) Notes on an outbreak of influenza at King Edward's schools for girls. *Br Med J* **1**, 418.

Brocklebank, J.T., Court, S.D.M., McQuillin, J. & Gardner, P.S. (1972) Influenza A infections in children. *Lancet* **2**, 497–500.

Broun, G.O., Oligschlaeger, D., Legier, M. *et al.* (1960) Studies of the epidemiology of influenza as demonstrated by serum pools. *Archiv Intern Med* **106**, 496–512.

Burch G.E., Walsh J.J. & Mogabgab W.J. (1959) Asian influenza—clinical picture. *AMA Archiv Intern Med* **103**, 696–707.

Burk, R.F., Schaffner, W. & Koenig, M.G. (1971) Severe influenza virus pneumonia in the pandemic of 1968–1969. *Archiv Intern Med* **127**, 1122–8.

Burnet, F.M., Stone, J.D. & Anderson, S.G. (1946) An epidemic of influenza B in Australia. *Lancet* 807–11.

Bury, J.S. (1900) A discussion on influenza as it affects the nervous system. *Br Med J* **2**, 877–84.

Buscho, R.O., Saxtan, D., Shultz, P.S., Finch, E. & Mufson, M.A. (1978) Infections with viruses and *Mycoplasma pneumoniae* during exacerbations of chronic bronchitis. *J Infect Dis* **137**, 377–83.

Busse, W.E. & Sosman, J.M. (1981) Altered luminol-dependent granulocyte chemiluminescence during *in vitro* incubation with an influenza vaccine. *Am Rev Resp Dis* **123**, 654–8.

Carilli, A.D., Gohd, R.S. & Gordon, W. (1964) A virologic study of chronic bronchitis. *New Engl J Med* **270**, 123–7.

Cartwright, K.A., Jones, D.M., Smith, A.J., Kaczmarski, E.B. & Palmer, S.R. (1991) Influenza A and meningococcal disease. *Lancet* **338**, 554–7.

Chin, T.D.Y., Mosley, W.H., Poland, J.D., Rush, D., Belden, E.A. & Johnson O. (1963) Epidemiologic studies of type B influenza in 1961–1962. *Am J Public Health* **53**, 1068–74.

Clark, P.S., Feltz, E.T., List-Young, B., Ritter, D.G. & Noble, G.R. (1970) An influenza B epidemic within a remote Alaska community. *J Am Med Assoc* **214**, 507–12.

Clemow, F.G. (1890) The epidemic in Russia. *Br Med J* **i**, 46–7.

Cockayne, E.A. (1918–1919) Heart block and bradycardia following influenza. *Quart J Med* **12**, 409.

Coffey, V.P. & Jessop, W.J.E. (1959) Maternal influenza and congenital deformities. *Lancet* **ii**, 935–8.

Cole, C.E.C. (1918) Preliminary report on the influenza epidemic at Bramshott in September–October, 1918. *Br Med J* **2**, 566–8.

Collinson, J., Nicholson, K.G., Cancio, E. *et al.* (1996) Effects of upper respiratory tract infections in patients with cystic fibrosis. *Thorax* **51**, 1115–22.

Connolly, A.M., Salmon, R.L. & Williams, D.H. (1993) What are the complications of influenza and can they be prevented? Experience from the 1989 epidemic of H3N2 influenza A in general practice. *Br Med J* **306**, 1452–4.

Connolly, M.G., Baughman, R.P., Dohn, M.N. & Linneman, C.C. (1994) Recovery of viruses other than cytomegalovirus from bronchoalveolar lavage fluid. *Chest* **105**, 1775–81.

Conover, P.T. & Roessman, U. (1990) Malformational complex in an infant with intrauterine influenza viral infection. *Archiv Pathol Lab Med* **114**, 535–8.

Conway, E.E., Haber, R.S., Gumprecht, J. & Singer, L.P. (1991) Toxic shock syndrome following influenza A in a child. *Crit Care Med* **19**, 123–5.

Conway, S.P., Simmonds, E.J. & Littlewood, J.M. (1992) Acute severe deterioration in cystic fibrosis associated with influenza virus infection. *Thorax* **47**, 112–14.

Corey, L., Rubin, R.J., Hattwick, M.A.W., Nobel, G.R. & Cassidy, E. (1976a) A nationwide outbreak of Reye's syndrome. *Am J Med* **61**, 615–25.

Corey, L., Rubin, R.J., Thompson, T.R. *et al.* (1976b) A nationwide outbreak of Reye's syndrome: its epidemiologic relationship to influenza B. *Am J Med* **61**, 204–8.

Corey, L., Rubin, R.J., Thompson, T.R. *et al.* (1977) Influenza B-associated Reye's syndrome: incidence in Michigan and potential for prevention. *J Infect Dis* **135**, 398–407.

Couch, R.B., Douglas, R.G., Fedson, D.S. *et al.* (1971) Correlated studies of a recombinant influenza-virus vaccine. III. Protection against experimental influenza in man. *J Infect Dis* **124**, 473–80.

Couch, R.B., Kasel, J.A., Gerin, J.L. *et al.* (1974) Induction of partial immunity to influenza by a neuraminidase-specific vaccine. *J Infect Dis* **129**, 411–20.

Couch, R.B., Englund, J.A. & Whimbey, E. (1997) Respiratory viral infections in immunocompetent and immunocompromised persons. *Am J Med* **102** (3A), 2–9.

Creighton, C. (1965) *A History of Epidemics in Britain*, Vols 1 & 2, 2nd edn. Frank Cass, London.

Crow, T.J., Done, D.J. & Johnstone, C. (1992) Schizophrenia is not due to maternal influenza in the second (or other) trimester of pregnancy (abstract) *Schizophrenia Res* **6**, 99–100.

Curwen, M., Dunnell, K. & Ashley, J. (1990) Hidden influenza deaths. *Br Med J* **300**, 896.

Curzon, P.G., Muers, M.F. & Rajah, S.M. (1983) Aplastic anaemia associated with influenza A infection. *Scand J Haematol* **30**, 232–4.

Davenport, F.M., Hennessy, A.V. & Francis, T. (1953) Epidemiologic and immunologic significance of age distribution of antibody to antigenic variants of influenza virus. *J Exp Med* **98**, 641–56.

Davis, L.E. & Kornfeld, M. (1980) Influenza A virus and Reye's syndrome in adults. *J Neurol Neurosurg Psych* **43**, 516–21.

Davis, L.E., Blisard, K.S. & Kornfeld, M. (1990) The influenza B mouse model of Reye's syndrome: clinical, virologic and morphologic studies of the encephalopathy. *J Neurol Sci* **97**, 221–31.

Davison, A.M., Thompson, D. & Robson, J.S. (1973) Intravascular coagulation complicating influenza A virus infection. *Br Med J* **i**, 654–65.

Delorme, L. & Middleton, P.J. (1979) Influenza A virus associated with acute encephalopathy. *Am J Dis Child* **133**, 822–4.

Dietzman, D.E., Schaller, J.G., Ray, C.G. & Reed, M.E. (1976) Acute myositis associated with influenza B infection. *Pediatrics* **57**, 255–8.

Dubowitz, V. (1958) Influenzal encephalitis. *Lancet* **i**, 140–1.

Dunbar, J.M., Jamieson, W.M., Langlands, J.H.M. & Smith, G.H. (1958) Encephalitis and influenza. *Br Med J* **i**, 913–15.

Dykes, R.C., Cherry, J.D. & Nolan, C.E. (1980) A clinical, epidemiologic, serologic, and virologic study of influenza C virus infection. *Archiv Intern Med* **140**, 1295-8.

Eadie, M.B., Stott, E.J. & Grist, N.R. (1966) Virological studies in chronic bronchitis. *Br Med J* **2**, 671-3.

Edward, D.G. (1941) Resistance of influenza virus to drying and its demonstration in dust. *Lancet* **ii**, 664-6.

Elting, L., Whimbey, E., Couch, R. *et al.* (1992) Influenza A infection in adult leukaemia patients. In: *Program and Abstracts of the 32nd Interscience Conference on Antimicrobial Agents and Chemotherapy*, p. 115, abstract 29. American Society for Microbiology, Washington D.C.

Embrey, R.P. & Geist, L.J. (1995) Influenza A pneumonitis following treatment of acute cardiac allograft rejection with murine monoclonal anti-CD3 antibody (OKT3) *Chest* **108**, 1456-9.

Engblom, E., Ekfors, T.O., Meurman, O.H., Toivanen, A. & Nikoskelainen J. (1983) Fatal influenza A myocarditis with isolation of virus from the myocardium. *Acta Med Scand* **213**, 75-8.

Erlenmeyer-Kimling, L., Folnegovic, Z., Hrabak-Zerjavic, V., Borcic, B., Folnegovic-Smalc, V. & Susser, E. (1994) Schizophrenia and prenatal exposure to the 1957 A2 influenza epidemic in Croatia. *Am J Psych* **151**, 1496-8.

Evans, K.M. & Kline, M.W. (1995) Prolonged influenza A infection responsive to rimantadine therapy in a human immunodeficiency virus-infected child. *Ped Infect Dis J* **14**, 332-4.

Fedrick, J. & Alberman, E.D. (1972) Reported influenza in pregnancy and subsequent cancer in the child. *Br Med J* **ii**, 485-8.

Feldman, S., Webster, R.G. & Sugg, M. (1977) Influenza A in children and young adults with cancer. *Cancer* **39**, 350-3.

Fildes, P., Baker, S.L. & Thompson, W.R. (1918) Provisional notes on the pathology of the present epidemic. *Br Med J* 697-700.

Finckh, E.S. & Bader, L. (1974) Pulmonary damage from Hong Kong influenza. *Austral & NZ J Med* **4**, 16-22.

Finklea, J.F., Sandifer, S.H. & Smith, D.D. (1969) Cigarette smoking and epidemic influenza. *Am J Epidemiol* **90**, 390-9.

Finland, M., Parker, F., Barnes, M.W. & Jolliffe, L.S. (1945) Acute myocarditis in influenza A infections. *Am J Med Sci* **209**, 455-68.

Finland, M., Ory, E.M., Meads, M. & Barnes, M.W. (1948) Influenza and pneumonia. *J Lab Clin Med* **33**, 32-46.

Flewett, T.H. & Hoult, J.G. (1958) Influenza encephalopathy and postinfluenza encephalitis. *Lancet* **ii**, 11-15.

Foster, D.A., Talsma, A., Furumotoo-Dawson, A. *et al.* (1992) Influenza vaccine effectiveness in preventing hospitalization for pneumonia in the elderly. *Am J Epidemiol* **136**, 296-307.

Foulkes, W., Rees, J. & Sewry, C. (1990) Influenza A and rhabdomyolysis. *J Infect* **21**, 303-4.

Foy, H.M., Cooney, M.K., Allan, I.D. & Albrecht, J.K. (1987) Influenza B in households: virus shedding without symptoms or antibody response. *Am J Epidemiol* **126**, 506-15.

Francis, T. (1940) A new type of virus from epidemic influenza. *Science* **92**, 405-6.

Francis, T. (1953) Influenza: the newe acquayantance. *Ann Intern Med* **39**, 203-21.

Frank, A.L., Taber, L.H., Wells, C.R., Wells, J.M., Glezen, W.P. & Paredes, A. (1981) Patterns of shedding of myxoviruses and paramyxoviruses in children. *J Infect Dis* **144**, 433-41.

Frank, A.L., Taber, L.H. & Wells, J.M. (1985) Comparison of infection rates and severity of illness for influenza A subtypes H1N1 and H3N2. *J Infect Dis* **151**, 73-80.

Franzen, D., Mertens, T., Waidner, T., Kruppenbacher, J., Hopp, H.W. & Hilger, H.H. (1991) Perimyocarditis in influenza A virus infection. *Klin Wochenschrift* **69**, 404-8.

Fry, J. (1958) Clinical and epidemiological features in a general practice. *Br Med J* **i**, 259-61.

Gamboa, E.T., Wolf, A., Yahr, M.D. *et al.* (1974) Influenza virus antigen in postencephalitic Parkinsonism brain. *Archiv Neurol* **31**, 228-32.

Gamboa, E.T., Eastwood, A.B., Hays, A.P., Maxwell, J. & Penn, A.S. (1979) Isolation of influenza virus from muscle in myoglobinuric polymyositis. *Neurology* **29**, 1323-35.

Garrett, R.R. (1918) Surgical emphysema due to a perforation of the left main bronchus. *Br Med J* 686.

Gaydos, J.C., Hodder, R.A., Top, F.H. *et al.* (1977) Swine influenza A at Fort Dix, New Jersey (January–February 1976). I. Case finding and clinical study of cases. *J Infect Dis* **136**, S356-62.

Gbadero, D.A., Johnson, A-W.B.R., Aderele, W.I. & Olaleye, O.D. (1995) Microbial inciters of acute asthma in urban Nigerian children. *Thorax* **50**, 739-45.

Gerber, G.J., Farmer, W.C. & Fulkerson, L.L. (1978) β-Hemolytic streptococcal pneumonia following influenza. *J Am Med Assoc* **240**, 242-3.

Gibson, T.C., Arnold, J., Craig, E. & Curnen, G.C. (1959) Electrocardiographic studies in Asian influenza. *Am Heart J* **57**, 661-68.

Giles, C. & Shuttleworth, E.M. (1957) Post-mortem findings in 46 influenza deaths. *Lancet* **ii**, 1224-5.

Gilroy, J. (1957) Asian influenza. *Br Med J* **2**, 997-8.

Glezen, W.P. (1982) Serious morbidity and mortality associated with influenza epidemics. *Epidemiol Rev* **4**, 25-44.

Glezen, W.P., Paredes, A. & Taber, L.H. (1980) Influenza in children: relationship to other respiratory agents. *J Am Med Assoc* **243**, 1345-9.

Goodpasture, E.W. (1919) The significance of certain pulmonary lesions in relation to the etiology of influenza. *Am J Med Sci* **158**, 863-70.

Gorell, J.M., Johnson, C.C. & Rybicki, B.A. (1994) Parkinson's disease and its comorbid disorders. *Neurology* **44**, 1865-8.

Gotch, O.H. & Whittingham, H.E. (1918) A report on the influenza epidemic of 1918. *Br Med J* 82–5.

Govan, A.D.T. & Macdonald, H.R.F. (1957) Influenza complicating heart disease in pregnancy. *Lancet* **ii**, 891.

Greco, T.P., Askenase, P.W. & Kashgarian, M. (1977) Postviral myositis: myxovirus-like structures in affected muscle. *Ann Intern Med* **86**, 193–4.

Griffiths, P.D., Ronalds, C.J. & Heath, R.B. (1980) A prospective study of influenza infections during pregnancy. *J Epidemiol Commun Health* **34**, 124–8.

Grist, N.R. (1955) Influenza A and C in Glasgow, 1954. *Br Med J* **2**, 994–7.

Grist, N.R. (1967) Viruses and chronic bronchitis. *Scot Med J* **12**, 408–10.

Gross, P.A., Quinnan, G.V., Rodstein, M. *et al.* (1988) Association of influenza immunization with reduction in mortality in an elderly population. *Archiv Intern Med* **148**, 562–5.

Guthrie, J., Forsyth, D.M. & Montgomery, H. (1957) Asiatic influenza in the middle east: an outbreak in a small community. *Lancet* **ii**, 590–2.

Hakosalo, J. & Saxen, L. (1971) Influenza epidemic and congenital defects. *Lancet* **ii**, 1346–7.

Hakulinen, T., Hovi, L., Karkinen-Jääskeläinen, M. & Penttinen K. (1973) Association between influenza during pregnancy and childhood leukaemia. *Br Med J* **iv**, 265–7.

Hall, C.B. & Douglas, R.G. (1975) Nosocomial influenza infection as a cause of intercurrent fevers in children. *Pediatrics* **55**, 673–7.

Hall, W.J., Douglas, R.G., Hyde, R.W., Roth, F.K., Cross, A.S. & Speers, D.M. (1976) Pulmonary mechanics after uncomplicated influenza A infection. *Am Rev Resp Dis* **113**, 141–7.

Hall, C.B., Douglas, R.G., Geiman, J.M. & Meagher, M.P. (1979) Viral shedding patterns of children with influenza B infection. *J Infect Dis* **140**, 610–13.

Halsey, N.A., Hurwitz, E.S., Meiklejohn, G. *et al.* (1980) An epidemic of Reye syndrome associated with influenza A (H1N1) in Colorado. *J Pediatr* **97**, 535–9.

Hanson, L.C., Weber, D.J., Rutala, W.A. & Samsa, G.P. (1992) Risk factors for nosocomial pneumonia in the elderly. *Am J Med* **92**, 161–6.

Hardy, J.M.B., Azarowicz, E.N., Mannini, A., Medearis, D.N. & Cooke, R.E. (1961) The effect of Asian influenza on the outcome of pregnancy, Baltimore 1957-1958. *Am J Public Health* **51**, 1182–8.

Harkness, G.A., Bentley, D.W. & Roghmann, K.J. (1990) Risk factors for nosocomial pneumonia in the elderly. *Am J Med* **89**, 457–63.

Hartshorn K.L. (1996) Etiology of bacterial superinfections complicating influenza virus infection. In: Brown, L.E., Hampson, A.W. & Webster, R.G. (eds) *Options for the Control of Influenza III*, pp. 499–508. Elsevier, Amsterdam.

Hattori, H., Kawamori, J., Takao, T. *et al.* (1983) Computed tomography in postinfluenzal encephalitis. *Brain Dev* **5**, 564–7.

Hawkins, S.A., Lyttle, J.A. & Connolly, J.H. (1987) Two cases of influenza B encephalitis. *J Neurol Neurosurg Psych* **50**, 1236–7.

Hayden, F.G., Treanor, J.J, Betts, R.F., Lobo, M., Esinhart, J.D. & Hussey, E.K. (1996) Safety and efficacy of the neuraminidase inhibitor GG167 in experimental human influenza. *J Am Med Assoc* **275**, 295–9.

Heikkinen, T., Ruuskanen, O., Waris, M., Ziegler, T., Arola, M. & Halonen, P. (1991) Influenza vaccination in the prevention of acute otitis media in children. *Am J Dis Child* **145**, 445–8.

Hers, J.F.P. (1966) Disturbances of the ciliated epithelium due to influenza virus. *Am Rev Resp Dis* **93**, 162–71.

Hers, J.F., Gosling, W.R.O., Masurel, N. & Mulder, J. (1957) Death from Asiatic influenza in the Netherlands. *Lancet* **2**, 1164–5.

Hers, J.F.P., Masurel, N. & Mulder, J. (1958) Bacteriology and histopathology of the respiratory tract and lungs of fatal Asian influenza. *Lancet* **ii**, 1141–3.

Hilleman, M.R., Werner, J.H. & Gauld, R.L. (1953) Influenza antibodies in the population of the USA: an epidemiological investigation. *Bull WHO* **8**, 613–31.

Hirschhorn, L.R., McIntosh, K., Anderson, K.G. & Dermody, T.S. (1992) Influenzal pneumonia as a complication of autologous bone marrow transplantation. *Clin Infect Dis* **14**, 786–7.

Hirst, G.K. (1941) The agglutination of red cells by allantoic fluid of chick embryos infected with influenza virus. *Science* **94**, 22–3.

Holland, W.W. (1957) A clinical study of influenza in the Royal Air Force. *Lancet* **ii**, 840–1.

Holt, P. & Kibblewhite, K. (1995) Acute polymyositis and myoglobinuric renal failure associated with influenza A infection. *NZ Med J* **108**, 463.

Hordvik, N.L., König, P., Hamory, B. *et al.* (1989) Effects of acute viral respiratory tract infections in patients with cystic fibrosis. *Ped Pulmonol* **7**, 217–22.

Horn, C.R., Wood, N.C. & Hughes, J.A. (1983) Invasive aspergillosis following post-influenza pneumonia. *Br J Dis Chest* **77**, 407–10.

Horner, F.A. (1958) Neurologic disorders after Asian influenza. *New Engl J Med* **258**, 983–5.

Horner, G.J. & Gray, F.D. (1973) Effect of uncomplicated, presumptive influenza on the diffusing capacity of the lung. *Am Rev Resp Dis* **108**, 866–9.

Hoult, J.G. & Flewett, T.H. (1960) Influenzal encephalopathy and post-influenzal encephalitis. Histological and other observations. *Br Med J* **i**, 1847–50.

Housworth, J. & Langmuir, A.D. (1974) Excess mortality from epidemic influenza, 1957–1966. *Am J Epidemiol* **100**, 40–8.

Howard, J.B., McCracken, G.H. & Luby, J.P. (1972) Influenza A2 virus as a cause of croup requiring tracheotomy. *J Pediatr* **81**, 1148–50.

Howells, C.H.L., Vesselinova-Jenkins, C.K., Evans, A.D. & James, J. (1975) Influenza vaccination and mortality from bronchopneumonia in the elderly. *Lancet* **i**, 381–3.

Hubert, B., Waitier, L., Garnerin, P. & Richardson, S. (1992) Meningococcal disease and influenza-like syndrome: a new approach to an old question. *J Infect Dis* **166**, 542–5.

Hurwitz, E.S. (1989) Reye's syndrome. *Epidemiol Rev* **11**, 249–53.

Hurwitz, E.S., Nelson, D.B., Davis, C., Morens, D. & Schonberger, L.B. (1982) National surveillance for Reye syndrome: a five year review. *Pediatrics* **70**, 895–900.

Hyman, A.S. (1927) Post-influenza bradycardia. *Archiv Intern Med* **40**, 120–7.

Influenza Committee of the Advisory Board to the D.G.M.S., France (1918) The influenza epidemic in the British Armies in France, 1918. *Br Med J* 505–9.

Jackson, W.P.U. (1946) Influenza B among West Indians: outbreaks in the Bahamas and in England. *Lancet* 631–5.

Jaimovich, D.G., Kumar, A., Shabino, C.L. & Formoli, R. (1992) Influenza B virus infection associated with non-bacterial septic shock-like illness. *J Infect* **25**, 311–15.

Jakeman, K.J., Rushdon, D.I., Smith, H. & Sweet, C. (1991) Exacerbation of bacterial toxicity to infant ferrets by influenza virus: possible role in sudden infant death syndrome. *J Infect Dis* **163**, 35–40.

Jamieson, W.M., Kerr, M., Green, D.M. *et al.* (1958) Some aspects of the recent epidemic of influenza in Dundee. *Br Med J* **1**, 908–13.

Jennings, R. (1968) Respiratory viruses in Jamaica: a virologic and serologic study. III. Haemagglutination-inhibiting antibodies to type B and C influenza viruses in the sera of Jamaicans. *Am J Epidemiol* **87**, 440–6.

Johanson, W.G., Pierce, A.K. & Sanford, J.P. (1969) Pulmonary function in uncomplicated influenza. *Am Rev Resp Dis* **100**, 141–6.

Jones, D.B. (1979) An association between sub-arachnoid haemorrhage and influenza A infection. *Postgrad Med J* **55**, 853–5.

Jordan, W.S., Denny, F.W., Badger, G.F. *et al.* (1958) A study of illness in a group of Cleveland families. XVII. The occurrence of Asian influenza. *Am J Hygiene* **68**, 190–212.

Karjalainen, J., Nieminen, M.S. & Heikkila, J. (1980) Influenza A1 myocarditis in conscripts. *Acta Med Scand* **207**, 27–30.

Kapila, C.C., Kaul, S., Kapur, S.C., Kalayanam, T.S. & Banerjee, D. (1958) Neurological and hepatic disorders associated with influenza. *Br Med J* **ii**, 1311–14.

Kark, J.D. & Lebiush, M. (1981) Smoking and epidemic influenza-like illness in female military recruits: a brief survey. *Am J Public Health* **71**, 530–2.

Kark, J.D., Lebiush, M. & Rannon, L. (1982) Cigarette smoking as a risk factor for epidemic A (H_1N_1) influenza in young men. *New Engl J Med* **307**, 1042–6.

Karpathios, T., Kostaki, M., Drakonaki, S. *et al.* (1995) An epidemic with influenza B virus causing benign acute myositis in ten boys and two girls. *Eur J Ped* **154**, 334–6.

Katagiri, S., Ohizumi, A. & Homma, M. (1983) An outbreak of influenza C influenza in a children's home. *J Infect Dis* **148**, 51–6.

Kaye, D., Rosenbluth, M., Hook, E.W. *et al.* (1962) Endemic influenza. II. The nature of the disease in the post-pandemic period. *Am Rev Resp Dis* **85**, 9–21.

Keane, W.R., Helderma, J.H., Luby, J., Gailiunas, P., Hull, A.R. & Kokko, J.P. (1978) Epidemic renal transplant rejection associated with influenza A Victoria. *Proc Clin Dialysis Transplant Forum* **8**, 232–6.

Kempe, A., Hall, C,B., MacDonald N.E. *et al.* (1989) Influenza in children with cancer. *J Pediatr* **115**, 33–9.

Kendell, R.E. & Kemp, I.W. (1989) Maternal influenza in the etiology of schizophrenia. *Archiv Gen Psych* **46**, 878–82.

Kerr, A.A., Downham, M.A.P.S., McQuillan, J. & Gardner, P.S. (1975) Gastric 'flu influenza B causing abdominal symptoms in children. *Lancet* **1**, 291–5.

Kessler, H.A., Trenholme, G.M., Vogelzang, N.J. *et al.* (1983) Elevated creatine phosphokinase levels associated with influenza A/Texas/1/77 infection. *Scand J Infect Dis* **15**, 7–10.

Khakpour, M., Saidi, A. & Naficy, K. (1969) Proved viraemia in Asian influenza (Hong Kong variant) during incubation period. *Br Med J* **4**, 208–9.

Kilbourne, E.D. (1959) Studies on influenza in the pandemic of 1957–1958. III. Isolation of influenza A (Asian strain) viruses from influenza patients with pulmonary complications. Details of virus isolation and characterization of isolates, with quantitative comparison of isolation methods. *J Clin Invest* **38**, 266–74.

Kilbourne, E.D. (1973) The molecular epidemiology of influenza. *J Infect Dis* **127**, 478–87.

Kim, H.W., Brandt, C.W., Arrobio, J.O., Murphy, B., Chanock, R.M. & Parrott, R.H. (1979) Influenza A and B infections in infants and young children during the years 1957–1976. *Am J Epidemiol* **109**, 464–79.

Klimek, J.J., Linenberg, L.B., Cole, S. *et al.* (1976) Fatal cases of influenza pneumonia with superinfection by multiple bacteria and herpes simplex virus. *Am Rev Resp Viruses* **113**, 683–8.

Klimov, A.I., Rocha, E., Hayden, F.G., Shult, P.A., Roumillat, L.F. & Cox, N.J. (1995) Prolonged shedding of amantadine-resistant influenza A viruses by immuno-deficient patients: detection by polymerase chain reaction-restriction analysis. *J Infect Dis* **172**, 1352–5.

Kobayashi, O., Sekiya, M. & Saitoh, H. (1992) A case of invasive broncho-pulmonary aspergillosis associated with influenza A (H3N2) infection. *Japanese J Thoracic Dis* **30**, 1338–44.

Kondo, S. & Abe, K. (1991) The effects of influenza virus infection on FEV1 in asthmatic children. *Chest* **100**, 1235–8.

Kovacs, B. (1985) Alteration of the blood-retina barriers in cases of viral retinitis. *Internat Ophthalmol* **8**, 159–66.

Krilov, L.R. & Swenson, P. (1985) Acute parotitis associated with influenza A infection. *J Infect Dis* **152**, 853.

Ksiazek, T.G., Olson, J.G., Irving, G.S., Settle, C.S., White, R. & Petrusso, R. (1980) An influenza outbreak due to A/USSR/77-like (H1N1) virus aboard a US navy ship. *Am J Epidemiol* **112**, 487–94.

Kunugi, H., Nanko, S. & Takei, N. (1992) Influenza and schizophrenia in Japan. *Br J Psych* **161**, 274–5.

Kurtz, J., Manvell, R.J. & Banks, J. (1996) Avian influenza virus isolated from a woman with conjunctivitis. *Lancet* **348**, 901–2.

Lamontagne, J.R. (1980) Summary of a workshop on influenza B viruses and Reye's syndrome. *J Infect Dis* **142**, 452–65.

Lamy, M.E., Pouthier-Simon, F. & Debacker-Willame, E. (1973) Respiratory viral infections in hospital patients with chronic bronchitis. *Chest* **63**, 336–41.

Langmuir, A.D., Worthen, T.D., Solomon, J., Ray, C.G. & Petersen, E. (1985) The Thucydides syndrome: a new hypothesis for the cause of the plague of Athens. *New Engl J Med* **313**, 1027–30.

Laraya-Cuasay, L.R., DeForest, A., Huff, D., Lischner, H. & Huang, N.N. (1977) Chronic pulmonary complications of early influenza virus infection in children. *Am Rev Resp Dis* **116**, 617–25.

Larson, H.E. & Blades, R. (1976) Impairment of human polymorphonuclear leukocyte function by influenza virus. *Lancet* **i**, 283.

Larson, H.E., Parry, R.P., Gilchrist, C., Liquetti, A. & Tyrrell, D.A.J. (1977) Influenza viruses and staphylococci *in vitro*: some interactions with polymorphonuclear leukocytes and epithelial cells. *Br J Exp Path* **58**, 281–88.

Larson, H.E., Parry, R.P. & Tyrrell, D.A.J. (1980) Impaired polymorphonuclear leukocyte chemotaxis after influenza virus infection. *Br J Dis Chest* **74**, 56–62.

Leck, I. & Stewart, J.K. (1972) Incidence of neoplasms in children born after influenza epidemics. *Br Med J* **iv**, 631–4.

Lewes, D., Rainford, D.J. & Lane, W.F. (1974) Symptomless myocarditis and myalgia in viral and *Mycoplasma pneumoniae* infections. *Br Heart J* **36**, 924–32.

Lewis, M., Kallenbach, J., Ruff, P., Zaltzman, M., Abramowitz, J. & Zwi, S. (1985) Invasive pulmonary aspergillosis complicating influenza A pneumonia in a previously healthy patient. *Chest* **87**, 691–3.

Lindsay, M.I., Herrmann, E.C., Morrow, G.W. & Brown, A.L. (1970) Hong Kong influenza: clinical, microbiologic, and pathologic features in 127 cases. *J Am Med Assoc* **214**, 1825–32.

Lipsky, B.A., Boyko, E.J., Inui, T.S. & Koepsell, T.D. (1986) Risk factors for acquiring pneumococcal infections. *Archiv Intern Med* **146**, 2179–85.

Little, R., White, M.R. & Hartshorn, K.L. (1994) Interferon-alpha enhances neutrophil respiratory burst responses to stimulation with influenza A and FMLP. *J Inf Dis* **170**, 802–10.

Liu, C. (1956) Rapid diagnosis of human influenza infection from nasal smears by means of fluorescein-labelled antibody. *Proc Soc Exp Biol Med* **92**, 883–7.

Ljungman, P. (1997) Respiratory virus infections in bone marrow transplant recipients: the European perspective. *Am J Med* **102** (3A), 44–7.

Ljungman, P., Andersson, J., Aschan, J.S. *et al.* (1993) Influenza A in immunocompromised patients. *Clin Infect Dis* **17**, 244–7.

Lloyd-Still, R.M. (1958) Psychosis following Asian influenza. *Lancet* **ii**, 20–1.

Louria, D.B., Blumenfeld, H.L., Ellis, J.T., Kilbourne, E.D. & Rogers, D.E. (1959) Studies on influenza in the pandemic of 1957–8. II. Pulmonary complications of influenza. *J Clin Invest* **38**, 213–65.

Lucke, B., Wright, T. & Kime, E. (1919) Pathologic anatomy and bacteriology of influenza. *Archiv Intern Med* **24**, 154–237.

Lui, K.-J. & Kendal, A.P. (1987) Impact of influenza epidemics on mortality in the United States from October 1972 to May 1985. *Am J Public Health* **77**, 712–16.

Luksza, A.R. & Jones, D.K. (1984) Influenza B virus infection complicated by pneumonia, acute renal failure and disseminated intravascular coagulation. *J Infect* **9**, 174–6.

Lynberg, M.C., Khoury, M.J., Lu, X. & Cocian, T. (1994) Maternal flu, fever, and the risk of neural tube defects: a population-based care-control study. *Am J Epidemiol* **140**, 244–55.

McConkey, B. & Daws, R.A. (1958) Neurological disorders associated with Asian influenza. *Lancet* **ii**, 15–17.

McConnochie, J.A. (1918) Haemorrhage in influenza. *Br Med J* 515.

MacDonald, N.E., Wolfish, N., McLaine, P., Phipps, P. & Rossier, E. (1986) Role of respiratory viruses in exacerbations of primary nephrotic syndrome. *J Pediatr* **108**, 378–82.

MacDonald, K.L., Osterholm, M.T., Hedberg, C.W. *et al.* (1987) Toxic shock syndrome. A newly recognised complication of influenza and influenza-like illness. *J Am Med Assoc* **257**, 1053–8.

McGregor, J.A., Burns, J.C., Levin, M.J., Burlington, B. & Meiklejohn, G. (1984) Transplacental passage of influenza A/Bangkok/(H3N2) mimicking amniotic fluid infection syndrome. *Am J Obstetr Gynecol* **149**, 856–9.

Magill, T.P. (1940) A virus from cases of influenza-like upper respiratory infection. *Proc Soc Exp Biol (New York)* **45**, 162–4.

Marrie, T.J., Durant, H. & Kwan, C. (1986) Nursing home acquired pneumonia: a case-control study. *J Am Geriatr Soc* **34**, 697–702.

Martin, C.J. (1918) An epidemic of fifty cases of influenza among the personnel of a base hospital, B.E.F., France. *Br Med J* 281–2.

Martin, C.M., Kunin, C.M., Gottlieb, L.S., Barnes, M.W., Liu. C. & Finland, M. (1959a) Asian influenza A in Boston, 1957–1958; observations in thirty-two influenza-associated fatal cases. *Archiv Intern Med* **103**, 515–31.

Martin, C.M., Kunin, C.M., Gottlieb, L.S. & Finland, M. (1959b) Asian influenza A in Boston, 1957–1958: severe staphylococcal pneumonia complicating influenza. *Archiv Intern Med* **103**, 532–42.

Mathur, U., Bentley, D.W. & Hall, C.B. (1980) Concurrent respiratory syncytial virus and influenza A infections in the institutionalized elderly and chronically ill. *Ann Intern Med* **93**, 49–52.

Mauch, T.J., Bratton, S., Myers, T., Krane, E., Gentry, S.R. & Kashtan, C.E. (1994) Influenza B virus infection in pediatric solid organ transplant recipients. *Pediatrics* **94**, 225–9.

Mednick, S.A., Machon, R.A., Huttunen, M.O. & Bonett, D. (1988) Adult schizophrenia following prenatal exposure to an influenza epidemic. *Archiv Gen Psych* **45**, 189–92.

Mednick, S.A., Machon, R.A., Huttunen, M.O. & Barr, C.E. (1990) Influenza and schizophrenia: Helsinki vs. Edinburgh. *Archiv Gen Psych* **47**, 875–6.

Meibalane, R., Sedmak, G.V., Sasidharan, P., Garg, P. & Grausz, J.P. (1977) Outbreak of influenza in a neonatal intensive care unit. *J Pediatr* **91**, 974–6.

Mellman, W.J. (1958) Influenza encephalitis. *J Pediatr* **53**, 292–7.

Middleton, P.J., Alexander, R.M. & Szymanski, M.T. (1970) Severe myositis during recovery from influenza. *Lancet* **ii**, 533–5.

Miller, R.F., Loveday, C., Holton, J., Sharvell, Y., Pate, G. & Brink, N.S. (1996) Community-based respiratory viral infections in HIV positive patients with lower respiratory tract disease: a prospective bronchoscopic study. *Genitourinary Med* **72**, 9–11.

Minor, T.E., Dick, E.C., Baker, J.W., Ouellette, J.J., Cohen, M. & Reed, C.E. (1976) Rhinovirus and influenza type A infections as precipitants of asthma. *Am Rev Resp Dis* **113**, 149–53.

Minow, R.A., Gorbach, S., Johnson, B.L. *et al.* (1974) Myoglobinuria associated with influenza A infection. *Ann Intern Med* **80**, 359–61.

Minuse, E., Willis, P.W., Davenport, F.M. & Francis, T. (1962) An attempt to demonstrate viremia in cases of Asian influenza. *J Lab Clin Med* **59**, 1016–19.

Monto, A.S. & Kioumehr, F. (1975) The Tecumseh study of respiratory illness. IX. Occurrence of influenza in the community, 1966–1971. *Am J Epidemiol* **102**, 553–63.

Monto, A.S., Ceglarek, J.P. & Hayner, N.S. (1981) Liver function abnormalities in the course of a type A (H1N1) influenza A outbreak: relation to Reye's syndrome. *Am J Epidemiol* **14**, 750–9.

Monto, A.S., Koopman, J.S. & Longini, I.M. (1985) The Tecumseh study of illness. XIII. Influenza infection and disease, 1976–1981. *Am J Epidemiol* **121**, 811–22.

Moore, G. (1977) Influenza and Parkinson's disease. *Public Health Rep* **92**, 79–80.

Morbidity and Mortality Weekly Report (1988) Increase in pneumonia mortality among young adults and the HIV epidemic—New York City, United States. *MMWR* **37**, 593–6.

Morens, D.M. & Littman, R.J. (1994) 'Thucydides syndrome' reconsidered: new thoughts on the 'plague of Athens'. *Am J Epidemiol* **140**, 621–8.

Morgan, D.A. & Chappell, A.G. (1977) Ventricular fibrillation in influenza myocarditis. *Br J Clin Pract* **31**, 192–4.

Morgensen, J.L. (1974) Myoglobinuria and renal failure associated with influenza. *Ann Intern Med* **80**, 362–3.

Moriuchi, H., Katsushima, N., Nishimura, H., Nakamura, K. & Numazaki, Y. (1991) Community-acquired influenza C virus infection in children. *J Pediatr* **118**, 235–8.

Morris, J.A., Kasel, J.A., Saglam, M., Knight, V. & Loda, F.A. (1966) Immunity to influenza as related to antibody levels. *New Engl J Med* **274**, 527–35.

Moser, M.R., Bender, T.R., Margolis, H.S. *et al.* (1979) An outbreak of influenza aboard a commercial airline. *Am J Epidemiol* **110**, 1–6.

Moss, S.E., Klein, R. & Klein, B.E.K. (1991) Cause-specific mortality in a population-based study of diabetes. *Am J Public Health* **81**, 1158–62.

Mullooly, J.P., Barker, W.H. & Nolan, T.F. (1986) Risk of acute respiratory disease among pregnant women during influenza A epidemics. *Public Health Rep* **101**, 205–11.

Muir, R. & Wilson, G.H. (1919) Influenza and its complications. *Br Med J* **i**, 3–5.

Murphy, H.H. (1891) Notes on influenza from some 200 cases, with complications and sequelae, showing infection, incubation, and behaviour of the contagion. In: Parsons, H.F. (ed.) *Report on the Influenza Epidemic of 1889–90*, pp. 305–9. Local Government Board, HMSO, London.

Murphy, B.R., Baron, S., Chalhub, E.G., Uhlendorf, C.P. & Chanock, R.M. (1973) Temperature-sensitive mutants of influenza virus. IV. Induction of interferon in the nasopharynx by wild-type and a temperature-sensitive recombinant virus. *J Infect Dis* **128**, 488–93.

Naficy, K. (1963) Human influenza infection with proved viraemia. *New Engl J Med* **269**, 964–6.

Nagai, T., Yagishita, A., Tsuchiya, Y., Asamura, S., Kurokawa, H. & Matsuo, N. (1993) Symmetrical thalamic lesions on CT in influenza A virus infection presenting with or without Reye syndrome. *Brain Dev* **15**, 67–73.

Nash, W.G. (1919) Surgical emphysema in a fatal case of influenza. *Br Med J* **i**, 9.

Newton, L. & Hall, S.M. (1993) Reye's syndrome in the British Isles: report for 1990/91 and the first decade of surveillance. *Communicable Dis Rep* **3**, R11–R16.

Nguyen-Van-Tam, J.S. & Nicholson, K.G. (1992) Influenza deaths in Leicestershire during the 1989–90 epidemic: implications for prevention. *Epidemiol Infect* **108**, 537–45.

Nichol, K.L., Margolis, K.L., Wouremna, J. & von Sternberg, T. (1996) Effectiveness of influenza vaccine in the elderly. *Gerontology* **42**, 274–9.

Nicholson, K.G. (1993) Immunisation against influenza among people aged over 65 living at home in Leicestershire during winter 1991–2. *Br Med J* **306**, 974–6.

Nicholson, K.G., Kent, J. & Ireland, D.C. (1993) Respiratory viruses and exacerbations of asthma in adults. *Br Med J* **307**, 982–6.

Nicholson, K.G., Stone, A.J., Botha, J.L. & Raymond, N.T. (1996) Effectiveness of influenza vaccine in reducing hospital admissions in people with diabetes. In: Brown, L.E., Hampson, A.W. & Webster, R.G. (eds) *Options for the Control of Influenza III*, pp. 113–18. Elsevier, Amsterdam.

Noble, R.L., Lillington, G.A. & Kempson, R.L. (1973) Fatal diffuse influenza pneumonia: premortem diagnosis by lung biopsy. *Chest* **63**, 644–6.

O'Callaghan, E., Gibson, T., Colohan, H.A. *et al.* (1991) Season of birth in schizophrenia: evidence for confinement of an excess of winter births to patients without a family history of mental disorder. *Br J Psych* **158**, 764–9.

Ohmit, S.E. & Monto, A.S. (1995) Influenza vaccine effectiveness in preventing hospitalization among the elderly during influenza type A and type B seasons. *Internat J Epidemiol* **24**, 1240–8.

Okuno, T., Takao, T., Ito, M., Mikawa, H. & Nakano, Y. (1982) Contrast enhanced hypodense areas in a case of acute disseminated encephalitis following influenza A virus. *Computer Radiol* **6**, 215–17.

Olsen, P.M., Horsleth, A. & Krasilnikoff, P.A. (1992) Varying clinical pictures among young children with influenza virus A infections. *Ugeskrift Laeger* **154**, 560–3.

Ong, E.L.C., Ellis, M.E., Webb, E.K. *et al.* (1989) Infective respiratory exacerbations in young adults with cystic fibrosis: role of viruses and atypical micro-organisms. *Thorax* **44**, 739–40.

Oseasohn, R., Adelsan, L. & Kaji, M. (1959) Clinicopathologic study of thirty-three fatal cases of Asian influenza. *New Engl J Med* **260**, 509–18.

Oswald, N.C., Shooter, R.A. & Curwen, M.P. (1958) Pneumonia complicating Asian influenza. *Br Med J* **ii**, 1305–11.

Paisley, J.W., Bruhn, F.W., Lauer, B.A. & McIntosh K. (1978) Type A2 influenza viral infections in children. *Am J Dis Child* **132**, 34–6.

Pallast, E.G.M., Jongbloet, P.H., Straatman, H.M. & Zielhuis, G.A. (1994) Excess seasonality of births among patients with schizophrenia and seasonal ovopathy. *Schizophrenia Bull* **20**, 269–76.

Parker, F., Jolliffe, L.S., Barnes, M.W. & Finland, M. (1946) Pathologic findings in the lungs of five cases from which influenza virus was isolated. *Am J Pathol* **22**, 797–819.

Parsons, H.F. (1891) *Report on the Influenza Epidemic of 1889–90*. Local Government Board, HMSO, London.

Partin, J.C., Partin, J.S., Schubert, W.K., Jacobs, R. & Saalfeld, K. (1976) Isolation of influenza virus from liver and muscle biopsy specimens from a surviving case of Reye's syndrome. *Lancet* **ii**, 599–602.

Patriarca, P.A., Weber, J.A., Parker, R.A. *et al.* (1985) Efficacy of influenza vaccine in nursing homes. Reduction in illness and complications during an influenza A (H3N2) epidemic. *J Am Med Assoc* **253**, 1136–9.

Perrotta, D.M., Decker, M. & Glezen, W.P. (1985) Acute respiratory disease hospitalizations as a measure of impact of epidemic influenza. *Am J Epidemiol* **122**, 468–76.

Petersdorf, R.G., Fusco, J.J., Harter, D.H. & Albrink, W.S. (1959) Pulmonary infections complicating Asian influenza. *Archiv Intern Med* **103**, 262–72.

Petersen, N.T., Hoiby, N., Mordhorst, C.H., Lind, K., Flensborg, E.W. & Bruun, B. (1981) Respiratory infections in cystic fibrosis patients caused by virus, chlamydia and mycoplasma—possible synergism with *Pseudomonas aeruginosa*. *Acta Paed Scand* **70**, 623–8.

Pinsker, K.L., Schneyer, B., Becker, N. & Kamholz, S.L. (1981) Usual interstitial pneumonia following Texas A2 infection. *Chest* **80**, 123–6.

Podosin, R.L. & Felton, W. L. (1958) The clinical picture of Far East influenza occurring at the fourth national boy scout jamboree. *New Engl J Med* **258**, 778–82.

Polak, M.F. (1959) Influenzasterfte in de herfst van 1957. *Nederlandische Tijdschrift Geneeskunde* **103**, 1098–109.

Potter, M.N., Foot, A.B.N. & Oakhill, A. (1991) Influenza A and the virus-associated haemophagocytic syndrome: cluster of three cases in children with acute leukaemia. *J Clin Pathol* **44**, 297–9.

Prechter, G.C. & Gerhard, A.K. (1989) Postinfluenza toxic shock syndrome. *Chest* **95**, 1153–4.

Preston, G. (1890) An outbreak of influenza on board the industrial training ship Mount Edgcumbe. *Br Med J* 477.

Pribble, C.G., Black, P.G., Bosso, J.A. & Turner, R.B. (1990) Clinical manifestations of exacerbations of cystic fibrosis associated with non-bacterial infections. *J Pediatr* **117**, 200–4.

Price, D.A., Postlethwaite, R.J. & Longson, M. (1976) Influenza virus A2 infections presenting with febrile convulsions and gastrointestinal symptoms in young children. *Clin Pediatr* **15**, 361–7.

Proby, C.M., Hackett, D., Gupta, S. & Cox, T.M. (1986) Acute myopericarditis in influenza A infection. *Quart J Med* **60**, 887–92.

Protheroe, S.M. & Mellor, D.H. (1991) Imaging in influenza A encephalitis. *Archiv Dis Childhood* **66**, 702–5.

Public Health Laboratory Service (1958) Deaths from Asian influenza, 1957. *Br Med J* **i**, 915–19.

Ramphal, R., Donnelly, W.H. & Small, P.A. (1980) Influenza pneumonia in pregnancy: failure to demonstrate transplacental transmission of influenza virus. *Am J Obstetr Gynecol* **138**, 347–8.

Ray, C.G., Icenogle, T.B., Minnich, L.L., Copeland, J.G. & Grogan, T.M. (1989) The use of intravenous ribavirin to treat influenza virus-associated acute myocarditis. *J Infect Dis* **159**, 829–36.

Ravenholt, R.T. & Foege W.H. (1982) 1918 influenza, encephalitis lethargica, Parkinsonism. *Lancet* **ii**, 860–4.

Reichmann, N., Kaufman, N. & Flatau, E. (1997) Acute effusive-constrictive pericarditis in influenza A. *Harefuah* **132**, 89–90.

Retailliau, H.F., Storch, G.A., Curtis, A.C., Horne, T.J., Scally, M.J. & Hattwick, M.A.W. (1979) The epidemiology of influenza B in a rural setting in 1977. *Am J Epidemiol* **109**, 639–49.

Risdall, R.J., McKenna, R.W., Nesbit, M.E. *et al.* (1979) Virus-associated haemophagocytic syndrome. *Cancer* **44**, 993–1002.

Robertson, G.M. & Elkins, F.A. (1890) Report of an epidemic of influenza (140 cases) occurring at the Royal Asylum, Morningside, Edinburgh. *Br Med J* 228–30.

Robertson, L., Caley, J.P. & Moore, J. (1958) Importance of *Staphylococcus aureus* in pneumonia in the 1957 epidemic of influenza A. *Lancet* 233–6.

Roldaan, A.C. & Masural, N. (1982) Viral respiratory infections in children staying in a mountain resort. *Eur J Resp Dis* **63**, 140–50.

Rolleston, J.D. (1919) Influenza. In: Coombs, C.F. & Short, A.R. (eds) *The Medical Annual: A Yearbook of Treatment and Practitioner's Index*, pp. 202–10. John Wright, Bristol.

Rott, R., Klenk, H.-D., Nagai, Y. & Tashiro, M. (1995) Influenza viruses, cell enzymes, and pathogenicity. *Am J Resp Crit Care Med* **152**, S16–S19.

Rowland, H.A.K. (1958) The influenza epidemic in Abadan. *Br Med J* **1**, 422–5.

Rowley, D.L. (1985) National Reye syndrome surveillance, 1982. *Pediatrics* **75**, 260–4.

Ruff, R.L. & Secrist, D. (1982) Viral studies in benign acute childhood myositis. *Archiv Neurol* **39**, 261–3.

Russell, E.J., Zimmerman, R.D., Leeds, N.E. & French, J. (1979) Reye syndrome: computed tomographic documentation of disordered intracerebral structure. *J Comp Ass Tom* **3**, 217–20.

Ruuskanen, O., Arola, M., Putto-Laurila, A. *et al.* (1989) Acute otitis media and respiratory virus infections. *Ped Infect Dis J* **8**, 94–9.

Ruutu, P., Vaheri, A. & Kosunen, T.U. (1977) Depression of human neutrophil motility by influenza virus *in vitro*. *Scand J Immunol* **6**, 897–906.

Safrin, S., Rush, M.S. & Mills, J. (1990) Influenza in patients with human immunodeficiency virus infection. *Chest* **98**, 33–7.

Saxen, L. Holmberg, P.C., Kurrpa, K., Kuosma, E. & Pyhälä, R. (1990) Influenza epidemics and anencephaly. *Am J Public Health* **80**, 473–5.

Scadding, J.G. (1937) Lung changes in influenza. *Quart J Med* **6**, 425–65.

Scheiblauer, H., Reinacher, M., Tashiro, M. & Rott, R. (1992) Interactions between bacteria and influenza A virus in the development of influenza pneumonia. *J Infect Dis* **166**, 783–91.

Schmaltz, A.A., Seitz, K.H., Schenck, W., Both, A. & Kraus, B. (1986) Restrictive cardiomyopathy as a late sequel of influenza A2 virus myocarditis. *Zeitschrift Kardiol* **75**, 605–8.

Schwarzman, S.W., Adler, J.L., Sullivan, R.J. & Marine, W.M. (1971) Bacterial pneumonia during the Hong Kong epidemic of 1968–1969. *Archiv Intern Med* **127**, 1037–41.

Serfling, R.E., Sherman, I.L. & Housworth, W.J. (1967) Excess pneumonia-influenza mortality by age and sex in three major influenza A2 epidemics, United States, 1957–58, 1960 and 1963. *Am J Epidemiol* **86**, 433–41.

Serie, C., Barme, M., Hannoun, C., Thibon, M., Beck, H. & Aquino, J.P. (1977) Effects of vaccination on an influenza epidemic in a geriatric hospital. *Dev Biol Stand* **39**, 317–21.

Sham, P.C., O'Callaghan, E., Takei, N., Murray, G.K., Hare, E.H. & Murray, R.M. (1992) Schizophrenia following prenatal exposure to influenza epidemics between 1939 and 1960. *Br J Psych* **160**, 461–6.

Shapiro, D. & Ferris, J. (1986) Influenza A and aspergillosis. *Chest* **89**, 318–19.

Shenouda, A. & Hatch, F.E. (1976) Influenza A viral infection associated with acute renal failure. *Am J Med* **61**, 697–702.

Shirono, K., Tsuda, H. & Akahoshi, I. (1996) Influenza-virus associated hemophagocytic syndrome in a patient with pernicious anemia. *Japanese J Clin Hematol* **37**, 511–13.

Silber, E.N. (1958) Respiratory viruses and heart disease. *Ann Intern Med* **48**, 228–41.

Simon, N.M., Rovner, R.N. & Berlin, B.S. (1970) Acute myoglobinuria associated with type A2 (Hong Kong) influenza. *J Am Med Assoc* **212**, 1704–5.

Skoner, D.P., Doyle, W.J., Seroky, J. & Fireman, P. (1996) Lower airway responses to influenza A virus in healthy allergic and non-allergic subjects. *Am J Resp Crit Care Med* **154**, 661–4.

Smith, W., Andrewes, C.H. & Laidlaw, P.P. (1933) A virus obtained from influenza patients. *Lancet* **i**, 66–8.

Smith, C.B., Kanner, R.E., Golden, C.A., Klauber, M.R. & Renzetti, A.D. (1980) Effect of viral infections on pulmonary function in patients with chronic obstructive pulmonary diseases. *J Infect Dis* **141**, 271–80.

Smith, A.P., Tyrrell, D.A.J., Al-Nakib, W. *et al.* (1989) Effects and after effects of the common cold and influenza on human performance. *Neuropsychobiology* **21**, 90–3.

Smith, A.P., Thomas, M., Brockman, P., Kent, J, & Nicholson, K.G. (1993) Effect of influenza B infection on human performance. *Br Med J* **306**, 760–1.

Smyth, A.R., Smyth, R.L., Tong, C.Y.W., Hart, C.A. & Heaf, D.P. (1995) Effect of respiratory virus infections including rhinovirus on clinical status in cystic fibrosis. *Archiv Dis Childhood* **73**, 117–20.

Soto, P.J., Broun, G.O. & Wyatt, J.P. (1959) Asian influenza pneumonitis. *Am J Med* **27**, 18–25.

Sperber, S.J. & Francis, J.B. (1987) Toxic shock syndrome during an influenza outbreak. *J Am Med Assoc* **257**, 1086–7.

Sprenger, M.J.W., Beyer, W.E.P., Kempen, B.M. & Mulder, P.G.H. (1993) Risk factors for influenza mortality? In: Hannoun, C., Kendal, A.P., Klenk, H.D., McMichael, A., Nicholson, K.G. & Oya, A. (eds) *Options for the Control of Influenza II*, pp. 15–23. Excerpta Medica, Amsterdam.

Stanley, E.D. & Jackson, G.G. (1966) Viraemia in Asian influenza. *Trans Assoc Am Physicians* **1**, 376–87.

Stanwell-Smith, R., Parker, A.M., Chakraverty, P., Soltanpoor, N. & Simpson, C.N. (1994) Possible association of influenza A with fetal loss: investigation of a cluster of spontaneous abortions and stillbirths. *CDR Rev* **4**, R28–R32.

Stevens, D., Burman, D., Clarke, S.K.R., Lamb, R.W., Harper, M.E. & Sarafian, A.H. (1974) Temporary paralysis after influenza B. *Lancet* **2**, 1354–5.

Stocks, P. (1935) The effect of influenza epidemics on the certified causes of death. *Lancet* **ii**, 386–95.

Stuart-Harris, C.H. (1961) Twenty years of influenza epidemics. *Am Rev Resp Dis* **83**, 54–61.

Stuart-Harris, C.H. & Schild, G.C. (eds) (1976) *Influenza, the Viruses and Disease*. Edward Arnold, London.

Sugaya, N., Nerome, K., Ishida, M. *et al.* (1992) Impact of influenza virus infection as a cause of pediatric hospitalization. *J Infect Dis* **165**, 373–5.

Sulkava, R., Rissanen, A. & Pyhälä, R. (1981) Post-influenzal encephalitis during the influenza A outbreak in 1979/1980. *J Neurol Neurosurg Psych* **44**, 161–3.

Susser, E., Lin, S.P. Brown, A.S. Luney, L.H. & Erlenmeyer-Kimling, L. (1994) No relation between risk of schizophrenia and prenatal exposure to influenza in Holland. *Am J Psych* **151**, 922–4.

Tablan, O.C., Anderson, L.J., Arden, N.H. *et al.* (1994) Guideline for prevention of nosocomial infection. Part 1. Issues on prevention of nosocomial pneumonia—1994. *Am J Infect Control* **22**, 247–92.

Takei, N., Sham, P., O'Callaghan, E., Murray, G.K., Glover, G. & Murray R.M. (1994) Prenatal exposure to influenza and the development of schizophrenia: is the effect confined to females? *Am J Psych* **151**, 117–19.

Talley, N.A. & Assumpcao, C.A.R. (1971) Disseminated intravascular clotting complicating viral pneumonia due to influenza. *Med J Austral* **2**, 763–6.

Tashiro, M., Ciborowski, P., Klenk, H.D., Pulverer, G. & Rott, R. (1987a) Role of a staphylococcal protease in the development of influenza virus pneumonia. *Nature* **352**, 536–7.

Tashiro, M., Ciborowski, P., Reinacher, M., Klenk, H.D., Pulverer, G. & Rott, R. (1987b) Synergistic role of staphylococcal proteases in the induction of influenza virus pathogenicity. *Virology* **157**, 421–30.

Taylor, J.W. (1919) Some experiences of the recent influenza epidemic in Bristol. *Br Med J* **i**, 153–4.

Taylor, R.M. (1949) Studies on survival of influenza virus between epidemics and antigenic variants of the virus. *Am J Public Health* **39**, 171–8.

Taylor, J.C., Ross, C.A.C & Stott, E.J. (1967) Influenza in the West of Scotland. *Br Med J* 406–8.

Tibbles, W. (1890) The epidemic of influenza in the rural sanitary district of Melton Mowbray. *Br Med J* 834–5.

Tillett, H.E., Smith, J.W.G. & Clifford, R.E. (1980) Excess morbidity and mortality associated with influenza in England and Wales. *Lancet* **i**, 793–5.

Tolan, R.W. (1993) Toxic shock syndrome complicating influenza in a child: case report and review. *Clin Infect Dis* **17**, 43–5.

Torrey, E.F., Rawlings, R. & Waldman, I.N. (1988) Schizophrenic births and viral diseases in two states. *Schizophrenia Res* **1**, 73–7.

Torrey, E.F., Bowler, A.E. & Rawlings, R. (1992) Schizophrenia and the 1957 influenza epidemic (abstract). *Schizophrenia Res* **6**, 100.

Troendle, J.F., Demmler, G.J., Glezen, W.P., Finegold, M. & Romano, M.J. (1992) Fatal influenza B pneumonia in pediatric patients. *Ped Infect Dis J* **11**, 117–21.

Urban, P., Chevrolet, J.C., Schifferli, J. & Cox, J. (1985) Invasive pulmonary aspergillosis associated with an acute influenza virus infection. *Revue Maladies Resp* **2**, 255–7.

Verel, D., Warrack, A.J.N., Potter, C.W., Ward, C. & Rickards, D.F. (1976) Observations on the A2 England influenza epidemic. *Am Heart J* **92**, 290–6.

Verhoef, J., Mills, E.L., Debets-Ossenkopp, Y. & Verbrugh, H.A. (1982) The effect of influenza virus on oxygen-dependent metabolism of human neutrophils. *Adv Exp Med Biol* **141**, 647–54.

Vullers, R., Bultmann, B., Fischer, H. & Haferkamp, O. (1980) Influenza A virus infection, a precipitating factor for the major heart attack. *Münchener Medizinische Wochenschrift* **122**, 1415–17.

Wakabyashi, Y., Nakano, T., Kikuno, T., Ohwada, T. & Kikawadfa, R. (1994) Massive rhabdomyolysis associated with influenza A infection. *Intern Med* **33**, 450–3.

Wald, T.G., Miller, B.A., Shult, P., Drinka, P., Langer, L. & Gravenstein, S. (1995) Can respiratory syncytial virus and influenza be distinguished clinically in institutionalized older persons? *J Am Geriatr Soc* **43**, 170–4.

Walsh, J., Burch, G.E., White, A., Mogabgab, W. & Dietlein, L. (1958) A study of the effects of type A (Asian strain) influenza on the cardiovascular system of man. *Ann Intern Med* **49**, 502–28.

Walsh, J.J., Dietlein, L.F., Low, F.N., Burch, G.E. & Mogabgab, W.J. (1961) Bronchotracheal response in human influenza. *Archiv Intern Med* **108**, 376–88.

Wang, E.E.L., Prober, C.G., Manson, B., Corey, M. & Levison, H. (1984) Association of respiratory viral infections with pulmonary deterioration in patients with cystic fibrosis. *New Engl J Med* **311**, 1653–8.

Warrell, M.J., Tobin, J.O. & Wald, N.J. (1981) Examination for influenza IgA and IgM antibodies in pregnancies associated with fetal neural-tube defects. *J Med Microbiol* **14**, 159–62.

Watson, C. (1900) Influenza. In: *Encyclopaedia Medica*, pp. 265–92. William Green & Sons, Edinburgh.

Watson, A.M. (1919) Influenza epidemic in Q.M.A.A.C. Hostel, Edinburgh. *Br Med J* **i**, 40–1.

Watson, C.G., Kucala, T., Tilleskjor, C. & Jacob, L. (1984) Schizophrenic birth seasonality in relation to the incidence of infectious diseases and temperature extremes. *Archiv Gen Psych* **41**, 85–90.

Weber, E.P. (1919) Spontaneous pneumothorax in the course of influenzal pneumonia. *Br Med J* **i**, 8–9.

Webster, R.G., Geraci, J., Petursson, G. & Skirnisson, K. (1981) Conjunctivitis in human beings caused by influenza A virus of seals. *N Engl J Med* **304**, 911.

Weinberg, R.J. & Nerney, J.J. (1983) Bilateral submacular haemorrhages associated with an influenza syndrome. *Ann Ophthalmol* **15**, 710–12.

Weingarten, S., Friedlander, M., Rascon, D., Ault, M., Morgan, M. & Meyer, R.D. (1988) Influenza surveillance in an acute-care hospital. *Archiv Intern Med* **148**, 113–16.

Weinstein, L (1976) Influenza: 1918, a revisit? *New Engl J Med* **294**, 1058–60.

Wells, C.E.C. (1971) Neurological complications of so-called 'influenza': a winter study in south-east Wales. *Br Med J* **1**, 369–73.

Whimbey, E., Elting, L.S., Couch, R.B. *et al.* (1994) Influenza A virus infections among hospitalized adult bone marrow transplant recipients. *Bone Marrow Transplant* **13**, 437–40.

Whimbey, E., Englund, J.A. & Couch, R.B. (1997) Community respiratory virus infections in immunocompromised patients with cancer. *Am J Med* **102** (3A), 10–18.

Whitaker, A.N., Bunce, I., & Graeme, E.R. (1974) Disseminated intravascular coagulation and acute renal failure in influenza A2 infection. *Med J Austral* **2**, 196–201.

Whittingham, H.E. & Sims, C. (1918) Some observations on the bacteriology and pathology of influenza. *Lancet* 865–71.

Wilkins, E.G.L., Nye, F., Roberts, C. & de Saxe, M. (1985) Probable toxic shock syndrome with primary staphylococcal pneumonia. *J Infect* **11**, 231–2.

Wilson, C.B. & Smith, R.C. (1972) Goodpasture's syndrome associated with influenza A2 virus infection. *Ann Intern Med* **76**, 91–4.

Wilson, W.J. & Steer, P. (1919) Bacteriological and pathological observations on influenza as seen in France during 1918. *Br Med J* 634–5.

Wilson, C.B. & Stein, A.M. (1969) Teratogenic potential of the Asian influenza. An extended study. *J Am Med Assoc* **210**, 336–7.

Winterbawer, R.H., Ludwig, W.R. & Hammer, S.P. (1977) Clinical course, management and long-term sequelae of respiratory failure due to influenza viral pneumonia. *Johns Hopkins Med J* **141**, 148–55.

Wirgman, C.W. (1918) An 'influenza' outbreak. Lancet 324–5.

Woodall, J., Rowson, K.E.K. & McDonald, J.C. (1958) Age and Asian influenza. *Br Med J* **4**, 1316–18.

Wright, P.F., Khaw, K.T., Oxman, M.N. & Scwachman, H. (1976) Evaluation of the safety of amantadine HCl and the role of respiratory viral infections in children with cystic fibrosis. *J Infect Dis* **134**, 144–9.

Wright, P.F., Ross, K.B., Thompson, J. & Karzon, D.T. (1977) Influenza A infections in young children. Primary natural infection and protective efficacy of live-vaccine induced or naturally acquired immunity. *New Engl J Med* **296**, 829–34.

Wright, P.F., Thompson, J. & Karzon, D.T. (1980) Differing virulence of H1N1 and H3N2 influenza strains. *Am J Epidemiol* **112**, 814–19.

Wright, P., Takei, N., Rifkin, L. & Murray, R.M. (1995) Maternal influenza, obstetric complications, and schizophrenia. *Am J Psychiatr* **152**, 1714–20.

Wynne-Griffith, G., Adelstein, A.M., Lambert, P.M. & Weatherall, J.A.C. (1972) Influenza and infant mortality. *Br Med J* **iii**, 553–6.

Yawn, D.H., Pyeatte, J.C., Joseph, J.M., Eichler, S.L. & Bunuel, R.G. (1971) Transplacental transfer of influenza virus. *J Am Med Assoc* **216**, 1022–3.

Yeldani, A.V. & Colby, T.V. (1994) Pathologic features of lung biopsy specimens from influenza pneumonia cases. *Human Pathol* **25**, 47–53.

Yousuf, H.M., Englund, J., Couch, R. *et al.* (1997) Influenza among hospitalized adults with leukaemia. *Clin Infect Dis* **24**, 1095–9.

Zamkoff, K. & Rosen, N. (1979) Influenza and myoglobinuria in brothers. *Neurology* **29**, 340–5.

Section 6
Immunology of Influenza

CHAPTER 20

Antibody-Mediated Immunity

David Brian Thomas, Andriani C. Patera, Christine M. Graham and Claire A. Smith

The major line of defence against influenza infection is mediated by neutralizing antibodies (Abs) directed against the viral membrane glycoprotein, haemagglutinin (HA). This is confirmed by the seasonal emergence of new variant viruses containing amino acid substitutions within the HA1 subunit, selected for by immune pressure of the neutralizing Ab response acting in concert with an error-prone RNA polymerase (Webster & Laver 1980; Ward & Dopheide 1981; Both *et al.* 1983; Wharton *et al.* 1989). This contrasts with cell-mediated immunity, frequently crossreactive between different virus subtypes, and in which T cells recognize proteolytically cleaved fragments of the more conserved internal proteins, such as the matrix protein or nucleoprotein, in association with major histocompatibility complex (MHC) class I or class II glycoproteins.

The HA of H3 subtype influenza viruses is a primary paradigm for studies of infection and immunity at the molecular level, due to the extensive structural information available from crystallographic studies (Wilson *et al.* 1981) and sequence data for the HA genes of variant viruses (Wiley *et al.* 1981). Moreover, the selection of laboratory variants, using neutralizing monoclonal antibodies (mAbs), have identified one, or at most two amino acid differences from the immunizing virus (Laver *et al.* 1979; Caton *et al.* 1982; Underwood 1984). The molecular location of these changes, in the membrane-distal ectodomain of the HA1 subunit, defines five major antigenic sites, designated A, B, C, D, E (Wiley *et al.* 1981; Wiley & Skehel 1987; Wharton *et al.* 1989) corresponding to surface exposed regions, proximal to the receptor binding pocket (Fig. 20.1). mAbs that bind to one or more of these sites inhibit viral attachment to terminal sialic acid residues of host membrane glycoproteins, and thereby prevent virus entry.

Since the technology for the production of human mAbs is still in its infancy, knowledge of the neutralizing Ab repertoire for HA has been deduced almost entirely from work with murine mAbs. Even so, it is reassuring to find that the amino acid residue changes, selected for by murine mAbs, have also featured in natural variant viruses, selected by the human Ab repertoire. There are some caveats required, however, in extrapolating from findings obtained with different species.

First, murine mAbs are established from naive donors following primary immunization and boosting (or very occasionally after infection) whereas the human population is subject to *recurrent* infection with antigenically distinct viruses. Concomitant immunity in the human to previous infection may compromise the repertoire to subsequent infection with a variant virus (the phenomenon of *original antigenic sin* that has been well documented: Fazekas de St. Groth & Webster 1966) resulting in crossreactive Ab responses, with reduced affinity. In contrast, murine mAbs are of moderate to high affinity.

Secondly, most studies in the mouse use immune splenocytes from a pool of three or more donors, on the reasoned assumption that the repertoires of genetically homogeneous, inbred mice are identical. But there may well be variation in the immune repertoire of individual inbred donors, as will be discussed below for MHC congenic mice.

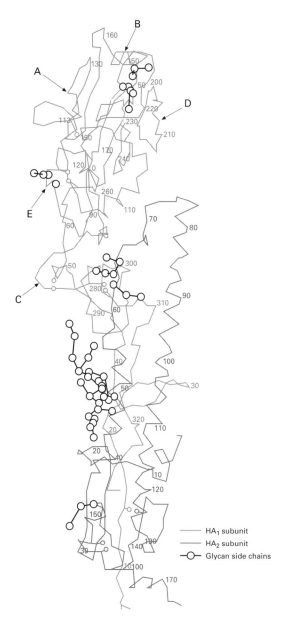

Fig. 20.1 Schematic representation of the bromelain-cleaved haemagglutinin (HA) monomer indicating the location of neutralizing antibody binding regions. The HA monomer consists of disulphide-linked HA$_1$ and HA$_2$ subunits. The N-linked glycan side chains are shown, and the antigenic regions are designated as A, B, C, D, E (after Wharton *et al.* 1989).

In this chapter we consider: (a) *immunodominance* in the neutralizing Ab responses of MHC congenic mice to natural infection, with particular emphasis on clonal analysis of *individual* donors with respect to Ab gene usage; (b) commonality in the location of neutralizing Ab and T$_H$ cell recognition sites on the HA molecule; and (c) a possible role of Ab affinity as a determinant of variant virus selection, with the preferential selection of receptor binding variants by low-affinity Abs.

Immunodominance in the neutralizing Ab repertoire

In the earlier studies of HA antigenicity, neutralizing mAbs were established from BALB/c mice following immunization and little attention was given to (possible) recruitment of a distinct Ab repertoire by natural intranasal infection, or to the influence of differences in host genetic background. This approach was invaluable, however, in identifying major antigenic sites of the HA$_1$ subunit (Fig. 20.1). Initially, some workers placed emphasis on the potential diversity of the Ab repertoire: Staudt and Gerhard (1983) estimated that the BALB/c response to immunization, and secondary challenge with A/PR/8/34 (H1N1 subtype), consisted of 1500 or more distinct paratopes. However, this estimate was based on serological assignment of mAb specificities, while direct sequencing of laboratory variants and assignment of recognition specificity to the three-dimensional structure of the bromelain-cleaved HA (B-HA) trimer considerably simplified the picture (Wiley *et al.* 1981) and advanced our understanding of HA antigenicity (Fig. 20.1). Underwood (1984), studying the secondary response of BALB/c mice immunized intraperitoneally with H3N2 subtype virus, found that the highest proportion of neutralizing mAbs was directed against the membrane-distal tip (site B), and the second most common site was the trimer interface, suggesting that the Ab repertoire might be skewed to one or two dominant sites.

Our aim, in this section, is to review work on the influence of host genetic background and a natural route of infection, on the neutralizing Ab repertoire of inbred and MHC congenic mice with a particular emphasis on immunodominance. CBA/Ca (H-2^k) or BALB/c (H-2^d) or MHC congenic BALB.K (H-2^k) mice infected intranasally with X31 (H3N2 subtype) exhibit typical signs of weight loss and reduced body temperature, and have been used to generate HA-specific hybridomas several months after the initial infection and final boost (Smith *et al.* 1991; Temoltzin-Palacios & Thomas 1994; Patera *et al.* 1995). They are representative therefore of a high-affinity, B memory cell response.

CBA/Ca repertoire (Smith *et al.* 1991)

A panel of hybridomas, established from three donors (JCB-2, JCB-3, JCB-4), was used to select X31 laboratory variants containing the indicated amino acid residue changes in the HA$_1$ subunit (Table 20.1). A noteworthy point was the frequent occurrence of variants containing the *same* single residue change, HA$_1$158 G→E, but with minor representation of variants with amino acid substitutions in other antigenic regions (HA$_1$63, HA$_1$144). HA$_1$158 G→E has featured in natural isolates (A/TEX/77 or A/BK/79) and is within a loop region formed by amino acids HA$_1$155–160 (site B, Fig. 20.1).

Secondly, natural infection of CBA/Ca mice recruited novel Ab specificities, not previously reported for mAbs obtained by immunization of BALB/c mice: Clone 5.1 selected a variant virus, HA$_1$165 N→S with the *loss* of an N-glycosylation site (Asn165 Val166 Thr167). Although the introduction of a carbohydrate side chain is known to alter HA antigenicity (e.g. HA$_1$ Asp63→Asn63 Cys64 Thr65) (Skehel *et al.* 1984), this is the first example of a reciprocal effect of carbohydrate removal on mAb recognition. The HA$_1$165 N-glycosylation site is highly conserved in H3 natural isolates. Clone 3.6.2 selected a novel residue change HA$_1$62 I→R (site E), not previously reported for X31 variants, selected by neutralizing mAb from BALB/c mice.

Thirdly, a majority of mAbs were of the IgG2a isotype, and this is consistent with the recruitment of a γ-interferon-secreting T$_H$1 type T-cell response during viral infection, that regulates class switching to this particular isotype (Mosmann & Coffman 1989).

BALB/c repertoire (Patera *et al.* 1995)

Immunodominance was also evident in this haplotype with the selection of the same laboratory variant (HA$_1$198 A→E) by mAbs from three different donors; and by the conspicuous absence of the HA$_1$158 G→E variant. As seen for the CBA/Ca repertoire, there was minor representation of other antigenic specificities (HA$_1$135, HA$_1$144, HA$_1$146; site A). HA$_1$198 is at the membrane-distal tip, proximal to the receptor binding pocket in an α-helical region, HA$_1$187–199, designated site B (Fig. 20.1).

BALB.K (H-2^k) repertoire (Patera *et al.* 1995)

To ascertain whether differences in Ab recognition specificity between CBA/Ca and BALB/c mice was related to MHC status, this study was extended to the MHC congenic strain, BALB.K. Here, there was *codominance*, with either the HA$_1$158 or HA$_1$198 variant being selected for by the neutralizing Ab repertoire of individual donors: for donor SFA7B, mAbs of different isotypes (IgM, IgA, IgG2a or IgG3) selected the same laboratory variant, HA$_1$158 G→E, whereas for donor SFA3B, HA$_1$198 A→E was the most frequently selected variant.

V region gene usage and B cell progenitor diversity

The prevalence of certain Ab recognition specificities following natural infection, as deduced from the sequencing of HA genes of laboratory variants which differed by the same residue change (HA$_1$158 G→E or HA$_1$198 A→E), could be due to either: (a) structural restriction in V region gene usage for Ab recognition specificity; or (b) the occurrence of a dominant B-cell clonotype within a given haplotype. Sequence analysis of heavy- and light-chain gene usage, and the deduced data on junctional region diversity, allowed us to obtain a genealogical profile of B cell progenitor frequency in the Ab repertoire of individual donors with respect to recognition specificity.

The primary recombination event during B-cell differentiation results in (D-J)$_H$ joining of heavy-

Table 20.1 Recognition specificity and isotype of neutralizing monoclonal antibodies (mAbs) established from individual CBA/Ca (H-2^k) or BALB/c (H-2^d) or congenic BALB.K (H-2^k) donors. Recognition specificity was determined by sequencing the haemagglutinin (HA) genes of *in ovo*, mAb-selected and cloned mutants of X31 which differed from wild-type by the indicated amino acid changes in the HA$_1$ subunit.

CBA/Ca donor

JCB-2			JCB-3			JCB-4		
B-cell hybridoma clone	Recognition specificity (HA$_1$)	mAb isotype	B-cell hybridoma clone	Recognition specificity (HA$_1$)	mAb isotype	B-cell hybridoma clone	Recognition specificity (HA$_1$)	mAb isotype
41.1	158 G→E	IgG2a	1.1	158 G→E	IgG2a	40.7	158 G→E	IgG3
7.3.2	63 D→N	IgM	8.1	158 G→E	IgG2a	35.4	158 G→E	IgG2a
29.1	158 G→E	IgG2a	4.3	158 G→E	IgG2b	2.1	158 G→E	IgG2a
37.1	158 G→E	IgA	3.6.2	62 I→R	IgG2a	3.1	158 G→E	IgG2a
5.1.1	158 G→E	IgG2a	3.6.2	63 D→N	IgG2a	4.3	158 G→E	IgG1
6.1	144 G→D	IgG2a	5.1	165 N→S	IgG2b	20.1	158 G→E	IgG2a
			7.1	63 D→N	IgG2a	12.1	158 G→E	IgG1
			8.2	158 G→E	IgG2a	29.1	144 G→D	IgG2a
			6.1	158 G→E	IgG2a			

BALB/c donor

CCB1B			CCB2B			CCB4B		
B-cell hybridoma clone	Recognition specificity (HA$_1$)	mAb isotype	B-cell hybridoma clone	Recognition specificity (HA$_1$)	mAb isotype	B-cell hybridoma clone	Recognition specificity (HA$_1$)	mAb isotype
6.1	198 A→E	IgG2a	9.1	144 G→D	IgG1	10.1	198 A→E	IgG1
11.1	198 A→E	IgG2a	3.1	144 G→D	IgG2a	14.3	198 A→E	IgG2a
12.1	198 A→E	IgG2a	2.1	198 A→E	IgG2b	2.1	198 A→E	IgG2a
5.1	198 A→E	IgG2b	5.1	198 A→E	IgG2b	6.1	198 A→E	IgG2a
17.1	135 G→E	IgG2b	7.1	198 A→E	IgG2b			
15.1	146 G→D	IgG2b	15.1	143 P→I 145 S→I	IgG3			
3.2	142 G→R	IgA						
10.1	198 A→E	IgA						

BALB.K donor

SFA2B			SFA3B			SFA7B		
B-cell hybridoma clone	Recognition specificity (HA$_1$)	mAb isotype	B-cell hybridoma clone	Recognition specificity (HA$_1$)	mAb isotype	B-cell hybridoma clone	Recognition specificity (HA$_1$)	mAb isotype
1.1	198 A→E	IgG2a	1.1	189 W→H	IgG1	6.1	135 G→E	IgG2a
7.2	198 A→E	IgG2a	3.1	198 A→E	IgG1	9.1	189 W→K	IgG2a
8.1	198 A→E	IgG2a	12.1	198 A→E	IgG1	19.1	158 G→E	IgG2a
9.1	198 A→E	IgG2b	2.1	198 A→E	IgG2a	3.1	198 A→E	IgG2b
3.1	198 A→E	IgG2b	10.1	198 A→E	IgG2a	11.1	158 G→E	IgG2b
2.1	158 G→E	IgG2b	4.1	158 G→E	IgG2a	5.1	158 G→E	IgG3
4.2	193 S→R	IgG2a	6.1	135 G→E	IgG2a	8.1	158 G→E	IgG3
5.2	205 S→Y	IgG2a	9.1	135 G→E	IgG2b	15.1	158 G→E	IgM
6.1	146 G→D	IgG2a	7.1	198 A→E	IgG2b	2.1	158 G→E	IgM
	158 G→V	IgG2a						
10.2	63 D→N	IgG2a	14.1	198 A→E		1.2	198 A→E	IgA
					IgG2b	7.1	198 A→E	IgA
						10.2	158 G→E	IgA

chain gene elements in the preprogenitor cell, and thereafter $(V-D-J)_H$ joining with heavy-chain commitment of the μ^+ progenitor cell. Following heavy- and light-chain association, the virgin IgM^+ cell may be triggered by encounter with antigen; and B-cell memory is established after IgM to IgG class switching and cognate recognition, in association with the antigen-specific $CD4^+$ T cell. Sequence analysis of $(VDJ)_H$ and $(VJ)_L$ gene usage by hybridomas of different isotypes provides an estimate

therefore of progenitor frequency in the individual's repertoire for a single antigenic site.

Initially, a comparison was made of B cell progenitor frequency in BALB.K mice, using hybridomas that recognized either HA_1158 or HA_1198. Consider the genealogical trees that we established for hybridomas from donor SFA7B, specific for HA_1158 (Fig. 20.2). This analysis illustrates the potential diversity of the B-memory repertoire for a single antigenic site, including the representation of

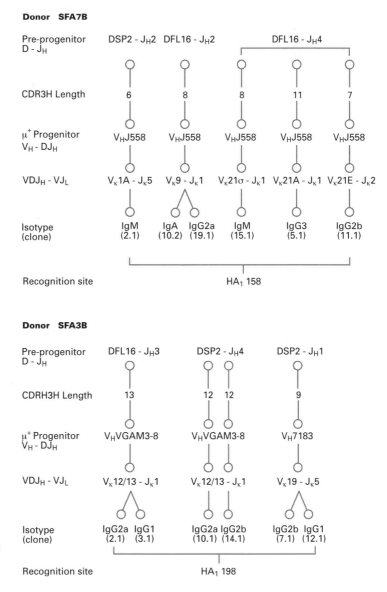

Fig. 20.2 Genealogical trees showing progenitor lineage, as deduced from heavy-chain and light-chain gene rearrangements of monoclonal antibodies from donor SFA7B or SFA3B. (From Patera *et al.* 1995, with permission from Wiley-VCH Verlag GmbH.)

most available isotypes (IgM, IgA, Ig2a, Ig2b, IgG3): six independent preprogenitor cells contributed to the repertoire as deduced from D_H-J_H joining, with restricted usage of the largest V_H family, J558, by all seven hybridomas and different CDR3H length. Light-chain gene usage was also diverse with six distinct $(V_\kappa$-$J_\kappa)_L$ associations. Hybridomas 2.1 and 15.1 were IgM Abs, and since the cell fusions were made several months after the initial infection (following IgM to IgG class switching), it is likely that both clones were recruited during a primary response to the secondary boost, 3 days before hybridoma fusion.

For donor SFA3B, six hybridomas representative of three major isotypes (IgG1, IgG2a and IgG2b) were from four independent μ^+ progenitor cells as deduced from the identity of their V_H and V_L genes and homologous CDR3H sequences. Clones 10.1 and 14.1 were from different progenitors and were distinguished in their CDR3H sequences and V_H usage. Clones (2.1 and 3.1) or (7.1 and 12.1) were sibling pairs derived from a common progenitor as shown by complete identity in heavy- and light-chain gene rearrangements. Genealogical analysis of hybridomas from donor SFA2B (data not presented) indicated that a minimum of four progenitors had generated the HA_1198 specific response.

Restricted V_L gene usage for CBA/Ca repertoire

The striking diversity of progenitor cells seen in the HA_1158 specific response of donor SFA7B (Fig. 20.2) contrasted with highly restricted gene usage by hybridomas from CBA/Ca donors with the same recognition specificity (Table 20.2; Patera *et al.* 1995). Seven hybridomas, established from JCB-2 or JCB-3 or JCB-4, used the *same* light-chain gene V_κ1A (K5.1) with various V_H genes. Moreover, there was a common association of D_H gene (DSP2.9) and J_H(2) gene elements and a remarkable constancy in CDR3H length, of six amino acids, for each of the seven hybridomas. But the number of B-cell progenitors varied between individuals: sequence homology between the JCB-3 clones indicated a common progenitor while a minimum of three μ^+ progenitors contributed to the memory response of donor JCB-4. The two hybridomas, from donor JCB-2, differed in both V_H and V_L gene usage, thereby defining two distinct progenitor cells.

In summary, the above genealogical data indicated that the observed immunodominance, or focusing of an individual's Ab repertoire to a single antigenic site, could not be accounted for by clonal dominance since a minimum of six progenitor cells contributed to the immune response, as seen for the HA_1158 specific hybridomas from donor SFA7B. Also, it is evident from these studies that no structural correlation exists between heavy- and light-chain gene usage and recognition specificity. Findings based on an analysis of hybridomas from CBA/Ca donors (Table 20.2) might suggest that light-chain gene usage accounted for the immunodominance of HA_1158 specific responses, since a majority of hybridomas used the same V_L gene, K5.1. Similarly, in the CBA/Ca repertoire, (Table

Table 20.2 Immunoglobulin gene usage by HA_1158-specific monoclonal antibody from individual CBA/Ca donors. CDR3H length was established from the deduced number of amino acid residues.

Donor	Clone	V_L family	V_L gene	J_κ gene	V_H family	D gene	CDR3H length	J_H gene	C_H isotype
JCB-2	5.1.1	V_κ1A	K5.1	4	V_H3609	DSP2.9	6	2	IgG2a
	29.1	V_κ19	βa)	4	V_HJ606	DSP2.9	11	1	IgG2a
JCB-3	6.1	V_κ1A	K5.1	1	V_HJ609	DSP2.9	6	2	IgG2a
	8.2	V_κ1A	K5.1	1	V_HJ606	DSP2.9	6	2	IgG2a
JCB-4	2.1	V_κ1A	K5.1	1	V_H10	DSP2.9	6	2	IgG2a
	3.1	V_κ1A	K5.1	2	V_H7183	DSP2.9	6	2	IgG2a
	4.3	V_κ1A	K5.1	1	V_H7183	DSP2.9	6	2	IgG1
	40.7	V_κ1A	K5.1	1	V_H7183	DSP2.9	6	2	IgG3

20.2), the constancy of CDR3H length with use of
the same D (DSP 2.9) and $J_H(2)$ elements might
suggest that the heavy chain conferred recognition
specificity. However, such structural correlates
were not evident in the BALB.K repertoire, where
there was diverse V_L usage and restricted V_H
family usage (for donor SFA7B) in the recognition
of HA_1158.

Earlier studies by Gerhard and colleagues
(Caton *et al.* 1986) of the Ab responses of BALB/c
mice to a (serologically) defined region of H1 subtype HA (site Ca, Caton *et al.* 1982) indicated
restricted V_κ gene usage in association with the
same V_H gene family (VH 7183) and the
expression of a dominant light-chain idiotype. In
subsequent studies by this group, the secondary
Ab repertoire, of a single BALB/c mouse, to antigenic site Sb was examined by sequence analysis
of a panel of mAbs that expressed a common idiotype (Clarke *et al.* 1990). The heavy chains were
encoded by a single V_H gene joined to a variety of
D_H and J_H elements, providing a minimum estimate of five clonal progenitor cells. From the constancy of CDR3H length between different mAbs,
and conserved residues at the $D-J_H$ junctions, it
was proposed that the heavy chain was important
in determining antigenic specificity. However,
further studies by these workers highlighted the
extensive diversity of V_H and V_L gene usage in
the Ab response to antigenic site Cb of A/PR/8/
34 (Kavaler *et al.* 1990).

What is evident, from all of these studies, is that
Ab recognition specificity does not correlate with
heavy- or light-chain gene usage since an apparent
correlation in one haplotype (HA_1158 specific
responses of CBA/Ca mice) is illusory and not
evident in an MHC congenic background (BALB.K
mice). As a result, no definitive conclusions can be
made concerning the structural basis of the
observed immunodominance; and neither can we
provide a cellular basis for the selection of diverse
clonotypes having a common recognition specificity. The finding that HA_1158 and HA_1198 specific
responses were codominant in BALB.K mice might
suggest that both MHC-linked, and background
genes were instrumental in a stochastic selection
process.

Commonality of B-cell and T$_H$-cell recognition sites

It is commonly agreed that the recognition repertoires of B cells (or Abs) and regulatory T-helper
(T_H) cells are distinct: neutralizing Abs recognize
conformational features of the native HA molecule whereas $CD4^+$ T_H cells recognize peptide
fragments, presented in association with MHC
class II molecules on the surface of an antigen
presenting cell. However, in a clonal analysis of
$CD4^+$ T-cell responses to HA, in three major
haplotypes ($H-2^b$, $H-2^d$, $H-2^k$), and following *natural infection* with X31 virus we found extensive
commonality in regions of the molecule recognized by both cell types.

Immunodominance, evident in the neutralizing
Ab responses of BALB/c mice for HA_1198 (Table
20.1), was mirrored in the focusing of T_H-cell
responses to this same region of the molecule
(Thomas *et al.* 1989). A majority of $CD4^+$ T-cell
clones, established from several BALB/c donors
following intranasal infection with X31, recognized
a synthetic peptide corresponding to the primary
sequence $HA_1186–205$; and failed to recognize
laboratory variants containing single amino acid
substitutions within this region of the molecule
($HA_1189, 193, 198, 199$). Moreover, a distinguishing
feature of $CD4^+$ T-cell responses to HA, following
natural infection, was the diversity of antigenic
peptides presented in association with a single
MHC class II restriction element (Thomas *et al.*
1989). We have established $I-A^d$-restricted T-cell
clones, from different individual donors, that
recognized synthetic peptides corresponding to the
primary sequences: $HA_158–73$, $HA_181–97$, $HA_1177–
199$, $HA_1186–205$ or $HA_1206–227$.

In the $H-2^k$ haplotype, $CD4^+$ T-cell clones also
focused on antigenic regions of HA1, as shown by
their recognition of synthetic peptides corresponding to the primary HA_1 sequences 54–63, 68–
83, 118–138, 226–245, 246–266 or 269–288 (Mills *et al.*
1986; Burt *et al.* 1989). These regions have featured
in antigenic drift of H3 subtype viruses, isolated
between 1969 and 1985 and T-cell clones were
sensitive, in their recognition of natural variants

(processed and presented as peptides by syngeneic antigen presenting cells), to substitutions within the primary sequence of the T-cell epitope. We have presented evidence that, in some instances, lack of variant virus recognition is a processing defect that can be reversed by site-specific mutagenesis of the MHC class II gene of the antigen presenting cell (Warren *et al.* 1990).

The HA2 subunit of the molecule is highly conserved between different natural isolates and Abs directed to this region of the molecule fail to neutralize viral infectivity. It is of some interest therefore that we failed to identify class II restricted (A^b or A^d or A^k) T-cell epitopes within HA2. Focusing of $CD4^+$ T-cell responses (during natural infection) to antigenic regions of HA_1, that are recognized by neutralizing Abs, might be a consequence of selective processing and presentation of antigenic peptides by the B memory cell.

T-cell receptor gene usage

Immunodominance, evident in neutralizing Ab responses to influenza infection in two major haplotypes ($H-2^d$, $H-2^k$), contrasted with the variety of antigenic peptides recognized by T_H clones in association with a single MHC class II restriction element. Even so, there was striking immunodominance in the individual's T-cell repertoire: a majority of T_H clones, from the same donor, recognized the same antigenic peptide, despite differences in their fine specificity for variant virus HA. Sequence analysis of T-cell receptor α- and β-chain genes, for T-cell clones from the same donor, indicated identical $(VDJ)_\beta$ and $(VJ)_\alpha$ rearrangements (Smith *et al.* 1994a,b). A single progenitor cell may have contributed therefore to the T-cell memory population. And there was no structural correlation between T-cell receptor gene usage and peptide specificity: T-cell clones, from different individuals but recognizing the same antigenic peptide, expressed distinct $(VDJ)_\beta$ rearrangements. It would seem that different cellular selection mechanism(s) account for the observed immunodominance in B-cell and T-cell responses during natural infection.

Receptor binding variant selection by low-affinity Abs

Crystallographic studies of B-HA complexed with sialyloligosaccharides (Weis *et al.* 1988) have established that the receptor binding site, which mediates virus attachment to terminal sialic acid residues of host cell surface glycoconjugates, is a shallow pocket of *conserved* amino acid residues near the membrane-distal tip of HA_1. Conservation of these residues in natural variant viruses is likely to be a functional restriction, since structural changes that affect receptor binding specificity would abrogate viral infectivity. Receptor binding variants of X31 are readily selected, however, by glycoprotein inhibitors, such as equine α_2-macroglobulin (present in horse serum), which contains sialyl α2,6-linked N-glycans. Such variants differ from wild-type virus by a single residue change, $HA_1$226 L→Q, and exhibit preferential binding for α2,3 sialyl glycoconjugates (Rogers *et al.* 1983). Here, we wish to consider examples of receptor binding variants that had been selected for by neutralizing Ab, and to conclude that a low-affinity Ab response may *preferentially* select such variant viruses, and be of some relevance to antigenic variation.

Most neutralizing mAbs, established from BALB/c mice following immunization or infection, are moderate- to high-affinity IgG Abs, and select laboratory variants with single amino acid substitutions within one of the major antigenic sites (Wharton *et al.* 1989). But receptor binding variants are obtained following selection with *subneutralizing levels* of polyclonal Abs (Fazekas de St. Groth 1977) or mAbs (Daniels *et al.* 1987; Yewdell *et al.* 1986; Temoltzin-Palacios & Thomas 1994). Receptor binding variants of influenza usually exhibit the following phenotype: (a) they are still recognized by the selecting Ab in ELISA, but fail to be neutralized; (b) they exhibit altered binding specificity in their recognition of sialyl α2,3- or α2,6-linked glycoconjugates; and (c) are resistant to inhibition of haemagglutination by horse serum glycoproteins. Yewdell *et al.* (1986) reported the selection of such a virus phenotype, using a mixture of mAbs specific for four antigenically defined sites of

A/PR/8/34, but at subneutralizing levels. It was suggested that the virus variants had a higher affinity for their receptor, based on their relative resistance to neuraminidase treatment of erythrocytes, in haemagglutination-inhibition assays. Daniels *et al.* (1987) reported an H3-specific mAb that was broadly crossreactive for natural isolates, and selected a receptor binding variant ($HA_1$193 S→N, 226 L→P) of X31, or alternatively a variant with deletions of residues $HA_1$224–230. These variants were recognized in ELISA, and showed altered specificity in haemagglutination assays with sialyl α2,3- or sialyl α2,6-derivatized erythrocytes. Temoltzin-Palacios and Thomas (1994), using subneutralizing levels of a mAb, specific for $HA_1$155 T→I of X31, selected a receptor binding mutant, $HA_1$190 E→D, 226 L→Q, that was still recognized in ELISA. Moreover, the initial X31 variant ($HA_1$155 T→I) exhibited altered receptor binding specificity for *N*-glycolylneuraminic acid residues, and was able to agglutinate horse erythrocytes, while X31 exhibited strict specificity for N-acetylneuraminic acid. In view of these findings, the question that we wished to address was whether low-affinity mAbs would preferentially select such a receptor binding phenotype.

Low-affinity mAb responses of human IgH transgenic mice

We employed a transgenic model system—mice bearing a human IgH gene minilocus and lacking a functional mouse IgH locus—to investigate the neutralizing Ab response under conditions in which an IgM to IgG class switch, and concomitant affinity maturation, was absent and in which V_H gene usage was restricted (Laeeq *et al.* 1997). The transgenic mouse line that we used contains a human IgH minilocus with V_H26 and D_H (D_{Q52}) and all of the J_H and secretory C_μ elements in association with an additional V_H (mouse V_H 186.2) and targeted disruption of the mouse C_μ membrane exon (Wagner *et al.* 1994).

Neutralizing mAbs, established from transgenic donors following X31 immunization, selected novel variant viruses with altered receptor binding specificity. The variant viruses contained residue changes *in both the receptor binding pocket and an antigenic site* ($HA_1$135 G→R, 225 G→D) or ($HA_1$145 S→N, 226 L→P); or alternatively residue changes proximal to the pocket that affected binding specificity: ($HA_1$135 G→R, 158 G→E) or ($HA_1$145 S→R, 158 G→E). Altered receptor binding specificity was indicated by the resistance of each variant virus to horse serum inhibition of haemagglutination, and by reduced binding to neoglycoproteins containing terminal sialyl α2,3-or α2,6-linked residues. A schematic representation of the receptor binding site is shown in Chapter 5 and the molecular locations of the residues that have featured in the receptor binding variants, described herein ($HA_1$135, 155, 190, 225, 226) are evident.

It should be emphasized that, in the human, IgM antibody responses to influenza virus infection may not have a significant role to play in immune protection, or selection of variant viruses. This is a consequence of the virus replicative cycle and the rapid IgM to IgG class switching following antigenic challenge. Influenza infection is restricted to the respiratory tract, due to a requirement for apical budding from epithelial cells into the bronchial lumen (Roth *et al.* 1983; Stephens *et al.* 1986). As a result, virus neutralization and clearance are mediated, for the most, part by secretory IgA and the transudation of serum IgG, both of which are of moderate to high affinity. However, in situations where immune responses are compromised, such as in the very young or the very old, a low-affinity IgG response might prevail. Morever, concomitant immunity to an earlier infection can recruit a crossreactive, heteroclitic response with reduced affinity for the challenge virus (Fazekas de St. Groth & Webster 1966).

In the interplay between frequency of mutations in the virus genome and selective pressure of neutralizing Ab responses there may well be a (reciprocal) role for Ab affinity and affinity of the virus for its receptor. Here, we have reported the preferential selection of receptor binding mutants by low-affinity (or subneutralizing levels of) mAbs; and such mutants can exhibit a higher affinity for sialyl-glycoconjugate receptors. Conversely, high-affinity Abs consistently select antigenic variants. Interestingly, recent H3 isolates (e.g. A/Beijing/

32/92) contain the same residue changes (HA$_1$190 E→D, 226 L→Q) that have occurred in a receptor binding variant of X31, selected by subneutralizing levels of mAb (Temoltzin-Palacios & Thomas 1994).

References

Both, G.W., Sleigh, M.J., Cox, N.J. & Kendal, A.P. (1983) Antigenic drift in influenza virus H3 haemagglutinin from 1968 to 1980. Multiple evolutionary pathways and sequential amino acid changes at key antigenic sites. *J Virol* **48**, 52–60.

Burt, D.S., Mills, K.H.G., Skehel, J.J. & Thomas, D.B. (1989) Diversity of the class II (I-A^k/I-E^k) restricted T-cell repertoire for influenza haemagglutinin and antigenic drift: six nonoverlapping epitopes on the HA$_1$ subject are defined by synthetic peptides. *J Exp Med* **170**, 383–97.

Caton, A.J., Brownlee, G.G., Yewdell, J.W. & Gerhard, W. (1982) The antigenic structure of the influenza virus A/PR/8/34 haemagglutinin (H1 subtype). *Cell* **31**, 417–27.

Caton, A.J., Brownlee, G.G., Staudt, L.M. & Gerhard, W. (1986) Structural and functional implications of a restricted antibody response to a defined antigenic region on the influenza virus haemagglutinin. *EMBO J* **5**, 1577–87.

Clarke, S., Rickert, R., Wloch, M.K., Staudt, L., Gerhard, W. & Weigert, M. (1990) The BALB/c secondary response to the Sb site of influenza virus haemagglutinin. Non-random silent mutation and unequal numbers of V$_H$ and V$_\kappa$ mutations. *J Immunol* **145**, 2286–96.

Daniels, R.S., Jeffries, S., Yates, P. *et al.* (1987) The receptor binding and membrane fusion properties of influenza virus variants selected using antihaemagglutinin monoclonal antibodies. *EMBO J* **6**, 1459–65.

Fazekas de St. Groth, S. (1977) Antigenic, adaptive and adsorptive variants of the influenza A haemagglutinin. In: Laver, R.G., Bachmayer, H. & Weil, R. (eds) *Topics in Infectious Diseases*, Vol. 3, pp. 25–48. Springer-Verlag, Vienna.

Fazekas de St., Groth, S. & Webster, R.G. (1966) Disquisitions on original antigenic sin. I. Evidence in man. *J Exp Med* **124**, 331–45.

Kavaler, J., Caton, A.J., Staudt, L.M., Schwartz, D. & Gerhard, W. (1990) A set of closely related antibodies dominates the primary antibody response to the antigenic site CB of the A/PR/8/34 influenza virus haemagglutinin. *J Immunol* **145**, 2312–21.

Laeeq, S., Smith, C.A., Wagner, S.D. & Thomas, D.B. (1997) Preferential selection of receptor-binding variants of influenza virus haemagglutinin by the neutralizing antibody repertoire of transgenic mice expressing a human immumoglobulin μ minigene. *J Virol* **71**, 2600–5.

Laver, W.G., Air, G.M., Webster, R.G., Gerhard, W., Ward, C.W. & Dopheide, T.A. (1979) Antigenic drift in type A influenza virus: sequence differences in the haemagglutinin of Hong Kong (H3N2) variants selected with monoclonal hybridoma antibodies. *Virology* **98**, 226–37.

Mills, K.H.G., Skehel, J.J. & Thomas, D.B. (1986) Extensive diversity in the recognition of influenza haemagglutinin by murine T helper clones. *J Exp Med* **163**, 1477–90.

Mossmann, T.B. & Coffman, R.L. (1989) TH1 and TH2 cells: different patterns of lymphokine secretion lead to different functional properties. *Annu Rev Immunol* **7**, 145–73.

Patera, A.C., Graham, C.M., Thomas, D.B. & Smith, C.A. (1995) Immunodominance with progenitor B cell diversity in the neutralizing antibody repertoire to influenza infection. *Eur J Immunol* **25**, 1803–9.

Rogers, G.N., Paulson, J.C., Daniels, R.S., Skehel, J.J., Wilson, I.A. & Wiley, D.C. (1983) Single amino acid substitutions in influenza haemagglutinin change receptor binding specificity. *Nature* **304**, 76–8.

Roth, M.G., Compans, R.W., Glusti, L. *et al.* (1983) Influenza virus haemagglutinin expression is polarised in cells infected with recombinant SV40 viruses carrying cloned haemagglutinin DNA. *Cell* **33**, 435–43.

Skehel, J.J., Stevens, D.J., Daniels, R.S. *et al.* (1984) A carbohydrate side chain on haemagglutinins of Hong Kong influenza viruses inhibits recognition by a monoclonal antibody *Proc Natl Acad Sci USA* **81**, 1779–83.

Smith, C.A., Barnett, B.C., Thomas, D.B. & Temoltzin-Palacios, F. (1991) Structural assignment of novel and immunodominant antigenic sites in the neutralizing antibody response of CBA/Ca mice to influenza haemagglutinin. *J Exp Med* **173**, 953–9.

Smith, C.A., Graham, C.M. & Thomas, D.B. (1994a) Immunodominance correlates with T cell receptor (αβ) gene usage in the Class II-restricted response to influenza haemagglutinin. *Immunology* **82**, 343–50.

Smith, C.A., Graham, C.M. & Thomas, D.B. (1994b) Productive rearrangement at both alleles of the T cell receptor β chain locus in CD4 T-cell clones specific for influenza haemagglutinin. *Immunology* **81**, 502–6.

Staudt, L.M. & Gerhard, W. (1983) Generation of antibody diversity in the immune response of BALB/c mice to influenza haemagglutinin. *J Exp Med* **157**, 687–704.

Stephens, E.B., Compans, R.W., Earl, P. & Moss, B. (1986) Surface expression of viral glycoproteins is polarised in epithelial cells infected with recombinant vaccinia viral vectors. *EMBO J* **5**, 237–45.

Temoltzin-Palacois, F. & Thomas, D.B. (1994) Modulation of immunodominant sites in influenza haemagglutinin compromise antigenic variation and select receptor-binding variant viruses. *J Exp Med* **179**, 1719–24.

Thomas, D.B., Burt, D.S., Barnett, B.C., Graham, C.M. & Skehel, J.J. (1989) B- and T-cell recognition of influenza haemagglutinin. *Cold Spring Harbor Symp Quant Biol* **LIV**, 487–95.

Wagner, S.D., Williams, G.T., Larson, T. *et al.* (1994) Antibodies generated from human immunoglobulin miniloci in transgenic mice. *Nucleic Acids Res* **22**, 1389–93.

Underwood, P.A. (1984). An antigenic map of the haemagglutinin of the influenza Hong Kong subtype (H3N2), constructed using mouse monoclonal antibodies. *Mol Immunol* **21**, 663–71.

Ward, C.W. & Dopheide, T.A. (1981) Evolution of the Hong Kong influenza A subtype. Structural relationship between the haemagglutinin from A/duck/Ukraine/63 (Hav7) and the Hong Kong haemagglutinins. *Biochem J* **195**, 337–40.

Warren, A.P., Pachedag, I., Benoist, C., Mathis, D. & Thomas, D.B. (1990) Defects in antigen presentation of mutant influenza haemagglutinins are reversed by mutations in the MHC Class II molecule. *EMBO J* **9**, 3849–56.

Webster, R.G. & Laver, W.G. (1980) Determination of the number of nonoverlapping antigenic areas on Hong Kong (H3N2) influenza virus haemagglutinin with monoclonal antibodies and the selection of variants with potential epidemiological significance. *Virology* **104**, 139–48.

Weis, W., Brown, J.H., Cusack, S., Paulson, J.C., Skehel, J.J. & Wiley, D.C. (1988) Structure of the influenza virus haemagglutinin complexed with its receptor, sialic acid. *Nature (Lond)* **333**, 426–31.

Wharton, S.A., Weis, W., Skehel, J.J. & Wiley, D.C. (1989) Structure, function and antigenicity of the haemagglutinin of influenza virus. In: Krug, R.M. (ed.) *The Influenza Viruses*, pp. 153–74. Plenum Press, New York and London.

Wiley, D.C. & Skehel, J.J. (1987) The structure and function of the haemagglutinin membrane glycoprotein of influenza virus. *Annu Rev Biochem* **56**, 365–94.

Wiley, D.C., Wilson, I.A. & Skehel, J.J. (1981) Structural identification of the antibody-binding sites of Hong Kong influenza haemagglutinin and their involvement in antigenic variation. *Nature (Lond)* **289**, 373–8.

Wilson, I.A., Skehel, J.J. & Wiley, D.C. (1981) Structure of the haemagglutinin membrane glycoprotein of influenza virus at 3 Å resolution. *Nature (Lond)* **289**, 366–73.

Yewdell, J.W., Caton, A.J. & Gerhard, W. (1986) Selection of influenza A virus adsorptive mutants by growth in the presence of a mixture of monoclonal anti-haemagglutinin antibodies. *J Virol* **57**, 623–8.

CHAPTER 21

Cell-Mediated Immune Response to Influenza Virus

Philip G. Stevenson and Peter C. Doherty

Experimental influenza virus infection of mice

Influenza virus has historically been a major cause of morbidity (Stuart-Harris 1979) and was thus one of the first human pathogens to be adapted to animal models for immunological investigation. The availability of defined virus strains and the accessibility of the murine immune system to experimental manipulation have since made the mouse model of influenza perhaps the most extensively characterized of any antiviral immune response (Ada & Jones 1986; Doherty et al. 1992). Although influenza viruses are not natural pathogens of mice, they do productively infect the murine respiratory epithelium (Sweet & Smith 1980). Influenza given intranasally under general anaesthesia establishes a pulmonary infection, and virus titres in the lung peak after 5–7 days. A virus-specific immune response is first detectable 3–5 days after infection (Stevenson et al. 1997a) and infectious virus is cleared within 7–10 days (Doherty et al. 1992). Except with highly virulent virus strains (Kawaoka 1991), or in severely immunocompromised mice (Wyde et al. 1983), productive infection remains essentially confined to the respiratory tract.

Influenza type A viruses are subject to considerable variation in their surface antigens, and antibody-mediated protection is confined to antigenically related viral subtypes (Webster et al. 1982). Interest in the antiviral cell-mediated immune response was thus stimulated at an early stage by the observation that it provides cross-reactive protection between serologically distinct virus subtypes (Schulman & Kilbourne 1965; Effros et al. 1977; Zweerink et al. 1977). Although hopes that this might form the basis of a vaccine protective against all influenza A subtypes have so far been unfulfilled, considerable advances have been made in understanding the processes underlying cell-mediated immunity.

CD8[+] T cells clear influenza virus infection from the lung

Influenza virus infection is lethal in athymic nude mice, which fail to clear virus from the lung (Wyde et al. 1977; Yap et al. 1979). Thus T-cell-mediated immunity is of vital importance in protecting against infection, and defences such as complement, natural killer (NK) cells and macrophages are by themselves insufficient. The search for an influenza virus vaccine has concentrated particular attention on identifying the critical protective T-cell subsets. Initial studies used an adoptive cell transfer of spleen cells, restimulated in vitro, to protect naive recipient mice against a lethal virus challenge. Transferrable protection was found to reside in the CD8[+] subset (Yap 1978), and CD8[+] cytotoxic T lymphocyte (CTL) clones grown in vitro were also effective (Taylor & Askonas 1986). CTL are thus a key antiviral defence, and their capacity to eliminate infected cells before new virions are produced is sufficient to clear virus from the lung. This is consistent with the predominance of CD8[+] T cells in the inflammatory infiltrate recoverable from infected lungs by bronchoalveolar lavage (BAL) (Allan et al. 1990).

Unlike the antiviral B-cell response, an effective

antiviral CTL response can be mounted in the absence of CD4$^+$ T-cell help. Mice either depleted of CD4$^+$ T cells by monoclonal antibody treatment (Lightman *et al.* 1987; Allan *et al.* 1990), or congenitally lacking these cells due to a targetted disruption of the major histocompatibility complex (MHC) class II locus (Bodmer *et al.* 1993; Tripp *et al.* 1995a), still clear virus with near-normal kinetics. Thus CTL are by themselves a sufficient defence, even in the absence of a CD4-dependent antibody response. In addition, B-cell-deficient mice depleted of CD4$^+$ T cells are still protected by CD8$^+$ T-cell immunity (Topham & Doherty 1998).

Mechanisms of CTL-mediated cytotoxicity

In accordance with the established principles of CTL recognition (Zinkernagel & Doherty 1975), influenza-specific cytotoxicity is exquisitely specific *in vivo*. Adoptively transferred CTL clear virus from the lung in an MHC-restricted manner (Wells *et al.* 1981), and show no evidence of bystander elimination of a concurrent infection with an unrelated virus (Lukacher *et al.* 1984). Experiments with Sendai virus, a similar respiratory pathogen, have shown that CTL clear virus from the lung only if the respiratory epithelial cells express MHC class I molecules (Hou 1995). Thus for CTL to be effective they must come into direct contact with the virus-infected target cells.

CTL have three major modes of cytotoxicity: perforin secretion, ligation of Fas on the target cell, and interferon-γ secretion (Kagi *et al.* 1995). The first two mechanisms both induce target cell apoptosis, and probably act via a final common pathway of cell suicide (Berke 1994). The effects of local high concentrations of interferon-γ are less well defined, and may act via macrophage activation to clear viral nucleic acid from infected cells without causing cell death (Guidotti & Chisari 1996). Interferon-γ does not contribute appreciably to CTL-mediated cytotoxicity *in vitro* (Lowin 1994). There is clearly a degree of redundancy between the different effector mechanisms, and a lack of just one does not necessarily lead to a major immune defect. Perforin is probably the most important

mediator of cytotoxicity, and is absolutely required to clear lymphochoriomeningitis virus infection (Kagi *et al.* 1994). In contrast, interferon-γ-deficient (Graham *et al.* 1993), perforin-deficient, and Fas-deficient mice can all clear influenza virus infection, although in the case of perforin or Fas deficiency this is delayed by 1–2 days. Recent experiments have shown that in the absence of a protective antibody response, perforin-deficient CTL must use Fas ligation to clear influenza virus from the mouse lung (Topham *et al.* 1997). Lethally irradiated, Fas-deficient mice reconstituted with perforin-deficient bone marrow and depleted of CD4$^+$ T cells do not clear virus infection, whereas irradiated Fas-positive recipients of perforin-deficient bone marrow or Fas-deficient recipients of normal bone marrow can do so. Thus, at least in these bone-marrow chimeric mice, interferon-γ secretion alone is an inadequate defence against influenza.

CD4$^+$ T cells promote a protective antiviral antibody response

Although CD8$^+$ T cells are sufficient for protection, this does not imply that they are also necessary. Unlike the non-cytopathic lymphochoriomeningitis virus, which can be cleared only by CTL (Assmann-Wischer *et al.* 1985), influenza is generally a cytopathic virus and thus passes through a cell-free stage when it is susceptible to neutralization by antibody (Palladino *et al.* 1995). Thus mice depleted of CD8$^+$ T cells by monoclonal antibody treatment (Ledbetter & Hertzenburg 1979), and β_2-microglobulin-deficient mice, which lack CD8$^+$ T cells (Zijlstra *et al.* 1990), still clear infectious influenza from the lung (Eichelberger *et al.* 1991a), although this process is noticeably impaired if a more virulent virus strain is used (Bender *et al.* 1992). Adoptively transferred CD4$^+$ T-cell clones can further protect athymic nude mice (which lack T cells), but not severe combined immunodeficient mice (which lack both T and B cells) against a lethal virus challenge (Scherle *et al.* 1992). This implies that a CD4-dependent antibody response can be protective in the absence of CD8$^+$ T cells, but that CD4$^+$ T cells are by themselves ineffective. This conclusion has since been further strengthened by the observations that in bone-marrow chimeric mice depleted of CD8[+] T cells and lacking MHC class II antigens on the respiratory epithelium, CD4[+] T cells can still be protective (Topham *et al.* 1996); whereas B-cell-deficient mice depleted of CD8[+] T cells survive influenza virus infection extremely poorly, if at all (Topham & Doherty 1998).

CD4[+] T cells are normally found in the BAL after intranasal infection (Allan 1990), where they make a major contribution to cytokine production, producing predominantly interferon-γ, a potent activator of macrophages (Sarawar *et al.* 1993). Treating β2-microglobulin-deficient mice with anti-interferon-γ antibody delays but does not prevent virus clearance (Sarawar & Doherty 1994). Although promoting a Th2-type CD4[+] T-cell response (IL-4 and IL-5 production) over a Th1-type (IL-2 and interferon-γ production) causes immunopathology in respiratory syncytial virus infection (Openshaw 1995), such a balance of cytokine production does not appear to be so critical with influenza. The major role of CD4[+] T cells is probably to provide B-cell help in the germinal centres of the draining lymph nodes, where interferon-γ promotes IgG2a production.

T-cell-mediated cytotoxicity always has the potential to be harmful rather than protective (Allan & Doherty 1985), and CTL-mediated protection against influenza is associated with a transient increase in lung pathology (Mackenzie *et al.* 1989). This effect has generally been more prominent with CD4[+] T cells (Liew & Russell 1983), perhaps because they are less efficient at clearing virus. Both CD4[+] and CD8[+] T cells can in some circumstances cause a deleterious immune pathology (Schiltknecht & Ada 1985; McLain *et al.* 1992), but the overwhelming conclusion is that both CD4[+] and CD8[+] T-cell-mediated immunity provides beneficial protection against influenza virus infection.

One more tantalizing footnote to influenza T-cell immunity in the lung is a possible role for γδ T cells. These are found in plentiful numbers towards the resolution of infection, but are not demonstrably virus-specific. No immune defect has been identified in their absence, and their precise function remains unknown (Doherty *et al.* 1992, 1996).

Quantitative measurement of the antiviral T-cell response

Antigen-specific immune responses are initiated in lymph nodes. The mediastinal lymph nodes become noticeably enlarged 3–5 days after intranasal influenza virus infection, and this increased cellularity is associated with both an appearance of virus-specific T-cell precursors and an accumulation of antigen non-specific T cells (Doherty *et al.* 1992). The key event in immune priming is viral antigen presentation to T cells by dendritic cells (Hamilton-Easton & Eichelberger 1995), and this process can be reproduced in tissue culture using purified cell populations (Macatonia *et al.* 1989; Nonacs *et al.* 1992). Primed CTL precursors then migrate from the lymph nodes to the lung, where they become fully activated effectors, and can be recovered by BAL 7–8 days after infection (Allan *et al.* 1990; Doherty *et al.* 1994). In contrast to pathogens such as lymphochoriomeningitis virus that replicate in lymphoid tissue (Oldstone *et al.* 1985), virus-specific CTL effectors are demonstrable in the draining lymph nodes or spleen only after infection with highly virulent influenza strains, and an analysis of antiviral immunity in these sites has depended chiefly upon an *in vitro* restimulation of specific precursor T cells (Doherty *et al.* 1992). Since bulk culture restimulations are only approximately quantitative, a limiting dilution format has proved the most useful method of following CTL populations. In this assay, single CTL precursors (pCTL) can be expanded by culture with an excess of growth factors and specific antigen to generate an effector cell population detectable by lysis of virus-infected target cells (Owen *et al.* 1982). Activated effector CTL themselves, which are directly cytotoxic *ex vivo*, are probably terminally differentiated and apparently lack the capacity to expand further *in vitro* (Doherty *et al.* 1992).

More recently, CD4[+] T-cell populations have been followed in a similar way by assaying IL-2 production in limiting dilution cultures (Doherty *et al.* 1996). Accurate quantification of the acute CD4[+] T-cell response is still difficult, but limiting dilution analysis has proved useful in following memory CD4[+] T-cell populations over time. CD4[+] T-cell responses may also be followed implicitly by antibody production, but the magnitude of the antibody response cannot easily be related to the number of responding T cells.

The T-cell population in the draining lymph nodes is dynamic

The increased cellularity of the mediastinal lymph nodes is associated with a considerable lymphocyte turnover. Based on flow cytometric analysis of cellular DNA content, up to 20% of the CTL in the lymph node are in cell cycle at the height of the response (Tripp *et al.* 1995b). Since this proportion far exceeds the number of virus-specific pCTL measurable by limiting dilution (less than 1% of CD8[+] T cells), there must be considerable stimulation of T cells without an apparent specificity for the infecting virus (bystander activation). A variety of cytokines are produced in the mediastinal lymph nodes after influenza virus infection (Sarawar & Doherty 1994), and as cytokines can be potent stimulators of memory T-cell proliferation even without specific antigenic stimulation (Tough *et al.* 1996), high local concentrations probably drive the proliferation of both virus-specific and non-specific T cells.

The virus-specific pCTL are clearly part of the cycling pool, and selective removal of the proliferating cells by bromodeoxyuridine incorporation and laser-induced apoptosis considerably reduces the numbers measurable by limiting dilution assay (Tripp *et al.* 1995a). However, pCTL numbers normally reach a stable level surprisingly soon after infection (Owen 1982), despite continued proliferation in the draining lymph nodes. Thus many specific pCTL must also be consumed, perhaps as terminally differentiated effector cells in the lung (Doherty *et al.* 1996). MHC class II-deficient mice, which lack CD4[+] T cells, generate normal levels of CTL effectors in the BAL and clear influenza virus infection with essentially normal kinetics (Bodmer *et al.* 1993), but show a considerable deficit in pCTL numbers in the lymph nodes and spleen (Tripp *et al.* 1995a). Although the production of virus-specific pCTL normally exceeds the consumption during viral clearance from the

lung, in the absence of CD4[+] T-cell-derived cytokines (Sarawar & Doherty 1994), the rate of pCTL consumption is presumably much closer to the rate of generation. It appears that from the initial lymph-node pool, many pCTL migrate to the lung to become terminally differentiated effectors, but a proportion of the excess survive to make up the memory population (Doherty *et al.* 1994).

Heterotypic immunity and T-cell memory

Despite the identification of an important role for CD8[+] T cells in the primary response to influenza virus infection, translating this into an effective vaccine by immune priming has proved problematic. The phenomenon originally observed was cross-protection after infection with serologically unrelated virus subtypes (heterotypic immunity) (Schulman & Kilbourne 1965). The survival of heterotypically immune mice correlates with a more rapid and potent CTL migration into the infected lung (Bennink *et al.* 1978), and *in vivo* T-cell depletion demonstrates that heterotypic immunity resides principally in the CD8[+] subset (Liang *et al.* 1994).

Determination of the molecular basis for CTL cross-protection demonstrated for the first time the nature of the viral antigen recognized by CTL, and substantiated the 'altered self' model established for CTL recognition of lymphochoriomenigitis virus (Zinkernagel & Doherty 1975). In contrast to the surface virion glycoproteins recognized by neutralizing antibodies, CTL-mediated cross-protection in C57BL/6 (H-2[b]) mice was found to be directed principally against the viral nucleoprotein (Townsend *et al.* 1984a; Yewdell *et al.* 1985). Virus-specific CTL clones recognized the nucleoprotein in transfected cell lines (Townsend *et al.* 1984b); truncated forms of the nucleoprotein could substitute for the whole molecule, as could short peptide fragments (Townsend *et al.* 1986); and an intracellular protein degradation pathway was identified as an essential part of MHC class I-restricted antigen presentation to CD8[+] CTL (Spies *et al.* 1992).

However, immunization with purified nucleoprotein or with a vaccinia virus recombinant expressing the nucleoprotein gene does not generate effective antiviral immunity (Andrew *et al.* 1987; Stitz *et al.* 1990). Although nucleoprotein-specific CD4$^+$ T cells can provide help for haemagglutinin-specific B cells (Scherle & Gerhard 1992), and even though immunization with a vaccinia virus recombinant expressing the influenza virus nucleoprotein generates a specific pCTL pool detectable by *in vitro* restimulation (Stitz *et al.* 1990), there is no effective protection against a lethal intranasal challenge. A viral nucleoprotein-expressing plasmid vector may yet prove to be a better vehicle for CTL immunization (Ulmer *et al.* 1993). As in any experimental model, the degree of immunity required for protection to be apparent depends critically upon the (generally arbitrary) challenge used. For example, immunization with a nucleoprotein-expressing vaccinia virus recombinant protects against the neurovirulent influenza virus A/WSN when it replicates slowly in the brain parenchyma, but not when it replicates rapidly in the cerebrospinal fluid (Stevenson *et al.* 1997b). In both cases the challenge is lethal without immunization, but one affords a greater window of opportunity for the memory CTL response to become effective. Claims as to the efficacy of cell-mediated immunity after various vaccination strategies thus have to be interpreted cautiously.

No immunization with an isolated viral component has proved as effective as heterotypic immunity in protecting against a lethal influenza virus challenge, perhaps because the nucleoprotein is only one of several major CTL targets (Bennink *et al.* 1987), or perhaps because factors other than merely the presence of antigen are important in stimulating a CTL response. As with CD4$^+$ T-cell-mediated cytokine production, the antigen non-specific antiviral defences stimulated by influenza virus infection, such as interferon-γ secretion and NK cell activation, probably play a large part in stimulating effective immunity (Kos & Engleman 1996). Interestingly, CD4-depleted, interferon-γ-deficient mice generate much lower levels of specific pCTL after Sendai virus infection than do those either γ-interferon deficient or CD4-depleted alone (Mo *et al.* 1997). Interferon-γ, perhaps derived from NK cells, may in some circumstances be able to sub-

stitute for CD4$^+$ T-cell-derived cytokines *in vivo*. Further dissection of the precise cytokine milieu during virus infection at the level of the single cell may enable us to identify more clearly the important factors in generating a potent CTL response.

The maintenance of T-cell memory

The problem of how the memory T-cell population can be maintained in a stable state of readiness against challenge without further antigenic stimulation is fundamental both to an understanding of immunological homeostasis and to a rational design of any vaccine. Viral RNA is not detectable by PCR amplification for longer than 2 weeks after intranasal influenza virus infection (Eichelberger *et al.* 1991b), and no persistent repository of viral antigen has been identified. This has made influenza a useful system with which to explore the maintenance of T-cell memory without the complication of further antigen-dependent T-cell activation. After intranasal infection, the frequency of influenza-specific pCTL in the total splenic pool is remarkably constant over the lifetime of the mouse. The same also appears to be true for CD4+ T cells, although these have been less extensively investigated (Doherty *et al.* 1996). Adoptive transfer studies have formally demonstrated in this and other systems that the maintenance of pCTL numbers after priming is independent of further stimulation by viral antigens (Hou *et al.* 1994; Lau *et al.* 1994; Mullbacher 1994). This has left the puzzle as to what exactly does maintain the memory pool. Memory T cells are clearly a dynamic population (Tough & Sprent 1994). They have a lower threshold of activation by antigen than their naive counterparts (Tabi *et al.* 1988; Pihlgren *et al.* 1996), and survive preferentially even in the absence of antigen (Tanchot *et al.* 1997). A recognition of crossreactive endogenous antigens (Beverley 1990) and an antigen-independent hyperresponsiveness to antigen-independent stimulation by cytokines (Tough *et al.* 1996) may both play a role in the maintenance of memory T-cell populations, although the importance of neither of these factors has been firmly established.

In contrast to the constant numbers of memory T-cell populations, there is evidence from influenza (Tripp *et al.* 1995c) and from other systems (Walker *et al.* 1995; Zimmermann *et al.* 1996) that the flow cytometric phenotype of memory cells gradually reverts back towards that of naive T cells. CD62L, which naive cells require to enter lymph nodes from the blood via high endothelial venules for immune priming (Gallatin *et al.* 1983), is shed by activated cells but is slowly regained by memory CTL, although the activation marker CD44 is maintained (Budd *et al.* 1987). The CD62L^{hi} CD44^{hi} CTL found late after influenza virus infection still respond to *in vitro* restimulation (Tripp *et al.* 1995c), but their effectiveness *in vivo* may be diminished. A decline in heterotypic immunity does occur in aged mice (Bender & Small 1993), but due to the limited lifespan of the laboratory mouse (about 2 years) it is difficult to distinguish a late diminution in immunological memory from more general senescent changes.

Systemic protection by heterotypic immunity

In humans, heterotypic immunity is initially effective (McMichael *et al.* 1983a), but apparently wanes over a 3–5-year period (McMichael *et al.* 1983b). However, the effectiveness of the memory CTL pool *in vivo* is difficult to assess. There is typically a lag phase of CTL recruitment before heterotypic immunity becomes fully effective, and it may protect only poorly against an acute transient illness, for example one confined to the upper respiratory tract. Indeed the very existence of influenza virus pandemics implies that heterotypic immunity does not provide long-lived protection against a productive infection. Instead there may be protection against systemic viral dissemination, which would be a more protracted process involving multiple rounds of viral replication. Such a protection against more severe disease is an important issue in influenza immunology, since viral pandemics may be associated with extensive pulmonary infection, systemic viral dissemination and neurological disease (Ravenholt & Foege 1982; Webster *et al.* 1982).

Protection against the neurovirulent influenza virus A/WSN is of particular interest in this regard. Sequence analysis of influenza recovered from a victim of the 1918 pandemic shows a close relationship between the neuraminidase of this virus and that of A/WSN (Taubenberger *et al.* 1997), in which it is the chief determinant of neurovirulence (Li *et al.* 1993). After intranasal immunization, memory pCTL do circulate effectively to other organs and protect against a subsequent lethal intracerebral challenge with A/WSN (Stevenson *et al.* 1996). In addition, if infection is limited to the immunoprivileged brain parenchyma, it does not elicit a primary immune response but is still eliminated by memory CTL (Stevenson *et al.* 1997b). The protective CTL migrate directly into the brain without further encountering viral antigens in lymphoid tissue, and thus without further activation (Stevenson *et al.* 1997c). Thus the heightened state of responsiveness measurable *in vitro* after immune priming is functionally important in the mouse model. But whether heterotypic immunity gives long-term protection against severe systemic disease in man cannot, in the absence of extensive epidemiological evidence, be conclusively determined.

Conclusions

Influenza virus infection of the murine respiratory tract has become the archetypal model of immunity to an acute monophasic illness. Although our knowledge is far from complete, this extensively investigated experimental system has provided many insights into how the immune system functions. Multiple effector mechanisms contribute to containing infection, and either CTL or antibody can be effective in an experimental setting. These normally act as synergistic partners: CTL eliminate virus-infected cells, while antibody neutralizes free virions before more cells are infected. CD4$^+$ T cells do not themselves have a significant direct effector role, but play a major part in coordinating the response; they are essential for antibody production and provide crucial cytokines to generate a large pCTL pool. Although antigen non-specific antiviral defences do not provide adequate protection in the absence of T cells, they probably do contribute to a maximally efficient response. The size of the T-cell memory pool appears to be 'set' early in infection and then maintained by unknown mechanisms, possibly involving antigen-independent stimulation by cytokines. However, memory CTL gradually lose activation markers with time, and this probably leads to a diminution in the effectiveness of the anamnestic response. What factors maintain the memory population and how these may be manipulated to generate more effective vaccination strategies remain key immunological questions which are likely to find answers in influenza viral immunology.

Acknowledgements

This study was supported by grant number 21765; travelling fellowship MRC (UK); and the American Lebanese Syrian Associated Charities (ALSAC).

References

Ada, G.L. & Jones, P.D. (1986) The immune response to influenza infection. *Curr Top Microbiol Immunol* **128**, 1–54.

Allan, J.E. & Doherty, P.D. (1985) Immune T cells can protect or induce fatal neurological disease in murine lymphocytic choriomeningitis. *Cell Immunol* **90** (2), 401–7.

Allan, W., Tabi, Z., Cleary, A. & Doherty, P.C. (1990) Cellular events in the lymph node and lung of mice with influenza: consequences of depleting CD4$^+$ T cells. *J Immunol* **144**, 3980–6.

Andrew, M.E., Coupar, B.E., Boyle, D.B. & Ada, G.L. (1987) The roles of influenza virus haemagglutinin and nucleoprotein in protection: analysis using vaccinia virus recombinants. *Scand J Immunol* **25** (3), 21–8.

Assmann-Wischer, U., Simon, M.M. & Lehmann-Grube, F. (1985) Mechanism of recovery from acute virus infection III. Subclass of T lymphocytes mediating clearance of lymphocytic choriomeningitis virus from the spleens of mice. *Med Microbiol Immunol* **174** (5), 249–56.

Bender, B.S. & Small, P.A. Jr (1993) Heterotypic immune mice loss protection against influenza virus infection with senescence. *J Infect Dis* **168** (4), 873–80.

Bender, B.S., Croghan, T., Zhang, L. & Small, P.A. (1992) Transgenic mice lacking class I major histocompatibility complex-restricted T cells have delayed viral clearance and increased mortality after influenza virus challenge. *J Exp Med* **175**, 1143–5.

Bennink, J., Effros, R.B. & Doherty, P.C. (1978) Influenzal pneumonia: early appearance of crossreactive T cells in lungs of mice primed with heterologous type A viruses. *Immunology* **35**, 503–9.

Bennink, J.R., Yewdell, J.W., Smith, G.L. & Moss, B. (1987) Anti-influenza virus cytotoxic T lymphocytes recognize the three viral polymerases and a nonstructural protein: responsiveness to individual viral antigens is major histocompatibility complex controlled. *J Virol* **61**, 1098–102.

Berke, G. (1994) The binding and lysis of target cells by cytotoxic lymphocytes: molecular and cellular aspects. *Annu Rev Immunol* **12**, 735–73.

Beverley, P.C. (1990) Is T-cell memory maintained by crossreactive stimulation? *Immunol Today* **11**, 203–5.

Bodmer, H., Obert, G., Chan, S., Benoist, C. & Mathis, D. (1993) Environmental modulation of the autonomy of cytotoxic T lymphocytes. *Eur J Immunol* **23**, 1649–54.

Budd, R.C., Cerottini, J.-C., Horvath, C. *et al.* (1987) Distinction of virgin and memory T lymphocytes: stable acquisition of the Pgp-1 glycoprotein concomitant with antigenic stimulation. *J Immunol* **138**, 3120–9.

Doherty, P.C., Allan, W. & Eichelberger, M. (1992) Roles of αβ and γδ T cell subsets in viral immunity. *Annu Rev Immunol* **10**, 123–51.

Doherty, P.C., Hou, S. & Tripp, R.A. (1994) CD8$^+$ T-cell memory to viruses. *Curr Opin Immunol* **6**, 545–52.

Doherty, P.C., Topham, D.J. & Tripp, R.A. (1996) Establishment and persistence of virus-specific CD4$^+$ and CD8$^+$ T-cell memory. *Immunol Rev* **150**, 23–44.

Effros, R.B., Doherty, P.C., Gerhard, W. & Bennink, J. (1977) Generation of both crossreactive and virus-specific T-cell populations after immunization with serologically distinct influenza A viruses. *J Exp Med* **145**, 557–68.

Eichelberger, M., Allan, W., Zijlstra, M., Jaenisch, R. & Doherty, P.C. (1991a) Clearance of influenza virus respiratory infection in mice lacking class I major histocompatibility complex-restricted CD8$^+$ T cells. *J Exp Med* **174**, 875–80.

Eichelberger, M., Wang, M., Allan, W., Webster, R. & Doherty, P.C. (1991b) Influenza virus RNA in the lung and lymphoid tissue of immunologically intact and CD4-depleted mice. *J Gen Virol* **72**, 1695–8.

Gallatin, W.M., Weissman, I.L. & Butcher, E.C. (1983) A cell-surface molecules involved in organ-specific homing of lymphocytes. *Nature* **304**, 30–4.

Graham, M.B., Dalton, D.K., Giltinan, D., Braciale, V.L., Stewart, T.A. & Braciale, T.J. (1993) Response to influenza infection in mice with a targeted disruption in the interferon gamma gene. *J Exp Med* **178** (5), 1725–32.

Guidotti, L.G. & Chisari, F.V. (1996) To kill or to cure: options in host defense against viral infection. *Curr Opin Immunol* **8**, 478–83.

Hamilton-Easton, A. & Eichelberger, M. (1995) Virus-specific antigen presentation by different subsets of cells from lung and mediastinal lymph nodes tissues of influenza virus-infected mice. *J Virol* **69**, 6359–66.

Hou, S. & Doherty, P.C. (1995) Clearance of Sendai virus by CD8$^+$ T cells requires direct targeting to virus-infected epithelium. *Eur J Immunol* **25** (1), 111–16.

Hou, S., Hyland, L., Ryan, K.W., Portner, A. & Doherty, P.C. (1994) Virus-specific CD8$^+$ T-cell memory determined by clonal burst size. *Nature* **369**, 652–4.

Kagi, D., Ledermann, B., Burki, K. *et al.* (1994) Cytotoxicity mediated by T cells and natural killer cells is greatly impaired in perforin-deficient mice. *Nature* **369**, 31–7.

Kagi, D., Ledermann, B., Burki, K., Zinkernagel, R.M. & Hengartner, H. (1995) Lymphocyte-mediated cytotoxicity *in vitro* and *in vivo*: mechanisms and significance. *Immunol Rev* **146**, 95–115.

Kawaoka, Y. (1991) Equine H7N7 influenza A viruses are highly pathogenic in mice without adaptation: potential use as an animal model. *J Virol* **65**, 3891–4.

Kos, F.J. & Engleman, E.G. (1996) Role of natural killer cells in the generation of influenza virus-specific cytotoxic T cells. *Cell Immunol* **173** (1), 1–6.

Lau, L.L., Jamieson, B.D., Somasundaram, T. & Ahmed, R. (1994) Cytotoxic T-cell memory without antigen. *Nature* **369**, 648–52.

Ledbetter, J.A. & Herzenberg, L.A. (1979) Xenogeneic monoclonal antibodies to mouse lymphoid differentiation antigens. *Immunol Rev* **47**, 63–90.

Li, S., Schulman, J., Itamura, S. & Palese, P. (1993) Glycosylation of neuraminidase determines the neurovirulence of influenza A/WSN/33 virus. *J Virol* **67**, 6667–73.

Liang, S., Mozdzanowska, K., Palladino, G. & Gerhard, W. (1994) Heterosubtypic immunity to influenza type A virus in mice. *J Immunol* **152**, 1653–61.

Liew, F.Y. & Russell, S.M. (1983) Inhibition of pathogenic effect of effector T cells by specific suppressor T cells during influenza virus infection in mice. *Nature* **304**, 541–3.

Lightman, S., Cobbold, S., Waldmann, H. & Askonas, B.A. (1987) Do L3T4$^+$ T cells act as effector cells in protection against influenza virus infection? *Immunology* **62**, 139–44.

Lowin, B., Hahne, M., Mattmann, C. & Tschopp, J. (1994) Cytolytic T-cell cytotoxicity is mediated through perforin and Fas lytic pathways. *Nature* **370**, 650–2.

Lukacher, A.E., Braciale, V.L. & Braciale, T.J. (1984) In vivo effector function of influenza virus specific cytotoxic T lymphocytes is highly specific. *J Exp Med* **160**, 814–16.

Macatonia, S.E., Taylor, P.M., Knight, S.C. & Askonas, B.A. (1989) Primary stimulation by dendritic cells induces antiviral proliferative and cytotoxic T-cell responses *in vitro*. *J Exp Med* **169**, 1255–64.

Mackenzie, C.D., Taylor, P.M. & Askonas, B.A. (1989) Rapid recovery of long histology correlates with clearance of influenza virus by specific CD8$^+$ cytotoxic T cells. *Immunology* **67** (3), 375–81.

McLain, L., Morgan, D.J. & Dimmock., N.J. (1992) Protection of mice from lethal influenza by defective interfering virus: T-cell responses. *J Gen Virol* **73**, 375–81.

McMichael, A.J., Gotch, F.M., Noble, G.R. & Beare, P.S. (1983a) Cytotoxic T-cell immunity to influenza. *New Engl J Med* **309**, 13–17.

McMichael, A.J., Gotch, F.M., Dongworth, D.W., Clark, A. & Potter, C.W. (1983b) Declining T-cell immunity to influenza, 1977–1982. *Lancet* **ii**, 762–4.

Mims, C.A. (1982) *The Pathogenesis of Infectious Disease*, 2nd edn. Academic Press, London.

Mitchell, D.M., McMichael, A.J. & Lamb, J.R. (1985) The immunology of influenza. *Br Med Bull* **41**, 80–5.

Mo, X.Y., Tripp, R.A., Sangster, M.Y. & Doherty, P.C. (1997) The cytotoxic T-lymphocyte response to Sendai virus is unimpaired in the absence of gamma interferon. *J Virol* **71** (3), 1906–10.

Mullbacher, A. (1994) The long term maintenance of cytotoxic T cell memory does not require persistence of antigen. *J Exp Med* **179**, 317–21.

Nonacs, R., Humborg, C., Tam, J.P. & Steinman, R.M. (1992) Mechanisms of mouse spleen dendritic cell function in the generation of influenza-specific, cytolytic T lymphocytes. *J Exp Med* **176**, 519–29.

Oldstone, M.B.A., Ahmed, R., Byrne, J., Buchmeier, M.J., Rivere, Y. & Southern, P. (1985) Virus and immune responses: lymphocytic choriomeningitis virus as a prototype model of viral pathogenesis. *Br Med Bull* **41**, 70–4.

Openshaw, P.J. (1995) Immunopathological mechanisms in respiratory syncytial virus disease. *Springer Sem Immunopath* **17** (2–3), 187–201.

Owen, J.A., Allouche, M. & Doherty, P.C. (1982) Limiting dilution analysis of the specificity of influenza-immune cytotoxic T cells. *Cell Immunol* **67**, 49–59.

Palladino, G., Mozdzanowska, K., Washko, G. & Gerhard, W. (1995) Virus-neutralizing antibodies of immunoglobulin G (IgG) but not of IgM or IgA isotypes can cure influenza virus pneumonia in SCID mice. *J Virol* **69**, 2075–81.

Pihlgren, M., Dubois, P.M., Tomkowiak, M., Sjogren, T. & Marvel, J. (1996) Resting memory CD8$^+$ T cells are hyperreactive to antigenic challenge *in vitro*. *J Exp Med* **184**, 2141–51.

Ravenholt, R.T. & Foege, W.H. (1982) 1918 influenza, encephalitis lethargica, parkinsonism. *Lancet* **ii**, 860–4.

Sarawar, S.R. & Doherty, P.C. (1994) Concurrent production of interleukin-2, interleukin-10, and gamma interferon in the regional lymph nodes of mice with influenza pneumonia. *J Virol* **68**, 3112–19.

Sarawar, S.R., Carding, S.R., Allan, W. *et al.* (1993) Cytokine profiles of bronchoalveolar ravage cells from mice with influenza pneumonia: consequences of CD4$^+$ and CD8$^+$ T-cell depletion. *Reg Immunol* **5**, 142–50.

Scherle, P.A. & Gerhard, W. (1992) Functional analysis of influenza-specific helper T-cell clones *in vivo*. T cells specific for internal viral proteins provide cognate help for B cell responses to haemagglutinin. *J Exp Med* **164** (4), 1113–28.

Scherle, P.A., Palladino, G. & Gerhard, W. (1992) Mice can recover from pulmonary influenza virus infection in the absence of class I-restricted cytotoxic T cells. *J Immunol* **148**, 212–17.

Schiltknecht, E. & Ada, G.L. (1985) *In vivo* effects of cyclosporine on influenza A virus infected mice. *Cell Immunol* **91**, 227–39.

Schulman, J.L. & Kilbourne, E.D. (1965) Induction of partial specific heterotypic immunity in mice by a single infection with influenza A virus. *J Bacteriol* **89**, 170–4.

Spies, T., Cerundolo, V., Colonna, M., Cresswell, P., Townsend, A. & Demars, R. (1992) Presentation of viral antigen by MHC class I molecules is dependent on a putative peptide transporter heterodimer. *Nature* **355**, 644–6.

Stevenson, P.G., Bangham, C.R.M. & Hawke, S. (1997c) Recruitment, activation and proliferation of CD8$^+$ memory T cells in an immunoprivileged site. *Eur J Immunol* **27**, 3259–68.

Stevenson, P.G., Hawke, S. & Bangham, C.R.M. (1996) Protection against lethal influenza virus encephalitis by intranasally primed CD8$^+$ memory T cells. *J Immunol* **157**, 3065–73.

Stevenson, P.G., Hawke, S., Sloan, D.J. & Bangham, C.R.M. (1997a) The immunogenicity of intracerebral virus infection depends on anatomical site. *J Virol* **71**, 145–51.

Stevenson, P.G., Freeman, S., Bangham, C.R.M. & Hawke, S. (1997b) *J Immunol* **159**, 1876–84.

Stitz, L., Schmitz, C., Binder, D., Zinkernagel, R., Paoletti, E. & Becht, H. (1990) Characterization and immunological properties of influenza A virus nucleoprotein (NP): cell-associated NP isolated from infected cells or viral NP expressed by vaccinia recombinant virus do not confer protection. *J Gen Virol* **71**, 1169–79.

Stuart-Harris, C.H. (1979) Epidemiology of influenza in man. *Br Med Bull* **35**, 3–8.

Sweet, C. & Smith, H. (1980) Pathogenicity of influenza virus. *Micro Rev* **44**, 303–30.

Tabi, Z., Lynch, F., Ceredig, R., Allan, J.E. & Doherty, P.C. (1988) Virus-specific memory T cells are Pgp-1$^+$ and can be selectively activated with phorbol ester and calcium ionophore. *Cell Immunol* **113**, 268–77.

Tanchot, C., Lemonnier, F.A., Perarnau, B., Freitas, A.A. & Rocha, B. (1997) Differential requirements for survival and proliferation of CD8 naive or memory T cells. *Science* **276**, 2057–62.

Taubenberger, J.K., Reid, A.H., Krafft, A.E., Bijwaard, K.E. & Fanning, T.G. (1997) Initial genetic characterization of the 1918 'Spanish' influenza virus. *Science* **275**, 1973–6.

Taylor, P.M. & Askonas, B.A. (1986) Influenza nucleoprotein-specific cytotoxic T-cell clones are protective in vivo. *Immunology* **58**, 417–20.

Topham, D.J. & Doherty, P.C. (1998) Clearance of an influenza A virus by CD4$^+$ T cells is inefficient in the absence of B cells. *J Virol* **72**, 882–5.

Topham, D.J., Tripp, R.A. & Doherty, P.C. (1997). CD8$^+$ T cells clear influenza virus by perforin or Fas-dependent processes. *J Immunol* **159**, 5197–200.

Topham, D.J., Tripp, R.A., Sarawar, S.R., Sangster, M.Y. & Doherty, P.C. (1996) Immune CD4$^+$ T cells promote the clearance of influenza virus from major histocompatibility complex class II -/- respiratory epithelium. *J Virol* **70** (2), 1288–91.

Tough, D.F. & Sprent, J. (1994) Turnover of naive- and memory-phenotype T cells. *J Exp Med* **179** (4), 1127–35.

Tough, D.F., Borrow, P. & Sprent, J. (1996) Induction of bystander T-cell proliferation by viruses and type I interferon *in vivo*. *Science* **272**, 1947–50.

Townsend, A.R.M. & Skehel, J.J. (1984a) The influenza A nucleoprotein gene controls the induction of both subtype-specific and crossreactive cytotoxic T cells. *J Exp Med* **160**, 552–63.

Townsend, A.R.M., McMichael, A.J., Carter, M.J., Huddleston, A. & Brownlee, G.G. (1984b) Cytotoxic T-cell recognition of the influenza nucleoprotein and haemagglutinin expressed in transfected mouse L cells. *Cell* **39**, 13–25.

Townsend, A.R.M., Rothbard, J., Gotch, F.M., Bahadur, G., Wraith, D. & McMichael, A.J. (1986) The epitopes of influenza nucleoprotein recognized by cytotoxic T lymphocytes can be defined with short synthetic peptides. *Cell* **44**, 959–68.

Tripp, R.A., Sarawar, S.R. & Doherty, P.C. (1995a) Characteristics of the influenza virus-specific CD8$^+$ T-cell response in mice homozygous for disruption of the H-2IA^b gene. *J Immunol* **155**, 2955–9.

Tripp, R.A., Hou, S., McMickle, A., Houston, J. & Doherty, P.C. (1995b) Recruitment and proliferation of CD8$^+$ T cells in respiratory virus infections. *J Immunol* **154**, 6013–21.

Tripp, R.A., Hou, S. & Doherty, P.C. (1995c) Temporal loss of the activated L-selectin-low phenotype for virus-specific CD8$^+$ memory T cells. *J Immunol* **154**, 5870–5.

Ulmer, J.B., Donnelly, J.J., Parker, S.E. *et al.* (1993) Heterologous protection against influenza by injection of DNA encoding a viral protein. *Science* **259**, 1745–9.

Walker, P.R., Ohteki, T., Lopez, J.A., MacDonald, H.R. & Maryanski, J.L. (1995) Distinct phenotypes of antigen-selected CD8 T cells emerge at different stages of an *in vivo* immune response. *J Immunol* **155**, 3443–52.

Webster, R.G., Laver, W.G., Air, G.M. & Schild, G.C. (1982) Molecular mechanisms of variation in influenza viruses. *Nature* **296**, 115–21.

Wells, M.A., Ennis, F.A. & Albrecht, P. (1981) Recovery from a viral respiratory infection. II. Passive transfer of immune spleen cells to mice with influenza pneumonia. *J Immunol* **126**, 1042–6.

Wyde, P.R., Couch, R.B., Mackler, B.F., Cate, T.R. & Levy, B.M. (1977) Effects of low- and high-passage influenza virus infection in normal and nude mice. *Infect Immun* **15** (1), 221–9.

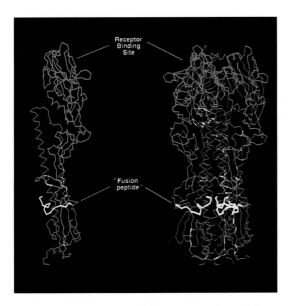

Plate 5.1 α-carbon tracing of the structure of one of the monomers of haemagglutinin and the BHA trimer. The HA$_1$ subunit is shown in blue and the HA$_2$ subunit in red. The locations of the receptor binding site and the fusion peptide, shown in white, are indicated.

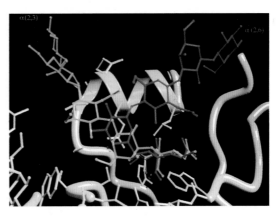

Plate 5.2 Diagrammatic representation of the receptor binding site of haemagglutinin bound to pentasaccharides with terminal sialic acid attached via either α-(2,3) or α-(2,6) linkage. The haemagglutinin is shown in yellow, the α-(2,3)-linked oligosaccharide in green, and the α-(2,6)-linked oligosaccharide in red. (Provided by Mike Eisen.)

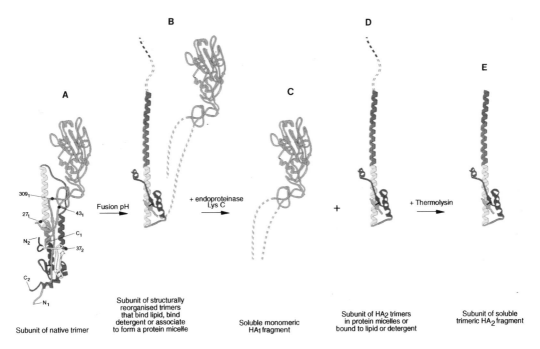

Plate 5.3 Diagrammatic representation summarizing the structural transitions which occur at the pH of membrane fusion. The structure on the left (A) shows a monomer of the native haemagglutinin trimer and indicates the positions of the N- and C-termini of each subunit, the positions at which Lys C (HA$_1$ residue 27) and thermolysin (HA$_2$ residue 37) cleave low pH haemagglutinin, and the positions (HA$_1$ residue 43 and HA$_2$ residue 309) at which the acid pH structure of the membrane-distal domains become disordered. The diagram (B) summarizes what is known of the acid pH structure based on the structure of Lys C tops (C) complexed with an Fab (Bizebard *et al.* 1995) and the structure (E) of TBHA$_2$ (Bullough *et al.* 1994). The broken lines indicate regions of unknown structure. (Reproduced from Skehel *et al.* 1995, with permission from Cold Spring Harbour Press.)

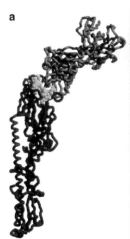 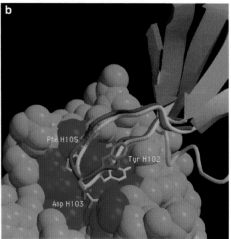

Plate 5.4 (a) Structure of Fab of HC19 complexed with haemagglutinin. Only a monomer of haemagglutinin is shown for clarity. HA_1 is in red and HA_2 in blue. The residues which comprise the receptor binding site are in yellow. The Fab molecule is in green. (b) Close up of the regions of contact between haemagglutinin and Fab 19. The H3 complimentarity-determining region is shown in yellow. The position it would occupy in the uncomplexed Fab is shown in red. The residues which constitute the receptor binding site are shown in purple. (Provided by Thierry Bizebard.)

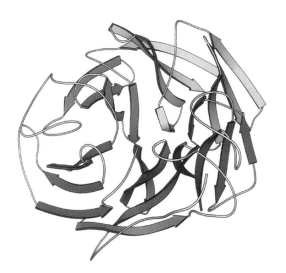

Plate 6.1 MOLSCRIPT (Kraulis 1991) drawing of the β-sheet propeller fold of influenza virus neuraminidase. Colour coding is progressively red to purple, highlighting the six β-sheets. The N-terminus is residue 82, to the rear of the figure and near the pronase cleavage site, which liberates soluble enzyme from the viral membrane. (Reproduced from Colman 1994, with permission from Cambridge University Press.)

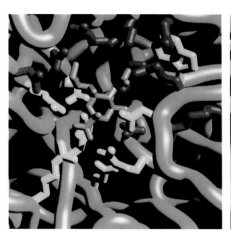 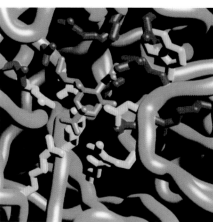

Plate 6.2

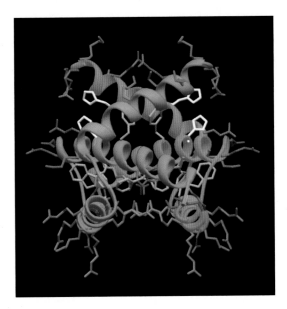

Plate 8.1 Three-dimensional structure of the dimeric RNA binding domain of the NS1 protein of influenza A virus: ribbon diagram. The N- and C-termini of each chain are indicated. Side chains of arginine (blue), lysine (green), histidine (grey), aromatic (yellow), aspartic acid (red), and glutamic acid (orange) residues are shown. One of the potential RNA binding domains is comprised of the basic (arginine- and lysine-rich) region at the bottom of the structure shown in this orientation. (Reproduced from Chien *et al.* 1997)

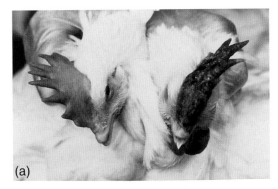

(a)

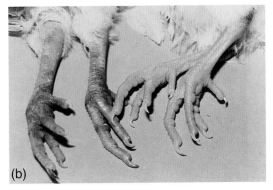

(b)

Plate 12.1 Chickens infected with highly pathogenic Chicken/Pennsylvania/83 (H5N2) influenza viruses. (a) Infected bird on right displays necrotic and oedematous comb with scabby lesions and swollen face caused by subcutaneous oedema 5–6 days after infection. (b) Infected bird on left shows haemorrhagic changes in subcutaneous tissue of the legs and feet 5–6 days after infection. (Reproduced from Webster & Kawaoka 1988, with permission from CRC Press.)

Plate 6.2 *(opposite)* Stereo image of the structure of sialic acid (green) bound in the active site of influenza virus neuraminidase. Amino acids conserved in all strains of influenza virus neuraminidase are coloured yellow and red, and the subset of those that are conserved between known viral and bacterial neuraminidase structures are coloured yellow (R118, D151, W178, E277, R292, R391, Y406, E425). W178 is not present in the proposed model for the parainfluenza virus HN protein. Of the red residues (E119, R152, R156, S179, D198, I222, R224, E227, E226, N294), D198 is Asn in N7 and N9 subtypes. The figure was generated with the HYDRASTER program, written by S. Watowich and L. Gross, based on work by D. Bacon and W. Anderson (RASTER3D) and R. Hubbard (HYDRA). (Reproduced from Colman 1994, with permission from Cambridge University Press.)

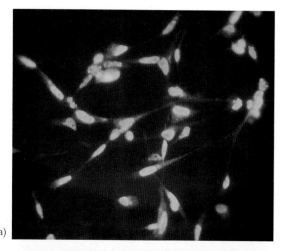

(a)

(b)

Plate 22.1 Immunofluorescence of influenza. (a) Primary chick embryo fibroblasts stained at 3 h post infection with influenza A H3N2 with monoclonal antibody to influenza nucleoprotein. (b) Uninfected control cells. Magnification × 400.

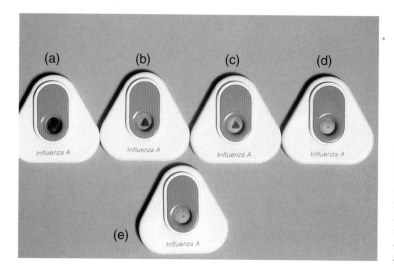

Plate 22.2 Rapid antigen detection of influenza A using a commercial membrane enzyme immunoassay which can be completed in 15 min. Samples (a), (b), (c) contain 10^6, 10^4, 5×10^3 pfu/ml of influenza virus, respectively. (d) is a clinical sample containing respiratory syncytial virus and (e) is a negative control sample.

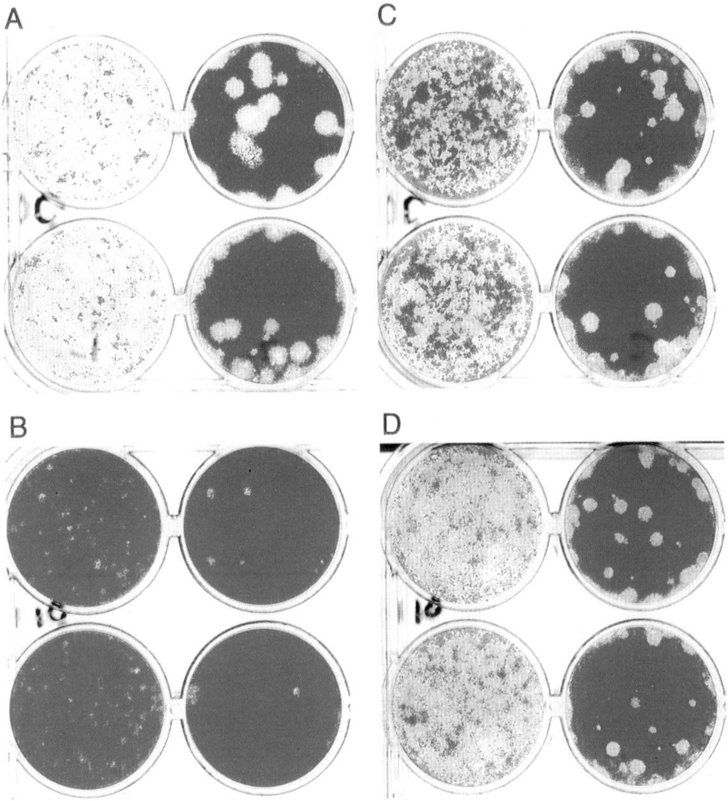

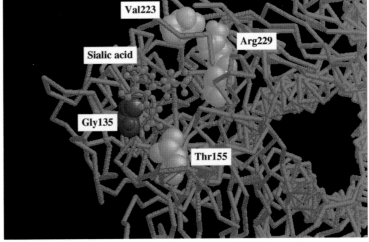

Plate 22.3 Plaque assay for amantadine resistance. MDCK cells infected with A / England / 292 / 95 (H3N2) (A and B) and A / England / 93 / 96 (H3N2) (C and D) stained at 72h post infection with 2% carbol fucshin. Cells were incubated with a semi-solid agar overlay containing 3 µg / ml TPCK-trypsin after inoculation, prior to staining. Amantadine at 1.0 µg / ml was incorporated into the overlay in (B) and (D). The reduction in plaque number and size of amantadine sensitive A / England / 292 / 95 is shown in (B), whereas A / England / 93 / 96 contains a Val to Ala substitution at position 27 of the M2 protein, conferring amantadine resistance (D).

Plate 36.1 Position of mutations in influenza A haemagglutinin selected by culture of virus in presence of zanamivir. Parental amino acids subject to mutation are shown (Gly 135, Thr 155, Val 223, Arg 229) which are close to the sialic acid binding site. (Redrawn from data of Weis *et al.* 1988, and viewed using RasMol; Sayle & Milner-White 1995.)

Wyde, P.R., Gilbert, B.E. & Levy, B.M. (1983) Evidence that T-lymphocytes are part of the blood-brain barrier to virus dissemination. *J Neuroimmunol* **5**, 47–58.

Yap, K.L., Ada, G.L. & McKenzie, I.F.C. (1978) Transfer of specific cytotoxic T lymphocytes protects mice inoculated with influenza virus. *Nature* **273**, 238–9.

Yap, K.L., Braciale, T.J. & Ada, T.L. (1979) Role of T-cell function in recovery from murine influenza infection. *Cell Immunol* **43**, 341–51.

Yewdell, J.W., Bennink, J.R., Smith, G.L. & Moss, B. (1985) Influenza A virus nucleoprotein is a major target antigen for crossreactive anti-influenza A virus cytotoxic T lymphocytes. *Proc Natl Acad Sci USA* **82**, 1785–9.

Zijlstra, J., Bix, M., Sinister, N.D., Loring, N.E., Raulet, J.M. & Jaenisch, D.H. (1990) Beta 2-microglobulin deficient mice lack CD4–8$^+$ cytolytic T cells. *Nature* **344**, 742–6.

Zimmermann, C., Brduscha-Riem, K., Blaser, C., Zinkernagel, R.M. & Pircher, H. (1996) Visualization, characterization, and turnover of CD8$^+$ memory T cells in virus-infected hosts. *J Exp Med* **183** (4), 1367–75.

Zinkernagel, R.M. & Doherty, P.C. (1975) H-2 compatibility requirement for T-cell-mediated lysis of target cells infected with lymphocytic choriomeningitis virus. *J Exp Med* **141**, 1427–36.

Zweerink, H.J., Courtneige, S.A., Skehel, J.J., Crumpton, M.J. & Askonas, B.A. (1977) Cytotoxic T cells kill influenza infected cells but do not distinguish between serologically distinct type A viruses. *Nature* **267**, 354–6.

Section 7
Laboratory Diagnosis
and Techniques

CHAPTER 22

Laboratory Diagnosis of Influenza

Maria Zambon

Introduction

Laboratory diagnosis of influenza infection is an important public health tool, given the proven ability of this viral infection to cause enormous morbidity and mortality. It also has a role to play in individual patient management and outbreak control. There are a number of different laboratory tests available for the diagnosis of influenza: some detect the presence of viral antigens, viral nucleic acid, virally infected cells or infectious virus particles in respiratory secretions; others are serological tests which rely on the detection of the host immune response to influenza infection. The application of different tests and testing strategies depends on the information required. The use of rapid diagnostic techniques such as antigen detection or direct immunofluorescence (DIF) is much more appropriate in primary care or hospital settings, where speed of diagnosis is the major concern, to allow both drug intervention and infection control, and antigenic information is of lesser importance. In this situation, sensitivity and specificity must be high to avoid false negative reactions, and the amount of specialized equipment and operator skill required should be minimized to allow widespread application of tests.

In contrast, a reference laboratory participating in or performing influenza surveillance requires a battery of tests at its disposal to allow the detailed antigenic characterization of isolates grown in both embryonated eggs and the most sensitive mammalian cell culture. Clearly, not all tests fulfil all desirable criteria (Table 22.1). One of the inherent dangers of relying too heavily on rapid diagnostic tests, despite their convenience and ease of use, is that they provide little or no antigenic information and usually do not allow isolation of influenza virus. For the forseeable future, optimum influenza vaccine formulation will continue to require detailed antigenic information on epidemic variants to ensure the best possible match between the current subunit vaccine and circulating strains. Thus characterization of influenza strains within national surveillance networks is required, which will entail maintenance of facilities and skill necessary for virus isolate characterization.

Type of clinical specimen

Mammalian influenza A viruses replicate primarily in the columnar epithelial cells of the respiratory tract (Loosli *et al.* 1953). The primary route of transmission is through airborne respiratory secretions. Avian influenza viruses replicate in both the respiratory and intestinal tract and virus is shed in the faeces. Faecal transmission is thought to be the major route of transmission from and between birds, and cloacal swabs are the sample of choice for avian influenza isolation (Webster *et al.* 1978).

Sampling of the human or mammalian respiratory tract for clinical virus isolation should attempt to maximize the harvest of virally infected epithelial cells. Nasopharyngeal washes or aspirates have a higher cellular content and are superior to nasopharyngeal swabs for human influenza virus isolation (Cruz *et al.* 1987). Throat swabs or throat washings are of limited use in the diagnosis of influenza since the majority of cells captured by this technique are squamous epithelia. However, a

Table 22.1 Advantages and disadvantages of diagnostic investigations.

Method	Time	Cost/ sample (£)	Skill	Task	Advantages	Disadvantages
Culture	2–7 days	10.00	+++	S, D	Whole virus Low cost	Requires infectious virus Skill Time Specialized equipment
Immunofluorescence	2–4 hours	10.00	+++	S, D	Speed	Requires intact cells Skill Lack of virus Specialized equipment
Antigen detection	15 minutes*– 2 hours	10–30.00*	+/–	S, P, D	No specialized facility Speed Low skill	Cost Lack of virus
RT-PCR	1–1½ days	75.00	+++++	S, D	Sensitivity Molecular analysis	Cost Skill Lack of virus Time Specialized equipment

S, surveillance; D, diagnostic laboratory; P, near patient testing; *, commercial cassette kit.

combined nose and throat swab can be a useful specimen for virus isolation. Furthermore, the convenience of nasopharyngeal swabs is a major factor in its selection. Nasopharyngeal aspirates, swabs and washes are all acceptable for culture, immunofluorescence (IF) and enzyme immuno-assays (EIA) for viral antigen detection. Endo-tracheal aspirates are also suitable for culture, EIA and IF, although they are not as good as bronch-oalveolar lavage (BAL) fluid which usually has a higher cellular content. Lung tissue derived from postmortem, open-lung or needle biopsy pro-cedures can be an excellent clinical sample for virus isolation and isolation of virus from lung tissue or BAL usually indicates lower tract infection.

Nasopharyngeal swabs should be cotton-, rayon- or dacron-tipped, plastic-coated or aluminium-shafted swabs. Wooden stick swabs should be avoided because of the potential for the pre-servatives used in the manufacture of wood to leach into transport media and inhibit subsequent cell culture, as has been demonstrated for other envel-oped viruses (Bettoli *et al.* 1982). Calcium alginate swabs should also be avoided as alginate may also be inhibitory to cell cultures (Bettoli *et al.* 1982). The

swab should be inserted deeply into the naso-pharynx, rotated vigorously to collect columnar epithelial cells, removed and replaced into viral transport medium (VTM). Swabs can either be left in VTM or agitated, fluid expressed from the swab and the swab removed. Nasopharyngeal aspirates are collected by placing fine-bore catheter tubing, connected to a mucous trap with vacuum suction, into the nostril past the anterior nares and applying suction. After removal of the catheter from the nose, VTM or saline is suctioned through the catheter from the nasal end, washing cellular material into the trap. Nasal washes are collected by instilling 1–2 ml of sterile PBS into the nares by using a catheter or fine bore tubing attached to a 5 ml syringe. The saline is immediately suctioned back into a syringe, yielding 1–2 ml of sample.

Transport

Transport conditions should be optimized to ensure maximal recovery of specimens. Specimens should be transported at 4°C or frozen at –70°C. The infectivity of enveloped viruses is generally rapidly destroyed at room temperature, although influenza is moderately stable compared to other respiratory viral pathogens such respiratory syncytial virus (RSV), and indeed can be recovered after up to 5 days from respiratory specimens sent by post (Ellis *et al.* 1997a). The VTM used can be critical in ensuring good virus recovery (Jensen & Johnson 1994). Ideally, VTM should include a balanced salt solution at neutral pH with protein stabilizers such as gelatin or bovine serum albumin (BSA), and antibiotics to reduce/inhibit growth of commensal or pathogenic bacteria. The use of bovine calf serum should be avoided in VTM used for transporting specimens for isolation of influenza, for reasons discussed below. Suitable media include Hanks' Balanced Salt Solution or Earles Minimal Essential Medium with veal infusion broth, or gelatin or BSA.

Cell culture

Characterization of the antigenic properties of influenza viruses recovered from clinical material amplified in either mammalian or avian tissue culture or embryonated eggs remains the cornerstone of worldwide influenza surveillance. Recent studies on the tropism of influenza viruses have helped to provide an understanding of the behaviour of natural isolates of influenza viruses in tissue culture and eggs and to refine strategies for isolation of influenza virus from clinical material.

Influenza viruses are able to replicate in a variety of primary, diploid and continuous cell cultures, although the susceptibility of most cell lines to influenza infection appears to be low (Dowdle & Schild 1975). Human influenza A (H1N1, H2N2 and H3N2) and B viruses preferentially attach to sialic acid with an α-(2,6) linkage to galactose (α-(2,6)-Gal) containing oligosaccharides, whereas avian and equine influenza A viruses preferentially attach to sialic acid with an α-(2,3) linkage to galactose (α-(2,3)-Gal) (Rogers & Paulson 1983). The receptor for influenza C has been identified as *N*-acetyl-9-O-acetylneuraminic acid (Neu5,9Ac2) (Rogers *et al.* 1986).

Primary monkey kidney (PMK) cells, which have a broad spectrum of susceptibility to many human viruses, are widely used in diagnostic laboratories for isolation of human influenza A and B viruses, although there are several problems associated with use of these cells. Whilst wild-type strains of influenza can be isolated using PMK cells, the titres of virus are usually lower than can be obtained from susceptible continuous cell lines. There is often batch-to-batch variation in sensitivity of the cells to influenza and frequent contamination with adventitious simian agents such as foamy viruses. Oncogene immortalized epithelial cell lines of PMK origin have been investigated for the culture of human influenza viruses but they have not proven superior to PMK cells or continuous cell lines (Clarke *et al.* 1996). The use of primary human epithelial tissue for culture of influenza viruses has been limited. Respiratory epithelium has not been easily accessible for studies of primary isolation of wild-type isolates, although this would clearly be a rational choice (reviewed by Wright *et al.* 1996). Cell lines derived from human ciliated columnar epithelial cells have been developed, but their use so far has been confined to the research setting (Endo *et al.* 1996). Primary chick embryo fibroblast cells are also suitable cells for the isolation of influenza viruses, although the growth of many human strains requires the addition of extraneous trypsin and in practice these cells are not routinely used for isolation work.

Mammalian epithelioid cells provide the most sensitive cell culture system for propagation *in vitro* of the largest number of human influenza A, B and C strains described to date. The most common of these in widespread use for influenza diagnosis is Madin–Darby canine kidney (MDCK), a continuous polarized cell line, first described in the 1970s, which has both α-(2,3) and α-(2,6) galactose-linked sialic acid on its cell surface (Tobita *et al.* 1975; Davies *et al.* 1978; Frank *et al.* 1979; Govorkova *et al.* 1996).

MDCK cells which differ in their functional and morphological characteristics have been described (Richardson *et al.* 1981; Simmons 1981). One of these morphological variants of MDCK cells lacks Neu5,9Ac2 on its cell surface and is resistant to influenza C virus (Schultze *et al.* 1996). Influenza C virus may otherwise be propagated in human malignant melanoma cell line HMV-II, of unknown receptor specificity (Moriuchi *et al.* 1990). Variation in susceptibility of MDCK subclones to other influenza A and B viruses has not been studied.

The distribution of sialic acid receptors on most mammalian cell lines has not been determined, and their influence on influenza virus attachment and replication is unclear. African green monkey kidney (Vero) cells contain predominantly α-(2,3) galactose-linked sialic acid on their cell surface, but are fully susceptible to human influenza A and B viruses (Govorkova *et al.* 1996). Therefore, the receptors present on the cell surface of mammalian cells are not the only determinant of susceptibility to influenza A and B.

Proteolytic activation of influenza virus

One of the general features of orthomyxo- and paramyxovirus replication is the necessity for post-translational cleavage of viral glycoproteins. The production of infectious progeny influenza virions following replication *in vitro* and *in vivo* is dependent on the post-translational cleavage of the major influenza glycoprotein haemagglutinin (HA) from its precursor form HA_0 to HA_1 and HA_2. HA from human influenza viruses cannot be cleaved by intracellular proteases during virus assembly in any of the continuous epithelioid cell lines described to date. Therefore, one of the major drawbacks of the use of continuous cell lines is the need to add extraneous proteolytic enzyme in order to ensure the cleavage of HA and multiple cycle viral replication. 1-Tosylamide-2-phenylethyl chloromethyl ketone-treated trypsin (TPCK-trypsin) is more stable at physiological temperatures and is currently the protease of choice.

Influenza virus replication in several continuous lines is impaired by the rapid inactivation of exogenous trypsin in the culture fluids due to the accumulation of a high molecular weight trypsin inhibitor synthesized by the cells (Kaverin & Webster 1995). Synthesis of the trypsin inhibitor varies in different cell cultures. In MDCK cells, it does not affect the growth of influenza virus but in other cell lines, e.g. Vero cells, there is impairment of multiple cycle replication of influenza (Kaverin & Webster

1995). Additionally, influenza replication is dependent on the seeding density of certain continuous cells, implying that cell-cycle control of influenza replication might be more tightly regulated in certain epithelial cells, compared with MDCK cells, in which replication of influenza is independent of seeding density (Kaverin & Klenk 1995). This may be relevant, as the synthesis of cellular proteases is also governed by the cell cycle (King *et al.* 1996). Study of A/WSN/33, a laboratory-adapted human H1N1 virus strain, indicates that cleavage of uncleaved HA can occur in MDBK (Madin–Darby bovine kidney) cells during entry of the virus into the endosome, without the need for addition of exogeneous trypsin (Boycott *et al.* 1994). Production of infectious human influenza strains in PMK cells also occurs in the absence of trypsin, although the sensitivity of batches of PMK cells may be improved by the addition of trypsin.

Cumulatively, these findings suggest that more continuous cell lines could be susceptible to influenza than has hitherto been recognized, but further work is required to characterize the nature and location of cellular protease enzymes involved in proteolytic activation of HA and into the manipulation of mammalian cell cultures in order to optimize conditions for growth of influenza.

It has been noted for some time that the presence of bovine calf serum post inoculation in cell cultures inhibits the production of infectious influenza virus (Dowdle & Schild 1975). This is likely to be due to the presence of inhibitors which inactivate the proteases responsible for cleavage of influenza or, alternatively, specific glycosylated macromolecules which inhibit receptor binding of influenza virus (see section on serological diagnosis). Moreover, cells which have been grown in medium which is bovine calf serum free for several passages yield higher titres of virus (Merten *et al.* 1996).

From the foregoing, it can be seen that optimum isolation of influenza, irrespective of the nature of the clinical specimen, will be achieved by using:
1 PMK cells washed with serum-free medium prior to inoculation and incubated in serum-free medium post inoculation; or

2 MDCK cells washed with serum-free medium prior to inoculation and incubated in serum-free medium, with the addition of TPCK-trypsin at concentrations of 1–3 µg/ml post inoculation; or
3 Vero cells washed in serum-free medium prior to inoculation and incubated in serum-free medium with the addition of TPCK-trypsin at a concentration of 1–2 µg/ml daily, post inoculation.

It has also been recognized that primary isolation is assisted by the use of a lower temperature of incubation such as 33°C, rolling tissue culture tubes and centrifugation of virus onto cell cultures.

Growth of influenza viruses in embryonated eggs

The superior growth of avian and equine influenza strains in embryonated avian eggs compared with cell culture means that the embryonated egg remains the system of choice for veterinary diagnostic work. Moreover, all known influenza strains undergo post-translational processing of haemagglutinin in the chick embryo, yielding infectious progeny virus. The virus yields of human influenza isolates from the cells lining the allantoic cavity of the egg are higher than in monolayer cultures of susceptible cells (including MDCK cells) if they are calculated per unit volume (e.g. plaque forming units [pfu] or haemagglutination units [HAU] per ml), but equivalent if calculated on a per cell basis. Partly for this reason, human influenza vaccines continue to be produced from virus grown in eggs. This in turn imposes constraints on international influenza surveillance since vaccine strain selection requires candidate strains to be primary isolates which have been made and passaged in eggs. Until cell-derived human influenza vaccines are in widespread use, isolation of human variants of influenza A and B will have to continue in embryonated eggs, despite increasing evidence for host cell selection of variants.

Human influenza viruses differ markedly in their ability to replicate in hens' eggs and in cell culture. In part, this reflects properties of the HA and neuraminidase (NA) surface proteins (Williams & Robertson 1993). There are many instances of selection of mutations in the HA of human virus isolates adapted to growth in different environments which appear to alter antigenicity (Rocha *et al.* 1993). In general, MDCK-grown human influenza A and B isolates are more antigenically homogenous than their egg-grown counterparts (Katz *et al.* 1990; Robertson *et al.* 1990), and more like the original clinical samples than egg-grown viruses (Robertson *et al.* 1985), a point which is particularly important in selection of strains for vaccine production. It must be ensured that properties of the egg-grown vaccine virus do not differ significantly from the original virus isolate. Clearly, for as long as influenza vaccines are produced in eggs, there will continue to be a need for primary isolation work in embryonated eggs, and influenza laboratories will need to grow virus in embryonated eggs and mammalian cell culture in parallel.

For maximum isolation in eggs, 10–11-day-old embryos are inoculated simultaneously intra-amniotically and intra-allantoically with clinical specimen. Eggs are incubated at 33–35° C for 3–4 days for mammalian isolates of influenza and at 37° C for avian isolates of influenza A, and samples of both amniotic and allantoic fluids are tested for the presence of virus. Reinoculation of the primary harvest material into the amniotic and allantoic cavity is recommended to try and recover human virus isolates with maximum sensitivity (blind passage). Influenza C only grows in the amniotic cavity of embryonated eggs.

Identification of virus growth

Influenza A viruses grow less vigorously in mammalian cell culture than influenza B viruses, which may reflect the host range adaptation of influenza A viruses—the human is the only host for influenza B. The cytopathic effect (CPE) of influenza A viruses in cell culture consists of slowly rounding degenerating cells, but may be absent or difficult to detect and is not pathognomonic. The production of CPE by wild-type isolates of influenza B is usually more reliable. Cells become more refractile and rounded and eventually fragment and detach (Fig. 22.1). The absence of a reliable, recognizable CPE in cell cultures inoculated with clinical specimens means that other methods of identifying virus-infected cell

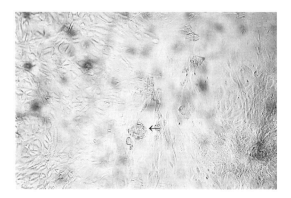

Fig. 22.1 Influenza cytopathic effect. Infection of primary monkey kidney cells with B/England/17/95 at 3 days post infection. Early foci of viral infection can be seen, with cells rounding and increasing in granularity. Magnification × 400.

cultures have to be used, e.g. haemagglutination, haemadsorption or immunostaining.

Haemagglutination and haemadsorption

The techniques of haemagglutination and haemadsorption remain as crucial in specialist influenza and routine diagnostic laboratories today as they were 50 years ago when the phenomenon of haemagglutination was first described by Hirst in 1941. In the presence of influenza, a suspension of red cells forms a lattice and fails to sediment (haemagglutinates). Influenza A, B and C viruses agglutinate red blood cells of several avian and animal species as they bind sialic acid on the surface of these cells. The ability to agglutinate erythrocytes from different species reflects the receptor specificity of influenza viruses, although the molecular basis for agglutination of erythrocytes has not been completely resolved (Ito *et al.* 1997). Site-directed mutation of the receptor binding site of the HA protein of H3N2 influenza affects the ability of HA protein to bind to red cells (Weis *et al.* 1988). Agglutination of erythrocytes can also alter on passage of influenza isolates, as seen by the change in haemagglutination profile during passage of human viruses in eggs, first reported as original–derived (O–D) variation (Burnet & Bull 1941).

From the time that agglutination was first observed, chicken, human or guinea-pig erythrocytes have commonly been used in this reaction. However, natural variation in field isolates of influenza A has led to alteration in ability of clinical isolates of human influenza to agglutinate particular species of red cells. For example, it has been noted that changes in the presumed receptor binding pocket of influenza H1N1 isolates are responsible for the loss of ability of recent isolates to agglutinate chicken erythrocytes (Morishita *et al.* 1996). Changes in the receptor binding residues in recent influenza A H3N2 viruses have also been noted, although the correlation between amino acid changes and binding specificity has not yet been identified (Lindstrom *et al.* 1996). With these findings in mind, the routine use of chick erythrocytes is no longer advisable for detection of human influenza A strains isolated after 1993, and turkey erythrocytes have been substituted in many influenza laboratories.

In the presence of viral HA in the cell membranes of infected cells, erythrocytes attach to the exposed glycoproteins, giving rise to the phenomenon of haemadsorption, where red cells are seen attaching to the surface of an infected cell monolayer. This technique is widely used in diagnostic laboratories to screen monolayers inoculated with clinical specimens for the presence of ortho- or para-myxoviruses. Cells infected with parainfluenza viruses and mumps also show haemadsorption with guinea-pig red cells. Identification of the virus responsible for haemadsorption is then performed either using haemadsorption inhibition tests with specific neutralizing antisera, or by immunostaining of infected cells using monoclonal antibodies. Guinea-pig cells are usually used for haemadsorption, as they are more sensitive for the detection of influenza than avian red cells. Mammalian erythrocytes lack a nucleus and are much smaller than avian erythrocytes; it is possible that the enhanced surface area to volume ratio of mammalian cells allows binding of more red cells by smaller amounts of virus, giving more obvious haemadsorption at lower titres of virus in cell culture (Fig. 22.2a). One of the major disadvantages of cell culture for the identification of influenza virus is the length of time needed to identify a culture-positive sample from

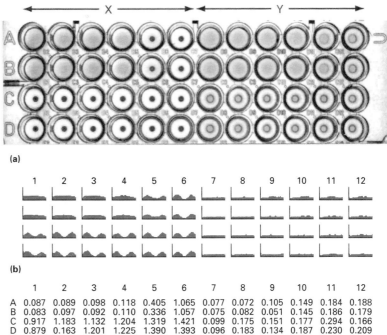

Fig. 22.2 Haemagglutination of influenza virus. (a) Rows A & B—titration of doubling dilutions of influenza A H3N2 virus from 1:5 to 1:160 by haemagglutination using turkey red cells (X) and guinea-pig red cells (Y). Rows C & D—negative controls. Note the incomplete settling patterns with guinea-pig red cells. (b),(c) Analysis of the haemagglutination pattern from (X) and (Y) using a plate reader and software (Dynatech MRX) giving automated reading (b) and hard copy read-out (c) of the graphical and numerical interpretation of the haemagglutination patterns in (a).

	1	2	3	4	5	6	7	8	9	10	11	12
A	0.087	0.089	0.098	0.118	0.405	1.065	0.077	0.072	0.105	0.149	0.184	0.188
B	0.083	0.097	0.092	0.110	0.336	1.057	0.075	0.082	0.051	0.145	0.186	0.179
C	0.917	1.183	1.132	1.204	1.319	1.421	0.099	0.175	0.151	0.177	0.294	0.166
D	0.879	0.163	1.201	1.225	1.390	1.393	0.096	0.183	0.134	0.187	0.230	0.209

standard isolation, on average 4–5 days. This has led to the development of methods for the detection of viral antigen expression in tissue culture using immunostaining methods.

Rapid culture assays

With the availability of well characterized and commercially available monoclonal antibodies, the detection of viruses in cultured cells by immunological methods 1–3 days after inoculation, prior to the development of a CPE, has found wide application in diagnostic virology. Tubes, shell vials, chamber slides or cell culture clusters may be used for this procedure.

Most commonly, MDCK cells are grown in shell vials or multiwell plates and when the cells are confluent, the growth medium is replaced by serum-free maintenance medium containing TPCK-trypsin. The use of 96 well plates for virus identification has obvious advantages of reduction in cost and ease of manipulation (Brumback *et al.* 1995; Brumback & Wade 1996; O'Neill *et al.* 1996).

Clinical specimens are inoculated in duplicate and centrifugation of the inoculum onto the cell culture is performed to improve the sensitivity of the assay (Seno *et al.* 1990). Cultures are incubated at 33–35° C for 12–72 h. Medium is removed and the cells are washed with PBS and fixed, using methanol or acetone. The fixed cells are incubated with a type-specific antibody, followed by an antispecies antibody conjugated with either a fluorescence or an enzyme indicator molecule. Cell cultures are viewed for specific staining using either a light or a fluorescence microscope. Influenza nucleoprotein (NP) antigen expression can be detected as early as 3 h post infection with this type of assay (Plate 22.1; see plate section facing p. 288). The sensitivity of rapid culture assays varies from 56 to 100% compared with standard isolation (Espy *et al.* 1986; Mills *et al.* 1989; Stokes *et al.* 1988; Ziegler *et al.* 1995) and can clearly be a useful rapid diagnostic test. Although such assays have clear utility in primary diagnostic work, the disadvantage of this type of assay is that viral antigen is not available for antigenic analysis, as required in surveillance of influenza, without reinoculation of the original specimen, although information about subtype can be obtained (Ziegler *et al.* 1995).

Subtyping influenza isolates

Differentiation between influenza A and B viruses and determination of the subtypes of influenza A viruses are the first steps in the characterization of newly isolated influenza viruses. This is traditionally done by haemagglutination-inhibition (HAI) tests with specific antisera raised in ferrets, sheep or chickens. HAI tests can also be used to identify novel

circulating variants, either by identification of a virus containing a novel subtype or by identification of a four-fold or greater reduction in reactivity to a particular antiserum (Table 22.2). Results of a reciprocal HAI test with ferret antisera on strains circulating in England in 1995–1997 are shown in Table 22.2(a). This clearly demonstrates the phenomenon of antigenic drift in influenza viruses. Viruses such as A/England/144/97, isolated in January 1997, react poorly with antisera raised to earlier prototype viruses (A/Beijing/32/92) compared with a virus such as A/England/67/94 isolated in 1994. A/England/268/96 does not react in HAI tests with

Table 22.2 Haemagglutination inhibition (HAI) testing of epidemic influenza A variants 1994–1997. HAI tests carried out using postinfection ferret antisera treated with receptor destroying enzyme and 8 haemagglutinin units of virus and 0.5% v/v turkey red cells.
(a) Antigenic drift. A virus which shows a four-fold or less reactivity with antisera raised to earlier antigens is considered to show significant antigenic drift; e.g. A/England/272/96 is antigenically similar to A/Wuhan/359/95, the influenza A H3N2 vaccine strain for 1996/97, but is a drift variant from A/England/301/95 which was isolated a few months earlier.
(b) Subtyping. The virus strain A/England/268/96 was recovered from a conjunctival swab and was initially identified as an influenza A virus by immunofluorescence using monoclonal antibodies directed to type-specific antigens on tissue culture cells which showed haemadsorption. A/England/268/96 does not react in HAI tests with antisera raised to human influenza A subtypes H1N1, H2N2 or H3N2, or influenza B. This clearly indicates that it had a novel HA for a human isolate. In this case, the HA was identified as H7, and it is surmised from the clinical history that transmission occurred directly from avians to a human (Kurtz *et al.* 1996).

Virus strain	A/Beijing/32/92	A/Shandong/9/93	A/Johannesburg/33/94	A/Wuhan/359/95
A/Beijing/32/92	**2560**	640	160	40
A/Shandong/9/93	640	**1280**	1280	80
A/Johannesburg/33/94	1280	640	**5120**	320
A/Wuhan/359/95	40	160	320	**1280**
A/England/67/94	2560	640	640	ND
A/England/301/95	1280	320	5120	160
A/England/272/96	640	1280	1280	5120
A/England/144/97	40	40	160	1280

(a)

Virus strain	A/Taiwan/ 1/86 (H1N1)	A/Singapore/ 1/57 (H2N2)	A/Johannesburg/ 33/94 (H3N2)	A/EquiPrague/ 56 (H7N7)	A/Fowl plague/ 34 (H7N1)	B/Panama/ 45/90
A/Taiwan/1/86	**5120**	< 10	< 10	< 10	< 10	< 10
A/Johannesburg/33/94	< 10	< 10	**2560**	< 10	< 10	< 10
A/Bury/1234/94 (H7N7)	< 10	< 10	< 10	1280	2560	< 10
A/EquiPrague/56 (H7N7)	< 10	< 10	< 10	**5120**	2560	< 10
A/England/268/96	< 10	< 10	< 10	1280	2560	< 10

(b)

ND, not done. Number in bold denotes homologous virus and its homologous antiserum.

sera raised to human influenza A subtypes or influenza B, but clearly reacts with antisera raised to viruses containing H7 HA, allowing unequivocal typing of the virus (Table 22.2b). However, such typing tests require large amounts of viral antigens.

Despite this, only a few attempts have been made to determine the subtype of influenza viruses by methods other than HAI, using polyclonal or monoclonal antibodies to stain infected cells (Fishaut *et al.* 1979; Johansson *et al.* 1979; Ziegler *et al.* 1995) or by using nucleic acid detection techniques (see below). These recent developments combine the sensitivity of virus isolation with speed of rapid diagnosis, take advantage of the advances which have occurred in rapid diagnosis of viral infections, and point the way for rapid subtyping identification where antigenic information is not crucial. One of the concerns involved in working with monoclonal antibodies to influenza is that the specificity of the monoclonal antibody will produce false negative reactions because of the rapid antigenic variation (antigenic drift) seen in influenza viruses, although this can be overcome by using a panel of antibodies (Ziegler *et al.* 1995).

Rapid diagnosis of influenza A and B

Immunofluorescence (IF) and enzyme immunosorbent assays (EIA) have been used for the direct identification of influenza virus on respiratory specimens containing exfoliated cells. Cells in a NPA or nasal wash or other respiratory sample are prepared by being washed several times in ice-cold buffer, resuspended and applied to microscope slides. After fixing in acetone, the cell preparation is reacted with commercially available specific antibodies. These are either directly conjugated to a fluorochrome (DIF), or reacted with a second antibody which is species-specific and conjugated to a fluorochrome (indirect IF). Polyclonal sera used as the detecting antibody often show unacceptably high levels of staining to cellular debris and bacteria (Shalit *et al.* 1985), and usually monoclonal antibodies are used to provide the appropriate sensitivity and specificity required of this test. Commonly, the commercially available monoclonal antibodies are to influenza proteins which are abundantly expressed and more conserved than the viral glycoproteins (conveniently, NP or M1) or to conserved regions of the HA protein. There does not appear to be much difference between the sensitivity of indirect IF and DIF (Table 22.3) although, theoretically, indirect IF should allow a greater signal amplification. When compared with influenza virus isolation, IF is 50–90% sensitive (Table 22.3). Clearly, the quality of the clinical sample is extremely important in the sensitivity of this test, and NPAs give the best results. DIF has the advantages of being able to assess specimen quality and test for multiple viruses in the same specimen, as well as being very rapid to perform. It is an extremely important test for the efficient detection of influenza in clinical samples in order to help determine clinical management (Arens *et al.* 1986). Recent advances in the performance of DIF include the use of microwave irradiation for accelerated staining of clinical specimens (Hite & Yuang 1996) and the inclusion of monoclonal antibody panels of different isotypes allowing multiple different fluorochromes to be included, thus allowing single cells to be stained for more than one pathogen (Murphy *et al.* 1996).

Rapid detection of viral antigen

A variety of tests such as radio- and fluoroimmunoassay, EIA and membrane EIA have been developed for the detection of influenza virus antigens either directly in clinical specimens or after amplification in cell culture (Sarkkinen *et al.* 1981; Walls *et al.* 1986; Chomel *et al.* 1992; Doller *et al.* 1992; Duverlie *et al.* 1992). These tests may be used either on solubilized cell lysates, on tissue culture supernatants 12–48 h following inoculation or directly on clinical specimens. Commonly, viral antigen is captured by a monoclonal antibody coated to the wells of microtitre plates, followed by detection by standard EIA. When evaluated against virus isolation in MDCK or PMK cells for detection of influenza directly in clinical specimens, assays of this format give a sensitivity of 50–80% and may take from 2 to 20 h to perform (Table 22.3). Maximum sensitivity is obtained by prolonging incubation of the specimen with the capture antibody and by using fluoroimmunoassay detection.

Table 22.3 Comparison of detection of influenza by different methods. Figures given in parentheses are authors' calculations of sensitivity compared with virus culture.

Study group	Location	Season	Number of samples	Culture (+)	IF (+)	Antigen detection	PCR	Study
Paediatric	USA	1991–92	190	23	24† (90%)	37 (100%)‡	—	Waner et al. 1991
Paediatric	USA	1991–92	81	20	12*/15† (65%*/75%†)	15 (75%)‡	—	Dominguez et al. 1993
Geriatric	USA	1991–92	160	46	49† (92.5%)	47 (100%)	—	Leonardi et al. 1994
All ages	France	1989–90	103	39	—	22 (56%)	—	Duverlie et al. 1992
Paediatric	Japan	?	63	22	—	—	48 (76%)	Morishita et al. 1992
Paediatric	Holland	1992–93	434	25	22* (88%)	—	25	Claas et al. 1993
All ages	Australia	1988–92	1703	67	—	58 (87%)	—	Kok et al. 1994
All ages	France	1990–91	1028	25	—	21 (84%)	—	Chomel et al. 1992
Adult	Czechoslovakia	1989–90	14	14	—	—	14 (100%)	Pisareva et al. 1992
All ages	Canada	1992–93	98	20	—	—	18 (90%)	Wright et al. 1995
Paediatric	USA	1992–93	72	20	—	20 (100%)‡	19 (95%)	Atmar et al. 1996
All ages	UK	1995–96	619	200	—	—	246 (90%)	Ellis et al. 1997b

* Direct immunofluorescence; † indirect immunofluorescence; ‡ commercial cassette kit.
IF, immunofluorescence; PCR, polymerase chain reaction.

Enzyme immunomembrane filter assays are also available commercially and require less than 15 min to complete (Todd *et al.* 1995; Johnson & Bloy 1993; Waner *et al.* 1991). NPAs and nasal washes work best in this assay although other respiratory samples can also be used. Specimens are diluted with a buffer containing detergent and mucolytic agent and are applied to a filter membrane. Viral antigens are non-specifically adsorbed to the membrane, which usually has a very high binding capacity, and detection is then with monoclonal antibodies and chromogens. A visible triangle on the filter membrane indicates a positive result (Plate 22.2; see plate section facing p. 288). Approximately 20 culture-positive cells or 1.5×10^3 pfu virus in suspension are required to give a positive result using this type of test. Comparison of the sensitivity of this kind of test with virus culture in MDCK or PMK ranges from 60 to 100% (Table 22.3). One of the advantages of this type of test is that it requires relatively little skill to perform and is only a little more complex than a home pregnancy test. Such tests have an obvious application in the diagnosis of influenza in the setting of general practice/physicians' offices and in the rapid identification of outbreaks in geriatric facilities and nosocomial outbreaks. However, one of the major disadvantages is the lack of virus isolate for antigenic characterization and the cost per unit of the commercial tests (Table 22.1). Moreover, weak positive staining of the filter has to be interpreted cautiously because all ELISA tests can give false positive reactions.

Detection of viral RNA

The detection of viral RNA in clinical specimens using hybridization has been performed with a moderate sensitivity (75%) on nasopharyngeal swabs (Havlickova *et al.* 1990) although this has proved to be a cumbersome technique and has not found wide application. In contrast, reverse transcriptase PCR (RT-PCR) is much more widely used in the diagnosis, typing and subtyping of influenza virus infection in clinical material or in tissue culture fluids. Appropriate selection of primers allows: type-specific identification of influenza viruses A, B or C (Yamada *et al.* 1991; Claas *et al.* 1992); subtype-specific identification of influenza A viruses (Zhang & Evans 1991); differentiation of high-growth reassortant vaccine donor genes from wild-type

strain genes (Klimov & Cox 1995); analysis of the origin of the RNA segments of a single virus strain (Adeyefa *et al.* 1994; Wentworth *et al.* 1997); and analysis of fixed archival material (Taubenberger *et al.* 1997). Although PCR offers the theoretical advantage of sensitivity and specificity of diagnosis and does not require infectious virus for detection, the necessity of a reverse transcriptase step influences the overall sensitivity of the technique.

Very few studies show a significant increase in detection rate of influenza in clinical specimens using RT-PCR compared with virus culture in MDCK cells (Table 22.3), which may reflect the inherent insensitivity of the reverse transcriptase stage of the reaction. Alternatively, the extraction methods used for the purification of RNA may also be critical in determining the overall sensitivity of the technique, as has been shown for the detection of RNA containing small round-structured viruses (Hale *et al.* 1996).

The appropriate combination of primer sets and optimization of PCR conditions allows the formulation of multiplex PCR for the detection of

Fig. 22.3 Multiplex polymerase chain reaction (PCR) for influenza A and B in clinical specimens. Multiplex nested PCR was performed directly from combined nose and throat swabs collected in virus transport medium. RNA was extracted from 100 µl of clinical specimens and reverse transcribed. cDNA was amplified in the presence of multiple nested primer sets targeted to the HA$_1$ portion of the haemagglutinin gene of influenza A and B capable of distinguishing between H1N1, H3N2 and influenza B (Zambon *et al.* 1996). Amplicons were analysed using agarose gel electrophoresis and ethidium bromide staining. Lanes 1–15, clinical samples sent through the post in 1995/1996 from the Royal College of General Practitioner influenza surveillance scheme in England & Wales; H1, H1N1 control; H3, H3N2 control; B, B control; –, negative control. (Reprinted from Zambon *et al.* 1996, 607–14, with kind permission from Elsevier Science – NL, Sara Burgerhartstraat 25, 1055 KV Amsterdam, the Netherlands.)

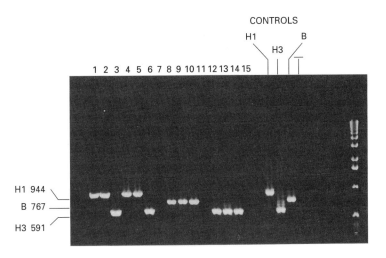

influenza A (H1N1 and H3N2) and B from clinical specimens in a single tube (Fig. 22.3) (Wright *et al.* 1995; Zambon *et al.* 1996) which is significantly more sensitive than virus culture when used on nose and throat swabs taken for surveillance of influenza (Ellis *et al.* 1997b). Alternatively, multisegment PCR, using primers which are complementary to the conserved 3′and 5′ sequences on each influenza RNA segment, allows the detection of all segments of a single influenza virus in a single tube (Wentworth *et al.* 1997). This has obvious use when attempting to identify parental genes in recombinant viruses.

Genetic analysis of epidemic virus variants

The sensitivity and specificity of RT-PCR have the capacity to revolutionize the molecular analysis of circulating influenza strains, improving the quality of the surveillance data available for the annual consideration of the composition of the influenza vaccine (Hampson & Cox 1996) and allowing more refined analysis of outbreaks of respiratory illness (Ellis & Zambon 1997). The ease of automated DNA sequencing applied to PCR products derived from isolates of influenza has greatly increased the amount of sequence data available. This allows detailed analysis of the molecular epidemiology of influenza virus, particularly the HA gene which contains the major antigenic sites of influenza, providing insights into the variation of influenza viruses infecting humans and the sequence changes associated with antigenic drift (Cox & Bender 1995; Ellis *et al.* 1995, 1997a). Moreover, the use of RT-PCR sequencing in the study of archival or post-mortem material has already achieved important results, as shown by the identification of the 1918 pandemic influenza virus strain by this technique (Taubenberger *et al.* 1997). Analysis of several small pieces of cDNA synthesized from RNA recovered from the lungs of a young soldier who died of influenza in 1919 has identified that the influenza HA, NA and NP genes are of swine origin, ending decades of speculation about this virus.

Careful selection of primers targeted to the HA gene allows other forms of molecular analysis of the PCR amplicons derived directly from clinical material. The combination of PCR and restriction digest analysis (PCR–restriction) is a powerful tool for providing information about the direction of genetic drift of the HA gene of viruses circulating in epidemic and non-epidemic periods without requiring detailed and laborious sequence analysis, and allows the investigation of many hundreds of strains in a very short period of time (Ellis *et al.* 1997a). PCR–restriction may also be used to differentiate between vaccine-like strains and circulating strains (Figs 22.4 and 22.5; Ellis *et al.* 1997b), and between drug-resistant and -sensitive genomes (Klimov *et al.* 1995). Thus the possibility of providing a profile of the genetic variability of influenza viruses during epidemic periods begins to be a reality, allowing better prediction of the emerging strains of influenza and a better match of vaccine strain to circulating strain (Cox & Regnery 1996).

Serological diagnosis of influenza

Serological detection of influenza virus infection is rarely useful in immediate clinical management. However, retrospective diagnosis may establish a clinical diagnosis in the absence of virus isolation, antigen detection or DIF detection. In addition, it may be a useful surveillance tool. Combined laboratory reports of serological detection of influenza provide good corroborative measures of the clinical indices of influenza and influenza activity. In the UK, this type of data provides an excellent, if delayed, marker of influenza epidemic activity, contributing to national surveillance data (Fig. 22.6; Hutchinson *et al.* 1995, 1996).

One of the difficulties with serological diagnosis of influenza is that it is necessary to evaluate paired serum samples. This is required because influenza infection is frequently a reinfection. There may already be pre-existing partial immunity to influenza, which is boosted by reinfection, and the results of single samples for influenza serology are unreliable using the most widely available tests, the complement fixation test (CFT) or haemagglutination inhibition (HAI). It is partly for this reason that testing for recent influenza infection by detection of IgM or other immunoglobulin isotypes has not yet had much impact on the serological diagnosis of influenza.

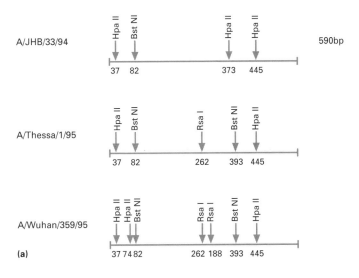

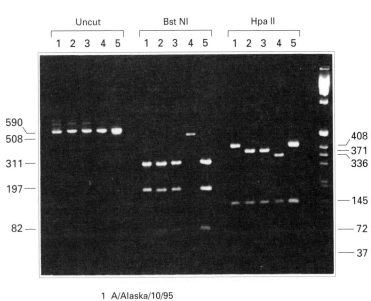

Fig. 22.4 Polymerase chain reaction (PCR) restriction analysis. (a) The cutting position of restriction enzymes Hpa II, Rsa I and Bst N1 on the 590bp amplicon generated by reverse transcriptase-PCR from the HA$_1$ segment of the haemagglutinin gene of three variants of influenza A H3N2 circulating between 1994 and 1997 is shown.
(b) Restriction digestion with Bst N1 to differentiate between A/JHB/33/94 (vaccine strain 1995/1996) and A/Thessa/1/95 and A/Wuhan/359/95 (vaccine strain 1996/1997) -like strains. Hpa II can discriminate between all three variants.

1 A/Alaska/10/95
2 A/Wuhan/359/95
3 A/Nanchang/933/95
4 A/Johannesburg/34/94
5 A/England/288/95 (A/Thessaloniki-like)

The earliest techniques for assessing serological responses to influenza virus were the classical neutralization tests using either cell monolayers and haemadsorption inhibition or plaque reduction (reviewed by Dowdle & Schild 1975). However, it was soon recognized that the results of HAI testing paralleled the results of the far more complex neutralization tests, but were much simpler and cheaper to perform (Hirst 1942). It was also noted that HAI titres gave a good correlate of protection in human sera (Hobson *et al.* 1972). Since then, the assessment of the protective capacity of an individual serum has been made using HAI titres, although CFTs are widely used in diagnostic

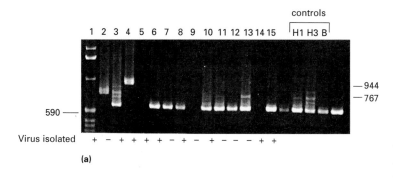

(a)

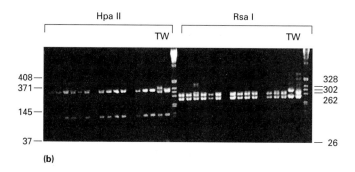

(b)

Fig. 22.5 Outbreak analysis. The first outbreak of influenza in the UK in the winter season of 1996/1997 occurred in the famous boys' boarding school in Harrow on the outskirts of London. Fifteen combined nose and throat swabs were taken from boys of 12–16 years of age. (a) Multiplex RT-PCR performed on the swabs confirmed that the outbreak of respiratory illness was due to influenza A H3N2 within 24 h. (b) Restriction digestion of the amplicons from the RT-PCR reaction in A, with the enzymes Hpa II and Rsa I, indicated that all of the viruses were A/Wuhan/359/95-like, which was subsequently confirmed by antigenic analysis of the viruses isolated from the swabs. The complete molecular analysis of this outbreak was available within 48 h of receipt of specimens, and was the first identification of A/Wuhan/359/95-like H3N2 viruses in the UK. W, A/Wuhan/359/95-like; T, A/Thessaloniki/1/95-like.

laboratories and provide a useful method of testing serum pairs against a number of potential antigens in order to assess serological profile. CFTs measure antibody responses to influenza NP, which is conserved. They are therefore helpful in differentiating type-specific antibodies to influenza A or B in humans and have an important role to play when new antigenic variants are circulating for which there are no specific reagents available, or when there has been cross-species transmission of influ-

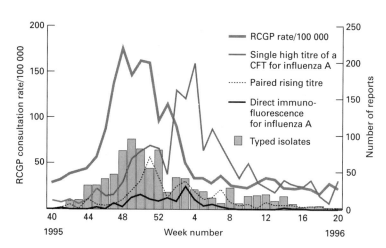

Fig. 22.6 Contribution of laboratory diagnosis of influenza A to national surveillance. Laboratory reports of influenza A to Communicable Disease Surveillance Centre from laboratories in England and Wales for the winter season 1995/1996. RCGP consultation rate is the incidence of 'influenza and influenza-like illness' derived from the weekly returns service of the Royal College of General Practitioners Research Unit, based on a sentinel physician network of approximately 95 general practices in England and Wales. Typed isolates are the isolates made by laboratories which are antigenically typed as either H3N2 or H1N1. CFT, complement fixation test; paired rising titre, four-fold or greater difference in paired sera with either CFT or haemagglutination inhibition for influenza A.

enza A subtypes. However, the rise in CFT titre following infection is slow, and the test itself is relatively insensitive and measures only the complement fixing classes of antibody. HAI and neutralization remain the gold standard for the assessment of serological responses to influenza and measure antibodies against subtype-specific and strain-specific antigens. Despite the tried and tested history of HAI testing and neutralization testing, both tests are susceptible to non-specific inhibitors, as described below.

Haemagglutination inhibition

The haemagglutination reaction between virus and erythrocyte is susceptible to inhibition. The most useful inhibition is that produced by influenza-specific antibody and it is used diagnostically in HAI assays which are used to assess the serological profile of individuals following influenza infection. The HAI antibody titre present in serum is probably the most useful correlate of protection from or susceptibility to influenza (Hobson *et al.* 1972) and is widely used in assessing vaccination responses (Fig. 22.7). Excellent review articles, which remain topical, on the practical considerations of diagnostic HAI serology for influenza are to be found in Dowdle and Schild (1975) and Dowdle *et al.* (1979). There are also non-specific inhibitors of haemagglutination present in the sera of various animals, termed α-, β- and γ-inhibitors (Krizanov & Rathova 1969). α- and γ-inhibitors are heat stable, sialylated glycoproteins that act by competing with cell receptors for binding to the viral haemagglutinin. γ-inhibitors have been identified in horse, pig and guinea-pig serum as α_2-macroglobulin (Ryan Poirier & Kawaoka 1991). However, human α_2-macroglobulin is only weakly active against influenza A H3N2. Rat serum, containing α_1-macroglobulin and murinoglobulin, is a potent inhibitor of influenza C haemagglutination (Herrler *et al.* 1985).

β-inhibitors are Ca^{2+}-dependent, non-sialylated, heat labile, mannose binding lectins and are present in high titre in bovine serum, as well as in mouse, guinea-pig, ferret and rabbit serum. It is also thought that β-inhibitors bind to carbohydrate residues on the HA molecule and inhibit access of

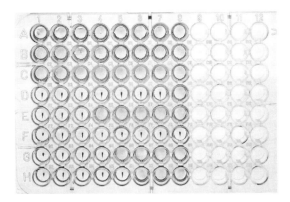

Fig. 22.7 Haemagglutination inhibition (HAI) testing of sera. Sera are pretreated with receptor destroying enzyme from *Vibrio cholerae* for 16 h at 37° C, prior to heat inactivation for 30 min at 56° C. Samples are serially diluted in phosphate buffered saline pH 7.4 in microtitre plates with V-shaped wells and eight agglutinating doses of virus antigen are added. Incubation for 1 h is then followed by the addition of 0.5% v/v turkey red cells and HAI titres are read after 30 min by inverting the plates to produce a streak, which increases the discrimination between true and false HAI titres. Doubling dilutions of sera from well 1–8 (reciprocal serum titres from 10 to 1280). A and B, pre- and postvaccination sera showing no HAI titres to A/Johannesburg/33/94, the H3N2 vaccine strain for 1995/1996; C and D, pre- and postvaccination sera showing a rise in HAI titre to A/Johannesburg/33/94 from < 10 (C) to 640 (D); E and F, pre- and postvaccination sera showing a boost in HAI titre to A/Johannesburg/33/94 from 40 (E) to > 1280 (F); G and H, pre- and postvaccination sera showing no significant change in HAI titre to A/Johannesburg/33/94 following vaccination from 80 (G) to 160 (H).

the virus to cell surface receptors (Anders *et al.* 1994, 1996). β-inhibitors are also resistant to periodate and neuraminidase treatment. The presence of such compounds in bovine serum provides a convenient explanation for the inhibitory effects of bovine serum on influenza growth in culture, although this has not yet been verified.

Interpretation of haemagglutination and HAI tests therefore requires recognition of these non-specific inhibitors of haemagglutination and the potential for false positives in HAI serology. Human sera are usually treated with receptor destroying enzyme from *Vibrio cholerae* prior to testing in HAI assay. This enzyme removes sialic acid from molecules present in sera which might prevent binding of virus to antibody by binding to HA_1. Partly because of the presence of non-specific inhibitors in serum and partly because HAI testing uses a biological 'read out', the HAI test, although a robust and well-used test, has many inherently unsatisfactory properties, not least of which is the lack of reproducibility between various different laboratories (Wood *et al.* 1994). The most common source of problems is inadequate destruction of non-specific inhibitors and variability of erythrocyte preparations. It is recommended that red cell suspensions be standardized by using haematocrit measurements or by measuring optical density. The performance of the HAI test is also influenced by the nature of the antigen. In particular, ether treatment of influenza B antigen enhances the reactivity of antisera in HAI testing several-fold, but may reduce the strain specificity of the test (Kendal & Cate 1983; Monto & Maassab 1981). Cell-culture derived antigens detect significant titre rises in HAI tests more frequently than do egg-grown antigens of the same virus strain (Pyhala *et al.* 1987). Further developments in standardizing and recording HAI tests are occurring with the use of customized software for reading HAI or HA results (Fig. 22.2b).

An alternative test based on the ability of influenza-specific antibodies to lyse antigen-coated red cells in the presence of complement—single radial haemolysis (SRH)—is recognized to be more reproducible and less error prone than HAI testing of sera (Wood *et al.* 1994), although it is less strain specific. However, there are significant disadvantages which include the necessity for high concentrations of purified antigen and uncertainty about the correlation between zone sizes seen in the SRH test and protection of particular sera. Standardization of SRH for assessment of susceptibility to influenza has not been possible in the way that standardization of SRH as a marker for immunity to rubella has been, mainly because of the constant necessity to keep updating the test antigens to take account of antigenic drift.

Attempts to determine IgM responses to influenza in serum using an antibody capture assay format and a red cell indicator detection system do not appear to have been widely made, although these offer a cheap and convenient method for assessing the IgM profile of sera (Goldwater *et al.* 1982) and have been very successful for detection of IgM to other virus infections (Hilfenhaus *et al.* 1993; Siqueira *et al.* 1994).

Neutralization assays

Classical neutralization methods based on plaque reduction or haemadsorption inhibition are laborious and take several days to complete. They are unsuitable for screening large numbers of serum samples. More recently developed neutralization-EIA (N-EIA) tests are suitable for the accurate titration of neutralizing antibodies in small quantities of serum (Okuno *et al.* 1990; Benne *et al.* 1994), and neutralizing antibody titres determined in this way correlate very well with titres obtained by HAI (Okuno *et al.* 1990). Assay formats of this type involve mixing serum and the virus strain of interest together for a short period, prior to transferring inoculum onto monolayers of MDCK cells in microtitre format, or mixing with cells in suspension (van der Water *et al.* 1993). Following standard adsorption and single-cycle or multiple-cycle replication, cells are fixed and stained for the presence of influenza viral antigens by EIA as described above, or the cytotoxicity index is calculated (van der Water *et al.* 1993). Neutralization activity can be calculated in two ways: as foci reduction, if an insoluble chromogen is used to stain cells (Okuno *et al.* 1990); or, alternatively, if a soluble substrate is used, spectrophotometric absorbance can be used to calculate an index of neutralizing activity of serum (Benne *et al.* 1994). One of the main concerns with this type of test is that monoclonal antibodies are used in the detection step, and it is necessary to ensure that antibodies react with new variants of influenza as described above.

Measurement of antibody subclasses

Comparison of HAI, CFT and EIA for the detection of influenza-specific antibody indicates that EIA can detect more antibody rises in serum than either of the other two tests, as would be expected (Julkunen et al. 1985), because not all serum antibodies are haemagglutination inhibiting and only a small proportion of antibodies are directed to the influenza NP. However, a satisfactory correlation between ELISA detection of IgG or IgG subclasses and protection from subsequent challenge with influenza infection has not been derived, despite several studies investigating this, using standard ELISA techniques and using split-virus antigen, whole-cell lysate or recombinant protein as antigen (Burlington *et al.* 1983; Harmon *et al.* 1989; Remarque *et al.* 1993).

Although a number of ELISA IgM tests for influenza have been described using egg, tissue culture and recombinant antigen (Harmon *et al.* 1989; Remarque *et al.* 1993; Rimmelzwaan *et al.* 1997), this kind of test also has not acquired widespread use in the diagnosis of influenza or the assessment of vaccine responses, probably because of the difficulty in assessing specificity of responses and the necessity to correlate with HAI titres in order to derive a measure of the protective capacity of individual sera. Similarly, several EIA formats for measuring influenza-specific IgA have been described (Remarque *et al.* 1993; Thompson *et al.* 1996; Rimmelzwaan *et al.* 1997) because of the interest in this molecule as an acute phase response to influenza infection and the possibility that mucosal IgA present in respiratory secretions may be a good correlate of protection from influenza (Rosen *et al.* 1970), although the optimum collection method for assessing mucosal IgA remains unclear. Thus the HAI titre of serum will continue to be a 'gold standard' for evaluation of susceptibility or protection from influenza for the forseeable future, although a reliable test for use on a single serum sample to diagnose recent infleunza infection is badly needed.

Immune electron microscopy

Electron microscopy (EM) has little place in the diagnosis of influenza infections, mainly due to the detection sensitivity of EM of approximately 10^6 particles per ml, a concentration of influenza virus seldom attained in respiratory secretions. However, the detection sensitivity of EM may be enhanced by the incorporation of an immune concentration step involving reaction of the respiratory secretion with a hyperimmune serum followed by ultracentrifugation and negative staining. Nevertheless, the sensitivity of this kind of technique still only approaches 50% of that achieved by virus culture (Ptakova & Tumova 1985).

Drug susceptibility testing

Amantadine and rimantadine are currently the only licensed drugs with proven antiviral activity against influenza. Isolation of drug-resistant variants has been described on numerous occasions and the conventional assay for drug susceptibility testing is the plaque reduction assay (Table 22.4), which assesses the susceptibility of multiple-cycle

Table 22.4 Methods for assessing drug resistance of virus isolates. MOI, multiplicity of infection.

Test	Advantages	Disadvantages
Plaque reduction	Gold standard Good for low volumes and low titres	Must titrate stock Labour intensive Slow Requires tissue culture Skill +++
Viral antigen detection ELISA	Good reproductibility Low-level antigen detected Can automate	IC_{50} is MOI dependent Need to develop ELISA Skill ++
Polymerase chain reaction hybridization	Do not require viable virus Rapid Sensitive Specific	Difficult to compare and quantitate genotype → phenotype?? Skill ++++

replication of influenza isolates to drugs included in the semisolid or solid overlay covering mono-layer cells infected at limiting dilution with virus (Hayden *et al.* 1980). The susceptibility of isolates may be defined by the reduction of infectious foci (pfu) seen following staining of the monolayer, and is usually expressed as an IC_{50} value (Plate 22.3; see plate section facing p. 288). This method is also used to assess the antiviral activity of novel anti-influenza drugs such as NA inhibitors, e.g. 4-guanidino-Neu-5Ac2en (GG167), and to test for susceptibility of naturally occurring isolates (von Itzstein *et al.* 1993).

However, plaque reduction is laborious and simpler alternatives for assessing the phenotype of viruses have been sought. These include single-cycle replication assays which rely on the detection of viral HA release using ELISA formats or inhibition of viral NP synthesis (Belshe *et al.* 1988; Ziegler *et al.* 1995). Cell monolayers in a microtitre plate format are inoculated with several input multi-plicities of virus and appropriate concentrations of drug, and virus replication is allowed to continue for up 16 h. The cells are fixed and virus antigen detected using soluble EIA substrates, or the supernatant fluid is sampled for the presence of viral haemagglutinin. Less than 50% inhibition of viral growth in the presence of defined concentra-tions of drug indicates resistant isolates. Assess-ment of the genotype of the isolate is then usually confirmed by sequencing of the relevant gene.

In the case of amantadine/rimantadine resis-tance, the mutations responsible for conferring resistance have been mapped to five residues in the transmembrane region of the viral M2 gene pro-duct. Differentiation of the mutations responsible for conferring resistance in particular isolates may be accomplished by RT-PCR restriction analysis of the M2 gene (Klimov *et al.* 1995) without requiring sequence analysis, which allows rapid screening of isolates. Analysis of M2 mutations associated with amantadine/rimantadine resistance would almost certainly be amenable to PCR mutation assays as have been documented for HIV and zidovudine resistance (Kaye *et al.* 1992), although these have not yet been described for influenza.

Resistance to GG167 *in vitro* has so far mainly been defined by resistance in multiple-cycle repli-cation assays (plaque assay) incorporating drug as part of the semisolid overlay. Genetic analysis of such resistant variants has used DNA sequencing to map mutations to at least one amino acid (posi-tion 119) in the NA molecule (Staschke *et al.* 1995). It has also been determined that mutation in the HA can affect the susceptibility to GG167 (Sahasra-budhe *et al.* 1996). Work in this area is still at a fairly early stage, and GG167 is in preliminary clinical trials. Therefore, abbreviated molecular methods for screening large number of viruses have not yet been described and further extensive characteriza-tion of the genetic determinants of resistance is required.

Conclusions

Each laboratory performing diagnosis of influenza will have particular priorities and expertise, which will influence the testing strategy chosen. Rapid methods of diagnosis such as DIF and commercial EIA antigen are likely to play an increasingly important role in patient and outbreak manage-ment and in deciding rational drug treatment, particularly in hospital laboratories. At the same time, the skills required to perform virological culture are likely to be undermined and the value of virus isolation underestimated, if only the immediate patient management is considered.

Whatever laboratory test is chosen for the diag-nosis of influenza, it is essential to remember the incredible capacity for genetic diversity among influenza viruses, particularly influenza A viruses, and every field isolate is a valuable resource in helping to understand genetic variation. Thus, wherever influenza is diagnosed and by whatever method, attempts should be made to identify the isolate antigenically, in order to provide minimal information about the type and subtype.

Characterization of influenza isolates is the cornerstone of successful WHO-sponsored global surveillance of influenza. In order to sustain improvements in strain selection for influenza vaccine manufacture and to derive population health gains from vaccination, antigenic and genetic characterization of field isolates are essential. Information about transmission of variants is also important, and the lack of spread of novel viruses may be crucial in limiting their pathogenic potential; for example, the documented transmission of an avian H7N7 virus (A/England/268/96) to a human in England in 1996 did not result in any secondary cases (Kurtz *et al.* 1996). Combining epidemiological, antigenic, genetic and phenotypic information pertaining to each field isolate offers the potential for powerful insights into the pathogenicity of influenza viruses in humans and will help to make the prediction of influenza pandemics less of a mediaeval star-gazing event, as occurred when influenza epidemics were first described in the 15th century, and more of a precise science in the 21st century.

References

Adeyefa, C.A.O., Quayle, K. & McCauley, J.W. (1994) A rapid method for the analysis of influenza virus genes: application to the reassortment of equine influenza genes. *Virus Res* **32**, 391–9.

Anders, E.M., Hartley, C.A., Reading, P.C. & Ezekowitz, R.A.B. (1994) Complement-dependent neutralization of influenza virus by a serum mannose binding lectin. *J Gen Virol* **75**, 615–22.

Anders, E.M., Reading, P.C., Morey, L.S. & Hartley, C.A. (1996) Role of mannose binding lectins in innate immunity to influenza. In: Brown, L.E., Hampson, A.W. & Webster, R.G. (eds) *Options for the Control of Influenza III*, pp. 244–9. ICS Elsevier, Amsterdam.

Arens, M.Q., Swierkosz, E., Schmidt, R.R., Armstrong, T. & Rivetna, K.A. (1986) Strategy for efficient detection of respiratory viruses in pediatric clinical specimens. *Diag Microbiol Infect Dis* **5**, 307–12.

Atmar, R.L., Baxter, B.D., Dominguez, E.A. & Taber, L.N. (1996) Comparison of reverse transcriptase PCR with tissue culture and other rapid diagnostic assays for detection of type A influenza virus. *J Clin Microbiol* **34**, 2604–6.

Belshe, R., Hall-Smith, M., Hall, C.B., Betts, R. & Hay, A.J. (1988) Genetic basis of resistance to rimantadine emerging during treatment of influenza virus infection. *J Virol* **65**, 1508–12.

Benne, C.A., Harmsen, M., de Jong, J.C. & Kraaljeveld, C.A. (1994) Neutralization enzyme immunoassay for influenza virus. *J Clin Microbiol* **32**, 987–90.

Bettoli, E.J., Brewer, P.M., Oxtoby, M.J., Zaidi, A.A. & Gauinam, M.E. (1982) The role of temperature and swab materials in the recovery of herpes simplex virus from lesions. *J Infect Dis* **145**, 399.

Boycott, R., Klenk, H.-D. & Ohuchi, M. (1994) Cell tropism of influenza virus mediated by haemagglutinin activation at the stage of virus entry. *Virology* **203**, 313–19.

Brumback, B.G. & Wade, C.D. (1996) Simultaneous rapid culture for four respiratory viruses in the same monolayer using a differential multicoloured fluorescent confirmatory stain. *J Clin Microbiol* **34**, 798–801.

Brumback, B.G., Cunningham, D.M., Morris, M.V. & Villavicencio, J.L. (1995) Rapid culture for influenza virus types A and B in 96 well plates. *Clin Diag Virol* **4**, 251–6.

Burlington, D.B., Clements, M.L. & Meikeljohn, G. (1983) Haemagglutination-specific antibody responses in immunoglobulins G, A and M isotypes as measured by enzyme-linked immunosorbent assay after primary or secondary infection of humans with influenza A virus. *Infect Immun* **41**, 540–5.

Burnet, F.M. & Bull, D.R. (1941) Changes in influenza virus associated with adaptation to passage in chick embryo. *Aust J Exp Biol Med Sci* **21**, 55–69.

Chomel, J.J., Remilleux, M.F., Marchand, P. & Aymard, M. (1992) Rapid diagnosis of influenza A. Comparison with ELISA immunocapture and culture. *J Virol Meth* **37**, 337–50.

Claas, E.J.C., Sprenger, M.J.W., Kleter, G.E.M., van Beek, R., Quint, W.G.V. & Masurel, N. (1992) Type-specific identification of influenza viruses A, B and C by the polymerase chain reaction. *J Virol Meth* **39**, 1–13.

Claas, E.C.J., von Milaan, A.J., Sprenger, M.J.W. *et al.* (1993) Prospective application of reverse transcriptase polymerase chain reaction for diagnosing influenza infections in respiratory samples from a children's hospital. *J Clin Microbiol* **31**, 2218–21.

Clarke, J.B., Chakraverty, P., Kreuzberg-Duffy, U. *et al.* (1996) Detection of human viruses using primary cells immortalised by oncogene transfection in comparison with primary cells and established cell lines. *J Med Virol* **50**, 176–80.

Cox, N. & Bender, C. (1995) Molecular epidemiology of influenza. *Sem Virol* **6**, 359–70.

Cox, N. & Regnery, H. (1996) Global influenza surveillance: tracking a moving target in a rapidly changing world. In: Brown, L.E., Hampson, A.W., Webster, R.G. (eds) *Options for the Control of Influenza III*, pp. 591–8. ICS Elsevier, Amsterdam.

Cruz, J.R., Quinonez, E., Ferandez, A. & Devalte, F. (1987) Isolation of viruses from nasopharyngeal secretions. Comparison of aspiration and swabbing as means of sample collection. *J Infect Dis* **156**, 415–16.

Davies, H.W., Appleyard, G., Cunningham, P. & Pereira, M.S. (1978) The use of a continuous cell line for the isolation of influenza viruses. *Bull WHO* **56**, 991–1993.

Doller, G., Schuy, W., Tijen, K.Y., Stekeler, B. & Gerth, H.-J. (1992) Direct detection of influenza virus antigen in nasopharyngeal specimens by direct enzyme immunoassay in comparison with quantitating virus shedding. *J Clin Microbiol* **30**, 866–9.

Dominguez, E.A., Taber, L.H. & Couch, R.B. (1993) Comparison of rapid diagnostic techniques for respiratory syncytial virus and influenza A virus respiratory infections in young children. *J Clin Microbiol* **31**, 2286–90.

Dowdle, W.R. & Schild, G.C. (1975) Laboratory propagation of human influenza viruses, experimental host range, and isolation from clinical material. In: Kilbourne, E.D. (ed.) *The Influenza Viruses and Influenza*, pp. 243–68. Academic Press, New York.

Dowdle, W.A., Kendal, A. & Noble, G.R. (1979) Influenza viruses. In: Lennette, E.H. & Schmidt, N.J. (eds) *Diagnostic Procedures for Viral Rickettsial and Chlamydial Infections*, 5th edn, pp. 585–609. American Public Health Association, Washington.

Duverlie, G., Houbart, L., Visse, B. *et al.* (1992) A nylon membrane enzyme immunoassay for rapid diagnosis of influenza A infection. *J Virol Meth* **40**, 77–84.

Ellis, J.S. & Zambon, M.C. (1997) Molecular analysis of an outbreak of influenza in the United Kingdom. *Eur J Epidemiol* **13**, 1–4.

Ellis, J.S., Chakraverty, P. & Clewley, J.P. (1995) Genetic and antigenic variation in the haemagglutinin of recently circulating human influenza A (H3N2) viruses in the United Kingdom. *Archiv Virol* **140**, 1889–904.

Ellis, J.S., Sadler, C.J., Laidler, P., Rebelo de Andrade, H. & Zambon, M.C. (1997a) Analysis of influenza A H3N2 strains isolated in England during 1995-6 using polymerase chain reaction restriction. *J Med Virol* **50**, 234–41.

Ellis, J.S., Sadler, C.S., Laidler, P.W. & Zambon, M.C. (1997b) Multiplex RT-PCR for surveillance of influenza A and B in England and Wales 1995/1996. *J Clin Microbiol* **35**, 2076–82.

Endo, Y., Carroll, K.N., Ikizler, M.R. & Wright, P. (1996) Growth of influenza A virus in primary differentiated epithelial cells derived from adenoids. *J Virol* **70**, 2055–8.

Espy, M.J., Smith, T.F., Harmon, M.W. & Kendal, A.P. (1986) Rapid detection of influenza virus by shell vial assay with monoclonal antibodies. *J Clin Microbiol* **24**, 677–9.

Fishaut, M., McIntosh, K. & Meiklejohn, G. (1979) Rapid subtyping of influenza A virus isolates by membrane fluorescence. *J Clin Microbiol* **9**, 269–73.

Frank, A.L., Couch, R.B., Griffis, C.A. & Baxter, B.D. (1979) Comparison of different tissue cultures for isolation and quantitation of influenza and parainfluenza viruses. *J Clin Microbiol* **10**, 32–6.

Goldwater, P.N., Webster, M. & Banatvala, J.E. (1982) Use of a simple new test for virus specific IgM to investigate an outbreak of influenza B in a hospitalised/aged community. *J Virol Meth* **4**, 9–18.

Govorkova, E.A., Murti, G., Meignier, B., de Taisne, C. & Webster, R.G. (1996) African Green Monkey Kidney (vero) cells provide an alternative host system for influenza A & B viruses. *J Virol* **70**, 5519–5524.

Hale, A.D., Green, J. & Brown, D.W. (1996) Comparison of four RNA extraction methods for the detection of small round structured viruses in faecal specimens. *J Virol Meth* **57**, 195–201.

Hampson, A.W. & Cox, N.J. (1996) Global surveillance for pandemic influenza: are we prepared? In: Brown, L.E., Hampson, A.W. & Webster, R.G. (eds) *Options for the Control of Influenza III*, pp. 50–9. ICS Elsevier, Amsterdam.

Harmon, M.W., Jones, I., Shaw, M. *et al.* (1989) Immunoassay for serological diagnosis of influenza type A using recombinant DNA produced nucleoprotein antigen and monoclonal antibody to IgG. *J Virol Meth* **27**, 25–30.

Hayden, F.G., Cote, K.M. & Douglas, R.G. Jr (1980) Plaque inhibition assay for drug susceptibility testing of influenza viruses. *Antimicrobial Agents Chemother* **17**, 865–70.

Havlickova, M., Pljusnin, A.Z. & Tumova, B. (1990) Influenza virus detection in clinical specimens. *Acta Virol* **34**, 446–56.

Herrler, G., Geyer, R., Muller, H.P., Stirms, S. & Klenk, H.D. (1985) Rat alpha 1 macroglobulin inhibits haemagglutination by influenza X virus. (1985) *Virus Res* **2**, 183–92.

Hilfenhaus, S., Cohen, B.J., Bates, C. *et al.* (1993) Antibody capture haemadherence tests for parvovirus B19-specific IgM and IgG. *J Virol Meth* **45**, 28–37.

Hirst, G.K. (1941) Agglutination of red cells by amniotic fluid of chick embryos infected with influenza virus. *Science* **94**, 22–3.

Hirst, G.K. (1942) The quantitative determination of influenza virus and antibodies by means of red cell agglutination. *J Exp Med* **75**, 47–64.

Hite, S.A. & Huang, Y.T. (1996) Microwave accelerated direct immunofluorescent staining for respiratory syncytial virus and influenza A virus. *J Clin Microbiol* **34**, 1819–20.

Hobson, D., Curry, R.C., Beare, A.S. & Ward-Gardner, A. (1972) The role of serum haemagglutination-inhibition antibody in protection against challenge virus infection with A2 and B viruses. *J Hygiene* **70**, 767–77.

Hutchinson, E.J., Joseph, C.A., Chakraverty, P., Zambon, M., Fleming, D.M. & Watson, J.M. (1995) Influenza surveillance in England & Wales October 1994–June 1995. *Commun Dis Rep Rev* **5**, R200–4.

Hutchinson, E.J., Joseph, C.A., Zambon, M., Fleming, D.M. & Watson, J.M. (1996) Influenza surveillance in England and Wales October 1995 to June 1996. *Commun Dis Rep Rev* **6**, R163-9.

Ito, T., Suzuki, Y., Mitnaul, L., Vines, A., Kida, H. & Kawaoka, Y. (1997) Receptor specificity of influenza A viruses correlates with the agglutination of erythrocytes from different animal species. *Virology* **227**, 493–9.

Jensen, C. & Johnson, F.B. (1994) Comparison of various transport media for viability maintenance of herpes simplex virus, respiratory syncytial virus, and adenovirus. *Diag Microbiol Infect Dis* **19**, 137–42.

Johansson, M.E., Grandien, M. & Arro, L. (1979) Preparation of sera for subtyping of influenza A viruses by immunofluorescence. *J Immunol Meth* **27**, 263–72.

Johnson, S.L.G. & Bloy, H. (1993) Evaluation of a rapid immunoassay for the detection of influenza A virus. *J Clin Microbiol* **31**, 142–3.

Julkunen, I., Pyhala, R. & Hovi, T. (1985) Enzyme immunoassay, complement fixation and haemagglutination inhibition tests in the diagnosis of influenza A and B virus infections. Purified haemagglutinin in subtype-specific diagnosis. *J Virol Meth* **10**, 75–84.

Katz, J.M., Wong, M. & Webster, R.G. (1990) Direct sequencing of the HA gene of influenza (H3N2) virus in original clinical samples reveals sequence identity with mammalian grown virus. *J Virol* **64**, 1808–11.

Kaverin, N.V. & Klenk, H.-D. (1995) The effect of cell density on influenza virus replication in CV-1 cells. *Mol Genet Microbiol Virol* **3**, 14–26.

Kaverin, N.V. & Webster, R.B. (1995) Impairment of multicycle influenza virus grown in Vero (WHO) cells by loss of trypsin activity. *J Virol* **69**, 2700–3.

Kaye, S., Loveday, C. & Tedder, R.S. (1992) A microtitre format point mutation assay: application to the detection of drug resistance in human immunodeficiency virus type-1 infected patients treated with zidovudine. *J Med Virol* **37**, 241–6.

Kendal, A.P. & Cate, T.R. (1983) Increased sensitivity and reduced specificity of haemagglutination inhibition tests with ether treated influenza B/Singapore/222/79. *J Clin Microbiol* **18**, 930–4.

King, R.W., Deshaies, R.J., Peters, J.M. & Kirschner, M.W. (1996) How proteolysis drives the cell cycle. *Science* **274**, 1652–8.

Klimov, A.I. & Cox, N.J. (1995) PCR restriction analysis of genome composition and stability of cold adapted reassortant live attenuated influenza vaccines. *J Virol Meth* **52**, 41–9.

Klimov, A.I., Rocha, E., Hayden, F.G., Shult, P.A., Roumillat, L.F. & Cox, N.J. (1995) Prolonged shedding of amantadine-resistant influenza A viruses by immunodeficient patients: detection by polymerase chain reaction-restriction analysis. *J Infect Dis* **172**, 1352–5.

Kok, T., Mickan, L. & Burrell, C.J. (1994) Routine diagnosis of seven respiratory viruses and *Mycoplasma pneumoniae* by enzyme immunoassay. *J Virol Meth* **50**, 87–100.

Krizanov, O. & Rathova, V. (1969) Serum inhibitors of myxoviruses. *Curr Top Microbiol Immunol* **47**, 125–51.

Kurtz, J., Manvell, R.J. & Banks, J. (1996) Avian influenza isolated from a woman with conjunctivitis. *Lancet* **348**, 901–2.

Leonardi, G.P., Leib, H., Birkhead, G.S., Smith, C., Costello, P. & Conron, W. (1994) Comparison of rapid detection methods for influenza A virus and their value in health care management of institutionalized geriatric patients. *J Clin Microbiol* **32**, 70–4.

Lindstrom, S., Sugita, S., Endo, A. *et al.* (1996) Evolutionary characterisation of recent human H3N2 influenza A isolates from Japan and China: novel changes in receptor binding domain. *Archiv Virol* **141**, 1349–55.

Loosli, G.C., Hamre, D. & Berlin, B.S. (1953) Airborne influenza A infections in immunised animals. *Trans Assoc Am Physicians* **66**, 222–30.

Merten, O.W., Hannoun, C., Manuguewa, J.C., Ventre, F. & Petres, S. (1996) Production of influenza virus in cell cultures for vaccine preparation. *Adv Exp Med Biol* **397**, 141–51.

Mills, R.D., Cain, K.J. & Woods, G.L. (1989) Detection of influenza by centrifugal inoculation of MDCK cells and staining with monoclonal antibodies. *J Clin Microbiol* **25**, 421–2.

Monto, A.S. & Maassab, H.F. (1981) Ether treatment of type B influenza virus antigen for the haemagglutination inhibition test. *J Clin Microbiol* **13**, 54–7.

Morishita, T., Kobayashi, S., Miyake, T. & Isomura, S. (1992) Rapid diagnosis of influenza infection by PCR method, detection of influenza virus HA gene in throat swab. *J Jap Assoc Infect Dis* **66**, 944–9.

Morishita, T., Nobusawa, E., Nakajima, K. & Kajima, S. (1996) Studies on the molecular basis for loss of the ability of recent influenza (H1N1) virus strains to agglutinate chicken erythrocytes. *J Gen Virol* **77**, 2499–506.

Moriuchi, H., Oshima, T., Nishimura, K., Nakamura, N., Katushima, N. & Numazaki, Y. (1990) Human malignant melanoma cell line (HMV-II) for isolation of influenza C and parainfluenza viruses. *J Clin Microbiol* **28**, 1147–50.

Murphy, P., Roberts, Z.M. & Waner, J.L. (1996) Differential diagnoses of influenza A virus, influenza B virus and respiratory syncytial virus infections by direct immunoflourescence using mixtures of monoclonal antibodies of different isotypes. *J Clin Microbiol* **34**, 1798–800.

Okuno, Y., Tanaka, K., Baba, K., Maeda, A., Kunita, N. & Ueda, S. (1990) Rapid focus neutralization test of influenza A and B viruses in microtiter system. *J Clin Microbiol* **28**, 1308.

O'Neill, H.J., Russell, J.D., Wyatt, D.E., McCaughey, C. & Coyle, P.V. (1996) Isolation of viruses from clinical specimens in microtitre plates with cells inoculated in suspension. *J Virol Meth* **62**, 169–78.

Pisareva, M., Bechtevera, T., Plyusinin, A., Dobretsova, A. & Kisselov, O. (1992) PCR amplification of influenza A specific sequences. *Archiv Virol* **125**, 313–18.

Ptakova, M. & Tumova, B. (1985) Detection of type A and B influenza viruses in clinical materials by immunoelectron microscopy. *Acta Virol* **29**, 19–24.

Pyhala, R., Pyhala, L., Valle, M. & Ano, K. (1987) Egg-grown and tissue-culture grown variants of influenza A (H3N2) virus with special attention to their use as antigens in seroepidemiology. *Epidemiol Infect* **99**, 745–53.

Remarque, E.J., van Beek, W.C.A., Ligthart, G.J. *et al.* (1993) Improvement of the immunoglobulin subclass response to influenza vaccine in elderly nursing home residents by the use of high-dose vaccines. *Vaccine* **11**, 649–54.

Richardson, J.C.W., Scalera, V. & Simmonds, N.L. (1981) Identification of two strains of MDCK cells which resemble separate nephron tubule segments. *Biochim Biophys Acta* **673**, 26–36.

Rimmelzwaan, G.F., Baars, M., van Beek, R. *et al.* (1997) Induction of protective immunity against influenza virus in a macaque model: comparison of conventional and ISCOM vaccines. *J Gen Virol* **78**, 757–65.

Robertson, J.S., Naeve, C.W., Webster, R.G., Bootman, J.S., Newman, R. & Schild, G.C. (1985) Alterations in haemagglutinin associated with adaptation of influenza B virus to growth in eggs. *Virology* **143**, 166–74.

Robertson, J.S., Bootman, J.S., Nicolson, C., Major, D., Robertson, E.W. & Wood, J.M. (1990) The haemagglutinin of influenza B virus present in clinical material is a single species identical to that of mammalian cell grown virus. *Virology* **179**, 35–40.

Rocha, E.P., Xu, X., Haut, E., Allen, J.R., Regnery, H. & Cox, N. (1993) Comparison of 10 influenza A (H1N1 and H3N2) sequences obtained directly from clinical specimens to those of MDCK cell and egg grown viruses. *J Gen Virol* **74**, 2513–18.

Rogers, G.N. & Paulson, V.C. (1983) Receptor determinants of human and animal influenza virus isolates: differences in receptor specificity of the H3 haemagglutinin based on species of origin. *Virology* **127**, 361–73.

Rogers, G.N., Herrler, G., Paulson, J.C. & Klenk, H.-D. (1986) Influenza C uses 9-O-acetyl-N-acetylneuraminic acid as a high-affinity receptor determinant for attachment to cells. *J Biol Chem* **261**, 5947–51.

Rosen, R.D., Butler, W.T., Waldmann, R.N. *et al.* (1970) The proteins in nasal secretions. II. A longitudinal study of IgA and neutralizing antibody levels in nasal washings from men infected with influenza virus. *J Am Med Assoc* **211**, 1157–61.

Ryan Poirier, K.A. & Kawaoka, Y. (1991) Distinct glycoprotein inhibitors of influenza A virus in different animal sera. *J Virol* **65**, 389–95.

Sahasrabudhe, A., Blick, T. & McKimm-Breschkim, J. (1996) Influenza virus variants resistant to GG167 with mutations in the haemagglutinin. In: Brown, L.E., Hampson, A.W. & Webster, R.G. (eds) *Options for the Control of Influenza III*, pp. 748–52. ICS Elsevier, Amsterdam.

Sarkkinen, H.K., Halonen, P.E. & Salmi, A.A. (1981) Detection of influenza A by radioimmunoassay and enzyme immunoassay from nasopharyngeal specimens. *J Med Virol* **7**, 213–20.

Schultze, B., Zimmer, G. & Herrler, G. (1996) Virus entry into a polarized epithelial cell line (MDCK): similarities and dissimilarities between influenza C virus and bovine corona virus. *J Gen Virol* **77**, 2507–14.

Seno, M.Y., Kanamoto, S., Takao, N., Takei, S., Fukuda, S. & Umisa, N. (1990) Enhancing effect of centrifugation on isolation of influenza virus from clinical specimens. *J Clin Microbiol* **28**, 1669–70.

Shalit, I., McKee, P.A., Beauchamp, H. & Waner, J.L. (1985) Comparison of polyclonal antiserum versus monoclonal antibodies for the rapid diagnosis of influenza A virus infections by immunofluorescence in clinical specimens. *J Clin Microbiol* **22**, 877–9.

Simmons, N.L. (1981) Ion transport in tight junctions of epithelial monolayers of MDCK cells. *J Membr Biol* **59**, 105–14.

Siqueira, M.M., Ferro, Z.A., Cohen, B.J., Brown, D.W.G. & Nascimento, J.P. (1994) IgM antibody capture haemadherence test (MACHAT) for the detection of measles-specific IgM. *J Virol Meth* **50**, 167–74.

Staschke, K.A., Colacino, J.M., Baxter, A.J. *et al.* (1995) Molecular basis for the resistance of influenza viruses to 4-guanidino-Neu 5 Ac2en. *Virology* **214**, 642–6.

Stern, H. & Tippett, K.C. (1963) Primary isolation of influenza viruses at 33 °C. *Lancet* **i**, 13.

Stokes, C.E., Bernstein, J.M., Kruger, S.A. & Hayden, F.G. (1988) Rapid diagnosis of influenza A and B by 24-hour fluorescent focus assays. *J Clin Microbiol* **26**, 1263–6.

Taubenberger, J.K., Reid, A.H., Krafft, A.E., Bijwaard, K.E. & Fanning, T.G. (1997) Initial genetic characterisation of the 1918 Spanish influenza virus. *Science* **275**, 1793–5.

Thompson, J., Pham, D.M., Werkhaven, J.A., Sannella, E., Ikizler, M. & Wright, P. (1996) Optimal collection and assay of upper respiratory specimens for determination of mucosal immune responses to influenza. In: Brown, Hampson & Webster (eds) *Options for the Control of Influenza III*, pp. 263–70. ICS Elsevier.

Tobita, K. (1975) Permanent canine kidney (MDCK) cells for isolation and plaque assay of influenza B viruses. *Med Microbiol Immunol* **162**, 23–7.

Tobita, K., Sugiura, A., Enomoto, C. & Furuyama, M. (1975) Plaque assay and primary isolation of influenza A viruses in an established line of canine kidney cells (MDCK) in the presence of trypsin. *Med Microbiol Immunol* **162**, 9–14.

Todd, S.J., Minnich, L. & Waner, J.L. (1995) Comparison of rapid immunofluorescence procedure with Test Pack RSV and Directigen Flu A for diagnosis of respiratory syncytial virus and influenza A virus. *J Clin Microbiol* **33**, 1650–1.

van der Water, C., van Dura, E.A., van der Stap, J.F.M.M., Brands, R. & Boersma, W.J.A. (1993) Rapid *in vitro* micro cytotoxicity tests for the detection and quantification of neutralizing antibodies to both viruses and toxins. *J Immunol Meth* **166**, 157–64.

von Itzstein, M., Wu, W.-Y., Kok, G.B. *et al.* (1993) Rational design of patent sialidase-based inhibitors of influenza virus replication. *Nature* **363**, 418–23.

Walls, H.H., Johansson, K.H., Harmon, M.W., Halonen, P.E. & Kendal, A.P. (1986) Time-resolved fluoroimmunoassay with monoclonal antibodies for rapid diagnosis of influenza infections. *J Clin Microbiol* **24**, 907–12.

Waner, J.L., Todd, S.J., Shalaby, N., Murphy, P. & Wall, L.V. (1991) Comparison of Directigen Flu-A with viral isolation and direct immunofluorescence for the rapid detection and identification of influenza A virus. *J Clin Microbiol* **29**, 479–82.

Webster, R.G., Yakling, M., Hinshaw, V.S., Bean, W.J. & Murti, K.G. (1978) Intestinal influenza: replication and characteristic action of influenza viruses in ducks. *Virology* **84**, 268–78.

Weis, W., Brown, J.H., Cusack, S., Paulson, J.C., Skehel, J.J. & Wiley, D.C. (1988) Structure of the influenza virus haemagglutinin complex with its receptor, sialic acid. *Nature* **333**, 426–31.

Wentworth, D.E., McGregor, M., Macklin, M.D., Neumann, V. & Hinshaw, V.S. (1997) Transmission of swine influenza virus to humans after exposure to experimentally infected pigs. *J Infect Dis* **175**, 7–15.

Williams, S.P. & Robertson, J.S. (1993) Analysis of the restriction to growth of non egg adapted human influenza virus in eggs. *Virology* **196**, 660–5.

Wood, J.M., Gaines-Das, R.E., Taylor, J. & Chakraverty, P. (1994) Comparison of influenza serological techniques by international collaborative study. *Vaccine* **12**, 167–74.

Wright, K.E., Wilson, G.A.R., Novosad, D., Dimock, C., Tan, D. & Weber, J.M. (1995) Typing and subtyping of influenza viruses in clinical samples by PCR. *J Clin Microbiol* **33**, 1180–4.

Wright, P.F., Ikizler, M., Carroll, K.N. & Endo, Y. (1996) Interactions of viruses with respiratory epithelial cells. *Sem Virol* **7**, 227–35.

Yamada, A., Imanishi, J., Nakajima, E., Nakajima, K. & Nakajima, S. (1991) Detection of influenza viruses in throat swab by using polymerase chain reaction. *Microbiol Immunol* **35**, 259–65.

Zambon, M.C., Ellis, J.S., Sadler, C.J. & Fleming, D.M. (1996) The use of multiplex PCR for typing and subtyping influenza viruses in a sentinel surveillance scheme in the UK. In: Brown, L.E., Hampson, A.W. & Webster, R.G. (eds) *Options for the Control of Influenza III*, pp. 607–14. ICS Elsevier, Amsterdam.

Zhang, W. & Evans, D. (1991) Detection and identification of human influenza viruses by polymerase chain reaction. *J Virol Meth* **33**, 165–89.

Ziegler, T., Hall, H., Sanchez-Fauquier, A., Gamble, W. & Cox, N. (1995) Type and subtype specific detection of influenza viruses in clinical specimens by rapid culture assay. *J Clin Microbiol* **33**, 318–22.

Section 8
Vaccines and Vaccine Development

CHAPTER 23

History of Inactivated Influenza Vaccines

John M. Wood and Michael S. Williams

Early events

It is remarkable that the first attempts to inject an influenza virus into humans were made only 2 years after the first isolation of human influenza virus from an infected ferret in 1933 (Smith *et al.* 1933). These studies, which were performed in the USA, were not originally designed to develop a vaccine, but were to investigate whether live influenza virus grown in chick embryos would infect humans and induce antibody after subcutaneous injection (Francis & Magill 1936). This pioneering work was done with A/PR/8/34 (H1N1) and it was observed that neutralizing antibodies developed in serum, peaked after 2 weeks and persisted for up to 6 months. The next significant step in developing a vaccine was the demonstration in 1936, that filtrates of influenza-infected mouse lungs, could induce protection in children when given by intramuscular injection (Stokes *et al.* 1937a). This observation was quickly confirmed 1 year later by a further study with PR8 virus in children (Stokes *et al.* 1937b). Although such studies would not be countenanced today, there were clearly some concerns about the safety of volunteers because attempts were made to inactivate the virus before further tests were performed. So it was in 1937, that Smith *et al.* (1938) prepared a formalin-treated filtrate of A/WS/33 (H1N1) virus from mouse lungs and attempted a controlled prophylactic study of the vaccine given by subcutaneous injection in the military in the UK. Unfortunately an influenza outbreak occurred before vaccination was complete so it was not possible to assess vaccine effectiveness. A second attempt at vaccination with inactivated virus was made 1 year later in the UK, but again there was no protective effect from the vaccine (Stuart-Harris 1945). This was followed by a series of studies using inactivated virus from either infected mouse lung or chick embryo tissue, but the results were again not very convincing. With the benefit of hindsight, the disappointing results were attributed to vaccine potency being too low or vaccine strains being inappropriate (Francis 1953). There was a suspicion that a more potent vaccine was needed and this led Hirst *et al.* (1942) to investigate the effect of vaccine dose on human immune response. They discovered that the most concentrated vaccines, produced by high speed centrifugation gave the highest serum antibody levels. At about this time, two significant discoveries were made, which greatly affected vaccine production. Burnett (1940) described growth of virus on the chorioallantoic membrane of hens' eggs and Hirst (1941) demonstrated that influenza virus would agglutinate red blood cells. Thus the scene was set for large-scale growth of virus in hens' eggs, purification of virus by adsorption to red blood cells and assessment of vaccine potency by haemagglutination. These techniques were used consistently during the next decade in the quest to demonstrate that vaccines were effective.

The US Army trials

In 1942, the Commission of Influenza of the US Armed Forces Board for the Investigation and Control of Influenza and other Epidemic Diseases in the Army, began a series of clinical studies using concentrated, inactivated influenza A and B vaccine. The first study was performed in about 8000 people and care was taken to use appropriate placebo control injections. The vaccine viruses were PR8 and B/Lee/40. They were concentrated by either freezing (which did not work well) or by adsorption to and elution from red cells, and then subsequent inactivation with formalin. Despite the fact that good antibody titres developed, there was very little influenza activity that winter, so no measure of effectiveness was possible. In 1943 a further trial was carried out in a series of army units throughout the USA (reviewed by Francis 1953). The vaccine contained PR8 and A/Weiss/43 (H1N1) as the influenza A strains and B/Lee/40 as the B component and equal numbers of test and control individuals (approximately 6000 each) were used. The vaccination was completed in October and by November, there was an epidemic of influenza A. In five of the nine units, the frequency of influenza-like illness in the controls was between 3.5 and 6 times more than the vaccinated groups and the incidence of hospitalized cases was 7.15% in the controls and only 2.2% in vaccinees. This was the first convincing proof that inactivated influenza vaccine given subcutaneously could protect (70–80% effectiveness) against natural influenza. As a result of this, the first licences for civilian vaccines were issued to several companies in the US in 1945. By this time, the entire US army was being vaccinated and an influenza B epidemic in the winter of 1945 gave further proof of vaccine effectiveness. One example was at the University of Michigan, where there were 600 vaccinated army personnel and 1100 unvaccinated navy personnel in a nearby unit (Francis *et al.* 1946). The incidence of flu-like illness was 9.9% (109 cases) in the navy and only 1.2% (seven cases) in the army (88% protection). Anecdotal evidence in many other units throughout the USA in 1945 suggested that army personnel had a much lower incidence of influenza than their navy counterparts (Francis 1953).

In the winter of 1947, the development of influenza vaccines suffered a major setback. A new influenza A (H1N1) variant, A/FM/1/47, appeared in Australia in 1946 and by 1947 had spread throughout the world. Following their earlier successes, vaccine was by that time, widely used throughout the world, but it proved to be singularly unsuccessful against the new virus: 11% protection at the University of Michigan (Francis *et al.* 1947); zero protection in the US army (Sartwell & Long 1948); and 35–50% protection in the UK (Mellanby *et al.* 1948). The results were so disappointing that one virologist was reported as saying that the recipients would have gained more benefit from eating the eggs used to make the vaccine (Hoyle 1968). The reason for such poor results was the antigenic difference between the epidemic strain A/FM/1 and vaccine strains PR8 and A/Weiss. The vaccines produced little or no antibody to A/FM/1, whereas excellent responses to the vaccine strain were seen. This prompted the US Commission on Influenza to recommend that a representative of the 1947 strains be included in subsequent vaccines. Thus, the unfortunate incident set in motion the process of vaccine strain selection which is such an important feature of modern vaccines.

Improvements in vaccine production

As discussed above, the first vaccines produced from chick embryos were too weak and it became apparent that virus concentration was needed. The use of red blood cell adsorption–elution from 1941 onwards and differential centrifugation, which was first introduced in 1936 (Elford & Andrewes 1936) were both equally effective. The latter method was scaled up for vaccine production in 1945 by the use of a Sharples centrifuge (Stanley 1945). This was essential as vaccination was becoming more widespread and large volumes of allantoic fluid had to be processed. By today's standards, however, the vaccines were relatively crude and they gave rise to significant local and systemic reactions. The introduction of the zonal centrifuge in the mid-1960s to separate influenza virus from contaminating egg protein, allowed preparation of highly purified influenza vaccines with significant reductions in vaccine reactogenicity (Reimer *et al.* 1966).

Although the newly purified vaccines were generally well tolerated, reactogenicity in young children remained a problem. It had been discovered in the late 1950s that virus particles could be disrupted with ether and they could induce haemagglutination inhibition (HI) antibody in animals (Davenport *et al.* 1959). Davenport then demonstrated that, not only were these split vaccines immunogenic in humans, but they also significantly reduced the incidence of febrile reactions (Davenport *et al.* 1964). Other splitting agents were also developed, such as Tween 80–ether mixtures (Brandon *et al.* 1967); cetyl trimethyl ammonium bromide (CTAB) and Triton N101 (Bachmayer 1975); sodium deoxycholate (Webster & Laver 1966) and tri(*n*-butyl) phosphate (Neurath *et al.* 1971). Each of these methods were shown to produce immunogenic vaccines and were developed commercially in different parts of the world: Tween 80–ether and tri(*n*-butyl) phosphate vaccines in the USA; CTAB, Triton N-101 and Tween 80–ether in Europe; and sodium deoxycholate in Australia. Split vaccines were first licensed in the USA in 1968 and since that time, numerous clinical trials have demonstrated that they were as immunogenic as whole virus vaccines and were less reactogenic, especially in children (reviewed by Potter 1982). This was particularly well demonstrated during the swine influenza campaign in the USA in 1976 (reviewed by Parkman *et al.* 1977; Wright *et al.* 1977), when the results of clinical trials led to the recommended use in children of split vaccine rather than whole virus vaccine. However, the trials also showed that split vaccines were not as immunogenic as whole virus vaccines in unprimed populations, such as young children and that a second booster dose was required. The worldwide success of split vaccines has continued to the present day and they are currently the most common type of influenza vaccine available.

A further technical improvement which developed from split vaccines, was the purification of haemagglutinin (HA) and neuraminidase (NA) surface antigens. The three most successful approaches were with Triton N101 (Brady & Furminger 1975), sodium or ammonium deoxycholate (Laver & Webster 1976) and CTAB (Bachmayer 1975) as splitting agents and further purification was by rate-zonal centrifugation on sucrose gradients. The resulting vaccine contained HA and

NA arranged as rosettes and only trace amounts of virus core proteins such as nucleoprotein. Following demonstration of immunogenicity in animal models, surface antigen vaccines were tested clinically and found to be immunogenic and very well tolerated, particularly in children (reviewed by Potter 1982). However, as with split vaccines, two doses of surface antigen vaccine were required to produce an adequate immune response in young children. Surface antigen vaccines were first licensed in the UK in 1980 and are now licensed in many countries.

During the 1980s and 1990s, various minor production changes were introduced, such as clarifying and depth filtration systems which greatly improved the efficiency of purification of vaccines.

Another major improvement in vaccine production was the introduction of high growth reassortants to increase virus yield (Kilbourne 1969). Typically, newly isolated influenza viruses grow poorly in hens' eggs and it would be extremely difficult to produce vaccine in sufficient quantity to meet modern demands from such strains. High-yielding viruses, such as PR8 can be used to produce reassortants with the external proteins from the newly isolated virus and the high growth characteristics of PR8. However, such techniques are at present limited to influenza A viruses only.

Adjuvants

Many different adjuvants have been explored over the past years, but only one, aluminium hydroxide, has ever been licensed for use in humans. The others—such as Freund's adjuvant, peanut oil, metabolizable oils such as A65 and Drakeol, muramyl dipeptides (MDP), liposomes and iscoms—have in one way or another not lived up to their potential or have been too reactogenic. The first of these to be tested in humans was based on Freund's incomplete adjuvant. When virus was emulsified in Arlacel A (mannide mono-oleate) and light mineral oil, it produced greatly enhanced antibody titres in humans so that only one-tenth of the usual amount of antigen need be used (Francis 1953). Although a prolonged follow-up study of American servicemen found no evidence of autoimmune disease or malignancies, studies in the UK demonstrated severe local reactions (Tyrrell 1976). Substitution of mineral oil with metaboliz-able oils such as Drakeol or peanut oil (A65), reduced the incidence of adverse reactions as seen in a series of studies using A65. Systemic reactions were rare, even in children, but the development of sterile but persistent abscesses in some vaccinees gave rise to concerns about long-term carcinogenic effects (Weibel *et al.* 1973).

The use of aluminium salts as adjuvants has been extensively investigated. In general, these adjuvants have been well tolerated, but their ability to enhance immune responses is questionable. In small animals, influenza virus subunits adsorbed to aluminium phosphate or aluminium hydroxide induce higher HI antibody titres than aqueous vaccine. However, when tested in humans, no differences could be detected (Davenport *et al.* 1968; Potter 1982). Thus, although aluminium salts have been licensed, there does not appear to be any advantage clinically, and they are not currently used.

The development of muramyl dipeptides and tripeptides, iscoms and liposomes has been more recent. In 1974, Lederer discovered in France that the adjuvant activity of Freund's complete adjuvant was a constituent of mycobacterial cell walls and an analogue, MDP could be synthesized chemically (Ellouz *et al.* 1974). The original MDP was found to be too pyrogenic for human use and subsequent work has focused on the development of more acceptable derivatives. Such analogues are most active when mixed together with lipid carriers, such as squalene or liposomes.

Liposomes were also discovered in 1974 (Allison & Gregoriadis 1974) and were shown to be immunologically active with a wide variety of antigens. They are small lipid membrane vesicles which can entrap proteins and adjuvants and augment immune responses. They are reviewed extensively in Chapter 30.

Iscoms or immunostimulating complexes, are cage-like structures with a diameter of about 35–40nm, originally formed as a complex between saponin and cholesterol (Morein *et al.* 1987). Although they had adjuvanting properties in mice, they were toxic for humans due to the saponin component. However, the discovery of a non-toxic component of saponin in 1991 has opened the way for clinical trials which are now in progress. It has been shown to be an effective adjuvant in equine influenza vaccines and is now licensed in Europe for use in horses (Mumford *et al.* 1994).

Intranasal vaccines

All vaccines described thus far have been administered by injection. There are, however, a number of attractions in developing a nasal vaccine: (i) it may reduce the incidence of local reactions; (ii) it may be a more acceptable route of administration than injections; and (iii) it may induce mucosal immunity which would be a significant improvement over conventional parenteral vaccines. A number of studies have been performed using nasal drops or sprays. In one such trial, volunteers received an inactivated A/England/42/72 (H3N2) vaccine and were later shown to be protected against challenge infection. However, the protection was weaker than that given by conventional vaccine and no serum antibody was detected (Potter *et al.* 1975). Results from other trials have sometimes confirmed efficacy (André *et al.* 1976) but at other times weak responses were seen (Beare *et al.* 1969). It is likely that a successful nasal vaccine will require a more efficient method of presentation to mucosal surfaces, e.g. iscoms, liposomes.

Vaccine standardization

Although vaccine standardization will be reviewed in a subsequent section, it is useful to examine the historical events in standardization leading up to the present day. Probably the most important aspect of vaccine standardization is potency. The early vaccines were ineffective due to lack of sufficient antigen and an *in vitro* test for HA activity was needed. The development of the haemagglutination test (Miller & Stanley 1944) allowed potency of vaccines to be measured in chick cell agglutination (CCA) units and this method was further refined by use of an international standard for haemagglutination (WHO 1968). However, even by the use of a standard, the results of the

CCA test could vary by up to two-fold between laboratories (Krag & Weis Bentzon 1971). A further drawback appeared with the advent of split and surface antigen vaccines, where the CCA test proved to be unreliable and not a good predictor of human immunogenicity. In the late 1970s two new techniques had been developed for measurement of vaccine potency, single radial immunodiffusion (SRD) (Schild *et al.* 1975) and rocket immuno-electrophoresis (RIE) (Mayner *et al.* 1977). Both

Table 23.1 Milestones in the development of influenza vaccines. CCA, chickcell agglutination; CTAB, cetyl trimethyl ammonium bromide; SRD, single radial immunodiffusion.

Year	Event	Reference
1933	Demonstration of virus transmission to ferrets	Smith *et al.* 1933
1935	Subcutaneous injection of PR8 virus grown in chick embryo induces neutralizing antibody in humans	Francis & Magill 1936
1936	Intramuscular injection of PR8 virus grown in mouse lungs conferred protection in humans	Stokes *et al.* 1937
1937	Subcutaneous injection into humans of formalin-inactivated WS virus grown in mouse lungs	Smith *et al.* 1938
1937	Growth of influenza virus in hens' eggs	Francis & Magill 1937
1940	Demonstration of chorioallantoic injection of eggs	Burnett 1940
1941	Agglutination of erythrocytes by influenza	Hirst 1941
1941	Purification of virus by adsorption and elution to erythrocytes	McClelland & Hare 1941
1943	Extensive clinical trials in USA showed vaccine was 70% effective	Francis 1953
1945	Vaccination of US Army showed consistent protection	Francis *et al.* 1946
1945	Sharples centrifuge introduced	Taylor *et al.* 1945
1945	License of first influenza vaccine in USA	No reference
1947	Vaccine failure due to antigenic drift	Francis *et al.* 1967
1964	Ether split virus induces neutralizing antibody but few adverse reactions in humans	Davenport *et al.* 1964
1966	Introduction of zonal centrifuge	Reimer *et al.* 1966
1966	Sodium deoxycholate split virus is non-pyrogenic and immunogenic in humans	Laver 1966
1968	International standard for CCA test	WHO 1968
1969	Development of high growth reassortants	Kilbourne 1969
1972	Virus split by tri (*n*-butyl) phosphate is safe and immunogenic in humans	Rubens *et al.* 1972
1975	SRD vaccine potency test developed	Schild *et al.* 1975
1976	Surface antigen vaccines produced by Triton N101 treatment or CTAB treatment	Brady & Furminger 1975
1976	CTAB surface antigen vaccine is safe and immunogenic in humans	Bachmayer *et al.* 1976
1976	Triton N101 surface antigen vaccine is safe and immunogenic in humans	Brady *et al.* 1976
1976	Surface antigen vaccine produced by ammonium deoxycholate is safe and immunogenic in humans	Laver & Webster 1976
1976	CCA test shown to be inadequate for testing split and surface antigen vaccines and SRD test clinically validated and subsequently adopted worldwide for all influenza vaccines	Ennis *et al.* 1977
1980	Licence of first surface antigen vaccine in UK	

techniques measure the concentration of HA antigen and can be used to measure the potency of whole virus, split and subunit vaccines. This was initially demonstrated by the large-scale clinical trials carried out in the US swine influenza vaccine campaign of 1976 (Ennis *et al.* 1977). Subsequent studies in 1978 (Wright *et al.* 1983) demonstrated that potency of vaccines measured by these techniques correlated much better with human reactogenicity and immunogenicity than vaccines measured by CCA tests. In general, SRD and RIE data agreed well. However, for some strains and manufacturing processes, RIE results proved to be inconsistent and did not agree with predicted results (i.e. protein values), perhaps due to electrical charge in the vaccine, affecting migration of HA under electrophoresis. Such results, together with unacceptable levels of RIE assay variability (Wood *et al.* 1981), resulted in only the SRD assay being currently used to standardize vaccines.

Conclusion

Most of the significant developments in influenza vaccines occurred over a 40-year period since the late 1930s (Table 23.1). Although no significant advances have been made during the past 17 years, a great deal of research and development has been taking place which may lead to further improvements in the vaccine. The virus may in future be grown in mammalian cells, which is potentially a more efficient and versatile production system than eggs, and from a regulatory standpoint, could result in a more defined product. Recombinant technologies coupled with modern expression systems (i.e. recombinant baculovirus) are being explored for vaccine production. New methods of antigen presentation (e.g. iscoms, liposomes, biodegradable microparticles) with or without adjuvant may be used for immunization at mucosal surfaces. A number of new adjuvants are under development and provided they are shown to be safe and immunologically active in humans, they could improve vaccine effectiveness. Finally, if the potential of DNA vaccines is realized in clinical trials and the safety issues can be resolved, influenza vaccines will be unrecognizable from the first crude vaccines in the 1930s.

References

Allison, A.C. & Gregoriadis, G. (1974) Liposomes as immunological adjuvants. *Nature* **252**, 252.

André, F.E., Uytterschaut, P., Niculescu, I.T.I. *et al.* (1976) Placebo-controlled double-blind clinical studies on the efficacy of different influenza vaccines assessed by experimental and natural infection. *Postgrad Med J* **52**, 319–20.

Bachmayer, H. (1975) Selective solubilization of haemagglutinin and neuraminidase: from influenza virus. *Intervirology* **5**, 260–72.

Beare, A.S., Hobson, D., Reed, S.E. & Tyrrell, D.A.J. (1969) Antibody responses to and efficacy of an inactivated spray vaccine. *Bull WHO* **41**, 549–51.

Brady, M.I. & Furminger, I.G.S. (1976) A surface antigen influenza vaccine I. Purification of haemagglutinin and neuraminidase proteins. *J Hygiene* **77**, 161–72.

Brandon, F.B., Cox, F., Lease, G.O., Timm, E.A., Quinn, E. & McLean, I.W. (1967) Respiratory virus vaccines III. Some biological properties of sephadex-purified ether-extracted influenza virus antigens. *J Immunol* **98**, 800–5.

Burnett, F.M. (1940) Influenza virus infection of the chick embryo lung. *Br J Exp Pathol* **21**, 147–53.

Davenport, F.M., Hennessy, A.V. & Askin, F.B. (1968) Lack of adjuvant effect of AlPO4 on purified influenza virus haemagglutinins in man. *J Immunol* **100**, 1139–40.

Davenport, F.M., Hennessy, A.V., Brandon, F.M., Webster, R.G., Barrett, C.D. & Lease, G.O. (1964) Comparisons of serologic and febrile responses in humans to vaccination with influenza A viruses or their haemagglutinins. *J Lab Clin Med* **63**, 5–13.

Davenport, F.M., Rott, R. & Schafer, W. (1959) Physical and biological properties of influenza virus components obtained after ether treatment. *Fed Proc* **18**, 563.

Elford, W.J. & Andrewes, C.H. (1936) Centrifugation studies: viruses of vaccinia, influenza and Rous sarcoma. *Br J Exp Pathol* **17**, 422–30.

Ellouz, F., Adam, A., Ciorbaru, R. & Lederer, E. (1974) Minimal structural requirements for adjuvant activity of bacterial peptidoglycan derivatives. *Biochem Biophys Res Comm* **59**, 1317–25.

Ennis, F.A., Mayner, R.E. & Barry, D.W. *et al.* (1977) Correlation of laboratory studies with clinical responses to A/New Jersey influenza vaccines. *J Infect Dis* **136** (suppl), 397–406.

Francis, T. (1953) Vaccination against influenza. *Bull WHO* **8**, 725–41.

Francis, T. & Magill, T.P. (1936) The incidence of neutralizing antibodies for human influenza virus in the serum of human individuals of different ages. *J Exp Med* **63**, 655–68.

Francis, T., Salk, J.E. & Bruce, W.M. (1946) The protective effect of vaccination against epidemic influenza B. *J Am Med Assoc* **131**, 275–8.

Francis, T., Salk, J.E. & Quilligan, J.J. (1947) Experience with vaccination against influenza in the spring of 1947. *Am J Public Health* **37**, 1013–16.

Hirst, G.K. (1941) Agglutination of red cells by allantoic fluid of chick embryos infected with influenza virus *Science* **94**, 22–3.

Hirst, G.K., Rikard, E.R., Whitman, L. & Horsfall, F.L. (1942) Antibody response of human beings following vaccination with influenza viruses *J Exp Med* **75**, 495–511.

Hoyle, L. (1968) *The Influenza Viruses.* Springer-Verlag, New York.

Kilbourne, E.D. (1969) Future influenza vaccines and use of genetic recombinants. *Bull WHO* **41**, 643–5.

Krag, P. & Weis Bentzon, M. (1971) The international reference preparation of influenza virus haemagglutinin (type A). *Bull WHO* **45**, 473–86.

Laver, W.G. & Webster, R.G. (1976) Preparation and immunogenicity of an influenza virus haemagglutinin and neuraminidase subunit vaccine. *Virology* **69**, 511–22.

Mayner, R.E., Blackburn, R.J. & Barry, E.W. (1977) Quantification of influenza vaccine haemagglutinin by immunoelectrophoresis. *Dev Biol Stand* **39**, 169–78.

Mellanby, H., Dudgeon, J.A., Andrewes, C.H. & Mackay, D.G. (1948) Vaccination against influenza A. *Lancet* **i**, 978–82.

Miller, G.L. & Stanley, W.M. (1944) Quantitative aspects of the red blood cell agglutination test for influenza virus. *J Exp Med* **79**, 185–95.

Morein, B., Lovgren, K., Hoglund, S. & Sundquist, B. (1987) The ISCOM: an immune stimulating complex. *Immunol Today* **8**, 333–8.

Mumford, J.A., Jessett, D., Dunleavy, U. *et al.* (1994) Antigenicity and immunogenicity of experimental equine influenza ISCOM vaccines. *Vaccine* **12**, 857–63.

Neurath, A.R., Rubin, B.A., Sillaman, J. & Tint, H. (1971) The effect of non-aqueous solvents on the quarternary structure of viruses: a procedure for the simultaneous concentration, purification and disruption of influenza viruses. *Microbios* **4**, 145–50.

Parkman, P.D., Hopps, H.E., Rastogi, S.C. & Meyer, H.M. (1977) Summary of clinical trials of influenza virus vaccines in adults. *J Infect Dis* **136** (suppl), 722–30.

Potter, C.W. (1982) Inactivated influenza virus vaccine. In: Beare, A.S. (ed.) *Basic and Applied Influenza Research*, pp. 116–58. CRC Press, Boca Raton.

Potter, C.W., Jennings, R., McLaren, C. & Clark, A. (1975) Immunity following intranasal administration of an inactivated, freeze-dried A/England/42/72 vaccine. *Arch Virol* **48**, 307–16.

Reimer, C.B., Baker, R.S., Newlin, J.E. & Havens, M.L. (1966) Influenza virus purification with the zonal ultracentrifuge. *Science* **152**, 1379–81.

Sartwell, P.E. & Long, A.P. (1948) Army experience with influenza 1946–47; epidemiological aspects. *Am J Hygiene* **47**, 135–41.

Schild, G.C., Wood, J.M. & Newman, R.W. (1975) A single radial immunodiffusion technique for the assay of haemagglutinin antigen. *Bull WHO* **52**, 223–30.

Smith, W., Andrewes, C.H. & Laidlaw, P.P. (1933) A virus obtained from influenza patients. *Lancet* **ii**, 66–8.

Smith, W., Andrewes, C.H. & Stuart-Harris, C.H. (1938) The immunization of human volunteers. *Special Rep Ser Med Res Council* **228**, 137–44.

Stanley, W.M. (1945) The preparation and properties of influenza virus vaccines concentrated and purified by differential centrifugation. *J Exp Med* **81**, 193–218.

Stokes, J., Chenoweth, A.D., Waltz, A.D., Gladen, R.G. & Shaw. (1937a) Results of immunization by means of active virus of human influenza. *J Clin Invest* **16**, 237–43.

Stokes, J., McGuiness, A.C., Langner, P.H. & Shaw, D. (1937b) Vaccination against epidemic influenza with active virus of human influenza. *Am J Med Sci* **194**, 757–68.

Stuart-Harris, C.H. (1945) Influenza epidemics and influenza viruses. *Br Med J* **1**, 251–7.

Tyrrell, D.A.J. (1976) Inactivated whole virus vaccine. In: Selby, P. (ed.) *Influenza: Virus, Vaccines and Strategy*, pp. 137–48. Academic Press, London.

Webster, R.G. & Laver, W.G. (1966) Influenza virus subunit vaccines: immunogenicity and lack of toxicity for rabbits of ether- and detergen-disrupted virus. *J Immunol* **96**, 596–605.

Weibel, R.E., McLean, A., Woodhour, A.F., Friedman, A. & Hilleman, M.R. (1973) Ten-year follow-up study for safety of adjuvant 65 influenza vaccine in man. *Proc Soc Exp Biol Med* **143**, 1053–6.

WHO (1968) 20th report of the WHO Expert Committee on Biological Standardization. *WHO Tech Rep Ser* **384**, 15–16.

Wood, J.M., Seagroatt, V., Schild, G.C., Mayner, R.E. & Ennis, F.A. (1981) International collaborative study of single radial immunodiffusion and immunoelectrophoresis techniques for the assay of haemagglutinin antigen of influenza virus. *J Biol Stand* **9**, 317–30.

Wright, P.F., Cherry, J.D., Hjordis, M.F. *et al.* (1983) Antigenicity and reactogenicity of influenza A/USSR/77 virus vaccine in children—a multicentered evaluation of dosage and safety. *Rev Infect Dis* **5**, 758–64.

Wright, P.F., Thompson, J., Vaughn, W.K., Folland, P.S., Sell, S.H.W. & Karzon, D.T. (1977) Trials of influenza A/New Jersey/76 virus vaccine in normal children: an overview of age-related antigenicity and reactogenicity. *J Infect Dis* **136** (suppl), 731–41.

CHAPTER 24

Vaccine Production

Ian G.S. Furminger

The isolation of influenza virus from humans in 1933 (Smith *et al.* 1933) opened up the possibility of producing a vaccine against the disease. The first vaccines were made from formalin-inactivated filtrates of influenza infected mouse lung. These gave rise to increased antibody to influenza on injection into humans but were never proven to prevent influenza (Andrews 1949). The first successful influenza vaccines were produced in the USA in 1945 using formalin-inactivated influenza virus grown in embryonated hens' eggs. Their efficacy was established in trials in 1943 showing about 70% protection against an H1N1 virus and this led to vaccine licensure in 1945 (Williams & Wood 1993). The vaccines were crude preparations of influenza virus in allantoic fluid and local and systemic adverse reactions were observed frequently (Salk 1948).

Subsequently efforts were made to purify influenza virus from allantoic fluid in an attempt to remove the pyrogenicity and systemic reactions produced by the earlier vaccines. For many years most vaccine was prepared by centrifugation of infected allantoic fluid in continuous flow Sharples centrifuges. The virus was pelleted on the rotor wall and although vaccines prepared in this way were much purer than before they still contained considerable amounts of egg-derived protein. It was not until the advent of larger scale ultracentrifuge rotors in 1966 that it was possible to purify commercial quantities of influenza virus in isopycnic gradients (Reimer *et al.* 1966). These earlier zonal centrifuges were soon replaced by the KII centrifuges that could be operated on a continuous basis (Reimer *et al.* 1967), and remain in use today.

Although very pure influenza virus was produced using the new technology, the whole virus vaccine still produced febrile reactions in both humans and rabbits (Peck 1968). This pyrogenicity was thought to come from extraneous membrane fragments from the host cells and/or the viral lipid membrane (Siegert & Braune 1964).

It was first shown by Hoyle *et al.* (1961) that influenza virus could be disrupted by diethyl ether which solubilizes the lipid membrane. Later it was shown that detergents such as sodium dodecyl sulphate (SDS) or sodium cholate (Webster & Laver 1966), Triton N101 (Corbel *et al.* 1970), Triton X100 (Scheid *et al.* 1972) and solvents such as tri(*n*-butyl) phosphate (Neurath *et al.* 1970) also disrupt influenza virus and that disruption of the influenza virus particle removes most of the febrile and other systemic reactions on inoculation (Neurath & Rubin 1971). Vaccines produced from disrupted highly purified influenza virus are called 'split vaccines' and they are still the most widely used vaccines today.

The main antigens required to produce a protective immunological response to influenza are the two surface glycoproteins, haemagglutinin and neuraminidase. 'Surface antigen' vaccines containing predominately haemagglutinin and neuraminidase were first produced in the mid-1970s (Brady & Furminger 1976a,b; Bachmayer 1975). They are the purest inactivated influenza vaccines and are widely used in many countries. Both 'split' and 'surface antigen' vaccines give very few adverse reactions and the pyrogenicity and other systemic reactions associated with the earlier whole virus vaccine have been reduced to negligible levels.

Although only inactivated influenza vaccines are licensed in Europe and the USA there has been considerable interest over the last 20 years in live influenza vaccines. These have been extensively used in Russia and are in clinical trial in the USA. The vaccines consist of allantoic fluid from embryonated hens' eggs infected with the attenuated strain of influenza virus. The vaccine is given either as drops or a spray by the nasal route.

Vaccine production

Whole virus vaccines

Although whole influenza virus vaccines are seldom used the production of purified virus in these vaccines represents an intermediate for the production of 'split' and 'surface antigen vaccines'. All influenza vaccines licensed in 1997 are produced from virus grown in embryonated hens' eggs. There are, however, vaccines in development that have been produced from influenza virus grown in cell culture (Brands *et al.* 1996) and from haemagglutinin produced by recombinant technique using baculovirus grown in insect cells (Treanor *et al.* 1996). These new techniques are discussed on p. 330.

The eggs used for vaccine production are from healthy flocks but the flocks are not specifically pathogen-free. It is assumed that the agent used to inactivate influenza virus will inactivate any extraneous agent present in the eggs. Manufacturers are required to validate their inactivation procedures to ensure that potential extraneous agents, such as, *Mycoplasma*, *Salmonella* and avian leucosis viruses are inactivated. The surface of eggs are contaminated with bacteria and most vaccine manufacturers wash the eggs with a disinfectant prior to inoculation to minimize contamination.

Embryonated hens' eggs are inoculated with seed virus after 10–11 days incubation at 37°C and then incubated for a further 2–3 days at 33–35°C depending on the virus strain.

Virus seed

The virus seed is one of the most important components of influenza vaccine production. The seed must be free from extraneous agents, possess the correct haemagglutinin and neuraminidase, and grow well. The growth is not only important from a commercial point of view, that may be measured by the number of doses per egg but also the higher the titre a virus grows to the easier it is to purify.

A decision is made in February of each year by the World Health Organization (WHO) on the strains to be incorporated into the following winter's vaccine. The manufacturers then receive strains that have been isolated in eggs from the control authorities. These are similar to the prototype strains and would be suitable for vaccine production. It is the manufacturers' responsibility to produce seed virus from the isolates sent to them. All seed viruses are isolated in eggs and it is assumed that if a manufacturer passages the virus at least three times at a low multiplicity of infection in specific pathogen-free (SPF) eggs, then any contaminating micro-organism will be diluted out to very low levels especially if it does not grow in eggs. The seeds are tested by serological methods to check that they have the correct haemagglutinin and neuraminidase antigens. They are also tested for the absence of bacteria, fungi and *Mycoplasma*.

Influenza viruses, that are traditionally isolated in embryonated eggs often do not replicate to high titre. Prior to the 1970s the viruses were passed many times for the empirical selection of a higher yielding virus. During passaging it was possible for the virus to change its antigenic structure. Since 1971, based upon studies about 10 years before (Kilbourne & Murphy 1960), genetic reassortment of new strains with a high yield donor virus have been employed to produce a fast growing virus of the desired antigenic composition (Kilbourne *et al.* 1971). The haemagglutinin and neuraminidase genes from the new A strains are reassorted with the genes coding for the other structural and nonstructural proteins from a fast growing strain such as A/PR/8/34. Both H1N1 and H3N2 reassortants have been used in inactivated influenza vaccine production. B virus reassortants have not been extensively used for producing inactivated vaccines. However, it is possible to produce them in the same way as for the A strains and they have been produced from cold-adapted live influenza virus vaccine master strains (Davenport *et al.* 1977).

After incubation during the virus growth stage the eggs are chilled at 4°C and the allantoic fluid harvested from healthy eggs. This is done either by candling the eggs prior to harvesting and/or examining the eggs, once the top has been removed. The aim is to eliminate any dead or contaminated eggs. The allantoic fluid is clarified usually by centrifugation and/or filtration.

It is at this point in the process that the methods used vary widely. Most manufacturers inactivate the virus after clarification but some leave the inactivation until later in the process and in some cases until just before the preparation of the monovalent pool. The two main inactivating agents used are formaldehyde and β-propiolactone.

The next stage in production is the purification of the influenza virus from the allantoic fluid. The two main approaches have been concentration by adsorption–elution procedures or centrifugation. Up until the early 1970s most producers used differential centrifugation in a Sharples Super-centrifuge with a low speed clarification of the resuspended virus pellet. This procedure was capable of concentrating the virus 10-fold and purifying the virus 100-fold with respect to protein content.

Another approach is to effect a partial purification and concentration by adsorption of the virus onto barium sulphate in the presence of potassium oxalate at 0–3°C pH 7.8–8.0. The barium sulphate with adsorbed virus is centrifuged off and the virus eluted (Reimer *et al.* 1966).

Towards the end of the 1960s zonal-centrifuge rotors were developed that were capable of purifying relatively large amounts of influenza virus by sucrose density gradient centrifugation. The first rotor used was Anderson's B-IV (Anderson *et al.* 1964; Reimer *et al.* 1966). This was used on a batch-wise process using virus, partially purified by either differential centrifugation or adsorption on to barium sulphate. The B-IV rotor was soon replaced by the B-XVI rotor in a KII centrifuge (Cline *et al.* 1966; Reimer *et al.* 1967). This rotor could be operated in a continuous mode and was capable of purifying influenza virus from allantoic fluid in one

step. However, the flow rate has to be fairly slow to achieve a good recovery and purification of virus. Most manufacturers carry out a concentration prior to sucrose density gradient centrifugation by either ultrafiltration, adsorption and elution, or differential centrifugation. The virus produced is 80–90% pure with respect to protein content. An electron micrograph of purified virus is shown in Fig. 24.1. Very little has changed over the last 20 years and purification of virus by sucrose density gradient centrifugation is still the method of choice used by most influenza vaccine manufacturers.

Whole virus vaccines are prepared by blending concentrates of appropriate virus strains to a standardized level of virus per strain per dose. Currently whole virus vaccines along with split and surface antigen vaccines all contain 15 µg haemagglutinin per strain per dose as measured by single radial immunodiffusion (Wood *et al.* 1977). Whole virus vaccines tend to be pyrogenic (Peck 1968) and are very little used these days. They have been superceded by split and surface antigen vaccines.

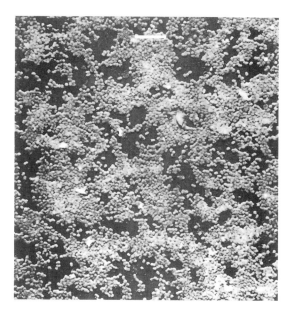

Fig. 24.1 An electron micrograph of purified influenza virus.

Split virus vaccines

The majority of split virus vaccines are produced by treating influenza virus that has been purified by sucrose density centrifugation with a detergent or solvent to disrupt the lipid membrane of the virus. Several methods are described in the literature and these are the basis of most of the methods used today.

The first disruption of influenza employed diethyl ether (Hoyle *et al.* 1961). It was not until 1966 when Webster and Laver demonstrated that the pyrogenicity of influenza virus was reduced by disruption of the influenza virus particle with SDS or sodium cholate that the desirability of using a split vaccine instead of a whole virus vaccine was realized. Similar results were obtained by Cromwell *et al.* (1969) using diethyl ether. The use of diethyl ether with the detergent Tween 80 was first described by Davenport *et al.* in 1964 and is still used today. This method has the disadvantage of requiring special precautions due to the explosive nature of ether. To overcome this Neurath *et al.* (1970) used the solvent tri(n-butyl) phosphate. Influenza virus was adsorbed from allantoic fluid on to calcium phosphate columns and the subunits eluted with tri(n-butyl) phosphate. Triton X100 (Scheid *et al.* 1972) and ammonium deoxycholate (Laver & Webster 1976) have also been used to prepare split vaccines.

Most of the splitting agents described above are still in use today. The actual methods used vary widely from one manufacturer to another but the aim is to have as pure a preparation as possible that is free from detergent at the end of the process. Thus virus purified by sucrose density centrifugation is often used as the starting material and the split product is not purified further. However, in some cases the split virus is further purified by ultracentrifugation using a batch-wise process. The solvents used are separated by phase separation. Ionic detergents such as ammonium dexycholate can be removed by dialysis whereas non-ionic detergents such as Triton X100 can be removed by salting out above their cloud point.

Surface antigen vaccines

During the early 1970s there was evidence to suggest that antibody to haemagglutinin and neuraminidase should be sufficient to produce a protective immune response against influenza (Slepushkin *et al.* 1971; Hobson *et al.* 1972; Dowdle *et al.* 1973). However, it was not until 1975 when Potter *et al.* demonstrated that a vaccine containing only haemagglutinin and neuraminidase protected against challenge in humans that this concept was established.

Laver and Valentine (1969) disrupted influenza virus with SDS and isolated haemagglutinin and neuraminidase subunits. When the SDS was removed the subunits aggregated to form rosettes showing a distinct but different morphology for the haemagglutinin and neuraminidase. Subsequently Brand and Skehel (1972) isolated crystalline haemagglutinin after treatment of influenza virus with the proteolytic enzyme bromelain. The bromelain cleaved the haemagglutinin molecule above the lipophylic end that is attached to the lipid membrane of the virus. Another approach was to solubilize the virus with the detergent Nonidet NP-40 and purify the subunits (Appleyard 1975). Neither of these vaccines were very immunogenic in humans and have not been licensed for human use.

Laver and Webster (1976) continued to work on surface antigen vaccines and described a method for producing a vaccine containing only haemagglutinin and neuraminidase. The production process contained many steps to obtain the purified antigens. This vaccine was experimental and has not been used on a wide scale in humans.

The two most successful surface antigen vaccines were developed by Bachmayer (1975) and Brady and Furminger (1976a,b). Both vaccines are licensed in many countries and are in widespread use. The Bachmayer method splits the virus with the cationic detergent trimethyl-cetyl-ammonium bromide. This method selectively removes the haemagglutinin and neuraminidase leaving the viral cores and lipid membrane behind. The subunits are separated from the viral cores in a batch-wise process by sucrose density gradient ultracentrifugation and the detergent is removed by dialysis (Bachmayer 1975).

Another successful approach involves the removal of haemagglutinin and neuraminidase by the non-ionic detergent Triton N101 (Brady & Furminger 1976a). In this method influenza virus, purified by sucrose density gradient centrifugation, is continuously passed through another sucrose density gradient containing Triton N101 which bands at the top of the gradient. As the virus enters the gradient it passes through the Triton N101 band where the haemagglutinin and neuraminidase are removed from the viral cores. The viral cores band at a higher sucrose density (48–52% w/w) than the surface antigen (20–30% w/w) (Fig. 24.2) The Triton N101 is removed from the surface antigens by salting out in the presence of phosphate. The separation of the viral cores from the surface antigens is shown in Fig. 24.2. Once the detergent has been removed the haemagglutinin and neuraminidase spikes aggregate to form rosettes (Fig. 24.3). The rosettes consist mainly of haemagglutinin or neuraminidase although rosettes containing both antigens are also found.

Composition of subunit and surface antigen vaccines

Subunit and surface antigen vaccines commercially available in the UK have been characterized by electron microscopy and SDS–polyacrylamide gel electrophoresis (SDS–PAGE) analysis (Renfrey &

Fig. 24.2 Splitting of influenza virus on a sucrose density gradient containing Triton N101 separating the cores and surface antigens. (From Brady & Furminger 1976a, with permission from Cambridge University Press.)

Watts 1994). It was found that the two surface antigen vaccines contained only about half the total protein content of the subunit vaccines. The lipid was also reduced in the surface antigen vaccines specially when produced according to Brady and Furminger (1976a) (Fig. 24.4). The latter vaccine was the only one in which the surface antigens appeared as rosettes by electron microscopy. With all the other vaccines the surface antigens were present in bilayer structures. In theory the rosettes have the potential to present the maximum intermolecular accessibility for epitope presentation although it is unknown what happens to the rosettes following injection. It has been reported (Pickering *et al.* 1992) that pyrogenicity may be related to the lipid content of influenza vaccine. However, clinical reactogenicity to surface antigen vaccine is low in children and young adults and there are very little differences between vaccine type (Bernstein & Cherry 1983).

Cell culture inactivated influenza vaccines

All commercially produced inactivated influenza vaccines have been propagated in embryonated hens' eggs. Influenza viruses grow well in eggs but the system lacks flexibility as it is dependent upon the supply of eggs. Hens have to be over 20 weeks old before they come into lay. Supplies of eggs are usually organized between January and July for the production of vaccine for the next winter in the Northern Hemisphere. Concern has been expressed that if a new pandemic strain should evolve

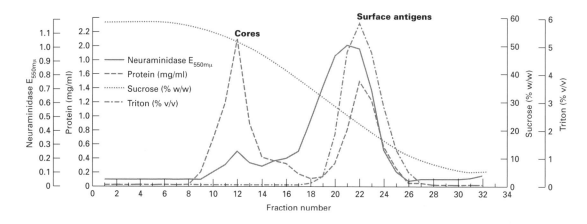

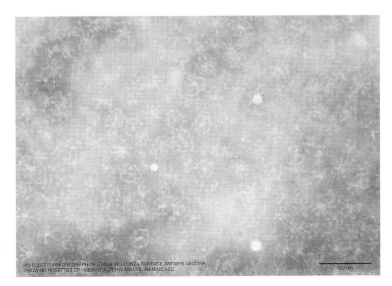

Fig. 24.3 An electron micrograph of a surface antigen vaccine prepared by splitting with Triton N101.

production would be limited to between these dates. These problems would be overcome if the virus could be propagated in cell culture. Several cell lines such as VERO, BHK-21 and MDCK (Madin-Darby canine kidney) have been examined for the growth of influenza virus. MDCK cells yield high titres of virus (up to 2000 HA units) in a short time (Merten *et al.* 1996). This yield is of the same order of magnitude as that obtained from the allantoic fluid of embryonated hens' eggs infected

with influenza virus. Thus a 100-l fermenter will produce a similar yield of virus as 10 000 eggs. MDCK cells have been grown on microcarriers in fermenters and infected with influenza virus. The virus produced has been used to produce a surface antigen vaccine using the method developed by Bachmayer *et al.* (1975). The vaccine was demonstrated to be safe and well tolerated in young healthy and elderly volunteers and to produce an adequate immune response (Brands *et al.* 1996).

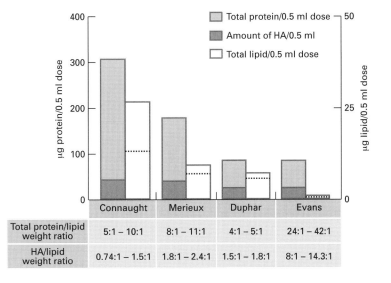

Fig. 24.4 A graphical representation of protein and lipid content of four commercially obtained influenza vaccines. HA, haemagglutinin. (Redrawn from Renfrey & Watts 1994 with permission from Elsevier Science Ltd., Kidlington, Oxfordshire UK.)

	Connaught	Merieux	Duphar	Evans
Total protein/lipid weight ratio	5:1 – 10:1	8:1 – 11:1	4:1 – 5:1	24:1 – 42:1
HA/lipid weight ratio	0.74:1 – 1.5:1	1.8:1 – 2.4:1	1.5:1 – 1.8:1	8:1 – 14.3:1

Production of influenza vaccine in recombinant systems

Influenza haemagglutinin has been expressed in insect cells by a recombinant baculovirus. Full length cDNA clones of the haemagglutinin of H3N2 and H1N1 viruses were inserted, and the uncleaved recombinant haemagglutinins were purified under non-denaturing conditions to greater than 95% purity. Vaccines containing 15 µg haemagglutinin per strain per dose produced an antibody response to the haemagglutinin in humans and were well tolerated (Powers *et al.* 1995; Treanor *et al.* 1996) but are still in development.

Vaccines produced by recombinant techniques could have the same advantage as those produced in tissue culture because they would not be dependent on large flocks of hens laying eggs. However, the inclusion of haemagglutinins and neuraminidases from three influenza strains in a vaccine would probably involve six separate systems for production.

Live virus vaccines

Live influenza vaccines have been used extensively in Russia and on an experimental basis in Europe and the USA. Up to the present time they have always been propagated in embryonated hens' eggs in the same way as for inactivated vaccines. The main difference in the production is that the live virus vaccines are not inactivated, so it is essential to ensure that they are free from extraneous agents. Thus the seeds and vaccines are produced in SPF eggs that are free from all common chicken pathogens.

The harvested allantoic fluid containing the virus has usually been used without further purification as the vaccine. The main emphasis has not been on the purity of the product, which is administered intranasally, but on safety testing to confirm the absence of any extraneous agents. The viruses have often been freeze dried to increase the stability.

Quality control of vaccines

Inactivated vaccines

The standards for influenza vaccines are laid down in detail in documents such as the *European Pharmacopoeia*. The main emphasis is on purity and standardization. The purity is demonstrated by SDS–PAGE analysis and tight limits on the levels of egg ovalbumin (not more than 1 µg per dose) and endotoxin (not more than 100 IU/dose). The vaccines must be free from infectious influenza virus and conform to the accepted standards for sterility for parenterally administered products. The antigen content of the vaccine is standardized at 15 µg of haemagglutinin per strain per dose. In Europe the potency of each year's formulation is monitored by observing the increase in haemagglutination inhibition antibodies after the administration of the vaccine to volunteers in a clinical trial.

Live vaccines

These vaccines are not licensed in western Europe or the USA although they are in an advanced state of clinical development. There are no formal regulations covering them. However, the main controls are on the levels of infectious virus of each of the strains in the vaccine and the proof of absence of any extraneous agents. These vaccines are controlled in a similar way to other live attenuated virus vaccines that are grown in chicken tissue such as measles, mumps and yellow fever.

Conclusion

Influenza vaccines have advanced considerably since crude preparations of inactivated influenza virus grown in eggs were used as vaccines. Modern vaccines consist of subviral preparations of highly purified influenza virus. In some cases the protective antigens, haemagglutinin and neuraminidase, are purified from the other viral proteins and lipids. Throughout the 50 years that influenza vaccines have been produced all commercially available approved vaccines have been prepared from influenza virus grown in embryonated hens' eggs.

There are now developments showing that it is feasible to grow influenza virus in large quantities in cell culture or by recombinant technology in insect cells. Vaccines prepared in these ways are in clinical trials and have demonstrated that it is possible to produce vaccine in an alternative system to eggs.

References

Anderson, N.G., Barringer, H.P., Babelay, E.F. & Fisher, W.D. (1964) The B-IV zonal centrifuge. *Life Sci* **3**, 667.

Andrews, C.H. (1949) Influenza in perspective. *Edinb Med J* **56**, 337–46.

Appleyard, G. (1975) Influenza subunit vaccines. *Int Virol* **3**, 76.

Bachmayer, H. (1975) Selective solubilisation of haemagglutinin and neuraminidase from influenza virus. *Intervirology* **5**, 260–72.

Bernstein, D.I. & Cherry, J.D. (1983) Clinical and antibody responses to influenza vaccines. *Am J Dis Child* **137**, 622–6.

Brady, M.I. & Furminger, I.G.S. (1976a) A surface antigen influenza vaccine. 1. Purification of haemagglutinin and neuraminidase. *J Hygiene* **77**, 161–72.

Brady, M.I. & Furminger, I.G.S. (1976b) A surface antigen influenza vaccine. 2 Pyrogenicity and antigenicity. *J Hygiene* **77**, 173–80.

Brand, C.M. & Skehel, J.J. (1972) Crystalline antigen from the influenza virus envelope. *Nature, New Biol* **238**, 145–7.

Brands, R., Palache, A.M. & van Scharrenburg, G.J.M. (1996) Madin-Darby canine kidney (MDCK) cells for the production of inactivated influenza vaccine. Safety characteristics and clinical results in the elderly. In: Brown, L.E., Hampson, A.W. & Webster, R.G. (eds) *Options for the Control of Influenza*, Vol. 3, pp. 683–93. Elsevier, Amsterdam.

Cline, G.B., Nunley, C.E. & Anderson, N.G. (1966) Improved continuous flow centrifugation with banding. *Nature* **212**, 487–9.

Corbel, M.J., Rondle, C.J.M. & Bird, R.G. (1970) Degradation of influenza virus by non-ionic detergent. *J Hygiene* **68**, 77–80.

Cromwell, H.A., Brandon, F.B., McLean, W.I. & Sadusk, J.F. (1969) Influenza immunisation *J Am Med Assoc* **210**, 1438–42.

Davenport, F.M., Hennessy, A.V., Brandon, F.M., Webster, R.G., Barrett, C.D. & Lease, G.O. (1964) Comparison of serologic and febrile responses in humans to vaccination with influenza A viruses or their haemagglutinins. *J Lab Clin Med* **64**, 5–13.

Davenport, F.M., Hennessy, A.V., Massab *et al.* (1977) Pilot studies on recombinant cold-adapted live type A and B influenza virus vaccines. *J Infect Dis* **136**, 17–25.

Dowdle, W.R., Mostow, S.R., Coleman, M.T. & Kaye, H.S. (1973) Inactivated influenza vaccines. 2. Laboratory indices of protection. *Postgrad Med J* **49**, 159–63.

Hobson, D., Curry, R.L., Beare, A.S. & Ward-Gardner, A. (1972) The role of serum haemagglutination-inhibiting antibody in protection against challenge infection with influenza A2 and B viruses. *J Hygiene* **70**, 767–77.

Hoyle, L., Horne, R.W. & Waterson., A.P. (1961) Structure and composition of myxoviruses. 11. Components released fron the virus particle by ether. *Virology* **13**, 448–59.

Kilbourne, E.D. & Murphy, J.S. (1960) Genetic studies of influenza viruses. I. Viral morphology and growth capacity as exchangeable genetic traits. Rapid in ova adaption of early passage Asian strains isolated by combination with PR8. *J Exp Med* **111**, 387–406.

Kilbourne, E.D., Schulman, J.L., Schild, G.S., Schoer, G., Swanson, J. & Bucher, D. (1971) Correlated studies of a recombinant influenza-virus vaccine. I. Derivation and characterization of virus and vaccine. *J Infect Dis* **124**, 449–62.

Laver, W.G. & Valentine, R.C. (1969) Morphology of the isolated haemagglutinin and neuraminidase subunits of influenza virus. *Virology* **38**, 105–19.

Laver, W.G. & Webster, R.G. (1976) Preparation and immunogenicity of an influenza virus haemagglutinin and neuraminidase subunit vaccine. *Virology* **69**, 511–22.

Merten, O.W., Hannoun, C., Manuguerra, J.C., Ventre, F. & Petres, S. (1996) Production of influenza virus in cell cultures for vaccine preparation. In: Cohen, S. & Shafferman, A. (eds) *Novel Strategies in Design and Production of Vaccines*, pp. 141–51. Plenum Press, New York.

Neurath, A.R. & Rubin, B.A. (1971) Viral structural components as immunogens of prophylactic value. In: Melnick, J.L. (ed.) *Monographs in Virology*, Vol. 4. Karger, Basle.

Neurath., A.R., Stasny, J.T., Rubin, B.A. *et al.* (1970) The effect of non-aqueous solvents on the quaternary structure of viruses: properties of haemagglutinin obtained by disruption of influenza viruses with tri (*n*-butyl)phosphate. *Microbios* **2**, 209–24.

Peck, F.B. (1968) Purified influenza virus vaccine, a study of viral reactivity and antigenicity. *J Am Med Assoc* **206**, 2277–82.

Pickering, J.M., Smith, H. & Sweet, C. (1992) Influenza virus pyrogenicity: central role of structural orientation of virion components and involvement of viral lipid and glycoproteins. *J Gen Virol* **73**, 1345–54.

Potter, C.W., Jennings, R., McLaren, C., Edey, D., Stuart-Harris, C.H. & Brady, M. (1975) A new surface-antigen adsorbed influenza virus vaccine II. Studies in a volunteer group. *J Hygiene* **75**, 353–62.

Powers, D.C., Smith, G.E., Anderson, E.L. *et al.* (1995) Influenza A virus vaccines containing recombinant H3 haemagglutinin are well tolerated and induce protective immune responses in healthy adults. *J Infect Dis* **171**, 1595–9.

Reimer, C.B., Baker, R.S., Newlin, T.E. & Havens, M.L. (1966) Influenza virus purification with the zonal centrifuge. *Science* **152**, 1379–81.

Reimer, C.B., van Baker, R.S., Frank, R.M., Newlin, T.E., Cline, G.B. & Anderson, N.G. (1967) Purification of large quantities of influenza virus by density gradient centrifugation. *J Virol* **1**, 1207–16.

Renfrey, S. & Watts, A. (1994) Morphological and biochemical characterisation of influenza vaccines commercially available in the UK. *Vaccine* **12**, 747–52.

Salk, J.E. (1948) Reactions to concentrated influenza virus vaccine. *J Immunol* **58**, 369–95.

Scheid, A., Caliguiri, L.A., Compans, R.W. & Choppin, P.W. (1972) Isolation of paramyxovirus glycoproteins. Association of both haemagglutinin and neuraminidase activities with the larger SV5 glycoprotein. *Virology* **50**, 640–52.

Siegert, R. & Braune, P. (1964) The pyrogen of myxoviruses. *Virology* **24**, 218–24.

Slepushkin, A.N., Schild, G.C., Beare, A.S., Chinn, S. & Tyrrell, D.A.J. (1971) Neuraminidase and resistance to vaccination with live influenza A Hong Kong vaccines. *J Hygiene* **69**, 571–8.

Smith, W., Andrews, C.H. & Laidlaw, P.P. (1933) A virus obtained from influenza patients. *Lancet* **ii**, 66–8.

Treanor, J.J., Betts, R.F., Smith, G.E. *et al.* (1996) Evaluation of a recombinant haemagglutinin expressed in insect cells as an influenza vaccine young and elderly adults. *J Infect Dis* **173**, 1467–70.

Webster, R.G. & Laver, W.G. (1966) Influenza virus subunit vaccines, immunogenicity and lack of toxicity for rabbits of ether- and detergent-disrupted virus. *J Immunol* **96**, 596–605.

Williams, M.S. & Wood, J.M. (1993) A brief history of inactivated influenza virus vaccine. In: Hannoun, C., Kendal, A. P., Klenk, H.D. & Ruben, F.L. (eds) *Options for the Control of Influenza*, Vol. 2, pp. 169–70. Elsevier, Amsterdam.

Wood, J.M., Schild, G.C., Newman, R.W. & Seagroatt, V. (1977) An improved single radial immunodiffusion technique for the assay of influenza haemagglutinin antigen. Application for potency determination of inactivated whole virus and subunit vaccines. *J Biol Stand* **5**, 237–47.

CHAPTER 25

Standardization of Inactivated Influenza Vaccines

John M. Wood

Introduction

There are three types of inactivated influenza vaccine currently available in the world: whole virus, split-product and surface antigen vaccines (Fig. 25.1). Viruses representing epidemiologically important influenza A (H1N1), A (H3N2) and B strains are grown in embryonated hens' eggs and the virus particles are subsequently purified and inactivated by chemical means before further processing.

One of the greatest challenges for vaccine manufacturers is to produce a safe and effective product despite the frequent changes in the vaccine strains. However, manufacturers are not alone in these endeavours. First, there are international requirements (WHO, European Pharmacopoeia, etc.) which form the benchmark for all aspects of vaccine quality; second, there are National Control Laboratories throughout the world that perform independent testing of vaccines; third, there are international standards that ensure comparability of quality control tests; and finally there is the WHO surveillance network of laboratories and international organizations which ensure that the most suitable vaccine strains are selected. In this chapter, some of the key considerations in standardization of influenza vaccine are discussed; one thing that should be borne in mind, however, is the limited time available to produce and standardize the product (8–9 months) before it is needed in the clinic.

Selection of vaccine strains

The first convincing evidence of the need to update vaccine strains was obtained in 1947 when a new influenza A (H1N1) variant, A/FM/1/47, spread throughout the world and the then current vaccines were seen to be ineffective. The lack of protection was attributed to an antigenically outdated strain in the vaccine. In April 1947 the WHO established a small committee to consider the problem. The resulting proposals made later the same year were that a World Influenza Centre (WIC) should be established which would collect and distribute information on influenza, coordinate laboratory work and train scientists. It would also work in close co-operation with several regional laboratories. The WIC was established at the National Institute for Medical Research in Mill Hill, UK and its first director was Dr C. H. Andrewes. This was the start of the WHO influenza programme (Payne 1953). Gradually a worldwide network was built up of WHO influenza laboratories, but it was quickly realized that one international centre was insufficient and a 'Strain Centre for the Americas' was established at the National Institutes of Health in Bethesda, Md, USA. The two international influenza centres collaborated closely to build up the surveillance network, and by 1953 there were 54 WHO influenza centres in 42 countries to provide viruses and information. The aims of the WHO influenza programme were initially to study influenza virus variation and epidemiology and to share the information worldwide. It soon became clear, however, that there was often enough time after identification of a new variant for the information to be put to practical use in countries not yet affected. By 1953, the WHO had begun to

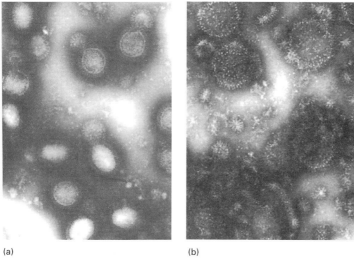

(a)

(b)

(c)

100 nm

Fig. 25.1 Electron micrographs of influenza vaccines. Vaccines are composed of: (a) whole-virus particles; (b) split-virus particles; and (c) subunit particles. The split-virus vaccine contains all the viral components whereas the subunit vaccine contains only haemagglutinin arranged in rosettes and neuraminidase arranged in cartwheel formations. Original magnification × 130 000.

inform governments about the correct choice of vaccine strains and a new and very important role had emerged for the WHO, which has continued to the present day.

There are currently 110 WHO influenza centres in 80 countries and their activities are coordinated by four Collaborating Centres for Influenza Reference and Research based in Mill Hill, UK, Atlanta, USA, Tokyo, Japan and Melbourne, Australia. Regular epidemiological surveillance information is reported to WHO headquarters by national public health authorities and virus samples are submitted by the WHO influenza centres to the four Collaborating Centres for antigenic analysis.

The WHO recommendation for influenza vaccine in the northern hemisphere is made in mid-February. Three types of information are assessed. First, antigenic and genetic data on viruses isolated worldwide are compared with data from strains isolated in previous years. Second, epidemiological data indicate whether new variants have the potential to spread and cause disease. Third, the ability of current vaccines to induce an antibody response in humans to the newly detected viruses is examined. The vaccine recommendation is published immediately by the WHO and it provides a basis for international standardization of vaccine strains. As an example of this process, we can examine the information from the influenza season 1996/97, which led to the vaccine recommendation for the season 1997/98. The predominant influenza activity in 1996/97 was caused by influenza A (H3N2) and influenza B viruses, but the circulating strains were not significantly different from vaccine strains. There was little influenza A (H1N1) activity worldwide, but the few isolates showed antigenic drift from the vaccine strain A/Texas/36/91. In addition, the representative recent A (H1N1) strain, A/Bayern/7/95, reacted weakly with post-vaccination antibody. Consequently, the WHO recommended a change in the A (H1N1) vaccine component to an A/Bayern/7/95-like strain but no change to the two other components, A/Wuhan/359/95 (H3N2)-like strain and B/Beijing/184/93-like strain (WHO 1997).

There is circumstantial evidence that significant influenza antigenic drift variants often emerge in China and there has been effort in recent years to establish extra Chinese surveillance sites. The success of the programme is illustrated by the increase in Chinese viruses available for analysis by the WHO and the number of Chinese variants included in recent vaccine recommendations (Cox & Regnery 1996).

One of the measures of success of the WHO surveillance programme is the high degree of match between WHO-recommended vaccine strains and those strains causing influenza in the world. In the 10-year period leading to the season 1996/97 there have been nine changes of the A (H3N2) strain, no changes of the A (H1N1) strain and four changes of the B strain, and there was a good match in 77% of cases (Table 25.1). This is a good record in view of the variability of influenza virus.

A recommendation for the southern hemisphere is usually made in September and occasionally at least one of the vaccine strains is different from those recommended in the northern hemisphere.

The strains recommended by the WHO are chosen by virtue of their antigenic and genetic characteristics, but there are often practical diffi-culties in their use as vaccine strains, because of either unacceptable passage history or poor growth in hens' eggs. In such cases alternative strains are selected, which have been isolated on approved egg substrates, or grow better in eggs and are antigenically similar to the WHO strains. For example, in 1995, the B/Beijing/184/93 strain was recommended by the WHO and it soon became clear that this virus grew very poorly in eggs. A panel of B/Beijing/184/93-like viruses was assembled and these viruses were examined by WHO laboratories and vaccine manufacturers worldwide. The data on virus growth from the European laboratories taking part in the investigation are reviewed in Table 25.2. It was apparent that B/Harbin/7/94 was the strain which was most suitable for vaccine production. The influenza A (H3N2) strain recommended by the WHO in 1995 was A/Johannesburg/33/94. It is now normal practice to attempt production of a high growth reassortant (Kilbourne 1969) in order to improve virus yield by use of a laboratory strain, such as A/PR/8/34 (H1N1). This process makes use of the fact that, during mixed infections with two influenza A viruses, their genes readily reassort into many different combinations. If one parental virus is a new wild-type strain and the other is PR8, it is possible to select progeny virus with genes coding for the surface glycoproteins of the wild-type virus and the remaining genes, either from PR8 alone or from both parents. Such a high growth reassortant virus would be expected to grow well in eggs yet resemble its wild-type parent antigenically. Two such reassortants, RESVIR-8 and NIB-34, were made from A/Johannesburg/33/94 and again there was a brief period of evaluation to judge their suitability for vaccine production. In haemagglutination-inhibition (HI) tests, both reassortants resembled A/Johannesburg/33/94 (Table 25.3). The reassortants were also examined by polymerase chain reaction (PCR) techniques (Robertson *et al.* 1992) for the identity and purity of their haemagglutinin (HA) and neuraminidase (NA) genes (Figs 25.2 and 25.3) and were found to contain only H3 and N2 genes derived from the A/Johannesburg/33/94 parent. In growth experiments, both RESVIR-8 and NIB-34 reassortants gave haemagglutination titres which were eight-

Table 25.1 Comparison of vaccine strains with concurrent epidemic strains. (Data obtained from *Weekly Epidemiological Record*, WHO.)

Virus subtype	Year	WHO vaccine recommendation	Epidemic strain
A (H1N1)	1987/88	Singapore/6/86	Singapore/6/86
	1988/89	Singapore/6/86	Singapore/6/86*
	1989/90	Singapore/6/86	Singapore/6/86*
	1990/91	Singapore/6/86	Singapore/6/86
	1991/92	Singapore/6/86	Singapore/6/86
	1992/93	Singapore/6/86	Singapore/6/86
	1993/94	Singapore/6/86	Singapore/6/86*
	1994/95	Singapore/6/86	Singapore/6/86*
	1995/96	Singapore/6/86	Singapore/6/86
	1996/97	Singapore/6/86	Singapore/6/86*
A (H3N2)	1987/88	Leningrad/360/86	**Sichuan/2/87†**
	1988/89	Sichuan/2/87	Sichuan/2/87 + Shanghai/11/87
	1989/90	Shanghai/11/87	Shanghai/11/87
	1990/91	Guizhou/54/89	**Beijing/353/89†**
	1991/92	Beijing/353/89	Beijing/353/89
	1992/93	Beijing/353/89	**Beijing/32/91†**
	1993/94	Beijing/32/92	**Shangdong/9/93†**
	1994/95	Shangdong/9/93	**Johannesburg/33/94†**
	1995/96	Johannesburg/33/94	Johannesburg/33/94
	1996/97	Wuhan/359/95	Wuhan/359/95
B	1987/88	Ann Arbor/1/96	**Beijing/1/87†**
	1988/89	Beijing/1/87	Beijing/1/87
	1989/90	Yamagata/16/88	Yamagata/16/88
	1990/91	Yamagata/16/88	Yamagata/16/88
	1991/92	Yamagata/16/88 or Panama/45/90	Yamagata/16/88 + Panama/45/90
	1992/93	Yamagata/16/88 or Panama/45/90	Yamagata/16/88
	1993/94	Panama/45/90	Panama/45/90
	1994/95	Panama/45/90	**Beijing/184/93†**
	1995/96	Beijing/184/93	Beijing/184/93*
	1996/97	Beijing/184/93	Beijing/184/93

* In these years there was little epidemic activity and the indicated strain is representative of those isolated.
† Strains in bold were antigenically different from vaccine strains.

fold higher than A/Johannesburg/33/94, but in small-scale virus purification experiments RESVIR-8 was superior to NIB-34 and was eventually chosen for vaccine production.

The above studies were performed throughout the European Union (EU) and the USA and there are mechanisms in each area to officially approve the choice of vaccine strains. In the USA, approval is given by the FDA Vaccines and Related Biological Products Advisory Committee, whereas in the EU, approval is given by an Influenza Working Party of the Committee for Proprietary Medicinal Products. However, such is the degree of colla-

boration, that similar strains are usually in use throughout the USA and the EU.

Vaccine potency

Since the HA protein is capable of stimulating a protective immune response to influenza virus infection, it is essential that influenza vaccines have HA antigenic activity. The original potency test for HA content was the chick cell agglutination (CCA) test, which was developed by Miller and Stanley (1944). The limitations of this test are described in Chapter 23. In the mid-1970s an improved test, the

Table 25.2 Growth of influenza B viruses in embryonated hens' eggs.

Virus strain	Egg allantoic fluids				Virus purification (mg protein/ 100 eggs)‡
	HA GMT*	No. of labs	Relative SRD titre†	No. of labs	
B/Beijing/184/93	56	6	+	2	4.3
B/Harbin/7/94	331	5	+++	2	5.7
B/Beijing/37/94	235	3	+++	1	Not tested
B/Bangkok/143/94	451	5	+	2	3.3
B/Bangkok/141/94	125	4	Not tested	—	Not tested
B/Shanghai/4/94	90	5	++	1	Not tested
B/Beijing/1/94	226	4	+++	1	Not tested

* Haemagglutination test, geometric mean titre.
† Single radial immunodiffusion (SRD) test using reagents for B/Panama/45/90.
‡ 100 eggs infected and virus purified by rate zonal ultracentrifugation on sucrose gradients.

single radial immunodiffusion (SRD) test was developed (Schild *et al.* 1975b) and this is the test that is now used worldwide to ensure standardization of vaccine potency. The test is based upon the reaction between HA and specific polyclonal serum in an agarose gel to produce a zone of precipitation. The size of the zone is dependent on HA concentration and vaccine potency is measured in micrograms of HA by means of a reference antigen with known HA concentration. A typical SRD test is shown in Fig. 25.4. The dose responses and vaccine potencies can be calculated either by means of a slope ratio analysis (Fig. 25.2), or alternatively by a parallel line analysis. The SRD test is influenza-subtype specific, so that each of the three vaccine strains can be measured independently in the final

Table 25.3 Antigenic characterization of reassortants RESVIR-8 and NIB-34.

Haemagglutination-inhibition reactions						
Virus	Postinfection ferret sera					
	A/Bj/32/92	A/Sh/9/93	A/Jhb/33/94	NIB-34	RESVIR-8	PR-8
A/Beijing/32/92	*800*	400	200	200	100	< 50
A/Shangdong/9/93	300	*1200*	1600	800	600	< 50
A/Johannesburg/33/94	100	400	*6400*	3200	3200	< 50
NIB-34 E4	50	300	6400	*3200*	3200	< 50
NIB-34 E6	100	400	6400	*3200*	3200	< 50
RESVIR-8 E7	100	400	6400	3200	*3200*	< 50
RESVIR-8 E9	100	300	6400	3200	*3200*	< 50
A/PR/8/34	< 50	< 50	< 50	< 50	< 50	*6400*

Neuraminidase-inhibition reactions		
Virus	Sera	
	Rabbit anti-N1	Sheep anti-N2
A/Johannesburg/33/94	20	100
NIB-34 E5	30	200
RESVIR-8 E8	< 10	100

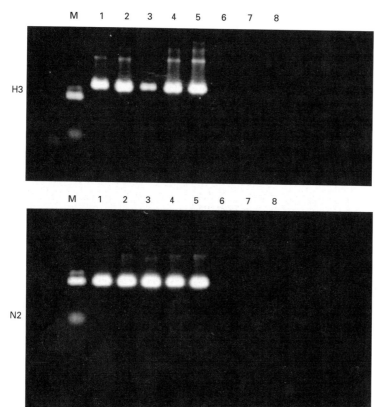

Fig. 25.2 Polymerase chain reaction (PCR) identity test of RESVIR-8 and NIB-34 reassortants. Two passage levels of NIB-34 (E4, track 2; E6, track 3) and of RESVIR-8 (E7, track 4; E9, track 5) and the parental virus A/Johannesburg/33/94 (track 1) were assessed for identity using PCR primers for H3 haemagglutinin and N2 neuraminidase. Tracks 6, 7 and 8 were negative controls; M, molecular weight markers. Both NIB-34 and RESVIR-8 were positive for H3 and N2 genes. (Reproduced by permission of Jim Robertson, NIBSC.)

trivalent vaccine. The test is dependent on strain-specific reagents (calibrated antigen and specific anti-HA serum) being available, so that each time a new vaccine strain is introduced, it is also necessary to update the SRD reagents.

When the SRD test was first developed, the dose of HA needed to induce a satisfactory immune response in primed individuals was found to be in the region of 7–20 µg HA per dose. Limits were set for vaccine potency, which differed from country to country. In recent years, however, most

vaccines in the world have contained 15 µg HA/strain/dose and this has been formally standardized in the EU since 1992 by a 'Note for Guidance on Harmonization of Requirements for Influenza Vaccines'.

The SRD test was adopted worldwide in the late 1970s, both as a result of inadequacies in the CCA test and also because numerous clinical trials have validated the test (Ennis *et al.* 1977; Pandemic Working Group of the MRC 1977; Nicholson *et al.* 1979) and an international collaborative study

Table 25.4 Comparative growth in hens' eggs of A/Johannesburg/33/94 (H3N2) and reassortants RESVIR-8 and NIB-34.

Virus strain	Egg allantoic fluids (haemagglutination titre)	Virus purification (mg protein/100 eggs)
A/Johannesburg/33/94	320	2.9
RESVIR-8	2560	18.0
NIB-34	2560	14.5

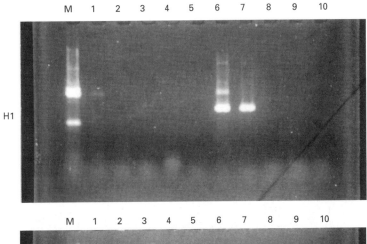

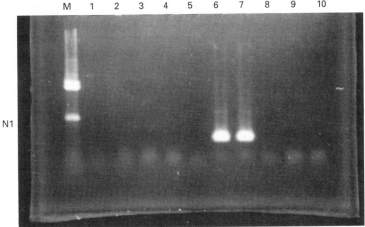

Fig. 25.3 Polymerase chain reaction (PCR) analysis of genetic purity of RESVIR-8 and NIB-34 reassortants. Two passage levels of NIB-34 (E4, track 4; E6, track 5) and of RESVIR-8 (E7, track 2; E9, track 3) and the two parental viruses A/Johannesburg/ 33/94 (track 1) and PR8 (10^{-7}–10^{-9} dilutions, tracks 6–8), were assessed using PCR primers for H1 haemagglutinin and N1 neuraminidase. Tracks 9 and 10 were negative controls; M, molecular weight markers. Both reassortants were negative for H1 and N1 genes. (Reproduced by permission of Jim Robertson, NIBSC.)

(Wood *et al.* 1981) demonstrated test reproducibility (geometric coefficient of variation between laboratories less than 10%). Over the past 20 years, the SRD test has been the cornerstone of vaccine potency standardization. Two EU collaborative studies in 1989 and 1990 (J.M. Wood, unpublished) have reaffirmed test reproducibility and numerous clinical studies have confirmed that the test measures immunologically active HA.

However, the test has not been without problems. Formaldehyde is commonly used to inactivate virus infectivity in vaccines, but under certain conditions it can interfere with diffusion of HA in the SRD test (Gandhi 1978), especially in combination with some Tween-ether split vaccines (Johannsen *et al.* 1983). Fortunately, most formaldehyde-inactivated vaccines are unaffected by

such interference and the SRD test can be used.

A second problem that has recently emerged is the influence of temperature on the SRD test. This was detected in 1994, when SRD tests of B/Harbin/ 7/94 vaccines gave higher HA values when the tests were performed at 37 °C than when they were performed at 20–25 °C (J.M. Wood, unpublished data). These results initiated an EU collaborative study to investigate this further. The study involved six laboratories, which tested vaccines prepared from five virus strains by five companies. The results are summarized in Fig. 25.5. In two laboratories (1 and 5), the higher assay temperature resulted in vaccine potencies that were up to 50% higher; in two laboratories (3 and 4), only small increases in vaccine potency were seen at the higher temperature; whereas in the remaining two

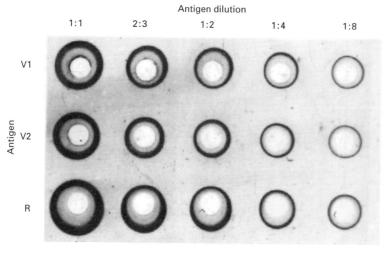

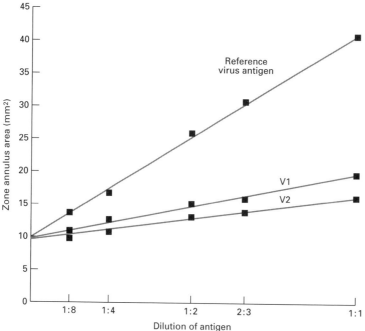

Fig. 25.4 Potency assay of inactivated influenza vaccine by single radial immunodiffusion (SRD). Dilutions of detergent-treated vaccine (V1 and V2) and reference antigen (R) were added to wells in agarose gels containing sheep antiserum to influenza virus haemagglutinin. SRD precipitin rings were measured and zone area was plotted against antigen dilution. Dose–response slopes were proportional to haemagglutinin concentration.

laboratories (2 and 6), lower potencies or only small increases were seen. The greatest increase in vaccine potency was 57%, for an A/Beijing/32/92 (H3N2) vaccine in laboratory 1. Overall there was no consistent pattern, but the study illustrated that temperature had a significant effect on the SRD test and should not be an assay variable. Thus, in 1994, the European Pharmacopoeia introduced new monographs for influenza vaccines, which required SRD tests to be performed at 20–25 °C.

Despite the fact that antibody to influenza virus NA is thought to play a role in protection by reducing the severity of infection (Couch *et al.* 1974), there are no NA potency requirements for vaccines. This is mainly due to two factors. First, the NA enzyme activity of some virus strains, notably

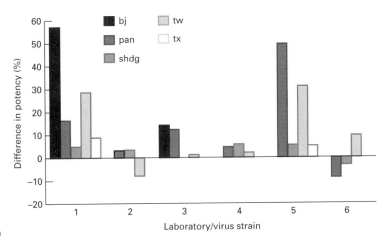

Fig. 25.5 European Union collaborative study on the effect of temperature on the single radial immunodiffusion (SRD) test. Six laboratories tested influenza vaccines prepared from A/Beijing/32/92 (H3N2) (bj), A/Shangdong/9/93 (H3N2) (shdg), A/Taiwan/1/86 (H1N1) (tw), A/Texas/36/91 (H1N1) (tx) and B/Panama/45/90 (pan) strains by SRD test at two temperatures, 20–25 °C and 37 °C. Laboratories 1 and 5 found higher vaccine potencies at 37 °C for most strains, whereas other laboratories found few differences. (Reproduced by permission of Alan Heath, NIBSC.)

A/New Jersey/8/76 (H1N1), does not survive vaccine processing. As the only accepted test for NA is for enzyme activity (Aymard-Henry *et al.* 1973), there is a clear need for an NA antigen test. Recently an ELISA capture assay for NA has been described (Aymard *et al.*, personal communication) and it would be useful to evaluate this test for vaccines. Second, there are conflicting reports on the immunogenicity of NA in vaccines. In US clinical studies of A/New Jersey/8/76 vaccines (Kendal *et al.* 1977), responses to NA were better than those to HA whereas the reverse was the case in the UK (Pandemic Working Group of the MRC 1977). More recently, Aymard *et al.* (1995) found low frequencies of antibody to NA after vaccination with influenza A (H3N2) strains, whereas in mice (Johannsson & Kilbourne 1990) and in humans (Kilbourne *et al.* 1995) purified NA is highly immunogenic. While the evidence is equivocal, it is clearly unwise at present to introduce vaccine potency requirements for NA and the approach taken in Europe is merely to demonstrate that the appropriate NA is present in the vaccine seed virus and monovalent vaccine.

Immunogenicity tests

Clinical trials of influenza vaccines are conducted every year in the EU for licensing purposes, and in other parts of the world regular trials also take place. The reason for such frequent trials is the continued need to assess immunogenicity of new vaccine strains. Clinical trials are also an important component of the WHO vaccine recommendation as discussed earlier.

In most clinical trials, vaccine immunogenicity is assessed by measuring serum antibody in haem-agglutination-inhibition (HI) tests. This test has been validated clinically, so that a serum HI titre of 1 : 40 is accepted as the 50% protective level of antibody (Hobson *et al.* 1972). Despite the universal acceptance of HI test results, there can be problems with test variability due to technical differences between laboratories, such as choice of erythrocytes; the method for treatment of serum to destroy non-specific inhibitors; and methods used to increase test sensitivity, such as ether treatment used for measurement of antibody to influenza B viruses (Kendal & Cate 1983). Within a laboratory, where conditions can be controlled, there is usually less than 10% variability in results of repeated HI tests (Noble *et al.* 1977; Wood *et al.* 1994). However, in one collaborative study where results from five laboratories were compared, the variability in HI test results was as high as 112% (Wood *et al.* 1994). The conclusion from this study was that use of a standard serum would improve HI reproducibility, but such measures would not be practicable, given the short lifespan of such a standard due to frequent changes in vaccine strains. It was suggested that exchange of serum panels between laboratories would be a more practical proposition, so that the magnitude of test differences could easily be seen and due allowances made. This is in fact the approach taken by WHO laboratories when they test sera in preparation for the annual vaccine recommendation.

An alternative serological test is the single radial haemolysis (SRH) test (Schild *et al.* 1975a). In this test, erythrocytes are first treated with influenza virus and then suspended in an agarose gel in the presence of guinea-pig complement. Antibody to influenza virus HA induces a zone of lysis, the size of which depends on the antibody titre. The SRH test has been validated clinically, so that a zone area of $50\,mm^2$ is equivalent to a 50% protective level (i.e. an HI titre of $1:40$) (Al-Khayatt *et al.* 1984). The test was compared with HI by collaborative study (Wood *et al.* 1974) and was found to be equally sensitive for measurement of antibody to influenza A virus but more sensitive for influenza B viruses. However, the most significant advantage was that it was much more reproducible between laboratories than the HI test. The SRH test has now been accepted by EU national authorities for use during annual clinical trials of influenza vaccine and certainly appears to offer some improvements in standardization of serological tests.

The protocols for annual EU vaccine clinical trials and the criteria for assessment of data have now been standardized within the EU. The main points are as follows.

Study population

Two groups of 50 healthy volunteers (18–60 years and over 60 years).

Trial procedure

Blood samples taken before and 3 weeks after one vaccine dose (0.5 ml by the intramuscular or subcutaneous route).

Monitoring and test procedures

Volunteers monitored for adverse reactions and sera tested for anti-HA antibody to the WHO reference strains by HI or SRH.

Criteria for assessment of vaccines

For each virus strain, at least one of the following criteria should be met:
1 Number of seroconversions or significant increases in anti-HA antibody titre greater than 40% (18–60 years) or 30% (over 60 years).
2 Mean geometric increase in titre greater than 2.5 (18–60 years) or 2.0 (over 60 years).
3 Proportion of subjects achieving an HI titre >40 or SRH titre $>25\,mm^2$ should be greater than 70% (18–60 years) or 60% (over 60 years).

Safety tests

It is essential that influenza vaccines are subject to a range of safety tests before they are used clinically. Some of the tests are those usually performed on many other medicinal products, such as abnormal toxicity test, sterility, endotoxin test. However, other tests are more specific to influenza vaccines.

The first of these is a test for avian leukosis and mycoplasmas in the seed virus, which is performed in some countries as these are possible adventitious agents from the egg substrate. In many countries there is also a requirement to demonstrate the efficiency of the virus splitting process used in vaccine production. This is because split-product vaccines have been shown to cause fewer adverse reactions than whole virus vaccines, particularly in children. If the splitting process is inefficient, the presence of whole virions may cause an unacceptable level of reactions in children. Therefore, whenever a new strain is introduced into a vaccine, it is important that the splitting process be revalidated. Similarly, for surface antigen vaccines, it is necessary to test for purity, to ensure that only low levels of internal virus proteins are present.

Standardization in the future

There are new challenges ahead with the next generation of influenza vaccines. Some of the existing methods of vaccine standardization may no longer be suitable, and new methods must be developed. In this section, I have considered some of the key issues with four new vaccine developments: adjuvants; vaccines produced from recombinant DNA technology; cell-culture vaccines; and DNA vaccines.

Adjuvants

1 There is evidence that some adjuvants interfere with the SRD potency test. New tests may be necessary, or alternative strategies for testing. In view of improved vaccine immunogenicity in the presence of adjuvants, less antigen may be needed and international requirements for vaccine potency may have to be changed.
2 There may be a need to monitor stability of the adjuvant in the presence of influenza antigens, e.g. binding efficiency, emulsion size.
3 Tests to monitor safety of adjuvants may be necessary.

Vaccines produced by recombinant DNA technology

In future, influenza virus proteins may be produced for use in vaccines by recombinant DNA technology using e.g. baculovirus, yeast or mammalian cell lines as expression systems. There are now EU guidelines for production and quality control of medicinal products derived by recombinant DNA technology (CPMP 1987) and the following are some of the points relating specifically to such products.
1 Gene products may deviate structurally, biologically or immunologically from their natural counterparts and they should be carefully monitored.
2 Potential contaminants of the final product may be influenced by the manufacturing process and they may not be contaminants normally associated with influenza vaccines.
3 The capacity of the purification procedure to remove unwanted host cell-derived proteins, nucleic acids, carbohydrates, viruses and other impurities should be validated.
4 Potency of the product should be monitored. Ideally, this should be done in a similar manner to conventional influenza vaccines.

Cell-culture vaccines

There is a great interest in moving towards growth of vaccine virus in cell-culture systems.
1 We should investigate mechanisms for providing influenza seed viruses grown exclusively in cells. In addition, the whole process of producing high-growth reassortants may need re-evaluation.
2 Growth of virus in cells may affect antigenic properties of the virus and possibly the SRD potency test.
3 International requirements for cell-culture-grown influenza vaccines are needed.

DNA vaccines

There is great progress being made in the field of DNA vaccines and influenza is one of the topics at the forefront of this research. However, DNA vaccines are so radically different from conventional vaccines that they pose special considerations in terms of safety. Robertson (1994) has outlined three major areas for concern.
1 Unexpected and untoward immunological consequences of the persistent expression of a foreign antigen, e.g. induction of tolerance, autoimmunity, anaphylaxis, hyperimmunity or autoaggression.
2 The potential for a transformation event by insertion into a host gene, e.g. a suppressor gene, or destabilization of a chromosome.
3 The formation of anti-DNA antibody similar to the situation with autoimmune diseases such as systemic lupus erythematosus.

In addition to the above safety concerns, some of the issues raised in connection with vaccines made by recombinant DNA technology will also apply to DNA vaccines.

Conclusion

Influenza vaccines are unique products and they present unique problems in vaccine standardization. During their 60-year history there has been an amazing degree of collaboration between academic institutions, WHO laboratories, government agencies and vaccine manufacturers to ensure that vaccines are safe and effective. Payne

(1953) recognized this many years ago, when he described the important achievement of the WHO surveillance system in harnessing the efforts of workers all over the world with no financial reward and often sacrifice of individual credit for their work. The spirit of this collaboration lives on today.

References

Al-Khayatt, R., Jennings, R. & Potter, C.W. (1984) Interpretation of responses and protective levels of antibody against attenuated influenza A viruses using single-radial-haemolysis. *J Hygiene (Cambridge)* **92**, 301–12.

Aymard, M., Odelin, M.F. & Million-Jolly, J. (1995) Immunité antigrippale. *Méd Mal Infect* **25**, 646–53.

Aymard-Henry, M., Coleman, M.T., Dowdle, W.R., Laver, W.G., Schild, G.C. & Webster, R.G. (1973) Influenza neuraminidase and neuraminidase-inhibition test procedures. *Bull WHO* **48**, 199–202.

Committee for Proprietary Medicinal Products ad hoc Working Party of Biotechnology/Pharmacy. (1987) Guidelines of the production and quality control of medicinal products derived by recombinant DNA technology. *Trends Biotech* **5**, 1–4.

Couch, R.B., Kasel, J.A., Gerin, J.L., Schulman, J.L. & Kilbourne, E.D. (1974) Induction of partial immunity to influenza by a neuraminidase-specific vaccine. *J Infect Dis* **129**, 411–20.

Cox, N.J. & Regnery, H.L. (1996) Global influenza surveillance: tracking a moving target in a rapidly changing world. In: Brown, L.E., Hampson, A.W. & Webster, R.G. (eds) *Options for the Control of Influenza III*, pp. 591–8. Elsevier, Amsterdam.

Ennis, F.A., Mayner, R.E., Barry, D.W. *et al.* (1977) Correlation of laboratory studies with clinical responses to A/New Jersey influenza vaccines. *J Infect Dis* **136**, 397–406.

Gandhi, S.S. (1978) The effect of formaldehyde treatment of influenza virus on the assay of its haemagglutinin antigen content by the single-radial-immunodiffusion (SRD) technique. *J Biol Standard* **6**, 121–6.

Hobson, D., Curry, R.C., Beare, A.S. & Ward-Gardner. (1972) The role of serum haemagglutination-inhibiting antibody in protection against challenge virus infection with A2 and B viruses. *J Hyg* **70**, 767–7.

Johannsen, R., Moser, H., Hinz, J., Friesen, H.-J. & Gruschkau, H. (1983) The quantification of the haemagglutinin content of influenza whole virus and tween-ether split vaccines. *J Biol Standard* **11**, 341–52.

Johansson, B.E. & Kilbourne, E.D. (1990) Comparative long-term effects in a mouse model system of influenza whole virus and purified neuraminidase vaccines followed by sequential infections. *J Infect Dis* **162**, 800–9.

Kendal, A.P. & Cate, T.R. (1983) Increased sensitivity and reduced specificity of haemagglutination-inhibition tests with ether-treated influenza B/Singapore/222/79. *J Clin Microbiol* **18**, 930–4.

Kendal, A.P., Noble, G.R. & Dowdle, W.R. (1977) Neuraminidase. Content of influenza vaccines and neuraminidase antibody response after vaccination of immunologically primed and unprimed populations. *J Infect Dis* **136**, 415–24.

Kilbourne, E.D. (1969) Future influenza vaccines and the use of genetic recombinants. *Bull WHO* **41**, 643–5.

Kilbourne, E.D., Couch, R.B., Kasel, J.A. *et al.* (1995) Purified influenza A virus N2 neuraminidase vaccine is immunogenic and non-toxic in humans. *Vaccine* **13**, 1799–803.

Miller, G.L. & Stanley, W.M. (1944) Quantitative aspects of the red blood cell agglutination test for influenza virus. *J Exp Med* **79**, 185–95.

Nicholson, K.G., Tyrrell, D.A.J., Harrison, P. *et al.* (1979) Clinical studies of monovalent inactivated whole virus and subunit A/USSR/77 (H1N1) vaccine: serological responses and clinical reactions. *J Biol Standard* **7**, 123–36.

Noble, G.R., Kaye, H.S., Yarbrough, W.B. *et al.* (1977) Measurement of haemagglutination-inhibiting antibody to influenza virus in the 1976 influenza vaccine program: methods and test reproducibility. *J Infect Dis* **136**, 429–34.

Pandemic Working Group of the Medical Research Council Committee on Influenza and Other Respiratory Virus Vaccines. (1977) Antibody responses and reactogenicity of graded doses of inactivated influenza A/New Jersey/76 whole virus vaccine in humans. *J Infect Dis* **136**, 475–83.

Payne, A.M.-M. (1953) The influenza programme of WHO. *Bull WHO* **8**, 755–74.

Robertson, J.S. (1994) Safety considerations for nucleic acid vaccines. *Vaccine* **12**, 1526–8.

Robertson, J.S., Nicolson, C., Newman, R. *et al.* (1992) High growth reassortant influenza vaccine viruses: new approaches to their control. *Biologicals* **20**, 213–20.

Schild, G.C., Pereira, M.S. & Chakraverty, P. (1975a) Single-radial-haemolysis: a new method for the assay of antibody to influenza haemagglutinin. *Bull WHO* **52**, 43–50.

Schild, G.C., Wood, J.M. & Newman, R.W. (1975b) A single-radial-immunodiffusion technique for the assay of influenza haemagglutinin antigen. *Bull WHO* **52**, 223–30.

WHO (1997) Recommended composition of influenza virus vaccine for use in the 1997–1998 season. *Weekly Epidemiol Rec* **72**, 57–61.

Wood, J.M., Seagroatt, V., Schild, G.C. *et al.* (1981) International collaborative study of single-radial-diffusion and immunoelectrophoresis techniques for the assay of haemagglutinin antigen of influenza virus. *J Biol Standard* **9**, 317–30.

Wood, J.M., Gaines-Das, R.E., Taylor, J. *et al.* (1994) Comparison of influenza serological techniques by international collaborative study. *Vaccine* **12**, 167–74.

CHAPTER 26

Vaccine Safety

Martin J. Wiselka

Historical perspective

The first influenza vaccines were developed in the 1940s. These early vaccines were derived from killed virus which had been cultured in allantoic fluid and concentrated to form the vaccine. The killed whole virus vaccines were found to be highly reactogenic due to the inclusion of contaminating pyrogens and other impurities (Salk 1948). The development of zonal centrifugation techniques allowed much larger quantities of virus to be highly purified with a significant reduction in the incidence of adverse reactions (Reimer *et al.* 1967).

Modern inactivated influenza vaccines were developed in the 1970s and have standardized antigenic components and purity. Current commercial influenza vaccines are multivalent and contain haemagglutinin and neuraminidase components derived from circulating strains of influenza A and B viruses. The antigenic composition of the vaccine is reviewed annually. Commercial vaccine preparations use either naturally occurring strains of influenza virus which replicate to high titre in allantoic fluid; or genetically stable reassortant viruses comprising the surface antigenic determinants of current epidemic strains and internal genes which facilitate high replication (Robertson *et al.* 1992). These are known as high growth reassortants. Resulting viruses are concentrated, purified and inactivated with formalin or β-propriolactone. Aluminium hydroxide adjuvant may also be incorporated into the final vaccine preparation. Although the amount of haemagglutinin in each dose of vaccine is standardized, the titre of neuraminidase is more variable as it has less stability during the manufacturing process and storage.

Three forms of inactivated vaccine are currently available: whole virus vaccines containing complete inactivated virus; split virus vaccine containing disrupted virus particles which are partially purified using organic solvents and detergents and separated by ultracentrifugation; and surface antigen (subunit) vaccine containing highly purified haemagglutinin and neuraminidase antigens. Antibodies to haemagglutinin and neuraminidase are the main determinants conferring protection against infection; however, reactogenicity is usually a result of internal virus components. Therefore whole virus vaccines tend to be associated with increased adverse effects compared to the newer subvirion preparations (Cate *et al.* 1977; Nicholson *et al.* 1979; Bernstein & Cherry 1983). The majority of published clinical experience on vaccine safety is derived from the use of licensed inactivated vaccines. Other types of vaccines which are currently being used or under investigation include recombinant haemagglutinin vaccines, oral administered inactivated vaccine and live attenuated temperature-sensitive vaccines.

Current guidelines for the use of influenza vaccine recommend that annual vaccination should be offered to high-risk individuals including elderly people, those with chronic medical conditions, and immunocompromised patients. Vaccine safety is of particular importance in these groups of vulnerable individuals. This chapter reviews the safety information available for the different vaccine formulations.

Safety of inactivated vaccines

Millions of doses of influenza vaccine are administered each year and the overall rate of reported adverse events following influenza vaccination is very low (Parkman *et al.* 1976; Cate *et al.* 1977; LaMontagne *et al.* 1983; Wiselka 1994; Morgan & King 1996). Between 1963 and 1991 the Committee of Safety of Medicines in the UK received 990 reports of possible adverse reactions to influenza vaccine (Watson *et al.* 1997). The majority of these were local effects at the site of administration. There is insufficient data to compare different types of vaccine and the causal relationship between symptoms and vaccination is often unclear in individual cases. Adverse effects of vaccine include local and systemic reactions and exacerbations of underlying medical conditions. These are summarized in Table 26.1.

Local and systemic effects

Local reactions occur with all injected vaccine preparations (Bernstein & Cherry 1983; Ruben 1987) and include tenderness at the site of injection which may be associated with erythema and induration. Systemic adverse effects are generally mild and include low-grade fever, myalgia and headache in the first 24–48 h after vaccination (Ruben 1987). Symptomatic treatment with acetaminophen (paracetamol) will control most adverse effects and has no effect on the immunological response to influenza vaccine (Gross *et al.* 1994).

Whole virus and split virus vaccines are associated with a similar incidence of systemic reactions in adults, however, children are more likely to develop systemic reactions after whole virus vaccines. Febrile convulsions are a particular concern in infants given whole virus vaccine (Ruben 1987). It is therefore recommended that split virus vaccines should be administered to children below the age of 12 years.

Several studies have investigated the incidence of adverse effects in particular groups of vaccinated subjects. A recent placebo-controlled study of influenza vaccination in 849 healthy working adults (Nichol *et al.* 1996) found that the incidence of systemic symptoms was similar in vaccine and placebo recipients, but there was a significant increase in the incidence of local soreness after vaccine. Local symptoms were usually mild, seldom affected normal activity and lasted less than 48 h. Logistic regression analysis showed that higher rates of systemic symptoms were associated with age under 40, female sex and concurrent upper respiratory tract illness.

A study of patients attending a 'walk-in flu-shot clinic' showed that vaccination was associated with an increase in flu-like symptoms over the following week. Symptoms were usually mild and did not affect normal activities (Margolis 1990). The subjects were a predominantly elderly population with two-thirds having underlying medical problems. This uncontrolled study was followed by a placebo-controlled, double-blind, cross-over trial of trivalent split-antigen vaccine in outpatients aged 65 or over (Margolis *et al.* 1990); 336 subjects, with a mean age of 76 years, completed the protocol. The incidence of systemic symptoms was found to be similar after vaccine or placebo; however, vaccination was again significantly associated with mild local soreness.

A double-blind, placebo-controlled study in 1806 elderly patients aged 60 or above gave similar results (Govaert *et al.* 1993). This study included 490 patients with underlying chronic medical conditions and showed no difference in the incidence of systemic reactions between vaccine and placebo groups, but vaccination was associated with an increased incidence of local effects. All adverse effects were described as mild and transitory and the incidence of systemic adverse effects was similar in those patients with and without other medical conditions.

A recent meta-analysis of 14 studies, including over 1800 vaccinees, investigated age and sex differences in the reactogenicity of influenza vaccine (Beyer *et al.* 1996). The results showed that fewer than 5% of elderly patients report any adverse effects, local reactions were reported more frequently by females, and previous history of vaccination or influenza did not affect the rate of reported reactions.

In conclusion, the incidence of reported adverse

Table 26.1 Adverse effects of influenza vaccine.

Adverse effect	Frequency	Association with vaccination	References
Inactivated vaccine			
Local erythema and tenderness	17–64%	Definite	Cate *et al.* 1977; Bernstein & Cherry 1983; Ruben 1987; Margolis 1990; Margolis *et al.* 1990; Govaert *et al.* 1993; Morgan & King 1996; Nichol *et al.* 1996
Fever and systemic symptoms	2–34%	Similar to placebo	Cate *et al.* 1977; Parkman *et al.* 1976; Bernstein & Cherry 1983; Ruben 1987; Margolis 1990; Margolis *et al.* 1990; Govaert *et al.* 1993; Morgan & King 1996; Nichol *et al.* 1996
Cutaneous reactions Pemphigoid, vasculitis, dermatomyositis Gianotti–Crosti syndrome	Case reports	Possible	Mader *et al.* 1993; Jani *et al.* 1994; Cambiaghi *et al.* 1995; Fournier *et al.* 1996
Uveitis	Case report	Possible	Knopf 1991
Allergic reactions Immediate or delayed anaphylaxis	Rare	Definite	Bierman *et al.* 1977
Fatal anaphylaxis	Case reports	Definite	Bierman *et al.* 1977
Neurological problems Guillain–Barré syndrome	1 : 100,000 (1976–77)	Probable for 1976–77 Swine flu vaccine	Langmuir *et al.* 1984; Roscelli *et al.* 1991; Safranek *et al.* 1991
Meningoencephalitis	Case reports	Possible	Rosenberg 1970; Gens & Beecham 1978; Guerrero & Retailleau 1979
Encephalopathy	Case reports	Possible	Warren 1956; Woods & Ellison 1968
Reversible paralysis	Case reports	Possible	Aggarwal *et al.* 1995
Exacerbations of chronic respiratory disease Increased bronchial reactivity to histamine or methacholine	Up to 90% of asthmatics	Definite	Ouellette & Reed 1965; Banks *et al.* 1985; Kava *et al.* 1987
Clinically significant exacerbations	0–2%	Probable	Bell *et al.* 1977; McIntosh *et al.* 1977; Knowles *et al.* 1981; Campbell & Edwards 1984; Kava & Laitenen 1985; Stenius-Aarniala *et al.* 1986; Albazzaz *et al.* 1987; Ghirga *et al.* 1991; Ong *et al.* 1991; Palache & Van der Velden 1992; Fox *et al.* 1995; Rothbarth *et al.* 1995; Park *et al.* 1996; Nicholson *et al.* 1998
Transient increase in viral load in HIV positive patients	Variable up to 90%	Probable	Yerly *et al.* 1994; O'Brien *et al.* 1995; Glesby *et al.* 1996; Rosok *et al.* 1996; Staprans *et al.* 1996

Continued

Table 26.1 *Continued*

Adverse effect	Frequency	Association with vaccination	References
Live attenuated vaccine			
Local symptoms	8%	Similar to placebo	Edwards *et al.* 1994
Fever and systemic symptoms	4–28% adults	Definite	Edwards *et al.* 1994; Gruber *et al.* 1996
	< 1% children		Rudenko *et al.* 1996
Exacerbations of chronic respiratory disease			
Increased bronchial reactivity to histamine or methacholine	Variable in asthmatics	Probable	Zeck *et al.* 1976; de Jongste *et al.* 1984; Watson *et al.* 1997
Clinically significant exacerbations	Nil documented		Miyazaki *et al.* 1993

effects is variable and depends on the vaccine preparation and the group of subjects who are vaccinated. Local reactions are experienced by 17–64% of vaccine recipients and 2–34% have systemic effects (see Table 26.1). Systemic reactions are more frequent in patients who have never previously received vaccine. A possible explanation for this finding is that patients with more severe reactions would decline further vaccination in subsequent years (Ruben 1987). The overall incidence of local and systemic adverse effects appears to decrease with advancing age. The reason for this is unclear but could be due to the subjects having had previous exposure to influenza antigens either following previous vaccination or naturally occurring illness (Margolis 1990; Govaert *et al.* 1993). Women report more local reactions than men, possibly due to increased subcutaneous fat leading to an increased proportion of women receiving subcutaneous rather than intramuscular injections (Nichol *et al.* 1996).

Unusual local reactions

Although current vaccines are well tolerated there are anecdotal case reports of unusually severe local reactions following vaccination including (i) bullous pemphigoid, which may be precipitated or exacerbated by influenza vaccine (Fournier *et al.* 1996); (ii) Gianotti-Crosti syndrome, a widespread, self-limiting, papular, erythematous rash,

usually associated with viral illness in children (Cambiaghi *et al.* 1995); (iii) dermatomyositis (Jani *et al.* 1994); and (iv) systemic vasculitis (Mader *et al.* 1993). Recurrent uveitis has also been reported following administration of influenza vaccine (Knopf 1991). The association of these immunological disorders with influenza vaccine is uncertain and a chance association is possible in view of the large number of patients receiving vaccine. Vaccine might trigger adverse effects through a direct effect of virus or vaccine products on the tissues or through immune activation resulting from influenza vaccination.

Allergic reactions

Commercial vaccines contain trace amounts of egg protein, formaldehyde and endotoxin together with preservative and any adjuvant in addition to inactivated virus. These other components may trigger allergic reactions in susceptible individuals. Contraindications to vaccination therefore include hypersensitivity to eggs, polymyxin or neomycin.

Severe allergic reactions following influenza vaccine are rare and are usually due to hypersensitivity to egg protein. The potential consequences of vaccinating hypersensitive individuals include immediate anaphylaxis and delayed reactions including erythema, pruritis, periorbital oedema, nasal congestion, bronchospasm and exacerbations of eczema (Bierman *et al.* 1977). Fatal anaphylaxis following influenza vaccination has been reported (Bierman *et al.* 1977).

Bierman *et al.* (1977) showed that the majority of children with documented sensitivity to eggs could be vaccinated successfully with no adverse effects. Sensitivity to a 1 in 100 dilution of vaccine, administered intradermally, was found to be a better guide to potential vaccine hypersensitivity than positive skin tests to egg proteins. High-risk patients who have a positive skin reaction to a 1 in 100 dilution of vaccine have been successfully desensitized using incremental challenges (Anolik *et al.* 1992). Murphy and Strunk (1985) showed that influenza vaccine could even be safely administered to asthmatic children with known hypersensitivity to egg proteins, and positive skin reactions both to egg protein and a 1 in 100 dilution of vaccine, by desensitization using a similar incremental challenge protocol.

Guillain–Barré syndrome

An increased incidence of Guillain–Barré syndrome (GBS) (polyradiculoneuritis) was observed during a vaccination programme against swine influenza in the USA in 1976–77. The vaccine used was the A/New Jersey/76 strain and 45 million doses were administered in the USA between October and December 1976. A case–control study indicated that the relative risk of developing GBS was increased approximately six-fold in vaccinees, with an incidence of around 1 in 100 000 vaccine recipients (Langmuir *et al.* 1984; Roscelli *et al.* 1991; Safranek *et al.* 1991). The increased risk was observed in a 6-week period following vaccination in adults. The epidemic curve of reported cases of GBS during this period strongly suggested a link with vaccination. There was a sharp peak in the number of cases with extensive weakness in the 7–14-day period after vaccination. This sharp peak of onset of symptoms after vaccination was not observed for patients with more limited weakness. It is thought that many of these milder cases were reflecting the usual background incidence of GBS and were probably unrelated to vaccination (Langmuir *et al.* 1984).

The exact cause of GBS remains controversial as the increased incidence of GBS was not observed in children under the age of 18, American military personnel, or in The Netherlands where over 1 million doses of an identical vaccine was administered during 1977 (Schonberger *et al.* 1979; Safranek *et al.* 1991). A significant increase in the number of cases of GBS has not been observed during subsequent vaccination campaigns (Hurwitz *et al.* 1981; Kaplan *et al.* 1982; Roscelli *et al.* 1991; MMWR 1994, 1996); however, the possibility remains that future vaccine strains might be associated with GBS or other rare adverse effects. Careful surveillance of potentially serious adverse effects of vaccination should therefore continue.

Other neurological conditions

Isolated cases have been reported where neurological problems have followed vaccination. The syndromes described include meningoencephalitis (Rosenberg 1970; Gens & Beecham 1978), encephalopathy (Warren 1956; Woods & Ellison 1968), and a reversible paralysis associated with anti-GD1b antibodies (Aggarwal *et al.* 1995). The incidence of meningoencephalitis during the period of intensive surveillance in 1976–77 was no greater than the background rate expected for these conditions (Guerrero & Retailleau 1979). In view of the millions of doses of vaccine administered annually these neurological adverse effects are exceedingly rare and may simply reflect a chance association rather than a true effect of vaccine.

Safety of inactivated influenza vaccine in patients with underlying medical conditions

Chronic respiratory disease

There is considerable information on the safety of influenza vaccine in patients with underlying respiratory disease. One of the earliest studies found that influenza vaccination was associated with increased sensitivity to methacholine which lasted for 72 h in nine of 10 asthmatic patients (Ouellette & Reed 1965). A further study showed an increase in airways sensitivity over the first 3 days after intramuscular influenza vaccination (Banks *et al.* 1985). In contrast, a small study in 27 asthmatic adults who were given saline or vaccine preparations found no significant increase in histamine-induced bronchial reactivity after administration of inactivated or live attenuated influenza virus vaccine (Kava *et al.* 1987).

Clinical studies in asthmatic children have shown that influenza vaccine is generally well tolerated (Bell *et al.* 1977; McIntosh *et al.* 1977; Ghirga *et al.* 1991). An uncontrolled study in 79 asthmatic children demonstrated a transient decrease in peak expiratory flow rate which was maximal at 48 h after vaccination (Bell *et al.* 1978). The mean decrease in morning peak flow was 12% and this reduction was associated with a significant increase in the use of bronchodilator medication. These changes were felt to be of relatively little clinical significance and the authors concluded that the benefits of vaccination in asthmatic children probably outweighed any minor adverse effects.

Park *et al.* (1996) recently investigated the safety and immunological response to trivalent subvirion vaccine in 109 children aged 6 months to 18 years with moderate to severe asthma. Fifty of the children were vaccinated during an acute exacerbation requiring oral steroid therapy! Although peak flows were not documented in this study the results showed that vaccination during an attack of asthma was not associated with an increased incidence of serious local or systemic adverse effects and oral steroid therapy did not attenuate the immunological response. The study concluded that influenza vaccine could be administered safely to children regardless of the condition of their asthma or concurrent therapy. These relatively small and uncontrolled studies suggest that inactivated influenza vaccines are generally safe and well tolerated in children with asthma.

Clinical studies of influenza vaccines in adult asthmatic patients have also shown that there is a very low incidence of clinically significant adverse effects (Campbell & Edwards 1984; Kava & Laitenen 1985; Stenius-Aarniala *et al.* 1986; Albazzaz *et al.* 1987; Palache & Van der Velden 1992; Rothbarth *et al.* 1995). Patients do sometimes report a worsening of their condition following vaccination; however, other respiratory viruses are often circulating in the community when influenza vaccine is administered. These viruses may cause

symptoms which are indistinguishable from influenza and are therefore responsible for some of the perceived vaccine failures or adverse effects (Nicholson *et al.* 1990; Ong 1992; Wiselka *et al.* 1992, 1993; Wiselka 1994). Nevertheless, there have been isolated case reports documenting sudden exacerbations of asthma following influenza vaccination (Daggett 1992; Hassan *et al.* 1992).

A multicentre, randomized, cross-over study in 262 adult asthmatic patients was recently organized in order to address these concerns regarding the safety of influenza vaccine (Nicholson *et al.* 1998). Trial participants received vaccine and placebo injections 2 weeks apart. The results showed that there were no significant differences between vaccine and placebo for all measures of severity of asthma including hospitalizations, general practitioner consultations, use of steroids and bronchodilator therapy. There were no significant differences in documented adverse effects resulting from split product or subvirion vaccines. Although mean peak flow recordings were similar following influenza vaccine or placebo, vaccine was associated with a significant deterioration in peak expiratory flow rate in a small number of subjects. Of 255 subjects with paired data, 8 had a reduction in peak expiratory flow rate of $\geq 30\%$ following vaccine, compared with none after placebo.

The conclusion from these studies and reports is that influenza vaccine is generally well tolerated in patients with asthma but vaccination may be associated with a clinically significant exacerbation in a small proportion of cases. Overall the benefits of vaccination in this group of patients are felt to outweigh any potential adverse effects.

There is less information on the effect of influenza vaccine in patients with other chronic respiratory diseases. Ong *et al.* (1991) found that administration of influenza vaccine over a 2-year period to 30 young adult patients with cystic fibrosis resulted in no significant adverse effects. No deterioration in peak flow or infective pulmonary exacerbations were demonstrated after vaccination. There is no evidence that vaccination is associated with an increased risk of adverse events in patients with chronic obstructive pulmonary disease (Knowles *et al.* 1981; Fox *et al.* 1995; Rothbarth *et al.* 1995).

Human immunodeficiency virus infection

Several groups have investigated the effect of influenza vaccination in patients with human immunodeficiency virus (HIV) and results have been conflicting. Some studies have shown that vaccination is associated with a transient increase in HIV RNA levels in most vaccine recipients (O'Brien *et al.* 1995; Rosok *et al.* 1996; Staprans *et al.* 1996), while other studies showed that vaccination had no effect on viral load (Yerly *et al.* 1994; Glesby *et al.* 1996). There are great variations in the response to vaccine between individual patients and the clinical stage of the patients, baseline viral load and concomitant therapy probably all play an important role in the response to vaccine. There is no evidence that vaccination leads to any long-term deterioration in patients with HIV (O'Brien *et al.* 1995; Glesby *et al.* 1996).

Renal failure and renal transplantation

Vaccination of adults and children with renal failure or following renal transplantation is associated with a relatively good antibody response and no increased incidence of adverse effects or worsening of renal function (Sheth *et al.* 1978; Grekas *et al.* 1993). Sheth *et al.* (1978) showed that the nature of renal disease in children and concomitant prednisolone therapy did not affect the response to vaccine. Approximately half of the children with nephrotic syndrome who were vaccinated had a transient mild increase in proteinuria, but this did not lead to any worsening of the renal disease and may simply have been a response to fever induced by the vaccine. Influenza vaccine did not affect serum creatinine or urinary protein and did not induce any evidence of graft rejection in transplant patients who were heavily immunosuppressed with prednisolone, azathioprine and cyclosporin (Grekas *et al.* 1993). It was therefore concluded that vaccination was safe in this group of patients.

Drug interactions with influenza vaccine

The interaction between influenza vaccine and theophyllines has been extensively investigated. Initial studies suggested that induction of interferon following influenza vaccine might alter theophylline metabolism, leading to a transient increase in theophylline levels (Renton *et al.* 1980). However, further studies have demonstrated that influenza vaccine has no clinically significant effect on the pharmacokinetics of theophyllines (Patriarca *et al.* 1983; Bukowsyj *et al.* 1984; Hannan *et al.* 1988).

Administration of influenza vaccine to patients anticoagulated with warfarin was shown to have no effect on the prothrombin time and did not lead to any increase in bleeding or other local side-effects (Patriarca *et al.* 1983; Raj *et al.* 1995).

The consequences of simultaneous administration of influenza and pneumococcal vaccine was investigated by Honkanen *et al.* (1996). Local and systemic reactions were more frequent in elderly subjects given combined vaccination compared to those receiving influenza vaccine alone and the pneumococcal vaccine was felt to be responsible for the majority of febrile reactions and other systemic effects. The adverse reactions following combined vaccination were not severe and the authors concluded that it was safe to administer influenza and pneumococcal vaccine together in this group of patients.

Live attenuated virus vaccines

Live attenuated, cold-adapted influenza vaccines have been developed as alternatives to the inactivated vaccines. These vaccines are produced by growing influenza virus for long periods at 25°C, or by a reassortment technique using haemagglutinin and neuraminidase genes from current circulating virus strains combined with the remaining genes derived from an attenuated cold-adapted strain (Kendal *et al.* 1981). These live attenuated viruses are therefore temperature sensitive and cold-adapted and replicate efficiently at 25–28°C but do not replicate at 37°C. They may be administered intranasally as they are able to replicate in the cooler nasal passages, but do not survive in the sinuses or lungs, except in very cold climates. Live attenuated influenza vaccines which are currently under development have combined haemagglutinin components of influenza virus with vaccinia or other carriers.

Theoretical adverse effects of live attenuated viruses include their ability to replicate in the pharynx, sinuses and lungs in cold climates and the possibility that the live vaccine strains may retain significant virulence (Oxford *et al.* 1978). This might be of particular importance in vulnerable and immunocompromised individuals who would normally benefit most from vaccination. There is also potential for further reassortment between live attenuated virus and other naturally occurring viruses which might result in the emergence of more virulent strains. Viral interference is another problem with bi- or trivalent vaccines and may result in a poor immunological response to some of the vaccine components (Murphy 1993). Clinical experience of live attenuated vaccines is limited in Europe and North America, although they have been used extensively in the countries of the former Soviet Union for over 30 years (Kendal *et al.* 1981).

Clinical studies of live attenuated virus vaccines

Edwards *et al.* (1994) compared the incidence of adverse reactions following live attenuated and inactivated vaccines in 5210 normal subjects of all ages over a 5-year period. The results showed that the live attenuated vaccine was associated with an increased rate of mild systemic symptoms, but significantly fewer local reactions than inactivated vaccine. The incidence of febrile reactions was similar for the two vaccines. A double-blind, placebo-controlled trial of monovalent and bivalent live attenuated vaccine in 182 seronegative infants aged 6–18 months found no significant differences in the rate of symptoms including fever and respiratory symptoms in the vaccine and placebo groups (Gruber *et al.* 1996).

The largest study of live attenuated, cold-adapted influenza vaccine was performed by Rudenko *et al.* (1996) who investigated nearly 130 000 children aged 3–14 years who had received mono-, di- and trivalent vaccines. The results showed that less than 1% of children reported febrile reactions following vaccination. Although the vaccines contain traces of chicken embryo protein

the vaccine did not induce an allergic response to chicken embryo proteins and immunoglobulin E (IgE) levels in vaccinated children remained in the normal range. The results of this exhaustive study confirmed that the live attenuated vaccines are associated with minimal adverse effects in children including those who are seronegative. Virological studies of type A reisolates obtained following vaccination confirmed that they were genetically stable and retained cold-adapted and temperature-sensitive phenotypes.

The safety of live attenuated vaccine in asthmatic children was investigated by Miyazaki *et al.* (1993) who vaccinated 19 institutionalized children with asthma and found that vaccination did not lead to any severe systemic reactions or exacerbations of asthma in this small group. Live vaccines appear to be particularly useful in children under the age of 6 months, where they are well tolerated and lead to significantly enhanced antibody responses compared to inactivated vaccine (Clements *et al.* 1996). Administration of live attenuated influenza vaccine to these young infants did not affect the immunogenicity of other childhood vaccines (Clements *et al.* 1996). The safety of live attenuated vaccines in very high-risk infants with congenital heart or pulmonary disease has not been fully evaluated (Murphy 1993).

Studies investigating the use of live attenuated vaccines in adults with asthma and chronic airways disease have yielded rather conflicting results on bronchial reactivity and respiratory symptoms (Zeck *et al.* 1976; Watson *et al.* 1997). De Jongste *et al.* (1984) found that bronchial responsiveness to histamine in asthmatic children was increased after administration of live attenuated influenza vaccine, but unaffected by inactivated vaccine. The release of histamine from leucocytes was not increased by immunization and the authors postulated that the increased bronchial reactivity probably resulted from epithelial damage caused by localized replication of the attenuated virus vaccine. Further large studies will be required before advocating live vaccines in patients with respiratory disease.

Novel vaccines

An orally administered, emulsion-inactivated

influenza vaccine has recently been developed (Avtushenko *et al.* 1996). The vaccine appears to induce a good local and systemic immunological response with no significant adverse effects.

A purified neuraminidase vaccine was administered to 88 subjects aged between 18 and 40 years in a dose-ranging study (Kilbourne *et al.* 1995). The antineuraminidase antibodies induced by the vaccine are not neutralizing and therefore do not prevent infection but viral replication and severity of infection are attenuated. The neuraminidase vaccine was well tolerated and no significant local or systemic reactions were reported in 88 vaccinated healthy volunteers (Kilbourne *et al.* 1995).

Influenza A vaccines incorporating highly purified haemagglutinin have recently been investigated in high-risk preterm babies (Groothuis 1994). Although antibody responses appeared to be slightly lower than the equivalent dose of split product vaccine the purified vaccine was not associated with any significant local or systemic adverse effects. Recombinant haemagglutinin has been produced using a baculovirus vector (Powers *et al.* 1995). Administration of a purified recombinant uncleaved H3 haemagglutinin vaccine to adult volunteers was found to cause fewer local adverse reactions than standard commercial subvirion vaccine (Powers *et al.* 1995). Antibody responses were equivalent to the subvirion vaccine and the recombinant vaccine was felt to offer advantages as it was less reactogenic. As the recombinant vaccine does not contain egg protein it might be particularly useful in allergic patients who are unable to tolerate standard vaccine preparations.

Conclusion

Safety of influenza vaccine is of crucial importance and large well-conducted studies have evaluated the adverse effects associated with inactivated and live attenuated vaccines. These studies have consistently demonstrated mild local and systemic reactions; however, current vaccines are generally well tolerated and serious or life-threatening adverse effects are vanishingly rare. Live attenuated vaccines and recombinant vaccines offer promise for the future and appear to be safe with

very few severe reactions reported in vaccinated subjects, including very young infants (Murphy 1993).

Concern over possible adverse effects is often cited by doctors as a reason not to vaccinate against influenza, but the perceived incidence of severe vaccine adverse effects is much greater than the actual incidence. Influenza vaccines have a good safety record and should not be withheld from high-risk individuals.

References

Aggarwal, A., Lacomis, D. & Guiliani, M.J. (1995) A reversible paralytic syndrome with anti-GD1b antibodies following influenza immunization. *Muscle Nerve* **18**, 1199–1201.

Albazzaz, M.K., Harvey, J.E., Grilli, E.A., Caul, EO. & Roome, A.P. (1987) Subunit influenza vaccination in adults with asthma: effect on clinical state, airway reactivity, and antibody response. *Br Med J* **294**, 1196–7.

Anolik, R., Spiegel, W., Posner, M. & Jakabovics, E. (1992) Influenza vaccine testing in egg-sensitive patients. *Ann Allergy* **68**, 69.

Avtushenko, S.S., Sorokin, E.M., Zoschenkova, N.Y., Zacharova, N.G. & Naichin, A.N. (1996) Clinical and immunological characteristics of the emulsion form of inactivated influenza vaccine delivered by oral immunization. *J Biotech* **44**, 21–8.

Banks, J., Bevan, C., Fennerly, A., Ebden, P., Walters, E.H. & Smith, A.P. (1985) Association between rise in antibodies and increase in airways sensitivity after intramuscular injection of killed influenza virus in asthmatic patients. *Eur J Resp Dis* **66**, 268–72.

Bell, T.D., Chai, H., Berlow, B. & Daniels, G. (1978) Immunisation with killed influenza virus in children with chronic asthma. *Chest* **73**, 140–5.

Bell, T.D., Leffert, F. & Mcintosh, K. (1977) Monovalent influenza A/New Jersey/76 virus vaccines in asthmatic children; pulmonary function and skin tests for allergy. *J Infect Dis* **136**, S612–15.

Bernstein, D.I. & Cherry, J.D. (1983) Clinical reactions and antibody responses to influenza vaccines. *Am J Dis Child* **137**, 622–6.

Beyer, W.E.P., Palache, A.M., Kerstens, R. & Masurel, N. (1996) Gender differences in local and systemic reactions to inactivated influenza vaccine, established by a meta-analysis of fourteen independent studies. *Eur J Clin Micro Infect Dis* **15**, 65–70.

Bierman, C.W., Shapiro, G.G., Pierson, W.E., Taylor, J.W., Foy, H.M. & Fox, J.P. (1977) Safety of influenza vaccination in allergic children. *J Infect Dis* **136**, S652–5.

Bukowsyj, M., Munt, P.W., Wigle, R. & Nakatsu, K. (1984) Theophylline clearance. Lack of effect of influenza vaccination and ascorbic acid. *Am Rev Respir Dis* **129**, 672–5.

Cambiaghi, S., Scarabelli, G., Pistritto, G. & Gelmetti, C. (1995) Gianotti-Crosti syndrome in an adult after influenza virus vaccination. *Dermatology* **191**, 340–1.

Campbell, B.G. & Edwards, R.L. (1984) Safety of influenza vaccination in adults with asthma. *Med J Aust* **140**, 773–5.

Cate, T.R., Kasel, J.A., Couch, R.B., Six, H.R. & Knight, V. (1977) Clinical trials of bivalent influenza A/New Jersey/76A/Victoria/75 vaccines in the elderly. *J Infect Dis* **136** (suppl), S518–25.

Clements, M.L., Makhene, M.K., Karron, R.A. *et al.* (1996) Effective immunization with live-attenuated influenza A virus can be achieved in early infancy. *J Infect Dis* **173**, 44–51.

Daggett P. (1992) Influenza and asthma. *Lancet* **339**, 367.

de Jongste, J.C., Degenhart, H.J., Neyens, H.J., Duiverman, E.J., Roatgeep, H.C. & Kerrebijn, K.F. (1984) Bronchial responsiveness and leucocyte reactivity after influenza vaccine in asthmatic patients. *Eur J Respir Dis* **65**, 196–200.

Edwards, K.M., Dupont, W.D., Westrich, M.K., Plummer, W.D., Palmer, P.S. & Wright, P.F. (1994) A randomized controlled trial of cold-adapted and inactivated vaccines for the prevention of influenza A disease. *J Infect Dis* **169**, 68–76.

Fournier, B., Descamps, V., Bouscarat, F., Crickx, B. & Belaich, S. (1996) Bullous pemphigoid induced by vaccination. *Br J Dermatol* **135**, 153–4.

Fox, R., French, N., Davies, L. *et al.* (1995) Influenza immunisation status and viral respiratory tract infections in patients with chronic airflow limitation. *Respir Med* **89**, 559–61.

Gens, R.D. & Beecham, H.J. (1978) Meningoencephalitis after influenza inoculation. *N Engl J Med* **299**, 721.

Ghirga, G., Ghirga, P., Rodino, P. & Prestl, A. (1991) Safety of the subunit influenza vaccine in asthmatic children, *Vaccine* **9**, 913–14.

Glesby, M.J., Hoover, D.R., Farzadegan, H. *et al.* (1996) The effect of influenza vaccination on human immunodeficiency virus type 1 load; a randomized, double-blind, placebo-controlled study. *J Infect Dis* **174**, 1332–6.

Govaert, T.M.E., Dinant, G.J., Aretz, K., Masurel, N., Sprenger, M.J.W. & Knottnerus, J.A. (1993) Adverse reactions to influenza vaccine in elderly people, randomised double blind placebo controlled trial. *Br Med J* **307**, 988–90.

Grekas, D., Alivanis, P., Kiriazopoulou, V. *et al.* (1993) Influenza vaccination on renal transplant patients is safe and serologically effective. *Int J Clin Pharm Ther Toxicol* **31**, 553–6.

Groothuis, J.R., Lehr, M.V. & Levin, M.J. (1994) Safety and immunogenicity of a purified haemagglutinin antigen in very young high-risk children. *Vaccine* **12**, 139–41.

Gross, P.A., Levandovski, R.A., Russo, C. *et al.* (1994)

Vaccine immune response and side effects with the use of acetaminophen with influenza vaccine. *Clin Diag Lab Immunol* **1**, 134–8.

Gruber, W.C., Belshe, R.B., King, J.C. *et al.* (1996) Evaluation of live attenuated influenza vaccines in children 6–18 months of age, safety, immunogenicity, and efficacy. *J Infect Dis* **173**, 1313–19.

Guerrero, I.C. & Retailleau, H.F. (1979) Increased meningoencephalitis after influenza vaccine. *N Engl J Med* **300**, 565.

Hannan, S.E., May, J.J., Pratt, D.S., Richtsmeier, W.J. & Bertino, J.S. (1988) The effect of whole virus vaccination on theophylline pharmacokinetics. *Am Rev Respir Dis* **137**, 903–6.

Hassan, W.U., Henderson, A.F. & Keaney, N.P. (1992) Influenza vaccination in asthma. *Lancet* **339**, 194.

Honkanen, P.O., Keistinen, T. & Kivela, S.L. (1996) Reactions following administration of influenza vaccine alone or with pneumococcal vaccine to the elderly. *Arch Int Med* **156**, 205–8.

Hurwitz, E.S., Schonberger, L.B. & Nelson, D.B. (1981) Guillain–Barré syndrome and the 1978–1979 influenza vaccine. *N Engl J Med* **304**, 1557–61.

Jani, F.M., Gray, J.P. & Lanham, J. (1994) Influenza vaccine and dermatomyositis. *Vaccine* **12**, 1484.

Kaplan, J.E., Katona, P. & Hurwitz, E.S. (1982) Guillain–Barré syndrome in the United States, 1979-1980 and 1980-1981. Lack of an association with influenza vaccine. *J Am Med Assoc* **248**, 698–700.

Kava, T. & Laitenen, L.A. (1985) Effects of killed and live attenuated influenza vaccine on symptoms and specific airway conductance in asthmatics and healthy subjects. *Allergy* **40**, 42–7.

Kava, T., Lindquist, A., Karjalainen, J. & Laitenen, L. (1987) Unchanged bronchial reactivity after killed influenza virus vaccine in adult asthmatics. *Respiration* **51**, 98–104.

Kendal, A.P., Maassab, H.F., Alexandrova, G.I. & Ghendon, Y.Z. (1981) Development of cold-adapted recombinant live, attenuated influenza A vaccines in the USA and USSR. *Antiviral Res* **1**, 339–65.

Kilbourne, E.D., Couch, R.B., Kasel, J.A. *et al.* (1995) Purified influenza A virus N2 neuraminidase vaccine is immunogenic and non-toxic in humans. *Vaccine* **13**, 1799–803.

Knopf, H.L. (1991) Recurrent uveitis after influenza vaccination. *Ann Ophthalmol* **23**, 213–14.

Knowles, G.K., Taylor, P. & Turner-Warwick, M. (1981) A comparison of antibody responses to Admune inactivated influenza vaccine in serum and respiratory secretions of healthy non-smokers, healthy cigarette smokers and patients with chronic bronchitis. *Br J Dis Chest* **75**, 283–90.

LaMontagne, J.R., Noble, G.R., Quinnan, G.V. *et al.* (1983) Summary of clinical trials of inactivated influenza vaccine. *Rev Infect Dis* **5**, 723–36.

Langmuir, A.D., Bregman, D.J., Kurland, L.T., Nathanson, N. & Victor, M. (1984) An epidemiologic and clinical evaluation of Guillain–Barré syndrome reported in association with the administration of swine influenza vaccines. *Am J Epidemiol* **119**, 841–97.

McIntosh, K., Foy, H.M., Modlin, J.F., Boyer, K.M., Hilman, B.C. & Gross, P.A. (1977) Multi-center two-dose trials of bivalent influenza A vaccines in asthmatic children aged 6–18 years. *J Infect Dis* **136**, S645–7.

Mader, R., Narendran, A., Lewtas, J. *et al.* (1993) Systemic vasculitis following influenza vaccination—report of three cases and literature review. *J Rheumatol* **20**, 1429–31.

Margolis, K.L. (1990) Frequency of adverse reactions after influenza vaccination. *Am J Med* **88**, 27–30.

Margolis, K.L., Nichol, K.L., Poland, G.A. & Pluhar, R.E. (1990) Frequency of adverse reactions to influenza vaccine in the elderly. A randomized, placebo controlled trial. *J Am Med Assoc* **264**, 1139–41.

Miyazaki, C., Nakayama, M., Tanaka, Y. *et al.* (1993) Imunization of institutionalized asthmatic children and patients with psychomotor retardation using live-attenuated cold-adapted reassortment influenza A H1N1, H3N2 and B vaccines. *Vaccine* **11**, 853–8.

MMWR Editorial (1994) Prevention and control of influenza. Part 1. Vaccines. Recommendations of the Advisory Committee on Immunization Practices (ACIP). *MMWR* **43**, 1–13.

MMWR (1996) Prevention and control of influenza. *MMWR* **45** (RR5), 1–24.

Morgan, R. & King, D. (1996) Influenza vaccination in the elderly. *Postgrad Med J* **72**, 339–42.

Murphy, B.R. (1993) Use of live attenuated cold-adapted influenza A reassortant virus vaccines in infants, children, young adults and elderly adults. *Infect Dis Clin Pract* **2**, 174–81.

Murphy, K.R. & Strunk, R.C. (1985) Safe administration of influenza vaccine in asthmatic children hypersensitive to egg proteins. *J Pediatr* **106**, 931–3.

Nichol, K.L., Margolis, K.L., Lind, A. *et al.* (1996) Side effects associated with influenza vaccination in healthy working adults. A randomized, placebo-controlled trial. *Arch Int Med* **156**, 1546–50.

Nicholson, K.G. *et al.* (1979) Clinical studies of monovalent inactivated whole virus and subunit A/USSR/77 (H1N1) vaccine, serological responses and clinical reactions. *J Biol Stand* **7**, 123–36.

Nicholson, K.G., Baker, D.J., Farquar, A., Hurd, D., Kent, J. & Smith, S.H. (1990) Acute upper respiratory tract viral illness and influenza immunization in homes for the elderly. *Epidemiol Infect* **105**, 609–18.

Nicholson, K.G., Nguyen-Van-Tam, J.S., Ahmed, A. *et al.* (1998) Comparison of the effects of inactivated influenza vaccines and placebo on respiratory symptoms, drug use, and pulmonary function in patients with asthma. A multicentre randomised cross over trial. *Lancet* **351**, 326–31.

O'Brien, W.A., Grovit-Ferbas, K., Namazi, A. *et al.* (1995) Human immunodeficiency virus type-1 replication can be increased in peripheral blood of seropositive patients after influenza vaccination. *Blood* **86**, 1082–9.

Ong, E.L.C. (1992) Influenza and asthma. *Lancet* **339**, 367–8.

Ong, E.L.C., Bilton, D., Abbott, J., Webb, K., McCartney, R.A. & Caul, E.O. (1991) Influenza vaccination in adults with cystic fibrosis. *Br Med J* **303**, 557.

Ouellette, J.J. & Reed, C.E. (1965) Increased response of asthmatic subjects to methacholine after influenza vaccine. *Allergy* **36**, 558–63.

Oxford, J.S., McGeoch, D.J., Schild, G.C., Beare, A.S. (1978) Analysis of virion RNA segments and polypeptides of influenza A virus recombinants of defined virulence. *Nature* **273**, 778–9.

Palache, A.M. & Van der Velden, J.W. (1992) Influenza vaccination in asthma. *Lancet* **339**, 741.

Park, C.L., Frank, A.L., Sullivan, M., Jindal, P. & Baxter, B.D. (1996) Influenza vaccination of children during acute asthma exacerbation and concurrent prednisolone therapy. *Pediatrics* **98**, 196–200.

Parkman, P.D., Gallasso, G.J., Top, F.H. & Noble, G.R. (1976) Summary of clinical trials of influenza vaccine. *J Infect Dis* **134**, 100–7.

Patriarca, P.A., Kendal, A.P., Stricof, R.L., Weber, J.A., Meissner, M.K. & Dateno, B. (1983) Influenza vaccination and warfarin or theophylline toxicity in nursing home residents. *N Engl J Med* **308**, 1601–2.

Powers, D.C., Smith, G.E., Anderson, E.L. *et al.* (1995) Influenza A virus vaccines containing purified recombinant H3 hemagglutinin are well tolerated and induce protective immune responses in healthy adults. *J Infect Dis* **171**, 1595–9.

Raj, G., Kumar, R. & McKinney, W.P. (1995) Safety of intramuscular influenza immunisation among patients receiving long-term warfarin anticoagulation. *Arch Int Med* **155**, 1529–31.

Reimer, C.B., Baker, R.S., van Frank, R.M. *et al.* (1967) Purification of large quantities of influenza virus by density gradient centrifugation. *J Virol* **1**, 1207–16.

Renton, K.W., Gray, J.D. & Hall, R.I. (1980) Decreased elimination of theophylline after influenza vaccine. *Canad Med Assoc J* **123**, 288–90.

Robertson, J.S., Nicholson, C., Newman, R., Major, D., Dunleavy, U. & Wood, J.M. (1992) High growth reassortant influenza vaccine viruses. New approaches to their control. *Biologicals* **20**, 213–20.

Roscelli, R.D., Bass, J.W. & Pang, L. (1991) Guillain–Barré syndrome and influenza vaccination in the US army, 1980–88. *Am J Epidemiol* **133**, 952–5.

Rosenberg, G.A. (1970) Meningoencephalitis following influenza vaccination. *N Engl J Med* **283**, 1209.

Rosok, B., Voltersvik, P., Bjerknes, R., Axelsson, M., Haaheim, L.R. & Asjo, B. (1996) Dynamics of HIV-1 replication following influenza vaccination of HIV+ individuals. *Clin Exp Immunol* **104**, 203–7.

Rothbarth, P.H., Kempen, B.M. & Sprenger, M.J.W. (1995) Sense and nonsense of influenza vaccination in asthma and chronic obstructive pulmonary disease. *Am J Respir Crit Care Med* **151**, 1682–6.

Ruben, F.L. (1987) Prevention and control of influenza. Role of vaccine. *Am J Med* **82** (suppl 6A), 31–4.

Rudenko, L.G., Lonskaya, N.I., Klimov, A.I., Vasilieva, R.I. & Ramirez, A. (1996) Clinical and epidemiological evaluation of a live, cold-adapted influenza vaccine for 3–14 year olds. *Bull WHO* **74**, 77–84.

Safranek, T.J., Lawrence, D.N., Kurland, L.T. *et al.* (the Expert Neurology Group) (1991) Reassessment of the association between Guillain–Barré syndrome and receipt of swine influenza vaccine in 1976–77. Results of a two states study. *Am J Epidemiol* **133**, 940–51.

Salk, J.E. (1948) Reactions to concentrated influenza virus vaccines. *J Immunol* **58**, 369–95.

Schonberger, L.B., Bregman, D.J., Sullivan-Bolyai, J.Z. (1979) *et al.* Guillain–Barré syndrome following vaccination in the National Influenza Immunization Program, United States, 1976–1977. *Am J Epidemiol* **110**, 105–23.

Sheth, K.J., Freeman, M.E., Eisenberg, C. & Sedmark, G.V. (1978) Influenza virus immunization. Antibody response and adverse effects in children with renal disease. *J Am Med Assoc* **239**, 2559–61.

Staprans, S.I., Hamilton, B.L., Follansbee, S.E. *et al.* (1996) Activation of virus replication after vaccination of HIV-1 infected individuals. *Clin Exp Immunol* **104**, 203–7.

Stenius-Aarniala, B., Huttunen, J.K., Phytala, R. *et al.* (1986) Lack of clinical exacerbations in adults with chronic asthma after immunisation with killed influenza virus. *Chest* **89**, 786–9.

Warren, W.R. (1956) Encephalopathy due to influenza vaccine. *Arch Int Med* **97**, 803–5.

Watson, J.M., Cordier, J.F. & Nicholson, K.G. (1997) Does influenza immunisation cause exacerbations of chronic airflow obstruction or asthma? *Thorax* **52**, 190–4.

Wiselka, M. (1994) Influenza, diagnosis, management, and prophylaxis. *Br Med J* **308**, 1341–5.

Wiselka, M.J., Kent, J., Cookson, J.B. & Nicholson, K.G. (1993) Impact of respiratory virus infection in patients with chronic chest disease. *Epidemiol Infect* **111**, 337–46.

Wiselka, M.J., Kent, J., Nicholson, K.G. & Stern, M. (1992) Influenza and asthma. *Lancet* **339**, 367–8.

Woods, C.A. & Ellison, G.W. (1968) Encephalopathy following influenza immunization. *J Pediatr* **65**, 745–8.

Yerly, S., Wuderli, W., Wyler, C.A. *et al.* (1994) Influenza immunization of HIV-1-infected individuals does not increase HIV-1 viral load. *AIDS* **8**, 1503–4.

Zeck, R., Solliday, N., Kehoe, N. & Berlin, B. (1976) Respiratory effects of live influenza virus vaccine. *Am Rev Respir Dis* **114**, 1061–7.

CHAPTER 27

Efficacy/Clinical Effectiveness of Inactivated Influenza Virus Vaccines in Adults

Kristin L. Nichol

Impact of influenza

Influenza is associated with a broad spectrum of illness and complications resulting in substantial morbidity and mortality throughout the world. It is estimated that 10–20% of people develop influenza each year (Couch 1993). The classic influenza syndrome experienced by about half of people with influenza is characterized by the abrupt onset of fever sore throat, non-productive cough and myalgias, with symptoms persisting for up to 1 week (Stuart-Harris 1961; LaForce et al. 1994). Unlike many other respiratory illnesses, influenza is not infrequently associated with profound malaise which may last several weeks and often results in restriction of activity (Sullivan et al. 1993). On average, each case of influenza is associated with 5–6 days of restricted activity, 3–4 days of bed disability, and about 3 days of work or school absenteeism (Kavet 1977). Approximately 40–50% of cases are medically attended (Kavet 1977; Couch 1993). The burden to society of influenza illness per se is therefore substantial (Congress of the US, Office of Technology Assessment 1981) and includes the human suffering associated with illness, lost productivity associated with impaired functioning while ill, and increases in school and work absenteeism. During large outbreaks this has resulted in significant disruption to everyday life (Piraino 1970).

The complications of influenza include secondary bacterial illnesses such as otitis media in children and bacterial pneumonia in elderly people (Cate 1987), exacerbations of underlying chronic cardiopulmonary conditions including chronic obstructive lung disease and congestive heart failure (McBean et al. 1993), and death (Collins & Lehmann 1953; Glezen 1982; Barker 1986; Lui & Kendal 1987). Among the elderly population, the risk for hospitalization from respiratory disease during an epidemic may approach 1 in 300 and the risk for dying 1 in 1500 (Couch 1993). In the USA, each year influenza is responsible for millions of work loss days and visits to the doctor (Kavet 1977; Congress of the US Office of Technology Assessment 1981; Sullivan et al. 1993), hundreds of thousands of hospitalizations (Couch 1993; Barker 1986), tens of thousands of excess deaths (Collins & Lehmann 1953; Glezen 1982; Lui & Kendal 1987) and billions of dollars in health-care costs (Williams et al. 1988; Fedson 1992).

Overview of inactivated influenza virus vaccines

Influenza virus vaccines represent the mainstay of efforts around the globe to prevent influenza and its complications. Inactivated vaccines have been gradually developed since the mid-1930s and were first licensed in the USA in 1945. In the 1970s, vaccine formulations were standardized for amount of antigen and types of antigen (usually two type A and one type B) contained in each year's vaccine (Williams & Wood 1993). Recommendations for the antigens to be included in each year's vaccine are made by the World Health Organization (WHO) in co-operation with national public health institutions based on international influenza surveillance data (Cox & Regenery1996). For central Europe, these recommendations are made to the European Union (EU) which then passes on the recommendations to the different national health centres (WHO 1996). In the USA, final recommendations are made by the Food and Drug Administration Vaccines and Related Biological Advisory Committee in collaboration with the Centers for Disease Control and Prevention (Centers for Disease Control and Prevention 1996). Vaccines as currently manufactured are either whole virus or split virus vaccines derived from egg-grown viruses. The whole virus vaccines contain intact, purified, formalin-treated virus. One form of split virus vaccine, the subvirion vaccine, is prepared by purifying chemically disrupted inactivated viruses. Another form of split virus vaccine, the purified surface antigen preparation, is prepared by chemically separating and purifying the surface antigens from the internal proteins of inactivated viruses.

Safety of inactivated influenza vaccines for adults

Early formulations of inactivated influenza virus vaccines were moderately reactogenic (Meiklejohn 1961; Slutzker *et al.* 1963; Davenport *et al.* 1964) but with the advent of improved rate-zonal centrifugation techniques in the late 1960s, subsequent inactivated influenza virus vaccines were found to be associated with substantially reduced rates of side-effects (Peck 1968; Mostow *et al.* 1969). In children, the whole virus formulations of inactivated influenza virus vaccine may be associated with higher rates of side-effects than with the split virus preparations. For this reason, split virus forms of the vaccine are preferred in children (Centers for Disease Control and Prevention 1997). In adults, however, no differences in reaction rates have been observed. Furthermore, recent placebo-controlled trials in elderly people (Margolis *et al.* 1990; Govaert *et al.* 1993) and healthy young adults (Nichol *et al.* 1996) have confirmed that systemic symptoms such as fever, headache and malaise do not occur more frequently following vaccination with split virus vaccines than after receipt of placebo injections. Local symptoms such as arm redness and soreness are experienced more frequently following vaccination, occurring in up to 25% of elderly patients

and 50% or more of younger, healthy adults. These local reactions, however, are generally mild and do not interfere with daily activities.

Following the swine influenza vaccination campaign in 1976, a serious adverse event which was observed following influenza vaccination was the occurrence of Guillain–Barré syndrome. (Safranek 1991). The increase in risk following vaccination was estimated to be approximately 1 per 100 000 persons vaccinated. Since 1976, there has been no clear association between Guillain–Barré syndrome and vaccination with inactivated influenza virus vaccines (Centers for Disease Control and Prevention 1997). Active surveillance programmes continue to monitor for the possibility of this and other serious side-effects which might be associated with vaccination. Even if Guillain–Barré syndrome were a true side-effect following vaccination, the extremely low absolute risk of contracting the illness is less than that for severe influenza that could be prevented by vaccination.

Concerns have recently been raised about another possible adverse effect of influenza vaccination, the impact of vaccination on viral load in people with human immunodeficiency virus (HIV) infection. While some studies have shown a transient increase in viral load following vaccination (O'Brien *et al.* 1995; Staprans *et al.* 1995; Rosok *et al.* 1996) others have not (Yerly *et al.* 1994; Glesby *et al.* 1996). None of the studies has documented a deterioration of clinical status or progression of HIV disease among vaccine recipients. Because people with HIV infection may be at increased risk for severe influenza illness and associated complications, many authorities recommend routine influenza vaccination for them (Centers for Disease Control and Prevention 1997).

Immunogenicity of inactivated influenza virus vaccines in adults

In adults, the whole virus and split virus forms of inactivated influenza virus vaccine are generally considered to have equivalent immunogenicity (La Montagne *et al.* 1983; Gross *et al.* 1987, 1988) and current recommendations support using either virus forms in adult populations (Centers for

Disease Control and Prevention 1997). Some researchers, however, have found evidence that whole virus preparations may be more (McElhaney *et al.* 1993, 1994) or less (Powers 1994) immunogenic than the split virus formulations of vaccine. When administered parenterally (usually intramuscularly) these vaccines induce local and systemic antibody production (Couch 1993; Brokstad *et al.* 1995). Both types of antibody provide protection against infection with the influenza virus, while systemic antibodies may also decrease the intensity of infection. The antibodies produced are type- and strain-specific and confer only varying degrees of protection against other influenza strains, depending on the degree of antigenic similarity between the strains. Cell-mediated immunity also plays an important role in preventing infection and reducing the severity of illness following vaccination.

Studies in healthy young adults confirm that inactivated vaccine induces a rapid systemic and local immune response (Brokstad *et al.* 1995) with up to 90% or more of normal subjects developing protective serum haemagglutination titres (Parkman *et al.* 1976; Wright *et al.* 1976; Cate *et al.* 1983; La Montagne *et al.* 1983; Quinnan *et al.* 1983; Beyer *et al.* 1986; Edwards *et al.* 1994) of ≥ 1 in 40 (Potter 1979) within 2 weeks of vaccination. Peak antibody levels develop within 4-6 weeks (Rastogi *et al.* 1995; Gross *et al.* 1996). Levels then wane over time, being about two-fold lower within 6 months (Cate *et al.* 1983). People with chronic medical conditions such as chronic renal failure (Jordan *et al.* 1973; Pabico *et al.* 1976; Grekas *et al.* 1993) and those who are immunocompromised, including solid organ transplant patients (Blumberg *et al.* 1996) and HIV-positive people (Huang *et al.* 1987; Nelson *et al.* 1988; Miotti *et al.* 1989) may have diminished responses to the vaccine. It has also been suggested that elderly people may also have a diminished response to the vaccine (Provinciali *et al.* 1994), though the results of some of these studies have been conflicting (Beyer *et al.* 1989). Underlying chronic medical conditions rather than age *per se* may be responsible for the lower antibody response seen in some of these studies (Gross *et al.* 1989). Healthy older people appear to have immune responses following vaccination similar to those seen in younger individuals (Gross *et al.* 1987; Gross *et al.* 1988). A recent study of 39 patients with chronic lung disease who were receiving corticosteroids showed that these patients also generated an adequate antibody response, with 84% showing a four-fold rise in antibody titre 1 month after vaccination (Kubiet *et al.* 1996).

Efficacy versus clinical effectiveness of vaccination

When interpreting the results of studies which assess the performance of influenza vaccine in decreasing outcomes, it is essential that several issues be considered. Firstly, the underlying efficacy of influenza vaccine depends on a number of factors. Unique among currently used immunizations, influenza vaccine must be administered each year because of the frequent antigenic changes in circulating strains of influenza viruses. The degree of protection afforded by any year's vaccine will depend on the degree of match between circulating virus strains and vaccine antigens as well as the individual's immune response to the vaccine and previous exposure to influenza antigens (Centers for Disease Control and Prevention 1997). In addition, the likelihood of an individual being exposed to influenza and developing infection will depend on the intensity of influenza activity for the season and in particular settings. Herd immunity may also influence the likelihood of outbreaks (Fox *et al.* 1971; Fox & Elveback 1975). This has been observed clinically in military populations (Davenport 1973), nursing homes (Patriarca *et al.* 1986; Arden *et al.* 1995; Potter *et al.* 1997), and in communities with high vaccination rates of children (Monto *et al.* 1970).

To evaluate the results of outcome studies critically and appropriately, it is also essential to distinguish between observed clinical effectiveness and underlying efficacy (Detsky & Naglie 1990; Fedson 1994). Efficacy refers to the reduction in outcomes evaluated in the context of the highly controlled circumstances of a clinical trial and which are specifically related to influenza, such as laboratory confirmed influenza. Conversely, clinical effectiveness refers to the observed reduction in clinically relevant but relatively non-specific clinical outcomes observed in a more 'real life' context. Only some of these outcomes may actually be related to influenza. For example, studies which assess the effectiveness of vaccination in reducing all pneumonia hospitalizations and deaths from all causes will include many outcomes which are not directly related to influenza. In a hypothetical study in which the observed decrease in outcomes from all causes (such as pneumonia hospitalizations) was 35% among vaccine recipients, the observed clinical effectiveness of vaccination would therefore be 35%. However, if only 40% of all outcomes were actually associated with influenza, then the underlying efficacy of the vaccine in reducing specifically influenza-related disease would be 35/40% or 87.5% (Fig. 27.1). Confusing clinical effectiveness for underlying efficacy results in a substantial underestimation of the actual performance of the vaccine (Fedson 1994). This potential dilution of estimates of vaccine efficacy is especially prominent when the proportion of study outcomes actually caused by influenza is low (Davenport 1973).

Efficacy of inactivated vaccine in young healthy adults

Studies of inactivated influenza virus vaccines among military recruits over 20–30 years of study have provided convincing evidence of the efficacy of vaccination in reducing cases of influenza illness in healthy young adults. They have established the estimates of vaccine efficacy in this group to be

about 70–90% during years when there is a good match between vaccine and circulating virus strains. Among recruits in the US army serial influenza vaccine field trials were carried out over a 30-year period (Davenport 1973). These randomized placebo-controlled trials typically involved thousands of recruits each year. During 14 study seasons, vaccine efficacy for reducing laboratory confirmed illness (culture or serological) was 80–90% for 7 of the study years, and approximately 70% for an additional 5 years. Vaccine efficacy was less than 50% for 2 years when there was a poor match between circulating and vaccine virus strains (Fig. 27.2). After implementing a routine influenza vaccination programme for recruits, the US army experienced a marked reduction in influenza outbreaks.

Similar field trials were carried out among recruits at the Lowry Air Force Base in Denver, between 1952 and 1971 (Meiklejohn 1983). These studies were carried out on groups of 1000–3000 subjects in which recruits were randomly assigned to receive typically monovalent vaccine or placebo. During 10 study seasons, vaccine efficacy in reducing laboratory confirmed influenza was between 72 and 95% for the seven seasons for which there was a good match between the vaccine and circulating virus strains. Vaccine efficacy was lower (60% or less) for the 3 years in which there was a poorer match between vaccine and circulating virus strains due to antigenic drift in two seasons and antigenic shift in one (see Fig. 27.2). The findings of these studies resulted in a policy of routine

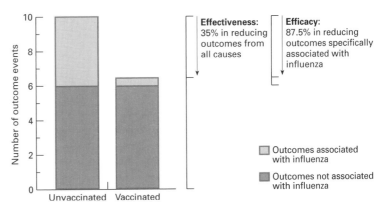

Fig. 27.1 Hypothetical example illustrating the relationship between clinical effectiveness and underlying efficacy. In this case, influenza vaccination was associated with a 35% reduction in all outcomes under evaluation (e.g. hospitalizations for pneumonia). But not all of the outcomes were actually related to influenza. Only 40% of them represented a complication of influenza. Thus, the underlying efficacy of the vaccine for preventing influenza-associated outcomes would be 35/40% = 87.5%.

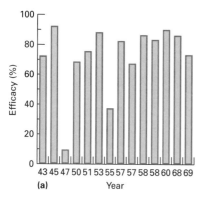
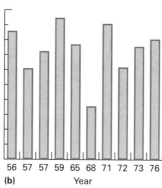

Fig. 27.2 Efficacy of influenza vaccination in healthy young adult populations. (a) US Army field trials. (b) US Air Force field trials. (Data adapted from Davenport 1973 and Meiklejohn 1983.)

influenza immunization for all recruits at the time of induction into the Air Force. This virtually eliminated outbreaks of influenza at the base.

Trials in healthy adult civilian populations have also demonstrated that influenza vaccine is highly efficacious. A clinical trial conducted in Australia in 1976 among medical students and staff demonstrated that vaccination was associated with an 80–90% reduction in laboratory confirmed cases of influenza illness (Hammond 1978). Similarly, placebo-controlled trials in the USA in the 1980s have also shown that immunization with inactivated influenza virus vaccines is associated with an efficacy of 65–80% or more in reducing culture or serologically confirmed influenza during years when there was a good match between vaccine and circulating virus strains (Keitel *et al.* 1986; Edwards *et al.* 1994; Couch *et al.* 1996) with lower rates of protection (40–60%) in years with mismatches between vaccine and epidemic virus antigens (Couch *et al.* 1996).

Clinical effectiveness of inactivated vaccine in healthy adults

The clinical effectiveness of influenza vaccination for such outcomes as respiratory illness and sick leave has also been assessed in a number of studies in healthy adults. These studies provide a glimpse of the health benefits vaccination might provide for a given population by evaluating the effect of vaccination on the kinds of clinical events encountered in everyday life. As discussed above, the estimates for clinical effectiveness of the vaccine derived from these studies must not be confused with estimates of underlying vaccine efficacy.

Controlled trials in the 1950s and 1960s in the UK demonstrated that influenza vaccination with monovalent or bivalent formulations of inactivated vaccine was associated with reductions of work absenteeism due to clinical influenza of 37% (Committee on Influenza and Other Respiratory Virus Vaccines 1964) to 40% (Committee on Clinical Trials of Influenza Vaccine 1953) during years when there was a good match between circulating virus and vaccine strains and no significant reduction during years when there was a poor match (Committee on Clinical Trials of Influenza Vaccine 1957; Committee on Influenza and Other Respiratory Virus Vaccines 1964). In the USA, a controlled trial among industrial employees during the 1968–69 season (Edmondson *et al.* 1971) showed that influenza vaccination with monovalent vaccine resulted in a 74–89% reduction in influenza-like illnesses. Vaccination was also associated with a 72% reduction in the number of influenza-related work absences and a 33% reduction in work loss days due to all illnesses (respiratory and non-respiratory). Similarly dramatic decreases in work absenteeism were seen in a controlled trial conducted in Australia during 1969 (Edmondson *et al.* 1970). In that study, vaccination with bivalent vaccine was associated with an 18.5% reduction in all respiratory illness and a 19.5% reduction in all illnesses. This translated into a 19% decrease in work loss episodes due to all respiratory illness which lasted 2 or more days and a 30% reduction in work loss episodes for all illnesses.

A 5-year study during the early 1970s among postal workers in the UK (Smith *et al.* 1979) also suggested that vaccination reduced sickness absences among vaccinated workers. However, baseline differences in absenteeism between the groups make the findings difficult to interpret. A more recent placebo-controlled trial among health-care workers failed to demonstrate a reduction in clinical illness or absenteeism (Weingarten 1988). This study, however, had a small sample size, and the study year (1985–86) was characterized by a poor match between circulating and vaccine virus strains.

Most recently, a placebo-controlled trial of 849 healthy working adults during the 1994–95 influenza season showed that influenza vaccination resulted in substantial health benefits for this population (Nichol *et al.* 1995). Immunization was associated with a 25% reduction in episodes of self-reported upper respiratory illness, a 43% reduction in sick leave due to all upper respiratory illness, and a 44% reduction in doctor's office visits for upper respiratory illness. These findings are quite similar to those from a randomized controlled trial conducted among employees of the Exxon Company in Houston, Texas. During the 1993–94 influenza A epidemic season, vaccination with the standard trivalent influenza vaccine was associated with an approximate 30% reduction in sickness-related work absenteeism of 1–3 days duration compared to the control group (D.M. Batey, Exxon, March 1997, personal communication).

While clinical trials represent the gold standard for evaluating the benefits of an intervention, observational studies may also shed light on the effectiveness of treatments. A prospective cohort study of university students during the 1971–72 season found that influenza vaccination was associated with a 69% reduction in clinically diagnosed influenza-like illnesses among students reporting to the university health service (Ruben *et al.* 1973). A retrospective cohort study of 2557 employees of a company in the UK during the 1990–91 season showed that, among vaccine recipients, there was a 54% reduction in influenza-like illness and a 50% reduction in sick leave due to influenza-like illness (Leighton *et al.* 1996). The results of these studies must be interpreted with some caution, however,

given their failure to adjust in their statistical analysis for baseline differences between vaccinated and unvaccinated subjects.

Efficacy and effectiveness in elderly people

Only a few trials have studied the efficacy of influenza vaccination in elderly populations for reducing laboratory confirmed outcomes. One of these was a randomized controlled trial conducted among elderly psychiatric patients during the 1968–69 season (Edmondson *et al.* 1971). In this study of 354 subjects, vaccination with monovalent inactivated vaccine was associated with a 62% reduction in laboratory confirmed influenza illness. A recent randomized double-blind placebo-controlled trial in 1838 subjects ages 60 and older in the Netherlands also assessed influenza vaccine efficacy in elderly people (Govaert *et al.* 1994). Vaccination during the 1991–92 season with a quadrivalent inactivated vaccine was associated with a 58% reduction in laboratory confirmed influenza illness.

Several trials in the 1960s evaluated the clinical effectiveness of influenza vaccination in reducing less specific, clinical outcomes which were not confirmed in the laboratory. A randomized controlled trial from 1964 to 1966 comparing monovalent A2 and B influenza vaccines among residents of a California retirement community (Stuart *et al.* 1969) found that vaccination was associated with a 96% reduction in febrile upper respiratory illnesses among subjects who had received vaccine during two consecutive seasons and a 38–55% reduction among people who had received the vaccine during a single season. Vaccination was also associated with a 50–70% reduction in hospitalizations. Another controlled trial in a retirement community in 1968–69 showed a 50–70% reduction in influenza-like illness (Schoenbaum *et al.* 1969). This study demonstrated that vaccination also reduced the severity and duration of symptoms associated with influenza illness.

Numerous observational studies have been conducted among elderly people which provide additional evidence for the clinical effectiveness of influenza immunization in both nursing home populations as well as among community living seniors. Taken together, these studies also suggest that influenza is directly or indirectly associated with a substantial proportion all episodes of respiratory illness, pneumonia, hospitalizations and deaths among elderly people. Much of this influenza-associated morbidity and mortality is undoubtedly often unrecognized as being related to influenza. These studies also highlight the dramatic health benefits at a population level which can be associated with immunization, despite the somewhat lower levels of vaccine efficacy seen in elderly populations when compared with younger adults.

Fig. 27.3 Clinical effectiveness of influenza vaccination in community living elderly. Data represent point estimates with 95% CI for the clinical effectiveness of the vaccine in reducing complications of influenza. (Data adapted from Foster *et al.* 1992; Fedson *et al.* 1993; Mullooly *et al.* 1994; Nichol *et al.* 1994; Fleming *et al.* 1995; Ohmit & Monto 1995; Nichol 1996; see also Table 27.1.)

Case–control and cohort studies from the USA, Canada and the UK have definitively established the health benefits of influenza vaccination in community living senior citizens over numerous seasons (Table 27.1 and Fig. 27.3). A case-control study conducted among elderly enrolees of the Kaiser Permanente Health Maintenance Organization in Portland, Oregon (Mullooly *et al.* 1994) evaluated the effectiveness of influenza vaccination in reducing hospitalizations for pneumonia and influenza and deaths. Pooled estimates for the nine seasons studied (1980–81 to 1988–89) showed that vaccination reduced hospitalization for pneumonia and influenza by 30% for high-risk elderly members and 40% for low-risk elderly members. Vaccination was also associated with a 33% reduction in pneumonia and influenza-related deaths among the high-risk subjects, although this latter did not quite reach statistical significance. Case–control studies from Manitoba for the epidemic years 1982–

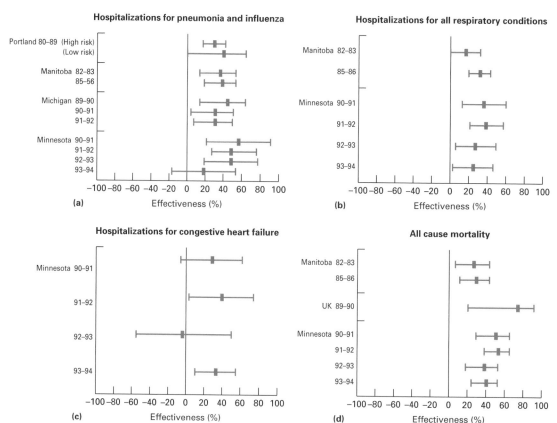

Table 27.1 Clinical effectiveness of influenza vaccination in reducing outcomes among non-institutionalized elderly.*

Outcome	Study	Design	Season(s)	Outbreak strains	Vaccine effectiveness (95% CI)
Hospitalizations for pneumonia and influenza	Portland	Case–control	1980–89	Mixed	30% (17–42%) (high-risk elderly)
					40% (1–64%) (low-risk elderly)
	Manitoba	Case–control	1982–83	H3N2	37% (15–53%)
		Case–control	1985–86	H3N2	39% (19–53%)
	Michigan	Case–control	1989–90	H3N2	45% (14–64%)
		Case–control	1990–91	B	31% (4–51%)
		Case–control	1991–92	H3N2	32% (7–50%)
	Minnesota	Cohort	1990–91	B	57% (21–91%)
		Cohort	1991–92	H3N2	52% (27–76%)
		Cohort	1992–93	B & H3N2	49% (19–78%)
		Cohort	1993–94	H3N2	19% (−17–54%)
Hospitalizations for all respiratory conditions	Manitoba	Case–control	1982–83	H3N2	17% (1–32%)
		Case–control	1985–86	H3N2	32% (20–43%)
	Minnesota	Cohort	1990–91	B	36% (13–59%)
		Cohort	1991–92	H3N2	39% (21–57%)
		Cohort	1992–93	B & H3N2	27% (6–48%)
		Cohort	1993–94	H3N2	25 (3–46%)
Hospitalizations for congestive heart failure	Minnesota	Cohort	1990–91	B	27% (−6–60%)
		Cohort	1991-92	H3N2	38% (2–72%)
		Cohort	1992–93	B & H3N2	−5% (−56–49%)
		Cohort	1993–94	H3N2	32% (9–54%)
Mortality (all causes)	Manitoba	Case–control	1982–83	H3N2	27% (7–42%)
		Case–control	1985–86	H3N2	30% (12–43%)
	UK	Cohort	1989–90	H3N2	75% (21–92%)
	Minnesota	Cohort	1990–91	B	51% (30–65%)
		Cohort	1991–92	H3N2	54% (39–65%)
		Cohort	1992–93	B & H3N2	39% (19–53%)
		Cohort	1993–94	H3N2	41% (25–53%)
Mortality (influenza associated)	UK	Case–control	1989–90	H3N2	41% (13–60%)

* Data have been adapted from Mullooly *et al.* 1994; Fedson *et al.* 1993; Foster *et al.* 1992; Ohmit & Monto 1995; Nichol *et al.* 1994; Nichol 1996; Fleming *et al.* 1995; Ahmed *et al.* 1995.

83 and 1985–86 (Fedson *et al.* 1993) have similarly shown that influenza vaccination of elderly people is associated with 37–39% reductions in hospitalizations for pneumonia and influenza. These studies also demonstrated that immunization was associated with 17–32% reductions in hospitalizations for all respiratory conditions and 27–30% reductions in deaths from all causes. Over the three seasons 1989–90 to 1991–92, serial case-control studies from Michigan (Foster *et al.* 1992; Ohmit & Monto 1995) likewise have found that immunization was 31–45% effective in reducing hospitalizations for pneumonia and influenza. Consecutive cohort studies from Minnesota for the years 1990–91 to 1993–94 (Nichol *et al.* 1994; Nichol 1996) have also shown that influenza vaccination is associated with

reductions in hospitalizations for pneumonia and influenza and for all respiratory conditions as well as a reduction in deaths from all causes. These studies have also demonstrated reductions in hospitalizations for congestive heart failure. The 4-year pooled estimates for vaccine effectiveness from the Minnesota serial cohort studies (Nichol 1996) are:

- 28% (95% CI 12–43%) for hospitalization for congestive heart failure
- 29% (95% CI 19–40%) for hospitalization for all respiratory conditions
- 39% (95% CI 26–56%) for hospitalization for pneumonia and influenza
- 44% (35–51%) for all causes of mortality.

The Minnesota studies also assessed reductions in outpatient visits associated with vaccination. Four-year pooled estimates for these categories were a 7% reduction (95% CI 2–13%) for outpatient visits for all respiratory conditions and a 16% reduction (95% CI 4–28%) in outpatient visits for pneumonia and influenza.

It is of interest to note that among the seasons included in these multiyear studies among community-living elderly people, several included both epidemic and non-epidemic years and influenza A and B seasons. The clinical effectiveness of influenza vaccination was shown not only during epidemic influenza A seasons, but also during non-epidemic influenza B seasons (Nichol *et al.* 1994; Ohmit & Monto 1995). This is not surprising as hospitalization rates for influenza-associated complications increase during non-epidemic seasons as well as during epidemic years (McBean *et al.* 1993).

In addition to the multiyear studies discussed above, two 1-year observational studies from the UK have also demonstrated that influenza vaccination has substantial effectiveness in elderly people. A cohort study of over 10 000 patients aged 55 and older from the computerized data bases of the Royal College of General Practitioners Research Unit in Birmingham (Fleming *et al.* 1995) showed that, during the 1989–90 epidemic, vaccination was associated with a 75% reduction in mortality. Similarly, a case–control study covering the same epidemic year and conducted in 36 district health authorities from five health regions in the England

(Ahmed *et al.* 1995) showed that vaccination reduced influenza-associated mortality by 41%.

Data from 20 cohort studies have been summarized in a recent meta-analysis (Gross *et al.* 1995). These studies have assessed the clinical effectiveness of influenza vaccination in reducing respiratory illness, pneumonia, hospitalizations, and death primarily among nursing home residents. Spanning the years 1965–66 to 1988–89, pooled estimates show that influenza vaccination is associated with a

- 56% (95% CI 39–68%) reduction in respiratory illness
- 53% (95% CI 35–66%) reduction in pneumonia cases
- 48% (95% CI 28–65%) reduction in hospitalizations
- 68% (95% CI 56–76%) reduction in death.

In the nursing home setting, vaccine effectiveness is also associated with the overall vaccination rate achieved in the nursing home. Vaccination rates of 80% or more for residents are associated with more effective degrees of herd immunity and lower rates of nursing home influenza outbreaks (Patriarca *et al.* 1986; Arden *et al.* 1995). Higher rates of vaccination among employees may also provide protection to nursing home residents (Potter *et al.* 1997).

Influence of repeated vaccinations on vaccine effectiveness

The influence of repeated vaccinations on the effectiveness of inactivated influenza vaccines has been a topic of discussion for nearly two decades. Two studies published in the 1970s by Hoskins *et al.* (1979) and Feery *et al.* (1979) called into question the benefits of annual vaccination. However, both studies suffered from methodological and interpretive flaws. The Hoskins study evaluated the effectiveness of inactivated influenza vaccine over several seasons at Christ's Church boarding school for boys. The findings of the Hoskins study are of uncertain significance (Nicholson 1993) because of misinterpretation of statistical significance (the attack rates in the previously vaccinated group, 29/134, did not differ significantly from attack rates in newly vaccinated students, 8/64, with $p = 0.18$ by chi square) and because of a poor match between vaccine and circulating virus strain during the main study season. Furthermore, the generalizability of a study assessing febrile respiratory illness among boys at a boarding school to other populations is uncertain. The study by Feery *et al.* evaluated the effectiveness of influenza vaccination among residents of a geriatric home during the 1975 season. Illness rates among the 154 volunteers (20%) did not differ from illness rates among 63 unvaccinated controls (19%). Severity of illness was, however, lower among vaccine recipients. One explanation offered for the apparent low rate of protection seen in the geriatric group was that the subjects were regular vaccinees. However, these results must also be interpreted with caution. The study had a small sample size and therefore limited power to detect a difference between the two groups; it also lacked randomization.

In contrast to the two studies discussed above, several recent studies have confirmed the effectiveness of repeated influenza vaccinations in adults. A 5-year trial in healthy adults from Houston evaluated first-time and multivaccinated subjects and compared them to placebo recipients (Keitel *et al.* 1986). Over the five study seasons (1983–87) multivaccinated subjects had similar or higher rates of protection than did their first-time vaccine recipient counterparts. Another placebo controlled trial in 1838 elderly subjects from the Netherlands found that previous vaccination was associated with higher rates of protection (relative risk [RR] for previously vaccinated subjects for serologically confirmed influenza 0.11 versus a RR of 0.56 for subjects not previously vaccinated) (Govaert *et al.* 1994). Finally, a case–control study in elderly patients from the UK also demonstrated higher rates of protection among previously vaccinated subjects (odds ratio [OR] for previously vaccinated subjects for influenza-related death 0.25 versus OR of 0.83 for first-time vaccine recipients) (Ahmed *et al.* 1995).

Cost-effectiveness of vaccination with inactivated influenza virus vaccine

Increasingly medical interventions are scrutinized to ensure that they not only provide health benefits to patients, but also that the economic implications of their use are also appropriate. Several studies from different countries have assessed the economic benefits associated with influenza vaccination of elderly people from the medical payer's perspective. The differences in direct medical care costs after subtracting the costs of vaccine and vaccine administration for a single influenza season have consistently shown that influenza vaccination of elderly people results in cost savings (Patriarca *et al.* 1987; Helliwell & Drummond 1988; Maucher & Gambert 1990; Centers for Disease Control and Prevention 1993; Mullooly *et al.* 1994; Nichol *et al.* 1994; Scott & Scott 1996). Other studies of the cost-effectiveness of influenza vaccination have evaluated the economic benefits per year of life saved or per year of healthy life gained. These studies have shown that influenza vaccination is also cost saving per healthy year of life gained (Riddiough *et al.* 1983), and that it is highly cost-effective at only US$145 per year of life saved (Centers for Disease Control and Prevention 1993). For healthy young working adults influenza vaccination is also likely to be highly cost-effective and may also be cost saving when accounting for both direct and indirect costs associated with illness and vaccination (Schoenbaum *et al.* 1976; Riddiough *et al.* 1983; Schoenbaum 1987; Yassi *et al.* 1991; Nichol *et al.* 1995; Levy 1996).

The actual economic benefits associated with influenza vaccination during a given season will depend on a number of factors including
- vaccine efficacy for a given season
- vaccination rates achieved
- costs of vaccine and administration
- influenza clinical attack rates for the season
- local health-care utilization patterns and costs
- the perspective taken for the economic analysis.
Nevertheless, existing data suggest that influenza vaccination compares favourably with other preventive and therapeutic interventions for adults. Few, if any other such interventions, may provide similar health benefits at such low cost or for similar savings (Russell 1992; Fedson 1994).

Conclusion

Influenza is a common disease worldwide, and each year is responsible for substantial morbidity and mortality. Inactivated influenza virus vaccines represent the primary means for preventing influenza and its complications. These vaccines are safe and immunogenic in adults. Most importantly, these vaccines clearly provide significant protection against influenza and its complications to both younger and older adult populations. In younger adults, inactivated vaccines are 70–90% efficacious in preventing laboratory confirmed influenza during seasons in which there is a good match between vaccine and circulating virus strains. In older adult populations, inactivated vaccines may have a somewhat lower efficacy. Nevertheless, they provide dramatic benefits in reducing the complications of influenza including hospitalizations for pneumonia and influenza, all respiratory conditions and congestive heart failure and in reducing deaths from all causes. Vaccination is also cost effective and even cost saving.

The challenge which now remains is to develop and implement effective strategies for optimal utilization of these vaccines. In the USA, despite long-standing national recommendations for their use, 40–50% or more of high-risk targeted populations fail to receive the vaccine each year (Centers for Disease Control and Prevention 1995a,b). Worldwide, influenza vaccine is underutilized, and national policies and recommendations for its use vary widely (Fedson *et al.* 1995; Nicholson *et al.* 1995). Factors which will contribute to enhancing delivery of these vaccines to the populations which stand to benefit include strong national policies and recommendations for their use, appropriate distribution and reimbursement systems, and effective administrative and organizational changes to clinical practice to ensure that vaccine is offered and administered to the targeted groups (Fedson 1992; Fiebach & Beckett 1994; Gyorkos *et al.* 1994). Only then will the promise of these highly effective vaccines be realized.

References

Ahmed, A.E.H., Nicholson, K.G. & Nguyen-Van-Tam, J.S. (1995) Reduction in mortality associated with influenza vaccine during 1989-90 epidemic. *Lancet* **346**, 591–5.

Arden, N., Monto, A.S. & Ohmit, S.E. (1995) Vaccine use and the risk of outbreaks in a sample of nursing homes during an influenza epidemic. *Am J Public Health* **85**, 399–401.

Barker, W.H. (1986) Excess pneumonia and influenza associated hospitalization during influenza epidemics in the USA, 1970-78. *Am J Public Health* **76**, 761–5.

Beyer, W.E.P., Palache, A.M., Baljet, M. & Masurel, N. (1989) Antibody induction by influenza vaccines in the elderly: a review of the literature. *Vaccine* **7**, 385–94.

Beyer, W.E.P., Teunissen, M.W.E., Diepersloot, R.J.A. & Masurel, N. (1986) Immunogenicity and reactogenicity of two doses of a trivalent influenza split vaccine. An open randomized study in healthy, unprotected, adult volunteers. *J Drug Ther Res* **11**, 369–74.

Blumberg, E.A., Albano, C., Pruett, T. *et al.* (1996) The immunogenicity of influenza virus vaccine in solid organ transplant recipients. *Clin Infect Dis* **22**, 295–302.

Brede, H.D. (1995) Influenza vaccines. *Int Arch Allergy Immunol* **108**, 318–20.

Brokstad, K.A., Cox, R.J., Olofsson, J. *et al.* (1995) Parenteral influenza vaccination induces a rapid systemic and local immune response. *J Infect Dis* **171**, 198–203.

Cate, T.R. (1987) Clinical manifestations and consequences of influenza. *Am J Med* **82** (suppl 6A), 15–19.

Cate, T.R., Couch, R.B., Parker, D. & Baxter, B. (1983) Reactogenicity, immunogenicity, and antibody persistence in adults given inactivated influenza virus vaccines, 1978. *Rev Infect Dis* **5**, 737–47.

Centers for Disease Control and Prevention (1993) Final results: Medicare influenza vaccine demonstration-selected states, 1988–1992. *MMWR* **42**, 601–4.

Centers for Disease Control and Prevention (1995a) Assessing adult vaccination status at age 50 years. *MMWR* **44**, 561–3.

Centers for Disease Control and Prevention (1995b) Influenza and pneumococcal vaccination coverage levels among people aged ≥ 65 years—USA, 1973–1993. *MMWR* **44**, 506–7, 513–15.

Centers for Disease Control and Prevention (1996) Update: influenza activity—USA and worldwide, 1995-96 season, and composition of the 1996-97 influenza vaccine. *MMWR* **45**, 326–9.

Centers for Disease Control and Prevention (1997) Prevention and control of influenza. *MMWR* **46** (RR-9).

Collins, S.D. & Lehmann, J. (1953) Excess deaths from chronic disease during influenza epidemics. *Public Health Monographs, US Public Health Service Publication*, no. 213, pp. 1–21. US Government Printing Office, Washington DC.

Committee on Clinical Trials of Influenza Vaccine (1953) Clinical trials of influenza vaccine. A progress report to the Medical Research Council by it Committee on Clinical Trials of Influenza Vaccine. *Br Med J* **2**, 1173–7.

Committee on Clinical Trials of Influenza Vaccine (1957) Clinical trials of influenza vaccine. Third progress report to the Medical Research Council by its Committee on Clinical Trials of Influenza Vaccine. *Br Med J* **2**, 1–7.

Committee on Influenza and Other Respiratory Virus Vaccines (1964) Clinical trials of oil-adjuvant influenza vaccines, 1960–3. Report to the Medical Research Council by its Committee on Influenza and Other Respiratory Virus Vaccines. *Br Med J* **2**, 267–71.

Congress of the US Office of Technology Assessment (1981) *Cost Effectiveness of Influenza Vaccination*, pp. 1–67. US Government Printing Office, Washington DC.

Couch, R.B. (1993) Advances in influenza virus vaccine research. *Ann NY Acad Sci* **685**, 803–12.

Couch, R.B., Keitel, W.A., Cate, T.R. *et al.* (1996) Prevention of influenza virus infections by current inactivated influenza virus vaccines. In: Brown, L.E., Hampson, A.W. & Webster, R.B. (eds) *Options for the Control of Influenza* Vol. 3, pp. 97–106. Elsevier, Amsterdam.

Cox, N.J. & Regnery, H.L. (1996) Global influenza surveillance: tracking a moving target in a rapidly changing world. In: Brown, L.E., Hampson, A.W. & Webster, R.G. (eds) *Options for the Control of Influenza*, Vol. 3, pp. 591–98. Elsevier Science, Amsterdam.

Davenport, F. (1973) Control of influenza. *Med J Aust* **1** (special suppl), 33–8.

Davenport, F.M., Hennessy, A.V., Brandon, F.M. *et al.* (1964) Comparisons of serologic and febrile responses in humans to vaccination with influenza A viruses or their hemagglutinins. *J Lab Clin Med* **63**, 5–13.

Detsky, A.S. & Naglie, I.G. (1990) A clinician's guide to cost-effectiveness analysis. *Ann Intern Med* **113**, 147–54.

Edmondson, K.W., Graham, S.M. & Warburton, M.F. (1970) A clinical trial of influenza vaccine in Canberra. *Med J Aust* **2**, 6–13.

Edmondson, W.P., Rothenberg, R., White, P.W. & Gwaltney, J.M. (1971) A comparison of subcutaneous, nasal, and combined influenza vaccination. II. Protection against natural challenge. *Am J Epidemiol* **93**, 480–6.

Edwards, K.M., Dupont, W.D., Westrich, M.K. *et al.* (1994) A randomized controlled trial of cold-adapted and inactivated vaccines for the prevention of influenza A disease. *J Infect Dis* **169**, 68–76.

Fedson, D.S. (1992) Clinical practice and public policy for influenza and pneumococcal vaccination of the elderly. *Clin Geriatr Med* **8**, 183–99.

Fedson, D.S. (1994) Influenza and pneumococcal vaccination of the elderly: newer vaccines and prospects for clinical benefits at the margin. *Prev Med* 751–5.

Fedson, D.S., Hannoun, C., Leese, J. *et al.* (1995) Influenza vaccination in developed countries, 1980–92. *Vaccine* **13**, 623–7.

Fedson, D.S., Wajda, A., Nicol, J.P. *et al.* (1993) Clinical effectiveness of influenza vaccination in Manitoba. *J Am Med Assoc* **270**, 1956–61.

Feery, B.J., Evered, M.G. & Morrison, E.I. (1979) Different protections rates in various groups of volunteers given subunit influenza virus vaccine in 1976. *J Infect Dis* **139**, 237–41.

Fiebach, N. & Beckett, W. (1994) Prevention of respiratory infections in adults. Influenza and pneumococcal vaccines. *Arch Intern Med* **154**, 2545–7.

Fleming, D.M., Watson, J.M., Nicholas, S. *et al.* (1995) Study of the effectiveness of influenza vaccination in the elderly in the epidemic of 1989–90 using a general practice database. *Epidemiol Infect* **115**, 581–9.

Foster, D.A., Talsma, A., Furumoto-Dawson, A. *et al.* (1992) Influenza vaccine effectiveness in preventing hospitalization for pneumonia in the elderly. *Am J Epidemiol* **136**, 296–307.

Fox, J.P. & Elveback, L.R. (1975) Herd immunity: changing concepts. In: Notkins, A.L. (ed.) *Viral Immunology and Immunopathology*, pp. 273–90. Academic Press, New York.

Fox, J.P., Elveback, L., Scott, W. *et al.* (1971) Herd immunity: basic concept and relevance to public health immunization practices. *Am J Epidemiol* **94**, 179–89.

Glesby, M.J., Hoover, D.R., Farzadegan, H. *et al.* (1996) The effect of influenza vaccination on human immunodeficiency virus type 1 load: a randomized, double-blind, placebo-controlled study. *J Infect Dis* **174**, 1332–6.

Glezen, W.P. (1982) Serious morbidity and mortality associated with influenza epidemics. *Epidemiol Rev* **4**, 25–44.

Govaert, T.M.E., Aretz, K., Masurel, N. *et al.* (1993) Adverse reactions to influenza vaccine in elderly people: a randomised double blind placebo-controlled trial. *Br Med J* **307**, 988–90.

Govaert T.M.E., Thijs, C.T.M.C.N., Masurel, N. *et al.* (1994) The efficacy of influenza vaccination in elderly individuals. A randomized double-blind placebo-controlled tria. *J Am Med Assoc* **272**, 1661–5.

Grekas, D., Alivanis, P., Kiriazopoulou, V. *et al.* (1993) Influenza vaccination in renal transplant patients is safe and serologically effective. *Int J Clin Pharm Ther Toxicol* **31**, 553–6.

Gross, P.A., Hermogenes, A.W., Sacks, H.S. *et al.* (1995) The efficacy of influenza vaccine in elderly people. A meta-analysis and review of the literature. *Ann Intern Med* **123**, 518–27.

Gross, P.A., Quinnan, G.V., Weksler, M.E. *et al.* (1988) Immunization of elderly people with high doses of influenza vaccine. *J Am Geriatr Soc* **36**, 209–12.

Gross, P.A., Quinnan, G.V., Weksler, M.E. *et al.* (1989) Relation of chronic disease and immune respone to influenza vaccine in the elderly. *Vaccine* **7**, 303–8.

Gross, P.A., Russo, C., Teplitzky, M. *et al.* (1996) Time to peak serum antibody response to influenza vaccine in the elderly. *Clin Diag Lab Immunol* **3**, 361–2.

Gross, P.A., Weksler, M.E., Quinnan, G.V. *et al.* (1987) Immunization of elderly people with two doses of influenza vaccine. *J Clin Microbiol* **25**, 1763–5.

Gyorkos, T.W., Tannenbaum, T.N., Abrahamowicz, A. *et al.* (1994) Evaluation of the effectiveness of immunization delivery methods. *Can J Public Health* **85** (suppl 1), 514–30.

Hammond, M.L., Ferris, A.A., Faine, S. *et al.* (1978) Effective protection against influenza after vaccination with subunit vaccine. *Med J Aust* **1**, 301–3.

Helliwell, B.E. & Drummond, M.F. (1988) The costs and benefits of preventing influenza in Ontario's elderly. *Can J Public Health* **79**, 175–9.

Hoskins, T.W., Davies, J.R., Smith, A.J. *et al.* (1979) Assessment of inactivated influenza-A vaccine after three outbreaks of influenza A at Christ's hospital. *Lancet* **1**, 33–5.

Huang, K.L., Ruben, F.L., Rinald, C.R. Jr *et al.* (1987) Antibody responses after influenza and pneumococcal immunization in HIV-infected homosexual men. *J Am Med Assoc* **257**, 2047–50.

Jordan, M.C., Rousseau, W.E., Tegtmeier, G.E. *et al.* (1973) Immunogenicity of inactivated influenza virus vaccine in chronic renal failure. *Ann Intern Med* **79**, 790–4.

Kavet, J.A. (1977) Perspective on the significance of pandemic influenza. *Am J Public Health* **67**, 1063–70.

Keitel, W.A., Cate, T.R. & Couch, R.B. (1986) Efficacy of sequential annual vaccination with inactivated influenza virus vaccine. *Am J Epidemiol* **127**, 353–64.

Kubiet, M.A., Gonzalez-Rothi, R.J., Cottey, R. & Bender, B.S. (1996) Serum antibody response to influenza vaccine in pulmonary patients receiving corticosteroids. *Chest* **110**, 367–70.

LaForce, F.M., Nichol, K.L. & Cox, N.J. (1994) Influenza: virology, epidemiology, disease, and prevention. *Am J Prev Med* **10** (suppl), 31–42.

La Montagne, J.R., Noble, G.R., Quinnan, G.V. *et al.* (1983) Summary of clinical trials of inactivated influenza vaccine—1978. *Rev Infect Dis* **5**, 723–6.

Leighton, L., Williams, M., Aubery, D. & Parker, S.H. (1996) Sickness absence following a campaign of vaccination against influenza in the workplace. *Occup Med* 146–50.

Levy, E. (1996) French economic evaluations of influenza and influenza vaccination. *PharmacoEconomic* **9**, 62–6.

Lui, K. & Kendal, A.P. (1987) Impact of influenza epidemics on mortality in the USA from October 1972 to May 1985. *Am J Public Health* **77**, 712–6.

McBean, A.M., Babish, J.D. & Warren, J.L. (1993) The impact and cost of influenza in the elderly. *Arch Intern Med* **153**, 2105–11.

McElhaney, J.E., Meneilly, G.S., Lechelt, K.E. *et al.* (1993) Antibody response to whole virus and split virus influenza vaccines in successful ageing. *Vaccine* **11**, 1055–60.

McElhaney, J.E., Meneilly, G.S., Lechelt, K.E. & Bleackley, R.C. (1994) Split virus influenza vaccines: do they provide adequate immunity in the elderly? *J Gerontol* **49**, M37–M43.

Margolis, K.L., Nichol, K.L., Poland, G.A. *et al.* (1990) Frequency of adverse reactions to influenza vaccine in the elderly. A randomized, placebo-controlled trial. *J Am Med Assoc* **264**, 1139–41.

Maucher, J.M. & Gambert, S.R. (1990) Cost-effective analysis of influenza vaccination in the elderly. *Age* **13**, 3–9.

Meiklejohn, G.N. (1961) Asian influenza vaccination: dosage, routes, schedules of inoculation, and reactions. *Am Rev Resp Dis* **83** (suppl), 175–7.

Meiklejohn, G. (1983) Viral respiratory disease at Lowry Air Force Base in Denver, 1952–1982. *J Infect Dis* **148**, 775–84.

Miotti, P.G., Nelson, K.E., Dallabetta, G.A. *et al.* (1989) The influence of HIV infection on antibody responses to a two-dose regimen of influenza vaccine. *J Am Med Assoc* **262**, 779–83.

Monto, A.S., Davenport, F.M., Napier, J.A. & Francis, T. (1970) Modification of an outbreak of influenza in Tecumseh, Michigan by vaccination of schoolchildren. *J Infect Dis* **122**, 16–25.

Mostow, S.R., Schoenbaum, S.C. & Dowdle, W.R. (1969) Studies with inactivated influenza vaccine purified by zonal centrifugation. I. Adverse reactions and serological responses. *Bull WHO* **41**, 525–30.

Mullooly, J.P., Bennett, M.D., Hornbrook, M.C. *et al.* (1994) Influenza vaccination programs for elderly people: cost-effectiveness in a health maintenance organization. *Ann Intern Med* **121**, 947–52.

Nelson, K.E., Clements, M.L., Miotti, P. *et al.* (1988) The influence of human immunodeficiency virus (HIV) infection on antibody responses to influenza vaccines. *Ann Intern Med* **109**, 383–8.

Nichol, K.L. (1996) Clinical effectiveness of influenza vaccine in community-living seniors. In: Brown, L.E., Hampson, A.W. & Webster, R.G. (eds) *Options for the Control of Influenza*, Vol. 3, pp. 119–22. Elsevier, Amsterdam.

Nichol, K.L., Lind, A., Margolis, K.L. *et al.* (1995) The effectiveness of vaccination against influenza in healthy, working adults. *N Engl J Med* **333**, 889–93.

Nichol, K.L., Margolis, K.L., Lind, A. *et al.* (1996) Side effects associated with influenza vaccination in healthy working adults. A randomized, placebo-controlled trial. *Arch Intern Med* **156**, 1546–50.

Nichol, K.L., Margolis, K.L., Wuorenma, J. & VonSternberg, T. (1994) The efficacy and cost effectiveness of vaccination against influenza among elderly people living in the community. *N Engl J Med* **331**, 778–84.

Nicholson, K.G. (1993) Annual vaccination: conclusions and recommendations. In: Hannoun, H.C., Kendal, A.P., Klenk, H.D. & Ruben, F.L. (eds), *Options for the Control of Influenza*, Vol. 2, pp. 451–5. Elsevier Science, Amsterdam.

Nicholson, K.G., Snacken, R. & Palache, A.M. (1995) Influenza immunization policies in Europe and the USA. *Vaccine* **13**, 365–9.

O'Brien, W.A., Grovit-Ferbas, K., Namazi, A. *et al.* (1995) Human immunodeficiency virus-type 1 replication can be increased in peripheral blood of seropositive patients after influenza vaccination. *Blood* **86**, 1082–9.

Ohmit, S.E. & Monto, A.S. (1995) Influenza vaccine effectiveness in preventing hospitalization among the elderly during influenza type A and type B seasons. *Int J Epidemiol* **24**, 1240–8.

Pabico, R.C., Douglas, R.G., Betts, R.F. *et al.* (1976) Antibody response to influenza vaccination in renal transplant patients: correlation with allograft function. *Ann Intern Med* **85**, 431–6.

Parkman, P.D., GAlasso, G.J., Top, F.H. & Noble, G.R. (1976) Summary of clinical trials of influenza vaccine. *J Infect Dis* **134**, 100–7.

Patriarca, P.A., Arden, N.H., Koplan, J.P. *et al.* (1987) Prevention and control of type A influenza infections in nursing homes. Benefits and costs of four approaches using vaccination and amantadine. *Ann Intern Med* **107**, 732–40.

Patriarca, P.A., Weber, J.A., Parker, R.A. *et al.* (1986) Risk factors for outbreaks of influenza in nursing homes. *Am J Epidemiol* **124**, 114–19.

Peck, F.B. (1968) Purified influenza virus vaccine: a study of viral reactivity and antigenicity. *J Am Med Assoc* **206**, 2277–82.

Piraino, F.F., Brown, E.M. & Krumbiegel, E.R. (1970) Outbreak of Hong Kong influenza in Milwaukee, winter of 1968–69. *Pub Health Rep* **85**, 140–50.

Potter, C.W. (1979) Determinants of immunity to influenza infection in man. *Br Med J* **35**, 69–75.

Potter, J., Stott, D.J., Roberts, M.A. *et al.* (1997) Influenza vaccination of health care workers in long-term care hospitals reduces the mortality of elderly patients. *J Infect Dis* **175**, 1–6.

Powers, D.C. (1994) Increased immunogenicity of inactivated influenza virus vaccine containing purified surgace antigen compared with whole virus in elderly women. *Clin Diag Lab Immunol* **1**, 16–20.

Provinciali, M., Di Stefano, G., Muzzioli, M. *et al.* (1994) Impaired antibody response to influenza vaccine in institutionalized elderly. *Ann NY Acad Sci* **717**, 307–14.

Quinnan, G.V., Schooley, R., Dolin, R. *et al.* (1983) Serologic responses and systemic reactions in adults after vaccination with monovalent A/USSR/77 and trivalent A/USSR/77, A/Texas/77, B/Hong Kong/72 influenza vaccines. *Rev Infect Dis* **5**, 748–57.

Rastogi, S., Gross, P.A., Bonelli, J. *et al.* (1995) Time to peak serum antibody response to influenza vaccine. *Clin Diag Lab Immunol* **2**, 120–1.

Riddiough, M.A., Sisk, J.E. & Bell, J.C. (1983) Influenza vaccination. Cost-effectiveness and public policy. *J Am Med Assoc* **249**, 3189–95.

Rosok, B., Voltersvik, P., Bjerknes, R. *et al.* (1996) Dynamics of HIV-1 replication following influenza vaccination of HIV+ individuals. *Clin Exp Immunol* **104**, 203–7.

Ruben, F.L., Akers, L.W., Stanley, E.D. & Jackson, G.G. (1973) Protection with split and whole virus vaccines against influenza. *Arch Intern Med* **132**, 568–71.

Russell, L.B. (1992) Opportunity costs in modern medicine. *Health Affairs* **11**, 162–9.

Safranek, T.J., Lawrence, D.N., Kurland, L.T. *et al.* (1991) Reassessment of the association between Guillain–Barré syndrome and receipt of swine influenza vaccine in 1976–1977: results of a two-state study. *Am J Epidemiol* **133**, 940–51.

Schoenbaum, S.C. (1987) Economic impact of influenza: the individual's perspective. *Am J Med* **82** (suppl 6A), 26–30.

Schoenbaum, S.C., McNeil, B.J. & Kavet, J. (1976) The swine-influenza decision. *N Engl J Med* **295**, 759–65.

Schoenbaum, S.C., Mostow, S.R., Dowdle, W.R. *et al.* (1969) Studies with inactivated influenza vaccines purified by zonal centrifugation. *Bull WHO* **41**, 531–5.

Scott, W.G. & Scott, H.M. (1996) Economic evaluation of vaccination against influenza in New Zealand. *PharmacoEconomic* **9**, 51–60.

Slutzker, B., Simon, W. & Saslaw, S. (1963) Reactions to polyvalent influenza virus vaccine in an aged population. *Am J Med Sci* **246**, 162–4.

Smith, J.W. & Pollard, R. (1979) Vaccination against influenza: a 5-year study in the post office. *J Hygiene* **83**, 157–70.

Staprans, S.I., Hamilton, B.L., Follansbee, S.E. *et al.* (1995) Activation of virus replication after vaccination of HIV-1-infected individuals. *J Exp Med* **182**, 1727–37.

Stuart, W.H., Dull, H.B., Newton, L.H. *et al.* (1969) Evaluation of monovalent influenza vaccine in a retirement community during the epidemic of 1965–1966. *J Am Med Assoc* **209**, 232–8.

Stuart-Harris, C.H. (1961) Twenty years of influenza epidemics. *Am Rev Resp Dis* **83** (part 2), 54–61.

Sullivan, K.M., Monto, A.S. & Longini, I.M. (1993) Estimates of the US health impact of influenza. *Am J Public Health* **83**, 1712–16.

Weingarten, S., Staniloff, H., Ault, M. *et al.* (1988) Do hospital employees benefit from the influenza vaccine? A placebo-controlled clinical trial. *J Gen Intern Med* **3**, 32–7.

WHO (1996) Recommended composition of influenza virus vaccines for use in the 1996–97 season. *WHO Weekly Epidemiol Rec* **71**, 57–64.

Williams, M.S. & Wood, J.M. (1993) A brief history of inactivated influenza virus vaccines. In: Hannoun, C., Kendal, A.P., Klenk, H.D. & Ruben F.L. (eds) *Options for the Control of Influenza*, Vol. 2, pp. 169–70. Excerpta Medica, Amsterdam.

Williams, W.W., Hickson, M.A., Kane, M.A. *et al.* (1988) Immunization policies and vaccine coverage among adults. The risk for missed opportunities. *Ann Intern Med* **108**, 616–25.

Wright, P.F., Dolin, R. & La Montagne, J.R. (1976) Summary of clinical trials of influenza vaccines. II. *J Infect Dis* **134**, 633–8.

Yassi, A., Kettner, J., Hammond, G. *et al.* (1991) Effectiveness and cost-effectiveness of an influenza vacci-nation program for health care workers. *Can J Infect Dis* **2**, 101–8.

Yerly, S., Wunderli, W., Wyler, C.A. *et al.* (1994) Influenza immunization of HIV-1-infected individuals does not increase HIV-1 viral load. *AIDS* **8**, 1503–4.

CHAPTER 28

Live Cold-Adapted, Reassortant Influenza Vaccines (USA)

Wendy A. Keitel and Pedro A. Piedra

Introduction

Epidemics of influenza circle the globe on an annual basis. In the USA alone, it is estimated that 20 000–40 000 deaths each year are the result of infections caused by influenza virus; the majority of these occur in the elderly and those with underlying conditions (Centers for Disease Control and Prevention 1996). Current strategies for the prevention of influenza using trivalent inactivated vaccines are targeted at high-risk populations in an attempt to protect these individuals from complications or death associated with influenza. Annual immunization of those at highest risk has had little or no impact on the occurrence of epidemic influenza, and alternative methods will be necessary in order to prevent influenza in large populations. Because the highest attack rates of influenza occur in children (Piedra & Glezen 1991) and children appear to be major 'spreaders' of influenza in the community (Jordan 1961), it is likely that routine immunization of children will be required to dampen or prevent influenza epidemics (Ada *et al.* 1987; Glezen 1996).

One possible approach to the control of influenza is the use of live, attenuated influenza virus vaccines administered intranasally. Several strategies for the production of attenuated vaccines failed to yield safe and immunogenic viruses (e.g. temperature-sensitive, or *ts* mutants; inhibitor-resistant strains; and host range variants) (Beare 1969; Chanock & Murphy 1979, 1980; Stuart-Harris 1980; Tolpin *et al.* 1982; Heilman & La Montagne 1990; Steinhoff *et al.* 1991). In contrast, cold-adapted (*ca*) reassortant (CR) viruses containing the six

internal genes of live, attenuated influenza A/Ann Arbor/6/60 (H2N2) or B/Ann Arbor/1/66, and the haemagglutinin (HA) and neuraminidase (NA) of contemporary wild-type (*wt*) influenza viruses appear to be reliably attenuated and immunogenic. Development of CR vaccines in the USA has continued over the past 30 years (Maassab & DeBorde 1985). The majority of this work has been supported by the US National Institutes of Health. The development and clinical evaluation of CR vaccines in the USA will be summarized in this chapter.

Development of attenuated vaccine viruses

The successful attenuation of several other viruses by means of cold adaptation provided the stimulus for developing a *ca* variant of influenza A virus for use as an attenuated donor strain for the production of vaccine viruses (Maassab 1967). Influenza A/Ann Arbor/6/60 (H2N2) virus was isolated from throat washings in primary chick kidney tissue cultures at 36° C. The virus was adapted to growth at 25° C by passaging at progressively lower temperatures. Virus which grew well at both 25° C and 33° C was then passaged repeatedly in tissue culture and in the allantoic cavity of embryonated hens' eggs at 25° C. The resulting *ca*, *ts* virus was shown to be avirulent when administered to human subjects (Kitayama *et al.* 1973). Similar methods were used to develop the attenuated influenza B virus donor strain, influenza B/Ann Arbor/1/66 (Maassab & DeBorde 1985; Alexandrova *et al.* 1990), although this *wt* parent was more temperature sensitive than the corresponding A/

Ann Arbor *wt* strain. Isolated clones of the master donor strains were selected by means of plaque purification (Maassab 1968).

The procedure for the production of CR vaccine viruses is shown schematically in Fig. 28.1 (Maassab *et al.* 1972; Murphy 1993). In brief, contemporary *wt* viruses which express the desired surface glycoproteins are cloned at 38–40° C (influenza A viruses) or 37° C (influenza B viruses), then plaque purified. Candidate vaccine viruses are generated by means of coinfection of tissue culture cells with the selected *wt* and *ca* donor viruses. This and all subsequent passages occur at 25–33° C. Progeny viruses are then grown in the presence of ferret antisera to the *ca* parent, which inhibits growth of viruses expressing the HA or NA of the attenuated donor. Plaque-purified clones of progeny viruses with the desired characteristics are selected for further evaluation (see below). Only viruses which grow to high titres at 33° C are considered for use as vaccine candidates. Selected clones of vaccine virus are grown in specific pathogen-free chick embryos, and allantoic fluid harvested from the eggs is stored at –60° C or below until use.

Phenotypic and genotypic characteristics of attenuated influenza A/Ann Arbor/6/60 and B/Ann Arbor/1/66, as well as the recombinant vaccine viruses, are outlined in Table 28.1 (Maassab & DeBorde 1985). Growth of the attenuated master strains and recombinants which acquire the six internal genes from the attenuated master strains is restricted at high temperatures. The number of plaques produced at higher temperatures is reduced significantly when compared to growth at 33° C (i.e., they are *ts*). The viruses grow equally well at 25° C and 33° C, reflecting their *ca* phenotype. Small plaque size and acid lability are additional *in vitro* characteristics of vaccine candidates. Intranasal inoculation of ferrets results in minimal or no clinical symptoms, and virus replication is restricted to the upper respiratory tract (Maassab 1969). Attenuation has also been demonstrated in mice, hamsters and infant rats (Mahmud *et al.* 1979; Tannock *et al.* 1984; Snyder *et al.* 1989).

Several general comments can be made regarding the attenuation of CR influenza vaccine viruses. A number of mutations located on each of the six

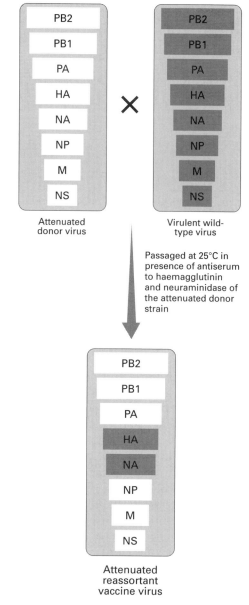

Fig. 28.1 Generation of cold-adapted reassortant influenza virus vaccines. Tissue culture cells are coinfected with attenuated donor virus (*ca* A/Ann Arbor/6/60 or *ca* B/Ann Arbor/1/66) and wild-type virus (influenza A [H3N2 or H1N1] or influenza B) and passaged in the presence of antiserum to the haemagglutinin and neuraminidase of the attenuated donor virus. Reassortants that contain the genes for the surface glycoproteins of the wild-type virus and the six non-surface genes from the attenuated donor (6/2 reassortants) are selected using plaque purification. (Adapted from Murphy 1993.)

Table 28.1 Biological and genetic properties of cold-adapted reassortant (CR) influenza A and B virus vaccines.

Phenotype	Characteristics	Gene(s) associated with indicated phenotype	
		CR influenza A viruses	CR influenza B viruses
Cold adaptation	Efficient growth at 25 °C and 33 °C	PA, PB2 (?)	
Temperature sensitivity	Restriction of growth at 37 °C to 39 °C	PB2, PB1 (?)	PA
Attenuation	Restricted replication in ferret and human respiratory tract; minimal to no illness produced	PB1, PB2, PA and M (gene constellation effect)	PA

internal genes inherited from the attenuated master strains have been identified. Although not all of these mutations confer attenuation, more than one gene contributes to the attenuation of both *ca* master strains. The polygenic nature of the attenuated phenotype is critical: attenuated *ts* vaccine candidates with point mutations reverted to virulence as a result of extragenic suppression and intragenic mutation (Murphy *et al.* 1980b), and point mutations resulted in enhanced virulence of an avian influenza virus (Webster *et al.* 1986). Multiple mutations confer increased stability on the attenuated phenotype. Attenuation of CR vaccine viruses also occurs as a result of gene–gene interactions, or the gene constellation effect (Subbarao *et al.* 1992).

Identification of the precise gene segments and mutations responsible for the *ca*, *ts* and attenuation phenotypes has been attempted using complementation–recombination assays, polyacrylamide gel electrophoresis, gene sequencing, oligonucleotide mapping and polymerase chain reaction amplification (Table 28.1) (Palese & Schulman 1976a,b; Kendal *et al.* 1977; Spring *et al.* 1977a,b; Cox & Kendal 1978; Kendal *et al.* 1981; Odagiri *et al.* 1982; Cox & Kendal 1984; Odagiri *et al.* 1986, 1987; Klimov & Cox 1995). The nucleotide sequences of the internal genes of both *ca* parents have been reported (Cox *et al.* 1988; DeBorde *et al.* 1988). For influenza A/Ann Arbor/6/60, 24 nucleotide differences between *wt* and *ca* viruses were found; 11 amino acid substitutions were predicted for proteins coded by these genes (Cox *et al.* 1988). Non-random reassortment of genes appears to occur during coinfection of cells with *wt* and *ca* master strains. In one study, only 4/64 possible combinations of internal genes were found (Cox *et*

al. 1979). Studies of single gene reassortant viruses, each of which inherited a single internal gene from the *ca* parent and the remaining genes from *wt* influenza A/Korea/1/82, indicated that the polymerase PA gene conferred the *ca* phenotype, and the PB2 and PB1 genes independently specified the *ts* phenotype (Snyder *et al.* 1988). In the same study, four genes from the *ca* donor were found to contribute to attenuation in humans: PA, M, PB2 and PB1. More recently, the roles of PB2 in conferring the *ts* phenotype and of the PA gene in conferring the *ca* phenotype have been questioned (Herlocher *et al.* 1996a,b). Additional studies using reverse genetics experiments should help to elucidate more precisely the genetic bases for the *ca*, *ts* and attenuated phenotypes. For *ca* influenza B/Ann Arbor/1/66, 105 nucleotide substitutions encoding 26 predicted amino acid substitutions were reported to be present in the six internal genes (DeBorde *et al.* 1988). The *ts* phenotype of influenza B/Ann Arbor/1/66 has been shown to be conferred by the PA gene, while attenuation and *ca* phenotypes appear to be polygenic (Donabedian *et al.* 1987, 1988).

Clinical trials of CR vaccine viruses

A summary of CR influenza vaccine viruses developed in the USA is shown in Table 28.2. Only viruses known to possess the six internal genes from the *ca* parent, and the HA and NA from the *wt* parent, are included. Although viruses which inherit less than six of the internal genes from the attenuated donor can be attenuated, safe, immunogenic and protective (Davenport *et al.* 1977; Moritz *et al.* 1980; Reeve *et al.* 1980; Murphy *et al.*

Table 28.2 Summary of cold-adapted reassortant (CR) influenza vaccine viruses (6/2 reassortants) tested in the USA: attenuation, infectivity, immunogenicity and protective efficacy.

Strain designation		Attenuated* vs. wild-type	Median HID†		Percentage shedding‡		Percentage with antibody response§		Efficacy¶		References
			Adults	Children	Adults	Children	Adults	Children	CR	WT	
A/H1N1 viruses											
A/Hong Kong/123/77	CR35	+	5.0	6.0	58	73	100	73	–**	+	Betts *et al.* 1985; Couch *et al.* 1986; Lazar *et al.* 1980; Murphy *et al.* 1980a, 1982; Wright *et al.* 1982; Zahradnik *et al.* 1983
A/California/10/78	CR37	+	6.1	3.5	48	31–100	92	57–89	+	+	Belshe & Van Voris 1984; Belshe *et al.* 1984; Clements & Murphy 1986; Clements *et al.* 1986a, b; Couch *et al.* 1986; Edwards *et al.* 1986; Feldman *et al.* 1985; Gorse *et al.* 1986, 1988; Johnson *et al.* 1985; Murphy *et al.* 1984; Treanor *et al.* 1990; Wright *et al.* 1985
A/Dunedin	CR64	–	5.3	–	22	–	56	60	–	–	Atmar *et al.* 1990; Edwards *et al.* 1994; Garcon *et al.* 1990; Gruber *et al.* 1990; Keitel *et al.* 1994; King *et al.* 1987; Piedra & Glezen 1991; Piedra *et al.* 1993
A/Texas/1/85	CR98	+	4.9	–	60	–	93	55	–	+	Atmar *et al.* 1990; Clover *et al.* 1991; Edwards *et al.* 1994; Piedra & Glezen 1991; Sears *et al.* 1988
A/Kawasaki/9/86	CR125	+	–	2.6	48–83	65–100	64–100	40–100	+	+	Atmar *et al.* 1990, 1995; Belshe *et al.* 1992; Clements *et al.* 1996; Edwards *et al.* 1994; Gorse *et al.* 1995, 1996; Gruber 1996; Gruber *et al.* 1993a, b, 1994, 1996; Karron *et al.* 1995; Keitel *et al.* 1993; Mbawuike 1996; Miyazaki *et al.* 1993; Piedra & Glezen 1991; Piedra *et al.* 1993; Powers *et al.* 1989, 1991, 1992; Steinhoff *et al.* 1991, 1993; Swierkosz *et al.* 1994; Tanaka 1993; Tomoda *et al.* 1994; Younger *et al.* 1994

A/Texas/36/91	—	—	—	—	—	6	—	16	—	+	King 1998; 1997; Treanor et al. 1996
A/H3N3 viruses											
A/Queensland/6/72	CR6	—	—	—	68	—	60	—	—	—	Davenport et al. 1977
A/Alaska/6/77	CR29	+	5.5	—	46	100	67	100	—	+	Clements et al. 1983; Couch et al. 1986; Keitel et al. 1984; Murphy et al. 1981, 1982; Wright et al. 1982
A/Peking/2/79	CR44	—	5.0	—	10	—	72	—	—	—	Betts et al. 1988
A/Washington/80	CR48	+	6.0	3.5	15	29–100	44–85	67–84	+	+	Belshe et al. 1984; Clements & Murphy 1986; Clements et al. 1984a, b, 1985, 1986a, b; Edwards et al. 1986; Feldman et al. 1985; Gorse & Belshe 1991; Gorse et al. 1986, 1988; Johnson et al. 1985, 1986; MRC Advisory Group 1984; Wagner et al. 1987; Wright et al. 1985
A/Korea/1/82	CR59	—	5.5	4.6	56	76–100	22–72	71–100	—	—	Anderson et al. 1989; Atmar et al. 1990; Belshe et al. 1992; Edwards et al. 1994; Garcon et al. 1990; Gorse & Belshe 1990, 1991; Gorse et al. 1991; Gruber et al. 1990; Piedra & Glezen 1991; Piedra et al. 1993
A/Bethesda/1/85	CR90	+	6.4	4.4	0–26	67	18–64	75	+	+	Atmar et al. 1990; Clover et al. 1991; Edwards et al. 1994; Keitel et al. 1993; Mbawuike et al. 1996; Piedra & Glezen, 1991; Piedra et al. 1993; Powers et al. 1991; Sears et al. 1988; Steinhoff et al. 1990, 1993; Treanor et al. 1990, 1992
A/Los Angeles/2/87	CR149	—	—	—	10–67	100	30–44	93–100	—	+	Atmar et al. 1995; Edwards et al. 1994; Gruber et al. 1993a, b, 1994, 1996; Keitel et al. 1993; Mbawuike et al. 1996; Miyazaki et al. 1993; Piedra et al. 1993; Swierkosz et al. 1994; Tanaka et al. 1993; Treanor et al. 1990

Continued

Table 28.2 Continued

Strain designation		Attenuated* vs. wild-type	Median HID†		Percentage shedding‡		Percentage with antibody response§		Efficacy¶		References
			Adults	Children	Adults	Children	Adults	Children	CR	WT	
A/Shanghai/11/87	CR159	–	–	–	–	–	–	–	–	–	Tanaka et al. 1993
A/Beijing/352/89		–	–	–	–	–	–	78–93	–	–	Gorse et al. 1995, 1996; Gruber 1996
A/Shangdong/9/93		–	–	–	–	–	–	92	–	+	Treanor et al. 1992
A/Johannesburg/33/94		–	–	–	–	43	–	90	–	–	King 1998
A/Wuhan/359/95		–	–	–	–	–	–	–	–	–	Belshe et al. 1997
Influenza B viruses											
B/Texas/1/84	CR87	+	5.4	4.5	100	60	59	60	+	–	Anderson et al. 1992; Atmar et al. 1990; Belshe et al. 1992; Keitel et al. 1990
B/Ann Arbor/1/86	CR117	+	6.4	2.5	28–100	90	20–66	84	–	+	Atmar et al. 1990; Clements et al. 1990; Edwards et al. 1991; Gruber et al. 1993a; Keitel et al. 1993; Miyazaki et al. 1993; Treanor et al. 1994
B/Yamagata/16/88	CR165	+	–	–	14	–	64	–	–	–	Atmar et al. 1995; Swierkosz et al. 1994; Tomoda et al. 1994; Treanor & Betts 1993; Treanor et al. 1994
B/Panama/45/90		–	–	–	–	52	–	50	–	+	King 1998; Treanor et al. 1992
B/Harbin/7/94		–	–	–	–	–	–	–	–	–	Belshe et al. 1997

* +, attenuated (less virulent than similar or lower doses of the homologous wild-type virus following experimental challenge of susceptible adults); † median human infectious dose = dose of virus ($TCID_{50}$) required to infect 50% of susceptible subjects; ‡ percentage of subjects with vaccine virus isolated from respiratory secretions following vaccination; § significant rise in serum haemagglutination-inhibition, neutralizing and/or ELISA antibody level following vaccination with one or two doses of vaccine; ¶ protection against infection and/or illness following experimental challenge with CR or wild-type (WT) virus, or upon exposure to naturally occurring WT influenza; **, not reported.

1981; Cate & Couch 1982; Monto *et al.* 1982; Keitel *et al.* 1986), their attenuation is less predictable (Murphy *et al.* 1979; Massaab *et al.* 1982). General requirements for the use of CR vaccine viruses for prevention of influenza in humans have been met; these include attenuation, genetic stability, non-transmissibility, safety, immunogenicity and protective efficacy. Reproducible attenuation of CR vaccines relative to the *wt* parental strains has been demonstrated repeatedly in experimental human challenge studies (Table 28.2). The safety, infectivity, immunogenicity and protective efficacy of CR vaccines when administered to adults and children are reviewed below.

Safety

CR influenza virus vaccines have been administered to approximately 9000 subjects between the ages of 2 months and > 80 years. When given to healthy adults at doses below 100 median human infectious doses (HID_{50}), the vaccines are well tolerated. Minor upper respiratory symptoms such as runny nose or scratchy throat during the week after vaccination typically develop in 5–10% of susceptible adults given monovalent vaccines, although a somewhat higher frequency of respiratory symptoms may occur in subjects who are fully susceptible to the vaccine virus based on serum neutralizing antibody levels (Keitel *et al.* 1990). Mild systemic reactions are reported in less than 5% of subjects in most studies, and fever is unusual. Vaccine viruses shed in respiratory secretions of adults have retained the *ca* and *ts* phenotypes (Maassab *et al.* 1994), and transmission to susceptible contacts has not been documented (Davenport *et al.* 1977; Murphy *et al.* 1980a; Clements *et al.* 1984b; Murphy *et al.* 1984; Couch *et al.* 1986). When bivalent CR influenza virus vaccines were administered to healthy subjects (mostly adults) who had not been selected for susceptibility to the vaccines, a 6–10% excess frequency in mild upper respiratory symptoms was seen in one study (Edwards *et al.* 1994); the frequencies of significant excess systemic complaints including muscle aching, headache and lethargy were 2%, 3% and 5%, respectively. The frequencies of fever, illness or

impaired activity were similar in subjects given monovalent or trivalent vaccine when compared with subjects given a placebo in another study (Atmar *et al.* 1995). Doses exceeding 100 HID_{50} have induced febrile or systemic reactions (Betts *et al.* 1988). Limited studies in groups of adults at high risk for complications associated with influenza, including elderly nursing home residents and patients with asthma, chronic obstructive pulmonary disease and other underlying conditions, have confirmed the favourable safety profile of mono- and bivalent CR vaccines; however, many of these patients were not fully susceptible to infection with the vaccine viruses (MRC Advisory Group 1984; Gorse *et al.* 1986, 1988, 1991; Powers *et al.* 1989, 1991; Atmar *et al.* 1990; Treanor *et al.* 1992, 1994). Deterioration in pulmonary function was not observed in several of these studies. Experimental coadministration of CR and *wt* influenza viruses to humans was safe (Younger *et al.* 1994), and CR virus suppressed replication of *wt* virus *in vitro* (Whitaker-Dowling *et al.* 1990) and clinical disease in ferrets (Whitaker-Dowling *et al.* 1991). CR vaccines have not been studied in pregnant women or in people with immune deficiencies.

Higher levels of replication of CR vaccine viruses in the respiratory tract of susceptible infants and children may allow for a greater possibility of reversion to more virulent viruses. Therefore, a critical test of safety for CR influenza vaccines was to demonstrate attenuation, genetic stability and non-transmissibility in seronegative children. Vaccination of seronegative children with monovalent CR influenza vaccines has been associated with minimal respiratory illness, and transmission of vaccine virus to close contacts has not been documented (Wright *et al.* 1982; Belshe & Van Voris 1984). Partial loss of the *ts* phenotype in Madin–Darby canine kidney (MDCK) cells was observed following vaccination of young children with CR influenza A/Alaska. However, *ts* and *ca* phenotypes were retained in primary chick tissue culture, and evaluation of one isolate in the ferret model system showed that it remained fully attenuated (Wright *et al.* 1982). Two isolates recovered from a child inoculated with CR influenza A/Korea showed partial loss of the *ts* phenotype in embryonated egg; both isolates remained fully attenuated in the ferret model (Anderson *et al.* 1989). Genetic stability as defined by retention of oligonucleotide markers of the CR donor strain was observed in nine out of 10 isolates obtained from seronegative children 5 or more days after vaccination (Cox & Kendal 1984). One isolate lost one and gained another oligonucleotide. These studies demonstrated the relatively high level of phenotypic and genetic stability of CR vaccine viruses. Subsequent studies have confirmed the safety and phenotypic stability of CR vaccine viruses when administered to infants and children as monovalent (Wright *et al.* 1982; Belshe & Van Voris 1984; Belshe *et al.* 1984; Feldman *et al.* 1985; Anderson *et al.* 1989; Steinhoff *et al.* 1990, 1991; Edwards *et al.* 1991; Anderson *et al.* 1992; Karron *et al.* 1995; Clements *et al.* 1996; Gruber *et al.* 1996), bivalent (Wright *et al.* 1985; Gruber *et al.* 1990; Clover *et al.* 1991; Piedra & Glezen 1991; Piedra *et al.* 1993; Gruber *et al.* 1996) or trivalent (Belshe *et al.* 1992; Gruber *et al.* 1993a; Swierkosz *et al.* 1994; King *et al.* 1997) preparations. Safety has also been observed in seropositive high-risk children with pulmonary disease (King *et al.* 1987; Miyazaki *et al.* 1993; Tanaka *et al.* 1993; Gruber *et al.* 1994). Vaccine doses of up to 10^7 TCID$_{50}$ (median tissue culture infectious doses) given as single or multiple doses have been associated with frequencies of respiratory illness that are comparable to those observed in placebo recipients. However, an excess of fever was seen in infants vaccinated with 10^7 TCID$_{50}$ of CR influenza A/Kawasaki (H1N1) virus (Clements *et al.* 1996). Transmission of CR vaccine viruses to close contacts has not been detected in these studies.

Infectivity and immunogenicity

Varying methods for the detection of virus shedding and serum and nasal wash antibody responses, as well as for ascertainment of the degree of susceptibility of subjects to the vaccine virus(es) prior to vaccination make direct comparisons of the results of the numerous clinical CR vaccine studies difficult. Nevertheless, several general comments can be made regarding the infectivity and immunogenicity of CR vaccines in humans. The dose of vaccine virus required to infect humans and to elicit detectable immune responses varies according to a number of factors, including age, prior exposure to related influenza viruses and pre-existing level of immunity. Intrinsic characteristics of the vaccine virus (specifically the viral glycoproteins) have been shown to be important determinants of immunogenicity in mice (Tannock *et al.* 1984; Tao *et al.* 1985). Composition of the inoculum (mono- vs. multivalent preparation) and method of delivery to the respiratory tract (Gruber *et al.* 1993b) are other factors which may affect the infectivity of CR vaccines.

The HID$_{50}$ for several monovalent CR influenza vaccines has been determined in adults and children with low to undetectable levels of serum antibody to the virus (Table 28.2). In each case, the dose of virus required to infect half of susceptible subjects was estimated based upon the occurrence of virus shedding in respiratory secretions and serum antibody responses. For healthy susceptible adults, the HID$_{50}$ ranges between $10^{4.9}$ and $10^{6.4}$ TCID$_{50}$ in MDCK tissue culture. In seronegative children, the HID$_{50}$ is usually at least 10-fold lower than that required to infect adults, and ranges between $10^{2.5}$ and $10^{4.6}$ TCID$_{50}$.

The pattern of vaccine virus shedding among healthy susceptible young adults is characterized by brief duration (usually 1–2 days) and low mean peak titres (< 0.1–2.0 log 10 TCID$_{50}$/ml). CR influenza A/H1N1 viruses have been detected in the respiratory secretions of most susceptible adults during the week after vaccination, but the shedding of CR influenza A/H3N2 vaccine viruses appears to be more variable (Table 28.2). Shedding of CR influenza B vaccine viruses has been detected in 16–100% of subjects (Clements *et al.* 1990; Keitel *et al.* 1990; Treanor & Betts 1993). Serum antibody responses are seen in most healthy susceptible young adults following vaccination with one or two doses containing $10^{6.5}$–10^8 TCID$_{50}$ of CR vaccine viruses (Table 28.2), although the benefit of administering a second dose 1 month after the initial dose to susceptible adults is unclear (Keitel *et al.* 1984; Couch *et al.* 1986; Nicholson *et al.* 1987). When virus shedding and serum antibody responses are both considered, infection rates exceed 75% in most studies.

Lower frequencies of virus shedding and/or serum antibody responses have been seen among subjects given attenuated influenza viruses in bivalent compared with monovalent vaccines (Potter *et al.* 1983; Couch *et al.* 1986), and evidence for interference based on the occurrence of reduced frequencies of virus shedding or serum antibody responses was observed in subjects given trivalent vaccine when compared with subjects given bivalent CR influenza A virus vaccine (Keitel *et al.* 1993). Evidence for non-specific resistance to infection with a heterotypic virus 1 month after initial vaccination was also reported in these studies. Heterotypic resistance to infection has also been observed in mice (Armerding *et al.* 1982; Tannock & Paul 1987). On the other hand, serum haemagglutinin-inhibition (HAI) antibody response

frequencies to the three vaccine viruses were similar among healthy unselected adults given a single dose of trivalent vaccine when compared with groups given the corresponding monovalent vaccines, suggesting that significant reductions in immunogenicity may not occur when individuals are susceptible to only one or two of the viruses in a trivalent vaccine (Atmar *et al.* 1995).

In infants 6 months of age and older who are seronegative to the vaccine strain, mean and peak titres of approximately 10^2 and 10^4 $TCID_{50}$/ml, respectively, are observed after vaccination with monovalent vaccines containing at least 10 HID_{50} (Belshe & Van Voris 1984; Steinhoff *et al.* 1990, 1991; Clements *et al.* 1996). Shedding of CR influenza vaccine viruses usually begins on days 1–3 after inoculation, and continues for a mean of 7–10 days

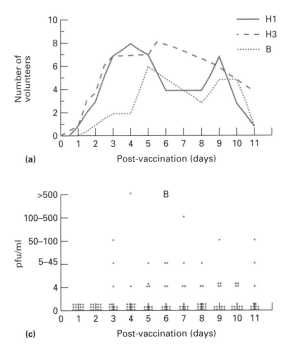

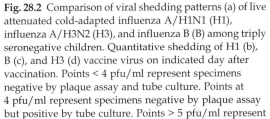

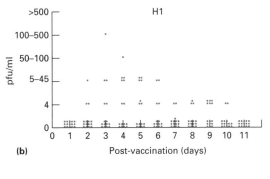

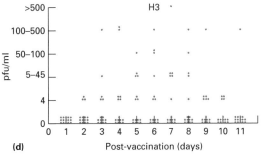

Fig. 28.2 Comparison of viral shedding patterns (a) of live attenuated cold-adapted influenza A/H1N1 (H1), influenza A/H3N2 (H3), and influenza B (B) among triply seronegative children. Quantitative shedding of H1 (b), B (c), and H3 (d) vaccine virus on indicated day after vaccination. Points < 4 pfu/ml represent specimens negative by plaque assay and tube culture. Points at 4 pfu/ml represent specimens negative by plaque assay but positive by tube culture. Points > 5 pfu/ml represent quantitative plaque counts by immunoperoxidase staining of plaque assays. Of the 17 seronegative children who received the live attenuated trivalent cold-adapted influenza vaccine, 10 shed H1, 13 shed H3, and 11 shed B vaccine virus. Out of 17 seronegative vaccinees 16 shed at least one of the vaccine virus strains. pfu, plaque forming units. (Reprinted from Belshe *et al.* 1992, with permission from the University of Chicago Press.)

(Fig. 28.2) Wright *et al.* 1982; Belshe & Van Voris 1984; Feldman *et al.* 1985; Steinhoff *et al.* 1990, 1991; Anderson *et al.* 1992; Belshe *et al.* 1992; Piedra *et al.* 1993). In one study, vaccine viruses were recovered from two subjects 18 and 21 days after vaccination, respectively (Piedra *et al.* 1993). Infection (virus shedding or antibody response) occurs in about 75% of monovalent vaccine recipients, and can vary for strains in multivalent preparations from 30 to 100% after a single dose. Infants under 6 months of age appear to be more resistant to infection with CR viruses: doses which normally produce a high rate of infection in older children have induced lower rates of infection in 2–4-month-old infants (Karron *et al.* 1995). An increase in dose from 10^6 to 10^7 TCID$_{50}$ can overcome this age-related reduction in infection rates (Steinhoff *et al.* 1991; Clements *et al.* 1996). One possible mechanism for reduced infectivity of the CR influenza virus vaccine in young infants is transplacentally acquired, influenza-specific antibody. In infants under 5 months of age, maternally acquired, influenza-specific antibody appears to protect against infection with naturally acquired influenza virus (Puck *et al.* 1980). In infants 6 months of age or older, low levels of influenza-specific antibody presumed to have been acquired transplacentally do not appear to interfere with the infectivity of CR influenza virus vaccine (Anderson *et al.* 1989; Piedra *et al.* 1993). No demonstrable effect on CR influenza virus vaccine infectivity has been observed due to heterosubtypic immunity (resistance to infection conferred by a prior immunity to an influenza virus belonging to another subtype), intercurrent viral infection, or concomitant administration of live polio virus vaccine (Piedra *et al.* 1993; Steinhoff *et al.* 1993; Clements *et al.* 1996).

Interference has been observed in children given multivalent CR influenza virus vaccines when compared with children given the corresponding monovalent vaccines. The frequency of shedding of CR influenza A/Kawasaki (H1N1) vaccine virus when given in combination with CR influenza A/ Bethesda (H3N2) was higher (6/6 infants) than when A/Kawasaki was given in combination with CR influenza A/Los Angeles (H3N2), in which case shedding of the H1N1 vaccine virus was not detected in any of the 10 infants. The A/Kawasaki virus dominated when given in combination with A/Bethesda, and the A/Los Angeles (H3N2) vaccine virus dominated in the second combination (Piedra *et al.* 1993). The dominance of a particular virus may be related in part to differences in the infectivity of the strains contained in the inoculum. In another study, the frequency of infection with the CR influenza B vaccine component based on virus shedding and serum antibody responses was significantly lower in triply seronegative subjects given a trivalent vaccine compared with those given the same dose of the B virus as a monovalent vaccine (Gruber *et al.* 1993a). Increasing the dose of the influenza B component resulted in an increased frequency of virus shedding in subjects given the trivalent vaccine; however, a delay in onset and reduced duration of shedding of CR influenza B vaccine virus were noted in comparison with subjects given the monovalent vaccine. Serum antibody responses to an influenza A/H1N1 vaccine in a bivalent preparation were lower than those observed following inoculation with the monovalent A/H1N1 vaccine in another study (Gruber *et al.* 1996). Vaccination with two doses of trivalent vaccine given 2 months apart increased the cumulative seroconversion rates against each of the vaccine strains to at least 80% in another group of seronegative infants and children (Swierkosz *et al.* 1994). Administration of two doses of a CR influenza virus vaccine containing a high dose of each of the virus strains may overcome the interference that may occur with multivalent preparations.

A direct correlation between viral shedding and induction of virus-specific serum antibody responses has been observed (Belshe & Van Voris 1984; Steinhoff *et al.* 1990, 1991; Edwards *et al.* 1991; Piedra *et al.* 1993; Swierkosz *et al.* 1994; Karron *et al.* 1995; Clements *et al.* 1996). Significant serum antibody responses occur in most seronegative children who are given at least 10 HID$_{50}$ of the vaccine virus and who shed virus after vaccination. The serum antibody response elicited is characteristic of a primary viral infection: serum IgG antibody peaks around 4–12 weeks, while IgA and IgM antibodies peak at 2 weeks and decline by 4–7 weeks (Murphy *et al.* 1982). Serum HAI and enzyme-linked immunoabsorbent assay (ELISA) IgG antibodies to the HA and NA were sustained for at least 12 months (Johnson *et al.* 1985). A similar pattern has been observed by studying the *in vitro* production of antibody by peripheral blood lymphocytes collected from children following vaccination (Edwards *et al.* 1986). Serum IgG1 is the predominant IgG subclass response to the surface HA protein (Garcon *et al.* 1990).

One goal of intranasal vaccination with replicating virus is to induce secretory and systemic immune responses that more closely resemble the immune responses induced by natural influenza virus infections. High frequencies of nasal secretory antibody responses are elicited following intranasal vaccination of susceptible subjects with CR influenza virus vaccines. IgA, IgG and/or IgM have been detected in nasal wash samples collected from both adults and children. Peak responses occur between 2 and 4 weeks after vaccination (Murphy *et al.* 1982; Clements & Murphy 1986). Although nasal wash antibody responses may persist for at least 1 year in some vaccinated children (Johnson *et al.* 1985), significant declines occur within 6 months in healthy and high-risk adults (Clements & Murphy 1986; Powers *et al.* 1989). The live virus vaccine preferentially induces IgA secretory antibody responses, but IgG responses are frequent; some of these IgG responses detected in nasal wash specimens appear to occur as a result of transudation of IgG from serum (Wagner *et al.* 1987). CR influenza virus vaccines have been shown to elicit significant nasal wash antibody responses even when given to adults with pre-existing serum antibody to the vaccine, and nasal wash antibody responses may occur in the absence of serum antibody responses (Clements *et al.* 1985; Gorse *et al.* 1988). In most studies, the frequency of nasal wash IgA antibody responses has been greater in persons given CR vaccine intranasally than in those given standard doses of inactivated vaccine parenterally (Zahradnik *et al.* 1983; Sears *et al.* 1988; Gorse *et al.* 1988, 1991). Conversely, serum antibody responses are stimulated more frequently with inactivated vaccine given parenterally.

Cell-mediated immune responses, particularly influenza virus-specific cytotoxic T lymphocytes (CTL), appear to be important for the recovery from influenza virus infection in animal models, although the role of CTL in human influenza is less well defined. Vaccination of young children and adults with live attenuated influenza virus vaccines has been shown to stimulate lymphocyte proliferation and interferon gamma secretion in response to *in vitro* incubation of peripheral blood mononuclear cells with inactivated virus (Lazar *et al.* 1980; Tomoda *et al.* 1995) and to enhance HLA-restricted virus-specific CTL in healthy and chronically ill older adults (Ennis *et al.* 1981, 1982; Gorse & Belshe 1990, 1991). Coadministration of CR vaccine intranasally and inactivated vaccine parenterally to elderly persons resulted in greater enhancement of CTL activity when compared to immunization with inactivated vaccine alone (Gorse *et al.* 1995). Infants with no prior influenza virus infection failed to develop MHC class I restricted, influenza A virus-specific CTL responses following vaccination with CR influenza virus vaccine, although induction of influenza A virus-specific CTL activity was observed following *wt* influenza A virus infection (Mbawuike *et al.* 1996). Multiple doses of vaccine may be necessary in order to induce antibody and cell-mediated immune responses similar to those which develop after natural influenza virus infection.

Efficacy

The protective efficacy of intranasal vaccination with CR influenza virus vaccines against artificial challenge with *wt* viruses (healthy adults) or CR vaccine viruses (adults and children), or against naturally occurring infection or disease associated with influenza has been demonstrated in a number of clinical trials conducted in a variety of populations (Table 28.2). Vaccination of susceptible adults with CR influenza A and B virus vaccines conferred 78–100% protection against influenza-associated illness following experimental challenge with homologous *wt* virus within 6 months after vaccination (Clements *et al.* 1990; Murphy 1993; Treanor *et al.* 1996); concomitant reductions in virus shedding also occurred in several studies. Significant protection against influenza virus shedding, infection or infection-associated illness caused by naturally occurring influenza has also been demonstrated (Couch *et al.* 1986; Edwards *et al.* 1994). In most cases, the level of protection conferred by CR vaccines has been comparable to that provided by inactivated vaccine during the first year after vaccination, although reductions in shedding after challenge with *wt* or CR vaccine virus have usually been greater in subjects vaccinated with CR viruses than in those given inactivated influenza virus vaccine parenterally (Clements *et al.* 1984a, 1986a; Johnson *et al.* 1986). Administration of CR vaccine to elderly nursing home residents in conjunction with intramuscular immunization with inactivated vaccine has been shown to enhance protection against influenza when compared to immunization with inactivated vaccine alone (Treanor *et al.* 1992); enhanced protection may in part be the result of improved mucosal antibody responses (Gorse *et al.* 1996). In contrast to inactivated influenza virus vaccines, where pre-existing serum antibody levels correlate well with protection against infection (Piedra & Glezen 1991), the correlate(s) of protection against infection conferred by vaccination with CR vaccines are less clearly defined. Serum and nasal antibodies (particularly IgA antibodies in nasal secretions) have both been shown to contribute to protection against challenge with *wt* virus or resistance to infection with vaccine virus (Clements *et al.* 1983, 1986b; Johnson *et al.* 1986; Powers *et al.* 1992), and protection may develop that is independent of evidence of infection with the vaccine virus based on virus shedding or serum antibody response (Betts *et al.* 1985).

Protection of healthy children against epidemic strains similar to the vaccine strain has been demonstrated with mono- and bivalent CR influenza virus vaccines (Wright *et al.* 1982; Belshe *et al.* 1984; Feldman *et al.* 1985). In most of these studies protection against infection was based on serological or illness data. Significant reductions in culture-confirmed infections have been shown in several studies (Piedra *et al.* 1990; Gruber *et al.* 1996). Efficacy was greatest in children under the age of 10 years when compared with older children

(Piedra *et al.* 1990; Clover *et al.* 1991; Piedra & Glezen 1991). Protection induced by vaccination with CR influenza virus vaccines may persist into a second season and may extend to viruses whose HA has 'drifted' from the HA of the vaccine strain (Couch *et al.* 1986; Clover *et al.* 1991; Piedra & Glezen 1991). Fewer data regarding protection conferred against naturally occurring influenza B virus infections are available, although protection of adults against experimental challenge with CR or *wt* virus has been demonstrated for three influenza B viruses (Clements *et al.* 1990; Keitel *et al.* 1990; Treanor *et al.* 1996). A pivotal efficacy study of trivalent CR influenza virus vaccine administered as a nasal spray to healthy 15–72-month-old children is in progress. The overall efficacy for prevention of influenza A/H3N2 and B was 93% during the first year of the trial (Belshe *et al.* 1997).

Unresolved questions

The foregoing data provide support for the concept that CR influenza virus vaccines are safe, immunogenic and protective against influenza; however, additional information would be useful in order to optimize and possibly expand their utility (Table 28.3). Variability in the infectivity or immunogenicity of CR vaccine strains has been observed (Table 28.2), and *in vitro* assays which would predict a high level of immunogenicity are desirable (Gruber *et al.* 1993a; Keitel *et al.* 1994). These assays might also provide information regarding the likelihood of viral interference in multivalent preparations, which can be overcome by means of adjusting the magnitude, sequence or

Table 28.3 Summary of unresolved questions related to the use of cold-adapted reassortant influenza virus vaccines.

Reasons for variability in infectivity/immunogenicity
Identification of reliable means for predicting viral interference in trivalent preparations
Definition of correlates of protection elicited by vaccination
Determination of optimal immunizing regimens in different age groups, including number of doses and schedule
Duration of protection
Breadth of heterotypic immunity induced by vaccination
Definition of target populations for vaccination

number of doses (Gruber 1996). The optimal interval for administration of multiple doses of vaccine needs to be determined if more than one dose is used. Identification of reliable correlates of protection conferred by vaccination would be useful in order to predict the efficacy of new vaccines. Definitive data regarding the duration of protection and the extent of protection provided against heterotypic (drifted) epidemic variants are not available.

Conclusion

The current strategy for prevention and control of influenza can reduce morbidity and mortality in high-risk groups, but the control of epidemic influenza in the community continues to elude us. Immunization of healthy children has the potential to dampen the impact of influenza among individuals and populations. The greatest benefit may be achieved by means of vaccinating healthy children. CR influenza virus vaccines administered intranasally may prove to be safe, effective and well-accepted alternatives to inactivated influenza virus vaccines for prevention of influenza in healthy adults, and valuable adjuncts to inactivated vaccine in order to enhance protection against influenza in certain high-risk populations.

References

Ada, G., Alexandrova, G., Couch, R.B. *et al.* (1987) Progress in the development of influenza vaccines: memorandum from a WHO meeting. *Bull WHO* **65** (3), 289–93.

Alexandrova, G.I., Maassab, H.F., Kendal, A.P. *et al.* (1990) Laboratory properties of cold-adapted influenza B live vaccine strains developed in the US and USSR, and their B/Ann Arbor/1/86 cold-adapted reassortant vaccine candidates. *Vaccine* **8**, 61–4.

Anderson, E.L., Belshe, R.B., Burk, B., Bartram, J. & Maassab, H.F. (1989) Evaluation of cold-recombinant influenza A/Korea (CR-59) virus vaccine in infants. *J Clin Microbiol* **27** (5), 909–14.

Anderson, E.L., Newman, F.K., Maassab, H.F. & Belshe, R.B. (1992) Evaluation of a cold-adapted influenza B/Texas/85 reassortant virus (CRB-87) vaccine in young children. *J Clin Microbiol* **30** (9), 2230–4.

Armerding, D, Rossiter, H., Ghazzouli, I. & Liehl, E. (1982) Evaluation of live and inactivated influenza A virus vaccines in a mouse model. *J Infect Dis* **145** (3), 320–30.

Atmar, R.L., Bloom, K., Keitel, W., Couch, R.B. & Greenberg, S.B. (1990) Effect of live attenuated, cold recombinant (CR) influenza virus vaccines on pulmonary function in healthy and asthmatic adults. *Vaccine* **8**, 217–24.

Atmar, R.L., Keitel, W.A., Cate, T.R., Quarles, J.M. & Couch, R.B. (1995) Comparison of trivalent cold-adapted recombinant (CR) influenza virus vaccine with monovalent CR vaccines in healthy unselected adults. *J Infect Dis* **172**, 253–7.

Beare, A.S. (1969) Laboratory characteristics of attenuated influenza viruses. *Bull WHO* **41**, 595–8.

Belshe, R., Lacuzio, D., Mendelman, P. & Wolff, M. (1997) Efficacy of a trivalent line attenuated intranasal influenza vaccine in children. (abstract). Presented at: *Infectious Diseases Society of America 35th Annual Meeting*, San Francisco.

Belshe, R.B. & Van Voris, L.P. (1984) Cold-recombinant influenza A/California/10/78 (H1N1) virus vaccine (CR-37) in seronegative children: infectivity and efficacy against investigational challenge. *J Infect Dis* **149** (5), 735–40.

Belshe, R.B., Van Voris, L.P., Bartram, J. & Crookshanks, F.K. (1984) Live attenuated influenza A virus vaccines in children: results of a field trial. *J Infect Dis* **150** (6), 834–40.

Belshe, R.B., Swierkosz, E.M., Anderson, E.L., Newman, F.K., Nugent, S.L. & Maassab, H.F. (1992) Immunization of infants and young children with live attenuated trivalent cold recombinant influenza A H1N1, H3N2, and B vaccine. *J Infect Dis* **165**, 727–32.

Betts, R.F., Douglas, R.G. Jr & Murphy, B.R. (1985) Resistance to challenge with influenza A/Hong Kong/123/77 (H1N1) wild-type virus induced by live attenuated A/Hong Kong/123/77 (H1N1) cold-adapted reassortant virus. *J Infect Dis* **151** (4), 744.

Betts, R.F., Douglas, R.G., Maassab, H.F., DeBorde, D.C., Clements, M.L. & Murphy, B.R. (1988) Analysis of virus and host factors in a study of A/Peking/2/79 (H3N2) cold-adapted vaccine recombinant in which vaccine-associated illness occurred in normal volunteers. *J Med Virol* **26**, 175–83.

Cate, T.R. & Couch, R.B. (1982) Live influenza A/Victoria/75 (H3N2) virus vaccines: reactogenicity, immunogenicity, and protection against wild-type virus challenge. *Infect Immun* **38** (1), 141–6.

Centers for Disease Control and Prevention (1996) Prevention and control of influenza: recommendations of the advisory committee on immunization practices (ACIP). *MMWR* **RR-5**, 1–24.

Chanock, R.M. & Murphy, B.R. (1979) Genetic approaches to control of influenza. *Perspect Biol Med* **22** (Part 2), S37–S48.

Chanock, R.M. & Murphy, B.R. (1980) Use of temperature-sensitive and cold-adapted mutant viruses in immunoprophylaxis of acute respiratory tract disease. *Rev Infect Dis* **2** (3), 421–32.

Clements, M.L. & Murphy, B.R. (1986) Development and persistence of local and systemic antibody responses in adults given live attenuated or inactivated influenza A virus vaccine. *J Clin Microbiol* **23** (1), 66–72.

Clements, M.L., O'Donnell, S., Levine, M.M., Chanock, R.M. & Murphy, B.M. (1983) Dose response of A/Alaska/6/77 (H3N2) cold-adapted reassortant vaccine virus in adult volunteers: role of local antibody in resistance to infection with vaccine virus. *Infect Immun* **40** (3), 1044–51.

Clements, M.L., Betts, R.F. & Murphy, B.R. (1984a) Advantage of live attenuated cold-adapted influenza A virus over inactivated vaccine for A/Washington/80 (H3N2) wild-type virus infection. *Lancet* **i**, 705–8.

Clements, M.L., Betts, R.F., Maassab, H.F. & Murphy, B.R. (1984b) Dose response of influenza A/Washington/897/80 (H3N2) cold-adapted reassortant virus in adult volunteers. *J Infect Dis* **149** (5), 814–15.

Clements, M.L., Tierney, E.L. & Murphy, B.R. (1985) Response of seronegative and seropositive adult volunteers to live attenuated cold-adapted reassortant influenza A virus vaccine. *J Clin Microbiol* **21** (6), 997–9.

Clements, M.L, Betts, R.F., Tierney, E.L. & Murphy, B.R. (1986a) Resistance of adults to challenge with influenza A wild-type virus after receiving live or inactivated virus vaccine. *J Clin Microbiol* **23** (1), 73–6.

Clements, M.L., Betts, R.F., Tierney, E.L. & Murphy, B.R. (1986b) Serum and nasal wash antibodies associated with resistance to experimental challenge with influenza A wild-type virus. *J Clin Microbiol* **24** (1), 157–60.

Clements, M.L, Snyder, M.H., Sears, S.D., Maassab, H.F. & Murphy, B.R. (1990) Evaluation of the infectivity, immunogenicity, and efficacy of live cold-adapted influenza B/Ann/Arbor/1/86 reassortant virus vaccine in adult volunteers. *J Infect Dis* **161**, 869–77.

Clements, M.L., Makhene, M.K., Karron, R.A. *et al.* (1996) Effective immunization with live attenuated influenza A virus can be achieved in early infancy. *J Infect Dis* **173**, 44–51.

Clover, R.D., Crawford, S., Glezen, W.P., Taber, L.H., Matson, C. & Couch, R.B. (1991) Comparison of heterotypic protection against influenza A/Taiwan/86 (H1N1) by attenuated and inactivated vaccines to A/Chile/83-like viruses. *J Infect Dis* **163**, 300–30.

Couch, R.B., Quarles, J.M., Cate, T.R. & Zahradnik, J.M. (1986) Clinical trials with live cold-reassortant influenza virus vaccines. In: Kendal, A.P. & Patriarca, P.A. (eds) *Options for the Control of Influenza*, pp. 223–41. Alan R. Liss, Inc, New York.

Cox, N.J. & Kendal, A.P. (1978) Effect of temperature on the order of electrophoretic migration of influenza virus neuraminidase and nucleoprotein genes in acrylamide gels lacking denaturing agents. *J Gen Virol* **40**, 229–32.

Cox, N.J. & Kendal, A.P. (1984) Genetic stability of A/Ann Arbor/6/60 cold-mutant (temperature sensitive) live

influenza virus genes: analysis by oligonucleotide mapping of recombinant vaccine strains before and after replication in volunteers. *J Infect Dis* **149** (2), 194–200.

Cox, N.J., Maassab, H.F. & Kendal, A.P. (1979) Comparative studies of wild-type and cold-mutant (temperature-sensitive) influenza viruses: non-random reassortment of genes during preparation of live virus vaccine candidates by recombination at 25° between recent H3N2 and H1N1 epidemic strains and cold-adapted A/Ann Arbor/6/60. *Virology* **97**, 190–4.

Cox, N.J., Kitame, F., Kendal, A.P., Kendal, A.P., Maassab, H.F. & Naeves, C. (1988) Identification of sequence changes in the cold-adapted, live attenuated influenza vaccine strain, A/Ann Arbor/6/60 (H2N2). *Virology* **167**, 554–67.

Davenport, F.M., Hennessy, A.V., Maassab, H.F. *et al.* (1977) Pilot studies on recombinant cold-adapted live type A and B influenza virus vaccines. *J Infect Dis* **136** (1), 17–25.

DeBorde, D.C., Donabedian, A.M., Herlocher, M., Naeve, C. & Maassab, H.F. (1988) Sequence comparison of wild-type and cold-adapted B/Ann Arbor/1/66 influenza virus genes. *Virology* **163**, 429–43.

Donabedian, A.M., DeBorde, D.C. & Maassab, H.F. (1987) Genetics of cold-adapted B/Ann/Arbor/1/66 influenza virus reassortants: the acidic polymerase (PA) protein gene confers temperature sensitivity and attenuated virulence. *Microb Pathogen* **3**, 97–108.

Donabedian, A.M., DeBorde, D.C., Cook, S., Smitka, C.W. & Maassab, H.F. (1988) A mutation in the PA protein gene of cold-adapted B/Ann/Arbor/1/66 influenza virus associated with reversion of temperature sensitivity and attenuated virulence. *Virology* **163**, 444–51.

Edwards, K.M., Snyder, P., Thompson, J.M., Johnson, P.R. & Wright, P.F. (1986) *In vitro* production of anti-influenza virus antibody after simultaneous administration of H3N2 and H1N1 cold-adapted vaccines in seronegative children. *Vaccine* **4**, 50–4.

Edwards, K.M., King, J.C., Steinhoff, M.C. *et al.* (1991) Safety and immunogenicity of live attenuated cold-adapted influenza B/Ann/Arbor/1/86 reassortant virus vaccine in infants and children. *J Infect Dis* **163**, 740–5.

Edwards, K.M., Dupont, W.D., Westrich, M.K., Plummer, W.D. Jr, Palmer, P.S. & Wright, P.F. (1994) A randomized controlled trial of cold-adapted and inactivated vaccines for the prevention of influenza A disease. *J Infect Dis* **169**, 68–76.

Ennis, F.A., Yi-Hua, Q., Riley, D. *et al.* (1981) HLA-restricted virus-specific cytotoxic T-lymphocyte responses to live and inactivated influenza vaccines. *Lancet* **ii**, 887–91.

Ennis, F.A., Yi-Hua, Q. & Schild, G.C. (1982) Antibody and cytotoxic T lymphocyte responses of humans to live and inactivated influenza vaccines. *J Gen Virol* **58**, 273–81.

Feldman, S., Wright, P.F., Webster, R.G. *et al.* (1985) Use of influenza A virus vaccines in seronegative children: live cold-adapted versus inactivated whole virus. *J Infect Dis* **152** (6), 1212–18.

Garcon, N.M., Groothuis, J., Brown, S., Lauer, B., Pietrobon, P. & Six, H.R. (1990) Serum IgG subclass antibody responses in children vaccinated with influenza virus antigens by live attenuated or inactivated vaccines. *Antiviral Res* **14**, 109–16.

Glezen, W.P. (1996) Emerging infections: pandemic influenza. *Epidemiol Rev* **18** (1), 64–76.

Gorse, G.J. & Belshe, R.B. (1990) Enhancement of anti-influenza cytotoxicity following influenza A virus vaccination in older, chronically ill adults. *J Clin Microbiol* **28** (11), 2539–50.

Gorse, G.J. & Belshe, R.B. (1991) Enhanced lymphoproliferation to influenza A virus following vaccination of older, chronically ill adults with live-attenuated viruses. *Scand J Infect Dis* **23**, 7–17.

Gorse, G.J., Belshe, R.B. & Munn, N.J. (1986) Safety of and serum antibody response to cold-recombinant influenza A and inactivated trivalent influenza virus vaccines in older adults with chronic diseases. *J Clin Microbiol* **24** (3), 336–42.

Gorse, G.J., Belshe, R.B. & Munn, N.J. (1988) Local and systemic antibody responses in high-risk adults given live-attenuated and inactivated influenza A virus vaccines. *J Clin Microbiol* **26** (5), 911–18.

Gorse, G.J., Belshe, R.B. & Munn, N.J. (1991) Superiority of live attenuated compared with inactivated influenza A virus vaccines in older, chronically ill adults. *Chest* **100** (4), 977–84.

Gorse, G.J., Campbell, M.J., Otto, E.E., Powers, D.C., Chambers, G.W. & Newman, F.K. (1995) Increased anti-influenza A virus cytotoxic T cell activity following vaccination of the chronically ill elderly with live attenuated or inactivated influenza virus vaccine. *J Infect Dis* **172**, 1–10.

Gorse, G.J., Otto, E.E., Powers, D.C., Chambers, G.W., Eickhoff, C.S. & Newman, F.K. (1996) Induction of mucosal antibodies by live attenuated and inactivated influenza virus vaccines in the chronically ill elderly. *J Infect Dis* **173**, 285–90.

Gruber, W.C. (1996) Factors important in ensuring immunogenicity of multivalent ca influenza vaccines in young children. In: Brown, L.E., Hampson, A.W. & Webster, R.G. (eds) *Options for the Control of Influenza III*, pp. 622–7. Elsevier Science B.V., Amsterdam.

Gruber, W.C., Taber, L.H., Glezen, W.P. *et al.* (1990) Live attenuated and inactivated influenza vaccine in school-age children. *Am J Dis Child* **144**, 595–600.

Gruber, W.C., Kirschner, K., Tollefson, S. *et al.* (1993a) Comparison of monovalent and trivalent live attenuated influenza vaccines in young children. *J Infect Dis* **168**, 53–60.

Gruber, W.C., Hinson, H.P., Holland, K.L., Thompson, J.M., Reed, G.W. & Wright, P.F. (1993b) Comparative trial of large-particle aerosol and nose drop administration of live attenuated influenza vaccines. *J Infect Dis* **168**, 1282–5.

Gruber, W.C., Campbell, P.W., Thompson, J.M., Reed, G.W., Roberts, B. & Wright, P.F. (1994) Comparison of live attenuated and inactivated influenza vaccines in cystic fibrosis patients and their families: results of a 3-year study. *J Infect Dis* **169**, 241–7.

Gruber, W.C., Belshe, R.B., King, J.C. *et al.* (1996) Evaluation of live attenuated influenza vaccines in children 6–18 months of age: safety, immunogenicity, and efficacy. *J Infect Dis* **173**, 1313–19.

Heilman, C. & La Montagne, J.R. (1990) Influenza: status and prospects for its prevention, therapy, and control. *Ped Clin N Am* **37** (3), 669–88.

Herlocher, M.L., Clavo, A.C. & Maassab, H.F. (1996a) Sequence comparisons of A/AA/6/60 influenza viruses: mutations which may contribute to attenuation. *Virus Res* **42**, 11–25.

Herlocher, M.L., Clavo, A.C., Treanor, J. & Maassab, H.F. (1996b) Phenotypic characteristics of A/AA/6/60 viruses and reassortants. In: Brown, L.E., Hampson, A.W. & Webster, R.G. (eds) *Options for the Control of Influenza III*, pp. 634–46. Elsevier Science B.V., Amsterdam.

Johnson, P.R., Feldman, S., Thompson, J.M., Mahoney, J.D. & Wright, P.F. (1985) Comparison of long-term systemic and secretory antibody responses in children given live attenuated, or inactivated influenza A vaccine. *J Med Virol* **17**, 325–35.

Johnson, P.R., Feldman, S., Thompson, J.M., Mahoney, J.D. & Wright, P.F. (1986) Immunity to influenza A virus infection in young children: a comparison of natural infection, live cold-adapted vaccine, and inactivated vaccine. *J Infect Dis* **154** (1), 121–7.

Jordan, W.S. Jr (1961) The mechanism of spread of Asian influenza. *Am Rev Resp Dis* **83** (Suppl. 2), 29–35.

Karron, R.A., Steinhoff, M.C., Subbarao, E.K. *et al.* (1995) Safety and immunogenicity of a cold-adapted influenza A (H1N1) reassortant virus vaccine administered to infants less than six months of age. *Ped Infect Dis J* **14**, 10–16.

Keitel, W.A., Cate, T.R. & Couch, R.B. (1984) Responses to large, small and booster doses of a live influenza A CR virus vaccine. (abstract). *The 24th Interscience Conference on Antimicrobial Agents and Chemotherapy*, Washington DC.

Keitel, W.A., Cate, T.R. & Couch, R.B. (1986) Evaluation of a cold-recombinant influenza B vaccine. In: Kendal, A.P. & Patriarca, P.A. (eds) *Options for the Control of Influenza*, pp. 287–91. Alan R. Liss, New York.

Keitel, W.A., Couch, R.B., Cate, T.R., Six, H.R. & Baxter, B.D. (1990) Cold recombinant influenza B/Texas/1/84 vaccine virus (CRB 87): attenuation, immunogenicity, and efficacy against homotypic challenge. *J Infect Dis* **161**, 22–6.

Keitel, W.A., Couch, R.B., Quarles, J.M., Cate, T.R., Baxter, B. & Maassab, H.F. (1993) Trivalent attenuated cold-adapted influenza virus vaccine: reduced viral shedding and serum antibody responses in susceptible adults. *J Infect Dis* **167**, 305–11.

Keitel, W.A., Couch, R.B., Cate, T.R. & Maassab, H.F. (1994) Variability of infectivity of cold-adapted recombinant influenza virus vaccines in humans. *J Infect Dis* **169**, 477.

Kendal, A.P., Cox, N.J., Murphy, B.R., Spring, S.B. & Maassab, H.F. (1977) Comparative studies of wild-type and 'cold-mutant' (temperature sensitive) influenza viruses: genealogy of the matrix (M) and non-structural (NS) proteins in recombinant cold-adapted H3N2 viruses. *J Gen Virol* **37**, 145–59.

Kendal, A.P., Maassab, H.F., Alexandrova, G.I. & Ghendon, Y. (1981) Development of cold-adapted recombinant live, attenuated influenza A vaccines in the USA and USSR. *Antiviral Res* **1**, 339–65.

King, J.C. Jr, Gross, P.A., Denning, C.R., Gaerlan, P.F., Wright, P.F. & Quinnan, G.V. Jr (1987) Comparison of live and inactivated influenza vaccine in high risk children. *Vaccine* **5**, 234–8.

King, J.C., Lagos, R., Bernstein, D.I. *et al.* Safety and immunogenicity of low and high doses of trivalent live cold-adapted influenza vaccine administered intranasally as drops of spray to healthy children. *J Infec Dis* (in press).

Kitayama, T., Togo, Y., Hornick, R.B. & Friedwald, W.T. (1973) Low-temperature-adapted influenza A2/AA/6/60 virus vaccine in man. *Infect Immun* **7** (1), 119–22.

Klimov, A.I. & Cox, N.J. (1995) PCR restriction analysis of genome composition and stability of cold-adapted reassortant live influenza vaccines. *J Virol Meth* **52**, 41–9.

Lazar, A., Okabe, N. & Wright, P.F. (1980) Humoral and cellular immune responses of seronegative children vaccinated with a cold-adapted influenza A/HK/123/77 (H1N1) recombinant virus. *Infect Immun* **27** (3), 862–6.

Maassab, H.F. (1967) Adaptation and growth characteristics of influenza virus at 25 °C. *Nature* **213**, 612–14.

Maassab, H.F. (1968) Plaque formation of influenza virus at 25 °C. *Nature* **219**, 645–6.

Maassab, H.F. (1969) Biologic and immunologic characteristics of cold-adapted influenza virus. *J Immunol* **102** (Vol. 3), 728–32.

Maassab, H.F. & DeBorde, D.C. (1985) Development and characterization of cold-adapted viruses for use as live virus vaccines. *Vaccine* **3**, 355–69.

Maassab, H.F., Kendal, A.P. & Davenport, F.M. (1972) Hybrid formation of influenza virus at 25 °C. *Proc Soc Exp Biol Med* **139**, 768–73.

Maassab, H.F., Kendal, A.P., Abrams, G.D. & Monto, A.S. (1982) Evaluation of a cold-recombinant influenza virus vaccine in ferrets. *J Infect Dis* **146** (6), 780–90.

Maassab, H.F., Shaw, M.W. & Heilman, C.A. (1994) Live influenza virus vaccine. In: Plotkin, S.A. & Mortimer, E.A. (eds) *Vaccines*, pp. 781–801. WB Saunders Company, Philadelphia.

Mahmud, M.I.A., Maassab, H.F., Jennings, R. & Potter, C.W. (1979) Influenza virus infection of newborn rats: virulence of recombinant strains prepared from a cold-adapted, attenuated parent. *Arch Virol* **61**, 207–16.

Mbawuike, I.N., Piedra, P.A., Cate, T.R. & Couch, R.B. (1996) Cytotoxic T-lymphocyte responses of infants after natural infection or immunization with live cold-recombinant or inactivated influenza A virus vaccine. *J Med Virol* **50**, 105–11.

Miyazaki, C., Nakayama, M., Tanaka, Y. *et al.* (1993) Immunization of institutionalized asthmatic children and patients with psychomotor retardation using live attenuated cold-adapted reassortant influenza A H1N1, H3N2 and B vaccines. *Vaccine* **11**, 853–8.

Monto, A.S., Miller, F.D. & Maassab, H.F. (1982) Evaluation of an attenuated, cold-recombinant influenza B virus vaccine. *J Infect Dis* **145** (1), 57–64.

Moritz, A.J., Kunz, C., Hofman, H., Liehl, E., Reeve, P. & Maassab, H.F. (1980) Studies with a cold-recombinant A/Victoria/3/75 (H3N2) virus. II. Evaluation in adult volunteers. *J Infect Dis* **142** (6), 857–60.

MRC Advisory Group on Pulmonary Function Tests in Relation to Live Influenza Vaccines (1984) Trials of live attenuated influenza virus vaccine in patients with chronic obstructive airways disease. *Br J Dis Chest* **78**, 236–47.

Murphy, B.R. (1993) Use of live attenuated cold-adapted influenza A reassortant virus vaccines in infants, children, young adults, and elderly adults. *Infect Dis Clin Pract* **2**, 174–81.

Murphy, B.R., Holley, H.P. Jr, Berquist, E.J. *et al.* (1979) Cold-adapted variants of influenza A virus: evaluation in adult seronegative volunteers of A/Scotland/840/74 and A/Victoria/3/75 cold-adapted recombinants derived from the cold-adapted A/Ann Arbor/6/60 strain. *Infect Immun* **23** (2), 253–9.

Murphy, B.R., Rennels, M.B., Douglas, R.G. *et al.* (1980a) Evaluation of influenza A/Hong Kong/123/77 (H1N1) *ts*-1A2 and cold-adapted recombinant viruses in seronegative adult volunteers. *Infect Immun* **29** (2), 348–55.

Murphy, B.R., Tolpin, M.D., Massicot, J.G., Kim, H.Y., Parrott, R.H. & Chanock, R.M. (1980b) Escape of a highly defective influenza A virus mutant from its temperature sensitive phenotype by extragenic suppression and other types of mutation. *Ann NY Acad Sci* **354**, 172–82.

Murphy, B.R., Chanock, R.M., Clements, M.L. *et al.* (1981) Evaluation of A/Alaska/6/77 (H3N2) cold-adapted recombinant viruses derived from A/Ann Arbor/6/60 cold-adapted donor virus in adult seronegative volunteers. *Infect Immun* **32** (2), 693–7.

Murphy, B.R., Nelson, D.L., Wright, P.F., Tierney, E.L., Phelan, M.A. & Chanock, R.M. (1982) Secretory and systemic immunological response in children infected with live attenuated influenza A virus vaccines. *Infect Immun* **36** (3), 1102–8.

Murphy, B.R., Clements, M.L., Madore, H.P. *et al.* (1984) Dose response of cold-adapted, reassortant influenza A/California/10/78 virus (H1N1) in adult volunteers. *J Infect Dis* **149** (5), 816.

Nicholson, K.G., Tyrrell, D.A.J., Oxford, J.S. *et al.* (1987) Infectivity and reactogenicity of reassortant cold-adapted influenza A/Korea/1/82 vaccines obtained from the USA and USSR. *Bull WHO* **65** (3), 2095–301.

Odagiri, T., DeBorde, D.C. & Maassab, H.F. (1982) Cold-adapted recombinants of influenza A virus in MDCK cells. I. Development and characterization of A/Ann Arbor/6/60 X A/Alaska/6/77 recombinant viruses. *Virology* **119**, 82–95.

Odagiri, T. Tosaka, A., Ishida, N. & Maassab, H.F. (1986) Biological characteristics of a cold-adapted influenza A virus mutation residing on a polymerase gene. *Arch Virol* **88**, 91–104.

Odagiri, T., Tanaka, T. & Tobita, K. (1987) Temperature-sensitive defect of influenza A/Ann Arbor/6/60 cold-adapted variant leads to a blockage of matrix polypeptide incorporation into the plasma membrane of the infected cells. *Virus Res* **7**, 203–18.

Palese, P. & Schulman, J.L. (1976a) Differences in RNA patterns of influenza A viruses. *J Virol* **17** (3), 876–84.

Palese, P. & Schulman, J.L. (1976b) Mapping of the influenza virus genome: identification of the hemagglutinin and the neuraminidase genes. *Proc Natl Acad Sci USA* **73** (6), 2142–6.

Piedra, P.A. & Glezen, W.P. (1991) Influenza in children: epidemiology, immunity, and vaccines. *Sem Ped Infect Dis* **2** (2), 140–6.

Piedra, P.A., Taber, L.H., Englund, J. & Glezen, W.P. (1990) Efficacy of cold recombinant (CR) influenza A vaccine in children is age dependent and associated with serotype antibody responses (abstract). 30th Interscience Conference Antimicrobial Agents and Chemotherapy. Atlanta, GA.

Piedra, P.A., Glezen, W.P., Mbawuike, I. *et al.* (1993) Studies on reactogenicity and immunogenicity of attenuated bivalent cold recombinant influenza type A (CRA) and inactivated trivalent influenza virus (TI) vaccines in infants and young children. *Vaccine* **11**, 718–24.

Potter, C.W., Jennings, R., Clark, A. & Ali, M. (1983) Interference following dual inoculation with influenza A (H3N2) and (H1N1) viruses in ferrets and volunteers. *J Med Virol* **11**, 77–86.

Powers, D.C., Sears, S.D., Murphy, B.R., Thumar, B. & Clements, M.L. (1989) Systemic and local antibody responses in elderly subjects given live or inactivated influenza A virus vaccines. *J Clin Microbiol* **27** (12), 2666–71.

Powers, D.C., Fries, L.F., Murphy, B.R., Thumar, B. & Clements, M.L. (1991) In elderly persons live attenuated influenza A virus vaccines do not offer an advantage over inactivated virus vaccine in inducing serum or secretory antibodies or local immunologic memory. *J Clin Microbiol* **29** (3), 498–505.

Powers, D.C., Murphy, B.R., Fries, M.F., Adler, W.H. & Clements, M.L. (1992) Reduced infectivity of cold-adapted influenza A/H1N1 viruses in the elderly: correlation with serum and local antibodies. *J Am Geriatr Soc* **40**, 163–7.

Puck, J.M., Glezen, W.P., Frank, A.L. & Six, H.R. (1980) Protection of infants from infection with influenza A virus by transplacentally acquired antibody. *J Infect Dis* **142** (6), 844.

Reeve, P., Almond, J.W., Felsenreich, V., Pibermann, M. & Maassab, H.F. (1980) Studies with a cold-recombinant A/Victoria/3/75 (H3N2) virus. I. Biologic, genetic, and biochemical characterization. *J Infect Dis* **142** (6), 850–6.

Sears, S.D., Clements, M.L., Betts, R.F., Maassab, H.F., Murphy, B.R. & Snyder, M.H. (1988) Comparison of live, attenuated H1N1 and H3N2 cold-adapted and avian–human influenza A reassortant viruses and inactivated virus vaccine in adults. *J Infect Dis* **158** (6), 1209–19.

Snyder, M.H., Betts, R.F., DeBorde, D. *et al.* (1988) Four viral genes independently contribute to attenuation of live influenza A/Ann Arbor/6/60 (H2N2) cold-adapted reassortant virus vaccines. *J Virol* **62** (2), 488–95.

Snyder, M.H., London, W.T., Maassab, H.F. & Murphy, B.R. (1989) Attenuation and phenotypic stability of influenza B/Texas/1/84 cold-adapted reassortant virus: studies in hamsters and chimpanzees. *J Infect Dis* **160** (4), 604–10.

Spring, S.B., Maassab, H.F., Kendal, A.P., Murphy, B.R. & Chanock, R.M. (1977a) Cold-adapted variants of influenza virus A. *Virology* **77**, 337–43.

Spring, S.B., Maassab, H.F., Kendal, A.P., Murphy, B.R. & Chanock, R.M. (1977b) Cold adapted variants of influenza A. II. Comparison of the genetic and biologic properties of ts mutants and recombinants of the cold adapted A/AA/6/60 strain. *Arch Virol* **55**, 233–46.

Steinhoff, M.C., Halsey, N.A., Wilson, M.H. *et al.* (1990) Comparison of live attenuated cold-adapted and avian–human influenza A/Bethesda/85 (H3N2) reassortant virus vaccines in infants and children. *J Infect Dis* **162**, 394–401.

Steinhoff, M.C., Halsey, N.A., Fries, L.F. *et al.* (1991) The A/Mallard/6750/78 avian–human, but not the A/Ann Arbor/6/60 cold-adapted, influenza A/Kawasaki/86 (H1N1) reassortant virus vaccine retains partial virulence for infants and children. *J Infect Dis* **163**, 1023–8.

Steinhoff, M.C., Fries, L.F., Karron, R.A., Clements, M.L. & Murphy, B.R. (1993) Effect of heterosubtypic immunity on infection with attenuated influenza A virus vaccines in young children. *J Clin Microbiol* **31** (4), 836–8.

Stuart-Harris, C. (1980) The present status of live influenza virus vaccine. *J Infect Dis* **142** (5), 784–93.

Subbarao, E.K., Perkins, M., Treanor, J.J. & Murphy, B.R. (1992) The attenuation of phenotype conferred by the M gene of the influenza A/Ann Arbor/6/60 cold-adapted virus (H2N2) on the A/Korea/82 (H3N2) reassortant virus results from a gene constellation effect. *Virus Res* **25**, 37–50.

Swierkosz, E.M., Newman, F.K., Anderson, E.L., Nugent, S.L., Mills, G.B. & Belshe, R.B. (1994) Multidose, live attenuated, cold-recombinant, trivalent influenza vaccine in infants and young children. *J Infect Dis* **169**, 1121–4.

Tanaka, Y., Ueda, K., Miyazaki, C. *et al.* (1993) Trivalent cold recombinant influenza live vaccine in institutionalized children with bronchial asthma and patients with psychomotor retardation. *Ped Infect Dis J* **12** (7), 600–5.

Tannock, G.A. & Paul, J.A. (1987) Homotypic and heterotypic immunity of influenza A viruses induced by recombinants of the cold-adapted master strain A/Ann Arbor/6/60-c. *Arch Virol* **92**, 121–33.

Tannock, G.A., Paul, J.A. & Barry, R.D. (1984) Relative immunogenicity of the cold-adapted influenza virus A/Ann Arbor/6/60 (A/AA/6/60-c.), recombinants of A/AA/6/60-c., and parental strains with similar surface antigens. *Infect Immun* **43** (2), 457–62.

Tao, S.J., Mak, N.K. & Ada, G.L. (1985) Sensitization of mice with wild-type and cold-adapted influenza virus variants: immune response to two H1N1 and H3N2 viruses. *J Virol* **53** (2), 645–50.

Tolpin, M.D., Clements, M.L., Levine, M.M. *et al.* (1982) Evaluation of a phenotypic revertant of the A/Alaska/77-*ts*-1A2 reassortant virus in hamsters and in seronegative adult volunteers: further evidence that the temperature-sensitive phenotype is responsible for attenuation of *ts*-1A2 reassortant viruses. *Infect Immun* **36** (2), 645–50.

Tomoda, T., Morita, H., Kurashige, T. & Maassab, H.F. (1995) Prevention of influenza by the intranasal administration of cold-recombinant, live-attenuated influenza virus vaccine: importance of interferon-γ production and local IgA response. *Vaccine* **13** (2), 185–90.

Treanor, J. & Betts, R.F. (1993) Evaluation of live attenuated cold-adapted influenza B/Yamagata/16/88 reassortant virus vaccine in healthy adults. *J Infect Dis* **168**, 455–9.

Treanor, J.J., Roth, F.K. & Betts, R.F. (1990) Use of live cold-adapted influenza A H1N1 and H3N2 virus vaccines in seropositive adults. *J Clin Microbiol* **28** (3), 596–9.

Treanor, J.J., Mattison, H.R., Dumyati, G. *et al.* (1992) Protective efficacy of combined live intranasal and inactivated influenza A virus vaccines in the elderly. *Ann Intern Med* **117** (8), 625–33.

Treanor, J., Dumyati, G., O'Brien, D. *et al.* (1994) Evaluation of cold-adapted, reassortant influenza B virus vaccines in elderly and chronically ill adults. *J Infect Dis* **169**, 402–7.

Treanor, J., Betts, R., Kotloff, K. *et al.* (1996) Evaluation of the efficacy of a trivalent intranasal live influenza vaccine for protection against experimental influenza challenge. Presented at: *The 4th Annual Workgroup Meeting on Improving the Performance of Influenza and Pneumococcal Vaccines in Older Adults*. Institute for Advanced Studies in Immunology and Aging, October 1996, Washington D.C.

Wagner, D.K., Clements, M.L., Reimer, C.B., Snyder, M., Nelson, D.L. & Murphy, B.R. (1987) Analysis of immunoglobulin G antibody responses after administration of live and inactivated influenza A vaccine indicates that nasal wash immunoglobulin G is a transudate from serum. *J Clin Microbiol* **25** (3), 559–62.

Webster, R.G., Kawaoka, Y. & Bean, W.J. (1986) Molecular changes in A/Chicken/Pennsylvania/83 (H5N2) influenza virus associated with acquisition of virulence. *Virology* **149**, 165–73.

Whitaker-Dowling, P., Lucas, W. & Younger, J.S. (1990) Cold-adapted vaccine strains of influenza A virus act as dominant negative mutants in mixed infections with wild-type influenza A virus. *Virology* **175**, 358–64.

Whitaker-Dowling, P., Maassab, H.F. & Younger, J.S. (1991) Dominant-negative mutants as antiviral agents: simultaneous infection with the cold-adapted live-virus vaccine for influenza A protects ferrets from disease produced by wild-type influenza A. *J Infect Dis* **164**, 1200–2.

Wright, P.F., Okabe, N., McKee, K.T. Jr, Maassab, H.F. & Karzon, D.T. (1982) Cold-adapted recombinant influenza A virus vaccines in seronegative young children. *J Infect Dis* **146** (1), 71–9.

Wright, P.F., Bhargava, M., Johnson, P.R., Thompson, J. & Karzon, D.T. (1985) Simultaneous administration of live, attenuated influenza A vaccines representing different serotypes. *Vaccine* **3**, 305–8.

Younger, J.S., Treanor, J.J., Betts, R.F. & Whitaker-Dowling, P. (1994) Effect of simultaneous administration of cold-adapted and wild-type influenza A viruses on experimental wild-type influenza infection in humans. *J Clin Microbiol* **32** (3), 750–4.

Zahradnik, J.M., Kasel, J.A., Martin, R.R., Six, H.R. & Cate, T.R. (1983) Immune responses in serum and respiratory secretions following vaccination with a live cold-recombinant (CR35) and inactivated A/USSR/77 (H1N1) influenza virus vaccine. *J Med Virol* **11**, 277–85.

CHAPTER 29

Cold-Adapted, Live Influenza Vaccines Developed in Russia

Yuri Ghendon

Cold-adapted donor strains

During 1961–1962, Alexandrova and Smorodintsev (1965) selected cold-adapted (*ca*) variants of influenza virus by passage of virus in chick embryos at low temperature.

ca strain A/Leningrad/134/17/57 (H2N2)

The *ca* strain A/Leningrad/134/17/57 (H2N2) (A/Len/17) was obtained by passage of wild influenza virus strain A/Leningrad/134/57 (H2N2) in chick embryos 20 times at 32°C and 17 times at 25°C (Alexandrova & Smorodintsev 1965). The *ca* strain replicated well in chick embryos at 25°C (ca_{25+} marker) but was unable to replicate at 40°C (ts_{40-} marker).

Studies in mice showed that pneumotropism and the detection of influenza virus in different organs of mice were decreased considerably with the *ca* variant in comparison with the wild parent virus (Medvedeva *et al.* 1991).

Detection of mutations in the genome

Taking into account the fact that temperature sensitivity (*ts*) of many animal viruses usually correlates with attenuation of virulence (Ghendon 1975), studies were carried out to detect *ts* lesions in genes of the influenza *ca* variant. Using reassortants of the *ca* variant with ts mutants of fowl plague virus, it was found that the A/Len/17 *ca* strain contained *ts* mutations in genes 1, 5 and 7 coding for PB2, NP and M proteins, and also in gene 4 coding for haemagglutinin (HA) (Ghendon *et al.* 1981; Medvedeva *et al.* 1991).

Direct evidence for the existence of multiple mutations in the genome of this *ca* virus was obtained by analysis of the nucleotide sequence of RNA segments of the viral genome. A total of 11 differences were found when the nucleotide sequence of the *ca* variant and parent wild strain were compared. Of these eight were deduced to encode amino acid (aa) substitutions in proteins PB2, PB1, PA, M1, M2 and NS2 (Klimov *et al.* 1992). Substitution of one aa was detected in the neuraminidase (NA) (Klimov *et al.* 1995b). The discrepancy between the detection of a mutation in the NP gene by the methods of reassortment and sequence analysis is explained by the fact that a *ts* mutation was already present in the NP gene of the wild virus parent (Medvedeva *et al.* 1991), and was preserved in the gene of the *ca* strain.

Clinical studies of A/Len/17 ca strain

Studies of clinical reactions to the A/Len/17 *ca* virus were conducted during the period 1961–1964, first in healthy adults and later in children 1–6 years of age. The vaccinees were immunized using two intranasal sprays, each containing 10^7 EID$_{50}$ of virus per dose, and separated by an interval of 2–3 weeks. This *ca* strain did not produce any serious adverse reactions in adults or children 3–6 years of age but caused unacceptable symptoms in young children 1–2 years of age. Altogether 92% of vaccinees exhibited a four-fold rise in titre of haemagglutination inhibition (HAI) antibody, and a distinct decrease in influenza attack rates was observed among vaccinees as compared to unvaccinated controls (Alexandrova *et al.* 1965).

ca strain A/Leningrad/134/47/57 (H2N2)

Given the reactions associated with the use of the *ca* strain of A/Len/17 in young infants, the decision was made to obtain a more attenuated *ca* strain. For this purpose the *ca* strain A/Len/17 was additionally passaged in chick embryos eight times at 28 °C and 22 times at 25 °C. It was then cloned by terminal dilution in chick embryos (Garmashova *et al.* 1984). The new variant A/Leningrad/134/47/57 (H2N2) (A/Len/47) was ca_{25+} and ts_{40-}, and the detection of influenza virus in various organs of mice infected with this *ca* strain was decreased considerably in comparison with the A/Len/17 *ca* strain (Medvedeva *et al.* 1984).

Detection of mutations in the genome

Reassortants of the *ca* strain with *ts*-sensitive mutants revealed the presence of ts mutations in genes 1, 2, 5, 7 and 8 (coding for PB2, PB1, NP, M and NS proteins, respectively) of the A/Len/47 *ca* strain (Ghendon *et al.* 1984b), and also in genes 4 and 6 coding for HA and NA (Medvedeva *et al.* 1991). A total of 17 differences in nucleotide sequence were found in seven segments of viral RNA when the wild parent and *ca* strain were compared. These nucleotide changes encode 11 aa substitutions in proteins PB2, PB1, PA, M1, M2, NP and NS2, and two aa substitutions in the NA (Klimov *et al.* 1992, 1995b).

The above data show that the genome of the A/Len/47 *ca* strain, which was passed 47 times at 'low' temperature, contains more mutations, including *ts* mutations, than the A/Len/17 *ca* strain which was passed 17 times only at 'low' temperature.

Clinical studies of A/Len/47 ca strain

Clinical studies of the A/Len/47 *ca* strain in 10 390 children 1–2 years of age, 28 963 children 3–6 years of age and 14 242 schoolchildren 7–14 years of age showed that this *ca* strain did not induce serious adverse reactions in children, including infants, and it remained immunogenic (Alexandrova 1971).

Ca strains of influenza B virus

Two *ca* variants of influenza B virus were selected as candidates for *ca* vaccine following the passage of influenza B virus in chick embryos at low temperature. The first *ca* strain, B/Leningrad/14/17/55 (B/Len/17), was obtained after 21 passages in chick embryos at 32 °C and 17 passages at 25 °C. The second *ca* strain, B/USSR/60/69, was obtained after 17 passages in chick embryos at 32 °C and 60 passages at 25 °C. Both *ca* strains were ca_{25+} and ts_{38-}. During clinical studies of these two *ca* strains in seronegative children, fever $\geq$ 37.5 °C was detected in 0.4–0.8% of children only, and four-fold rises in HAI antibody titre were observed in 81–87% of vaccinees (Alexandrova & Smorodintsev 1965; Alexandrova *et al.* 1990).

Cold-adapted reassortants

Studies with *ca* variants of influenza A and B viruses have shown that *ca*-attenuated reassortants which inherit five or six genes coding for non-glycosylated proteins from the *ca* parent strain and genes for the HA and NA from contemporary wild influenza virus can be obtained rapidly. Thus the *ca* strains have the potential to act as donors of attenuation for the production of new vaccines that are required in the presence of antigenic drift.

The following method is used to obtain *ca* reassortant vaccines from *ca* donor strains and contemporary wild influenza virus. Chick embryos are infected with equal doses of a *ca* donor of attenuation and 'native' or partially heat-inactivated wild influenza virus and are incubated at 32–34 °C for 18 h (or 48 h if heat-treated virus is used). Allantoic fluids are harvested and pooled and then passed two to three times in chick embryos at 25–28 °C in the presence of antiserum specific to the *ca* donor strain. Virus is then cloned two to three times by terminal dilution in chick embryos at 25 °C or 32 °C (Polezhaev *et al.* 1980; Medvedeva *et al.* 1983).

Analysis of the genome composition of *ca* reassortant

After cloning, reassortants with ca_{25+} and $ts_{38/40-}$

markers are selected and their genome composition is analysed by RNA–RNA hybridization (Ghendon *et al.* 1979). *ca* reassortants which inherit five or six genes coding for non-glycosylated proteins from the *ca* donor strain and genes encoding the HA and NA from the contemporary wild influenza virus are considered as candidate *ca*-reassortant vaccine strains and are evaluated in volunteers.

The number and location of *ts* mutations in genes inherited from *ca* donor strains have been identified for several reassortants. Such analyses are considered important since they ensure that genes associated with attenuation in the *ca* donor are stable and are present in the reassortants. For four reassortants *ts* mutations were detected by reassortment tests with *ts* mutants in three to five genes inherited from the *ca* donor strains which corresponded to those in the parent genes. In another reassortant the *ts* mutation in gene 5 (NP) disappeared. Interestingly, in three reassortants a new *ts* mutation in gene 3 (PA) was detected which was not present in the gene from the parent *ca* strain (Ghendon *et al.* 1984a; Medvedeva *et al.* 1984).

Recently, a rapid method to analyse the genome composition and stability of mutations in *ca* reassortants has been developed. The new technique provides information on the presence or absence of mutations in *ca* reassortants within 10 h (Klimov & Cox 1995).

Clinical studies of reassortants obtained using the A/Len/17 *ca* donor strain

Clinical trials using *ca* reassortants obtained by crossing the A/Len/17 *ca* donor strain with wild H3N2 or H1N1 strains of influenza A have been carried out in groups of healthy young adults. No reassortant induced serious adverse reactions in vaccinees and all reassortants were immunogenic. A rise of HAI antibody titre was found in about 80% of vaccinees (Alexandrova *et al.* 1979; Polezhaev *et al.* 1982). It was shown, however, that the immunogenicity of *ca*-reassortant vaccine correlates with the dose of vaccine virus. The immunogenicity was poor using a dose of $10^{5.0}$ $EID_{50}/0.2$ ml and the optimal dose was $10^{7.0}$–$10^{7.5}$ EID_{50} (Alexandrova *et al.* 1979). The reactogenicity and immunogenicity of eight

ca reassortants, obtained by crossing A/Len/17 or A/Leningrad/9/37/46 *ca* donor strains with wild influenza A/H1N1 or A/H3N2 viruses which inherited from *ca* donor strains one to six genes coding for non-glycosylated proteins, were investigated in healthy young adult volunteers. All reassortants, irrespective of the number of genes inherited from the *ca* parent strains, were non-reactogenic to vaccinees, including those who had no antibodies to the HA and NA before immunization. Even the reassortant which inherited only one gene (M gene) containing a *ts* mutation from the *ca* parent strain was non-reactogenic. Analysis of the immunogenicity of the reassortants showed that the percentage of vaccinees who developed ≥ four-fold increases in HAI antibody titre was more or less the same irrespective of the reassortant used (Ghendon *et al.* 1981).

A study of the safety and immunogenicity of a *ca* reassortant obtained by crossing A/Len/17 *ca* donor strain with wild influenza virus strain A/Korea/1/82 (H3N2) was undertaken in the UK on behalf of the WHO by Nicholson *et al.* (1987). Healthy young adult volunteers received two intranasal inoculations with $10^{7.5}$ EID_{50} of the reassortant separated by an interval of 4 weeks. The reassortant was well tolerated by vaccinees; 70% of seronegative volunteers produced HAI antibody after the first dose and 84% seroconverted after the second. The HAI antibody titre increased in 85% of subjects with initial titres of ≤ 1 : 40 after the first dose and in 92% after the second. Even in vaccinees with an initial titre of more than 1 : 40, the *ca* reassortant increased the HAI antibody titre in 56% after the first dose and in 80% after the second.

Recently a trivalent *ca*-reassortant vaccine was prepared using A/Len/17 and B/USSR/60/69 *ca* donor strains. About 400 nursing home residents aged 60 years and older received live trivalent vaccine, inactivated vaccine, live vaccine in combination with inactivated vaccine, or a placebo. Side-effects did not differ significantly when the groups vaccinated with live or inactivated vaccines were compared. Serum HAI antibody and nasal antiviral IgA antibody responses were higher among vaccinees who received the combination of live *ca* and inactivated vaccines as compared to those receiving either vaccine alone (Rudenko *et al.* 1996b).

ca-reassortant A/H1N1 and A/H3N2 vaccines that were prepared using the A/Len/17 *ca* donor of attenuation were used widely to vaccinate workers in the former USSR from 1977 onwards (Zhdanov 1986). Unfortunately there were no control field trials to assess the protective efficacy of these *ca*-reassortant vaccines among adults.

Clinical studies of *ca* reassortants obtained using the A/Len/47 *ca* donor strain

Reassortants obtained from the A/Len/47 *ca* donor strain were evaluated in young adults, school-children and infants. All *ca* reassortants that were studied (A/H1N1 and A/H3N2) were found to be both safe and immunogenic among vaccinees of all ages (Alexandrova *et al.* 1986; Rudenko *et al.* 1996a).

The immunogenicity of one and two doses of monovalent *ca* reassortant vaccines (A/H1N1 and A/H3N2) has been studied in children 7–15 years of age. Overall a single dose of *ca* vaccine induced a $\geq$ four-fold rise of HAI antibody titre in 61% of children whose initial antibody titre was < 1 : 16 and in 23–27% of children whose initial antibody titre was 1 : 32–1 : 64. After two doses a $\geq$ four-fold rise in antibody titre was found in 81–86% and 31–36% of vaccinees, respectively (Alexandrova *et al.* 1984). More recently Vorobiev *et al.* (1991) showed that an A/H1N1 *ca*-reassortant vaccine stimulated a cyto-toxic cell-mediated immune response in healthy young adults.

Clinical studies of *ca* reassortants obtained using the influenza B *ca* donor strain

The first influenza B *ca* reassortants were obtained by crossing the B/Len/17 *ca* donor strain with wild influenza B/England/2608/76. The reassortants inherited genes coding for PB2, PB1, PA, NP and M proteins from the *ca* parent and those coding for the HA, NA and NS proteins from the wild parent. These reassortants were found to be safe among young seronegative adults, but the immunogenicity of these influenza B reassortants was lower in comparison with the parent *ca* donor strain (Med-vedeva *et al.* 1983). Subsequently the B/Len/17 *ca*

donor strain was crossed with wild influenza B/Ann Arbor/1/86; the composition of the genome of this reassortant was as in the previous study. This *ca* reassortant was found to be safe in children 3–7 years of age and a rise in titre of neutralizing anti-body was detected in 58% of seronegative children after the first dose and in 72% after the second. Among seronegative children 8–15 years of age, 31% developed an antibody response after the first dose and 42% after the second. Among children with an initial antibody titre > 1 : 20, 17% developed an increase in antibody after the first dose and 29% responded to two doses (Obrosova-Serova *et al.* 1990).

Bivalent *ca* reassortant vaccine

Because A/H1N1 and A/H3N2 *ca* reassortants contained five or six genes from the same *ca* parent, it was anticipated that coinfection might be possible with slight interference only. This was confirmed in a study using chick embryos coinfected with two *ca* reassortants, A/H1N1 and A/H3N2 (Alexandrova *et al.* 1984).

Vaccination of children 3–15 years of age with either monovalent or bivalent *ca*-reassortant vac-cines was carried out using the A/Len/47 *ca* donor strain. Fever > 37.5 °C occurred in less than 1.0% of those who received monovalent or bivalent vaccine. H1 and H3 components of bivalent *ca* vaccine were just as immunogenic as each of the monovalent *ca* vaccines (Alexandrova *et al.* 1984).

Subsequently a bivalent *ca*-reassortant vaccine containing influenza B and influenza A/H1N1 (obtained using the B/Len/17 and A/Len/47 *ca* donor strains) was investigated in 3–14-year-old children. Few reactions occurred and the safety profile of this bivalent vaccine did not differ from those of monovalent vaccines. Analysis of immu-nogenicity showed that the *ca* A/H1N1 monovalent vaccine induced HAI antibody in 68.9% of sero-negative children and in 72.2% of those with a prevaccination antibody titre of > 1 : 20. As a com-ponent of bivalent vaccine the H1N1 component evoked antibody responses in 78.5% of seronegative children and 68.7% of those with antibody. The influenza B monovalent vaccine induced antibody in 45.6% of seronegative children; similarly, as a component of the bivalent vaccine, it evoked a response in 41.9% (Rudenko *et al.* 1991).

ca-reassortant trivalent vaccine

Studies of the safety and immunogenicity of trivalent *ca*-reassortant vaccines containing influenza A/H1N1, A/H3N2 and influenza B reassortants were undertaken. The vaccines were well tolerated by seronegative (HAI antibody < 1:20) children 3–14 years of age and no serious adverse reactions were observed in groups of children who were vaccinated with mono- or trivalent vaccines. The immune responses to the H1 and H3 reassortants in mono- and trivalent vaccines were comparable. A four-fold rise in antibody titre to the H1 component was found in 61% of children who received monovalent vaccine and in 63.3% of those who were given trivalent vaccine. Similarly, a four-fold rise in antibody to the H3 component occurred in 73.3% of recipients of monovalent vaccine and in 69.8% of those receiving trivalent vaccine. The immunogenicity of the influenza B reassortant in monovalent vaccine was slightly higher than in trivalent vaccine — four-fold rises in 54.5% vs. 43.7%, respectively. The geometric mean HAI antibody titres after vaccination were in the range 1:30–1:50 for all components and were virtually identical in recipients of monovalent or trivalent vaccines (Rudenko *et al.* 1996a).

In another study (Rudenko *et al.* 1993), children 7–14 years of age who had HAI antibody titres of less than 1:20 were given *ca*-trivalent reassortant vaccine. The vaccine was well tolerated and fever > 37.6 °C occurred in 0.6% of vaccinees only. This vaccine induced four-fold rises of antibody to the H1 component in 51.2% of vaccinees, to the H3 component in 64.0%, and to the influenza B component in 42.9%.

Safety of *ca* vaccine

Adverse reactions

The above data show that mono-, bi- and trivalent *ca*-reassortant vaccines are all well tolerated by adults and children and do not induce any serious adverse reactions. Studies of the safety of *ca*-reassortant vaccines (Alexandrova *et al.* 1984, 1986; Rudenko *et al.* 1993, 1996a) revealed that the incidence of transient febrile reactions of more than 37.6 °C was approximately 0.7–1.0%. There was no increase in the incidence of systemic or nasopharyngeal reactions in vaccinees in comparison to those receiving the placebo. The low incidence of clinical reactions to *ca* vaccines was also confirmed independently by polyclinic physicians who were involved in the studies. Full blood counts, blood biochemistry and urine analysis were carried out before and 3 days after the first dose of vaccine, and 3 days and 1 month after the second dose. The circulating IgE concentration was also determined in order to detect subclinical allergic reactions. Epidemiological methods were used to examine vaccine safety based on analysis of somatic and infectious diseases other than influenza (12 diseases in all) among vaccinees and non-vaccinated control children for up to 6 months after immunization. The results of the haematological and biochemical tests revealed no abnormalities among vaccinees as compared with those who received the placebo. The incidence of common complaints other than influenza were comparable among children who received vaccine and those who received the placebo. No allergic reactions were detected in vaccinated children (Rudenko *et al.* 1996a).

Genetic stability of *ca* vaccine

Several influenza A/H1N1 and A/H3N2 *ca*-reassortant vaccines were passed five times in chick embryos at 32 °C; each one completely retained the *ts* phenotype of the initial *ca* reassortant (Ghendon *et al.* 1984a; Medvedeva *et al.* 1990).

The stability of *ts* mutations in individual genes of virus isolates from children who received *ca*-reassortant vaccines derived from the A/Len/47 *ca* donor strain was investigated. A total of 23 isolates were obtained 48 h after vaccination from children in Kaliningrad (see p. 396). The *ca*-reassortant vaccines each originally contained *ts* mutations in five genes from the *ca* donor strain. All 14 isolates from children who were vaccinated with the A/H1N1 *ca*-reassortant vaccine and all nine isolates from children who were vaccinated with the A/H3N2 vaccine retained *ts* mutations in all genes in which *ts* mutations were detected originally (Ghendon *et al.* 1984a).

In another study isolates were obtained from children 3–6 years of age following vaccination with influenza A/H1N1 and A/H3N2 *ca* reassortants. Eighty isolates were obtained, 52 on days 1–4, 16 on days 5–7 and 12 on days 8–12 after vaccination. All 80 isolates retained their ca_{25+} and ts_{40-} phenotype. However, when they were analysed further, some isolates obtained late after vaccination lost one of the five original *ts* mutations, mostly in genes coding for proteins PB2 and PB1, rarely in genes coding for NP and NS, and never in the gene coding for the M protein (Medvedeva *et al.* 1990).

As noted above, 14 mutations (11 coding) were detected in the genome of A/Len/47 *ca* donor strain (Klimov *et al.* 1992). Preservation of these mutations in the genome of isolates obtained from children 2, 5 and 8 days after vaccination (Novgorod studies, see p. 396) was examined using sequence analysis. The sequence data demonstrated that all nine coding mutations selected for examination were conserved in the genome of all 11 isolates investigated (Klimov *et al.* 1995a).

The genetic stability of A/Len/17 *ca*-reassortant vaccines used to immunize the elderly (Klimov *et al.* 1996) has also been studied by sequence analysis. The isolates retained a high degree of genetic stability of mutations originally present in the *ca* donor strain. However, genetic variability within genes coding for M and NP proteins was observed in some isolates from vaccinated schoolchildren which is attributed to heterogeneity within the A/Len/17 *ca* donor strain. It is the author's view that cloning of this *ca* donor strain or strong selection and comprehensive analysis of *ca* reassortants is required for the preparation of *ca* vaccines using A/Len/17 *ca* virus as a donor strain.

The data presented above clearly show that *ca*-reassortant vaccines are highly stable genetically as *ts* mutations reversed rarely and only in one of several genes containing such mutations. The possession of multiple mutations in the genome of *ca* donor strains, and the ability to transfer genes with these mutations to contemporary wild influenza viruses by reassortant, facilitates the regular production of *ca* reassortants with reproducible biological properties and minimal chance of reverting to virulence, even though the actual basis for attenuation is unknown.

Transmission of *ca* influenza virus vaccine

The potential for transmission of *ca* influenza virus vaccine was studied in a kindergarten in children 3–6 years of age. Twenty-two children were vaccinated with *ca*-reassortant vaccine and 18 children in the same kindergarten received a placebo. Nasal swabs were obtained from all children on days 1, 2, 3, 7 and 18 after the first dose of vaccine and on days 1 and 3 after the second. Eleven influenza virus strains were isolated from vaccinated children. No virus was isolated from contact children who received the placebo (Rudenko *et al.* 1996a). These data indicate that the *ca* influenza virus did not spread from vaccinees to susceptible contacts.

Efficacy of *ca*-reassortant vaccines

A large field trial of bivalent *ca*-reassortant vaccine, which was derived from the A/Len/47 *ca* donor strain, was carried out in Kaliningrad during 1982–1983. Nearly 30 000 3–15-year-old children were given two doses of vaccine containing A/H1N1 and A/H3N2 reassortants, or a placebo. The bivalent live vaccine was completely attenuated for children, causing transient febrile reactions in fewer than 1%. The immunogenicity of the vaccine was high. Four-fold rises of antibody to the H1 component of vaccine were detected in 93.2% of vaccinees and to the H3 component in 70.8% (Alexandrova *et al.* 1984). During the 4 months after vaccination, when there were epidemics of influenza A/H1N1 and A/H3N2, the incidence of influenza-like illnesses was 50% lower in the vaccinees than in the children who received the placebo (Alexandrova *et al.* 1986).

A similar study was carried out in 21 000 schoolchildren aged 7–14 years of age in Novgorod during 1989–1990 and 1990–1991. The children received either live *ca*-reassortant vaccine (derived from A/Len/47), inactivated vaccine or a placebo

(Rudenko *et al.* 1993). The *ca* vaccines were bivalent during the first year, containing A/H1N1 and A/H3N2 components. During the second year they were trivalent, containing an influenza B *ca* reassortant in addition. The inactivated vaccines were whole virus preparations produced from influenza virus strains similar antigenically to the wild influenza virus parents of the *ca*-reassortant vaccines.

Analysis of symptoms during 1990–1991 in groups of about 300 vaccinees showed the presence of transient febrile reactions in 0.6% of those who received the live vaccine, 1.8% of those given inactivated vaccine, and 0.7% of those who received the placebo.

During the first year of the study an outbreak of influenza was caused by an A/H3N2 virus; during the second year outbreaks were caused by influenza A/H1N1 and influenza B viruses. During the 1989–1990 season, the live *ca* vaccine was 30.0% effective in preventing respiratory influenza-like illness in children 7–10 years of age; the inactivated vaccine was 24.2% effective. In older children (11–14 years) the effectiveness of the live *ca* vaccine was significantly higher (51.9%) than that of the inactivated vaccine (19.6%). During the epidemiological season of 1990–1991 the effectiveness of the live *ca* vaccine in 7–10-year-old children was 39.5%, significantly higher than the 27.3% effectiveness seen with the inactivated vaccine. In the 11–14-year-old children the difference between the two vaccines was not statistically significant.

The effect of vaccination on the occurrence of influenza in unvaccinated contacts was also examined in the above study. The analysis showed that the live *ca* vaccine, but not inactivated vaccine, was associated with reduced transmission of wild influenza virus in the school, indirectly protecting the unvaccinated students and staff. This 'herd immunity' effect is an important goal of national vaccination strategies in which children are regularly vaccinated (Rudenko *et al.* 1993).

Conclusion

The data presented in this chapter have shown that three *ca* donor strains have been developed in Russia: first, the A/Leningrad/134/17/57 (H2N2) *ca* strain, which has 10 mutations (eight coding) in five genes and *ts* mutations in three genes coding for non-glycosylated proteins; second, the more attenuated *ca* strain A/Leningrad/134/47/57 (H2N2), which has 14 mutations (11 coding) in six genes and *ts* mutations in five genes coding for non-glycosylated proteins; and third, an attenuated *ca* influenza B virus. The results of clinical trials of A/Len/17 and A/Len/47 *ca* strains indicate the advisability of having two *ca* donor strains, with different levels of attenuation, for the preparation of *ca* reassortant vaccines for children and adults. This is considered important not only for reasons of safety but also for vaccine immunogenicity.

The immunogenicity and efficacy of live vaccines depend on the ability of attenuated virus to replicate in vaccinees and to present those viral proteins to the host immune system that are responsible for the induction of immunity. *ca* vaccines that are sufficiently attenuated for children may replicate well in children whose immunity to influenza is low, but may prove to be too attenuated for adults and fail in adults to induce adequate immunity. Conversely a *ca* strain that is able to replicate in adults may cause adverse reactions in young children, many of whom do not possess antibody to influenza virus (as occurred during a study with the *ca* strain A/Len/17; see p. 396).

The safety of mono-, bi- and trivalent *ca* reassortant vaccines was demonstrated in clinical studies and field trials. In one study we observed that one *ca* reassortant, which inherited only a single gene (M) containing a *ts* mutation from the *ca* parent strain, was both safe and immunogenic (see p. 396). Nonetheless, analysis of both *ca* donor strains, A/Len/17 and A/Len/47, revealed the presence of multiple mutations in most genes coding for non-glycosylated proteins. Since there are no data showing which mutation or combination of mutations is responsible for the attenuation, it is considered most important that candidate *ca*-reassortant vaccines should have mutations in no less than five genes coding for non-glycosylated proteins. It is suggested that the possession of multiple mutations throughout the genome should confer full attenuation and reduce the likelihood of reversion to virulence during replication in vaccinees.

On the basis of the foregoing scientific and clinical data it can be concluded that the *ca* donor strains developed in Russia and the reassortant vaccines are safe, genetically stable, non-transmissible immunogenic and efficacious in children and adults. It has been established that *ca* reassortants can be delivered as trivalent intranasal vaccines, and that the possession of *ca* and *ts* markers and nucleotide mutations are available to monitor vaccine shedding in the field. *ca* influenza vaccines can be produced in an acceptable substrate, they do not require concentration or purification of the virus and should be less expensive than current inactivated influenza vaccines. Taking into consideration the ease of vaccine production and administration to adults and children, live *ca* influenza vaccines represent an optimal preparation for mass prophylaxis. Indeed, live *ca* vaccine may be the most appropriate means for the control of an influenza pandemic, when rapid vaccine production and implementation of mass immunization is crucial. Moreover, with a global programme of immunization, it is conceivable that comprehensive immunization of children (who represent the principal vectors of infection) could reduce the impact of infection in those most at risk of the complications of influenza through herd immunity.

It can be concluded that *ca*-reassortant live influenza vaccines will have an important role in the prophylaxis of influenza.

References

Alexandrova, G. (1971) Basic trends in vaccination of children against influenza by use of live vaccine. In: *Proc. Symp. on Live Influenza Vaccines*, pp. 121–30. Yugoslav. Acad. Sci. Arts, Zagreb.

Alexandrova, G. & Smorodintsev, A. (1965) Obtaining of an additionally attenuated vaccinating cryophilic influenza strain. *Rev Roum Inframicrobiol* **2**, 179–89.

Alexandrova, G., Mikutskaya, B., Pleshanova, N. & Smorodintsev, A. (1965) Reactive and immunogenic properties and epidemiologic efficacy of further attenuated influenza virus vaccinal strains obtained in preschool children. *Vopr Virusol* **10**, 67–73 [in Russian].

Alexandrova, G., Garmashova, L., Golubev, D. *et al.* (1979) Experience in selection of safe thermosensitive recombinants of influenza A virus. *Vopr Virusol* **24**, 342–6 [in Russian].

Alexandrova, A., Polezhaev, F., Budilovsky, G. *et al.* (1984) Recombinant cold-adapted attenuated influenza A vaccines for use in children: reactogenicity and antigenic activity of cold-adapted recombinants and analysis of isolates from the vaccinees. *Infect Immun* **44**, 734–9.

Alexandrova, G., Budilovsky, G., Koval, T. *et al.* (1986) Study of live recombinant cold-adapted influenza bivalent vaccine of type A for use in children: an epidemiological control trial. *Vaccine* **4**, 114–18.

Alexandrova, G., Maassab, H., Kendal, A. *et al.* (1990) Laboratory properties of cold-adapted influenza B live vaccine strains developed in the US and USSR, and their B/Ann Arbor/1/86 cold-adapted reassortant vaccine candidate. *Vaccine* **8**, 61–4.

Garmashova, L., Polezhaev, F. & Alexandrova, G. (1984) Cold-adapted A/Leningrad/134/47/57 (H2N2) strain, a specific donor of attenuation of live influenza vaccine for children, and recombinants produced on its base. *Vopr Virusol* **29**, 28–31 [in Russian].

Ghendon, Y. (1975) *Molecular Genetics of Animal Viruses*. Medicina, Moscow.

Ghendon, Y., Klimov, A., Blagoveshenskaya, O. & Ghenkina, D. (1979) Investigation of recombinants of human influenza and fowl plague viruses. *J Gen Virol* **43**, 183–91.

Ghendon, Y., Klimov, A., Alexandrova, G. & Polezhaev, F. (1981) Analysis of genome composition and reactogenicity of recombinants of cold-adapted and virulent virus strains. *J Gen Virol* **53**, 215–24.

Ghendon, Y., Klimov, A., Lisovskaya, A., Alexandrova, G. & Medvedeva, T. (1984a) Molecular-genetic analysis of the cold-adapted strain, a donor of attenuation for live influenza vaccine for children, of the recombinants produced on its basis, and isolates from vaccinated children. *Vopr Virusol* **29**, 22–8 [in Russian].

Ghendon, Y., Polezhaev, F., Lisovskaya, K., Medvedeva, T. & Klimov, A. (1984b) Recombinant cold-adapted attenuated influenza A vaccines for use in children: molecular-genetic analysis of the cold-adapted donor and recombinants. *Infect Immun* **44**, 730–3.

Klimov, A. & Cox, N. (1995) PCR restriction analysis of genome composition and stability of cold-adapted reassortant live influenza vaccine. *J Virol Meth* **52**, 41–9.

Klimov, A., Cox, N., Yotov, W., Rocha, E., Alexandrova, G. & Kendal, A. (1992) Sequence changes in the live attenuated, cold-adapted variants of influenza A/Leningrad/134/57 (H2N2) virus. *Virology* **186**, 795–7.

Klimov, A., Egorov, A., Gushina, M. *et al.* (1995a) Genetic stability of cold-adapted A/Leningrad/134/47/57 (H2N2) influenza virus: sequence analysis of live cold-adapted reassortant vaccine strains before and after replication in children. *J Gen Virol* **76**, 1521–5.

Klimov, A., Romanova, Y., Egorov, A. *et al.* (1995b) Nucleotide sequences of the neuraminidase gene of influenza A/Leningrad/134/57 (H2N2) virus and two of its live, attenuated, cold-adapted variants. *Virus Genes* **10**, 95–8.

Klimov, A., Rudenko, L., Egorov, A. *et al.* (1996) Genetic stability of Russian cold-adapted live attenuated reassortant influenza vaccines. In: Brown, L., Hampson, A. & Webster, R. (eds) *Options for the Control of Influenza III*, pp. 129–36. Elsevier, Amsterdam.

Medvedeva, T., Gordon, M., Ghendon, Y., Klimov, A. & Alexandrova, G. (1983) Attenuated influenza B virus recombinants obtained by crossing of B/England/2608/76 virus with cold-adapted B/Leningrad/14/17/55 strain. *Acta Virol* **27**, 311–17.

Medvedeva, T., Lisovskaya, K., Polezhaev, F., Garmashova, L., Alexandrova, G. & Ghendon, Y. (1984) Location of *ts* defects in the genome of cold-adapted recombinant influenza A virus vaccine strains. *Acta Virol* **28**, 204–11.

Medvedeva, T., Romanova, Y., Gushina, M. *et al.* (1990) *Ts*-phonotype of reisolates from children vaccinated with live cold-adapted influenza type A vaccine. *Vopr Virusol* **35**, 101–5 [in Russian].

Medvedeva, T., Kudryavtseva, V., Zhikhareva, P., Romashkina, V., Alexandrova, G. & Klimov, A. (1991) Mutations in the genes coding for haemagglutinin and neuraminidase in cold-adapted variants of influenza A/Leningrad/134/57 (H2N2) virus. *Vopr Virusol* **36**, 96–100 [in Russian].

Nicholson, K., Tyrrell, D., Oxford, J. *et al.* (1987) Infectivity and reactogenicity of reassortant cold-adapted influenza A/Korea/1/82 vaccines obtained from the USA and USSR. *Bull WHO* **65**, 295–301.

Obrosova-Serova, N., Slepushkin, A., Kendal, A. *et al.* (1990) Evaluation in children of cold-adapted influenza B live attenuated intranasal vaccine prepared by reassortment between wild-type B/Ann Arbor/1/86 and cold-adapted B/Leningrad/14/55 viruses. *Vaccine* **8**, 57–60.

Polezhaev, F., Garmashova, L., Rumovsky, V., Alexandrova, G. & Smorodintsev, A. (1980) Peculiarities of obtaining attenuated thermosensitive recombinants of influenza A virus at the end of the H3N2 epidemic cycle. *Acta Virol* **24**, 273–8.

Polezhaev, F., Garmashova, L., Koval, T., Taranova, G., Topuria, N. & Alexandrova, G. (1982) Attenuated *ts* recombinants of influenza virus A/USSR/77 (H1N1) variety obtained by crossing with a cold-adapted donor of attenuation A/Leningrad/134/47/57 (H2N2) virus. *Acta Virol* **26**, 221–6.

Rudenko, L., Ramires, A., Barro, M. *et al.* (1991) Vaccination properties of live recombinant influenza types A and B used separately and in combination in children of 3–14 years. *Vopr Virusol* **36**, 472–4 [in Russian].

Rudenko, L., Slepushkin, A., Monto, A. *et al.* (1993) Efficacy of live attenuated and inactivated influenza vaccines in schoolchildren and their unvaccinated contacts in Novgorod, Russia. *J Infect Dis* **168**, 881–7.

Rudenko, L., Lonskaya, N., Klimov, A. *et al.* (1996a) Clinical and epidemiological evaluation of a live, cold-adapted influenza vaccine for 3–14 year olds. *Bull WHO* **74**, 77–84.

Rudenko, L., Arden, N., Gzigorieva, E. *et al.* (1996b) Safety and immunogeneity of Russian live-attenuated and US inactivated trivalent influenza vaccines in the elderly. In: Brown, L., Hampson, A. & Webster, R. (eds) *Options for the Control of Influenza III*, pp. 572–8. Elsevier, Amsterdam.

Vorobiev, K., Rudenko, L., Islamova, N. *et al.* (1991) Immune response formation in volunteers immunized with a live recombinant influenza vaccine. *Vopr Virusol* **36**, 475–7 [in Russian].

Zhdanov, V. (1986) Live influenza vaccines in USSR: development and practical application. In: Kendal, A. & Patriarka, P. (eds) *Options for the Control of Influenza*, UCLA Symposia on Molecular and Cellular Biology, no. 36, pp. 193–205. A. & R. Liss, New York.

CHAPTER 30

Liposomal Presentation of Influenza Antigens

Reinhard Glück and Alfred Wegmann

Liposomes

Liposomes are lipid membrane particles that can serve as vehicles or delivery systems for vaccine antigens and/or immunostimulators such as lipopolysaccharide (LPS), lipid A, monophosphoryl lipid A (MPL), muramyldipeptide (MDP) and its derivatives and cytokines (Gupta *et al.* 1993; Alving 1993; Alving *et al.* 1992, 1993). Over the past 20 years, liposomes have been found to act as adjuvants with a number of antigens (van Rooijen 1990; Alving 1991, 1993; Alving *et al.* 1992, 1993; Antimisiaris *et al.* 1993; Gupta *et al.* 1993; Pietrobon 1995). Liposomes are usually made up of biodegradable materials such as phospholipids and were originally developed as carriers for drugs or other biologically active substances. Both humoral and cell-mediated immune responses have been elicited by liposomes (Pietrobon 1995). Immunostimulators such as MPL, LPS and MDP when encapsulated within liposomes show enhanced adjuvanticity with reduced side-effects. Adjuvanticity of liposomes appears to be due to depot formation at the site of injection and efficient presentation of antigen to macrophages (van Rooijen 1992; Fortin & Therien 1993).

Until recently, liposome technology has been concerned with vesicles composed of phospholipids. One type of liposome (Novasome® vesicle) has been used commercially for more than 3 years as a safe and potent immunological adjuvant for two poultry vaccines approved by the US Department of Agriculture (Gupta *et al.* in press). These liposome vesicles, composed of dioxyethylene cetyl ether, cholesterol and oleic acid, were evaluated with human vaccine antigens (tetanus and diph-theria toxoids) in rabbits and mice (Gupta *et al.* in press). Tetanus and diphtheria toxoids encapsulated in or mixed with these liposomes elicited antitoxin levels similar to those elicited by antigens given with Freund's complete adjuvant (FCA) or adsorbed onto aluminium adjuvants. Liposomal tetanus toxoid preparations, particularly those with encapsulated MPL/squalene or squalene alone, consistently elicited higher levels of IgG2a and IgG2b antibodies (Gupta *et al.* in press).

Another type of liposome referred to as a virosome or fusogenic liposome is created by inserting virus fusion proteins into a liposome bilayer. These preparations exhibit superior adjuvant/carrier properties when used to deliver an encapsulated antigen (Glück *et al.* 1994).

Immunological presentation of liposomal influenza antigens

The viral glycoprotein haemagglutinin (HA) has been the subject of considerable study because of its role as the major antigen against which a protective immune response is directed. The majority of the influenza virion protein is in the HA spikes which are distributed evenly on the surface of the virus particles. It is this glycoprotein that allows the virus to attach to specific receptors on the cell surface and causes endosomal fusion of the virion and cell membranes during entry. The surface HA spikes are trimers of HA_1–HA_2 units. The HA_1 monomer has a globular membrane-distal domain of anti-parallel β-sheets which contains the sialic acid-containing receptor binding site. The regions of antigenic variation are clustered within five regions of this distal portion of the molecule. HA is anchored in the viral membrane through a single membrane-spanning hydrophobic segment located near the COOH terminus of the HA_2 polypeptide chain (Tsurudome *et al.* 1992). This hydrophobic segment is responsible for the major binding of HA spikes to the liposomal phospholipid vesicles.

Influenza virus infects a cell by fusion of the viral membrane with the endosomal membrane after entry of the virus particles through receptor-mediated endocytosis (Brunner *et al.* 1991; Tsurudome 1992; Weber *et al.* 1994; Durrer *et al.* 1996). The same process occurs with respect to the interaction between infectious virus and the immune system. It was therefore of special importance to preserve this fusogenic property of HA during solubilization of viral components, purification from core proteins and reconstitution to the subunit virosomal formulation. The spike protein molecules are quantitatively incorporated in a single population of virosomes of uniform buoyant density and appear at the surface of the membrane. These virosomes display haemagglutination activity and a strictly pH-dependent haemolytic activity; they fuse with erythrocyte ghosts, as revealed by a fluorescence resonance energy transfer assay; the rate and pH dependence of fusion are essentially the same as those of the intact virus; and HA-containing virosomes also fuse with cultured cells (BHK-21) either at the level of the endosomal membrane or directly with the cellular plasma membrane upon brief exposure to low pH. Furthermore it was possible to show (Bender *et al.* 1995) that inactivated influenza virus vaccines with preserved fusion activity of HA elicited strong human $CD8^+$ cytolytic cell responses when presented on dendritic cells. Only vaccine with HA which retained its fusogenic activity was optimally effective and accessed the cytoplasm of dendritic cells.

Viral neuraminidase (NA) is an exoglycosidase that hydrolyses terminal sialic acid residues from any glycoconjugate, including viral glycoprotein. Virion NA spikes are tetramers of the NA molecules that are anchored in the lipid bilayer by an N-terminal hydrophobic amino acid sequence (Shaw *et al.* 1992). Unlike HA, the lipophilic region of NA will spontaneously insert in the liposomal bilayer

membrane during the detergent removal process. It was recently shown that inhibition of the NA activity (e.g. through antibodies) leads to the reduction of influenza infectivity in man (Powers *et al.* 1996).

According to current immunological dogma, cells that express class II major histocompatibility complex (MHC) molecules are responsible for the initial presentation of antigen to helper T lymphocytes (Th) during induction of immunity (Alving 1992). Helper T cells are characterized by the presence of CD4 molecules on the cell surface. The CD4 molecule is part of an immunoadhesion receptor complex that specifically recognizes the combination of the autologous class II MHC and the particular peptide antigen or antigen fragment bound to the MHC on the surface of the antigen presenting cells (APC). The binding of the receptor on the $CD4^+$ Th to the peptide–MHC II complex on the APC triggers a 'conversation' between the Th and the APC in the form of secretion of a complex array of mediators and lymphokines, including membrane-bound and secreted interleukin-1 (IL-1) from macrophages and interferon-γ (IFN-γ) and interleukin-2 (IL-2) from T cells. The conversation between activated macrophage APCs and Th results in the initiation of a process of recruitment of numerous types of specific progenitor T lymphocytes and B lymphocytes leading to proliferation of specific B- or T-cell clones expressing specific immunity (e.g. antibody production or cytotoxic T lymphocytes (CTLs)) against the antigen that was originally taken up by the APC.

MHC molecules have a hydrophobic region that can span lipid bilayer membranes and it might be expected that they could be influenced by membrane lipid composition. Several studies have shown that immunological presentation involving class II MHC antigens can be strongly diminished or blocked by treatment of APCs with phospholipase A_2 or phospholipase C. This indicates that phospholipids on the APC may be critically important for functional activity of the class II MHC molecules.

In a mouse model, the incorporation of influenza HA_2 (from A/USSR/90/77 (H1N1)) into egg-yolk purified phosphatidylcholine (PC) liposomes together with DNP-Cap-PE (DNP-aminocaproyl-phosphatidylethanolamine) induced an IgG response to the HA peptides and elicited a shift from an IgM response for DNP (as seen with liposomes without HA_2) to an IgG response to DNP involving all IgG subclasses (Garçon & Six 1991). When the HA_2 antigens present on the surface of the liposomes were detached by bromelaine, the IgG response to DNP remained unaffected. This suggests that HA_2 situated within the liposomal membrane is active as a Th epitope. Complementary experiments revealed that the liposomal device also elicited a memory response for DNP. It was concluded that the liposomes containing the viral HA had provided a T-cell dependent effect for the T-cell independent DNP antigen.

Several preclinical and clinical studies which are referred to in the two following sections have confirmed that virosomal presentation of influenza subunit antigens efficiently enhance the stimulation of cellular immunity.

Production of a commercialized influenza virosome vaccine

At the Swiss Serum & Vaccine Institute, Berne, influenza seed virus is inoculated into 11-day-old embryonated hens' eggs from flocks under veterinary control. The inoculated eggs are incubated for a further 50–60 h at 33–35 °C, depending on the strain. During this period, they are illuminated for a second time (after 40 h) to eliminate dead eggs. After incubation the eggs are cooled overnight at 1–4 °C; they are then opened under laminar flow and the allantoic fluid is aspirated into sterile steel tanks. After centrifugation the virus suspension is filtered by step filtration, through a filter of 0.65 μm and 0.22 μm, directly into a new 200 l steel tank. The filtered virus suspension is concentrated about four-fold with a molecular filter system (polysulphone membranes), and then purified and concentrated sucrose density-gradient ultracentrifugation. The virus-containing fraction is diluted and dialysed against phosphate buffered saline (PBS) pH 7.4 to reduce the sugar content to less than 1%. Subsequently, inactivation is performed with beta-propiolactone (BPL) at a final concentration of 1 : 2000. Inactivated concentrates are tested for HA content by the single radial diffusion test (SRD), sterility,

absence of replicating virus (inactivity), total protein, thiomersal, residual BPL, ovalbumin and endotoxin.

Three monovalent influenza bulks, currently H1N1, H3N2 and B, are pooled and used as the starting material for the manufacture of the influenza subunit virosomes. The pool is pelleted in a fixed-angle ultracentrifuge at about $60\,000 \times g$ for 1 h. The supernatant contains residual soluble proteins and is discarded. The pellet is dissolved in 100 mM octaethylene glycol (OEG) solution and the viruses are thereby disintegrated. Subsequently, the influenza glycoproteins and the viral envelope phospholipids are separated from other virus constituents by a further fixed-angle ultracentrifugation at $100\,000 \times g$ for 1 h. This time the supernatant is processed further and the pellet is discarded. This double ultracentrifugation makes use of the various properties of the unwanted constituents so that a particularly high degree of purity is achieved. After the first ultracentrifugation, dissolved unwanted constituents (e.g. solubilized viral and egg substrate proteins) in the supernatant are discarded. After the second ultracentrifugation the other unwanted non-solubilized constituents are pelleted and discarded and the purified supernatant is further processed. After this purification of the glycoproteins and envelope phospholipids, the lecithin is added and solubilized.

The safety of the egg lecithin is particularly important here, since it is of natural origin and the suspension is not subjected to further inactivation. The lecithin from egg yolk (phosphatidylcholine) is obtained from the company *Lipoid* in Germany, and is used by other producers of pharmaceutical products for parenteral use. Chemical analysis of the composition, particle size measurement, solubility measurements and tests for microbiological purity are performed by the manufacturer. The manufacture of the egg lecithin has been validated with regard to virus elimination. This validation was performed in cooperation with the Freie Universität Berlin, Germany: the initial solution was spiked with Newcastle disease virus, avian adenovirus (serotype I celovirus) and avian reovirus. None of these viruses could be recovered from the product after manufacture.

Liposomes carrying the influenza subunits at the surface are formed spontaneously during the removal of the OEG detergent by chromatography. As shown by electron micrographic studies, the distribution of influenza subunits at the liposomal surface is not regular, which means that some of the vesicles are more densely spiked than others (Fig. 30.1). The detergent-free suspension containing virosomal influenza subunits is passed through a 5 mcm filter in order to separate the chromatographic matrix substance from the suspension. The filtered pool is subsequently tested for HA content, purity, absence of detergent, and phospholipid, and then diluted with PBS–NaCl pH 7.4 to yield the final bulk.

Preclinical investigations with hemagglutinin–neuraminidase subunit unilamellar virosomal vaccines

Unilamellar virosomal subunit vaccine containing influenza HA and NA incorporated into bilayer structures closely resembles whole virus influenza vaccine (Figs 30.1 & 30.2). A series of preclinical studies have recently been performed in animals to establish the efficacy of liposomal vaccines in eliciting antibody and T-cell mediated immune responses.

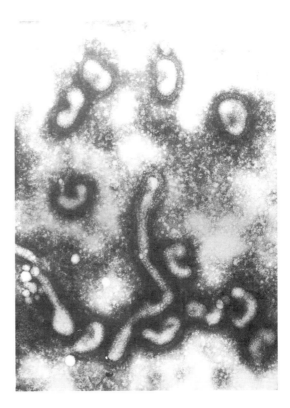

Fig. 30.2 Transmission electron micrograph of whole virus influenza vaccine bulk A/Singapore/6/86, negatively stained with phosphatungstate. Magnification × 100 000. (Source: Th. Wyler, Institute of Zoology, University of Berne, Switzerland.)

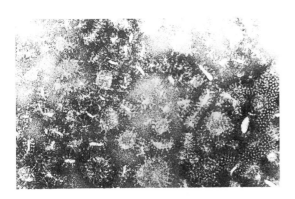

Fig. 30.1 Transmission electron micrograph of virosomal influenza vaccine (liposomes which show haemagglutinin and neuraminidase spikes at their surface), negatively stained with phosphatungstate. Magnification × 100 000. (Source: Th. Wyler, Institute of Zoology, University of Berne, Switzerland.)

In one study (Gregoriadis *et al.* 1992), reconstituted influenza virus (A/PR/8 strain) envelopes (RIVE) and influenza virus (A/Sichuan/87 (H3N2) strain) surface antigens were entrapped in dehydration–rehydration vesicles (DRV liposomes) composed of egg PC or distearoyl phosphatidylcholine (DSPC DRV) and equimolar (32 μmol) cholesterol. Balb/c mice injected intramucularly with PC or DSPC DRV liposomes containing 0.1 and 1.0 μg RIVE exhibited primary (higher dose only) and secondary responses (IgG1) which were significantly higher than those obtained in mice injected with identical amounts of non-entrapped RIVE. Significantly higher secondary responses were also observed for the IgG2a and IgG2b subclasses. In experiments designed to assess the effectiveness of DRV liposomes as a carrier of influenza virus antigens in a potential vaccine, hamsters were immunized intramuscularly with 0.1, 0.5 and 5.0 µg of free or liposome-entrapped influenza A/Sichuan/87 surface antigens. Results showed increased haemagglutination inhibition (HI) antibody levels in terms of both primary (0.5 and 5.0 µg doses) and secondary (all doses) responses in the sera of animals treated with the liposomal formulations.

In continuation of these investigations the immunogenicity and protective efficacy of an influenza A subunit vaccine preparation administered to mice in an aqueous form, or presented as immunostimulatory complexes (ISCOMs), liposomes or FCA, were assessed in comparative studies with infectious virus (Ben-Ahmeida *et al.* 1993). The ISCOM is a cage-like structure with a diameter of 30–40 nm into which antigens can be incorporated. It consists of glycosides of the adjuvant Quil A, cholesterol, the antigen, and in most cases phospholipids, such as phosphatidylcholine or -ethanolamine. Quil A is a preparation from the bark of *Quillaja saponaria* Molina, consisting of a refined mixture of closely related saponins. Quil A has potent adjuvant activity and is widely used as an adjuvant in veterinary vaccines. The adjuvant activity is related to the triterpene glycosides. The typical cage-like structure is formed by Quil A–cholesterol micelles, which are held together through hydrophobic interactions. Both intranasal and parenteral routes of administration were assessed. An enzyme-linked immunosorbent assay (ELISA) was used to measure nasal wash and serum antibody responses in groups of unprimed mice, while protection was determined by the recovery of homologous influenza virus from mouse nasal washes and lung homogenates following challenge infection by the intranasal route. The results showed that parenteral administration of the influenza antigen preparations induced variable levels of both local and systemic antibodies at weeks 3, 7 and 22 post immunization. Although the greatest levels of antibody and protection were elicited in mice following live virus infection, formulation of influenza surface HA and NA proteins into ISCOMs or liposomes elicited high and persistent antibody responses and provided relatively

good protection of the upper and lower respiratory tracts of these animals. The results also showed a relatively poor effect of subunit antigen preparations in promoting humoral immune responses and protection, irrespective of the nature of their presentation, when given by the intranasal route.

In another preclinical study (Nerome *et al.* 1990), muramyldipeptide (MDP) (6-0-(2-tetradecyl-hexadecanoyl)-N-acetylmuramyl-L-isoglutamine) was incorporated into liposomes with HA and NA molecules of influenza virus. Electron microscopic examination revealed that HA and NA subunits were attached to the inner and outer surfaces of lamellar structures of the liposomes, probably through their hydrophobic ends. The addition of cholesterol resulted in greater stability of the liposomes, which were similar in size and shape to native influenza virus particles. These liposomes enhanced the immunogenicity of HA in mice, such that the levels of antibody induced were about 16-fold higher than those of subunit HA vaccine alone. Results of proliferation tests with spleen cells from mice and guinea-pigs were consistent with the immunopotentiation of HA by liposomes. In addition, the higher antibody levels produced in mice, immunized with the HA and MDP-containing liposomes (MDP virosomes), were maintained for at least 6 months. Enhancement of the cellular immune response, measured by delayed-type hypersensitivity reactions, was also observed in the guinea-pigs immunized with MDP virosome vaccine. Preliminary tests with splenocytes from mice immunized with different vaccines also indicated that the MDP virosome vaccine induced cytotoxic T-cell activity in these mice. This study revealed that the formation of liposomes with MDP enhanced the level and persistence of circulating antibody and enhanced cellular immunity in guinea-pigs and mice.

Clinical investigations with haemagglutinin–neuraminidase subunit unilamellar virosomal vaccines

Kaji *et al.* (1992) carried out phase I clinical trials using virosomal influenza vaccines containing various amounts of HA and NA and different concentrations of MDP as an adjuvant. Seventy-seven volunteers received the vaccines which contained HA and NA from A/Yamagata/120/86 (H1N1), A/Fukuoka/C29/86 (H3N2) and B/Nagasaki/1/87 strains of influenza. The MDP-adjuvanted vaccine induced higher HA antibody titres against A/Yamagata (H1N1) and A/Fukuoka (H3N2) strains than non-adjuvanted vaccine. However, adjuvanted and non-adjuvanted vaccines containing HA and NA from B/Nagasaki were poorly immunogenic. Local adverse reactions occurred more frequently after injection of MDP-adjuvanted vaccine.

The safety and immunogenicity of another virosomal influenza vaccine presenting a unilamellar structure was evaluated in comparison with commercial whole virus and subunit vaccines in elderly people (Glück *et al.* 1994). The virosomal vaccine contained HA and NA from H1N1 and H3N2 strains of influenza A and influenza B which were incorporated into the membrane of liposomes composed of phosphatidylcholine (PC). A total of 126 residents of a nursing home, aged 63–102, were randomized to receive one of the

vaccines. All three vaccines were well tolerated. The serological data obtained by HI are presented in Tables 30.1 (seroconversion) and 30.2 (geometric mean HA antibody titre and range). The virosome formulation evoked the highest geometric mean titres in addition to significantly higher ($p = 0.039$–0.0016) seroconversion rates (i.e. $\geq$ four-fold rise in antibody titre) to all three vaccine components. Moreover, the percentage of vaccinees who achieved titres of $\geq 1:40$ was significantly higher ($p = 0.035$–0.0017) for the H1N1 and B/Yamagata strains following immunization with the virosome formulation. Immunization with the virosome formulation did not result in a significant rise in anti-PC antibodies.

Interestingly, immunization of elderly as well as young individuals performed in another study with the same unilamellar virosomal influenza vaccine resulted in a greater enhancement of mononuclear cell proliferation after influenza virus stimulation *in vitro* than did immunization with whole-cell influenza vaccine (Saurwein-Teissl *et al.* 1996). Preliminary studies performed with the uni-

Table 30.1 Seroconversion rates following vaccination with whole virus, virosome and subunit influenza vaccines i.e. $\geq$ four-fold titre rise/total (%).

Vaccine	H1N1 Singapore		H3N2 Beijing		B/Yamagata	
Whole virus	19/32 (59)		19/32 (59)		14/32 (44)	
		$p = 0.009$		$p = 0.039$		$p = 0.031$
Virosome	52/63 (83)		50/63 (79)		42/63 (67)	
		$p = 0.0019$		$p = 0.0033$		$p = 0.0016$
Subunit	14/31 (45)		16/32 (52)		10/31 (32)	

Table 30.2 Geometric mean haemagglutinin antibody titres and ranges following vaccination with whole virus, virosome and subunit influenza vaccines.

Vaccine	H1N1 Singapore		H3N2 Beijing		B/Yamagata	
	Pre	Post	Pre	Post	Pre	Post
Whole virus	2.9	29.1*	25.2	130*	3.4	16.3*
	(0–80)	(0–320)	(0–160)	(10–640)	(0–20)	(0–640)
Virosome	2.4	44.2*	20.6	142*	2.4	17.5*
	(0–80)	(0–640)	(0–320)	(20–2560)	(0–40)	(0–320)
Subunit	1.8	14*	26.4	121*	2.9	11.4*
	(0–40)	(0–320)	(0–160)	(10–5120)	(0–40)	(0–160)

* Denotes values which are significant ($p < 0.01$) as compared with baseline values.

lamellar phosphatidylcholine-phosphatidylethano-
lamine (PC-PE) virosomal influenza vaccine administered by intranasal application have also
demonstrated encouraging results consisting of
increased serum HA antibody levels of the IgG as
well as of the IgA class (R. Glück, unpublished
data). In the autumn of 1997 a liposomal influenza
subunit vaccine was registered in Switzerland by
the Swiss Serum & Vaccine Institute, Berne, following extensive clinical testing. By June 1997 the
immunogenicity, tolerability and safety of the Swiss
liposomal vaccine had been evaluated in over 1100
subjects (including 113 children) recruited into nine
clinical trials conducted in three countries. All trials
used the liposomal product, in most instances at a
standard dosage of 15 µg HA for each virus strain,
administered as a single 0.5 ml intramuscular
injection. As shown in Table 30.3, the liposomal
vaccine was well tolerated in comparison with
whole virus vaccine, and was in general more
immunogenic than other vaccines (Table 30.4). As
shown in Table 30.4, a single 0.5 ml dose of the
virosomal vaccine evoked a higher seroconversion
rate in comparison with commercially available
subunit and whole virus product vaccines in adults,
but not in children. However, an acceptable protective serum antibody level was reached by all
types of vaccine. In a further study, the concomitant
administration of diphtheria and tetanus toxoids
with liposomal influenza vaccine to elderly subjects
did not modify the antibody response or the
frequency of adverse effects to the anti-influenza
vaccine (and, importantly, the antibody responses
to the diphtheria and tetanus toxoid components
were not adversely affected either).

Clinical investigation of a unilamellar virosomal vaccine combining three influenza virus antigens and five further viral and bacterial antigens

A clinical study of the efficacy and reactogenicity of
different antigen combinations including hepatitis
A, hepatitis B, tetanus and diphtheria toxoid as well
as three strains of influenza type A and B was
published by Mengiardi *et al.* in 1995. The reactogenicity and immunogenicity of the combined

vaccine injected into one group of volunteers were
compared with those of the corresponding single
vaccines simultaneously applied at five different
sites in the other group of volunteers. All antigens
were bound to the liposome surface and liposomal
vesicles were separated from unconjugated antigens using ultrafiltration or sucrose density ultracentrifugation. The combined virosomal vaccine
contained the following antigens: hepatitis A antigen 500 radioimmunoassay (RIA) units, hepatitis B
surface antigen (HBsAg) 10 µg; diphtheria toxoid 1
Lf; tetanus toxoid 10 Limus flocculation (Lf);
influenza antigen A/Singapore (6/86)-like (H1N1)
antigen 15 µg; A/Beijing (353/89)-like (H3N3)
antigen 15 µg; and B/Yamagata (16/88)-like antigen 15 µg. The vaccines used for separate injection
had the same antigen content and were adsorbed
onto aluminium adjuvant (Di, Te, HBs).

While the antibody responses to diphtheria toxoid, tetanus toxoid and the three influenza antigens
were similar among vaccinees given either the
combined or separate vaccine formulations, the HBs
antibody titre failed to increase and the hepatitis A
antibody response was substantially impaired using
the combined virosomal vaccine. A lack of HBs
antibody production was to be expected after a
single vaccination. However, the impaired hepatitis
A antibody increase proved to be the result of an
antigenic suppression which was prevented by
halving the diphtheria and tetanus toxoid content of
the combined vaccine without impairing the
immune response to the toxoids. Table 30.5 shows
that the seroconversion rates and the geometric
mean titres (GMTs) were similar for influenza A and
B antigens given either as (a trivalent) influenza
vaccine or in combination with hepatitis A and B
antigens and diphtheria and tetanus toxoids.

Summary

Preliminary investigations indicate that unilamellar
liposomes act as optimal adjuvants for enhancing
antibody and T-cell mediated immune responses,
including those for influenza subunit antigens.
Studies in man have shown that unilamellar virosomal influenza vaccines induce higher seroconversion rates to the HA than conventional

Table 30.3 Incidence of local and systemic reactions after whole virus vaccine, subunit vaccine and virosomal vaccine. Adverse reactions/total volunteers (%). n.d., no data.

Study number	Age of volunteers (years)	Local reaction			Total adverse events			Cough			Headache		
		Whole virus	Subunit	Virosomal	Whole virus	Subunit	Virosomal	Whole virus	Subunit	Virosomal	Whole virus	Subunit	Virosomal
9009	≤54	30/104 (29)	n.d.	13/105 (12)	21/104 (20)	n.d.	30/105 (29)	4/104 (4)	n.d.	6/105 (6)	14/104 (13)	n.d.	12/105 (11)
9225	63–102	none	4/34 (12)	1/38 (3)	4/32 (13)	2/31 (6)	3/63 (5)	3/32 (9)	1/31 (3)	3/63 (5)	1/32 (3)	none	none
9311	≥65	n.d.	1/2 (50)	1/9 (11)	n.d.	2/2 (100)	9/9 (100)	n.d.	none	3/38 (8)	n.d.	2/34 (5)	none
9410	≥1–≤6	n.d.	11/18 (61)	18/31 (58)	n.d.	13/18 (72)	27/31 (87)	n.d.	2/2 (100)	5/9 (55)	n.d.	none	none
9410	>6–33	n.d.			n.d.				9/18 (50)	15/31 (48)		6/18 (33)	15/31 (48)
9414	≥18–<60	15/46 (33)	n.d.	12/56 (21)	1/46 (2)	n.d.	1/56 (2)	none	n.d.	none	none	n.d.	none
9414	≥60	11/48 (23)	n.d.	16/56 (28)	1/48 (2)	n.d.	none	none	n.d.	none	none	n.d.	none
9435	≥2–≤11	n.d.	8/12 (67)	8/13 (61)	n.d.	4/12 (33)	3/13 (23)	n.d.	1/12 (8)	1/13 (8)	n.d.	none	
9435	≥6–≤12	n.d.	7/12 (58)	5/12 (42)	n.d.	3/12 (25)	6/12 (50)	n.d.	1/12 (8)	1/12 (8)	n.d.	none	2/12 (17)

Table 30.4 Overview of comparative clinical studies with whole virus, subunit and virosomal influenza vaccines showing seroconversion rates i.e. ≥ four-fold titre rise/total volunteers (%). n.d., no data.

Study number	Methodology	Age of volunteers (years)	Number ≥ four-fold rise/total (%)								
			H1N1			H3N2			B		
			Whole virus	Subunit	Virosomal	Whole virus	Subunit	Virosomal	Whole virus	Subunit	Virosomal
9009	Double blind	≤54	50/95 (53)	n.d.	65/91 (71)	49/95 (52)	n.d.	65/91 (71)	42/95 (44)	n.d.	52/91 (57)
9225	Double blind	63–102	19/32 (59)	14/31 (45)	52/63 (83)	19/32 (59)	16/32 (52)	52/63 (83)	14/32 (44)	10/31 (32)	42/63 (67)
9311	Double blind	≥65	n.d.	13/34 (38)	27/38 (71)	n.d.	22/34 (65)	36/38 (95)	n.d.	14/34 (41)	23/38 (61)
9410	Open, randomized	≥1–≤6	n.d.	1/1 (100)	8/9 (89)	n.d.	0/1 (0)	5/9 (56)	n.d.	1/1 (100)	7/9 (78)
9410	Open, randomized	>6–33	n.d.	15/18 (83)	26/31 (84)	n.d.	12/18 (67)	20/31 (65)		13/18 (72)	16/31 (52)
9414	Double blind	≥18–<60	26/46 (57)	n.d.	35/56 (63)	31/46 (67)	n.d.	35/56 (63)	20/46 (44)	n.d.	22/56 (40)
9414	Double blind	≥60	32/48 (67)	n.d.	34/52 (65)	30/48 (63)	n.d.	34/52 (65)	28/48 (58)	n.d.	31/52 (60)
9435	Double blind	≥2–≤11	n.d.	10/12 (83)	10/11 (91)	n.d.	9/12 (75)	10/11 (100)	n.d.	11/12 (92)	9/11 (82)
9435	Double blind	≥6–≤12	n.d.	10/11 (91)	11/11 (100)	n.d.	8/11 (73)	11/11 (100)	n.d.	9/11 (82)	7/11 (64)

Table 30.5 Influenza haemagglutinin inhibition antibody titres on days 0 and 28. Group A (n = 23) received the liposomal combined vaccine while group B (n = 23) received single injections with the corresponding monovaccine. GMT, geometric mean titre.

	Day 0		Day 28	
	Group A (combined)	Group B (monovaccine)	Group A (combined)	Group B (monovaccine)
A/Singapore H1N1				
Seroconversion (%)			20/23 (86.9)	22/23 (95.6)
GMT	12	10	300	226
*p**	0,87		0,27	
A/Beijing H3N2				
Seroconversion (%)			21/23 (91.3)	20/23 (86.9)
GMT	34	31	525	411
*p**	0,71		0,40	
B/Yamagata				
Seroconversion (%)			21/23 (91.3)	19/23 (82.6)
GMT	10	8	94	165
*p**	0,58		0,11	

* Mann–Whitney–Wilcoxon test.

vaccines and are well tolerated. When several viral and toxoid antigens including those of three influenza virus strains were incorporated into the same unilamellar virosome, the capacity of the influenza virus antigens to induce high HA antibody titres was not impaired.

References

Alving, C.R. (1991) Liposomes as carriers of antigens and adjuvants. *J Immunol Meth* **140**, 1–13.

Alving, C.R. (1992) Immunologic aspects of liposomes: presentation and processing of liposomal protein and phospholipid antigens. *Biochim Biophys Acta* **1113**, 307–22.

Alving, C.R. (1993) Lipopolysaccharide, lipid A, and liposomes containing lipid A as immunologic adjuvants. *Immunobiology* **187**, 430–46.

Alving, C.R., Verma, J.N., Rao, U. *et al.* (1992) Liposomes containing lipid A as a potent non-toxic adjuvant. *Res Immunol* **143**, 197–8.

Alving, C.R., Detrick, B., Richards, R.L., Lewis, M.G., Shaffemann, A. & Eddy, G.A. (1993) Novel adjuvant strategies for experimental malaria and AIDS vaccines. In: Bystryn, J., Ferrone, S. & Livingston, P. (eds) *Specific Immunotherapy of Cancer with Vaccines*. New York. *Ann NY Acad Sci* **690**, 265–75.

Antimisiaris, S.G., Jayasekera, P. & Gregoriadis, G. (1993) Liposomes as vaccine carriers. Incorporation of soluble and particulate antigens in giant vesicles. *J Immunol Meth* **166**, 271–80.

Ben-Ahmeida, E.T.S., Gregoriadis, G., Potter, C.W. & Jennings, R. (1993) Immunopotentiation of local and systemic humoral immune responses by ISCOMs, liposomes and FCA: role in protection against influenza A in mice. *Vaccine* **11**, 1302–9.

Bender, A., Bui, K.B., Feldman, M.A.V., Larsson, M. & Bhardwaj, N. (1995) Inactivated influenza virus, when presented on dendritic cells, elicits human CD8[+] cytolytic T cell responses. *J Exp Med* **182**, 1663–71.

Brunner, J., Zugliani, C. & Mischler, R. (1991): Fusion acitivity of influenza virus PR8/34 correlates with a temperature-induced conformational change within the hemagglutinin ectodomain detected by photochemical labeling. *Biochem* **30**, 2432–8.

Durrer, P., Galli, C., Hoenke, S. *et al.* (1996) H+-induced membrane insertion of influenza virus hemagglutinin involves the HA_2 amino-terminal fusion peptide but not the coiled coil region. *J Biol Chem* **271** (23), 13417–21.

Fortin, A. & Therien, H.M. (1993) Mechanism of liposome adjuvanticity: an *in vivo* approach. *Immunobiology* **188**, 316–22.

Garçon, N.M.J. & Six, H.R. (1991) Universal vaccine carrier. Liposomes that provide T-dependent help to weak antigens. *J Immunol* **146**, 3697–702.

Glück, R. & Althaus, B. (1995) Immunogenität einer neuen liposomalen Influenzavakzine. Abstract of Annual Meeting Swiss Soc Internat Medicine, Montreux 1995, abstract no. P298. *Schweiz Med Wschr* **125** (Suppl. 69), 745.

Glück, R., Mischler, R., Finkel, B. *et al.* (1994) Immunogenicity of new virosome influenza vaccine in the elderly people. *Lancet* **344**, 160–3.

Gregoriadis, G., Tan, L., Ben-Ahmeida, E.T.S. & Jennings, R. (1992) Liposomes enhance the immunogenicity of reconstituted influenza virus A/PR/8 envelopes and the formation of protective antibody by influenza virus A/Sichuan/87 (H3N2) surface antigen. *Vaccine* **10**, 747–53.

Gupta, R.K., Relyveld, E.H., Lindblad, E.B., Bizzini, B., Ben-Efraim, S. & Gupta, C.K. (1993) Adjuvants—a balance between toxicity and adjuvanticity. *Vaccine* **11**, 293–306.

Gupta, R.K., Varanelli, C., Wallach, D.F.H, Griffin, P. & Siber, G.R. (in press) Adjuvant properties of non-phospholipid liposomes (Novasomes®) in experimental animals for human vaccine antigens. *Vaccine*.

Kaji, M., Kaji, Y., Kaji, M. *et al.* (1992) Phase I clinical tests on influenza MDP-virosome vaccine (KD-5382). *Vaccine* **10**, 663–7.

Mengiardi, B., Berger, R., Just, M. & Glück, R. (1995) Virosomes as carriers for combined vaccines. Vaccine **13**, 1306–15.

Nerome, K., Yoshioka, Y., Ishida, M. *et al.* (1990) Development of a new type of influenza subunit vaccine made by muramyldipeptide-liposome: enhancement of humoral and cellular responses. *Vaccine* **8**, 503–9.

Pietrobon, P.J.F. (1995) Liposome design and vaccine development. In: Powell, M.F., & Newman, M.J. (eds) *Vaccine Design: The Subunit and Adjuvant Approach*, pp. 347–61. Plenum Publishing Corporation, New York.

Powers, D., Kilbourne, E.D. & Johansson, B.E. (1996) Neuraminidase-specific antibody responses to inactivated influenza virus vaccine in young and elderly adults. *Clin Diag Lab Immunol* **3** (5), 511–16.

Saurwein-Teissl, M., Steger, M.M., Glück, R., Cryz, S. & Grubeck-Loebenstein, B. (1996) *In vitro* studies on the stimulatory effects of a new virosome influenza vaccine on T cells from young and old healthy individuals. In: *Symposium of Oesterreichische Gesellschaft für Allergologie und Immunologie*. Vienna, November 21–3, 1996.

Shaw, M.W., Arden, N.H. & Maassab, H.F. (1992) New aspects of influenza viruses. *Clin Microbiol Rev* **5** (1), 74–92.

Tsurudome, M., Glück, R., Graf, R., Falchetto, R., Schaller, U. & Brunner, J. (1992): Lipid interactions of the hemagglutinin HA_2 NH_2-terminal segment during influenza virus-induced membrane fusion. *J Biol Chem* **267** (28), 20225–32.

van Rooijen, N. (1990) Liposomes as carrier and immunoadjuvant of vaccine antigens. In: Mizrahi, A. (ed.) *Bacterial Vaccines, Advances in Biotechnological Processes*, Vol. 13, pp. 255–79. Wiley-Liss, New York.

van Rooijen, N. (1992) Liposomes as an *in vivo* tool to study and manipulate macrophage function. 41st Forum in Immunology. *Res Immunol* **143**, 177–256.

Weber, T., Paesold, G., Galli, C., Mischler, R., Semenza, G. & Brunner, J. (1994) Evidence for H^+-induced insertion of influenza hemagglutinin HA_2 N-terminal segment into viral membrane. *J Biol Chem* **269** (28), 18353–8.

CHAPTER 31

DNA Vaccination: a Potential Future Strategy

Robert G. Webster

Summary

Immunization with purified DNA is a powerful new technique for inducing immune responses. It has been less than 10 years since the first demonstration, which used influenza as the model system, of the induction of protective immunity by this approach. The concept of DNA immunization is very simple and involves insertion of the gene encoding the antigen of choice into a bacterial plasmid and injection of the plasmid into the host where the antigen is expressed, and where it induces humoral and cellular immunity. The most effective routes and methods for DNA immunization are bombardment with particles coated with DNA ('gene gun' technique), followed by the intramuscular and intradermal routes. DNA immunization technology has the potential to induce immunity to all antigens that can be completely encoded in DNA, which therefore include all protein, but not carbohydrate, antigens. The available information supports the notion that DNA immunization results in presentation of antigens to the host's immune system in a natural form, like that achieved with live attenuated vaccines.

Some potential advantages of DNA immunization are that it (i) mimics live attenuated vaccination while eliminating the possibility of contamination with undesirable adventitious agents from the culture system; (ii) provides correct major histocompatibility class (MHC) I presentation of antigen; (iii) allows concurrent administration of multiple DNA-encoded antigens and/or cytokines; (iv) provides genetic stability of immunizing plasmid; (v) may increase the rapidity with which new vaccines with genetic identity are generated; (vi) may allow creation of vaccines for agents that cannot be grown in culture; (vii) obviates the need for a 'cold chain' for vaccines in developing countries; and (viii) may permit modulation of the immune response. The perceived risks of DNA immunization include (i) the integration of the plasmid into the host genome; (ii) the induction of anti-DNA antibodies and autoimmunity; and (iii) the induction of tolerance. Each of these potential advantages and disadvantages will be addressed in this chapter.

DNA immunization is in its infancy, and many questions remain to be answered. The efficiency of transfection of host cells is low but sufficient to induce immunological responsiveness. The DNA plasmid is retained in the transfected cells in an unintegrated form for the life of the cell, the majority of transfected cells are eliminated but residual expression has been detected for longer periods.

Because the initial human trials are still in progress, it is currently too early to predict the future use of DNA vaccines in human immunization programmes. Providing that the perceived risks do not materialize, DNA immunization will likely be particularly advantageous for rapidly changing vaccines when antigenic drift and shift occurs in influenza in humans. The biotechnology age will increase our sophistication in the design, delivery and use of DNA vaccines to modulate both desirable and undesirable aspects of the immune response, and DNA immunization will ultimately be the approach for the majority of vaccines.

Introduction

The eradication of smallpox, the control and likely eradication of poliomyelitis, and the control of measles have been achieved through vaccination, and the associated cost–benefit amounts to billions of pounds per year. The quest to control a large number of infectious diseases continues, as vaccines are not available for most of these, and conventional strategies are unlikely to produce the necessary reagents. The preparation of vaccines for influenza presents a unique problem, for each year we have to 'reinvent the wheel' and select the most appropriate strain, prepare high growth reassortants, and manufacture and standardize new vaccine(s) before the onset of the influenza season. This process is necessary because influenza viruses lack proof-reading mechanisms to control the accuracy of the replication of their genomes (Holland *et al.* 1992) and therefore show continuous antigenic drift.

Each February, the World Health Organization (WHO) collaborating laboratories meet to review information obtained from more than 110 laboratories worldwide and decide which strains best represent those that are likely to be dominant in the next year. Experience at reviewing the data and some good guesswork has resulted in surprisingly good matches with the influenza virus that has become dominant in recent years. This process takes up to 6 months, and because the viruses in nature continue to evolve, the vaccine strain used can be as much as a year out of date by the time the vaccine is delivered to humans. Therefore, although the development of a 'new' vaccine each year is remarkable, in terms of virus variability, even this pace is too slow. This lag can pose serious problems when preparing for an influenza pandemic, especially in the worst-case scenario of reappearance of a highly pathogenic 'Spanish-type influenza'. DNA immunization may offer certain advantages over conventional vaccine strategies of inactivated intact virus or subunit vaccines.

This chapter discusses the design of plasmids for DNA immunization, the features of the immune response(s) induced, modulation of that response, safety considerations and the efficacy of DNA-based vaccines. The potential advantages and dis-advantages will be evaluated. Although this chapter will focus on studies on DNA immunization to influenza, this strategy is applicable to most infectious diseases and cancer.

DNA immunization—the strategy

The concept of DNA immunization is very simple and is based on the fact that DNA encodes the genetic information for all protein antigens. DNA encoding the antigen(s) of choice for influenza viruses—including haemagglutinin (HA), neuraminidase (NA) and nucleoprotein (NP)—are inserted into a plasmid, which is injected into the host. Host cells then express the virion proteins instead of virus particles (Fig. 31.1). These proteins are in the correct configuration to induce both antibody and cell-mediated immune responses and protective immunity.

The first report of protective immunity induced by DNA of an infectious agent (in this case, influenza) was published in 1993 (Robinson *et al.* 1993; Ulmer *et al.* 1993), and this technology was quickly applied to a wide range of infectious agents (Table 31.1). The routes of inoculation used for DNA immunization include intramuscular, intradermal, and gene-gun delivery to the skin (Wolff *et al.* 1990; Tang *et al.* 1992; Fynan *et al.* 1993). One of the most effective methods for potentiating the efficiency of transfection is the use of a gene-gun to shoot DNA-coated gold beads directly into cells (Yang *et al.* 1990). The most dramatic effect of particle bombardment with DNA was found on induction of immunity after DNA transfer to the epidermis (Fynan *et al.* 1993): as little as 0.04 µg of a plasmid containing the HA of influenza A/PR/8/ 34 (H1N1) provided 100% protection of mice from challenge after one immunization. Other novel methods for delivering plasmid DNA into host cell include the use of highly attenuated *Shigella* (Sizemore *et al.* 1995). The advantages of this system are that the *Shigella* vector is designed to deliver DNA to the colonic mucosa and is therefore suitable for oral or mucosal immunization. Delivery of DNA-encoded antigens to the mucosal immune system will likely permit immunization with multiple antigens simultaneously.

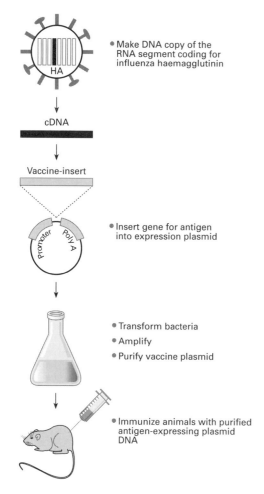

Fig. 31.1 Schematic illustration of the preparation of a DNA vaccine containing influenza virus haemagglutinin. (From Webster & Robinson, 1997, with permission from Adis International.)

The construct used for DNA immunization

A DNA copy of the RNA segment of influenza virus encoding, for example, the HA protein is inserted into a bacterial plasmid (see Fig. 31.1). The gene product should not be toxic to these cells, as has been found with some viral proteins (Ertl *et al.* 1995). This circular plasmid, which can replicate in bacteria, contains control elements including a strong eukaryotic promoter of cytomegalovirus (CMV early promoter), intron A and sequences

encoding a tissue plasminogen activator (tPA), which enables expression of the HA protein in the B cells of a mammalian host (Fig. 31.2). Other characteristics that are desirable in expression vectors for DNA immunization include: (i) high copy number; and (ii) lack of replication or integration into the host chromosome. The medium which contains the plasmid DNA for vaccination must be free of any contamination, particularly toxic or inherently antigenic substances such as endotoxins and antibiotics. The aim is to express (in mammalian cells) high levels of a gene product defining antigenic domains that will stimulate the desired immune response and modulate it when necessary. The low efficiency of direct gene transfer with plasmid DNA (only 1–2% of mouse muscle cells are transfected; Davis *et al.* 1993b) makes high-level expression necessary.

A range of viral enhancers have been successfully used in vectors for direct DNA immunization

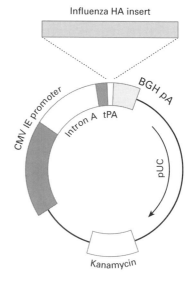

Fig. 31.2 Schematic illustration of a typical plasmid used for DNA vaccination. The double-stranded plasmid DNA derived from bacteria contains a strong eukaryotic promoter from human cytomegalovirus (CMV immediate early promoter, CMVIE promoter), intron A, sequences encoding a tissue plasminogen activator leader (tPA), a cloning site for inserting the gene of interest, the bovine growth hormone polyadenylation sequence (BGHpA), and a selectable marker (kanamycin). (From Webster & Robinson, 1997, with permission from Adis International.)

Table 31.1 Early examples of induction of immunity to infectious agents by DNA immunization. CTL, cytotoxic T lymphocyte.

Virus	Gene	Animal	Antibodies	Cell-mediated response	Protection	Comment	References
Influenza (H7N7), (H1N1)	Haemagglutinin Nucleoprotein	Chicken, mouse	Yes	CTLs to nucleoprotein	Protection from challenge	Homologous and heterologous protection	Robinson et al., 1993; Ulmer et al., 1993; Fynan et al., 1993
Herpes bovine	BHV/1 glycoprotein	Mice, cattle	ELISA antibodies	NT	Reduced virus shedding in calves	Seroconversion in both mice and cattle	Cox et al., 1993
Hepatitis B	HBsAg	Mice	High levels of circulating antibodies	Strong CTL responses	NT	Superior to recombinant protein immunization	Davis et al., 1993a
Rabies	Rabies glycoprotein	Mice	Neutralizing antibodies	Virus-specific CTLs	Protection from lethal challenge	Full response involving TC and Th	Xiang et al., 1994
HIV	Env, Gag, Pol, Rev	Mice, monkeys	Antibodies to gp 160 and gp 41	Lymphocyte proliferation and CTLs	NT	Cross clade antibody activity, no challenge	Coney et al., 1994
Malaria, Plasmodium yoelii	Circumsporozite protein (PyCSP)	Mice	High levels of antibodies	Strong CTL responses	Yes	Nine of 16 mice protected superior to irradiated sporozoite immunization	Hoffman et al., 1994
Mycobacterium leprae	Heat shock mileprae (MLhsP65)	Mice	NT	CD4 and CD8 T-cell responses	Yes	Adoptive transfer of immunity with CD8 cells	Lowrie et al., 1994
LCMV	Nucleoprotein/Glyoprotein	Mice	Antiviral antibodies	Virus-specific CTLs	Reduced virus titres	Less efficacious than recombinant vaccinia expressed antigens	Zarozinski et al., 1995; Yokoyama et al., 1995; Martins et al., 1995
Herpes	Glycoprotein B	Mice	HSV specific antibody of IgC-2a isotype	Adoptive transfer with CD4+ cells No CD8+ response	Protection against persistent infection	Immunity similar to infectious virus	Manickan et al., 1995

including those of SV40, retrovirus, polyoma, papilloma as well as a variety of cellular enhancers. The highest levels of expression in a wide range of mammalian cells and host animals has been obtained with the enhancer from human CMV (Cheng *et al.* 1993).

In addition to expression of large amounts of protein for DNA immunization, the plasmid also requires short oligonucleotide immunostimulatory sequences (Sato *et al.* 1996). These sequences include a transcriptional unit that directs antigen synthesis and an adjuvant unit in the plasmid backbone that elicits the production of type 1 interferon and interleukin-12 (IL-12) in the transfected cells and antibody-producing cells (APCs).

The mechanism of DNA uptake by cells has not been resolved. In muscle cells, it has been proposed that DNA is taken up through the T tubules (Wolff *et al.* 1992). When administered by the particle bombardment method, DNA is delivered directly into the cells, and transfected skin-derived dendritic cells localize in the draining lymph nodes (Condon *et al.* 1996). Overall, the efficiency of transfecting cells after direct DNA administration is very low. However, for immunological priming and maintenance, a small number of cells transiently expressing antigen may be ideal.

Although plasmid DNA that enters a host cell might conceivably be integrated into the cell chromosome at low frequency, available evidence indicates that neither integration nor replication actually occurs (Nichols *et al.* 1995). The administered plasmid DNA seems to transiently reside as an extrachromosomal element in the nucleus of the transfected cell, where the gene it carries can be transcribed and translated. Plasmid DNA has been detected for several months after inoculation into liver or muscle. Indeed, DNA of bacterial origin retains methylation patterns characteristic of bacteria rather than the mammalian host in which it is being maintained.

This unintegrated plasmid DNA remains in the transfected cells for the life of the cell. With intradermal inoculation, the transfected cells are shed within days of inoculation, whereas intramuscularly inoculated myocytes are longer lasting. In one study, plasmid DNA containing the NP gene of

influenza A virus (VIJNeo-NP) persisted for at least 18 weeks in mouse muscle before decreasing over time (Nichols *et al.* 1995).

General features of DNA immunization

A review of the early literature (see Table 31.1) reveals that DNA immunization, like infection, initiates both antibodies and cell-mediated immune responses. Influenza virus has served as a model system to understand the mechanism(s) by which DNA vaccines induce immunity. These mechanisms are as follows.

Induction of protective immunity to influenza in mice and chickens

In addition to demonstrating the efficacy of DNA immunization in mice and chickens, the initial studies with influenza established that the efficiency of transfection does not necessarily determine the efficacy of vaccination (Fynan *et al.* 1993; Robinson *et al.* 1993; Ulmer *et al.* 1993). Thus, whereas intramuscular injection leads to maximum expression of saline solutions containing DNA, intradermal administration was as efficacious in inducing immunity. These studies indicate that proper antigen presentation is probably more important than high levels of expression. The high immunogenicity of DNA that has been delivered by gene gun to the epidermis of mice seems to be due to the presence of Langerhans' cells, which can present transfected antigens to the T helper (Th) compartment of the immune system. These studies also established the induction of both Th and B-cell immunity by DNA immunizations, thereby setting the stage for its further development.

Induction of crossreactive (heterotypic) immunity to influenza viruses

Influenza viruses show continuous antigenic drift, which makes it necessary to change human vaccine strains almost every year to keep abreast of antigenic changes in the HA and NA. The NP of influenza virus, one of the antigenically conserved internal proteins, is important in the induction of crossreactive cytotoxic T lymphocytes (CTLs) (see Chapter 21) and recovery from infection, but it does not provide significant protection from initial infection.

The demonstration that DNA immunization with the NP of influenza A provides heterotypic immunity between different subtypes of influenza A in mice (Montgomery *et al.* 1993; Ulmer *et al.* 1993) is important if this phenomenon is shown to extend to animals naturally infected with influenza, including humans, pigs, horses and chickens. Studies on the preclinical efficacy of contemporary human vaccine strains in ferrets and non-human primates suggest that DNA expression vectors encoding HA and internal proteins were more efficient than were conventional-inactivated or subvirion vaccines (Donnelly *et al.* 1995). Preliminary studies with DNA vaccine to the NP of A/PR/8/34 (H1N1) in mice failed to provide protection from homologous challenge (Robinson *et al.* 1997), indicating that more studies are needed to determine if heterotypic immunity induced by NP to influenza applies across all subtypes and in naturally infected hosts. Other studies by Fu *et al.* (1997) have identified an immunorecessive CTL epitope on influenza NP that may require intensive immunization for induction. This finding may explain the discrepancy between these studies. Further experiments are needed to demonstrate heterotypic immunity clearly, but if the promise of heterotypic immunity is fulfilled, then DNA immunization may revolutionize the control of influenza.

Induction of long-term B-cell immunity to influenza in mice

Comparative studies of conventional and DNA vaccines to influenza virus have established that DNA vaccination is equivalent to live vaccination in protecting mice from challenge (Justewicz *et al.* 1995; Boyle *et al.* 1996). Two doses of intradermal gene-gun administered DNA vaccine provided 100% protection, as did a live virus vaccine, whereas a subunit vaccine provided only 70% protection. The APCs localized in the spleen and bone marrow after vaccination; after challenge these cells were found in the lymph nodes draining the lungs. CD4$^+$ cells were vital for induction of APCs, because treatment with anti-CD4$^+$ antibody completely abolished AFCs from all compartments. The immunity induced by DNA immunization was maintained in the spleen and bone marrow for at least 1 year. Because repeated challenge with live influenza virus resulted in mobilization of AFCs to the lymphoid tissues associated with the respiratory tract, DNA immunization of mice provides long-term (perhaps life-long) immunity to the homologous virus (Justewicz *et al.* 1996). Studies in ferrets and non-human primates (Donnelly *et al.* 1995) confirm that DNA immunization is more effective than conventional influenza virus subunit vaccines.

Broadening of the antibody response to the HA of influenza virus

Preliminary evidence suggests that DNA immunization may more effectively induce crossreactive antibody than does vaccination with live influenza virus. Immunization of ferrets with DNA encoding the HA of A/PR/8/34 (H1N1) induced antibodies that crossreacted with A/Swine/Shope/30 (H1N1) (Webster *et al.* 1994). This crossreaction was not found after natural infection of ferrets. These studies indicate the potential for inducing high-affinity antibodies. In addition, these preliminary results warrant further study, for if crossreactive antibodies are induced, it may be possible to reduce the frequency at which influenza vaccine strains are changed.

Modulation of the antibody isotype by DNA immunization

There is increasing evidence that DNA immunization permits the investigator to modulate the immune response by targeting a Th1 or Th2 response. Th1 responses lead to cell-mediated immune killing of infected cells and production of neutralizing antibody production, whereas Th2 responses induce immunoglobulin E (IgE) and allergic responses. Because the bacterial DNA used for immunization induces cytokines, the plasmid vector can alter the intensity and character of the immune response. One such cytokine is interferon-γ (IFN-γ), a central mediator of cellular immune reactions that can promote responsiveness by up regulating the expression of class II molecules. Furthermore, IFN-γ participates in the interplay of Th1/Th2 cells and can shift the balance away from a Th2 response. At present, the full range of cytokines induced by bacterial DNA is unknown, and it is unclear whether the action of this molecule is to promote responsiveness in general or steer the immune system in the direction of Th1 responsiveness (Pisetsky *et al.* 1995).

Intramuscular or intradermal DNA vaccination of mice with the HA of influenza virus induced primarily IgG-2a antibodies, whereas gene-gun immunization produces mainly IgG-1 antibodies. Therefore, different methods of delivering gene vaccines can influence the isotype of the antibodies produced (Feltquate *et al.* 1997). Intramuscular immunization may result in Th1-like responses, due to the predominance of IgG-2a antibodies, CTL activity, and IFN-γ production and to the lack of IL-4 release. In contrast, gene-gun immunization appears to elicit a Th2 response (Fuller & Haynes 1996). Studies on the antibody isotypes induced in mice after DNA immunization with plasmid DNA encoding the circumsporozite protein of *Plasmodium yoelli* revealed an isotype switch from IgG-1 to IgG-2a (Mor *et al.* 1995). Isotype switching has important implications for therapeutic manipulation of the immune system, particularly in regard to allergies and autoimmunity.

Manipulation of the immune response with cytokine genes

In addition to altering the character of the immune response, the cytokines induced by the plasmids used for DNA immunization can alter the intensity of the response (Pisetsky *et al.* 1995). Cytokines play a central role in the immune response by promoting the activation of specific and non-specific effector mechanisms. Inoculation of mice with vectors that expressed granulocyte-macrophage colony-stimulating factor (GM-CSF) and the rabies glycoprotein enhanced the B- and T-helper cell activity to rabies virus, whereas concurrent inoculation with an additional plasmid expressing IFN-γ resulted in a decreased immune response (Xiang & Ertl 1995).

Coexpression of other cytokines, including IL-6 (Ramshaw *et al.* 1996), has also been shown to augment the immune response to DNA vaccines encoding the HA of influenza viruses. Therefore, inoculation of mixtures of plasmids that encode antigen or cytokines or of polycistronic vectors that express both may improve the efficacy of DNA immunization. Most importantly, DNA immunization has the potential for yielding further insight into the interplay of antigen and cytokine in the modulation of immune responses.

Safety considerations

All vaccines must be safe, effective, inexpensive, heat-stable, able to induce long-lasting immunity and simple to administer (Ada 1994). At the first WHO symposium on nucleic acid vaccines, DNA immunization was described as providing 'arguably the greatest advantage over the use of purified recombinant-derived protein antigens, especially in the many cases in which it has proved difficult or impossible to produce a complex viral or parasitic antigen in a native form using traditional recombinant techniques *in vitro*' (Schödel *et al.* 1994). The introduction of genetic information into mammalian hosts raises several safety concerns. The three safety concerns discussed here include (i) the formation of anti-DNA antibodies; (ii) the unexpected and untoward consequences of persistent expression of a foreign antigen; and (iii) the potential for causing transformation (Robertson 1994).

Anti-DNA antibodies

Most of the information about anti-DNA antibodies stems from studies on autoimmune diseases such as systemic lupus erythematosus (SLE). Antibodies against single-stranded (ss) DNA, double-stranded (ds) RNA, polyribonucleotides, ribonucleoproteins (RNP), and ribosomes are found at high levels in the sera of patients with SLE (Koffler *et al.* 1969). Autoantibodies after DNA immunization could arise as a consequence of polyclonal B-cell expansion and/or antigen-driven B-cell activation and selection, but neither is likely sufficient by itself for the development of autoimmunity. In addition, although antibodies to ssDNA can be experimentally induced in mice, it is exceedingly difficult to raise antibodies to native dsDNA. In fact, in these cases the antigen is usually denatured ssDNA, often coupled to a carrier, and not the original native DNA.

Studies to date indicate that there is no evidence for antibody induction against the DNA even after repeated injections (Parker *et al.* 1995) of mice or humans (Nabel *et al.* 1993). To provide rigorous testing of the immunogenicity of plasmid DNA, mice prone to autoimmunity (B/W) and controls (BALB/c) were immunized with a plasmid encoding the glycoprotein of *P. yoelii* (Mor *et al.* 1995). The patterns of the immune responses in both strains were similar, and there was no evidence that the B/W mice produced anti-DNA antibodies that interfered with vaccine effectiveness. Therefore, the formation of anti-DNA antibodies and the induction of autoimmune disease are considered to be unlikely consequences of the administration of plasmid DNA.

Altered immune state

Events that may lead to an altered immune state include the induction of tolerance, autoimmunity, anaphylaxis, hyperimmunity and autoaggression. Studies in neonatal mice with a vector that expressed the rabies virus glycoprotein induced B- and T-cell responses, with no evidence of induction of tolerance (Wang *et al.* 1997). At the present time, each of these consequences remain theoretical considerations. Thus far, no evidence suggests that these possible scenarios are practical concerns (Robertson 1994).

Transformation

Theoretically, the introduction of extraneous DNA could lead to the formation of tumour cells through the insertion into or deactivation of a suppressor gene (Griffiths 1995). Disruption of a tumour suppressor gene through the insertion of extraneous DNA can occur in one of three ways: by random integration, homologous recombination or retrovirus-mediated insertion. The most likely means in the present context is random integration. DNA transfected into actively growing cell cultures by a variety of means can integrate either randomly or by homologous recombination (Hasty *et al.* 1991), with random insertion being the more frequent event, even when good homology exists. Whether similar integration occurs in non-dividing muscle cells after injection of DNA vaccine plasmids or in cells from other tissues by incidental exposure has not been definitively determined. For DNA vaccines, the likelihood of insertion should be devoid of sequences known to promote insertion into the human chromosome.

Nichols *et al.* (1995) used polymerase chain reaction (PCR) analysis to look for sequences from an influenza NP-DNA vaccine plasmid (VIJneo-NP) in genomic DNA purified from the quadriceps muscle and 12 other tissues of immunized mice. These studies demonstrated that no integration could be detected at 3, 6, 12 and 18 weeks after the injection of 100 µg vaccine into each quadricep muscle. The level of sensitivity (1–7.5 plasmid copies per 150 000 nuclei) indicated that the frequency of any induced mutation would be approximately three orders of magnitude less than that of spontaneous mutation. Using data from the transfection and infection of cell cultures with retroviruses, Temin (1990) created a worst-case scenario of the risk of transformation after DNA immunization. According to those calculations, the probability of a harmful effect from injected DNA was three orders of magnitude less than that for spontaneous mutation.

Although direct inoculation of oncogene DNA can induce tumours, the risk of induction of tumours by plasmids specifically designed for DNA immunization is several orders of magnitude below that associated with spontaneous mutation rate of human DNA. Additional testing for integration is needed before DNA vaccines will be generally accepted for use in people. In addition, the risk/benefit ratios will have to be weighed in the context of specific diseases.

Regulatory considerations

The factors affecting the development and certification of DNA vaccines have been discussed in an excellent article by Maurice Hilleman (1995). A major consideration is close co-operation between the parties developing these vaccines and the regulatory authorities who have the authority for approving the content, quality and safety of the product and the clinical testing of candidate vaccines. Experience with live virus vaccines can provide insight into safety and benefits that are relevant to DNA vaccines. As Hilleman points out, 'It is perhaps a great benefit to mankind that the safety of live viral vaccines was established during an era of lesser technical and regulatory complexities'. It is most encouraging that DNA-based vaccines for influenza and for human immunodeficiency virus (HIV) are in clinical trials (Conference Report 1996).

Mechanisms of induction of immunity to DNA immunization

In part, live attenuated vaccines are so effective because they activate CD8$^+$ and CD4$^+$ precursor cells that give rise to the major antiviral effector cells: the MHC class I-restricted CTLs and the class II-restricted Th cells (Braciale 1993). The reason for this resides in the cell biology of the synthesis, assembly, and transport of the MHC class I molecule. The effective specific immune response to viral and parasitic diseases that is induced by DNA immunization involves both cell-mediated and antibody-mediated immunity. The available information supports the idea that like live attenuated vaccines, DNA immunization results in presentation of antigens in a natural form to the host immune system (Fig. 31.3). One model for the priming of humoral and cellular immune responses by DNA vaccines reflects the distinct pathways of MHC class I and II antigen-processing in cell culture (see Fig. 31.3). Immune responses are thought to occur when antigen that is encoded by the plasmid-containing myocyte or kerotinocyte is released by secretion or cell death. The antigens are then taken up by macrophages and B cells, thereby initiating a Th-dependent antibody response.

The mechanism of induction of immune responses in naive animals after DNA immunization is still largely unresolved. The ability to manipulate the immune response with specifically designed plasmids affords the potential of up- or downregulating various components of the

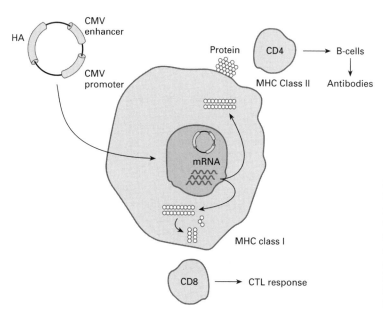

Fig. 31.3 Immune responses induced by DNA immunization. The immune responses induced are similar to those after infection with live attenuated viruses and induce both antibody and cell-mediated immune responses. CMV, cytomegalovirus; HA, haemagglutinin; MHC, major histocompatibility complex; CTL, cytotoxic T lymphocyte.

immune response as required. Including sequences that are mitogenic and provide adjuvant effects may stimulate desired responses, whereas elimination from vaccine plasmids of sequences that promote autoimmune responses or undesired cellular responses may be equally possible. Elucidating the mechanisms by which DNA immunization induces immunity will likely reap far-reaching benefits.

Future directions

We are at the very dawn of the DNA vaccine era. The optimal plasmid construct for DNA immunization of humans probably has not yet been designed, and the role of immunostimulatory sequences in the antigenic DNA and the influence of its methylation status have not been established. For use in humans, the selectable marker (kanamycin) cannot be used and must be replaced. One question that remains to be answered for influenza viruses is 'How will long-lasting immunity to DNA vaccines influence the immune response to subsequent vaccination (or infection) with variants of that subtype?' Will an 'original sin' response be detrimental? This potential disadvantage of DNA immunization needs to be addressed in future studies.

Of immediate practical importance is the need to manufacture vaccines rapidly in response to the next influenza pandemic, and distributing and administering vaccines to an increasing world population will continue to be an enormous logistic problem. Our as-yet limited knowledge of DNA vaccination technology already suggests that DNA vaccines may greatly alleviate these concerns. Understanding the mechanisms by which plasmid DNA is taken up and expressed and the means to manipulate the multiple parameters involved in B- and T-cell responses may lead us to discover strategies for directing the immune response to conserved but currently non-antigenic regions of the influenza HA and NA. Providing that DNA vaccines meet the safety requirements discussed previously, this method of immunization will likely play an important role in future strategies to control influenza and many other infectious diseases.

Acknowledgements

This work was supported by Public Health Service grants AI-08831 from the National Institute of Allergy and Infectious Diseases and the Cancer Centre Support (CORE) grant CA-21765 and by the American Lebanese Syrian Associated Charities (ALSAC).

References

Ada, G.L. (1994) Vaccines and immune responses. In: Webster, R.G. and Granoff, A. (eds) *Encyclopedia of Virology*, pp. 1503–7. Academic Press.

Boyle, C.M., Morin, M., Webster, R.G. & Robinson, H.L. (1996) Role of different lymphoid tissues in the initiation and maintenance of DNA-raised antibody responses to the influenza virus H1 glycoprotein. *J Virol* **70**, 9074–8.

Braciale, T.J. (1993) Naked DNA and vaccine design. *Trends Microbiol* **1**, 323–4.

Cheng, L., Ziegelhoffer, P.R. & Yang, N.-S. (1993) *In vivo* promoter activity and transgene expression in mammalian somatic tissues evaluated by using particle bombardment. *Proc Natl Acad Sci USA* **90**, 4455–9.

Condon, C., Watkins, S.C., Celluzzi, C.M., Thompson, K. & Falo, L.D. Jr (1996) DNA-based immunization by *in vivo* transfection of dendritic cells. *Nature Med* **2**, 1122–7.

Coney, L., Wang, B., Ugen, K.E. *et al.* (1994) Facilitated DNA inoculation induces anti-HIV-1 immunity *in vivo*. *Vaccine* **12**, 1545–50.

Conference Report (1996) First humans receive naked DNA vaccine. *AIDS Weekly Plus* **1**, 5.

Cox, G., Zamb, T.J. & Babiuk, L.A. (1993) Bovine herpesvirus 1: immune responses in mice and cattle injected with plasmid DNA. *J Virol* **67**, 5664–7.

Davis, H.L., Michel, M. & Whalen, R. (1993a) DNA-based immunization induces continuous secretion of hepatitis B surface antigen and high levels of circulating antibody. *Hum Mol Genet* **2**, 1847–51.

Davis, H.L., Whalen, R.G. & Demeneix, B.A. (1993b) Direct gene transfer into skeletal muscle *in vivo*: Factors affecting efficiency of transfer and stability of expression. *Hum Gene Ther* **4**, 151–9.

Donnelly, J.J., Friedman, A., Martinez, D. *et al.* (1995) Preclinical efficacy of a prototype DNA vaccine: enhanced protection against antigenic drift in influenza virus. *Nat Med* **1**, 583–7.

Ertl, H.C.J., Verma, P., He, Z. & Xiang, Z.Q. (1995) Plasmid vectors as anti-viral vaccines. *Ann NY Acad Sci* **772**, 77–87.

Feltquate, D.M., Webster, R.G. & Robinson, H.L. (1997) Different TH cell types and antibody isotypes generated by saline and gene gun DNA immunization. *J Immunol* **158**, 2278–84.

Fu, T.-M., Friedman, A., Ulmer, J.B., Liu, M.A. & Donnelly, J.J. (1997) Protective cellular immunity: Cytotoxic T-lymphocyte responses against dominant and recessive epitopes of influenza virus nucleoprotein induced by DNA immunization. *J Virol* **71**, 2715–21.

Fuller, D.H. & Haynes, J.R. (1996) A qualitative progression in HIV type 1 glycoprotein 120-specific cytotoxic cellular and humoral immune responses in mice receiving a DNA-based glycoprotein 120 vaccine. *AIDS Res Hum Retroviruses* **10**, 1433–41.

Fynan, E.F., Webster, R.G., Fuller, D.H., Haynes, J.R., Santoro, J.C. & Robinson, H.L. (1993) DNA vaccines: Protective immunizations by parenteral, mucosal, and gene-gun inoculations. *Proc Natl Acad Sci USA* **90**, 11478–82.

Griffiths, E. (1995) Assuring the safety and efficacy of DNA vaccines. *Ann NY Acad Sci* **772**, 152–63.

Hasty, P., Rivera-Perez, J. & Bradley, A. (1991) The length of homology required for gene targeting in embryonic stem cell. *Mol Cell Biol* **11**, 5586–91.

Hilleman, M.R. (1995) DNA vectors: precedents and safety. *Ann NY Acad Sci* **772**, 1–14.

Hoffman, S.L., Sedegah, M. & Hedstrom, R.C. (1994) Protection against malaria by immunization with *Plasmodium yoelii* circumsporozoite protein nucleic acid vaccine. *Vaccine* **12**, 1529–33.

Holland, J.J., De La Torre, J.C. & Steinhauer, D.A. (1992) RNA virus populations as quasispecies. *Curr Topics Microbiol Immunol* **176**, 1–20.

Justewicz, D.M., Morin, M.J., Robinson, H.L. & Webster, R.G. (1995) Antibody-forming cell response to virus challenge in mice immunized with DNA encoding the influenza virus hemagglutinin. *J Virol* **69**, 7712–17.

Koffler, D., Carr, R.I., Agnello, V. *et al.* (1969) Antibodies to polynucleotides: distribution in human serums. *Science* **166**, 1648–9.

Lowrie, D.B., Tascon, R.E., Colston, M.J. *et al.* (1994) Towards a DNA vaccine against tuberculosis. *Vaccine* **12**, 1537–40.

Manickan, E., Rouse, R.J.D., Yu, Z. *et al.* (1995) Genetic immunization against herpes simplex virus. Protection is mediated by CD4$^+$ T lymphocytes. *J Immunol* **155**, 259–65.

Martins, L.P., Lau, L.L. & Asano, M.S. (1995) DNA vaccination against persistent viral infection. *J Virol* **69**, 2574–82.

Montgomery, D.L., Shiver, J.W., Leander, K.R. *et al.* (1993) Heterologous and homologous protection against influenza A by DNA vaccination: Optimization of DNA vectors. *DNA Cell Biol* **12**, 777–83.

Mor, G., Klinman, D.M., Shapiro, S. *et al.* (1995) Complexity of the cytokine and antibody response elicited by immunizing mice with *Plasmodium yoelii* circumsporozoite protein plasmid DNA. *J Immunol* **155**, 2039–46.

Nabel, G.J., Nabel, E.G., Yang, Z.Y. *et al.* (1993) Direct gene transfer with DNA-liposome complexes in melanoma: expression, biologic activity, and lack of toxicity in humans. *Proc Natl Acad Sci USA* **90**, 11307–11.

Nichols, W., Ledwith, B., Mann, S. & Troilo, P.J. (1995) Potential DNA vaccination into host cell genome. *Ann New York Acad Sci* **772**, 30–9.

Parker, S.E., Vahlsing, L.H., Serfilippi, L.M. *et al.* (1995) Cancer gene therapy using plasmid DNA: safety evaluation in rodents and non-human primates. *Hum Gene Ther* **6**, 575–90.

Pisetsky, D.S., Reich, C., Crowley, S.D. *et al.* (1995) Immunological properties of bacterial DNA. *Ann NY Acad Sci* **772**, 152–63.

Ramshaw, I.A., Leong, K.H., Ramsay, A.J. & Boyle, D.B. (1996) Induction of protective immunity against influenza virus using DNA and recombinant avipoxvirus vectors. In: Brown, L.E., Hampson, A.W. and Webster R.G. (eds) *Options for the Control of Influenza III*, pp. 772–6. Elsevier Science.

Robertson, J.S. (1994) Safety considerations for nucleic acid vaccines. *Vaccine* **12**, 1526–8.

Robinson, H.L., Boyle, C.A., Feltquate, D.M., Morin, M.J., Santoro, J.C. & Webster, R.G. (1997) DNA immunization for influenza virus: Studies using hemagglutinin and nucleoprotein-expressing DNAs. *J Infect Dis* **176**, S50–55.

Robinson, H.L., Hunt, L.A. & Webster, R.G. (1993) Protection against a lethal influenza virus challenge by immunization with a haemagglutinin-expressing plasmid DNA. *Vaccine* **11**, 957–60.

Sato, Y., Roman, M., Tighe, H. *et al.* (1996) Immunostimulatory DNA sequences necessary for effective intradermal gene immunization. *Science* **273**, 352–4.

Schodel, F., Aguado, M.-T. & Lambert, P.-H. (1994) Introduction: nucleic acid vaccines. *Vaccine* **12**, 1491–2.

Sizemore, D.R., Branstrom, A.A. & Sadoff, J.C. (1995) Attenuated Shigella as a DNA delivery vehicle for DNA-mediated immunization. *Science* **270**, 299–302.

Tang, D.-C., DeVit, M. & Johnston, S.A. (1992) Genetic immunization is a simple method for eliciting an immune response. *Nature* **356**, 152.

Temin, H.M. (1990) Overview of biological effects of addition of DNA molecules to cells. *J Med Virol* **31**, 13–17.

Ulmer, J.B., Donnelly, J.J., Parker, S.E. *et al.* (1993) Heterologous protection against influenza by injection of DNA encoding a viral protein. *Science* **259**, 1745–9.

Wang, Y., Xiang, Z., Pasquini, S. & Ertl, H.C.J. (1997) Immune response to neonatal genetic immunization. *Virology* **228**, 278–84.

Webster, R.G., Fynan, E.F., Santoro, J.C. & Robinson, H.L. (1994) Protection of ferrets against influenza challenge with a DNA vaccine to the hemagglutinin. *Vaccine* **12**, 1495–8.

Webster, R.G. & Robinson, H.L. (1997) *BioDrugs* **4**, 273–92.

Wolff, J.A., Dowty, M.E., Jiao, S. *et al.* (1992) Expression of naked plasmids by cultured myotubes and entry of plasmids into T tubules and caveolae of mammalian skeletal muscle. *J Cell Sci* **103**, 1249–59.

Wolff, J.A., Malone, R.W., Williams, P. *et al.* (1990) Direct gene transfer into mouse muscle *in vivo*. *Science* **247**, 1465–8.

Xiang, Z. & Ertl, H.C.J. (1995) Manipulation of the immune response to a plasmid-encoded viral antigen by coinoculation with plasmids expressing cytokines. *Immunity* **2**, 129–35.

Xiang, Z.Q., Spitalnik, S., Tran, M., Wunner, W.H., Cheng, J. & Ertl, H.C.J. (1994) Vaccination with a plasmid vector carrying the rabies virus glycoprotein gene induces protective immunity against rabies virus. *Virology* **199**, 132–40.

Yang, N.-S., Burkholder, J., Roberts, B. *et al.* (1990) *In vivo* and *in vitro* gene transfer to mammalian somatic cells by particle bombardment. *Proc Natl Acad Sci USA* **87**, 9568–72.

CHAPTER 32

New Approaches to Vaccination

Pamuk Bilsel and Yoshihiro Kawaoka

The currently licensed influenza vaccine in use is an inactivated influenza vaccine. The inactivated vaccine is administered intramuscularly by injection, and stimulates primarily humoral immunity which is moderately protective and relatively short lived (reviewed in Kilbourne 1993). Influenza vaccination is 70–90% effective in preventing influenza-like illness in young healthy adults when the vaccine antigens closely match the circulating influenza virus strains. However, the efficacy of the inactivated vaccine in the prevention of influenza-like illness is suboptimal in children and in elderly people. Influenza virus infection and its complications are life-threatening in elderly people due to decreased immunological response and other high-risk groups with respiratory problems (Patriarca *et al.* 1985; Foster *et al.* 1992; Govaert *et al.* 1994; Nichol *et al.* 1994). Therefore, new approaches to influenza vaccines have been to either improve the efficacy of the currently licensed inactivated vaccine or the use of live attenuated virus vaccines.

Because of the limitations of the current vaccines, research efforts have been directed mainly towards the development of more potent adjuvants to augment the immunogenicity of inactivated influenza virus vaccines and the development of live attenuated influenza vaccines that may provide longer lasting protection (reviewed in Clements 1992). Live attenuated virus vaccines administered intranasally, would induce local, mucosal, cell-mediated and humoral immunity, thus providing longer lasting protection than that seen following injection of the inactivated vaccine. Previous approaches to the development of attenuated influenza donor strains have been to take advan-

tage of the segmented RNA genome of influenza viruses and allow reassortment to occur between wild-type human and attenuated influenza viruses. Host range mutants generated from reassortment of human and avirulent avian influenza viruses have been evaluated as prototype vaccine candidates but have failed either because of genetic instability or the inability to attenuate reproducibly every wild-type strain. Temperature-sensitive mutants of H3N2 viruses were found to be attenuated and were used to generate reassortants with current human viruses; however, again the attenuation of reassortants were not predictable (Murphy *et al.* 1982; Tolpin *et al.* 1982; Snyder *et al.* 1986; Clements *et al.* 1992; Murphy 1992).

One of the more promising efforts of the traditional approaches has been the development of the live attenuated cold-adapted influenza vaccines, which is proceeding as a vaccine for use in humans (Maassab *et al.* 1993). The cold-adapted virus is genetically stable owing partly to the multigenic requirement for the attenuated phenotype and shown to be repeatedly safe (Snyder *et al.* 1988; Herlocher *et al.* 1993). Local antibody response to virus replication, specifically immunoglobulin A (IgA) antibody production, at the site of administration is the major mechanism by which this vaccine affords protection against influenza. However, although this vaccine appears to be efficacious in children and young adults, it may be too attenuated to stimulate an ideal immune response in elderly people who have been exposed to many influenza virus infections during their lifetimes (Gorse *et al.* 1991, 1996; Powers *et al.* 1991, 1992; Shaw *et al.* 1992).

Therefore, there have been continuous attempts

at vaccine development to achieve better efficacy in all vulnerable population groups who are vaccinated — especially the elderly population. In the context of the many unsuccessful attempts at vaccine development, there is a need for a more rational approach to vaccine design that involves the sequential introduction of specific, defined attenuating mutations into a virus to produce a donor strain that is satisfactorily attenuated and that exhibits a stable attenuated phenotype during replication *in vivo* (Clements 1992).

The recently developed reverse genetics techniques for influenza viruses has enabled the construction of influenza A viruses that contain altered genomes (Enami *et al.* 1990). The ability to introduce attenuation characteristics into the viral genome holds the promise for developing a live attenuated influenza virus for vaccination. This chapter will focus on the use of reverse genetics to define molecular determinants of attenuation for influenza viruses and discuss development of vaccine candidates using the technique. There is also a section on the use of adjuvants in conjunction with the inactivated vaccine that has been shown to be effective in the elderly population and the use of expressed influenza proteins that have been shown to stimulate a protective immune response in animals.

Reverse genetics (ribonucleoprotein transfection)

Previously, the only method for exchanging genes in influenza viruses was to rely on reassortment between two different virus strains by coinfecting cells. Because of the segmented nature of the influenza virus genome, the progeny virions could receive RNA segments from either parental strain. Such reassortment, however, only leads to the exchange of naturally occurring genes in influenza viruses (Garcia-Sastre & Palese 1993a). Recent development of reverse genetic techniques using the ribonucleoprotein (RNP) transfection system allows the replacement of influenza virus genes with *in vitro* generated recombinant RNA molecules (Enami & Palese 1991). Negative-strand RNA viruses have been refractory to genetic

manipulation because the genomic RNA of these viruses is not itself infectious. When viral RNA is synthesized *in vitro* and introduced into cells the negative-sense viral RNA is not translated in the transfected cell and therefore cannot initiate infection. However, Luytjes *et al.* (1989) developed an RNP transfection method in which the *in vitro* generated RNA transcripts are coated with viral nucleoprotein (NP) and polymerase proteins that act as biologically active RNPs in the transfected cell. A brief outline of the method follows and is shown in Fig. 32.1.

The RNP transfection method can be divided into four steps.

1 Preparation of RNA: plasmid DNA coding for an influenza virus segment is transcribed into negative-sense RNA in an *in vitro* transcription reaction.

2 Encapsidation of the RNA: the transcribed RNA is then mixed with gradient purified NP and polymerase proteins isolated from disrupted influenza virus to form a biologically active RNP complex.

3 Transfection and rescue of the encapsidated RNA: the artificial ribonucleocapsid is transfected to the cells previously infected with a helper influenza virus that contains a different gene from the one being rescued. The helper virus will amplify the transfected RNA.

4 Selection of transfected gene: because both the helper virus and the transfectant containing the rescued gene are in the culture supernatant, an appropriate selection system is necessary to isolate the virus bearing the transfected gene. The different selection systems that have been used to rescue influenza genes are discussed below. For a review of the variations that have been developed of the RNP transfection method for the genetic manipulation of negative-stranded RNA viruses, see Luo & Palese 1992; Seong & Brownlee 1992; Garcia-Sastre & Palese 1993a, 1993b; Liu & Air 1993; Seong 1993).

Influenza A rescue systems

The selection system allows generation of novel transfectant influenza viruses with specific biological and molecular characteristics. There are

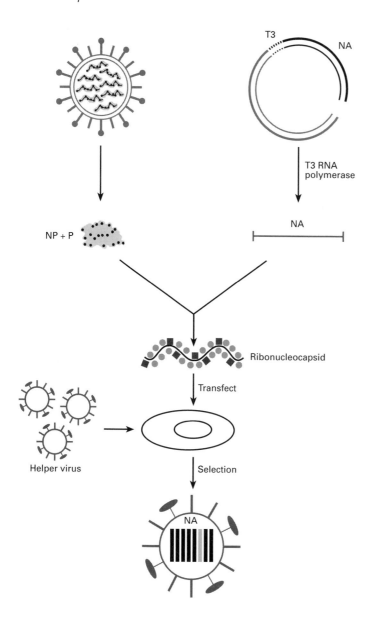

Fig. 32.1 Schematic drawing of the reverse genetics procedure. NA, neuraminidase; NP, nucleoprotein; P, protein. (From Bilsel & Kawaoka 1994, with permission from R&W Publications.)

only a small number of influenza A virus strains for which genetic determinants of host range and virulence are known which limits the number of viruses and genes amenable to genetic manipulation (Murphy & Webster 1990). The choice of mutations that can be introduced into a transfectant virus is restricted by the availability of an efficient selection system. These can be in the form of host range mutants, in which growth of the transfectant

is selected and the helper is restricted; temperature-sensitive mutants, where the transfectant can grow in what is the non-permissive temperature for the helper virus; or antibodies and drugs that inhibit the growth of the helper virus. Described below are the prevalent selection methods that have been used to rescue influenza A virus genes into transfectant viruses. Different systems allow for different genes to be rescued, but as technologies improve, multiple mutations in multiple genes can be introduced into one virus. Introducing multiple attenuating mutations into the virus genes would yield more stably attenuated mutants that could serve as donor strains for vaccine viruses that contain the haemagglutinin (HA) and neuraminidase (NA) of current strains.

Host range selection systems

NA. The concept of introducing mutations into the virus genome and obtaining infectious virus from a cDNA clone was first demonstrated by the rescue of the NA gene of A/WSN/33 (H1N1) (WSN) virus (reviewed in Garcia-Sastre & Palese 1993a). Influenza A virus containing the WSN NA gene can form plaques in Madin–Darby bovine kidney (MDBK) cells in the absence of trypsin (Schulman & Palese 1977). Conversely, WSN human kidney (HK) cells, which differs from WSN only in its NA being derived from A/HK/1/68 (H3N2) virus, does not form plaques in MDBK cells without trypsin. Thus, the WSN–HK virus is a host range mutant that provides a selection system for WSN NA in MDBK cells. Therefore, when an *in vitro* synthesized WSN NA gene was RNP transfected into helper WSN–HK-infected cells, viruses containing the transfected NA gene were selected by plaquing on MDBK cells without trypsin (Enami *et al.* 1990). This MDBK selection system has turned out to be a very efficient selection system, enabling numerous WSN NA genes that contain engineered mutations to be rescued into transfectant viruses. The WSN NA has been studied extensively (Enami & Palese 1991). The NA stalk has been altered to contain foreign epitopes, had additional residues inserted or deleted (Castrucci *et al.* 1992, 1994). Most alterations have mildly altered the biological properties of the resulting transfectant virus but some have shown drastic phenotypic effects (Luo *et al.* 1993). Deletion of the NA stalk has resulted in a host-range mutant that can be used as a helper virus itself (Castrucci & Kawaoka 1993). Alterations in the cytoplasmic tail and transmembrane domains have revealed more about the functions of the protein and have also served as examples of attenuation (Bilsel *et al.* 1993; Garcia-Sastre & Palese 1995; Mitnaul *et al.* 1996).

Influenza viruses containing a gene with altered non-coding sequences were first generated by Muster *et al.* (1991). A transfectant virus (NA/B-NS) was obtained in which the non-coding region of the NA gene was derived from the non-structural (NS) gene of influenza B virus. This virus was attenuated in mice due to the NA gene not being replicated as efficiently as wild-type which was reflected in its lower packaging rate into virions (Luo *et al.* 1992). This serves as a prototype for attenuation by mutagenizing the non-coding regions of a given protein and can be applied for other genes as rescue systems become available.

PB2. Subbarao *et al.* (1993) first described the rescue of an attenuating mutation on a non-surface protein. An avian-human influenza A virus PB2 single-gene reassortant virus (with an avian influenza A virus PB2 gene) that replicates efficiently in avian tissue but poorly in mammalian cells was used as a helper virus to rescue a transfected human influenza A virus PB2 gene. The human influenza A PB2 gene transfectant is selected because the avian influenza A virus PB2 gene restricts viral replication in mammalian cells in culture. This system was first used to rescue a wild-type PB2 gene of A/AA/60 virus, followed by a mutant derivative that had a single amino acid substitution at 265 introduced that conferred a temperature-sensitive (ts) and attenuated (att) phenotype to the transfectant virus. The transfectant virus was immunogenic and protected hamsters from subsequent challenge with wild-type virus. The rescue of an internal virus polymerase protein, PB2, into influenza A virus paves the way to introducing additional mutations to achieve the right balance between immunogenicity and attenuation of a viral vaccine candidate.

Antibody selection

The surface glycoproteins of influenza virus, HA and NA, are embedded in the viral envelope and can interact with antibodies. Antibodies to the HA neutralize virus replication and this has been exploited in the rescue of different subtypes of influenza HA into transfectant viruses. Negative selection is based on using neutralizing antibodies that are directed against the HA of the helper virus to suppress its replication (Muster *et al.* 1994; Zurcher *et al.* 1994). Positive selection uses antibodies against the transfected HA to 'capture' transfectants that contain the transfected HA (Horimoto & Kawaoka 1994).

Negative selection. A selection based upon antibody screening was used to introduce new epitopes into the HA molecule. Specifically, the HA epitope of the A/WSN (H1N1) virus was replaced by that of the H2 or H3 subtype. Mice immunized with the chimaeric virus, carrying the six amino acid loop of the H3 subtype of the A/HK strain, produced antibody responses against both the HK and the WSN virus.

In addition to HA epitopes of different virus subtypes, Li *et al.* (1992) have obtained different transfectant influenza A viruses with chimaeric HAs containing epitope derived from the V3 loop of the human immunodeficiency virus type 1 (HIV-1) glycoprotein (gp120) and the epitope of the circumsporozoite protein of *Plasmodium yoelii* (Li *et al.* 1992; Li *et al.* 1993a, 1993b).

Positive selection. An antibody-mediated virus trapping system for the rescue of Ty/Ont HA (H5) using antibodies against both the helper virus (H1) HA and the H5 HA was developed by Horimoto and Kawaoka (1994). Tissue culture plates coated with anti-H5 antibodies were incubated with the transfection supernatant to trap the viruses with the H5 HA. MDCK cell suspension containing trypsin was added after the unbound virus was washed out. Trapped viruses then undergo multiple cycles of replication while further propagation of the helper virus was prevented by antibody to the H1 molecule in the tissue culture supernatant. Using this selection system, transfectant viruses were generated that contained mutations in the HA cleavage site and assessed for virulence. This selection system can be used effectively to rescue the surface glycoproteins, HA and NA of influenza virus.

Temperature-sensitive helper viruses

The first gene to be rescued by a temperature-sensitive helper virus was the NS gene. A temperature-sensitive host-range influenza virus strain with a 36 nucleotide deletion in the NS gene (Snyder *et al.* 1990) was used to rescue a transfected wild-type NS gene at the non-permissive temperature.

Temperature-sensitive mutants have had limited use as helper viruses, mainly because their high reversion rates and leakiness have made isolation of transfectants problematic. Li *et al.* (1995) developed an RNP transfection method based on electroporation that has allowed the successful use of temperature-sensitive mutants to rescue NP and matrix genes of influenza virus. Temperature-sensitive viruses of A/WSN/33, ts51 and ts56, were used to rescue the matrix and NP genes, respectively.

Electroporation was used as a means of introducing the artificial RNPs into MDBK-infected cells and was found to increase the transfection efficiency relative to the diethylaminoethanol (DEAE)–dextran method. The greater efficiency of electroporation is suggested to result from the decrease in titre of the helper virus, presumably due to the observed cell damage after electroporation which increases the ratio of the transfectant to helper virus. An impediment to rescue of internal genes has been the low transfection efficiency combined with a requirement for a strong selection system for the transfectant gene since most of the virus in the transfection supernatant will be helper virus. Another improvement, a two-step modification of the RNP transfection method, has allowed for a chimaeric matrix gene (between fast-growing WSN and slow-growing Aichi) to be rescued by ts51 virus, although at low efficiency (Yasuda *et al.* 1994).

Amantadine resistance

A reverse genetics system has been developed for the matrix gene using amantadine resistance as a selection criteria (Castrucci & Kawaoka 1995). This selection system was used to examine the importance of the carboxyl terminal residues of the M2 protein of influenza A virus in virus replication. Attempts to generate viruses with either five or 10 residues deleted were unsuccessful; however, a mutant with a carboxyl-terminal Glu deletion (COOH-1) was rescued with an efficiency comparable to that of viruses with the parental matrix gene. The COOH-1 mutation was stable during virus replication in ferrets and retained sufficient immunogenicity to protect ferrets against subsequent challenge with wild-type virus. Although the level of attenuation of COOH-1 in ferrets was limited, the rescue system should facilitate efforts to identify attenuating mutations in the matrix gene products. Amantadine resistance is not a characteristic that is desirable in the final vaccine strain but as a selection system it can be used to create matrix gene based host-range mutants which could be used in the generation of amantadine-sensitive transfectant viruses.

Influenza B virus reverse genetics

Although influenza A and B viruses are very similar to one another, there are differences in *cis*-acting signals, coding strategies, proteins, host ranges, and biological properties which have been less studied than for the A viruses. Therefore, the reverse genetics of influenza B has lagged behind the A viruses. Thus far, there has been rescue of an HA protein using monoclonals against the helper virus HA to neutralize helper virus growth (Barclay & Palese 1995). Also mutants containing deletions in the 5′ non-coding region of the HA gene have been rescued implying that this region of the genome is flexible in sequence and length. There are no described host-range mutants or characterized temperature-sensitive mutants or drug resistance for influenza B viruses.

Reverse genetics in the generation of viral vaccine candidates

Attenuating mutations can be introduced into the non-coding or coding regions of HA and NA genes of influenza viruses (as discussed above) but the HA and NA cannot be used to confer attenuation because the vaccine viruses must contain the HA and NA genes of the new epidemic virus to be useful in immunization.

Attenuating mutations must be located in the genes which encode the internal proteins of the virus. This 'master donor' strain could be used on an annual basis to generate attenuated vaccines containing the HA and NA genes corresponding to current viruses. Temperature sensitivity has been a desired phenotype in such candidates because the vaccine virus would be restricted in replication in the lower respiratory tract yet would retain ability to grow in the cooler upper respiratory tract and potentially stimulate a protective immune response (Maassab *et al.* 1993). There has been a correlation between the temperature sensitivity phenotype and attenuation phenotype to some degree (Richman & Murphy 1979).

The use of PB2 reverse genetics for influenza A virus vaccine development now allows the optimization of attenuation by stepwise addition of attenuating mutations to one gene segment until a satisfactory level of attenuation has been reached (Subbarao *et al.* 1993). The biological properties of transfectant viruses containing the mutant genes can be evaluated directly *in vivo* to assess the effect of each serially added mutation at every stage of development (Subbarao *et al.* 1995). Before being considered for human testing, an attenuated vaccine strain must be safe, immunogenic and genetically stable (Clements 1992). Three approaches taken with the PB2 gene to generate such vaccine strains are described below. The mutagenesis approach and positions of the mutations are different to allow different candidates as are the animal model systems and genetic stability assays used.

First, Subbarao *et al.* (1995) have made an effort to sequentially add previously defined PB2 temperature-sensitive mutations to the PB2 gene segment and hope that it can be transferred to currently circulating wild-type strains by reassortment and reproducibly confer attenuation in different wild-type backgrounds.

Second, Parkin *et al.* (1996) have used a charged cluster to alanine mutagenesis approach to attenuate the PB2 gene. Third, the cap binding function of

PB2 is the target of mutagenesis in the hopes of generating a stably attenuated viral vaccine candidate (Parkin *et al.* 1997). The immunogenicity and safety of the vaccine strains are tested in different animal models. Several assays for testing genetic stability are also described.

Use of PB2 selection system to generate vaccine candidates

Subbarao *et al.* (1993) (see above) have demonstrated the feasibility of using the PB2 host-range system to rescue a PB2 gene bearing a site-directed mutation into a transfectant virus. The PB2 gene of A/AA/60 mutated at position 265, a mutation previously observed in the cold-adapted donor virus, was shown to confer the temperature-sensitive and attenuation phenotype to the transfectant virus (Subbarao *et al.* 1993). The strategy for developing a viral vaccine candidate was to introduce temperature-sensitive mutations sequentially into this PB2 gene already bearing a temperature-sensitive mutation and show a progressive increase in temperature sensitivity and attenuation. Temperature-sensitive mutations previously identified (aa112 556 658) in different influenza A viruses were introduced by reverse genetics into the wild-type influenza AA PB2 gene to see if it conferred the temperature-sensitive phenotype in this background. Although specific single mutations resulted in only a very modest increase in temperature sensitivity and attenuation, a successive increase in the level of temperature sensitivity and attenuation was achieved by the addition of a second and third temperature-sensitive mutation to the PB2 gene segment that already contained the aa265 mutation (Subbarao *et al.* 1995). In this way, it was possible to produce two triple mutants (mt265 + 112 + 658 and mt265 + 112 + 556) that were further restricted in replication *in vitro* at elevated temperatures compared to the single or double mutants.

The mutant PB2 transfectant viruses were found to be attenuated for replication in hamsters. The level of temperature sensitivity of transfectant viruses correlated significantly with the peak level of virus replication in the upper and lower respiratory tracts of hamster, indicating that the

level of temperature sensitivity achieved by site-directed mutagenesis was the predominant determination of attenuation.

Immunization of hamsters with virus containing three temperature-sensitive mutations in the PB2 gene induced haemagglutination inhibiting antibodies and protected hamsters against wild-type virus challenge. The lower respiratory tract was protected by the highly defective triple mutant viruses. The upper respiratory tract of the hamsters were not protected, presumably because hamsters clear virus faster than humans. The longer duration of influenza virus replication in the human upper respiratory tract should induce a greater mucosal antibody response and is anticipated to be sufficiently immunogenic in humans (Subbarao *et al.* 1995).

The stability of the temperature-sensitive phenotype was assayed after prolonged replication in immunocompromised mice. This *in vivo* model would presumably be comparable to influenza virus vaccine strain replication in fully susceptible seronegative humans. Two of the three double mutants exhibited complete stability of the temperature-sensitive phenotype after prolonged replication in the immunocompromised host. Genetic stability testing of these PB2 mutants have also given an indication as to what gene constellations may be targeted in trying to make a final vaccine donor strain. However, PB2 temperature-sensitive revertants did appear and have developed suppressor mutations in the PA gene (Subbarao *et al.* 1995).

In contrast to using previously defined temperature-sensitive mutations, Parkin *et al.* (1996) have exploited the PB2 system to generate a vaccine donor strain by a clustered charge to alanine mutagenesis approach. The underlying principle in this approach is the prediction that charged amino acids are candidates for being involved in interpeptide interactions since they are frequently on the surface of proteins (Chotia 1976; Janin 1979). Mutagenesis of these charged amino acids to uncharged ones, such as alanine, would not disrupt the overall structure or stability of the protein but may give rise to proteins that function only at low temperature (Wiskerchen & Muesing 1995). Eight clusters of charged amino acids in the PB2 protein of A/LA/2/87 (H3N2) were mutagenized by changing the charged amino acids to uncharged alanine. Of the six mutants that could be rescued, five were temperature sensitive with some displaying small plaque phenotype at low temperature. All of the temperature-sensitive mutants were attenuated in mice compared with wild-type virus, but the degree of attenuation in mice did not always correlate with the shut-off temperature in tissue culture. Some of the PB2 mutants generated by clustered charge to alanine substitutions failed to replicate in mouse lungs to a detectable level despite high shut-off temperatures in MDCK cells. These results suggest that temperature-sensitive mutants generated by clustered charge mutagenesis exposed sites which affect not only thermosensitivity but also, independently, *in vivo* replication (Parkin *et al.* 1996).

Two of the Ala mutants that were attenuated in mice were used to infect ferrets. Ferrets have been used extensively to test the reactogenicity of candidate influenza vaccine strains since they show several signs of influenza virus infection which are shared with humans, such as fever and coryza (Maassab *et al.* 1982). ALA 1 (39°C shut-off) and ALA 6 (small plaque, 40°C shut-off) were chosen because of the apparent difference between the shut-off temperature in MDCK cells and attenuated phenotype in mice. ALA 1 grew to wild-type levels in ferret nasal turbinates, was not detectable in lungs, and induced a strong febrile response. Thus, the phenotype of ALA 1 in ferrets was similar to wild-type control in spite of being attenuated in the mouse lung. ALA 6 grew less well than wild-type in nasal turbinates of ferrets, was not detected in lungs, and did not induce fever. This virus was attenuated in ferrets, even though it was not very temperature sensitive in MDCK cells (40°C shut-off) (Parkin *et al.* 1996). These results clearly suggest that the determinants for evaluating vaccine candidates are still in their infancy.

The third approach that differs from the mutagenesis approaches described above to generate a stable attenuated mutant is to target essential functional sites within a viral protein which interacts directly with a host factor (Parkin *et al.* 1997).

Such mutations are less likely to be suppressed by a second mutation in a viral gene, compared to mutations in residues that interact with another viral protein or RNA. Host proteins do not display the genetic plasticity that RNA viruses do, therefore the effects of such mutations would be more stable. Parkin *et al.* (1997) attempted to do this by targeting the cap binding function of the viral polymerase subunit, PB2. The tryptophan residues in PB2 were mutated to phenylalanine since tryptophan residues have been implicated in binding of cellular cap binding protein, eIF-4E, to the cap structure (Altmann *et al.* 1988).

PB2 genes rescued that contained a single mutation were mildly affected with regard to temperature sensitivity in MDCK cells. Replication of these transfectants in mice did not reveal any attenuating effects. Therefore, combination mutants were created to lower the shut-off temperature in order to achieve an acceptable level of attenuation in mice. Transfectant viruses containing multiple mutations in their PB2 genes were examined for their ability to replicate in the respiratory tract of mice. Mutants (5ts and 3ts/3WF) with five and six mutations, respectively, had shut-off temperatures of 38°C but were not detected in mouse lungs at all. Two triple mutant viruses which had shut-off temperatures of 40°C in tissue culture grew very poorly in mice lungs. These results imply that the restriction of replication is due to factors other than thermosensitivity since the core temperature of the mouse is 37°C. Virulence and reactogenicity in ferrets correlated with that seen in mice.

The candidate vaccine strains were put through three assays for genetic stability.

1 Replication in immunodeficient mice: prolonged virus replication in nude mice for 14 days (approximates duration of virus shedding in completely susceptible humans) (Subbarao *et al.* 1995; Wright *et al.* 1975).

2 Tissue culture stress test: successive growth at elevated temperatures in cell culture, test previously used to isolate temperature-sensitive revertants of temperature-sensitive candidates (Murphy *et al.* 1982; Treanor *et al.* 1994).

3 Multiple passage through ferrets: temperature-sensitive phenotype of virus assessed in tissue culture after serial passage in ferrets.

Of the candidate vaccine strains, only 3ts/3WF was genetically stable in all three assays. Other viruses were found to lose their temperature sensitivity in at least one of the three different assays. These results demonstrate that influenza A viruses generated by rational design have the potential to serve as live attenuated vaccines in humans. Temperature sensitivity in tissue culture, attenuation in the respiratory tracts of mice and ferrets, immunogenicity in mice and ferrets as well as reactogenicity in ferrets have served well as markers in generating vaccine candidates (Parkin *et al.* 1997). However, as in the three situations above where candidates have been evaluated, there is not yet a correlation between the effect of a given mutation and its phenotype. Only as more candidates are generated can such a consensus be formed and lead to determining what is predictive of the human situation.

Immunomodulators to improve inactivated influenza vaccine

Current vaccines are less effective in the elderly population, therefore the use of adjuvants with intranasal administration of the inactivated vaccine has been the approach taken to enhance the immune response (Clements 1992). The immunostimulators described below are summarized in Table 32.1.

Dehydroepiandrosterone

One of the factors involved in immunosenescence is dehydroepiandrosterone (DHEA), an abundantly secreted, weak androgenic adrenocortical steroid hormone (Danenberg *et al.* 1995). Concentrations of DHEA decline after the third decade of life, reaching 10–20% of the peak level in the elderly population. The precise biological role of DHEA is not known, but it is thought to have immunomodulating activity. DHEA administration to mice reverse some of the typical phenomena of immunosenescence. Recently, DHEA treatment was found effective in augmenting the response to immunization of old mice with recombinant hepatitis B vaccine. These experiments were planned to study the effects of DHEA treatment on the efficacy of old mice immunization against influenza, as measured by the titre of antibodies and the protection against exposure with live influenza virus. Older subjects, either mice or human, respond poorly to influenza vaccine. Decreased humoral antibody response in old mice has been previously shown to be associated with increased susceptibility to pulmonary infection with influenza. Danenberg *et al.* (1995) have demonstrated that administration of DHEA to old mice combined with inactivated influenza vaccine, augments the humoral response against influenza. Following inoculation with live virus, an effective protection against pulmonary infection was achieved. It is suggested that DHEA may augment the immunization of old mice to viral vaccines by reducing interferon-γ (IFN-γ) levels, delaying the rapid clearance of virus and permitting proper immunization.

MF59

Tween/Span stabilized emulsion used in combination with influenza vaccine results in

Table 32.1 Immunomodulators to improve inactivated influenza vaccine.

Adjuvant	Reference
DHEA: augments humoral response in old mice to viral vaccine	Danenberg *et al.* 1995
MF59: enhanced immunogenicity against H3N2 and B components, not H1N1	Ott *et al.* 1995; Martin *et al.* 1996
QS21: enhance immunogenicity against H3N2 initially, against H3N2 and B upon repeated vaccination	Ronco 1996

significantly higher antibody titres to vaccine (Ott *et al.* 1995). MF59 is shown to have an enhancing effect in the immunogenicity of H3N2 and B components but not H1N1 component of vaccine (Martin 1996).

QS21

Saponin-derived fraction that is added to current inactivated flu vaccine was shown to stimulate response to the H3N2 component of inactivated vaccine but showed no difference in response to H1N1 or B virus (Ronco 1996).

Expressed influenza virus proteins

Haemagglutinin

Influenza virus HA and other gene products can be expressed efficiently at the cell surface and present themselves appropriately in the context of host histocompatibility antigens so that they can elicit both humoral and cell-mediated immune responses. The HA recombinant vaccinia virus produces a predominantly subtype-specific cytotoxic lymphocyte (CTL) response while the NP recombinant induces a broad cross-type specific CTL response (Endo *et al.* 1991). Vaccinia virus and fowlpox virus are two systems being used. Fowlpox virus differs from vaccinia virus in that it does not replicate in non-avian species. This suggests that recombinants derived from fowlpox might be much less virulent in immunocompromised human hosts and would be less likely to be transmitted to unvaccinated contacts or to revert to virulence than vaccinia virus recombinants. HA expressed in insect cells by a recombinant baculovirus has shown protective efficacy against natural viral challenge. High dose in elderly people correlated with higher serum antibody response (Treanor *et al.* 1996).

M2

Because the M2 is so abundantly expressed in virus-infected cells, it is a good target for influenza virus-specific CTL. The M2 protein was expressed by a baculovirus recombinant and its potential to induce protective immunity in Balb/c mice was tested (Slepushkin *et al.* 1995). Vaccination of mice with partially purified baculovirus recombinant expressed M2 shortened the duration of virus shedding and protected mice from lethal virus challenge. Serum antibody was detected in mice. These results demonstrated the potential to induce heterosubtypic immunity to type A influenza viruses by vaccinating with a conserved transmembrane protein. Vaccinated mice were protected from lethal challenge with a heterologous virus. The mechanism by which anti-M2 antibody plays a role in the protective effect is not clear, as it has not been demonstrated that serum from M2 vaccinated mice can limit virus infectivity *in vitro* or transfer immunity as has Mab. However, the mechanism is currently under investigation. It is postulated that the anti-M2 response may involve complement-dependent cytolytic antibody or antibody-dependent cell-mediated cytotoxicity.

Future directions

Inactivated and cold-adapted influenza virus vaccines are 6 : 2 reassortant viruses which derive the two glycoprotein genes from the circulating wild-type strains and the six non-GP genes from the master donor strain. Due to the antigenic variability of influenza virus, influenza vaccines are updated on an annual basis to represent the HA and NA of the circulating epidemic strain. This antigenic drift problem associated with influenza vaccines cannot be addressed by expressed influenza proteins or stimulating the immune response with adjuvants. Reverse genetics will allow one to adjust the attenuation of a vaccine strain and enable selection of a live vaccine strain optimally suited for any target population. New rescue systems are being developed for influenza viruses with developments toward helper free systems (Garcia-Sastre *et al.* 1994; Mena *et al.* 1994, 1996; Percy *et al.* 1994; Pleschka *et al.* 1996) that will be combined with the molecular information being gained about influenza viruses. Reverse genetics, in due time, will be used to generate genetically engineered live influenza A and B vaccine strains.

References

Altmann, M., Edery, I., Trachsel, H. & Sonenberg, N. (1988) Site-directed mutagenesis of the tryptophan residues in yeast eukaryotic initiation factor 4E. *J Biol Chem* **263**, 17229–32.

Barclay, W.S. & Palese, P. (1995) Influenza B viruses with site-specific mutations introduced into the HA gene. *J Virol* **69**, 1275–9.

Bilsel, P., Castrucci, M.R. & Kawaoka, Y. (1993) Mutations in the cytoplasmic tail of influenza A virus neuraminidase affect incorporation into virions. *J Virol* **67**, 6762–7.

Bilsel, P. & Kawaoki, Y. (1994) Generation of a stably attenuated influenza virus by reverse genetics. In: *Equine Infectious Diseases VII, Proceedings of the 7th International Conference.* R&W Publications, Newmarket.

Castrucci, M.R., Bilsel, P. & Kawaoka, Y. (1992) Attenuation of influenza A virus by insertion of a foreign epitope into the neuraminidase. *J Virol* **66**, 4647–53.

Castrucci, M.R., Hou, S., Doherty, P.C. & Kawaoka, Y. (1994) Protection against lethal lymphocytic choriomeningitis virus (LCMV) infection by immunization of mice with an influenza virus containing an LCMV epitope recognized by cytotoxic T lymphocytes. *J Virol* **68**, 3486–90.

Castrucci, M.R. & Kawaoka, Y. (1993) Biologic importance of neuraminidase stalk length in influenza A virus. *J Virol* **67**, 759–64.

Castrucci, M.R. & Kawaoka, Y. (1995) Reverse genetics system for generation of an influenza A virus mutant containing a deletion of the carboxyl-terminal residue of M2 protein. *J Virol* **69**, 2725–8.

Chotia, C. (1976) The nature of the accessible and buried surfaces in proteins. *J Mol Biol* **105**, 1–14.

Clements, M.L. (1992) Influenza vaccines. In: Ellis, R.W. (ed.) *Vaccines: New Approaches to Immunological Problems*, pp. 129–50. Butterworth-Heinemann, Boston.

Clements, M.L., Subbarao, E.K., Fries, L., Karron, R.A., London, W.T. & Murphy, B.R. (1992) Use of single-gene reassortant viruses to study the role of avian influenza A virus genes in attenuation of wild-type human influenza A virus for squirrel monkeys and adult human volunteers. *J Clin Microbiol* **30**, 655–62.

Danenberg, H.D., Ben-Yehuda, A., Zakay-Rones, Z. & Friedman, G. (1995) Dehydroepiandroesterone (DHEA) treatment reverses the impaired immune response of old mice to influenza vaccination and protects from influenza infection. *Vaccine* **13**, 1445–8.

Enami, M., Luytjes, W., Krystal, M. & Palese, P. (1990) Introduction of site-specific mutations into the genome of influenza virus. *Proc Natl Acad Sci USA* **87**, 3802–5.

Enami, M. & Palese, P. (1991) High-efficiency formation of influenza virus transfectants. *J Virol* **65**, 2711–13.

Endo, A., Itamura, S., Iinuma, H. *et al.* (1991) Homotypic and heterotypic protection against influenza virus infection in mice by recombinant vaccinia virus expressing the haemagglutinin or nucleoprotein gene of influenza virus. *J Gen Virol* **72**, 699–703.

Foster, D.A., Talsma, A., Furumoto-Dawson, A. *et al.* (1992) Influenza vaccine effectiveness in preventing hospitalization for pneumonia in the elderly. *Am J Epidemiol* **136**, 296–307.

Garcia-Sastre, A., Muster, T., Barclay, W.S., Percy, N. & Palese, P. (1994) Use of a mammalian internal ribosomal entry site element for expression of a foreign protein by a transfectant influenza virus. *J Virol* **68**, 6254–61.

Garcia-Sastre, A. & Palese, P. (1993a) Genetic manipulation of negative-strand RNA virus genomes. *Ann Rev Microbiol* **47**, 765–90.

Garcia-Sastre, A. & Palese, P. (1993b) Infectious influenza viruses from cDNA-derived RNA: reverse genetics. In: Carrasco, L., Sonenberg, N. & Wimmer, E. (eds) *Regulation of Gene Expression in Animal Viruses*, pp. 107–14. Plenum, New York.

Garcia-Sastre, A. & Palese, P. (1995) The cytoplasmic tail of the neuraminidase protein of influenza A virus does not play an important role in the packaging of this protein into viral envelopes. *Virus Res* **37**, 37–47.

Gorse, G.J., Belshe, R.B. & Munn, N.J. (1991) superiority of live attenuated compared with inactivated influenza A virus vaccines in older, chronically ill adults. *Chest* **100**, 977–84.

Gorse, G.J., Otto, E.E., Powers, D.C., Chambers, G.W., Eickhoff, C.S. & Newman, F.K. (1996) Induction of mucosal antibodies by live attenuated and inactivated influenza virus vaccines in the chronically ill elderly. *J Infect Dis* **173**, 285–90.

Govaert, T.M., Thijs, C.T., Masurel, N., Sprenger, M.J., Dinant, G.J. & Knottnerus, J.A. (1994) The efficacy of influenza vaccination in elderly individuals. A randomized double-blind placebo-controlled trial. *J Am Med Assoc* **272**, 1661–5.

Herlocher, M.L., Maassab, H.F. & Webster, R.G. (1993) Molecular and biological changes in the cold-adapted 'master strain' A/AA/6/60 (H2N2) influenza virus. *Proc Natl Acad Sci USA* **90**, 6032–6.

Horimoto, T. & Kawaoka, Y. (1994) Reverse genetics provides direct evidence for a correlation of hemagglutination cleavability and virulence of an avian influenza A virus. *J Virol* **68**, 3120–8.

Janin, J. (1979) Surface and inside volumes in globular proteins. *Nature* **277**, 491–2.

Kilbourne, E.D. (1993) Inactivated influenza vaccines. In: Plotkin, S.A. and Mortimer, E.A. (eds) *Vaccines*, pp. 565–81. Saunders, Philadelphia.

Li, S., Polonis, V., Isobe, H. *et al.* (1993a) Chimeric influenza virus induces neutralizing antibodies and cytotoxic T cells against human immunodeficiency virus type 1. *J Virol* **67**, 6659–66.

Li, S., Rodrigues, M., Rodriguez, D. *et al.* (1993b) Priming with recombinant influenza virus followed by administration of recombinant vaccinia virus induces CD8[+] T-cell-mediated protective immunity against malaria. *Proc Natl Acad Sci USA* **90**, 5214–18.

Li, S., Schulman, J.L., Moran, T., Bona, C. & Palese, P. (1992) Influenza A virus transfectants with chimeric hemagglutinins containing epitopes from different subtypes. *J Virol* **66**, 399–404.

Li, S., Xu, M. & Coelingh, K. (1995) Electroporation of influenza virus ribonucleoprotein complexes for rescue of the nucleoprotein and matrix genes. *Virus Res* **37**, 153–61.

Liu, C. & Air, G.M. (1993) Selection and characterization of a neuraminidase-minus mutant of influenza virus and its rescue by cloned neuraminidase gene. *Virology* **194**, 403–7.

Luo, G., Bergmann, M., Garcia-Sastre, A. & Palese, P. (1992) Mechanism of attenuation of a chimeric influenza A/B transfectant virus. *J Virol* **66**, 4679–85.

Luo, G., Chung, J. & Palese, P. (1993) Alterations of the stalk of the influenza virus neuraminidase: deletions and insertions. *Virus Res* **29**, 141–53.

Luo, G. & Palese, P. (1992) Genetic analysis of influenza virus. *Curr Opin Genet Dev* **2**, 77–81.

Luytjes, W., Krystal, M., Enami, M., Parvin, J.D. & Palese, P. (1989) Amplification, expression, and packaging of a foreign gene by influenza virus. *Cell* **59**, 1107–13.

Maassab, H.F., Kendal, A.P., Abrams, G.D. & Monto, A.S. (1982) Evaluation of a cold-recombinant influenza virus vaccine in ferrets. *J Infect Dis* **146**, 780–90.

Maassab, H.F., Shaw, M.W. & Heilman, C.A. (1993) Live influenza virus vaccine. In: Plotkin, S.A. & Mortimer, E.A. (eds) *Vaccines*, pp. 781–801. Saunders, Philadelphia.

Martin, J.T. (1996) Enhanced immunogenicity of Chiron Biocine adjuvanted influenza vaccine in the elderly. In: Brown, L.E., Hampson, A.W. & Webster, R.G. (eds) *Options for the Control of Influenza*, Vol. 3, pp. 647–52. Elsevier, Amsterdam.

Mena, I., de la Luna, S., Albo, C. *et al.* (1994) Synthesis of biologically active influenza virus core proteins using a vaccinia virus T7 RNA polymerase expression system. *J Gen Virol* **75**, 2109–14.

Mena, I., Vivo, A., Perez, E. & Portela, A. (1996) Rescue of a synthetic chloramphenicol acetyltransferase RNA into influenza virus-like particles obtained from recombinant plasmids. *J Virol* **70**, 5016–24.

Mitnaul, L.J., Castrucci, M.R., Murti, K.G. & Kawaoka, Y. (1996) The cytoplasmic tail of influenza A virus neuraminidase (NA) affects NA incorporation into virions, virion morphology, and virulence in mice but is not essential for virus replication. *J Virol* **70**, 873–9.

Murphy, B.R. (1992) Use of live, attenuated cold-adapted influenza A reassortant virus vaccines in infants, children, young adults, and elderly adults. *Infect Dis Clin Pract* **2**, 174–81.

Murphy, B.R., Markoff, L.J., Hosier, N.T., Massicot, J.G. & Chanock, R.M. (1982) Production and level of genetic stability of an influenza A virus temperature-sensitive mutant containing two genes with temperature-sensitive mutations. *Infect Immun* **37**, 235–42.

Murphy, B.R. & Webster, R.G. (1990) Orthomyxoviruses. In: Fields, B.N., Knipe, D.M. *et al.* (eds) *Virology*, Vol. I, 2nd edn, pp. 1091–152. Raven Press, New York.

Muster, T., Guinea, R., Trkola, A. *et al.* (1994) Cross-neutralizing activity against divergent human immunodeficiency virus type 1 isolates induced by the gp41 sequence ELDKWAS. *J Virol* **68**, 4031–4.

Muster, T., Subbarao, E.K., Enami, M., Murphy, B.R. & Palese, P. (1991) An influenza A virus containing influenza B virus 5′ and 3′ non-coding regions on the neuraminidase gene is attenuated in mice. *Proc Natl Acad Sci USA* **88**, 5177–81.

Nichol, K.L., Margolis, K.L.Wuorenma, J. & Von Sternberg, T. (1994) The efficacy and cost-effectiveness of vaccination against influenza among elderly persons living in the community. *N Engl J Med* **331**, 778–84.

Ott, G., Barchfel, G.L. & Van Nest, G. (1995) Enhancement of humoral response against human influenza vaccine with the simple submicron oil/water emulsion adjuvant MF59. *Vaccine* **3**, 1557–62.

Parkin, N.T., Chiu, P. & Coelingh, K.L. (1996) Temperature-sensitive mutants of influenza A virus generated by reverse genetics and clustered charged to alanine mutagenesis. *Virus Res* **46**, 31–44.

Parkin, N.T., Chiu, P. & Coelingh, K.L. (1997) Genetically engineered live attenuated influenza A virus vaccine candidates. *J Virol* **71**, 2772–8.

Patriarca, P.A., Weber, J.A., Parker, R.A. *et al.* (1985) Efficacy of influenza vaccine in nursing homes. Reduction in illness and complications during an influenza A (H3N2) epidemic. *J Am Med Assoc* **253**, 1136–9.

Percy, N., Barclay, W.S., Garcia-Sastre, A. & Palese, P. (1994) Expression of a foreign protein by influenza A virus. *J Virol* **68**, 4486–92.

Pleschka, S., Jaskunas, S.R., Engelhardt, O.G., Zurcher, T., Palese, P. & Garcia-Sastre, A. (1996) A plasmid-based reverse genetics system for influenza A virus. *J Virol* **70**, 4188–92.

Powers, D.C., Fries, L.F., Murphy, B.R., Thumar, B. & Clements, M.L. (1991) In elderly persons live attenuated influenza A virus vaccines do not offer an advantage over inactivated virus vaccine in inducing serum or secretory antibodies or local immunologic memory. *J Clin Microbiol* **29**, 498–505.

Powers, D.C., Murphy, B.R., Fries, L.F., Adler, W.H. & Clements, M.L. (1992) Reduced infectivity of cold-adapted influenza A H1N1 viruses in the elderly: correlation with serum and local antibodies. *J Am Geriatr Soc* **40**, 163–7.

Richman, D.D. & Murphy, B.R. (1979) The association of the temperature-sensitive phenotype with viral attenuation in animals and humans: implications for the development and use of live virus vaccines. *Rev Infect Dis* **1**, 413–33.

Ronco, J. (1996) *New Influenza Vaccines Workshop 12*. Symposium reports for the options for the control of influenza III meeting, Australia.

Schulman, J.L. & Palese, P. (1977) Virulence factors of influenza A viruses: WSN virus neuraminidase required for plaque production in MDBK cells. *J Virol* **24**, 170–6.

Seong, B. (1993) Influencing the influenza virus: genetic analysis and engineering of the negative-sense RNA genome. *Infect Agents Dis* **2**, 17–24.

Seong, B.L. & Brownlee, G.G. (1992) A new method for reconstituting influenza polymerase and RNA *in vitro*: a study of the promoter elements for cRNA and vRNA synthesis *in vitro* and viral rescue *in vivo*. *Virology* **186**, 247–60.

Shaw, M.W., Arden, N.H. & Maassab, H.F. (1992) New aspects of influenza viruses. *Clin Microbiol Rev* **5**, 74–92.

Slepushkin, V.A., Katz, J.M., Black, R.A., Gamble, W.C., Rota, P.A. & Cox, N.J. (1995) Protection of mice against influenza A virus challenge by vaccination with baculovirus expressed M2 protein. *Vaccine* **13**, 1399–402.

Snyder, M.H., Betts, R.F., DeBorde, D. *et al.* (1988) Four viral genes independently contribute to attenuation of live influenza A/Ann Arbor/6/60 (H2N2) cold-adapted reassortant virus vaccines. *J Virol* **62**, 488–95.

Snyder, M.H., Clements, R.F., Betts, R. *et al.* (1986) Evaluation of live avian–human reassortant influenza A H3N2 and H1N1 virus vaccines in seronegative adult volunteers. *J Clin Microbiol* **23**, 852–7.

Snyder, M.H., London, W.T., Maassab, H.F., Chanock, R.M. & Murphy, B.R. (1990) A 36 nucleotide deletion mutation in the coding region of the NS1 gene of an influenza A virus RNA segment 8 specifies a temperature-dependent host range phenotype. *Virus Res* **15**, 69–84.

Steinhoff, M.C., Halsey, N.A., Fries, L.F. *et al.* (1991) The A/Mallard/6750/78 avian–human but not the A/Ann Arbor/6/60 cold-adapted, influenza A/Kawasaki/86 (H1N1) reassortant virus vaccine retains partial virulence for infants and children. *J Infect Dis* **163**, 1023–8.

Subbarao, E.K., Kawaoka, Y. & Murphy, B.R. (1993) Rescue of an influenza A virus wild-type PB2 gene and a mutant derivative bearing a site-specific temperature-sensitive and attenuating mutation. *J Virol* **67**, 7223–8.

Subbarao, E.K., Park, E.J., Lawson, C.M., Chen, A.Y. & Murphy, B.R. (1995) Sequential addition of temperature-sensitive missense mutations into the PB2 gene of influenza A transfectant viruses can effect an increase in temperature sensitivity and attenuation and permits the rational design of a genetically engineered live influenza A virus vaccine. *J Virol* **69**, 5969–77.

Tolpin, M.D., Clements, M.L., Levine, M.M. *et al.* (1982) Evaluation of a phenotypic revertant of the A/Alaska/77-temperature-sensitive-1A2 reassortant virus in hamsters and in seronegative adult volunteers: further evidence that the temperature-sensitive phenotype is responsible for attenuation of temperature-sensitive-1A2 reassortant viruses. *Infect Immun* **36**, 645–50.

Treanor, J., Perkins, M., Battaglia, R. & Murphy, B.R. (1994) Evaluation of the genetic stability of the temperature-sensitive PB2 gene mutation of the influenza A/Ann Arbor/6/60 cold-adapted vaccine virus. *J Virol* **68**, 7684–8.

Treanor, J.J., Betts, R.F., Smith, G.E. *et al.* (1996) Evaluation of a recombinant hemagglutinin expressed in insect cells as an influenza vaccine in young and elderly adults. *J Infect Dis* **173**, 1467–70.

Wiskerchen, M. & Muesing, M.A. (1995) Identification and characterization of a temperature-sensitive mutant of human immunodeficiency virus type 1 by alanine scanning mutagenesis of the integrase gene. *J Virol* **69**, 597–601.

Wright, P.F., Sell, S.H., Shinozaki, T., Thompson, J. & Karzon, D.T. (1975) Safety and antigenicity of influenza A/HongKong/68-ts-1 (E) (H3N2) vaccine in young seronegative children. *J Pediatr* **87**, 1109–16.

Yasuda, J., Bucher, D.J. & Ishihama, A. (1994) Growth control of influenza A virus by M1 protein: analysis of transfectant viruses carrying the chimeric M gene. *J Virol* **68**, 8141–6.

Zurcher, T., Luo, G. & Palese, P. (1994) Mutation at palmitylation sites of the influenza virus affect virus formation. *J Virol* **68**, 5748–54.

CHAPTER 33

Children as a Target for Immunization

William C. Gruber

Inactivated influenza vaccine has been consistently shown to protect adult populations against influenza illness in randomized clinical trials; these studies support the use of vaccine and promise economic benefits. Recommendations resulting from these studies target influenza vaccines at elderly people and populations with cardiopulmonary disease. However, current use of vaccines has done little to forestall yearly epidemics and may not provide adequate protection for high-risk groups (Nguyen-van-Tam & Nicholson 1992). What then is the best strategy for preventing influenza morbidity and epidemic spread?

Monto and Ohmit have recently highlighted (Monto & Ohmit 1996) that a proper understanding of the ability of influenza vaccine to protect relies on the ability to distinguish vaccine efficacy versus effectiveness; efficacy is an experimental determination most commonly derived from a randomized trial while effectiveness determines the value of the intervention as it is actually used. This chapter presents arguments to suggest that the effectiveness of influenza immunization might be improved by broadening its use to include children. Specifically, universal immunization of children not only offers prospects for control of paediatric influenza morbidity, but also may serve to reduce the severity of influenza epidemics in the community at large. The advent of nasally delivered live attenuated influenza vaccines avoids the unappealing prospect of yearly influenza 'shots', and makes a universal immunization policy practical.

Rationale for targeting children to receive influenza vaccine

Influenza attack rates and illness morbidity are high in children. Influenza A epidemics generally occur every 1–2 years and influenza B circulates widely every 3–4 years; both A and B viruses may cocirculate in a given season. Not surprisingly, young children have been observed to experience more than one influenza illness in a single season (Frank et al. 1983b).

Morbidity due to influenza in children can be significant. Influenza attack rates can be 40% or more in school-aged children, which is higher than the 10–20% rate observed in young adult populations (Glezen & Denny 1973; Fox et al. 1982a,b). Influenza-associated hospitalizations for acute respiratory disease in children less than 5 years of age (42.7/100 000) are second only to hospitalization rates of the elderly population (Glezen 1993). The young infant appears to be at greatest risk for hospitalization. This is in part because presenting symptoms during the first 2 months of life often mimic those of bacterial sepsis (Glezen et al. 1980b; Dagan & Hall 1984). Outbreaks of influenza imitating sepsis often associated with apnoea have occurred in neonatal intensive care units (Meibalane et al. 1977).

Children in the 2-month to 2-year-old age group experience influenza illness with features in common to those of other virus infections, notably respiratory syncytial virus (RSV), adenovirus and parainfluenza (Glezen et al. 1980; Huq et al. 1990). Influenza infection is symptomatic in over two-thirds of these young children and is more commonly associated with laryngotracheobronchitis, bronchopneumonia and pneumonia than in older children and adults (Murphy *et al.* 1981; Wright *et al.* 1981; Liou *et al.* 1987). Evidence of pulmonary involvement occurs in 10–50% of symptomatic illness in these young children. Most episodes of bronchopneumonia are mild and associated with complete recovery. However, pneumonia due to influenza can also be fatal in otherwise healthy children (Downham *et al.* 1975; Liou *et al.* 1987; Troendle *et al.* 1992).

Influenza-associated croup syndromes tend to be more severe than those associated with parainfluenza virus, the more common cause. In influenza-associated tracheobronchitis, secretions are tenacious and the fever is typically higher. Airway compromise is often more severe and may be complicated by bacterial superinfection (Edwards *et al.* 1983; Belshe 1986).

Children 2–5 years of age may have relatively mild, afebrile upper respiratory influenza illness (Frank *et al.* 1979; Wright *et al.* 1980). More commonly, primary infection in the preschool-aged child manifests as a febrile upper respiratory illness with a lower respiratory component, often tracheobronchitis. During one influenza epidemic, 50% of closely followed children were infected and of these, 63% were symptomatic with high fever, systemic toxicity and lower respiratory symptoms (Wright *et al.* 1977a). H1N1-associated illness appears to be less severe than that of H3N2 (Wright *et al.* 1980), and influenza B epidemics have generally been associated with lower mortality rates than influenza A outbreaks. Studies in families have regularly indicated a high incidence of fever and respiratory symptoms in children (Glezen & Denny 1973; Glezen *et al.* 1980a; Frank *et al.* 1985; Glezen *et al.* 1987).

Evaluations which have sought to determine the burden of respiratory illness have consistently noted a peak frequency of paediatric visits to primary care physicians in a health maintenance organization during the influenza season (Glezen *et al.* 1987). The impetus for keeping children out of the doctor's office can be expected to grow as capitated managed care assumes a larger and larger share of the health-care market.

Children with underlying cardiopulmonary disease are at increased risk for more severe influenza disease (Mullooly & Barker 1982; Wang *et al.* 1984). Children with cystic fibrosis complicated by influenza infection have lower expiratory flow and decreased Schwachman scores in comparison with children infected with other respiratory viruses (Pribble *et al.* 1990). Children with cystic fibrosis and influenza infection also experience increased hospitalization rates and respiratory illness morbidity in comparison to uninfected cystic fibrosis patients (Gross *et al.* 1993). Influenza can be associated with life-threatening pneumonia in immunocompromised children, such as children with solid organ transplants (Mauch *et al.* 1994). High influenza attack rates of influenza infection and high morbidity might be expected in influenza-naive human immunodeficiency virus (HIV)-positive infants and children, yet there are no series which report exceptional morbidity or mortality in this population. Safrin *et al.* (1990) reported a series of five adult HIV cases, in whom the morbidity of influenza infection seemed no worse than for healthy subjects.

Targeting influenza intervention to high-risk populations has current priority in policy. However, the high-risk paediatric population may represent only a fraction of children hospitalized for influenza. In one urban study only 13% of children under 5 years of age who were hospitalized during influenza epidemics in 1985–90 had a high-risk condition for which influenza vaccination is recommended (Glezen 1993).

Bacterial superinfection is a major complication of influenza illness. Of influenza infections 10–50% have associated acute otitis media (Henderson *et al.* 1982), many of which have a bacterial aetiology. Pneumonia mortality, primarily due to pneumococcal secondary infection, is tied intimately to influenza virus epidemics (Glezen *et al.* 1987). *Staphylococcus aureus* may serve to enhance cleavage and virulence of influenza (Tashiro *et al.* 1987). *Staphylococcus aureus* secondary infection may manifest as a croup-like illness or pneumonia (Edwards *et al.* 1983). *Staphylococcus aureus* infections at sites other than the lung have been identified following influenza infection, and toxic shock syndrome is a recognized complication (MacDonald *et al.* 1987; Gruber & Pietsch 1988). Some observations have linked severe invasive *Neisseria meningitides* infection to influenza epidemics (Harrison *et al.* 1991; Hubert *et al.* 1992). This has important implications for the paediatric patient, since the highest meningococcal attack rates are observed in children (Samuelsson *et al.* 1991).

Infection of preschool and school-aged children appears to drive community influenza A and B epidemics (Fig. 33.1) (Longini *et al.* 1982). As early as 1920 (Armstrong & Hopkins 1921), the epidemic curve for influenza illness has been shown to peak in schoolchildren several days before the community peak. Contemporary studies continue to indicate that school absenteeism in the winter months precedes other signs of an influenza epidemic in the community (Glezen & Couch 1978). What accounts for the role of children as a driving force in influenza epidemics? High attack rates and prolonged shedding of influenza in young children make infants and young children particularly effective in the spread of influenza (Glezen & Couch 1978; Frank *et al.* 1979, 1981, 1983a). Adults typically shed influenza virus for only a few days after infection, and titres of recovered virus are often lower than those of children. In contrast, influenza virus replication is detectable 1–3 days after infection, and often persists 10 days to 2 weeks in young children (Frank *et al.* 1981). These observations are true for both wild-type virus infections as well as those following attenuated vaccines for H3N2, H1N1 and B influenza viruses (Wright *et al.* 1982, 1985; Belshe *et al.* 1984; Clements *et al.* 1984, 1990; Gruber *et al.* 1993; Swierkosz *et al.* 1994). Hence, the relative immunological naiveté of the paediatric patient, rather than the virulence of a particular influenza strain appears to play the greater role in ensuring prolonged shedding.

It is understandable that household contacts of an influenza-infected child might have a greater risk of acquiring influenza illness than adults without children. In the Houston Family Study, the presence of a child in the home was associated with a greater risk of influenza infections in adults, than in households without children (Frank et al. 1985). A broad and effective intervention strategy in children might be expected to reduce wintertime paediatric outpatient morbidity, paediatric hospi-

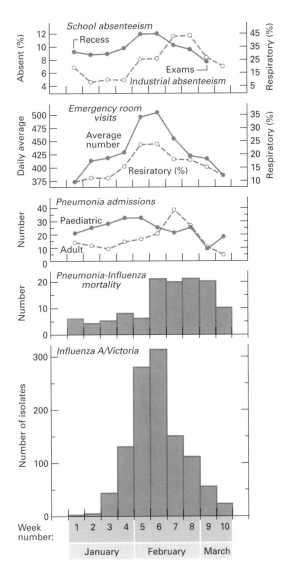

Fig. 33.1 Interpandemic influenza in the Houston area 1974–76, which demonstrates high attack rates in children prior to spread of influenza in the community. (From Glezen & Couch 1978 with permission from the Massachusetts Medical Society.)

talizations, and possibly impact community spread of disease.

Immunity

Targeting influenza vaccination of children only makes sense if children can develop immunity that will protect against childhood disease and community spread after subsequent exposure to wild-type strains. As discussed elsewhere in this volume, the changeable nature of the influenza haemagglutinin thwarts this effort. Complete protection for influenza A subtypes and B is often transient and limited to strains to which adults and children have been previously exposed, either by vaccine or live virus antigen. Reinfection rates have been noted to be as low as 2–12% and as high as 67% for influenza A and B viruses in populations of closely followed children (Hall *et al.* 1973; Frank *et al.* 1979, 1983, 1987; Fox *et al.* 1982b; Glezen 1993). The degree of antigenic drift, socioeconomic status, crowding and exposure to risk contribute to disease susceptibility (Frank *et al.* 1979; Frank & Taber 1983). Children suffer the added disadvantage of limited opportunity for exposure and priming of the immune response early in life. Several studies have noted inadequate haemagglutination inhibition, neutralization, or enzyme-linked immunoadsorbent assay (ELISA) antibody responses after single or two doses of inactivated vaccine (Wright *et al.* 1977b, 1983; Groothuis *et al.* 1991, 1994; Piedra *et al.* 1993). Otherwise healthy children less than 2 years of age with culture defined influenza infection and typical illness may fail to make specific antibody to the infecting serotype. Hence, young children require several years of exposure to influenza epidemics or a priming dose of vaccine to assure reliable response to all three vaccine antigens after inactivated vaccine administration (Bernstein *et al.* 1982). Reinfections are more common with haemagglutination-inhibition (HAI) antibody titres of ≥1 in 32 and may be age dependent, with younger children at greater jeopardy for inadequate protective response against rechallenge. Young children have been shown to boost local immunoglobulin A (IgA) responses to influenza A subtypes, after repeated exposure to influenza (Johnson *et al.* 1986). Although the actual contribution of secretory IgA antibody to influenza protection in children is speculative and largely based on experience in the mouse (Ben Ahmeida *et al.* 1992; Novak *et al.* 1993), its presence has generally been favoured. To ensure protection of infants and children against influenza, influenza vaccines must be immunogenic after a single dose or must be given as two doses prior to wild-type influenza exposure.

Current status of paediatric influenza vaccines and prospects for universal immunization

Trivalent inactivated influenza vaccines containing H1N1, H3N2, and B antigens are currently used for the prevention of influenza. These vaccines are currently formulated as whole virus vaccines (containing intact formalin-treated virus) or split virus vaccines (containing formalin-treated virus disrupted to solubilize the lipid envelope). Whole virus vaccines are slightly more immunogenic in children, but they are associated with an unacceptably high number of local and febrile reactions (Marine & Stuart-Harris 1976). In the USA, trivalent split virus vaccines are recommended for immunization of children less than 13 years of age (Table 33.1). The current USA strategy of annual influenza immunization targets high-risk children 6 months of age or older and their care providers, as noted in Table 33.2. Because of the inconsistency of protection in young children after a single exposure to influenza A or B antigens, two doses of trivalent inactivated vaccine administered 1 month apart are recommended as initial immunization for children younger than 9 years of age. Inactivated influenza provided 50–80% protection against febrile influenza H1N1, H3N2 or B illness, when administered to all children in a cohort of families under active surveillance (Gruber *et al.* 1990; Clover *et al.* 1991; Glezen *et al.* 1993). Protection was highest in children 10–18 years of age. Even two doses of vaccine may fail to be reliably immunogenic in young infants; Groothuis noted variable responses with different H1N1, H3N2 and B antigens in seronegative high-risk infants under 2 years of age (Groothuis *et al.* 1991). Responses to A/Mississippi/1/85 (H3N2) reached 93% after two doses of vaccine containing this antigen but less than 50% of subjects responded to A/Sichuan/360/86 (H3N2) after receiving two doses of vaccine containing this antigen. Responses to several other H1N1 and B antigens did not reach 50%. The

Table 33.1 Recommended schedule for intramuscular administration of influenza vaccine. (See Anonymous 1994.)

Age	Vaccine*	Dose (ml)†	No. of doses‡
6–35 months	Split virus only	0.25	1–2
3–8 years	Split virus only	0.5	1–2
9–12 years	Split virus only	0.5	1
> 12 years	Whole or split virus	0.5	1

* Split virus vaccine is given to young children because of the lower potential for producing febrile reactions; may also be labelled 'subvirion', or 'purified surface antigen'. The preferred site for administration is the deltoid for older children, and the anterolateral aspect of the thigh in infants and young children.
† Doctors should refer to product insert for possible changes in dosage in future years.
‡ Two doses are recommended if the child is receiving influenza vaccine for the first time.

prospect of annual influenza shots, repeated doses for initial immunization, and incomplete protection afforded by inactivated vaccine has proved a daunting challenge to the expansion of current immunization practice. Intranasally administered, live attenuated influenza vaccines offer promise of overcoming these limitations.

Live attenuated reassortant vaccines are in development which recombine the internal protein genes of a cold-adapted parent with wild-type haemagglutinin and neuraminidase genes (Massab 1967). The derivation and development of these vaccines are discussed in Chapters 28 and 29. These vaccines are administered intranasally by drops or spray. Single strain cold-adapted vaccines are reliably non-reactogenic, and immunogenic in children after a single dose (Wright *et al.* 1982; Belshe *et al.* 1984; Edwards *et al.* 1991). Seroconversions after monovalent preparations containing at least 10^6 $TCID_{50}$ of virus range from 60 to 100% in seronegative children. Immunogenicity of H1N1 vaccines have generally lagged their H3N2 and B counterparts, but have generally exceeded 60%. Bivalent (H1N1, H3N2) and trivalent (H1N1, H3N2, B) cold-adapted vaccines are safe, but immunogenicity of individual vaccine strains often is reduced when they are combined. Reductions in both H1N1 and B virus immunogenicity have been

Table 33.2 Recommendations for influenza immunization in children. (See Anonymous 1994.)

High-risk children with the following medical conditions should be immunized annually
Cystic fibrosis, asthma or other chronic pulmonary disease
Haemodynamically significant cardiac disease
Immunosuppressive therapy
Sickle-cell anaemia and other haemoglobinopathies

High-risk children with the following medical conditions may be at increased risk of complicated influenza illness and may benefit from annual immunization
HIV infection
Diabetes mellitus
Chronic renal disease
Chronic metabolic diseases
Recipients of long-term aspirin therapy (e.g. rheumatoid arthritis, Kawasaki's disease)

Close contacts of high-risk patients who meet the following criteria should be considered for annual immunization
Hospital personnel in contact with paediatric patients
Household contacts of high-risk patients including siblings and primary caretakers
Children in households with high-risk adults

observed in populations of seronegative children 6–18 months of age, after a single dose of multivalent vaccines containing these strains (Belshe *et al.* 1992; Gruber *et al.* 1993). The responses to individual components of multivalent vaccines are not always predictable. Simultaneous nasal inoculation of ferrets with attenuated H1N1 and H3N2 influenza virus resulted in influenza H3N2 infection in all animals, but H1N1 infection was reduced compared to the rate of infection in ferrets inoculated with H1N1 alone (Potter *et al.* 1983). Simultaneous nasal inoculation of adult volunteers yielded the opposite finding; H1N1 infection reduced the likelihood of H3N2 infection (Potter *et al.* 1983). The same cold-adapted H1N1 virus strain when used in combination with different H3N2 or B viruses may demonstrate significant differences in immunogenicity in seronegative children. Results after administration of the same cold-adapted H1N1 antigen (A/Kawasaki/9/86) from two different manufacturers and in combination with two different H3N2 antigens have produced seroconversions as low as 40% and as high as 73% (Gruber *et al.* 1996, 1997). In addition, dose–response studies have been performed in children as young as 2 months of age. It appears that in seronegative influenza-naive children less than 6 months of age, immunogenicity of cold-adapted influenza vaccines are reduced in comparison to responses in older children (Karron *et al.* 1995; Gruber *et al.* 1997). Results of these investigations and ongoing trials suggest that the following factors will be important in assuring immunogenicity of multivalent cold-adapted influenza vaccines in children:

• age of the vaccine recipient and pre-existing serological status
• doses of component cold-adapted influenza strains
• antigen used in measurement of vaccine response
• vaccine manufacturer.

Fortunately, high or repetitive doses of trivalent cold-adapted vaccine appear to circumvent limitations imposed by these factors (Gruber *et al.* 1993; Swierkosz *et al.* 1994; Clements *et al.* 1996)

How well do cold-adapted influenza vaccines perform in protecting children against wild-type influenza illness? These vaccines compare favourably with inactivated vaccines in their ability to protect healthy children against influenza. Reductions in influenza infection or illness have averaged 50–80% after single or yearly doses of cold-adapted influenza vaccine (Clover *et al.* 1991; Rudenko *et al.* 1993; Edwards *et al.* 1994; Gruber *et al.* 1994). In one study, protection against influenza associated otitis media was observed (Gruber *et al.* 1996). Serologically defined infection occurred in less than 10% of children with cystic fibrosis whose entire family received cold-adapted vaccine over 3 years; rates were comparable to rates observed in an accompanying family cohort of trivalent inactivated vaccine recipients (Gruber *et al.* 1994). In one trial, cold-adapted vaccine protection against H1N1 infection appeared to persist for 2 years, but trivalent inactivated vaccine did not induce such durable protection (Clover *et al.* 1991; Glezen *et al.* 1993).

It appears that cold-adapted vaccines hold promise for protection of immunized children against influenza morbidity. However, does administration of vaccine to children offer the prospect of reducing the impact of influenza in the community? There are several examples to suggest that broad immunization can extend protection to the unvaccinated. Immunization of all school-aged children with inactivated vaccine was effective in reducing the severity of a community outbreak of influenza A in Tecumseh, Michigan (Monto *et al.* 1970). A broad immunization campaign which included children between 1 and 5 years of age demonstrated evidence of protection against spread of influenza A/Hong Kong (H3N2); a 68% reduction in H3N2 influenza attack rates was observed in heavily immunized communities (Warburton *et al.* 1972). Although similar data are lacking for cold-adapted influenza vaccines, several observations provide support for the use of cold-adapted vaccine for broad immunization.

Japanese and Russian live attenuated influenza A and B vaccines have been produced by similar recombinant technology to that used for development of American cold-adapted vaccines. Japanese vaccines were shown to protect against institutional spread of influenza among children with mental retardation or asthma (Miyazaki *et al.* 1993). Russian live attenuated influenza A and B vaccines have been reported to reduce absenteeism due to respiratory illness by up to 50% in populations of schoolchildren. Protection against winter respiratory illness during the influenza epidemic appeared to extend to children and school staff who were unimmunized (Rudenko *et al.* 1993, 1996; Slepushkin *et al.* 1993; Khan *et al.* 1996).

Other approaches to protection of children include use of DNA vaccines (Chapter 31), use of adjuvants to alter cell-mediated immunity or antibody response, and maternal immunization. Each of these experimental approaches has merit and deserves further investigation. Immunization of pregnant women with passive transfer of protective antibody deserves special mention. This strategy may ensure protection of small high-risk infants prior to their own vaccination. Significantly higher IgG antibodies to maternal influenza vaccine antigens have been identified in cord and infant serum after maternal immunization in the third trimester when compared to antibody levels of unimmunized mothers (Englund *et al.* 1993).

At a recent international conference devoted to options for control of influenza, there was little support for general immunization of young children with inactivated vaccine, but members did support the principle of general immunization with an efficacious live attenuated influenza virus vaccine (Potter 1993). If multivalent cold-adapted vaccines can reliably protect against influenza illness for each component strain, the opportunity for broader immunization of children and adults will be at hand. A large efficacy trial of trivalent cold-adapted influenza vaccine has recently been conducted in over 1000 children in the winter of 1996–97 in the USA. Results from this trial will likely dictate the future for this vaccine. Public acceptance of a nasally delivered, attenuated influenza vaccine, its ease of delivery, potential prevention of community spread, and potential reduction of costly doctor's visits in the managed health-care environment will determine its public health future (Karzon 1993). A satisfactory live attenuated influenza vaccine would warrant consideration of a universal immunization policy for healthy children.

References

Anonymous. (1994) Influenza. In: Peter, G. (eds) *1994 Red Book: Report of the Committee on Infectious Diseases*, pp. 275–83. American Academy of Pediatrics, Elk Grove Village, IL.

Armstrong, C. & Hopkins, R. (1921) An epidemiological study of the 1920 epidemic of influenza in an isolated rural community. *Public Health Rep* **36**, 1671–702.

Belshe, R. (1986) Viral respiratory disease in the intensive care unit. *Heart Lung* **15**, 222–6.

Belshe, R., Swierkosz, E., Anderson, E., Newman, F., Nugent, S. & Massab, H. (1992) Immunization of infants and young children with live attenuated trivalent cold-recombinant influenza A H1N1, H3N2, and B vaccine. *J Infect Dis* **165**, 727–32.

Belshe, R., Van Voris, L., Bartram, J. & Crookshanks, F. (1984) Live attenuated influenza A virus vaccines in children: results of a field trial. *J Infect Dis* **150**, 834–40.

Ben Ahmeida, E., Jennings, R., Erturk, M. & Potter, C. (1992) The IgA and subclass IgG responses and protection in mice immunised with influenza antigens administered as ISCOMS, with FCA, ALH or as infectious virus. *Arch Virol* **125**, 71–86.

Bernstein, D., Zahradnik, J., DeAngelis, C. *et al.* (1982) Influenza immunization in children and young adults. *Am J Dis Child* **136**, 513–17.

Clements, M., Betts, R. & Murphy, B. (1984) Advantage of live attenuated cold-adapted influenza A virus over inactivated vaccine for A/Washington/80 (H3N2) wild-type virus infection. *Lancet* **i**, 705–8.

Clements, M., Makhene, M., Karron, R. *et al.* (1996) Effective immunization with live attenuated influenza A virus can be achieved in early infancy. Paediatric Care Centre. *J Infect Dis* **173**, 44–51.

Clements, M., Snyder, M., Sears, S., Massab, H. & Murphy, B. (1990) Evaluation of the infectivity, immunogenicity, and efficacy of live cold-adapted influenza B/Ann Arbor/1/86 reassortant virus vaccine in adult volunteers. *J Infect Dis* **161**, 869–77.

Clover, R., Crawford, S., Glezen, W., Taber, L., Matson, C. & Couch, R. (1991) Comparison of heterotypic protection against influenza A/Taiwan/86 (H1N1) by attenuated and inactivated vaccines to A/Chile/83-like viruses. *J Infect Dis* **163**, 300–4.

Dagan, R. & Hall, C. (1984) Influenza A virus infection imitating bacterial sepsis in early infancy. *Paediatr Infect Dis* **3**, 218–21.

Downham, M., Gardner, P., McQuillin, J. *et al.* (1975) Role of respiratory viruses in childhood mortality. *Br Med J* **1**, 235–9.

Edwards, K., Dundon, M. & Altemeier, W. (1983) Bacterial tracheitis as a complication of viral croup. *Paediatr Infect Dis* **2**, 390–1.

Edwards, K., Dupont, W., Westrich, M., Plummer, W., Palmer, P. & Wright, P. (1994) A randomized controlled trial of cold-adapted and inactivated vaccines for the prevention of influenza A disease. *J Infect Dis* **169**, 68–76.

Edwards, K., King, J., Steinhoff, M. *et al.* (1991) Safety and immunogenicity of live attenuated cold-adapted influenza B/Ann Arbor/1/86 reassortant virus vaccine in infants and children. *J Infect Dis* **163**, 740–5.

Englund, J., Mbawuike, I., Hammill, H., Holleman, M., Baxter, B. & Glezen, W. (1993) Maternal immunization with influenza or tetanus toxoid vaccine for passive antibody protection in young infants. *J Infect Dis* **168**, 647–56.

Fox, J., Cooney, M., Hall, C. & Foy, H. (1982a) Influenza virus infections in Seattle families, 1975–1979. II. Pattern of infection in invaded households and relation of age and prior antibody to occurrence of infection and related illness. *Am J Epidemiol* **116**, 228–42.

Fox, J., Hall, C., Cooney, M. & Foy, H. (1982b) Influenza virus infections in Seattle families, 1975–1979. I. Study design, methods and the occurrence of infections by time and age. *Am J Epidemiol* **116**, 212–27.

Frank, A. & Taber, L. (1983) Variation in frequency of natural reinfection with influenza A viruses. *J Med Virol* **12**, 17–23.

Frank, A., Taber, L., Glezen, W., Geyer, E., McIlwain, S. & Paredes, A. (1983a) Influenza B virus infections in the community and the family. The epidemics of 1976–1977 and 1979–1980 in Houston, Texas. *Am J Epidemiol* **118**, 313–25.

Frank, A., Taber, L., Glezen, W., Paredes, A. & Couch, R. (1979) Reinfection with influenza A (H3N2) virus in young children and their families. *J Infect Dis* **140**, 829–36.

Frank, A., Taber, L. & Porter, C. (1987) Influenza B virus reinfection. *Am J Epidemiol* **125**, 576–86.

Frank, A., Taber, L. & Wells, J. (1983b) Individuals infected with two subtypes of influenza A virus in the same season. *J Infect Dis* **147**, 120–4.

Frank, A., Taber, L. & Wells, J. (1985) Comparison of infection rates and severity of illness for influenza A subtypes H1N1 and H3N2. *J Infect Dis* **151**, 73–80.

Frank, A., Taber, L., Wells, C., Wells, J., Glezen, W. & Paredes, A. (1981) Patterns of shedding of myxoviruses and paramyxoviruses in children. *J Infect Dis* **144**, 433–41.

Glezen, W. (1993) Anatomy of an urban influenza epidemic. In: Hannoun, C., Klenk, H., Kendal, A. & Ruben, F. (eds) *Options for the Control of Influenza*, Vol. 2, pp. 11–14. Excerpta Medica, New York.

Glezen, W. & Couch, R. (1978) Interpandemic influenza in the Houston area, 1974–76. *N Engl J Med* **298**, 587–92.

Glezen, W., Couch, R., Taber, L. *et al.* (1980a) Epidemiologic observations of influenza B virus infections in Houston, Texas, 1976–1977. *Am J Epidemiol* **111**, 13–22.

Glezen, W., Decker, M., Joseph, S. & Mercready, R. (1987) Acute respiratory disease associated with influenza epidemics in Houston, 1981–1983. *J Infect Dis* **155**, 1119–26.

Glezen, W. & Denny, F. (1973) Epidemiology of acute lower respiratory disease in children. *N Engl J Med* **288**, 498–505.

Glezen, W., Paredes, A. & Taber, L. (1980b) Influenza in children. Relationship to other respiratory agents. *J Am Med Assoc* **243**, 1345–9.

Glezen, W., Taber, L. & Gruber, W. *et al.* (1993) Family studies of vaccine efficacy in children: comparison of protection provided by inactivated and attenuated influenza vaccines. In: Hannoun, C., Kendall, A., Klenk, H. & Ruben, F. (eds) *Options for the Control of Influenza*, Vol. 2, pp. 435–7. Excerpta Medica, New York.

Groothuis, J., Lehr, M. & Levin, M. (1994) Safety and immunogenicity of a purified haemagglutonin antigen in very young high-risk children. *Vaccine* **12**, 139–41.

Groothuis, J., Levin, M., Rabalais, G., Meiklejohn, G. & Lauer, B. (1991) Immunization of high-risk infants younger than 18 months of age with split product influenza vaccine. *Paediatrics* **87**, 823–8.

Gross, P., Denning, C., Gaerlan, P. *et al.* (1993) Benefit of annual influenza immunization in patients with cystic fibrosis. In: Hannoun, C., Klenk, H., Kendal, A. & Ruben, F. (eds) *Options for the Control of Influenza*, Vol. 2, pp. 417–21. Excerpta Medica, New York.

Gruber, W., Belshe, R., King, J. *et al.* (1996) Evaluation of live attenuated influenza vaccines in children 6–18 months of age: safety, immunogenicity, and efficacy. National Institute of Allergy and Infectious Diseases, Vaccine and Treatment Evaluation Program and the Wyeth-Ayerst cold-adapted Influenza Vaccine Investigators Group. *J Infect Dis* **173**, 1313–19.

Gruber, W., Campbell, P., Thompson, J., Reed, G., Roberts, B. & Wright, P. (1994) Comparison of live attenuated and inactivated influenza vaccines in cystic fibrosis patients and their families: results of a 3-year study. *J Infect Dis* **169**, 241–7.

Gruber, W., Darden, P., Still, J. *et al.* (1997) Evaluation of bivalent live attenuated influenza A vaccines in children 2 months to 3 years of age: safety, immunogenicity and dose–response. *Vaccine* **15**, 1379–84.

Gruber, W., Kirschner, K., Tollefson, S. *et al.* (1993) Comparison of monovalent and trivalent live attenuated influenza vaccines in young children. *J Infect Dis* **168**, 53–60.

Gruber, W. & Pietsch, J. (1988) Toxic shock syndrome due to *Staphylococcus aureus* enterocolitis. *Paediatr Infect Dis J* **7**, 71–2.

Gruber, W., Taber, L. & Glezen, W. *et al.* (1990) Live attenuated and inactivated influenza vaccine in school-age children. *Am J Dis Child* **144**, 595–600.

Hall, C., Cooney, M. & Fox, J. (1973) The Seattle virus watch. IV. Comparative epidemiologic observations of infections with influenza A and B viruses, 1965–69, in families with young children. *Am J Epidemiol* **98**, 365–89.

Harrison, L., Armstrong, C., Jenkins, S. *et al.* (1991) A cluster of meningococcal disease on a school bus following epidemic influenza. *Arch Int Med* **151**, 1005–9.

Henderson, F., Collier, A., Sanyal, M. *et al.* (1982) A longitudinal study of respiratory viruses and bacteria in the etiology of acute otitis media with effusion. *N Engl J Med* **306**, 1377–83.

Hubert, B., Watier, L., Garnerin, P. & Richardson, S. (1992) Meningococcal disease and influenza-like syndrome: a new approach to an old question. *J Infect Dis* **166**, 542–5.

Huq, F., Rahman, M., Nahar, N. *et al.* (1990) Acute lower respiratory tract infection due to virus among hospitalized children in Dhaka, Bangladesh. *Rev Infect Dis* **12** (suppl 8), S982–7.

Johnson, P., Feldman, S., Thompson, J., Mahoney, J. & Wright, P. (1986) Immunity to influenza A virus infection in young children: a comparison of natural infection, live cold-adapted vaccine, and inactivated vaccine. *J Infect Dis* **154**, 121–7.

Karron, R., Steinhoff, M., Subbarao, E. *et al.* (1995) Safety and immunogenicity of a cold-adapted influenza A (H1N1) reassortant virus vaccine administered to infants less than 6 months of age. *Paediatric Infect Dis J* **14**, 10–16.

Karzon, D. (1993) Cold-adapted live vaccines: conclusions and recommendations. In: Hannoun, C., Klenk, H., Kendal, A. & Ruben, F. (eds) *Options for the Control of Influenza*, Vol. 2, pp. 445–8. Excerpta Medica, New York.

Khan, A., Polezhaev, F., Vasiljeva, R. *et al.* (1996) Comparison of US inactivated split virus and Russian live attenuated, cold-adapted trivalent influenza vaccines in Russian schoolchildren. *J Infect Dis* **173**, 453–6.

Liou, Y.Barbour, S., Bell, L. & Plotkin, S. (1987) Children hospitalized with influenza B infection. *Paediatr Infect Dis J* **6**, 541–3.

Longini, I., Koopman, J., Monto, A. & Fox, J. (1982) Estimating household and community transmission parameters for influenza. *Am J Epidemiol* **115**, 736–51.

MacDonald, K., Osterholm, M., Hedberg, C. *et al.* (1987) Toxic shock syndrome. A newly recognized complication of influenza and influenza-like illness. *J Am Med Assoc* **257**, 1053–8.

Marine, W. & Stuart-Harris, C. (1976) Reactions and serologic responses in young children and infants after administration of inactivated monovalent influenza A vaccine. *J Paediatr* **88**, 26–30.

Massab, H. (1967) Adaptation and growth characteristics of influenza virus at 25°C. *Nature* **213**, 612–14.

Mauch, T., Bratton, S., Myers, T., Krane, E., Gentry, S. & Kashtan, C. (1994) Influenza B virus infection in paediatric solid organ transplant recipients. *Paediatr* **94**, 225–9.

Meibalane, R., Sedinak, G., Sasidharan, P. *et al.* (1977) Outbreak of influenza in a neonatal intensive care unit. *J Paediatr* **91**, 974–6.

Miyazaki, C., Nakayama, M., Tanaka, Y. *et al.* (1993) Immunization of institutionalized asthmatic children and patients with psychomotor retardation using live attenuated cold-adapted reassortment influenza A H1N1, H3N2 and B vaccines. *Vaccine* **11**, 853–8.

Monto, A., Davenport, F., Napier, J. & Francis, T. (1970) Modification of an outbreak of influenza in Tecumseh, Michigan by vaccination of school children. *J Infect Dis* **122**, 16–25.

Monto, A. & Ohmit, S. (1996) Effectiveness evaluation of inactivated influenza vaccines: methods and results. In: Brown, L., Hampson, A. & Webster, R. (eds) *Options for the Control of Influenza*, Vol. 3, pp. 93–6. Elsevier, Amsterdam.

Mullooly, J. & Barker, W. (1982) Impact of type A influenza on children: a retrospective study. *Am J Public Health* **72**, 1008–16.

Murphy, T., Henderson, F., Clyde, W., Collier, A. & Denny, F. (1981) Pneumonia: an 11-year study in a paediatric practice. *Am J Epidemiol* **113**, 12–21.

Nguyen-van-Tam, J. & Nicholson, K. (1992) Influenza deaths in Leicestershire during the 1989–90 epidemic: implications for prevention. *Epidemiol Infection* **108**, 537–45.

Novak, M., Moldoveanu, Z., Schafer, D., Mestecky, J. & Compans, R. (1993) Murine model for evaluation of protective immunity to influenza virus. *Vaccine* **11**, 55–60.

Piedra, P., Glezen, W., Mbawuike, I. *et al.* (1993) Studies on reactogenicity and immunogenicity of attenuated bivalent cold recombinant influenza type A (CRA) and inactivated trivalent influenza virus (TI) vaccines in infants and young children. *Vaccine* **11**, 718–24.

Potter, C.W. (1993) Vaccination of infants and children: conclusions and recommendations. In: Hannoun, C., Klenk, H., Kendal, A. & Ruben, F. (eds) *Options for the Control of Influenza*, Vol. 2, pp. 449–50. Excerpta Medica, New York.

Potter, C., Jennings, R., Clark, A. & Ali, M. (1983) Interference following dual inoculation with influenza A (H3N2) and (H1N1) viruses in ferrets and volunteers. *J Med Virol* **11**, 77–86.

Pribble, C., Black, P., Bosso, J. & Turner, R. (1990) Clinical manifestations of exacerbations of cystic fibrosis associated with non-bacterial infections. *J Paediatr* **117**, 200–4.

Rudenko, L., Lonskaya, N., Klimov, A., Vasilieva, R. & Ramirez, A. (1996) Clinical and epidemiological evaluation of a live, cold-adapted influenza vaccine for 3–14-year-olds. *Bull WHO* **74**, 77–84.

Rudenko, L., Slepushkin, A., Monto, A. *et al.* (1993) Efficacy of live attenuated and inactivated influenza vaccines in schoolchildren and their unvaccinated contacts in Novgorod, Russia. *J Infect Dis* **168**, 881–7.

Safrin, S., Rush, J. & Mills, J. (1990) Influenza in patients with human immunodeficiency virus infection. *Chest* **98**, 33–7.

Samuelsson, S., Gustavsen, S. & Ronne, T. (1991) Epidemiology of meningococcal disease in Denmark, 1980–1988. *Scand J Infect Dis* **23**, 723–6.

Slepushkin, A., Obrosova-Serova, N., Bursteva, E. *et al.* (1993) Results of several controlled trials of live cold-adapted influenza A (H3N2) and influenza B vaccines for children in Moscow, 1987–1990. In: Hannoun, C., Klenk, H., Kendal, A. & Ruben, F. (eds) *Options for the Control of Influenza*, Vol. 2, pp. 79–83. Excerpta Medica, New York.

Swierkosz, E., Newman, F., Anderson, E., Nugent, S., Mills, G. & Belshe, R. (1994) Multidose, live attenuated, cold-recombinant, trivalent influenza vaccine in infants and young children. *J Infect Dis* **169**, 1121–4.

Tashiro, M., Ciborowski, P., Klenk, H.D., Pulverer, G. & Rott, R. (1987) Role of *Staphylococcus* protease in the development of influenza pneumonia. *Nature* **325**, 536–7.

Troendle, J., Demmler, G., Glezen, W., Finegold, M. & Romano, M. (1992) Fatal influenza B virus pneumonia in paediatric patients. *Paediatr Infect Dis J* **11**, 117–21.

Wang, E., Prober, C., Manson, B., Corey, M. & Levison, H. (1984) Association of respiratory viral infections with pulmonary deterioration in patients with cystic fibrosis. *N Engl J Med* **311**, 1653–8.

Warburton, M., Jacobs, D., Langsford, W. & White, G. (1972) Herd immunity following subunit influenza vaccine administration. *Med J Australia* **2**, 67–70.

Wright, P., Bhargava, M., Johnson, P., Thompson, J. & Karzon, D. (1985) Simultaneous administration of live, attenuated influenza A vaccines representing different serotypes. *Vaccine* **3**, 305–8.

Wright, P., Cherry, J., Foy, H. *et al.* (1983) Antigenicity and reactogenicity of influenza A/USSR/77 virus vaccine in children—a multi-centred evaluation of dosage and safety. *Rev Infect Dis* **5**, 758–64.

Wright, P., Okabe, N., McKee, K., Massab, H. & Karzon, D. (1982) Cold-adapted recombinant influenza A virus vaccines in seronegative young children. *J Infect Dis* **146**, 71–9.

Wright, P., Ross, K., Thompson, J. *et al.* (1977a) Influenza A infections in young children. *N Engl J Med* **296**, 829–34.

Wright, P., Thompson, J. & Karzon, D. (1980) Differing virulence of H1N1 and H3N2 influenza strains. *Am J Epidemiol* **112**, 814–19.

Wright, P., Thompson, J., McKee, K., Vaughn, W., Sell, S. & Karzon, D. (1981) Patterns of illness in the highly febrile young child: epidemiologic, clinical, and laboratory correlates. *Pediatrics* **67**, 694–700.

Wright, P., Thompson, J., Vaughn, W. *et al.* (1977b) Trials of influenza A/New Jersey/76 virus vaccine in normal children: an overview of age-related antigenicity and reactogenicity. *J Infect Dis* **136**, S731–41.

CHAPTER 34

National Immunization Policies and Vaccine Distribution

David S. Fedson

Over the past quarter century, one factor that has had a major impact on thinking about health care in developed countries has been the recognition that there are large geographical variations in the rates of use of medical and surgical services (Wennberg & Gittelsohn 1982). In most instances, these variations have little if any relationship to the underlying rates of the diseases for which their use is intended. Why they occur is poorly understood, and attempts to explain them on the basis of 'clinical uncertainty' or 'practice style' are incomplete and unsatisfactory. Nonetheless, not knowing 'which rate is right' has not prevented decision makers from undertaking programmes to limit the use of services thought to be overused and not worthwhile.

Almost all studies showing geographical variations in health-care delivery have focused on expensive medical and surgical treatments. By comparison, little attention has been given to geographical variations in inexpensive preventive services such as adult vaccination. If anything, these services are more likely to be underutilized than overutilized. Recently, however, a group of investigators has gathered historical information comparing influenza vaccine distribution and vaccination recommendations and reimbursement in 22 countries (Fedson *et al.* 1995, 1997). Not surprisingly, large variations in the levels of influenza vaccine use and differences in national recommendations and reimbursement policies have been demonstrated. A steady increase in vaccine use has also occurred in most of these countries, especially in recent years. This chapter reviews these findings.

In order to compare influenza vaccination among countries, the number of doses of influenza vaccine distributed annually was determined for each country during the period 1980–95. This information was obtained from the ministries of health or regulatory agencies in all countries except Canada, where it was obtained directly from the vaccine manufacturers. Rates were calculated for the number of doses of vaccine distributed per 1000 total resident population per year. The results are shown in the Fig. 34.1 (Fedson *et al.* 1997). They show that in any given year there were substantial differences in the levels of influenza vaccine distributed among the 22 countries. For example (and excluding Japan, whose special circumstances are discussed below), in 1985 none of the countries used more than 100 doses per 1000 population, and vaccine distribution levels ranged from 14 doses (Denmark) to 99 doses (Iceland) per 1000 population, a seven-fold difference. In 1990, the variation in vaccine use between countries was even greater: 13 doses (Austria) compared with 158 doses (Spain) per 1000 population; a 12-fold difference. What is also evident from Fig. 34.1 is that over the period surveyed, influenza vaccine use increased in most countries, especially during the 1990s. Thus, in 1995, 12 of 21 countries (excluding Japan) used 100 doses of influenza vaccine per 1000 population, and distribution levels ranged from 48 doses (Ireland) to 239 doses (USA) per 1000 population. In spite of this overall increase, there was still an almost five-fold difference between the countries with the lowest and highest rates of vaccine distribution.

Recommendations for influenza vaccination also varied among countries (Fedson *et al.* 1995, 1997; Nicholson *et al.* 1995). The major features of these policies are shown in Table 34.1. In 1995, six of the 22

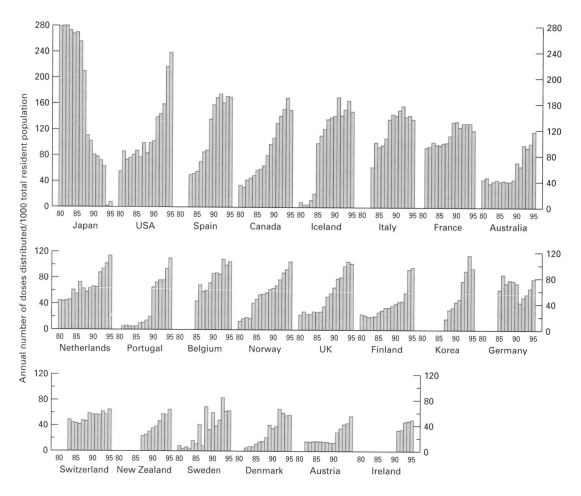

Fig. 34.1 Influenza vaccine distribution in 22 countries, 1980–95. The annual numbers of doses of influenza vaccine distributed per 1000 total population are shown by the solid bars. For some countries, data for the early years were not available, and no solid bars are shown for these years. (Redrawn from Fedson 1997, with permission from Elsevier Science Ltd, Kidlington, Oxfordshire, UK.)

countries did not recommend influenza vaccination for elderly persons above a certain age, usually (65 years). With the exception of Japan, all countries recommended influenza vaccination for patients with cardiopulmonary disorders, and almost all included those with metabolic diseases and immunological disorders. However, five countries did not specifically mention nursing home residents, and 12 countries did not recommend influenza vaccination for health-care workers.

Reimbursement policies for influenza vaccination of recommended groups also varied among countries (Table 34.2) (Fedson *et al.* 1995, 1997). The major difference was whether vaccination was paid for by national or social health insurance (including vaccination provided free of charge in public clinics) or paid for directly by those who were vaccinated. Table 34.2 also shows whether influenza vaccination was recommended for all elderly persons in each country, and lists the countries according to the number of doses of influenza vaccine distributed in 1995. As can be seen, countries whose health-care systems required individuals to pay for vaccination had lower rates of vaccine use than those with some form of public reimbursement, Iceland being the only exception. In addition, countries that did not recommend

Table 34.1 Recommendations for influenza vaccination in 22 countries, 1995.

Recommendation	Countries with recommendation
All elderly persons*	All countries except the Netherlands, UK, Finland, Sweden, Denmark and Japan
Cardiopulmonary diseases	All countries except Japan
Metabolic diseases (especially diabetes mellitus)	All countries except Norway, Finland, Denmark and Japan
Immunological disorders	All countries except New Zealand, Sweden and Japan
Nursing home residents	All countries except Italy, the Netherlands, Finland, Sweden and Japan
Health-care workers	All countries except Spain, France, Australia, the Netherlands, Portugal, Norway, United Kingdom, Finland, Sweden, Denmark, Ireland and Japan

* All persons ≥ 65 years of age except for France (≥ 70 years), Belgium (≥ 60 years and Iceland (≥ 60 years).

influenza vaccination for all elderly persons often had lower rates of vaccine use.

It would be difficult to argue that variations among countries in influenza vaccine use, vaccination recommendations or vaccination reimbursement reflect different levels of knowledge about the impact of influenza on human health or the clinical effectiveness of influenza vaccination. This knowledge is widely available and shared among all countries studied. Several other reasons must account for the observed differences. They include differences in the basic structure of the health-care system, the organization of medical practice by generalist and specialist doctors, the extent to which primary care services are provided by public agencies, and the activities of professional organizations and the vaccine manufacturers in conducting public and professional education programmes for influenza vaccination. More general economic, political and historical factors also play a role in determining vaccine use, although it is difficult to quantify their effects. No doubt individual factors that are important in one country are less so in other countries. Sometimes, one or two decision makers have been responsible for major changes in influenza vaccination in a given country. The importance of many of these factors is illustrated by a brief summary of some of the changes that have

occurred with influenza vaccination in different countries since 1980.

UK and Ireland

Influenza vaccine use began to increase in the UK in 1988 and reached a level of 102 doses per 1000 population in 1995. During this period, the Chief Medical Officer's annual letter to doctors regarding influenza vaccination was supplemented by programmes for public and professional education that were supported by the vaccine manufacturers. In addition, increased attention to the health impact of influenza following the large outbreak of disease in 1989–90 (Fleming *et al.* 1990; Ashley *et al.* 1991; Nguyen-Van-Tam & Nicholson 1992), studies of vaccine uptake (Nicholson *et al.* 1987; Nicholson 1993; Nguyen-Van-Tam & Nicholson 1993) and case–control studies of vaccination effectiveness (Ahmed *et al.* 1995; Fleming *et al.* 1995; Ahmed *et al.* 1997) contributed to an increasing awareness of the importance of influenza vaccination. Although vaccination recommendations targeted only persons with recognized at-risk conditions, the National Health Service provided reimbursement for all doses of vaccine delivered. A recent study of influenza vaccination in Gwent county in Wales showed that in 1994–95 the overall rate of vaccine

Table 34.2 Influenza vaccination reimbursement in 22 countries and its relationship to vaccination recommendations for elderly persons and vaccine use.

Country	Reimbursement for vaccination of recommended groups by national or social health insurance	Vaccination recommended for all elderly persons*	Number of doses of influenza vaccine distributed per 1000 population in 1955
USA	Yes	Yes	239
Spain	Yes	Yes	170
Canada	Yes	Yes	150
Iceland	—†	Yes‡	148
Italy	Yes	Yes	136
France	Yes	Yes§	119
Australia	Yes	Yes	117
The Netherlands	Yes	—	114
Portugal	Yes	Yes	110
Belgium	Yes¶	Yes‡	105
Norway	Yes	Yes	105
UK	Yes	—	102
Finland	Yes	—	96
Korea	—	Yes	95
Germany	Yes	Yes	80
Switzerland	—	Yes	64
New Zealand	—	Yes	64
Sweden	—	—	63
Denmark	—	—	56
Austria	—	Yes	54
Ireland	—	Yes	48
Japan	—	—	8

* ≥ 65 years in age unless otherwise specified.
† Indicates no.
‡ ≥ 60 years in age.
§ ≥ 70 years in age.
¶ In Belgium, 40% of the cost of vaccination is reimbursed.

use was closely similar to that for the UK as a whole (Fedson & Litt 1996). However, vaccine use by individual general practitioners varied from approximately 30 doses to more than 270 doses per 1000 persons enrolled in these doctors' practices. Furthermore, while less than half of persons in at-risk groups were vaccinated, 25% of those vaccinated were not included in the groups for whom vaccination was recommended. Whether the UK should expand its recommendation for influenza vaccination to include all elderly persons continues to be actively debated. Nonetheless, with no change in policy, influenza vaccine use doubled during the period 1989–95. In contrast, during the same period the rate of influenza vaccine use in Ireland was little more than half that in the UK. Unlike the UK, Irish recommendations included all elderly persons, but no public reimbursement was provided.

France

Since the early 1980s France has had a relatively high level of influenza vaccine use. One reason for this is the annual programme for public and professional education conducted by the Groupe d'Etude et d'Information sur la Grippe (GEIG) (Saliou 1996). In addition, in 1985 the major social health insurance agency and private health insurers agreed to pay for vaccinating all persons ≥ 75 years in age and younger persons with at-risk conditions. The age limit was lowered to 70 years in 1988 and full reimbursement was assumed by the social health insurance system. In the autumn, each person ≥ 70 years in age receives by mail a voucher for one dose of influenza vaccine. The vaccine is obtained from a pharmacist and taken to a doctor for administration. Surveys indicate that vaccination coverage in persons ≥ 75 years in age rose from 30% in 1979 to 70% in 1995 (Saliou 1996). Systems for influenza surveillance are well developed in France (Costagliola *et al.* 1995; Quenel *et al.* 1994), and epidemiological data suggest that vaccination has had a substantial impact in preventing influenza-associated mortality (Carrat & Valleron 1995).

Belgium and the Netherlands

During the period 1988–95, both Belgium and the Netherlands almost doubled their use of influenza vaccine. Although public reimbursement for vaccination was available in both countries (in Belgium it covered only 40% of vaccination costs), only Belgium recommended vaccination for all elderly persons (≥ 60 years). In 1996, however, a study showing influenza vaccination would be cost-effective for all elderly persons led the Netherlands to adopt an age-based (≥ 65 years) vaccination policy. This was followed by a sharp increase in vaccine use in 1996–97 (M.J.W. Sprenger, personal communication 1997).

The Nordic countries

The importance of individual decision makers for influenza vaccination is illustrated by Iceland, where in 1985 the Director General of Health decided that influenza vaccination would be recommended for persons ≥ 60 years in age. Although patients had to pay for vaccination themselves, vaccine use rose dramatically, and it remained above 140 doses per 1000 population each year after 1990. Among the other four Nordic countries, only Norway managed to reach (in 1995) a level of vaccine use above 100 doses per 1000 population. Norway also had both a recommendation that included all elderly persons and public reimbursement for vaccination. In the other three Nordic countries, influenza vaccination was recommended only for at-risk persons, and only Finland provided

public reimbursement. All had lower rates of vaccine use than Iceland and Norway. However, in 1993 vaccination recommendations in Finland began to be interpreted more broadly. Also, government purchase of vaccine for administration to medically defined at-risk individuals in public health centres increased. As a result, vaccine distribution more than doubled during the period 1993–95. Finland extended its vaccination recommendations to include all elderly persons in 1996. This decision, and a public health campaign to improve influenza awareness, led to a further increase in vaccine use in 1996–97.

Germany, Switzerland and Austria

The use of influenza vaccine remained relatively low in Germany, Austria and Switzerland up through 1995. The data shown for Germany for the years prior to 1991 include both East and West Germany. After reunification, vaccine use fell from 87 doses per 1000 population in 1990 to 43 doses per 1000 population in 1991, reflecting the discontinuation of vaccination programmes for workers in the former East Germany. Vaccine use for all Germany then rose to 85 doses in 1995. Austria had one of the lowest levels of influenza vaccine use throughout the study period, although levels gradually improved starting in 1991. Switzerland's modest levels of vaccine use in the 1980s showed little increase in the early 1990s. All three countries had recommendations for vaccinating all elderly persons, but only Germany provided public reimbursement for vaccination. In 1996, Switzerland began to provide similar reimbursement through its social health insurance system.

Italy, Spain and Portugal

Among all countries in Western Europe, Italy and Spain (along with Iceland) have been the leading users of influenza vaccine. Italy's lead appeared as early as 1984, and starting in 1988 Italy used ≥ 136 doses per 1000 population each year. In Spain, vaccine use increased gradually during the 1980s; rose abruptly to 136 doses per 1000 population in 1989 and remained at levels ≥ 158 doses per 1000 population thereafter. In both countries, influenza vaccinations were provided without charge by local public health clinics. In Italy, at least half of all influenza vaccinations were given by public centres. In Spain, public vaccination programmes were introduced in 1989; and these programmes accounted for virtually all of the growth in vaccine use in the 1990s. In Portugal, vaccine use was initially low but increased substantially in 1990; reaching a level of 110 doses per 1000 population in 1995. An educational programme for doctors conducted by a group of pulmonary specialists played an important role in increasing awareness of influenza vaccination.

Australia and New Zealand

After a decade in which the annual level of vaccine use in Australia was ≤ 46 doses per 1000 population, utilization began to increase in 1990; reaching 117 doses per 1000 population in 1995. An important contributor to this increase was the annual influenza awareness campaign co-ordinated by staff of the World Health Organization (WHO) Collaborating Centre for Influenza Reference and Research in Melbourne and sponsored by the vaccine manufacturers. Equally important were efforts of community-based coalitions such as the Vaccine Promotion Group in South Australia (Fedson & Litt 1996). The impact of this multifaceted public and professional influenza awareness programme was reflected in an increase in vaccination rates among persons ≥ 65 years in age from 28% in 1990 to 63% in 1995. Compared with Australia, influenza vaccine use in New Zealand was much lower throughout this period, although it gradually increased in the 1990s.

Japan and Korea

Among developed countries, the experience with influenza vaccine in Japan was unique. Influenza vaccination programmes were initiated for Japanese schoolchildren in 1962 in order to prevent transmission of infection to older adults (Hirota & Kaji 1994; Hirota *et al*. 1996). In 1976, vaccination of schoolchildren aged 3–18 years was made com-

pulsory. As a result, high vaccination rates (equivalent to 80%) were achieved in the early 1980s, as reflected in vaccine distribution levels equivalent to 280 doses per 1000 population annually. The rates began to fall in the mid-1980s when doubts were raised about the effectiveness of these programmes. In 1992 only 18% of children were vaccinated and 2 years later influenza was dropped from the list of diseases targeted by national vaccination programmes. In subsequent years, very little influenza vaccine was produced or distributed in Japan, reflecting the absence of any recommendation for vaccinating older and/or at-risk adults. Throughout this period there was little awareness among Japanese health professionals or the public that influenza is a health threat to adults, or that influenza vaccination is beneficial. Unlike Japan, South Korea showed a steady increase in its use of influenza vaccine starting in the late 1980s. Vaccination was recommended for all elderly persons, although no public reimbursement was provided. It was generally believed that most of the vaccine was used for older adults, although there were no solid data to support this view. It is possible that some of the influenza vaccine used each year was given to children for the same reasons it was once given to children in Japan.

USA and Canada

The use of influenza vaccine in the USA and Canada throughout the period 1980–95 was similar in spite of fundamental differences in their health-care systems (Fedson 1995). Vaccination recommendations in the two countries were virtually identical, but until 1993 only Canada provided public reimbursement for vaccination. Vaccine distribution in Canada was largely determined by provincial health departments which purchased approximately 90% of all vaccine distributed throughout the country. The health departments then supplied vaccine free-of-charge to doctors for administration to patients. Doctors were allowed to submit claims to provincial health insurance agencies for reimbursement of their charges for vaccine administration. Although vaccine use increased steadily throughout the 1980s, the rate of growth increased in 1988 following the introduction of programmes for public and professional education co-ordinated by the Lung Association of Canada and sponsored by the vaccine manufacturers. In 1990, when the level of vaccine use was 107 doses per 1000 population, the vaccination rate among elderly persons was estimated to be 45% (Duclos & Hatcher 1993). A government-sponsored consensus conference in 1992 served to further increase influenza awareness throughout Canada (Canadian Consensus Conference on Influenza 1993). In the USA, no federal reimbursement was provided for vaccination before 1993 (Fedson 1995) and, except for a few public programmes paid for by state or local governments, the costs of vaccination were paid for by patients themselves. Vaccine use began to increase in the 1990s, in part due to the federal government's Medicare Influenza Vaccine Demonstration (Centers for Disease Control and Prevention 1993) and other programmes to increase public awareness and professional education. It increased even more dramatically after implementation of Medicare reimbursement starting in 1993, and by 1995 vaccine use had reached a level of 239 doses per 1000 population. In that year, vaccination rates among persons ≥ 65 years in age were estimated to have reached approximately 60% (Centers for Disease Control and Prevention 1996).

Conclusion

This brief review shows that expressing influenza vaccine use as the number of doses distributed per 1000 population provides a convenient way to follow changes in individual countries over time and to compare different countries in the same year. Using this approach, a long-term increase in vaccine use within a country can easily be displayed, and in specific years large-scale differences (often five- to 10-fold or more) between countries can be shown. Nonetheless, there are limitations to this approach. For example, if it is assumed that all persons ≥ 65 years in age are (or should be) the major target group for influenza vaccination, it must be remembered that the proportion of the total population in each country accounted for by elderly persons will vary. For 21 of the 22 countries

(excluding the Republic of Korea) surveyed above, in 1995 these proportions ranged from 11.2% in Iceland to 17.3% in Sweden (Division of Health Situation and Trend Assessment 1996). In other words, on a population basis the proportion of elderly persons in Sweden was slightly more than 50% greater than that in Iceland. If it is assumed that similar proportions of the vaccine distributed were given to elderly persons in these two countries, the relative differences in overall vaccine distribution levels (148 doses and 63 doses per 1000 population in Iceland and Sweden, respectively) would underestimate the much larger difference in actual vaccination rates for elderly persons. More dramatically, if in 1995 similar proportions of the vaccine distributed in Korea and in the other developed countries were given to elderly persons, because only 5.6% of the Korean population was ≥ 65 years in age, the 95 doses of vaccine distributed per 1000 total population would represent a rate of vaccination in elderly Koreans that exceeded the vaccination rates for elderly persons in all other countries except in the USA. It is highly unlikely that this actually happened, and more likely that much of the influenza vaccine distributed in Korea was given to children, as suggested earlier. These examples illustrate the importance of not assuming that because a country has a high level of vaccine distribution it has a similarly high level of vaccine coverage among target groups such as the elderly. High levels of vaccine distribution could just as easily indicate more widespread vaccination of younger, non at-risk individuals. Thus, knowing levels of vaccine distribution is not a substitute for independent surveys that track vaccination rates in elderly persons and other at-risk groups. Such data are available for very few countries.

It is still uncertain whether vaccination policies and the presence or absence of public reimbursement are the primary factors affecting influenza vaccination. The differences in vaccine distribution levels in different countries in a given year suggest that reimbursement is the more important of the two (see Table 34.2). However, because long-term increases in vaccine distribution have been repeatedly demonstrated in individual countries without any changes in recommendations or reimbursement policies, other factors are probably of equal if not greater importance. In many ways, vaccine distribution levels (or, if known, vaccination rates) represent useful 'social biopsies'. Properly interpreted, they suggest economic, historical and cultural factors that determine how people in a county regard one another and, in particular, how they regard the elderly. Much can be learned from the macroepidemiology of influenza vaccine distribution levels, recommendations and reimbursement policies. However, this knowledge must be complemented by a similar understanding of the microepidemiology of influenza vaccination at the level of smaller institutions (e.g. hospitals, clinics) and individual doctors and their patients. Better understanding of both will ensure that the demonstrated benefits of influenza vaccination reach an ever larger number of people.

Acknowledgement

The author gratefully acknowledges the contributions of the following individuals to this work: Ann-Marie Ahlbom, Franz Ambrosch, Klaus Brø Jorgensen, Pierre-Etienne Cambillard, Jann Cloetta, Isabella Donatelli, Alan W. Hampson, Claude Hannoun, Yoshio Hirota, Lance C. Jennings, James Kiely, Jane Leese, Hanne Nøkleby, Olafur Olafsson, Helena Rebelo de Andrade, Francisco Salmerón, Hak-Kyoon Shin, René Snacken, Marc J.W. Sprenger, Raymond A. Strikas and Martti Valle. In 1996, the European Scientific Working Group on Influenza assumed the responsibility for continuing the survey of influenza vaccination.

References

Ahmed, A.H., Nicholson, K.G. & Nguyen-Van-Tam, J.S. (1995) Reduction in mortality associated with influenza vaccination during the 1989–90 epidemic. *Lancet* **346**, 591–5.

Ahmed, A.H., Nicholson, K.G., Nguyen-Van-Tam, J.S. & Pearson, J.C.G. (1997) Effectiveness of influenza vaccine in reducing hospital admissions during the 1989–90 epidemic. *Epidemiol Infect* **118**, 27–33.

Ashley, J., Smith, T. & Dunnel, K. (1991) Deaths in Great Britain associated with the influenza epidemic of 1989/90. *Population Trends*. Office of Population Censuses and Surveys, London, HMSO **65**, 16–20.

Canadian Consensus Conference on Influenza. (1993) *Canad J Infect Dis* **4**, 251–6.

Carrat, F. & Valleron, A.J. (1995) Influenza mortality among the elderly in France, 1980–90: how many deaths may have been avoided through vaccination? *J Epidemiol Commun Health* **49**, 419–25.

Centers for Disease Control and Prevention. (1993) Final results: Medicare influenza vaccine demonstration—selected states, 1988–92. *MMWR* **42**, 601–4.

Centers for Disease Control and Prevention (1996) Pneumococcal and influenza vaccination levels among adults ≥ 65 years. United States, 1993. *MMWR* **45**, 853–9.

Costagliola, D., Flahaut, A., Galinec, D., Garnerin, P.H., Menares, J. & Valleron, A.J. (1995) A routine tool for detection and assessment of epidemics of influenza-like syndromes in France. *Am J Public Health* **81**, 97–9.

Division of Health Situation and Trend Assessment (1996) *Demographic Data for Health Situation Assessment and Projection, 1996*, pp. 91–176. World Health Organization, Geneva.

Duclos, P. & Hatcher, J. (1993) Epidemiology of influenza vaccination in Canada. *Canad J Public Health* **84**, 311–15.

Fedson, D.S. (1995) Influenza and pneumococcal vaccination in Canada and the United States, 1980–93: what can the two countries learn from each other? *Clin Infect Dis* **20**, 1371–6.

Fedson, D.S., Hannoun, C., Leese, J. *et al.* (1995) Influenza vaccination in 18 developed countries, 1980–92. *Vaccine* **13**, 623–7.

Fedson, D.S., Hirota, Y., Shin, H.K. *et al.* (1997) Influenza vaccination in 22 developed countries, an update to 1995. *Vaccine* **15**, 1506–11.

Fedson, D.S. & Litt, J. (1996) Implementation of vaccine policy. In Brown, L.E., Hampson, A.W. & Webster, R.G (eds) *Options for the Control of Influenza III*, pp. 140–8. Elsevier, Amsterdam.

Fleming, D.M., Crombie, D.L., Norbury, C.A. & Cross, K.W. (1990) Observations on the influenza epidemic of November/December 1989. *Br J Gen Pract* **40**, 495–7.

Fleming, D.M., Watson, J.M., Nicholas, S., Smith, G.E. & Swan, A.V. (1995) Study of the effectiveness of influenza vaccination in the elderly in the epidemic of 1989–90 using a general practice database. *Epidemiol Infect* **115**, 581–9.

Hirota, Y., Fedson, D.S. & Kaji, M. (1996) Japan lagging in influenza jabs (letter). *Nature* **380**, 18.

Hirota, Y. & Kaji, M. (1994) Scepticism about influenza vaccine efficacy in Japan (letter). *Lancet* **344**, 408–9.

Nguyen-Van-Tam, J.S. & Nicholson, K.G. (1992) Influenza deaths in Leicestershire during the 1989–90 epidemic: implication for prevention. *Epidemiol Infect* **108**, 537–45.

Nguyen-Van-Tam, J.S. & Nicholson, K.G. (1993) Influenza immunization: vaccine offer, request and uptake in high risk patients during the 1991/92 season. *Epidemiol Infect* **111**, 347–55.

Nicholson, K.G. (1993) Immunization against influenza among people aged over 65 living at home in Leicestershire during winter 1991–2. *Br Med J* **306**, 974–6.

Nicholson, K.G., Snacken, R. & Palache, A.M. (1995) Influenza immunization policies in Europe and the United States. *Vaccine* **13**, 365–9.

Nicholson, K.G., Wiselka, M.J. & May, A. (1987) Influenza vaccination of the elderly: perceptions and policies of general practitioners and outcome of the 1985–6 immunization program in Trent, UK. *Vaccine* **5**, 302–6.

Quenel, P., Dab, W., Hannoun, C. & Cohen, J.M. (1994) Sensitivity, specificity and predictive value of health service based indicators for the surveillance of influenza A epidemics. *Int J Epidemiol* **23**, 849–55.

Saliou, P. (1996) The influenza study and information group: an original French construct for influenza control information. In: Brown, L.E., Hampson, A.W. & Webster, R.G (eds) *Options for the Control of Influenza III*, pp. 579–83. Elsevier, Amsterdam.

Wennberg, J. & Gittelsohn, A. (1982) Variations in medical care among small areas. *Sci Am* **246**, 120–34.

Section 9
Antivirals

CHAPTER 35

Amantadine and Rimantadine

Fred Y. Aoki

Amantadine and rimantadine are important, equally efficacious alternatives to vaccine for the prevention of influenza A illness. When prescribed for therapy, they ameliorate a spectrum of influenza-specific symptoms and thereby exceed the symptomatic benefits of antipyretics and analgesics. Amantadine was the first of this pair of compounds to be licensed. It was approved for prophylaxis of H2N2 (Asian) influenza A infection in the USA in 1966, and for prophylaxis and treatment of all influenza A infections in 1976. Its efficacy and safety in young healthy adults has been established beyond question. However, its narrow toxic-to-therapeutic ratio has made precise dosing imperative. In spite of considerable evaluation including analysis of its clinical pharmacokinetics, it has been difficult to define optimal dose schedules for individuals in cohorts which are at highest risk for development of complications of influenza A infection, such as the elderly and those with chronic cardiopulmonary, renal and other diseases in whom amantadine disposition may be, or is, altered. This has limited the wider use of amantadine. The acceptance of rimantadine, which had been widely used for influenza prophylaxis in the USSR, as an equally effective and better tolerated alternative to amantadine promised to enhance clinicians' ability to use drugs to control influenza A virus infection. This expectation has, however, been diminished by the increasing awareness of the importance of shared amantadine and rimantadine resistance that emerges frequently and rapidly during clinical use of these agents in infected individuals. The two agents are considered together.

Structure and chemistry

Amantadine is a symmetrical, thermally stable C-10 primary amine with a cage-like structure. As a hydrochloride salt it is water soluble with a pKa of 10.14 (Perrin & Hawkins 1972). Following the report of its antiviral effect (Davies *et al.* 1964), a systematic study was undertaken to identify structure–activity relationships and to discover more potent agents with a broader spectrum of action (Aldrich *et al.* 1971). Molecules with useful antiviral activity against non-influenza viruses were not identified. Substitution of the amino group by a variety of molecules reduced the anti-influenza activity of amantadine, indicating the importance of a basic nitrogen for activity (Runti & Sciortino 1968). Altering the cage structure demonstrated the importance of the adamantane nucleus for retention of activity (Lundahl *et al.* 1972).

Substitutions at R sites in structures shown in Fig. 35.1a,b,c and d (Aldrich *et al.* 1971) yielded a maximum 60% increase in potency as assessed by determination of AVl_{50} in a mouse model of lethal influenza A (swine) pneumonia. AVl_{50} was the dose (mg/kg) which reduced mortality by a half-log (3.2-fold) following a standard intranasal inoculum of 20-LD_{50} doses of virus (Whitney *et al.* 1970). Substitutions at the R site in Fig. 35.1c yielded three compounds whose AVl_{50} was the lowest observed, 1.4 mg/kg, three-fold lower than that of amantadine (4.6 mg/kg). One of these three congeners was rimantadine, whose greater potency *in vitro* and *in vivo* was described shortly thereafter (Tsunoda *et al.* 1965).

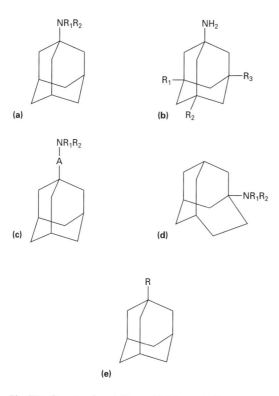

Fig. 35.1 Structural variations of (a) (amantadine hydrochloride; $R_1R_2 = H_2 - HCl$) synthesized to elucidate structure–activity relationships and to identify other antiviral molecules. Variations in the structure in (c) (A = CHCH₃; $R_1R_2 = H_2HCl$) yielded rimantadine hydrochloride. (Reprinted from Aldrich *et al.* 1971, with permission from the American Chemical Society.)

Hundreds of other amantadine congeners have been synthesized and evaluated for antiviral activity (Whitney *et al.* 1970; Lundahl *et al.* 1972; van Hes *et al.* 1972; Vaczi *et al.* 1973) with only modest success. The best of these congeners, spiroamantadine (1′-methyl-spiro (adamantane-2,3′-pyrrolidine) maleate) was three times as potent as amantadine in the mouse bioassay described above. However, in controlled trials in susceptible healthy volunteers, well-tolerated doses of 70 and 120 mg/day started 2 days prior to and 46 h after intranasal challenge had only modest prophylactic and therapeutic effects, respectively (Beare *et al.* 1972; Arroyo *et al.* 1975). These results appeared not to support further clinical evaluation.

Other alicyclic compounds resembling amanta-dine have been evaluated as agents for the treatment of influenza. A cyclononane containing a primary amine hydrochloride and thus resembling amantadine was five times as active as amantadine against H3H2 viruses *in vitro* and more active than amantadine for prophylaxis in mice (Swallow 1984). In volunteer challenge studies it provided 72 and 91% protection and reduced viral shedding at doses of 100 or 200 mg/day compared with placebo. Nasal washing and serum drug concentrations 24 h after first and last doses of 200 mg/day were at least 100 µg/L, which was the minimum concentration that inhibited the challenge virus. Given therapeutically beginning 6–15 h after onset of symptoms, 200 mg/day was minimally more effective than placebo in reducing virus excretion or clinical symptom score at day 3 and 4, respectively (Al-Nakib *et al.* 1986). Cyclo-octylamine hydrochloride, a cyclic amine with a similar spectrum of antiviral activity and mode of action as amantadine was as effective against influenza virus infections in mice, ferrets and rhesus monkeys (Hoffman 1973). In human volunteers, intranasal therapy with cyclooctylamine solution initiated 2 days prior to virus challenge produced only incomplete protection compared to placebo (Togo *et al.* 1972). Its efficacy compared to amantadine or rimantadine has not been reported.

Spectrum

In vitro

Neumayer *et al.* (1965) first described the antiviral activity of amantadine in tissue culture and *in ovo* in detail. Tsunoda *et al.* (1965) shortly thereafter reported the *in vitro* antiviral spectrum of rimanta-dine. Amantadine was not toxic to cells in culture at a maximum concentration of 25 µg/ml whereas toxic effects were uniformly observed at 100 µg/ml. Rimantadine 36 µg/ml but not 24 µg/ml was slightly toxic to cells (Tsunoda *et al.* 1965). Consistent, potent antiviral activity was demonstrated against influenza A, A1 and A2 virus strains. Subsequently, all other known human influenza A group viruses were reported to be sensitive to amantadine (Hayden *et al.* 1980a; Belshe *et al.* 1989), as were some avian (Kato &

Eggers 1969) and equine influenza A strains (Kaye & Robinson 1967). Tsunoda *et al.* (1965) initially reported, and Tisdale and Bauer (1977) confirmed, that rimantadine inhibited influenza A and was as much as twice as potent as amantadine on a weight basis. Belshe *et al.* (1989) extended these observations to H1N1 and H3N2 strains isolated between 1978 and 1988 and observed that rimantadine was on average eight-fold more potent than amantadine. Most sensitive influenza A strains are inhibited by < 1 µg/ml of rimantadine and amantadine in a plaque reduction assay (Hayden *et al.* 1980a; Belshe *et al.* 1989).

Other viruses causing respiratory disease (parainfluenza types 1–3, influenza B) as well as nonrespiratory disease (pseudorabies, Rous, Esh and mouse sarcoma, arena and lymphocytic choriomeningitis virus) have been reported to be sensitive to amantadine (reviewed in Hoffman 1973; Hayden *et al.* 1980a) or rimantadine (respiratory syncytial virus, rubeola) (Tsunoda *et al.* 1965) or both drugs (rubella). However, the activity is limited to tissue culture systems at concentrations (10–100 µg/ml) that cannot tolerably be attained *in vivo*. Other viruses causing respiratory disease that are insensitive to amantadine include rhinovirus and adenoviruses.

In vivo

Oxford reviewed the limitations of studying laboratory animals with experimental influenza A infection as models of human infection and concluded that no single species is ideal for this purpose (1977). However, studies of amantadine and rimantadine in mice and ferrets have generally correlated with results in humans. Both drugs were effective for prophylaxis and treatment by oral, intraperitoneal, subcutaneous and intranasal (aerosol) administration. Amantadine was effective when given prophylactically as a single dose 1 h before infection or as late as 72 h, but not 96 h, after infection (Grunert *et al.* 1965). Rimantadine was more effective than amantadine in mice when lung consolidation, mortality, lung virus concentration and haemagglutination inhibition (HAI) antibodies were evaluated (Tsunoda *et al.* 1965; Schulman 1968). Rimantadine was much more effective than aman-

tadine in preventing treated mice from transmitting infection to untreated contact mice and in protecting contact mice (Schulman 1968). In chickens, amantadine and rimantadine administered in the same concentration in water beginning at the time of intranasal instillation of an avian influenza A virus were equally effective in preventing death (Webster *et al.* 1985). In chickens, amantadine 0.01% supplied in drinking water produced concentrations in serum of 354 ng/ml, similar to levels observed in humans ingesting 200 mg/day by mouth (see Table 35.3). Amantadine was effective in preventing lethal infection in horses (Bryans *et al.* 1966) and turkeys (Lang *et al.* 1970) caused by influenza A equine and turkey viruses, respectively.

Although amantadine inhibited the following viruses *in vitro*, it was not effective in mice with infection due to influenza B, pseudorabies (Grunert *et al.* 1965) or Friend leukaemia virus (Mirand *et al.* 1965), in ferrets infected with rubella (Cusamano *et al.* 1965), in chickens with Rous sarcoma virus (Oker-Blom & Andersen 1967) or rhesus monkeys with experimental rubella infection (Stephenson *et al.* 1965).

The data indicate that human influenza A viruses are relatively more sensitive to rimantadine than to amantadine and much more susceptible than other viruses to these agents. In mice and ferrets, rimantadine is more effective than amantadine for prophylaxis and treatment. In chickens infected with avian influenza A/Chicken/Pennsylvania/1370/83 (H5N2) virus infection, the drugs were equiefficacious. The relative insusceptibility of noninfluenza A viruses to amantadine is paralleled by a lack of effectiveness of this agent *in vivo* in animals or chickens.

Mechanism of action

In the first report on the inhibitory effect of amantadine on influenza A virus replication in cell culture, 40 µg/ml amantadine completely prevented plaque formation when added prior to infection but only reduced plaque size when added up to 3 days after infection (Neumayer *et al.* 1965). Rimantadine shares the same mechanism of action (Bukrinskaya 1982).

At concentrations greater than $100\,\mu mol/l$ (> $15\,\mu g/ml$), amantadine retards the acid-pH triggered conformational change of cleaved haemagglutinin (HA) into a form that facilitates intracytoplasmic fusion of the viral and endosomal membranes. This non-specific effect is shared by other weak bases (Ohkuma & Poole 1978) and occurs at high amantadine and rimantadine concentrations that are not attained tolerably *in vivo*. It probably accounts for the inhibitory effect of amantadine and rimantadine against influenza B and C, and a variety of other enveloped RNA viruses such as paramyxoviruses, togaviruses and retroviruses (see above).

In contrast, low concentrations of amantadine and rimantadine (< $5\,\mu mol/l$ (< $0.75\,\mu g/ml$)) exert a strain-specific inhibitory effect on the replication of sensitive influenza A viruses. The primary determinant of drug susceptibility is the M_2 matrix protein although the HA also affects the sensitivity of some influenza A viruses.

M_2 protein, the product of a spliced transcript of genome segment 7 (Lamb *et al.* 1981), is a 97 amino acid integral membrane protein (Lamb *et al.* 1985). M_2 forms a homotetramer that is a minor component of influenza virions (23–60 copies per virion; Lamb *et al.* 1985) compared to HA and neuraminidase (NA) but is abundantly expressed (10^6–10^7 molecules) on the surface of virus-infected cells. On the plasma membrane of infected cells M_2 spans the membrane once and is orientated such that the 23 N-terminal residues are disposed extracellularly with a 54 residue C-terminal cytoplasmic domain. A hydrophobic 19 amino acid sequence which is highly conserved among all human, swine, equine and avian strains of influenza spans the plasma membrane.

M_2 serves as an acid pH-activated ion channel (Pinto *et al.* 1992) whose function is inhibited by both amantadine (Wang *et al.* 1993) and rimantadine (Chizhmakov *et al.* 1996). Although commonly assumed, there are no data to indicate that amantadine or rimantadine bind to the pore region of the M_2 ion channel itself. Rather, the drugs appear to act as allosteric blockers that bind to the M_2 protein and in doing so, cause conformational change in the pore-forming region that interferes with proton transfer through the ion channel across the membrane of the virus or endosome (Wang *et al.* 1993).

For all susceptible influenza virus strains, the block occurs at an early stage in replication, between the steps of virus penetration by viropexis (with a possible role for fusion) (Dourmashkin & Tyrrell 1974) and uncoating. It is hypothesized that amantadine and rimantadine inhibit acid activation of the M_2 ion channel that normally results in acidification of the interior of the virion with resultant dissociation of the M_1 matrix protein from the ribonucleoprotein complex (uncoating) so that transport of the ribonucleoprotein complex to the nucleus that is a requisite step for genomic transcription, translation and assembly, cannot occur. In addition to this effect that is observed with all amantadine- and rimantadine-sensitive influenza strains, a second, late, inhibitory effect is also observed on some avian influenza strains that have an HA that is cleaved intracellularly and have a high pH optimum of fusion. The drugs cause premature conformational change in the HA in the trans-Golgi complex during transport of HA to the cell surface. The drugs thereby impair expression of HA at the surface and interfere with virus release (Ruigrok *et al.* 1991).

Resistance

Resistance of influenza A viruses to amantadine and rimantadine *in vitro* was described in the initial reports of the antiviral effects of these drugs (Cochran *et al.* 1965; Tsunoda *et al.* 1965). Resistance could be obtained after as little as one passage in tissue culture (Cochran *et al.* 1965) but induction of a stable resistant phenotype required selection in the presence of a high concentration of drug (Ilyenko 1975). This was thought to reflect a growth advantage of the susceptible parent strain in the absence of compound. Drug-resistant strains were also readily obtained by passage in treated mice (Oxford *et al.* 1970), being observed after one passage in lung tissue from one of 12 treated mice and eight of 12 mice after three passages. The mean *in vitro* susceptibility increased from 0.3 to $3.4\,\mu g/ml$ and $25\,\mu g/ml$ after one and three passages, respectively. Although it was initially reported that amantadine-resistant virus selected by *in vitro* culture of influenza A virus in the presence of amantadine retained most of its sensitivity to rimantadine (Tsunoda *et al.* 1965), such viruses are now considered to be completely crossresistant (Belshe *et al.* 1989). In 1981, two strains of H_3N_2 virus that were relatively resistant to amantadine and rimantadine were identified among 21 isolates from the Berlin epidemic, demonstrating the circulation of resistant strains in nature for the first time (Heider *et al.* 1981).

RNA sequencing of many of these amantadine- and rimantadine-resistant strains has demonstrated that the genetic basis of resistance is a single nucleotide change in the M_2 protein, resulting in an amino acid substitution at position 26, 27, 30, 31 or 34 in the membrane-spanning region of M_2 (Hay *et al.* 1986). This knowledge of the genetic basis of drug resistance is compatible with the results of genetic reassortment studies in which transfer of RNA segment 7 coding for the M gene (M_1 and M_2 proteins) from resistant to sensitive strains during dual infections results in transfer of the drug-resistant phenotype (Appleyard 1977). However, other reassortment studies suggest that for some strains, the NA, nucleoprotein (NP) (Scholtissek & Faulkner 1979) and HA genes (Hay *et al.* 1985) also contribute to drug susceptibility or resistance.

The molecular basis of the change in susceptibility to amantadine and rimantadine caused by these mutations is not known. Structurally, introduction of a more polar or charged amino acid may alter the disposition of the M_2 protein in the membrane while other changes may affect M_2 protein–amantadine binding without affecting protein association. Functionally, cloned drug-resistant mutant M_2 expressed in *Xenopus laevis* oocytes produced ionic currents that were resistant to the drug (Pinto *et al.* 1992). It is postulated that this thereby obviates drug-induced interference with pH-activated intracellular steps in influenza virus replication.

Combination antiviral treatments

In vitro studies indicate that combinations of two inhibitors of influenza A virus produce consistently enhanced inhibitory therapeutic effects compared to each component used alone (Table 35.1). Limited studies of two drug combinations in mice with experimental influenza infection demonstrate similar therapeutic effects (Petrova *et al.* 1982; Zhirnov 1987). No studies have demonstrated antagonism. Whether combined medication can produce synergic prophylactic or therapeutic antiviral effects, reduced toxicity or delay emergence of resistant strains is not yet known but the potential for such benefits mandates further study.

Table 35.1 Anti-influenza virus activity of antiviral combinations *in vitro*.

Antiviral combination	Virus	Duration of culture (h)	Cell culture	References
Amantadine + Chick interferon	A/WSN/H1N1	24–72	Chick embryo	Lavrov *et al.* (1968)
Rimantadine + ribavirin	A/Fowl Plague	20	Chick embryo	Galegov *et al.* (1977)
Rimantadine + ribavirin	A/Texas/77/H3N2, A/USSR/77/H1N1	24	Madin–Darby canine kidney	Hayden *et al.* (1986)
Amantadine + ribavirin	A/Alaska/77/H3N2	28	Ferret tracheal ring	Burlington *et al.* (1983)
Rimantadine or ribavirin + rIFN-α2	A/Aichi/68/H3N2, A/England/80/H1N1	24–48	Primary Rhesus monkey kidney	Hayden *et al.* (1984)
Amantadine or rimantadine + ribavirin, interferon, zanamivir, or 2′-deoxy-2′-fluoroguanosine	A/Virginia/87/H1N1, A/Virginia/88/H3N2			Madren *et al.* (1995)

Clinical effectiveness

The clinical effectiveness of amantadine and rimantadine is limited to influenza A virus infection. Amantadine did not prevent illness due to induced parainfluenza type 1 infection in adult volunteers (Smith *et al.* 1967). Neither amantadine nor rimantadine prevented influenza B infection in adults (Taylor-Dickinson *et al.* 1967) or children (Clover *et al.* 1986). The use of these agents as adjuncts to vaccine for prophylaxis of influenza A virus infection and for treatment of established influenza A virus illness has been established in children and adults in a number of clinical settings, including the community, the home environment and institutions.

Prophylaxis

Amantadine and rimantadine have repeatedly been shown to be effective in preventing illness during experimental challenge with influenza A viruses in young healthy adults or natural infection with wild virus strains in the community in young healthy adults and children. An antiviral effect has been demonstrated by reduced recovery of virus. During natural influenza A infection, both amantadine (Reuman *et al.* 1989b) and rimantadine (Clover *et al.* 1991) have been demonstrated to reduce immunoglobulin A (IgA) secretory antibody response in nasal mucus but not the circulating HAI antibody response. Their effectiveness in protecting individuals who are at increased risk of premature death during influenza A epidemics has been limited to studies in elderly subjects.

The model of experimentally induced influenza A virus infection in healthy adult volunteers has been useful in demonstrating the relationship between amantadine dose, prophylactic efficacy and plasma concentrations (Aoki *et al.* 1985; Reuman *et al.* 1989a) and to test the utility of a loading dose to accelerate the development of protection. Dose–response studies suggest that the slope of the curve is relatively flat from 50 to 200 mg/day and that efficacy may decline, unexpectedly, at doses greater than 300 mg/day (Aoki *et al.* 1985). Steady-state trough plasma amantadine concentrations are (mean + SD) 77 + 52 – 110 +

39 ng/ml (50 mg/day), 184 $\pm$ 79 ng/ml (100 mg/day), and 302 $\pm$ 80 – 404 $\pm$ 209 ng/ml (200 mg/day). A loading dose of 300 mg amantadine for 1 (Stanley *et al.* 1965) or 2 days (Bloomfield *et al.* 1970) followed by 200 mg/day appeared to be no more protective than 200 mg/day (reviewed by Hoffman 1973). The inability to demonstrate the clinical utility of a pharmacokinetically correct loading dose may have been in part due to inconsistent amantadine absorption. In a crossover study of 200 mg amantadine followed by 100 mg twice daily versus 100 mg twice daily alone in nine healthy volunteers, plasma amantadine concentration at 12 h after the first dose was 339 $\pm$ 247 (mean $\pm$ SD) versus 147 $\pm$ 107 ng/ml (p = NS, Wilcoxon signed rank test; Aoki, F.Y. and Sitar, D.S. 1981). Five of nine and zero of nine in the two groups, respectively, had serum amantadine concentrations greater than or equal to 300 ng/ml at 12 h. Results of representative studies of the range of doses of amantadine and rimantadine tested for prevention of experimentally induced influenza illness are presented in Table 35.2a.

Prophylaxis of individuals in the community during influenza A outbreaks

Placebo-controlled trials have repeatedly demonstrated the protective efficacy of both amantadine and rimantadine against naturally occurring outbreaks of influenza A virus infection due to H1N1, H2N2 and H3N2 subtype viruses in young adults and children (Table 35.2b). Amantadine and rimantadine taken daily reduce influenza illness rates by 50–90% (Jackson *et al.* 1967; Maugh 1979; Oxford & Galbraith 1980; Bektimirov *et al.* 1985; Table 35.2b). Reasons for the almost two-fold variation in efficacy are not known. However, serum HAI antibody titres probably are a factor since protective efficacy has been demonstrated to be directly related to titre (Quilligan *et al.* 1966; Smorodintsev *et al.* 1970b). Conversely, chemoprophylactic efficacy may be less in seronegative populations during exposure to new pandemic or epidemic subtypes of virus (H3N2: Oker-Blom *et al.* 1970; H2N2: Wendel *et al.* 1966; H1N1: Monto *et al.* 1979). This may reflect a greater virulence of such

Table 35.2 (a–c) Representative controlled trials illustrating the relationship between amantadine and rimantadine daily dose and protective efficacy compared with placebo against induced or natural influenza A virus infection.

(a) Induced influenza A illness in healthy, young adults.

Drug and duration	Study population (*n*)	Daily dose (mg)	Percentage ill	Efficacy in preventing illness vs. placebo (%)*	Reference
Amantadine 8 days	20	50	20	66	Reuman *et al.* (1989a)
	20	100	15	74	
	19	200	11	82	
	19	Placebo	58		
Amantadine 8 days	22	100	9	78	Sears & Clements (1987)
	22	Placebo	41		
Amantadine 11 days	19	100	47	39	Smorodintsev *et al.* (1970b)
	19	200	53	39	
	31	Placebo	90	—	
Rimantadine 11 days	27	400	26	70	Dawkins *et al.* (1968)
	28	Placebo	86		
Rimantadine 7 days	10	50	10	89	Zlydnikov *et al.* (1971)
	20	Placebo	95		
Rimantadine 7 days	90	100	18	78	Zlydnikov & Romanov (1972)
	118	Placebo	81		
Rimantadine 1 dose	10	200	N/A	45	Zlydnikov *et al.* (1972)
	20	Placebo	N/A		

(b) Natural influenza A infection in healthy individuals in the community.

Drug and duration	Study population (*n*)	Daily dose (mg)	Percentage ill	Efficacy in preventing illness vs. placebo (%)*	Reference
Amantadine 30 days	3885	100	4	53	Smorodintsev *et al.* (1970a)
	2498	Placebo	8		
Amantadine 7 weeks	136	200	6	71	Monto *et al.* (1979)
	139	Placebo	20		
Amantadine 6 weeks	113	200	2	91	Dolin *et al.* (1982)
	132	Placebo	21		
Rimantadine 6 weeks	133	200	3	85	Dolin *et al.* (1982)
	132	Placebo	21		
Rimantadine 6 weeks	112	100	1	86	Brady *et al.* (1990)
	110	Placebo	6		
Rimantadine 30 days	659	50–100	N/A	82	Zlydnikov 1981
	391	Placebo	N/A		
Rimantadine 35–48 days	41 + 29	Children < 10 years 5 mg/kg/day max 150; children > 10 years 200	0	100	Clover *et al.* (1986) Crawford *et al.* (1988)
	35 + 27	Placebo	17 + 24		

Continued

Table 35.2 *Continued*

(c) Children in boarding schools or institutions; adults in hospitals and prisons.

Drug and duration	Study population (*n*)	Daily dose (mg)	Percentage ill	Efficacy in preventing illness vs. placebo (%)	Reference
Amantadine 16 weeks	Children 8–19 years				Finklea *et al.* (1967)
	139	1–2.5	0.6	92	
	154	Placebo	8		
Amantadine 9 days	Children 12–18 years				Rose (1983)
	126	100	17	70	
	382	Placebo	57		
Amantadine 14 days	Children 13–19 years				Payler & Purdham (1984)
	267	100	1	90	
	269	Placebo	11		
Amantadine 64 days	Children mean age 8.1 years				Quilligan *et al.* (1966)
	126	35–140	10	69	
	43	Placebo	30		
Amantadine 10–14 days	Adult prisoners				Wendel *et al.* (1966)
	439	200	1	74	
	355	Placebo	4		
Amantadine mean 14–16 days	Adult inpatients				O'Donoghue *et al.* (1973)
	50	200	0	80	
	61	Not treated	11		
Rimantadine 6–7 weeks	Elderly nursing home residents				Dolin *et al.* (1983)
	39	200	10	63	
	44	Placebo	27		

* Confirmed by virus isolation or serologically.

strains. Finally, pharmacokinetic factors also probably contribute as reflected in variation in plasma drug concentration at a given dose. At a dose of 200 mg/day, intra- and interindividual variation in steady-state trough plasma amantadine concentrations were 1.5-fold and 2.2-fold, respectively (Aoki, F.Y. & Sitar, D.S. 1979), similar to the two-fold interindividual variation in maximum plasma concentration of amantadine and rimantadine observed in six young adults (Hayden *et al.* 1985).

In two studies in households, rimantadine administered to only the children in a household was 100% effective in preventing confirmed influenza A illness compared to placebo (Clover *et al.* 1986; Crawford *et al.* 1988). Moreover, rimantadine prophylaxis of children reduced proved influenza A illness rates in the parents of the children 58% compared to placebo.

When compared directly, the 200 mg daily doses of amantadine and rimantadine currently recommended for young healthy adults in the USA were equally efficacious in preventing influenza-like illness in 65–78% of volunteers and laboratory-confirmed illness, in 85–91% (Dolin *et al.* 1982). In the former USSR, the optimal daily dose of rimantadine was considered to be 50 mg (Zlydnikov *et al.* 1981).

Prophylaxis of residents of institutions

Amantadine and rimantadine have been demonstrated to be efficacious in controlled trials in children and adults residing in closed populations including boarding schools, prisons, acute and chronic care hospitals (Table 35.2c). Several uncontrolled studies suggest that mass chemoprophylaxis of elderly residents of nursing homes with amantadine interrupts influenza A outbreaks (Leeming 1969; Arden *et al.* 1988; Staynor *et al.* 1994) or reduced mortality (Libow *et al.* 1996). Continuing disease in staff members not given chemoprophylaxis (Atkinson *et al.* 1986) underscores the need for inclusion of staff as well as residents in such programmes. Rimantadine ought to be as effective as amantadine and perhaps better tolerated than amantadine (see below), but no data have yet been published on its comparative effectiveness in interrupting influenza transmission in nursing home residents and staff.

Post-exposure prophylaxis in households

The concept of preventing spread of influenza A illness by postexposure prophylaxis of household contacts with amantadine and rimantadine has been demonstrated in controlled trials (Galbraith *et al.* 1969a; Bricaire *et al.* 1990). Chemoprophylaxis of contacts but not index cases for 10 days with amantadine or rimantadine reduced confirmed influenza A illness by 74 and 70%, respectively. Conversely, when the index case was treated simultaneously, both drugs were ineffective (Galbraith *et al.* 1969b; Hayden *et al.* 1989). Failure of prophylaxis in the latter study was confirmed to be due to emergence of drug-resistant virus in the treated index case and it was the likely explanation

for the failure in the 1969 study of Galbraith *et al.* as well. This strategy has potential utility in settings other than households and deserves wider use when vaccine is unavailable, intolerable or likely to be ineffective due to a poor antigenic match with an outbreak strain.

Treatment of acute influenza illness

Amantadine and rimantadine appear to be equally efficacious for the treatment of acute uncomplicated influenza illness due to a variety of subtypes in children, young adults and elderly individuals. Equivalence has, however, only been formally demonstrated in young adults (Van Voris *et al.* 1981). In one of the earliest therapy trials, amantadine initiated in the first 48 h of acute H3N2 influenza illness and continued for 7 days at a dose of 200 mg/day for adults and a dose adjusted for age in children, reduced the mean duration of fever from a total of 4.7 days in placebo recipients to 3.5 (children) to 4.0 days (adults) and reduced the maximum temperature observed (Kitamoto 1968). Subsequently, the therapeutic effects of amantadine and rimantadine have been evaluated in 15 and five other studies, respectively, in young adults (reviewed by Floor-Wieringa *et al.* 1967; Rabinovich *et al.* 1969; Wingfield *et al.* 1969; Hornick *et al.* 1970; Hoffman 1973; Galbraith 1975; Little *et al.* 1976, 1978; Van Voris *et al.* 1981; Younkin *et al.* 1983; Hayden & Monto 1986; Hayden *et al.* 1991), and two and four other studies, respectively, in children (Kitamoto 1968, 1971; Galbraith *et al.* 1971; Clover *et al.* 1986; Hayden 1986; Hall *et al.* 1987; Thompson *et al.* 1987) and one study each in elderly subjects (Betts *et al.* 1987). The therapeutic benefits have thereby been observed to extend to include accelerated amelioration of influenza-specific symptoms (Younkin *et al.* 1983) and signs (Togo *et al.* 1970), and more rapid overall functional improvement (Van Voris *et al.* 1981). In addition, the duration or titre of virus excreted in upper airway secretions declines more rapidly in amantadine- and rimantadine-treated adults (Knight *et al.* 1970; Van Voris *et al.* 1981). In children treated with rimantadine for 5 days (6.6 mg/day up to 150 mg/day for those less than 9 years of age and 200 mg/day for older children) virus titre was reduced but the duration of virus excretion in treated children was longer by a mean of 1 day than in placebo recipients (Hall *et al.* 1987). Finally, peripheral airways patency is restored more rapidly by amantadine than placebo treatment (Little *et al.* 1976). The therapeutic effect of amantadine (and likely, rimantadine) exceeds that of aspirin in adults (Younkin *et al.* 1983). Rimantadine was not more effective than acetaminophen in children (median 4–6 years, range 1–12) but mild illness and the young age of the subjects may have precluded a rigorous analysis of symptoms as a treatment parameter (Thompson *et al.* 1987). Overall, the data are consistent with a specific but limited treatment effect of amantadine and rimantadine in acute uncomplicated influenza in healthy individuals.

It is not certain that the therapeutic effects of amantadine and rimantadine will persist if more than 48 h elapse before initiation of therapy or be enhanced if a higher dose is used or a loading dose is initially administered, but limited data suggest that these strategies will not likely enhance the utility of amantadine and rimantadine for influenza therapy. Knight *et al.* (1970) reported that in subjects ill for more than 48 h before treatment, there was a more rapid decline in virus titre in throat secretions and that some respiratory symptoms and signs resolved more rapidly than in patients ill for less than 48 h, but this report requires confirmation. Rimantadine 300 mg/day for 10 days was no more effective than 200 mg/day amantadine (Wingfield *et al.* 1969; Van Voris *et al.* 1981 observed no difference between 200 mg/day amantadine compared to rimantadine). A modified rimantadine loading dose of 300 mg on day 1 followed by the recommended therapeutic dose of 200 mg/day (Hayden & Monto 1986) appeared to be no different to 200 mg/day in other studies.

Additional concerns about the therapeutic effect of amantadine and rimantadine include uncertainty about its utility in patients with serious or life-threatening influenza infection such as primary viral pneumonia, and the emergence of drug-resistant viruses during therapy. No controlled studies have been conducted to determine whether amantadine or rimantadine will be beneficial in treatment of complicated severe influenza A infection. However, in an uncontrolled study, amantadine 400–500 mg/day was associated with 55% survival of 11 patients with primary influenza pneumonia (Couch 1976). In case reports, combined use of amantadine plus aerosolized (Kirshon *et al.* 1988; Embrey & Geist 1995) or intravenous ribavirin (Hayden *et al.* 1996) was associated with a successful outcome in patients with acute influenza pneumonia.

Amantadine- and rimantadine-resistant (Hall *et al.* 1987; Hayden *et al.* 1989) viruses have been isolated from 10 to 27% of normal patients within 4–5 days of initiation of therapy (reviewed in Hayden & Hay 1992). In immunocompromised patients, influenza A virus can cause prolonged (17–58 days) illness (Safrin *et al.* 1990) with prolonged (9 weeks) virus excretion during rimantadine therapy (Evans & Kline 1995). During amantadine therapy in two recipients of allogeneic bone marrow transplants, each patient excreted two genotypically different amantadine-resistant strains of H3N2 influenza A virus (Klimov *et al.* 1995). In immunocompromised patients, amantadine and rimantadine resistance may be even more common than in normal hosts. Since resistant strains are stable genotypically, transmissible and cause treatment-resistant disease, their recognition has highlighted the need for more research as to their clinical importance and means for obviating their appearance and controlling the disease they cause. No consensus currently exists on how amantadine and rimantadine therapeutic use should be modified, if at all, to minimize this problem (Hayden & Couch 1993).

Clinical pharmacokinetics

Much is known about the clinical pharmacokinetics of amantadine and rimantadine (see Table 35.3) but our knowledge is incomplete (Aoki & Sitar 1988; Wills 1989; Wintermeyer & Nahata 1995). Elimination of both drugs from plasma is consistent with a first-order kinetic process. Amantadine and rimantadine tissue distribution data in animals (Bleidner *et al.* 1965; Uchiyama & Shibuya 1969;

Table 35.3 Clinical pharmacokinetic characteristics of amantadine and rimantadine in healthy adults.

Kinetic parameter*	Amantadine		Rimantadine	
	Young	Elderly	Young	Elderly
Relative oral bioavailability (%)	62–93[1]	53[2]–100[3]	75–93[4,5]	N/A†
T_{abs} (h)	0.6 ± 0.5[4]	1.3 ± 0.8[4]	0.6 ± 0.5[4]	1.2 ± 1.5[4]
T_{max} (h)	3.2 ± 2.0[1,4,6]	4.3 ± 2.5[3,4]	4.6 ± 2.1[4]	4.0 ± 2.4[4]
Vd_{ss} (l/kg) at 200 mg/day	6.1 ± 2.1[4,6]	3.6 ± 1.1[4]	18.4 ± 0.6[4,7,8]	11.5 ± 2.9[4]
Plasma protein binding (%)	67	N/A	40	N/A
Clearance (ml/min/kg)				
plasma or total	5.0 ± 2.1[4,6]	2.0 ± 0.9[3,4]	6.1 ± 1.9[4,7]	4.7 ± 2.0[4]
renal	6.4 ± 3.7[6]	2.0 ± 1.1[3]	1.2 ± 0.4[7]	N/A
non-renal	0[6]	0[3]	6.4 ± 1.4[7]	N/A
Urinary excretion of unchanged drug (%)	62–93[1]	53[2]–100[3]	22 ± 8[5]	N/A
Plasma $t_{1/2}$ (h)	14.8 ± 6.2[1,4,6]	26.1 ± 9.7[3,4]	29.1 ± 9.7[7,8,9,12,13,14]	36.5 ± 14.5[4]
Therapeutic range (ng/ml)				
$C_{max,ss}$				
200 mg/day	475 ± 110[6]	—	416 ± 108[9]	447 ± 108[10]
100 mg/day	—	362 ± 158[3]	—	—
$C_{trough,ss}$				
200 mg/day	302 ± 80[11]	—	300 ± 75[9]	310 ± 87[10]
100 mg/day	—	301 ± 75[3]	—	—

* T_{abs}, absorption half-life; T_{max}, time to peak plasma concentration; Vd_{ss}, apparent volume of distribution at steady state; $t_{1/2}$, elimination half-life; $C_{max,ss}$, maximum concentration in plasma at steady state; $C_{trough,ss}$, plasma concentration just prior to a dose at steady state (minimum concentration).
† N/A, not available.
[1] Bleidner *et al.* (1965); [2] Montanari *et al.* (1975); [3] Aoki & Sitar (1985); [4] Hayden *et al.* (1985); [5] Rubio *et al.* (1988); [6] Aoki (unpublished data 1979); [7] Capparelli *et al.* (1988); [8] Wills *et al.* (1987a); [9] Wills *et al.* (1987c); [10] Tominack *et al.* (1988); [11] Aoki *et al.* (1985); [12] Wills *et al.* (1987b); [13] Wills *et al.* (1987d); [14] Atmar *et al.* (1990).

Spector 1988) and limited data in humans (amantadine in brain and cerebrospinal fluid; Brenner *et al.* 1989; Kornhuber *et al.* 1995) suggest that these drugs distribute into multiple anatomical compartments. However, no data from studies of their concentrations in plasma over time following bolus intravenous injection have been available to permit characterization of the kinetic model, possibly multicompartmental, that best describes their behaviour in humans. Accordingly, formulae that make the most conservative assumptions (one-compartment open model, Aoki *et al.* 1979, or a non-compartmental model) have been used to calculate their kinetic characteristics. Predictions about rimantadine accumulation (Tominack *et al.* 1988) and amantadine loading doses (Aoki, F.Y. and Sitar, D.S., unpublished data, 1979) based on these calculations have been reasonably accurate.

The most noteworthy similarity in amantadine and rimantadine pharmacokinetics is the comparable maximum and minimum (trough) plasma concentration at steady-state associated with equiefficacious, currently recommended prophylactic doses.

The most noteworthy differences between amantadine and rimantadine concern their apparent volume of distribution at steady-state (Vd_{ss}), elimination half-life from plasma (see Table 35.3) and the mode of their clearance from plasma. Amantadine Vd_{ss} is weakly inversely related to dose (Aoki & Sitar 1988); the relationship between rimantadine Vd_{ss} and dose is not known. At the same dose, 200 mg/day, the mean Vd_{ss} of both drugs is 1.6–1.7-fold less in healthy elderly than in young adults while that of rimantadine is two- to three-fold greater than that of amantadine in the same age group. The physioanatomical basis of this difference is not known.

Amantadine mean plasma half-life is almost two-fold greater in healthy elderly subjects than in young adults, whereas that of rimantadine is not different between these two healthy age groups. Rimantadine mean plasma half-life in young healthy adults is two-fold greater than that of amantadine. The mean + SD plasma half-life of rimantadine in healthy children 5–8 years of age, 24.8 + 9.4 h, is similar to that of adults (Anderson *et al.* 1987).

Amantadine is eliminated from plasma wholly by renal tubular secretion and glomerular filtration (Aoki & Sitar 1988), whereas rimantadine is eliminated by hepatic metabolism (approximately 65%), renal metabolism (20%) and renal excretion of unchanged drug (15%) (Capparelli *et al.* 1988). Amantadine half-life and renal clearance are inversely related to creatinine clearance (Cl_{cr}) and urine pH (Geuens & Stevens 1967), respectively. For patients with Cl_{cr} 10–50 ml/min, amantadine half-life (h) = 99.7 – 1.53 × (Cl_{cr} ml/min) (from Horadam *et al.* 1981; Wu *et al.* 1982). Rimantadine half-life is not affected by mild to moderate renal dysfunction (Wills 1989). In patients with dialysis-dependent renal failure, amantadine and rimantadine half-life (mean ± SD) are 200 ± 36 h (Horadam *et al.* 1981) and 47.1 ± 13.4 h (Capparelli *et al.* 1988), respectively. Amantadine dose needs to be reduced proportionate to the degree of renal dysfunction when Cl_{cr} declines below 80 ml/min (Wu *et al.* 1982), whereas rimantadine dose needs to be reduced (by one-half) only in those with severe renal insufficiency (Capparelli *et al.* 1988).

Rimantadine undergoes extensive hydroxylation, conjugation and glucuronidation (Rubio *et al.* 1988) prior to renal excretion. The metabolites do not possess antiviral activity (Manchand *et al.* 1990). They accumulate in the presence of renal disease, apparently without clinical consequence (Wills 1989). Chronic stable liver disease did not alter rimantadine pharmacokinetics (Wills *et al.* 1987a). Dose reduction to 100 mg/day is recommended, however, for patients with severe hepatic disease. From 5 to 15% of amantadine undergoes metabolic transformation, mostly *N*-acetylation (Köppel & Tenczer 1985). No correlation was demonstrated between N-acetyltransferase-2 acetylator phenotype and amantadine acetylation (Hoff *et al.* 1991).

In nasal mucus of healthy subjects, rimantadine concentrations are on average 1.5 times greater than in plasma (Hayden *et al.* 1985; Tominack *et al.* 1988), whereas amantadine concentrations are only 0.5 times as great (Hayden *et al.* 1985). Since both drugs are equally effective at the same dose (Dolin *et al.* 1982), the relevance of these observations to antiviral effect is unclear. Amantadine concentration in cerebrospinal fluid is 52–96% of concurrent levels in serum (Fahn *et al.* 1971; Brenner *et al.* 1989; Kornhuber *et al.* 1995). In brain tissue of patients treated chronically with a median dose of 200 mg/day, amantadine was uniformly distributed throughout the brain at a mean concentration of 30 548 ng/ml (Kornhuber *et al.* 1995). Rimantadine is transported across the blood–brain barrier of rats at 10 times the rate of amantadine (Spector 1988) so that rimantadine concentrations in brain may be even greater than those of amantadine. This could account in part for the greater Vd_{ss} of rimantadine than amantadine (see Table 35.3). Nicotine and cotinine, its metabolite, increase rat renal tubular accumulation of amantadine, presumably by interfering with cationic tubular secretory transport (Wong *et al.* 1992) but no effect of chronic smoking on amantadine renal clearance was observed in volunteers (Wong *et al.* 1995).

Few clinically significant interactions have been demonstrated during concurrent administration of amantadine or rimantadine and other drugs. Amantadine administered with triamterene and hydrochlorothiazide caused central nervous system (CNS) toxicity and a 50% increase in plasma amantadine concentration in a child (Wilson & Rajput 1983). Trimethroprim-sulphamethoxazole given with amantadine caused toxic delirium attributed to inhibition of renal tubular amantadine secretion (Speeg *et al.* 1989). Quinine and quinidine reduced amantadine renal clearance 27–32% in male volunteers (Gaudry *et al.* 1993). No clinically important consequences arose from 11 to 18% changes in rimantadine clearance or plasma concentrations during concomitant administration of therapeutic doses of cimetidine (Holazo *et al.* 1989), aspirin or acetaminophen (Wills 1989).

Adverse effects

Preclinical toxicological testing indicates that amantadine is essentially free of pharmacodynamic effects at antiviral doses. It lacks anti-inflammatory, antipyretic and teratogenic properties (Vernier *et al.* 1969). At doses in excess of five times those producing antiviral effects in animals, CNS stimulatory effects and variable cardiovascular system (CVS) effects are observed which are dose-related and reversible. CNS effects are evidenced by tremors, myoclonic jerks and clonic convulsions. In mice, amantadine is 100 times less potent than D-amphetamine in stimulating spontaneous motor activity. The exact CNS locus and mechanism of these effects are not known. Non-competitive inhibition of excitatory N-methyl-D-aspartate receptors (Parsons *et al.* 1995) by amantadine and release of dopamine from central neurones, particularly residual, intact dopaminergic terminals in patients with Parkinson's disease (Lang 1984) may account for some of the toxic side-effects as well as its therapeutic effects in such patients. CVS effects of amantadine at high doses include ventricular extrasystoles with bigeminal pulse and reduced myocardial contractility, likely related to alterations in synthesis, release and uptake of norepinephrine (Von Voighander & Moore 1971). Preclinical toxicological characteristics of rimantadine have not been described, but a reference to the nine-fold greater acute oral LD_{50} of rimantadine (6400 mg versus 700 mg for amantadine) (Scott *et al.* 1978) is consistent with its better tolerance in humans. Adverse effects of amantadine and rimantadine in humans are consistent with expectations from these toxicology studies. Thus, the principal adverse reactions to amantadine involve the CNS and rimantadine appears better tolerated.

Placebo-controlled, double-blind trials in all age groups demonstrate that both amantadine and rimantadine cause dose-related adverse effects but are generally well tolerated. In case reports, additional uncommon adverse reactions have been described. Finally, observations of patients with iatrogenic or self-administered overdose complete the profile of amantadine and rimantadine side-effects. In controlled trials in healthy young adults, amantadine doses of less than 100 mg/day cause no more adverse effects than placebo. Amantadine 100 mg/day causes significantly more CNS side-effects than placebo: sleep deterioration or malaise (1.14% versus 0, respectively; Smorodintsev *et al.* 1970a). Amantadine 200 mg/day caused an excess of headache (8.7 versus 3.4%, respectively; Oker-Blom *et el.* 1970), nervousness (7.7 versus 2.1%, respectively) or mental depression (13.4 versus 6.4%, respectively; Monto *et al.* 1979), as well as the sleep difficulty or nervousness observed at 100 mg/day (30 versus 15%; Reuman *et al.* 1989a). In one study, amantadine caused more dyspepsia (3.3%) than placebo (1.6%) (Smorodintsev *et al.* 1970a).

Rimantadine tends to cause more gastrointestinal side-effects than placebo in comparative trials: abdominal pain (8 versus 2%, respectively; Hayden *et al.* 1989), and gastritis, nausea and vomiting, diarrhoea or abdominal pain (8.6 versus 4.0%; $0.10 < p < 0.20$, respectively; Bricaire *et al.* 1990).

Placebo-controlled, double-blind trials of amantadine and rimantadine prophylaxis in elderly healthy adults have demonstrated side-effects comparable in nature and incidence to those observed in young healthy adults (Petterson *et al.* 1980; Soo 1989; Monto *et al.* 1995).

In placebo-controlled trials comparing amantadine and rimantadine efficacy and tolerance concurrently, amantadine 200 mg/day caused more CNS side-effects than rimantadine 200 mg/day or placebo (13 versus 6% versus 4%, respectively; Dolin *et al.* 1982). In healthy working adults given amantadine or rimantadine at a dose of 300 mg/day or placebo, CNS side-effects were reported in 33, 9 and 9%, respectively, and sleep disturbance in 39, 13 and 7.5%, respectively (Hayden *et al.* 1981). The greater incidence of side-effects in amantadine recipients correlated with higher mean plasma concentrations at 4 h after the first dose. At similar plasma concentrations, no difference in side-effects between drugs was demonstrable (Hayden *et al.* 1983). Reports of inability to concentrate were supported by the observation of inferior performances in tasks requiring sustained attention by subjects given amantadine but not rimantadine or placebo (Hayden *et al.* 1983). At a dose of amantadine 400 mg/day, 25% (Tyrrell *et al.* 1965) to nearly

100% (Jackson *et al.* 1967) of subjects experienced 'malaise, tremors and insomnia' or 'toxic effects', respectively.

Amantadine and rimantadine side-effects usually appeared within 2–3 h of drug ingestion in the first 2–4 days of treatment and often became tolerable at lower doses even if the drug was continued or disappeared in less than 6 h if the drug at higher doses was discontinued (Jackson *et al.* 1967; Monto *et al.* 1979; Hayden *et al.* 1981; Bryson *et al.* 1982).

In subjects of all ages who were given rimantadine, the incidence of adverse effects was greater in treatment studies than in prophylaxis trials, likely because of concurrent symptoms of influenza (Soo 1989). Amantadine tolerance in treatment studies of brief duration (see above) may also have been adversely affected by concurrent acute influenza A illness (Galbraith 1975; Van Voris *et al.* 1981; Younkin *et al.* 1983).

In case reports, seizures have been reported at therapeutic doses in individuals with convulsive disorders administered amantadine (Atkinson *et al.* 1986) or rimantadine (Bentley *et al.* 1989). During amantadine administration worsening or relapse of pre-existing psychiatric disorders (Hausner 1980; Nestelbaum *et al.* 1986; Stewart 1987), evocation of mania (Rego & Giller 1989) or pathological jealousy (McNamara & Durso 1991) have been described. Amantadine treatment of Parkinson's disease was associated with livido reticularis in 10 of 18 and 36 of 40 patients (Shealy *et al.* 1970; Vollum *et al.* 1971) and heart failure has been attributed to amantadine cardiomyopathy (Parkes *et al.* 1977; Vale & Maclean 1977). Sudden but reversible vision loss occurred in a 67-year-old man during prolonged amantadine prophylaxis (Pearlman *et al.* 1977).

Iatrogenic or self-administered overdoses of amantadine cause CNS and cardiac irritability as predicted from preclinical toxicology studies (see above), as well as anticholinergic effects not predicted by studies in animals (Gerlak *et al.* 1970). Toxic manifestations such as psychosis (Fahn *et al.* 1971), hallucinations (Armbruster *et al.* 1974), depression and confusion (Ing *et al.* 1979), and disinhibition with aggressive behaviour (Rizzo *et al.*

1973) were associated with plasma amantadine concentrations from 680 to 4400 ng/ml (reviewed by Aoki & Sitar 1988), and, in iatrogenic cases, were attributable to administration of relatively high doses in patients with renal dysfunction. Malignant cardiac arrythmia (Sartori *et al.* 1984) or complex ventricular ectopic heart beats (Pimental & Hughes 1991) have been described in cases of amantadine overdose. Anticholinergic effects of amantadine overdose in man are reversed with physostigmine (Casey 1978).

References

Aldrich, P.E., Hermann, E.C., Meier, W.E. *et al.* (1971) Structure-activity relationships of compounds related to 1-adamantamine. *J Med Chem* **14**, 535–41.

Al-Nakib, W., Higgins, P.G., Willman, J. *et al.* (1986) Prevention and treatment of experimental influenza A virus infection in volunteers with a new antiviral 1C1 130 685. *J Antimicrobial Chemother* **18**, 119–29.

Anderson, E.L., Van Voris, L.P., Bartram, J., Hoffman, H.E. & Belshe, R.B. (1987) Pharmacokinetics of a single dose of rimantadine in young adults and children. *Antimicrobial Agents Chemother* **31**, 1140–2.

Aoki, F.Y. & Sitar, D.S. (1985) Amantadine kinetics in healthy elderly men: implications for influenza prevention. *Clin Pharmacol Ther* **37**, 137–44.

Aoki, F.Y. & Sitar, D.S. (1988) Clinical pharmacokinetics of amantadine hydrochloride. *Clin Pharmacokinet* **14**, 35–51.

Aoki, F.Y., Sitar, D.S. & Ogilvie, R.I. (1979) Amantadine kinetics in healthy young subjects after long-term dosing. *Clin Pharmacol Ther* **26**, 729–36.

Aoki, F.Y., Stiver, H.S., Sitar, D.S., Boudreault, A. & Ogilvie, R.I. (1985) Prophylactic amantadine dose and plasma concentration–effect relationships in healthy adults. *Clin Pharmacol Ther* **37**, 128–36.

Appleyard, G. (1977) Amantadine-resistance as a genetic marker for influenza viruses. *J Gen Virol* **36**, 249–55.

Arden, N.H., Patriarca, P.A., Fasano, M.B. *et al.* (1988) The roles of vaccination and amantadine prophylaxis in controlling an outbreak of influenza A (H3N2) in a nursing home. *Arch Int Med* **148**, 865–8.

Armbruster, K.F.W., Rahn, A.C., Ing, T.S., Halper, I.S. & Dyama, J.H. (1974) Amantadine toxicity in a patient with renal insufficiency. *Nephrology* **13**, 183–6.

Arroyo, M., Beare, A.S., Reed, S.E. & Craig, J.W. (1975) A therapeutic study of an adamantane spiro compound in experimental influenza A infection in man. *J Antimicrobial Chemother* **1** (suppl), 87–93.

Atkinson, W.L., Arden, N.H., Patriarca, P.A., Leslie, N., Kung-Jong, L. & Gohd, R. (1986) Amantadine prophylaxis during an institutional outbreak of type A (H1N1) influenza. *Arch Int Med* **146**, 1751–6.

Atmar, R.L., Greenberg, S.B., Quarles, J.M. *et al.* (1990) Safety and pharmacokinetics of rimantadine small-particle aerosol. *Antimicrobial Agents Chemother* **34**, 2228–33.

Beare, A.S., Hall, T.S. & Tyrrell, D.A.J. (1972) Protection of volunteers against challenge with A/Hong Kong/68 influenza virus by a new adamantane compound. *Lancet* **i**, 1039–40.

Bektimirov, T.A., Douglas, R.G. Jr, Dolin, R., Galasso, G.J., Krylov, V.F. & Oxford, J. (1985) Current status of amantadine and rimantadine as anti-influenza-A agents: memorandum from a WHO Meeting. *Bull WHO* **63**, 51–6.

Belshe, R.B., Burk, B., Newman, F., Cerrutti, R.L. & Sim, I.S. (1989) Resistance of influenza A virus to amantadine and rimantadine: results of one decade of surveillance. *J Infect Dis* **159**, 430–5.

Bentley, D.W., Karki, S.D. & Betts, R.F. (1989) Rimantadine and seizures (letter). *Ann Int Med* **110**, 323–4.

Betts, R.F., Treanor, J.J., Graman, P.S., Bentley, D.W. & Dolin, R. (1987) Antiviral agents to prevent or treat influenza in the elderly. *J Respir Dis* **8** (suppl), S56–9.

Bleidner, W.E., Harmon, J.B., Hewes, W.E., Lynes, T.E. & Hermann, E.C. (1965) Absorption, distribution and excretion of amantadine hydrochloride. *J Pharmacol Exp Ther* **150**, 484–90.

Bloomfield, S.S., Gaffney, T.E. & Schiff, G.E. (1970) A design for the evaluation of antiviral drugs in human influenza. *Am J Epidemiol* **91**, 568–74.

Brady, M.T., Sears, S.D., Pacini, D.L. *et al.* (1990) Safety and prophylactic efficacy of low-dose rimantadine in adults during an influenza A epidemic. *Antimicrobial Agents Chemother* **34**, 1633–6.

Brenner, M., Haass, A., Jacobi, P. & Schimrigk, K. (1989) Amantadine sulfate in treating Parkinson's disease: clinical effects, psychometric tests, and serum concentrations. *J Neurol* **236**, 153–6.

Bricaire, F.C., Hannoun, C. & Boissel, J.P. (1990) Prevention of influenza A: effectiveness and tolerance of rimantadine hydrochloride. *Presse Med* **19**, 69–72.

Brown, E.R. & Gordon, P. (1971) NPT-10381: suppression of mouse influenza mortality, morbidity and replication of virus antigen. *Federation Proceedings* **30**, p. 242 (abstract 279).

Bryans, J.T., Zent, W.W., Grunert, R.R. & Boughton, D.C. (1966) 1-adamantanamine hydrochloride prophylaxis for experimentally induced A/equine 2 influenza virus infection. *Nature* **212**, 1542–4.

Bryson, Y.J., Monaham, C., Pollack, M. & Shields, W.D. (1982) A prospective double-blind study of side-effects associated with the administration of amantadine for influenza A virus prophylaxis. *J Infect Dis* **141**, 543–7.

Bukrinskaya, A.G., Vorkunova, N.D., Kornilayeva, G.V., Narmanbetova, R.A. & Vorkunova, G.K. (1982) Influenza virus uncoating in infected cells and effect of rimantadine. *J Gen Virol* **60**, 49–59.

Burlington, D.B., Meikeljohn, G. & Mostow, S.R. (1983) Anti-influenza A activity of combinations of amantadine and ribavirin in ferret trachea ciliated epithelium. *J Antimicrobial Chemother* **11**, 7–14.

Capparelli, E.V., Stevens, R.C., Chow, M.S.S., Izard, M. & Wills, R.J. (1988) Rimantadine pharmacokinetics in healthy subjects and patients with end-stage renal failure. *Clin Pharmacol Ther* **43**, 536–41.

Casey, D.E. (1978) Amantadine intoxication reversed by physostigmine (letter). *N Engl J Med* **298**, 516.

Chizhmakov, I.V., Geraghty, F.M., Ogden, D.C., Hayhurst, A., Antonion, M. & Hay, A.J. (1996) Selective proton permeability and pH regulation of the influenza virus M2 channel expressed in mouse erythroleukemia cells. *J Physiol* **494**, 329–36.

Clover, R.D., Crawford, S.A., Abell, T.D., Ramsey, C.N. Jr, Glezen, W.P. & Couch, R.B. (1986) Effectiveness of rimantadine prophylaxis of children within families. *Am J Dis Child* **140**, 706–9.

Clover, R.D., Waner, J.L., Becker, L. & Davis, A. (1991) Effect of rimantadine on the immune response to influenza A infections. *J Med Virol* **34**, 68–73.

Cochran, K.W., Maassab, H.F., Tsunoda, A. & Berlin, B.S. (1965) Studies on the antiviral activity of amantadine hydrochloride. *Ann NY Acad Sci* **130**, 432–9.

Couch, R. (1976) National Institute of Allergy and Infectious Disease: antiviral agents in influenza — summary of influenza workship VIII. *J Infect Dis* **134**, 516–27.

Crawford, S.A., Clover, R.D., Abell, T.D., Ramsey, C.N. Jr, Glezen, W.P. & Couch, R.B. (1988) Rimantadine prophylaxis in children: a follow-up study. *Pediatr Infect Dis J* **7**, 379–83.

Cusumano, C.L., Sever, J.L., Schiff, G.M. & Heubner, R.J. (1965) Effect of amantadine HCl on rubella virus in tissue culture and in ferrets. *Clin Res* **13**, 41.

Davies, W.L., Grunert, R.R., Haff, R.F. *et al.* (1964) Antiviral activity of 1-adamantanamine (amantadine). *Science* **144**, 862–3.

Dawkins, A.T. Jr, Gallager, L.R., Togo, Y., Hornick, R.B. & Harris, B.A. (1968) Studies on induced influenza in man. II. Double-blind study designed to assess the prophylactic efficacy of an analogue of amantadine hydrochloride. *J Am Med Assoc* **203**, 93–7.

Dolin, R., Betts, R.F., Treanor, J.J. *et al.* (1983) Rimantadine prophylaxis of influenza in the elderly. In: *Program and Abstracts of the 23rd Interscience Conference on Antimicrobial Agents and Chemotherapy, Washington DC, American Society of Microbiology*, p. 210, abstract 691.

Dolin, R., Reichman, R.C., Madore, H.P., Maynard, R., Linton, P.N. & Webber-Jones, J. (1982) A controlled trial of amantadine and rimantadine in the prophylaxis of influenza A infection. *N Engl J Med* **307**, 580–4.

Dourmashkin, R. & Tyrrell, D.A.J. (1974) Electron microscopic observations on the entry of influenza virus into susceptible cells. *J Gen Virol* **24**, 129–41.

Embrey, R.P. & Geist, L.J. (1995) Influenza A pneumonitis following treatment of acute cardiac allograft rejection with murine monoclonal anti-CD3 antibody (OKT3). *Chest* **108**, 1456–9.

Evans, K.D. & Kline, M.W. (1995) Prolonged influenza A infection responsive to rimantadine therapy in a human immunodeficiency virus-infected child. *Pediatr Infect Dis J* **14**, 332–4.

Fahn, S., Craddock, G. & Kumin, G. (1971) Acute toxic psychosis from suicidal over-dosage of amantadine. *Arch Neurol* **25**, 45–8.

Finklea, J.F., Hennessy, A.V. & Davenport, F.M. (1967) A field trial of amantadine prophylaxis in naturally occurring acute respiratory illness. *Am J Epidemiol* **85**, 403–12.

Floor-Wieringa, A.Geuens, H. & Van Strik, R. (1967) Prophylactic and therapeutic clinical trials with 1-adamantane amine hydrochloride during influenza A2 epidemics. *Proc 5th Int Cong Chemother, Vienna* **4**, 333–46.

Galbraith, A.W. (1975) Therapeutic trials of amantadine (Symmetrel) in general practice. *J Antimicrobial Chemother* **1**, 81–8.

Galbraith, A.W., Oxford, J.S., Schild, G.C., Potter, C.W. & Watson, G.I. (1971) Therapeutic effect of 1-adamantanamine hydrochloride in naturally occurring influenza A2/Hong Kong infection. *Lancet* **ii**, 113–15.

Galbraith, A.W., Oxford, J.S., Schild, G.C. & Watson, G.I. (1969a) Protective effect of 1-adamantanamine hydrochloride on influenza A2 infections in the family environment. *Lancet* **ii**, 1026–8.

Galbraith, A.W., Oxford, J.S., Schild, G.C. & Watson, G.I. (1969b) Study of 1-adamantanamine hydrochloride used prophylactically during the Hong Kong influenza epidemic in the family environment. *Bull WHO* **41**, 677–82.

Galegov, G.A., Pushkarskaya, N.L., Obrosova-Serova, N.P. & Zholanov, V.M. (1977) Combined action of ribavirin and rimantadine in experimental myxovirus infection. *Experientia* **33**, 905–6.

Gaudry, S.E., Sitar, D.S., Smyth, D.D., McKenzie, J.K. & Aoki, F.Y. (1993) Gender and age as factors in the inhibition of renal clearance of amantadine by quinine and quinidine. *Clin Pharmacol Ther* **54**, 23–7.

Gerlak, R.P., Clark, R., Stump, J.M. & Vernier, V.G. (1970) Amantadine-dopamine interaction. *Science* **169**, 203–4.

Geuens, H.F. & Stephens, R.L. (1967) Influence of the pH of the urine on the rate of excretion of 1-adamantanamine. *5th International Congress of Chemotherapy. Vienna, June 26 – July 1, 1967*, pp. 703–13. Verlag der Wiener Medizinischen Akademie, Vienna.

Grunert, R.R., McGahen, J.W. & Davies, W.L. (1965) The *in vivo* antiviral activity of 1-adamantanamine (Amantadine) 1. Prophylactic and therapeutic activity against influenza viruses. *Virology* **26**, 262–9.

Hall, C.B., Dolin, R., Gala, C.L. *et al.* (1987) Children with influenza A infection: Treatment with rimantadine. *Pediatrics* **80**, 275–82.

Hausner, R.S. (1980) Amantadine-associated recurrence of psychosis. *Am J Psychiatr* **137**, 240–2.

Hay, A.J., Wolstenholme, A.J., Skehel, J.J. & Smith, M.H. (1985) The molecular basis of the specific anti-influenza action of amantadine. *EMBO J* **4**, 3021–4.

Hay, A.J., Zambon, M.C., Wolstenholme, A.J., Skehel, J.J. & Smith, M.H. (1986) Molecular basis of resistance of influenza A viruses to amantadine. *J Antimicrobial Chemother* **18** (suppl B), 19–29.

Hayden, F.G. (1986) Combinations of antiviral agents for treatment of influenza virus infections. *J Antimicrobial Chemother* **18** (suppl B), 77–83.

Hayden, F.G. & Anderson, B.A. (1981) Influenza A strain differences in antiviral effects of rimantadine and ribavirin combinations. *Clin Res* **29**, 868A.

Hayden, F.G., Belshe, R.B., Clover, R.D., Hay, A.J., Oakes, M.G. & Soo, W. (1989) Emergence and apparent transmission of rimantadine-resistant influenza A virus in families. *N Engl J Med* **321**, 1696–702.

Hayden, F.G., Cote, K.M. & Douglas, R.G. Jr (1980a) Plaque inhibition assay for drug susceptibility testing of influenza viruses. *Antimicrobial Agents Chemother* **17**, 865–70.

Hayden, F.G. & Couch, R. (1993) Clinical and epidemiological importance of influenza A viruses resistant to amantadine and rimantadine. In: Hannoun, H.C. (ed.) *Options for the Control of Influenza*, pp. 333–41. Elsevier Science, Amsterdam.

Hayden, F.G., Douglas, R.G. Jr & Simons, R. (1980b) Enhancement of activity against influenza viruses by combinations of antiviral agents. *Antimicrobial Agents Chemother* **18**, 536–41.

Hayden, F.G., Gwaltney, J.M. Jr, Van De Castle, R.L., Adams, K.F. & Giordani, B. (1981) Comparative toxicity of amantadine hydrochloride and rimantadine hydrochloride in healthy adults. *Antimicrobial Agents Chemother* **19**, 226–33.

Hayden, F.G. & Hay, A.J. (1992) Emergence and transmission of influenza A viruses resistant to amantadine and rimantadine. *Curr Topics Microbiol Immunol* **176**, 119–30.

Hayden, F.G., Hoffman, H.E. & Spyker, D.A. (1983) Differences in side-effects of amantadine hydrochloride and rimantadine hydrochloride relate to differences in pharmacokinetics. *Antimicrobial Agents Chemother* **23**, 458–64.

Hayden, F.G., Minocha, A., Spyker, D.A. & Hoffman, H. (1985) Comparative single-dose pharmacokinetics of amantadine hydrochloride and rimantadine hydrochloride in young and elderly adults. *Antimicrobial Agents Chemother* **28**, 216–21.

Hayden, F.G. & Monto, A.S. (1986) Oral rimantadine hydrochloride therapy of influenza A virus H3N2 subtype infection in adults. *Antimicrobial Agents Chemother* **29**, 339–41.

Hayden, F.G., Sable, C.A., Connor, J.D. & Lane, J. (1996) Intravenous ribavirin by constant infusion for serious influenza and parainfluenza virus infection. *Antiviral Ther* **1**, 51–6.

Hayden, F.G., Schlepushkin, A.N. & Pushkarskaya, N.L. (1984) Combined interferon-α 2, rimantadine hydrochloride, and ribavirin inhibition of influenza virus replication *in vitro*. *Antimicrobial Agents Chemother* **25**, 395–400.

Hayden, F.G., Sperber, S.J., Belshe, R.B., Clover, R.D., Hay, A.J. & Pyke, S. (1991) Recovery of drug-resistant influenza A virus during therapeutic use of rimantadine. *Antimicrobial Agents Chemother* **35**, 1741–7.

Heider, H., Adamczyk, B., Presber, H.W., Schroeder, C., Feldblum, R. & Indulen, M.K. (1981) Occurrence of amantadine- and rimantadine-resistant influenza A virus strains during the 1980 epidemic. *Acta Virol* **25**, 395–400.

Hoff, H.R., Sitar, D.S. & Aoki, F.Y. (1991) Acetylator phenotype does not predict acetylation of amantadine in man. *Manitoba Med* **61**, 164–8.

Hoffman, C.E. (1973) Amantadine HCl and related compounds. In: Carter, W.A. (ed.) *Selective Inhibitors of Viral Functions*, pp. 199–211, CRC Press, Cleveland, Ohio.

Holazo, A.A., Choma, N., Brown, S.Y., Lee, L.F. & Wills, R.J. (1989) Effect of cimetidine on the disposition of rimantadine in healthy subjects. *Antimicrobial Agents Chemother* **33**, 820–3.

Horadam, V.W., Sharp, J.G., Smilack, J.D. *et al.* (1981) Pharmacokinetics of amantadine hydrochloride in subjects with normal and impaired renal function. *Ann Int Med* **94**, 454–8.

Hornick, R.B., Togo, Y., Mahler, S. & Iezzoni, D. (1970) Evaluation of amantadine hydrochloride in the treatment of A2 influenzal disease. *Ann NY Acad Sci* **173**, 10–19.

Ilyenko, V.I. (1975) The study of formation of amantadine- and rimantadine-resistant variants of influenza. *Voprosy Virusol* **2**, 199–202.

Ing, T.S., Daugirdas, J.T., Soung, L.S., Klawans, H.L. & Mahurker, S.D. (1979) Toxic effects of amantadine in patients with renal failure. *Canad Med Assoc J* **120**, 695–8.

Jackson, G.G., Stanley, E.D. & Muldoon, R.L. (1967) Chemoprophylaxis of viral respiratory diseases. *First International Conference on vaccines against viral and rickettsial diseases in man*. Pan American World Health Organization Scientific Publication **217**, 595–603.

Kato, N. & Eggers, H.J. (1969) Inhibition of uncoating of fowl plaque virus by 1-adamantanamine hydrochloride. *Virology* **37**, 632–41.

Kaye, H.S. & Robinson, R.Q. (1967) Inhibition *in vitro* and *in vivo* of equine influenza virus by amantadine hydrochloride (Symmetrel). *Bacteriol Proc* **162**.

Kirshon, B., Faro, S., Zurawin, R.K., Samo, T.C. & Carpenter, R.J. (1988) Favorable outcome after treatment with amantadine and ribavirin in a pregnancy complicated by influenza pneumonia. *J Reprod Med* **33**, 399–401.

Kitamoto, O. (1968) Therapeutic effectiveness of amantadine hydrochloride in influenza A2. Double blind studies. *Jap J Tubercul* **15**, 17–26.

Kitamoto, O. (1971) Therapeutic effectiveness of amantadine hydrochloride in naturally occurring Hong Kong influenza—double-blind studies. *Jap J Tubercul Chest Dis* **17**, 1–8.

Klimov, A., Rocha, E., Hayden, F.G., Shult, P.A., Roumillat, L.F. & Cox, N.J. (1995) Prolonged shedding of amantadine-resistant influenza A viruses by immunodeficient patients: detection by polymerase chain reaction-restriction analysis. *J Infect Dis* **172**, 1352–5.

Knight, V., Fedson, D., Baldini, J., Douglas, R.G. & Couch, R.B. (1970) Amantadine therapy of epidemic influenza A2 (Hong Kong). *Infect Immun* **1**, 200–4.

Köppel, C. & Tenczer, J. (1985) A revision of the metabolic disposition of amantadine. *Biomed Mass Spectrom* **12**, 499–501.

Kornhuber, J., Quack, G., Dansz, W. *et al.* (1995) Therapeutic brain concentrations of the NMDA receptor antagonist amantadine. *Neuropharmacology* **34**, 713–21.

Lamb, R.A., Lai, C.-J. & Choppin, P.W. (1981) Sequences of mRNA's derived from genome RNA segment 7 of influenza virus: colinear and interrupted mRNA's code for overlapping proteins. *Proc Natl Acad Sci USA* **78**, 4170–4.

Lamb, R.A., Zebedee, S.L. & Richardson, C.D. (1985) Influenza virus M2 protein is an integral membrane protein expressed on the infected cell-surface. *Cell* **40**, 627–33.

Lang, A.E. (1984) Treatment of Parkinson's disease with agents other than levodopa and dopamine agonists: controversies and new approaches. *Canad J Neurol Sci* **11**, 210–20.

Lang, G., Narayan, O. & Rouse, B.T. (1970) Prevention of malignant avian influenza by 1-adamantanamine hydrochloride. *Archiv Gesamte Virusfors* **32**, 171–84.

Lavrov, S.V., Eremkina, E.I., Orlova, T.G., Galegov, G.A., Soloviev, V.D. & Zhdanov, V.M. (1968) Combined inhibition of influenza virus reproduction in cell culture using interferon and amantadine. *Nature* **217**, 856–7.

Leeming, J.T. (1969) Amantadine hydrocholoride and the elderly (letter). *Br Med J* **1**, 313–14.

Libow, L.S., Neufeld, R.R., Olson, E., Breuer, B. & Starer, P. (1996) Sequential outbreak of influenza A and B in a nursing home: Efficacy of vaccine and amantadine. *J Am Geriatr Soc* **44**, 1153–7.

Little, J.W., Hall, W.J., Douglas, R.G. Jr, Hyde, R.W. & Speers, D.M. (1976) Amantadine effect on peripheral airways abnormalities in influenza. *Ann Int Med* **85**, 177–82.

Little, J.W., Hall, W.J., Douglas, R.G. Jr, Mudholkar, G.S., Speers, D.M. & Patel, K. (1978) Airway hyperreactivity and peripheral airway dysfunction in influenza A infection. *Am Rev Respir Dis* **118**, 295–303.

Lundahl, K., Schut, J., Schlatmann, J.L.M.A., Paerels, G.B. & Peters, A. (1972) Synthesis and antiviral activities of adamantane spiro compounds. 1. Adamantane and analogous spiro-3'-pyrrolidines. *J Med Chem* **15**, 129–32.

McNamara, P. & Durso, R. (1991) Reversible pathologic jealousy (Othello syndrome) associated with amantadine. *J Geriatr Psychiatr Neurol* **4**, 157–9.

Madren, L.K., Shipman, C. Jr & Hayden, F.G. (1995) *In vitro* inhibitory effects of combinations of anti-influenza agents. *Antiviral Chem Chemother* **6**, 109–13.

Manchand, P.S., Cerrutti, R.L., Martin, J.A. *et al.* (1990) Synthesis and antiviral activity of metabolites of rimantadine. *J Med Chem* **33**, 1992–5.

Maugh, III T.H. (1979) Panel urges wide use of antiviral drug. *Science* **206**, 1058–60.

Mirand, E.A.Back, A. & Grace, J.T. Jr (1965) Studies of 1-adamantananine against Friend virus disease in mice. *Exp Med Surg* **23**, 239–42.

Montanari, C., Ferrari, P. & Bavazzano, A. (1975) Urinary excretion of amantadine by the elderly. *Eur J Clin Pharmacol* **8**, 349–51.

Monto, A.S., Gunn, R.A., Bandyk, M.G. & King, C.L. (1979) Prevention of Russian influenza by amantadine. *J Am Med Assoc* **241**, 1003–7.

Monto, A.S., Ohmit, S.E., Hornbuckle, K. & Pearce, C.L. (1995) Safety and efficacy of long-term use of rimantadine for prophylaxis of Type A influenza in nursing homes. *Antimicrobial Agents Chemother* **29**, 2224–8.

Neumayer, E.M., Haff, R.F. & Hoffman, C.E. (1965) Antiviral activity of amantadine hydrochloride in tissue culture and *in vivo*. *Proc Soc Exp Med Biol* **119**, 393–6.

Nestelbaum, Z., Siris, S.G., Rifkin, A. *et al.* (1986) Exacerbation of schizophrenia associated with amantadine. *Am J Psychiatr* **143**, 1170–1.

O'Donaghue, J.M., Ray, C.G., Terry, D.W. Jr & Beaty, H.N. (1973) Prevention of nosocomial influenza infection with amantadine. *Am J Epidemiol* **97**, 276–85.

Ohkhuma, S. & Poole, B. (1978) Fluorescence probe measurement of the intralysomal pH in living cells and the pertubation of pH by various agents. *Proc Natl Acad Sci USA* **75**, 3327–31.

Oker-Blom, N. & Andersen, L. (1967) Inhibition of Rous sarcoma virus and chicken leucosis virus by 1-adamantanamine hydrochloride. *Acta Pathol Microbiol Scand* **187** (suppl), 79–80.

Oker-Blom, N., Hovi, T., Leinikki, P., Palosuo, T., Petterson, R. & Suni, J. (1970) Protection of man from natural infection with influenza A2 Hong Kong virus by amantadine: a controlled field trial. *Br Med J* **iii**, 676–8.

Oxford, J.S. (ed.) (1977) Animal models of influenza virus infection as applied to the investigation of antiviral compounds. In: *Chemoprophylaxis and Virus Infections of the Respiratory Tract*, pp. 1–26. CRC Press, Cleveland, Ohio.

Oxford, J.S. & Galbraith, A. (1980) Antiviral activity of amantadine: a review of clinical and laboratory data. *Pharmacol Ther* **11**, 181–262.

Oxford, J.S., Logan, L.S. & Potter, C.W. (1970) *In vivo* selection of an influenza A2 strain resistant to amantadine. *Nature, London* **226**, 82–3.

Parkes, J.D., Marsden, C.D. & Price, P. (1977) Amantadine-induced heart failure (letter). *Lancet* **i**, 904–5.

Parsons, C.G., Quack, G., Bresink, I. *et al.* (1995) Comparison of the potency, kinetics and voltage-dependency of a series of uncompetitive NMDA receptor antagonists *in vitro* with anticonvulsive and motor impairment activity *in vivo*. *Neuropharmacology* **34**, 1239–58.

Payler, D.K. & Purdham, P.A. (1984) Influenza prophylaxis with amantadine in a boarding school. *Lancet* **i**, 502–4.

Pearlman, J.T., Kadish, A.H. & Ramseyer, J.C. (1977) Vision loss associated with amantadine hydrocholoride (letter). *Arch Neurol* **34**, 199–200.

Perrin, D.D. & Hawkins, I. (1972) The dissociation constant of 1-aminoadamantane cation. *Experientia* **28**, 880.

Petrova, I.G., Balashov, V.I., Pushkarskaya, N.L., Terskikh, I.I., Lidek, M.Y. & Gdegov, G.A. (1982) Investigation on the effectiveness of rimantadine and ribamide combination administered in aerosol on experimental influenza infection in white mice. *Voprosy Virusol* **27**, 440–3.

Petterson, R.F., Hellstrom, P.-E., Penttinen, K.R. *et al.* (1980) Evaluation of amantadine in the prophylaxis of influenza A (H1N1) virus infection in a controlled field trial among young adults and high-risk patients. *J Infect Dis* **142**, 377–83.

Pimental, L. & Hughes, B. (1991) Amantadine toxicity presenting with complex ventricular ectopy and hallucinations. *Pediatr Emerg Care* **7**, 89–92.

Pinto, L.H., Hodsinger, L.J. & Lamb, R.A. (1992) Influenza virus M2 protein has ion channel activity. *Cell* **69**, 517–28.

Quilligan, J.J. Jr, Hirayama, M. & Baernstein, H.D. Jr (1966) The suppression of A2 influenza in children by the chemoprophylactic use of amantadine. *J Pediatr* **69**, 572–5.

Rabinovich, S., Baldini, J.T. & Bannister, R. (1969) Treatment of influenza. The therapeutic efficacy of rimantadine HCl in a naturally occurring influenza A outbreak. *Am J Med Sci* **257**, 328–35.

Rego, M.D. & Giller, E.L. Jr (1989) Mania secondary to amantadine treatment of neuroleptic-induced hyperprolactinemia. *J Clin Psychiatr* **50**, 143–4.

Reuman, P.D., Bernstein, D.I., Keefer, M.C., Young, E.C., Sherwood, J.R. & Schiff, G.M. (1989a) Efficacy and safety of low dosage amantadine hydrochloride as prophylaxis for influenza A. *Antiviral Res* **11**, 27–40.

Reuman, P.D., Bernstein, D.J., Keeley, S.P., Young, E.C., Sherwood, J.R. & Schiff, G.M. (1989b) Differential effect of amantadine hydrochloride on the systemic and local immune response to influenza A. *J Med Virol* **27**, 137–41.

Rizzo, M., Biandrate, P., Tognoni, G. & Morselli, P.A. (1973) Amantadine in depression: relationship between behavioural effects and plasma levels. *Eur J Clin Pharmacol* **5**, 226–8.

Rose, H.J. (1983) Use of amantadine in influenza: a second report. *J Roy Coll Gen Pract* **33**, 651–3.

Rubio, F.R., Fukuda, E.K. & Garland, W.A. (1988) Urinary metabolites of rimantadine in humans *Drug Metab Disp Biol Fate Chem* **16**, 773–7.

Ruigrok, R.W.H., Hirst, E.M.A. & Hay, A.J. (1991) The specific inhibition of influenza A virus maturation by amantadine: an electron microscopic examination. *J Gen Virol* **72**, 191–4.

Runti, C. & Sciortino, T. (1968) Potenziali antivirali: I acilderivati superiori di basi tiopuriniche e dell'amantidina: adamantanoilderivati. *Farm Ed Sci* **23**, 106–13.

Safrin, S., Rush, J.D. & Mills, J. (1990) Influenza in patients with human immunodeficiency virus infection. *Chest* **98**, 33–7.

Sartori, M., Pratt, C.M. & Young, J.B. (1984) Torsade de pointe. Malignant cardiac arryhmia induced by amantadine poisoning. *Am J Med* **77**, 388–91.

Scholtissek, C. & Faulkner, G.P. (1979) Amantadine-resistant and -sensitive influenza A strains and recombinants. *J Gen Virol* **44**, 807–15.

Schulman, J.L. (1968) Effect of 1-amantanamine hydrochloride (amantadine HCl) and methyl-1-adamatanethylamine hydrochloride (rimantadine HCl) on transmission of influenza virus infection in mice. *Proc Soc Exp Biol Med* **128**, 1173–8.

Scott, G.H., Stephen, E.L. & Berendt, R.F. (1978) Activity of amantadine, rimantadine, and ribavirin against swine influenza in mice and squirrel monkeys. *Antimicrobial Agents Chemother* **13**, 284–8.

Sears, S.D. & Clements, M. (1987) Protective efficacy of low-dose amantadine in adults challenged with wild-type influenza A virus. *Antimicrobial Agents Chemother* **31**, 1470–3.

Shealy, C.N., Weeth, J.P. & Mercier, D. (1970) Livedo reticularis in patients with Parkinsonism receiving amantadine. *J Am M Assoc* **212**, 1522–3.

Smith, C.B., Purcell, R.H. & Chanock, R.M. (1967) Effect of amantadine hydrochloride on parainfluenza type 1 virus infections in adult volunteers. *Am Rev Respir Dis* **95**, 689–92.

Smorodintsev, A.A., Karpuchin, G.I., Zlydnikov, D.M. *et al.* (1970a) The prospect of amantadine for prevention of influenza A in humans (effectiveness of amantadine during influenza A2/Hong Kong epidemics in January-February 1969 in Leningrad). *Ann NY Acad Sci* **173**, 44–73.

Smorodintsev, A.A., Zlydnikov, D.M., Kiseleva, A.M., Romanov, J.A., Kazantsev, A.P. & Rumovsky, V.I. (1970b) Evaluation of amantadine in artificially induced A2 and B influenza. *J Am Med Assoc* **213**, 1448–54.

Soo, W. (1989) Adverse effects of rimantadine: summary from clinical trials. *J Respir Dis* **10** (suppl), 26–31.

Spector, R. (1988) Transport of amantadine and rimantadine through the blood–brain barrier. *J Pharmacol Exp Ther* **244**, 516–19.

Speeg, K.V., Leighton, J.A. & Maldonado, A.L. (1989) Case report: toxic delirium in a patient taking amantadine and trimethoprim-sulfamethoxazole. *Am J Med Sci* **298**, 410–12.

Stanley, E.D., Muldoon, R.E., Akers, L.W. & Jackson, G.G. (1965) Evaluation of antiviral drugs: the effect of amantadine on influenza in volunteers. *Ann NY Acad Sci* **130**, 44–51.

Staynor, K., Foster, G., McArthur, M., McGeer, A., Petric, M. & Simor, A.E. (1994) Influenza A outbreak in a nursing home: the value of early diagnosis and the use of amantadine hydrochloride. *Canad J Infect Control* **9**, 109–11.

Stephenson, J.A., Artenstein, M.S., Parkman, P.D., Beuscher, E.L. & Druzd, A.D. (1965) Effect of amantadine hydrochloride on rubella virus infection in the rhesus monkey. *Antimicrobial Agents Chemother* **5**, 548–52.

Stewart, J.T. (1987) Adverse behavioral effects of amantadine therapy in Huntington's disease. *South Med J* **80**, 1324–5.

Swallow, D.L. (1984) Antiviral agents 1978–83. In: Jucker, E. (ed.) *Progress in Drug Research*, pp. 127–95. Birkhauser Verlag, Berlin.

Taylor-Dickinson, P.C., Chang, T.-W. & Weinstein, L. (1967) Effects of amantadine on influenza B and measles virus infection in children. *Antimicrobial Agents Chemother*, 521-6.

Thompson, J., Fleet, W., Lawrence, E., Pierce, E., Morris, L. & Wright, P. (1987) A comparison of acetaminophen and rimantadine in the treatment of influenza A infection in children. *J Med Virol* **21**, 249–55.

Tisdale, M. & Bauer, D.J. (1977) The relative potencies of anti-influenza compounds. *Ann NY Acad Sci* **284**, 254–63.

Togo, Y., Hornick, R.B., Felitti, V.J. *et al.* (1970) Evaluation of therapeutic efficacy of amantadine in patients with naturally occurring A2 influenza. *J Am Med Assoc* **211**, 1149–56.

Togo, Y., Schwartz, A.R., Tominaga, S. & Hornick, R.B. (1972) Cyclo-octylamine in the prevention of experimental human influenza. *J Am Med Assoc* **220**, 837–41.

Tominack, R.L., Wills, R.J., Gustavson, L.E. & Hayden, F.G. (1988) Multiple-dose pharmacokinetics of rimantadine in elderly adults. *Antimicrobial Agents Chemother* **32**, 1813–19.

Tsunoda, A.Maasab, H.F., Cochran, K.W. & Eveland, W.C. (1965) Antiviral activity of α-methyl-1-adamantane-methylamine hydrochloride. *Antimicrobial Agents Chemother*, **5**, 553–60.

Tyrrell, D.A.J., Bynoe, M.L. & Hoorn, B. (1965) Studies of the antiviral activity of 1-adamantanamine. *Br J Exp Pathol* **46**, 370–5.

Uchiyama, M. & Shibuya, M. (1969) Distribution and excretion of ^{3}H-amantadine HCl. *Chem Pharmacol Bull* **17**, 841–3.

Vaczi, L., Hankovszky, O.H., Hideg, K. & Hadhazy, G. (1973) Antiviral effect of 1-aminoadamatane derivatives *in vitro. Acta Microbiol Acad Sci Hungar* **20**, 241–7.

Vale, J.A. & Maclean, K.S. (1977) Amantadine-induced heart failure (letter). *Lancet* **i**, 548.

Van Hes, R.Smit, A., Kratt, T. & Peters, A. (1972) Synthesis and antiviral activities of adamantane spino compounds. *J Med Chem* **15**, 132–6.

Van Voris, L.P., Betts, R.F., Hayden, F.G., Christmas, W.A. & Douglas, R.G. Jr (1981) Successful treatment of naturally occurring influenza A/USSR/77/H1N1. *J Am Med Assoc* **245**, 1128–31.

Vernier, V.G., Harmon, J.B., Stump, J.M., Lynes, T.E., Marvel, J.P. & Smith, D.H. (1969) The toxicologic and pharmacologic properties of amantadine hydrochloride. *Toxicol Applied Pharmacol* **15**, 642–65.

Vollum, D., Parkes, J.D. & Doyle, D. (1971) Livedo reticularis during amantadine treatment. *Lancet* **i**, 627–8.

Von Voighander, P.E. & Moore, K.E. (1971) Dopamine release from the brain *in vivo* by amantadine. *Science* **174**, 408–10.

Wang, C., Takeuchi, K., Pinto, L.H. & Lamb, R.A. (1993) Ion channel activity of influenza A virus M2 protein: characterization of the amantadine block. *J Virol* **67**, 5585–94.

Webster, R.G., Kawoska, Y., Bean, W.J., Beard, C.W. & Brugh, M. (1985) Chemotherapy and vaccination: a possible strategy for the control of highly virulent influenza virus. *J Virol* **55**, 173–6.

Wendel, H.A., Synder, M.T. & Pell, S. (1966) Trial of amantadine in epidemic influenza. *Clin Pharmacol Ther* **7**, 38–42.

Whitney, J.G., Gregory, W.A., Kauer, K.C. *et al.* (1970) Antiviral agents. I. Bicyclo[2.2.2] octan- and -oct-2-enamines. *J Med Chem* **13**, 254–60.

Wills, R.J. (1989) Update on rimantadine's clinical pharmacokinetics. *J Respir Dis* **10** (suppl), 20–5.

Wills, R.J., Belshe, R., Tomlinson, D. *et al.* (1987a) Pharmacokinetics of rimantadine hydrochloride in patients with chronic liver disease. *Clin Pharmacol Ther* **42**, 449–54.

Wills, R.J., Choma, N.Buopane, G., Lin, A. & Keigher, N. (1987b) Relative bioavailability of rimantadine HCl tablet and syrup formulations in healthy subjects. *J Pharm Sci* **76**, 886–8.

Wills, R.J., Farolino, D.A., Choma, N. & Keigher, N. (1987c) Rimantadine pharmacokinetics after single and multiple doses. *Antimicrobial Agents Chemother* **31**, 826–8.

Wills, R.J., Rodriguez, L.C., Choma, N. & Oakes, M. (1987d) Influence of a meal on the bioavailability of rimantadine HCl. *J Clin Pharmacol* **27**, 821–3.

Wilson, T.W. & Rajput, A.H. (1983) Amantadine-dyazide interaction. *Canad Med Assoc J* **129**, 974–5.

Wingfield, W.L., Pollack, D. & Grunert, R.R. (1969) Therapeutic efficacy of amantadine HCl and rimantadine HCl in naturally occurring influenza A2 respiratory illness in man. *N Engl J Med* **281**, 579–84.

Wintermeyer, S.M. & Nahata, M.C. (1995) Rimantadine: a clinical perspective. *Ann Pharmacother* **29**, 299–310.

Wong, L.T.Y., Sitar, D.S. & Aoki, F.Y. (1995) Chronic tobacco smoking and gender as variables affecting amantadine disposition in healthy subjects. *Br J Clin Pharmacol* **39**, 81–4.

Wong, L.T.Y., Smyth, D.D. & Sitar, D.S. (1992) Interference of renal organic cation transport by (−) (+) nicotine at concentrations documented in plasma of habitual tobacco smokers. *J Pharmacol Exp Ther* **261**, 21–5.

Wu, M.J., Ing, T.S., Soung, L.S., Daugirdas, J.T., Hano, J.E. & Gandhi, V.C. (1982) Amantadine hydrochloride pharmacokinetics in patients with impaired renal function. *Clin Nephrol* **17**, 19–23.

Younkin, S.W., Betts, R.F., Roth, F.K. & Douglas, R.G. Jr (1983) Reduction in fever and symptoms in young adults with influenza A/Brazil/78 H1N1 infection after treatment with aspirin or amantadine. *Antimicrobial Agents Chemother* **23**, 577–82.

Zhirnov, O.P. (1987) High protection of animals lethally infected with influenza virus by aprotinin-rimantadine combination. *J Med Virol* **21**, 161–7.

Zlydnikov, D.M., Alexandrova, G.I., Romanov, Y.A., Rumovsky, V.I. & Vasyljev, V.G. (1972) Dependence of the prophylactic effect of amantadine and rimantadine on the intensity of local and general immunity. In: Plander, E.M. (ed.) *Inhibitors of Viral Activity*, pp. 93–7. Zinatne, Riga.

Zlydnikov, D.M., Kubar, O.I., Kovaleva, T.P. & Kamforin, L.E. (1981) Study of rimantadine in the USSR: a review of the literature. *Rev Infect Dis* **3**, 408–21.

Zlydnikov, D.M. & Romanov, Y.A. (1972) The results of a clinical study of the prophylactic anti-influenza efficacy of amantadine and rimantadine. In: Smorodintsev, A.A. (ed.) *Chemoprophylaxis and Chemotherapy of Influenza*, pp. 71–6. Leningrad.

Zlydnikov, D.M., Romanov, Y.A., Lebedeva, V.K., Elkin, V.M. & Rumovsky, V.I. (1971) Comparative study of the prophylactic efficacy of amantadine and rimantadine. In: Zlydnikov, D.M. (ed.) *Chemoprophylaxis of Influenza with Amantadine*, pp. 209–20. Leningrad.

CHAPTER 36

Inhibitors of Influenza Virus Neuraminidase

Charles R. Penn

Inhibitors of the influenza (A and B) virus neura-minidase were first described in the early 1970s, but it was the development of zanamivir (4-guanidino-Neu5Ac2en, GG167), first described in 1993 by von Itzstein *et al.* that established the neuraminidase as a credible target for antiviral therapy. Since then there has been a resurgence of interest in the development of new inhibitors of influenza virus, but zanamivir is the first neuraminidase inhibitor to have been evaluated for efficacy in human trials. Most of this chapter is therefore devoted to a review of zanamivir, but other inhibitors are discussed briefly.

The evolution of inhibitors of influenza virus neuraminidase can be considered in three phases. In the first, a series of inhibitors, based on *N*-acetylneuraminic acid (sialic acid), was described that were non-selective inhibitors of the enzyme class. The second phase was the introduction of specificity for influenza virus neuraminidase (exemplified by zanamivir). In the third (current) phase, inhibitors with pharmacokinetics suitable for oral dosing are sought.

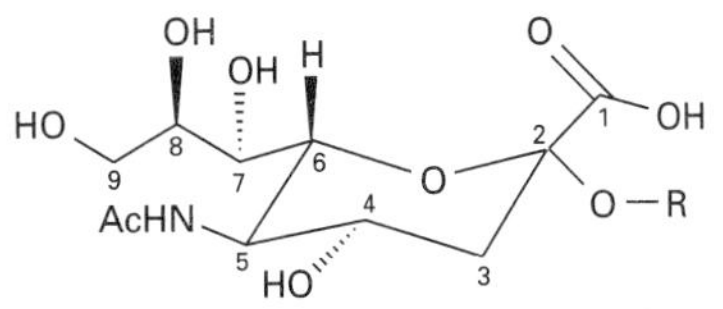

First-generation inhibitors—non-specific inhibition

The first neuraminidase inhibitors to be described were analogues of the substrate sialic acid (see Fig. 36.1), and have the common feature of dehy-dration at the C2,C3 position. The prototype inhibitor 2-deoxy-2,3-dehydro-*N*-acetylneuraminic acid (also known as DANA, or Neu5Ac2en) (Fig. 36.2) together with a series of C5 substituted analogues were described by Meindl and co-

Fig. 36.1 Chemical structure of *N*-acetylneuraminic acid (as the α-sialoside) showing carbon atom numbering.

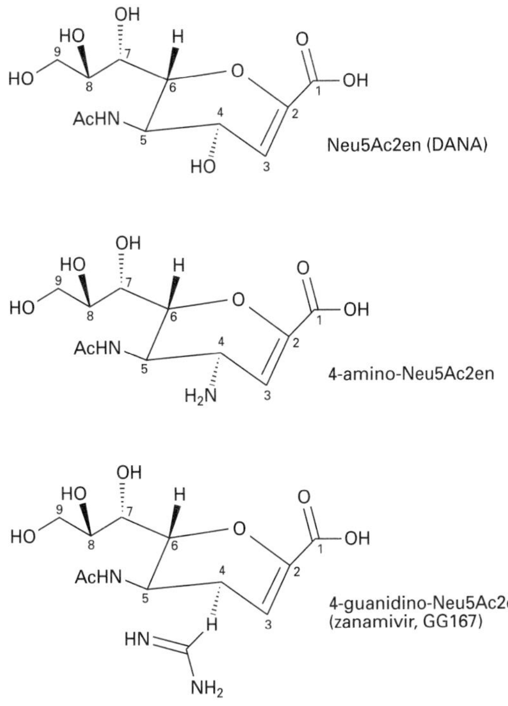

Fig. 36.2 Chemical structure of 2,3 dehydrated analogues of *N*-acetylneuraminic acid (sialic acid).

workers (Meindl & Tuppy 1969; Meindl *et al.* 1974; Palese *et al.* 1974).

The dehydration at C2,C3 introduces planarity at C2, such that the molecule resembles the sialosyl cation which is believed to be a transition state during catalysis (Chong *et al.* 1992; Taylor & von Itzstein 1993), and Neu5Ac2en is thus a non-specific inhibitor of all viral, bacterial and mammalian 2,3- and 2,6-neuraminidases examined to date. This lack of selectivity of inhibition is one of the reasons that these molecules, although effective inhibitors of the influenza A and B virus neuraminidase at micromolar concentrations, were not considered as candidates for antiviral therapy. The other reason was a lack of demonstrable efficacy in animal models of infection (Palese & Schulman 1977). This may be attributable either to insufficient potency against the viruses in culture, since Neu5Ac2en is about 10-fold less active against influenza A viruses in culture than amantadine (Woods *et al.* 1993), or to poor pharmacokinetics, since Neu5Ac2en is rapidly cleared via the kidneys and distributes poorly into tissues (Nohle *et al.* 1982). Indeed the latter authors commented that 'It seems, according to the results reported here, not very promising to apply Neu5Ac2en as a sialidase inhibitor *in vivo*, as this substance is so rapidly excreted after oral and intravenous administration', although antiviral activity in a murine and ferret models of respiratory infection was subsequently demonstrated by intranasal but not systemic administration (von Itzstein *et al.* 1993).

A number of other chemically diverse molecules have been described that inhibit influenza virus neuraminidase, though none of these have been developed as antiviral agents. These include the siastatins and some plant flavanoids (reviewed by Bamford 1995).

Second-generation inhibitors— introducing specificity

A breakthrough in the exploitation of neuraminidase as a target for antiviral therapy came with the description of C4-modified analogues of Neu5Ac2en (von Itzstein *et al.* 1993, 1994). The synthesis of these molecules was a direct result of the determination by X-ray crystallography of the structure of the viral neuraminidase and its interaction with the substrate sialic acid (Varghese *et al.* 1983, 1992; see Chapter 6), which revealed that the hydroxy group at C4 on the substrate was positioned close to two acidic residues in the active site of the neuraminidase (glutamates 119 and 227). Substitution of the 4-OH in the prototype inhibitor by the more basic amino- and guanidino groups (see Fig. 36.2) results in a 20- or 500-fold increase in the inhibition of influenza neuraminidase, respectively (von Itzstein *et al.* 1993; see also Table 36.1). 4-guanidino-Neu5Ac2en (zanamivir) is a particularly effective inhibitor that is now known to be equally effective against both influenza A and B virus neuraminidases (Hart & Bethell 1995) despite earlier reports that indicated some difference in the activity against the two virus types (Holtzer *et al.* 1993; Pegg & von Itzstein 1994). Zanamivir is an extremely potent inhibitor of the influenza virus neuraminidase, exhibiting inhibition constants (K_is) of 10^{-10}–10^{-9}M, and this has been explained in part by expulsion of a water molecule from the enzyme active site, leading to slow-binding kinetics of inhibition. This slow binding, combined with such

Table 36.1 Inhibition of influenza and human neuraminidase (sialidase) by Neu5Ac2en and C4/substituted analogues (data from von Itzstein *et al.* 1993).

Inhibitor	Influenza A virus* (A/Tokyo/3/67)	Influenza B virus* (B/Hong Kong/3/91)	Human placental sialidase†
Neu5Ac2en	1×10^{-6}	—	1.2×10^{-5}
4-amino-Neu5Ac2en	5×10^{-8}	—	9.3×10^{-3}
4-guanidino-Neu5Ac2en (zanamivir)	2.0×10^{-10}	7.0×10^{-10}	1.0×10^{-3}

* K_i (M).
† IC_{50} (M).

low K_is, necessitates complex analysis of the inhibition kinetics (see von Itzstein *et al.* 1993; Hart & Bethell 1995), which may account for some of the differences in results reported initially.

The introduction of these 4-substitutions, as well as conferring substantially greater affinity for the viral enzyme than the 4-hydroxy parent (Neu5Ac2en), also introduces considerable specificity as the affinity for enzymes other than influenza virus neuraminidase is much reduced. Thus zanamivir does not effectively inhibit other viral or bacterial neuraminidase (Holtzer *et al.* 1993) nor is it an effective inhibitor of a human neuraminidase (sialidase) (von Itzstein *et al.* 1993; see Table 36.1).

Zanamivir is also a very effective inhibitor of influenza viruses in cell culture. Concentrations of 5–15 nmol/l inhibit by 50% plaque formation by standard laboratory passaged influenza A and B viruses in Madin–Darby canine kidney (MDCK) cells (Woods *et al.* 1993; Fig. 36.3). Higher concentrations are required to prevent plaque formation by some other clinical isolates that have not been laboratory passaged, although the neuraminidases of these viruses are inhibited as effectively as any other isolate by zanamivir. This does not appear to be specific to zanamivir, but to neuraminidase inhibition generally, since the same effect is observed with Neu5Ac2en (DANA). One of

these apparently less sensitive isolates (A/Stockholm/24/90) has also been evaluated in a murine model of infection (Woods *et al.* 1993), and found to be as sensitive to inhibition by zanamivir as the most sensitive laboratory passaged isolates. The most probable explanation for this variability in sensitivity to neuraminidase inhibition in cell culture (but not in other assays), is that isolates of influenza virus differ in their dependence on neuraminidase for growth in the MDCK cells (although still highly dependent on the neuraminidase for growth *in vivo* and therefore likely to be sensitive to such inhibitors in clinical use). The properties of these viruses are similar to those with altered haemagglutinin that have been selected by laboratory passage in the presence of zanamivir (see below), and the basis for the phenotype may therefore be similar (Table 36.2).

Zanamivir inhibits a wide range on influenza viruses in cell culture, including (in contrast to amantadine and rimantadine) both influenza A and B viruses, as well as examples of all nine known neuraminidase A subtypes using avian influenza viruses (Thomas *et al.* 1994; Gubareva *et al.* 1995). Although MDCK cells are a standard system for measuring the growth of influenza viruses, they can be grown in other cells and zanamivir inhibits growth of both influenza A and B viruses in explant

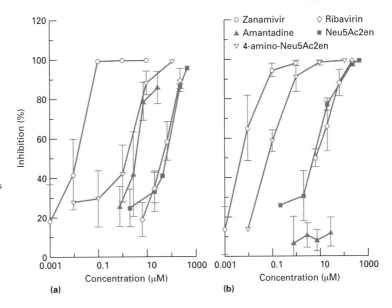

Fig. 36.3 Inhibition of plaque formation by different concentrations of zanamivir, 4-amino-Neu5Ac2en, Neu5Ac2en, amantadine and ribavirin. Influenza viruses used were A/Singapore/1/57 (a) and B/Victoria/102/85 (b). (Redrawn from von Itzstein *et al.* 1993, with permission from Macmillan Magazines Ltd.)

Table 36.2 Summary of properties on zanamivir.

Property	Reference
Potent inhibitor of influenza A and B neuraminidases	von Itzstein *et al.* 1993; Hart & Bethell 1995
Ineffective inhibitor of other neuraminidases (sialidases)	von Itzstein *et al.* 1993; Holtzer *et al.* 1993
Potent and selective inhibitor of influenza A and B viruses *in vitro*	von Itzstein *et al.* 1993; Woods *et al.* 1993; Hayden *et al.* 1994
Inhibits influenza viruses of all known neuraminidase subtypes	Thomas *et al.* 1994; Gubareva *et al.* 1995
Effective in animal models by respiratory application	Ryan *et al.* 1994, 1995
More potent than amantadine, rimantadine or ribavirin *in vitro* and in animal models	Woods *et al.* 1993; von Itzstein *et al.* 1993, Hayden *et al.* 1994; Ryan *et al.* 1994
Rapid renal clearance, without metabolism, low tissue penetration	Ryan *et al.* 1994; Hayden *et al.* 1996a
Effective in preventing and moderating infection in experimental human infections	Hayden *et al.* 1996c, 1996a; Walker *et al.* 1997
Reduces duration of illness when used to treat naturally acquired influenza	Hayden *et al.* 1996b, 1997

culture of human respiratory epithelium, a cell culture system that most closely resembles the natural site of replication in humans (Hayden *et al.* 1994). As expected from the enzyme specificity described above, zanamivir is ineffective as an inhibitor of parainfluenza viruses *in vitro*, although such viruses do have a neuraminidase (Woods *et al.* 1993).

As mentioned above, early efforts to demonstrate efficacy in animal models of infection with Neu5Ac2en and its C5-substituted analogues were not successful.

This may have been due to a combination of the relatively modest potency of these compounds (the antiviral activity of Neu5Ac2en *in vitro* is about one-tenth that of amantadine and similar to ribavirin; Woods *et al.* 1993), and to rapid clearance (Nohle *et al.* 1982). Zanamivir has been evaluated in several different animal models of influenza infection, and is very effective against models that mimic the respiratory infection when given by direct application to the respiratory tract. Thus, doses of 0.027 mg/kg twice a day given intranasally to mice infected with influenza A virus reduce replication

by 90%, considerably higher doses of amantadine (3.51 mg/kg) and ribavirin (33.9 mg/kg) were required to achieve the same effect under the same experimental conditions (von Itzstein *et al.* 1993). Similarly zanamivir is more effective than ribavirin at reducing replication of influenza B virus in the same model (Ryan *et al.* 1994). Zanamivir is also extremely effective by both intranasal administration (von Itzstein *et al.* 1993; Ryan *et al.* 1995) and aerosol inhalation (R. Fenton *et al.*, unpublished observations) in ferrets infected with either influenza A or B virus. The ferret is an excellent model of influenza infection in humans, with an acute self-limiting upper respiratory tract infection with increased nasal discharge, virus shedding into the respiratory tract and pyrexia. In this model zanamivir significantly reduces virus shedding, and pyrexia at doses down to 0.05 mg/kg twice daily, significantly better than ribavirin or amantadine. Zanamivir was effective when treatment started either before infection or shortly after, and virus replication did not resume when treatment was stopped after 5 days.

In contrast to the data summarized above, zanamivir is less effective when given systemically (orally or by intraperitoneal injection). In infected mice doses of over 100 mg/kg are required to demonstrate any reduction in viral replication (von Itzstein *et al.* 1993; Ryan *et al.* 1994). These observations are explained by the pharmacokinetic profile of zanamivir, which like Neu5Ac2en, is characterized by rapid renal clearance, poor oral availability and poor tissue penetration (volume of distribution equates with extracellular water) (Ryan *et al.* 1994; Hayden *et al.* 1996a). Thus very high systemic doses of zanamivir would be required to achieve an effective concentration in the extracellular airway (where the neuraminidase is active), and antiviral activity *in vivo* can best be achieved by administering the inhibitor directly to the respiratory tract. This stratagem has the additional benefits of very low systemic exposure to drug (leading to an enhanced safety profile), and the potential for more immediate effect on virus replication.

Consistent with the pharmacokinetic profile described above, zanamivir is also less effective against systemic influenza infections. Although in humans influenza virus infection is confined to the respiratory tract, in other species (notably some avian species) some strains of the virus will spread beyond the site of infection and cause a systemic, often lethal, infection. McCauley *et al.* (1995) and Gubareva *et al.* (1995) have shown that zanamivir has only a partial effect on the course of such infections, and in most cases, even at high doses (up to 1.5 mg/kg intratracheally) failed to protect chickens from lethal influenza infection. In these experiments infection was also by the intratracheal route. However, since influenza virus infection in humans is confined to the cells lining the respiratory tract airway, these observations on systemic infections in animal models are unlikely to be of clinical relevance.

Experimental infection of healthy human volunteers by influenza virus is a well-documented and established means of early evaluation of potential therapies or vaccines (see Chapter 39), and can give an early indication of the potential benefits and uses of such agents. Zanamivir has been evaluated in this way by Hayden *et al.* (1996a, 1996c). In four studies, zanamivir at different doses and dosing frequency, was given to volunteers by intranasal drops or spray, starting either before or after intranasal challenge with an influenza A virus (A/Texas/91). Zanamivir was found to be very effective in rapidly reducing virus shedding (measured in nasal washes) following the start of treatment (Fig. 36.4a), thus demonstrating for the first time that a neuraminidase inhibitor can have an antiviral effect in humans. When dosing of zanamivir was started after infection, infection rates were similar in both drug and placebo groups, but measures of fever, total symptom score and some other measures of illness were significantly reduced in the groups receiving zanamivir (Fig. 36.4b). The impact of zanamivir on infection and symptoms was even greater when treatment was started before the infection (prophylaxis), with an infection rate of 13% in the zanamivir group compared to 73% in the placebo group (Hayden *et al.* 1996c). In the same study groups zanamivir almost completely protected subjects from febrile illness (95% effective), and significantly reduced other indicators of illness (Fig. 36.4c).

Similar studies using an influenza B virus have confirmed that zanamivir can be effective in preventing and moderating influenza B infections (Hayden *et al.* 1996b). Zanamivir also reduced the development of middle ear pressure abnormalities (commonly associated with influenza) in these experimental infections (Walker *et al.* 1997).

The above studies in volunteer subjects provided the first formal proof that inhibition of influenza virus neuraminidase, a new therapeutic concept, could prevent or ablate clinical influenza in humans. This concept has been further substantiated by the results from phase II clinical trials conducted with zanamivir in patients with naturally acquired influenza. In 173 patients with confirmed influenza given zanamivir, the median length of time to alleviation of symptoms was one day shorter (four days vs. five days) than in 89 patients given placebo, but up to three days shorter (four days vs. seven days, $p \leq 0.01$) in certain subgroups (Hayden *et al.* 1997). Zanamivir was well tolerated in all clinical studies to date (Hayden *et al.* 1996a,b,c, 1997).

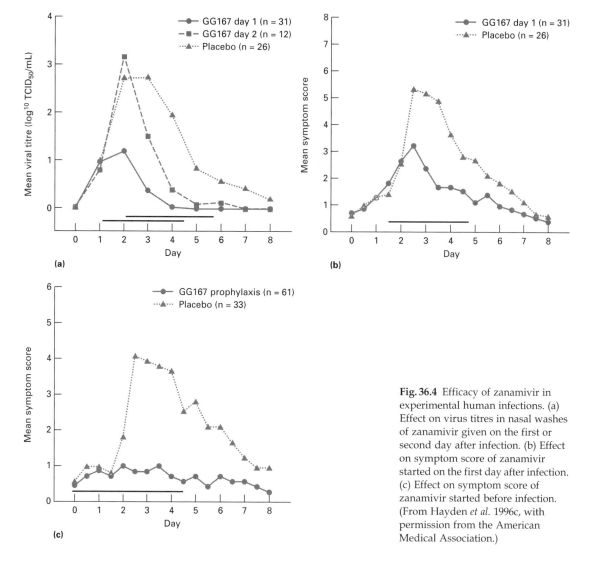

Fig. 36.4 Efficacy of zanamivir in experimental human infections. (a) Effect on virus titres in nasal washes of zanamivir given on the first or second day after infection. (b) Effect on symptom score of zanamivir started on the first day after infection. (c) Effect on symptom score of zanamivir started before infection. (From Hayden *et al.* 1996c, with permission from the American Medical Association.)

Resistance

The emergence of viruses resistant to an inhibitor is a normal evolutionary event that will unsurprisingly occur once a selective pressure is applied, and has been demonstrated for almost every antiviral agent that has so far been described. The issue is not whether such viruses can be isolated, but whether they have any impact on the clinical utility of the antiviral agent. In some cases (e.g. acyclovir) the mutations that confer resistance to inhibition may impair virus growth

or pathogenicity so that they do not readily occur (Field & Biron 1994). In others, such as treatment of human immunodeficiency virus (HIV) infection with 2′-deoxy-3′-thiacytidine (3TC) and azidothymidine (AZT), mutations conferring resistance to one drug restore sensitivity to the other so that a treatment benefit is maintained (Kuritzkes *et al.* 1996). For the first-generation inhibitors of influenza A viruses (amantadine and rimantadine), the selection of resistant viruses is of clinical relevance and is associated with treatment failure (Hayden 1994).

Influenza viruses with reduced sensitivity to zanamivir have been isolated in several laboratories following tissue culture passage of virus in the presence of drug. To date there have been no reports of resistant viruses emerging as a result of clinical use of zanamivir, suggesting that zanamivir may be less susceptible to development of resistance than is the case for amantadine/rimantadine. The properties of those viruses that have been isolated in laboratory culture (for which two mechanisms have emerged) support this proposition, as discussed below.

Changes in neuraminidase

In the first of these two mechanisms, mutations occur in the neuraminidase gene that result in amino acid substitutions in the active site of the enzyme. Changes have been described at amino acid position 119 where the glutamate that normally occurs is changed to glycine (Blick *et al.* 1995; Staschke *et al.* 1995), asparagine or alanine (Gubareva *et al.* 1996) and also at amino acid 292 (arginine to lysine, Gubareva *et al.* 1997). At least some of these changes lead to instability of the neuraminidase, other changes in the enzyme properties and/or impaired growth of the virus (McKimm-Breschkin *et al.* 1996a,c; Gubareva *et al.* 1997), and this may explain why such viruses have not been observed during the early clinical studies with zanamivir experiments (Hayden *et al.* 1996a), despite their isolation from *in vitro*.

Changes in haemagglutinin

A less expected development has been the isolation of influenza A viruses with altered haemagglutinin (McKimm-Breschkin *et al.* 1996b; Penn *et al.* 1996; Sahasrabudhe *et al.* 1996). Several mutations have been described, most of which are close to the sialic acid binding site (at Thr 155, Val 223, Arg 229 and Gly 135; Plate 36.1, facing page 288) though one at a more distal location has also been described (at Gly 75; Gubareva *et al.* 1996). Similar changes in haemagglutinin have also been found in an influenza B virus cultured in the presence of zanamivir (Asn 145 Ser and Asn 150

Ser; Staschke *et al.* 1995). The precise mechanism whereby changes in haemagglutinin reduce sensitivity *in vitro* to zanamivir is not fully understood, but is likely to arise from an alteration to the interaction between haemagglutinin and the receptor sialic acid. Thus a reduction in affinity for the receptor may compensate for the loss of neuraminidase (receptor destroying) activity through inhibition. This hypothesis is supported by observations that some of these haemagglutinin variants show a reduced affinity for red blood cells (evidence of reduced receptor affinity; Sahasrabudhe *et al.* 1996), and the proximity of most of these changes to the sialic acid binding site. These viruses would therefore have a reduced dependence on neuraminidase, consistent with the observation that these viruses are less sensitive to all neuraminidase inhibitors including Neu5Ac2en (DANA), and yet have no change in neuraminidase sequence.

An additional observation with one of these haemagglutinin variants (a derivative of A/Singapore/1/57 with a change at Gly 135) is that altered virus retains sensitivity to zanamivir in a murine model of infection, comparable to that of the parental wild-type virus. This is very similar to the phenotype of the natural isolate A/Stockholm/24/90 described above. The precise mechanisms whereby changes in haemagglutinin may confer a reduced dependence *in vitro* but not *in vivo* have yet to be determined but the balance between the receptor binding properties of haemagglutinin, and the receptor-destroying activities of the neuraminidase, may be crucial in maintaining the viability of influenza virus in its natural environment.

A further inference from these data is that such compensatory changes in haemagglutinin are unlikely to impact on the clinical utility of neuraminidase inhibitors such as zanamivir, although any correlation between *in vitro* and *in vivo* observations on resistance phenotypes should be made with caution. That such variants have not so far been observed following experimental human infections and clinical trials conducted to date (Hayden *et al.* 1996a) supports the contention that such viruses may not be readily selected.

Third-generation inhibitors-changing pharmacokinetics

By the end of 1996 zanamivir was still the only neuraminidase inhibitor to be evaluated for clinical efficacy, but several other similar molecules have been described. These all contain two key features seen with zanamivir: basic substitutions at C4 (or equivalent), that confer specificity for influenza viruses, and a double bond that gives the planar conformation to C2 seen in most neuraminic acid based inhibitors. Since zanamivir is an extremely effective and selective inhibitor of the influenza virus neuraminidase, effort has been directed towards synthesis of molecules that might be effective orally (i.e. with a different pharmacokinetic profile).

A range of molecules based on the original Neu5Ac2en template have been described, including C4-disubstituted (Groves & von Itzstein 1996), C5- and C6-truncated analogues (Bamford *et al.* 1995; Starkey *et al.* 1995), phosphonates (White *et al.* 1995) and sulphur isosteres (Kok *et al.* 1996), though none of these inhibitors offer any particular advantage over zanamivir. Similarly, changing the ring structure to an aromatic ring (benzoic acid derivatives), although yielding enzyme inhibitors, has not resulted in molecules with potency comparable to zanamivir (Singh *et al.* 1995).

None of the above molecules offer the prospect of substantially altered pharmacokinetics. However, two groups have described molecules with lipophilic side chains replacing the glycerol side chain at C6. Smith *et al.* (1996) and Sollis *et al.* (1996) have described some C6 carboxamide derivatives of Neu5Ac2en that are very potent inhibitors of influenza neuraminidase, that, with the less polar side chain at C6 have the potential for higher oral

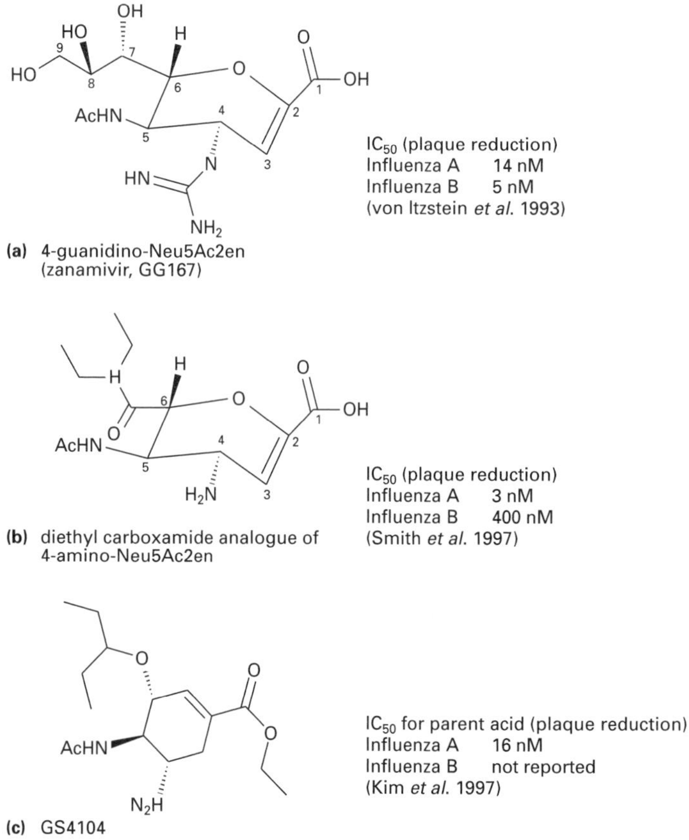

IC$_{50}$ (plaque reduction)
Influenza A   14 nM
Influenza B   5 nM
(von Itzstein *et al.* 1993)

(a) 4-guanidino-Neu5Ac2en (zanamivir, GG167)

IC$_{50}$ (plaque reduction)
Influenza A   3 nM
Influenza B   400 nM
(Smith *et al.* 1997)

(b) diethyl carboxamide analogue of 4-amino-Neu5Ac2en

IC$_{50}$ for parent acid (plaque reduction)
Influenza A   16 nM
Influenza B   not reported
(Kim *et al.* 1997)

(c) GS4104

Fig. 36.5 Chemical structures of two lipophilic analogues of Neu5Ac2en (b,c), compared with that of zanamivir (a). Inhibition of plaque formation by influenza A and B virus reported for each inhibitor is also shown.

bioavailability and efficacy (Fig. 36.5b). However, molecules of this type show greater inhibition of influenza A neuraminidase than that of influenza B viruses (Smith *et al.* 1996; Sollis *et al.* 1996). In the second, a similar lipophilic side chain has been introduced into a carbocyclic analogue of Neu5Ac2en (Kim *et al.* 1997). An ethyl ester of one of the molecules from this series (designated GS4104, Fig. 36.5c), is reported to have the desired pharmacological properties and to be effective orally in animal models of influenza infection (Kim *et al.* 1997).

Conclusion

Neuraminidase inhibitors offer a new prospect for treatment and control of influenza. This concept has been established with zanamivir, a potent inhibitor of both influenza A and B viruses that has been shown to prevent and limit illness in experimental influenza, and to reduce illness in naturally acquired infections.

References

Bamford, M. (1995) Neuraminidase inhibitors as potential anti-influenza drugs. *J Enzyme Inhib* **10**, 1–16.

Bamford, M., Castro Pichel, J., Husman, W., Patel, B., Storer, R. & Weir, N. (1995) Synthesis of 6-, 7- and 8-carbon sugar analogues of potent anti-influenza 2,3-didehydro-2,3-dideoxy-N-acetylneuraminic acid derivatives. *J Chem Soc Perkin Trans* **1**, 1181–8.

Blick, T., Tiong, T., Sahasrabudhe, A. *et al.* (1995) Generation and characterization of an influenza neuraminidase variant with decreased sensitivity to the neuraminidase-specific inhibitor 4-guanidino-Neu5Ac2en. *Virology* **214**, 475–84.

Chong, A., Pegg, M., Taylor, N. & von Itzstein, M. (1992) Evidence for a sialosyl cation transition-state complex in the reaction of sialidase from influenza virus. *Eur J Biochem* **207**, 335–43.

Field, A. & Biron, K. (1994) 'The end of innocence' revisited: resistance of herpesviruses to antiviral drugs. *Clin Microbiol Rev* **7**, 1–13.

Groves, R. & von Itzstein, M. (1996) Synthesis of C4-disubstituted analogues of N-acetylneuraminic acid. *J Chem Soc Perkin Trans* **1**, 2817–21.

Gubareva, L., Bethell, R., Hart, G., Murti, K., Penn, C. & Webster, R. (1996) Characterization of mutants of influenza A virus selected with the neuraminidase inhibitor 4-guanidino-Neu5Ac2en. *J Virol* **70**, 1818–27.

Gubareva, L., Penn, C. & Webster, R. (1995) Inhibition of replication of avian viruses by the neuraminidase inhibitor 4-guanidino-2,4-dideoxy-2,3-dehydro-N-acetyl-neuraminic acid. *Virology* **212**, 323–30.

Gubareva, L., Robinson, M., Bethell, R. & Webster, R. (1997) Catalytic and framework mutations in the neuraminidase active site of influenza viruses resistant to 4-guanidino-Neu5Ac2en (GG167). *J Virol* **71**, 3385–90.

Hart, G. & Bethell, R. (1995) 2,3-Didehydro-2, 4-dideoxy-4-guanidino-N-acetyl-D-neuraminic acid (4-guanidino-Neu5Ac2en) is a slow-binding inhibitor of sialidase from both influenza A virus and influenza B virus. *Biochem Mol Biol Int* **36**, 695–703.

Hayden, F. (1994) Amantadine and rimantadine resistance in influenza A viruses. *Curr Opin Infect Dis* **7**, 674–7.

Hayden, F., Lobo, M., Hussey, E. & Eason, C. (1996a) Efficacy of intranasal GG167 in experimental human influenza A and B virus infection. In: Brown, L.E., Hampson, A.W. & Webster, R.G. (eds) *Options for the Control of Influenza*, Vol. 3, pp. 718–25. Elsevier Science, Amsterdam.

Hayden, F., Osterhaus, A., Treanor, J. *et al.* (1996b) Phase II studies of the therapeutic efficacy and safety of GG167 in uncomplicated influenza. *36th Interscience Conference on Antimicrobial Agents and Chemotherapy*, p. 171, Abstract H45. American Society for Microbiology, Washington DC.

Hayden, F., Treanor, J., Betts, R., Lobo, M., Esinhart, J. & Hussey, E. (1996c) Safety and efficacy of the neuraminidase inhibitor GG167 in experimental human influenza. *J Am Med Assoc* **275**, 295–9.

Hayden, F., Osterhaus, A., Treanor, J. *et al.* (1997) Efficacy and safety of the neuraminidase inhibitor zanamivir in the treatment of influenza virus infections. *N Engl J Med* **337**, 874–80.

Hayden, F., Rollins, B. & Madren, L. (1994) Anti-influenza virus activity of the neuraminidase inhibitor 4-guanidino-Neu5Ac2en in cell culture and in human respiratory epithelium. *Antiviral Res* **25**, 123–31.

Holzer, C., von Itzstein, M., Jin, B., Pegg, M., Stewart, W. & Wu, W-Y. (1993) Inhibition of sialidases from viral, bacterial and mammalian sources by analogues of 2-deoxy-2, 3-didehydro-N-acetylneuraminic acid modified at the C4 position. *Glycocon J* **10**, 40–4.

Kim, C., Lew, W., Williams, W *et al.* (1997) Influenza neuraminidase inhibitors possessing a novel hydrophobic interaction in the enzyme active site: design, synthesis, and structural analysis of carbocyclic sialic acid analogues with potent anti-influenza activity. *J Am Chem Soc* **119**, 681–90.

Kok, G., Campbell, M., Mackey, B. & von Itzstein, M. (1996) Synthesis and biological evaluation of sulphur isosteres of the potent influenza virus sialidase inhibitors 4-amino-4-deoxy- and 4-deoxy-4-guanidino-Neu5Ac2en. *J Chem Soc Perkin Trans* **1**, 2811–15.

Kuritzkes, D., Quinn, J., Benoit, S. *et al.* (1996) Drug resistance and virologic response in NUCA 3001, a randomized trial of lamivudine (3TC) versus zidovudine (ZDV) versus ZDV plus 3TC in previously untreated patients. *AIDS* **10**, 975–81.

McCauley, J., Pullen, L., Forsyth, M., Penn, C. & Thomas, G.P. (1995) 4-guanidino-Neu5Ac2en fails to protect chickens from infection with highly pathogenic avian influenza virus. *Antiviral Res* **27**, 179–86.

McKimm-Breschkin, J., Blick, T., Sahasrabudhe, A. *et al.* (1996a) Influenza virus variants with decreased sensitivity to 4-amino and 4-guanidino-Neu5Ac2en. In: Brown, L.E., Hampson, A.W. & Webster, R.G. (eds) *Options for the Control of Influenza*, Vol. 3, pp. 726–34. Elsevier Science, Amsterdam.

McKimm-Breschkin, J., Blick, T., Sahasrabudhe, A. *et al.* (1996b) Generation and characterization of variants of NWS/G70C influenza virus after *in vitro* passage in 4-amino-Neu5Ac2en and 4-guanidino-Neu5Ac2en. *Antimicrobial Agents Chemother* **40**, 40–6.

McKimm-Breschkin, J., McDonald, M., Sahasrabudhe, A., Blick, T. & Colman, P. (1996c) Mutation in the influenza virus neuraminidase gene resulting in decreased sensitivity to the neuraminidase inhibitor 4-guanidino-Neu5Ac2en leads to indstability of the enzyme. *Virology* **225**, 240–2.

Meindl, P., Bodo, G., Palese, P., Schulman, J. & Tuppy, H. (1974) Inhibition of neuraminidase activity by derivatives of 2-deoxy-2, 3-dehydro-*N*-acetylneuraminic acid. *Virology* **58**, 457–63.

Meindl, P. & Tuppy, H. (1969) 2-deoxy-2, 3-dehydrosialic acids. I. Synthesis and properties of 2-deoxy-2, 3-dehydro-*N*-acetylneuraminic acids and their methyl esters. *Monatshafte Chem* **100**, 1295–306.

Nohle, U., Beau, J.-M. & Schauer, R. (1982) Uptake, metabolism and excretion of orally and intravenously administered, double-labelled *N*-glycolylneuraminic acid and single-labelled 2-deoxy-2, 3-dehydro-*N*-acetylneuraminic acid in mouse and rat. *Eur J Biochem* **126**, 543–8.

Palese, P. & Schulman, J. (1977) Inhibitors of viral neuraminidase as potential antiviral drugs. In: Oxford, J.S. (ed.) *Chemoprophylaxis* and *Virus Infections of Respiratory Tract*, pp. 189–205. CRC Press, Cleveland.

Palese, P., Schulman, J., Bodo, G. & Meindl, P. (1974) Inhibition of influenza and parainfluenza replication in tissue culture by 2-deoxy-2, 3-dehydro-*N*-trifluoro-acetylneuraminic acid (FANA). *Virology* **59**, 490–8.

Pegg, M. & von Itzstein, M. (1994) Slow-binding inhibition of sialidase from influenza virus. *Biochem Mol Biol Int* **34**, 851–8.

Penn, C., Bethell, R., Fenton, R., Gearing, K., Healy, N. & Jowett, A. (1996) Selection of influenza virus with reduced sensitivity *in vitro* to the neuraminidase inhibitor GG167 (4-guanidino-Neu5Ac2en). In: Brown, L.E., Hampson, A.W. & Webster, R.G. (eds) *Options for the*

Control of Influenza, Vol. 3, pp. 735–40. Elsevier Science, Amsterdam.

Ryan, D. M., Ticehurst, J., Dempsey, M. & Penn, C. (1994) Inhibition of influenza virus replication in mice by GG167 (4-guanidino-2, 4-dideoxy-2, 3-dehydro-N-acetylneuraminic acid) is consistent with extracellular activity of viral neuraminidase. *Antimicrobial Agents Chemother* **38**, 2270–5.

Ryan, D.M., Ticehurst, J. & Penn, C. (1995) GG167 (4-guanidino-2, 4-dideoxy-2, 3-dehydro-*N*-acetylneuraminic acid) is a potent inhibitor of influenza virus in ferrets. *Antimicrobial Agents Chemother* **39**, 2583–4.

Sahasrabudhe, A., Blick, T. & McKimm-Breschkin, J. (1996) Influenza variants resistant to GG167 with mutations in the haemagglutinin. In: Brown, L.E., Hampson, A.W. & Webster, R.G. (eds) *Options for the Control of Influenza*, Vol. 3, pp. 748–52. Elsevier Science, Amsterdam

Sayle, R. & Milner-White, E. (1995) Rasmol: biomolecular graphics for all. *Trends Biochem Sci* **20**, 333–79.

Singh, S., Jedrzejas, M., Air, G. *et al.* (1995) Structure based inhibitors of influenza virus sialidase. A benzoic acid lead with novel interaction. *J Med Chem* **38**, 3217–25.

Smith, P., Sollis, S., Howes, P. *et al.* (1996) Novel inhibitors of influenza sialidases related to GG167 structure-activity, crystallographic and molecular dynamic studies with 4H-pyran-2-carboxylic acid 6-carboxamides. *Bioorganic Med Chem Lett* **6**, 2931–6.

Sollis, S., Smith, P., Howes, P., Cherry, P. & Bethell, R. (1996) Novel inhibitors of influenza sialidase related to GG167 synthesis of 4-amino and guanidino 4H-pyran-2-carboxylic acid-6-propylamides—selective inhibitors of influenza A virus sialidase. *Bioorganic Med Chem Lett* **6**, 1805–8.

Starkey, I., Mahmoudian, M., Noble, D. *et al.* (1995) Synthesis and influenza virus sialidase inhibitory activity of the 5-desacetamido analogue of 2, 3-didehydro-2, 4-dideoxy-4-guanidinyl-*N*-acetylneuraminic acid (GG167). *Tetrahedron Lett* **36**, 299–302.

Staschke, K., Coacino, J., Baxter, A. *et al.* (1995) Molecular basis for the resistance of influenza viruses to 4-guanidino-Neu5Ac2en. *Virology* **214**, 642–6.

Taylor, N. & von Itzstein, M. (1993) Molecular modelling studies on ligand binding to sialidase from influenza virus and the mechanism for catalysis. *J Med Chem* **37**, 616–24.

Thomas, P., Forsyth, M., Penn, C. & McCauley, J. (1994) Inhibition of the growth of influenza viruses *in vitro* by 4-guanidino-2, 4-dideoxy-*N*-acetylneuraminic acid. *Antiviral Res* **24**, 351–6.

Varghese, J., Laver, W. & Colman, P. (1983) Structure of the influenza virus glycoprotein antigen neuraminidase at 2.9A resolution. *Nature* **303**, 35–40.

Varghese, J., McKimm-Breschkin, J., Caldwell, J., Kortt, A. & Colman, P. (1992) Structure of the complex between influenza virus neuraminidase and sialic acid, the viral receptor. *Proteins Struct Funct Genet* **14**, 327–32.

von Itzstein, M., Wu, W-Y. & Jin, B. (1994) The synthesis of 2, 3-didehydro-2, 4-dideoxy-4-guanidinyl-N-acetyl-neuraminic acid. *Carbohydrate Res* **259**, 301–5.

von Itzstein, I., Wu, W-Y., Kok, G. *et al.* (1993) Rational design of potent sialidase-based inhibitors of influenza virus replication. *Nature* **363**, 418–23.

Walker, J., Hussey, E., Treanor, J., Moltalvo, A. & Hayden, F. (1997) Effects of the neuraminidase inhibitor GG167 on otological manifestations of experimental human influenza. *J Infect Dis* **176**, 1417–22.

Weis, W., Brown, J., Cusack, S., Paulson, J., Skehel, J. & Wiley, D. (1988) Structure of the influenza haemagglutinin complexed with its receptor, sialic acid. *Nature* **333**, 426–31.

White, C., Janakiraman, M., Laver, W. *et al.* (1995) A sialic acid-derived phosphonate analogue inhibits different strains of influenza virus neuraminidase with different efficiencies. *J Mol Biol* **245**, 623–34.

Woods, J., Bethell, R., Coates, J. *et al.* (1993) 4-Guanidino-2, 4-dideoxy-2, 3-dehydro-N-acetylneuraminic acid is a highly effective inhibitor both of the sialidase (neuraminidase) and of growth of a wide range on influenza A and B viruses *in vitro*. *Antimicrobial Agents Chemother* **37**, 1473–9.

CHAPTER 37

Alternative Influenza Antiviral Agents

Robert Lambkin and John S. Oxford

Introduction

Influenza A and B viruses have a substantial impact in the community in terms of both morbidity and mortality; they also have a substantial economic consequence (Stuart-Harris *et al.* 1984). In 1989/90 over 29 000 people died of influenza or the complications thereof in UK (Ashley *et al.* 1991). It is perhaps rather unusual that two separate scientific meetings, supported not by pharmaceutical companies, but by the National Institute of Health and the World Health Organization (WHO), urged more extensive use in the community of the two licensed antivirals amantadine and rimantadine. Influenza vaccination is recommended in the UK and Europe for 'at-risk' groups, i.e. people with a relatively high chance of serious illness, and in the USA for a wider group, namely the over 65s. However, a number of vaccinees fail to respond to the vaccine (Lambkin *et al.* 1997). In addition, even the induction of what might be considered a protective antibody titre against the virus does not guarantee that an individual will not become infected and suffer illness. Vaccination of the 'at-risk' groups and even prophylactic treatment with amantadine cannot always prevent high mortality rates in nursing homes (Morens & Rash 1995). Lastly the ever-present risk of a pandemic outbreak of influenza A (PHLS Response to a pandemic of influenza: An action plan) with the potential for subsequent high mortality and the long lead time for influenza vaccine supplies (greater than 1 year) leave no doubt that the development of new and efficacious compounds effective against influenza A and B viruses is urgently required. More con-

sideration could be given to the molecular pathology of influenza in humans. Where exactly does the virus replicate and how are the recognized clinical symptoms of headache and myalgia caused? Are these symptoms the consequence of cytokines released during viral replication and could antiviral drugs alleviate them or not? Could influenza virus be a more neurological virus than has been previously considered and if so will the existing antivirals act in the central nervous system? Exactly how does a virus like influenza cause the important (at least for the patient) symptoms of a sore throat and cough: by direct lysis of cells in the throat or more indirectly? It is clear therefore that there are many important questions to be answered and it is our consideration that as the science of antivirals evolves so important scientific medical questions will be resolved.

In this chapter we have reviewed both recent and historical literature in order to highlight possible opportunities for the design or development of new compounds. We have broken down the infectious cycle of influenza virus into arbitrary steps and we discuss compounds that may be able to inhibit the virus at each stage. It would be anticipated that with a highly mutable virus such as influenza potentially drug-resistant viruses would already exist or could thereafter be selected. Even with the advent of exciting new antineuraminidase drugs (von Itzstein *et al.* 1996) molecules acting at different points of the life cycle are required. Under these circumstances, as with other quasispecies RNA viruses such as the human immunodeficiency virus (HIV) (Oxford *et al.* 1996), combination chemoprophylaxis could be explored. The recent identification of potent anti-NA (antineuraminidase) compounds (Woods *et al.* 1993; Ryan *et al.* 1995; von Itzstein *et al.* 1996) has resurrected interest in specific enzymes of influenza virus as targets.

An overview of the infectious cycle of influenza virus

The infectious cycle of influenza A virus provides many possible targets for therapeutic intervention. The viral replicative cycle, lasting 6–7 h in susceptible cells of the upper and lower respiratory tract, can be divided into the following eight stages:

1 virus attachment;
2 virus entry;
3 virus uncoating;
4 primary transcription of input vRNA;
5 replication of vRNA and secondary transcription;
6 translation of viral mRNAs to produce viral proteins;
7 post-translational modification of viral proteins;
8 assembly of viral structural components and release of progeny virus.

Stages 1–3 are shown schematically in Fig. 37.1 and stages 4–8 are shown in Fig. 37.3.

Stage 1: Virus attachment to host cells

The most obvious target for an influenza antiviral agent would appear to be the initial attachment of the virus to the cell membrane. An agent capable of preventing this attachment stage would prevent the primary infection, but this approach has not been easily achieved with other viruses, e.g. soluble CD4 and HIV. In practical terms the compounds would have to be used prophylactically so as to be present in nasal and throat washes (and possibly tears) to prevent initial interaction between virus and cell. It is conceivable though that later therapeutic intervention might also reduce virus spread and virus-induced symptoms.

Another alternative would be to destroy the influenza A virus before it has the opportunity to attach to the host cell. Virucidal compounds that destroy the virus on contact have been identified and these may well be an area suitable for further development (Oxford 1994). Influenza A virus infection is initiated by the attachment of the haemagglutinin (HA) to oligosaccharides bearing *N*-acetylneuraminic acid (sialic acid) in the terminal position (Gottschalk 1957). Sialic acid residues are

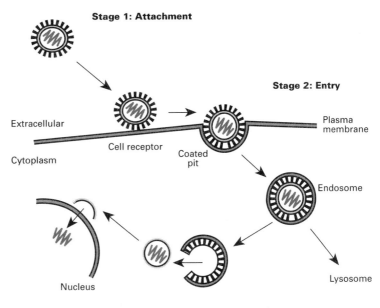

Fig. 37.1 Influenza A virus infectious cycle stages 1–3 (From Outlaw & Dimmock 1993, with permission from Academic Press.)

found on a wide range of glycolipids and/or glycoproteins present in cell membranes, thus giving the influenza virus a diverse range of potential target cells. The receptor binding pocket on the influenza A virus HA most studied (the H3N2 subtype) is a depression at the distal end of the molecule and is thought to be highly conserved amongst influenza A viruses (Wiley & Skehel 1987).

The identification or design of compounds that are capable of preventing attachment of the HA to the sialic acid residues has been greatly helped by analyses of the three dimensional structure of the H3 subtype of the HA (Wiley *et al.* 1981). In particular, the determination of the structure when complexed with an antibody (Bizebard *et al.* 1995) has supplied a comprehensive understanding of the interactions that occur, allowing the design of potential inhibitors. The influenza HA is a type 1 membrane protein with an N-terminal signal sequence, an ectodomain of 500 residues, a transmembrane domain of 27 residues and a C-terminal cytoplasmic domain of 10 residues. The HA spike is a homotrimer with trimer assembly occurring in the endoplasmic reticulum.

Inhibitors of viral attachment to the host cell membrane

Viruses such as HIV have a choice of receptors on cells (Deng & Nickoloff 1994) and therefore decoy compounds often have to be relatively complex mixtures. With influenza there is some evidence for a second receptor binding site on the HA which may complicate the initial binding process. However, the main receptor binding site is a pocket located at the distal end of each monomer and the residues forming the pocket are largely conserved between subtypes. Contact between the 5-N-acetyl group of neuramic acid at Tyr-153 and Gly-134 of the pocket play an important role in receptor binding (Weiss *et al.* 1988).

In the search for substances interfering with receptor binding, various neuraminic acid analogues have been tested. In most of these compounds only low affinity for HA has been observed. However, substitution of the carboxyl oxygen in the N-acetyl group by sulphur resulted in increased HA affinity and such substances inhibited influenza replication (Itoh *et al.* 1995).

These inhibitors could act in one of three ways:
- by sterically blocking the HA binding site with a compound that competes with the sialic acid on the cell surface binding site or binds near to this site;
- by forming complexes with the sialic acid groups on the surface of the target cells thus rendering them inaccessible to the HA on the virion; or
- by preventing access of the HA binding site to the sialic acid moiety by some non-specific mechanism. Until recently attempts to block the binding of the HA to sialic acid residues were not particularly successful as early compounds based on derivatives of sialic acid were of low potency. An example is the methyl ether derivative, Neu5Ac2Me; however, this compound has a poor dissociation constant of 2–3 mM (Sauter *et al.* 1989; Watowich *et al.* 1994). The addition of hydrophobic substitutes increased the dissociation constant to 40 μM (Toogood *et al.* 1991). Bivalent sialic acid ligands have been shown to have some effect on the binding of influenza to the host cell (Glick *et al.* 1991). It has been observed that the binding of the α-sialoside reconstituted in liposomes is greater than for the monomer alone. Liposomes constructed from sialoside lipid that are then polymerized are particularly potent and can inhibit influenza virus haemagglutination of red blood cells at picomolar concentrations (Spevak 1993). It has been proposed that this is due to the polymeric nature of the interaction (Ellens *et al.* 1990). Working on this assumption, another group (Lees *et al.* 1994) synthesized compounds that presented multiple copies of ligands, derivatives of sialic acid and its analogues. These bound to the influenza A virus HA in competition with the substrate ~ 3–10^3 μM (Glick & Toogood 1991; Glick *et al.* 1991) and it is believed that compounds act by binding intertrimerically. However, far more potent compounds are produced if the sialic acid residues are incorporated onto polymeric templates (Sabesan *et al.* 1992; Roy *et al.* 1993; Spevak *et al.* 1993; Lees *et al.* 1994; Mammen *et al.* 1995). The nature of the template is important in determining the efficacy of the compound, with the presence of hydrophobic constituents in the template increasing the affinity of the compound for the virus receptor binding site. Additionally if the sialic acid residues are spaced

55 Å apart (that is, the same distance apart that they occur naturally on the cell membrane) the potency of the compound is further increased (Glick *et al.* 1991). The most effective compound produced in this way had a 100-fold higher avidity for whole virions than the monovalent ligand. These polymeric compounds inhibited the haemagglutination of red blood cells with an IC_{50} of 0.6 nM at 36 °C (Mammen *et al.* 1995). Currently the only published data describe *in vitro* assays and *in vivo* studies have yet to be published.

The most potent compounds produced to date that block the binding of the virus receptor pocket and the receptor itself have been polyacrylamide derivatives incorporating sialic acid (Lees *et al.* 1994; Mammen *et al.* 1995). Although the most probable mechanism of inhibition is a combination of the polyvalent interaction and steric interference, a mechanism based solely on polyvalent interaction cannot be ruled out. Sulphated polysaccharides and polysulphates are known to be inhibitory to a range of enveloped viruses including influenza, and such inhibitory molecules are frequently extracted from medicinal plants and seaweeds. Witirouw *et al.* (1994) describes a galactan sulphate extracted from the red seaweed which blocks viral adsorption to cell membranes. But although these natural polysaccharides products are potent viral inhibitors *in vitro*, little data are available on *in vivo* antiviral effects and toxicity and bioavailability.

Stage 2: Virus entry

Mammalian cells internalize extracellular particles which are > 200 nm in diameter by phagocytosis and particles less than ~ 200 nm in diameter by pinocytosis (Marsh 1984). Pinocytosis is further divided into adsorptive (receptor-mediated) endocytosis and fluid-phase pinocytosis.

Influenza virus is about 120 nm in diameter and is believed to enter cells by adsorptive endocytosis (Dourmashkin & Tyrrell 1970; Matlin *et al.* 1981; reviewed by: Marsh 1984; Patterson & Oxford 1986). Virus is usually endocytosed in coated pits. Viral entry is rapid with a $t_{1/2}$ of about 10 minutes (Martin *et al.* 1981; Yoshimura *et al.* 1982), but this is dependent on both the virus strain and the cell type.

The low pH required for membrane fusion of the endosome and virus may also be important in later uncoating stages and this may well provide a useful target for anti-influenza compounds; these will be discussed later. However, as yet, there are no potential therapeutic compounds that act directly to prevent endocytosis of the virus. Indeed as endocytosis is an essential function for any cell it would seem at first sight to be extremely difficult to design a highly selective compound with a satisfactory therapeutic index.

Stage 3: Influenza virus uncoating

It has been suggested that influenza virus undergoes a two-stage uncoating process (Bukrinskaya *et al.* 1982a,b).

1 Primary uncoating in which the viral lipid membrane fuses with the endosomal lipid membrane, in the cell cytoplasm.

2 Secondary uncoating in which the viral matrix protein is removed from the ribonucleoprotein (RNP) complex thus enabling release of viral RNA, which enters the nucleus of the cell.

Primary uncoating

Once the virus is inside the cell the endosomal vesicle pH is lowered by an ATP-dependent proton pump and the subsequent fusion of the viral and endosomal membranes is rapid and efficient (Davey *et al.* 1985). In the low-pH environment of the endosome the membrane fusion activity of the HA is triggered. The optimal range for this is pH 5–6.4 (Daniels 1985), but varies somewhat with the strain of influenza virus. The conformational change that occurs in the HA at low pH causes the HA1 globular head to lose its trimeric structure (Doms *et al.* 1985; Gething *et al.* 1986) although the stem remains trimeric (Ruigrok *et al.* 1988). The remarkable study of Bullough *et al.* (1994) described crystallization of the low-pH bromelain-released portion of HA_2 and showed dramatic movement of the structure transporting the fusion peptide over a distance of at least 100 Å towards the host cell membrane. This flexibility may play a role in the fusion mechanism. Conformational change exposes

10 uncharged hydrophobic amino acids in the N-terminal sequence of the HA_2 (Skehel & Waterfield 1975). In the neutral conformation these are buried in a hydrophobic cleft at the interface between the monomers (Ruigrok *et al.* 1986a,b). This decapeptide is also homologous with the N-terminus of the fusion (F) protein of Sendai virus (Skehel & Waterfield 1975; Scheid & Choppin 1977). The precise mechanism of fusion or the catalytic role of the fusion motif of HA_2 is still not entirely clear (Stegmann 1994).

The intracellular fusion of the virus with the endosomal membrane releases a subviral particle (SVP) — i.e. the RNP in conjunction with the M proteins — into the cytoplasm where secondary uncoating occurs. Obviously this is a vital stage of the virus life cycle and provides an opportunity for anti-influenza drugs to act.

Prevention of acidification of the endosome can be achieved crudely by the use of bases to buffer the lowering pH, e.g basic amine derivatives. Chloroquine and norakin are both believed to act in this way (Shibata *et al.* 1983). As yet, however, there are no possible compounds that are capable of blocking this stage and acting therapeutically *in vivo*.

Inhibition of virus cell fusion

Fusion mediated by the HA is a vital step in the life cycle of the virus, but there is still an unclear understanding of the role of the different portions of the HA. For example, Kemble *et al.* (1994) reported that the transmembrane domain is required for fusion, whilst there is additional evidence that the cytoplasmic tail may also be involved.

A series of sulphonic acid polymers have been shown to be potent and selective inhibitors of influenza A virus (Ikeda *et al.* 1994). These compounds inhibit the replication of influenza A virus in both HeLa (at a concentration of 0.15 μg/ml) and Madin–Darby canine kidney (MDCK) cells (at a concentration of 4.0 μg/ml). The compounds are non-toxic to the cells at concentrations greater than 1000 μg/ml. The mode of antiviral action of the sulphonic acid polymers is believed to be the inhibition of virus–cell fusion. The prototype sulphonic acid polymer poly 2-acrylamido-2-methyl-1-propanesulphonic acid (PAMPS) when administered intranasally (at the time of infection) to mice as a single dose of 10 or 50 mg per kg of body weight completely inhibited influenza A virus replication in the lungs. In addition, virus-associated lung consolidation in immunocompetent mice was reduced and SCID (severe combined immune deficient) mice were completely protected against influenza A virus-associated mortality. However, when it was administered 1 h before or after virus inoculation, no protective effect was observed at a dose of 10 or 100 mg/kg.

The plant flavonoid 5,7,4'-trihydroxy-8-methoxyflavone (F36), which is extracted from the roots of *Scutellaria baicalensis*, significantly reduced the single cycle replication of influenza virus from 4 h to 12 h in a dose-dependent manner (Nagai *et al.* 1995). F36 acted by inhibiting the fusion of A/PR8 with the endosome when added between 0 and 2 h after infection. Interestingly F36 also appears to act by preventing budding of the progeny virus from the cell when it is added 3 h post incubation. It is believed that the flavonoid acts at this stage by inhibiting the NA and thus prevents the elution of the virus from neuraminic acid molecules on the host cell. NA inhibitors are considered in more detail in Chapter 36.

Prevention of the conformational change of the HA

An alternative point of action for anti-influenza drugs would be to disrupt the structure of the HA earlier in the viral life cycle. The conformational change in HA is irreversible and if the target membrane is absent then the HA becomes both fusion and receptor binding incompetent (Stegmann *et al.* 1987).

Dextran sulphate with molecular weights of 8000 and 500 000 has been shown to be an effective inhibitor of a range of viruses. With regard to influenza virus it prevents fusion of influenza virus with red blood cells (RBC) (Krumbiegel *et al.* 1992). The polymer strongly inhibited the low pH-induced fusion. Virus–RBC fusion was completely blocked by the high molecular weight dextran sulphate at concentrations of 0.5 mg/ml. The polymer was only inhibitory when added at early stages of the fusion reaction, but the pH-induced conformational change of the HA was not affected by dextran sulphate as measured by its susceptibility to proteolytic digestion. Removal of dextran sulphate after the low pH-requiring stages allowed the system to fuse at neutral pH indicating that the inhibitory effect requires the continuous presence of dextran sulphate during the fusion reaction. It is currently unclear at what stage dextran sulphate acts, although it may interfere with the low pH-requiring conformational changes leading to formation of the 'prefusion complex'. If dextran sulphate is not present, presumably the complex is sufficiently stable by this stage that dextran sulphate is no longer effective (Krumbiegel *et al.* 1992).

Secondary uncoating

The release of RNPs from their association with the viral M1 structural protein requires a lowering of pH (Zhirnov 1990) and this acidity is essential for successful infection (Martin & Helenius 1991a,b). It has been proposed that the ion channel activity of the influenza M2 protein is important in lowering the pH surrounding the subviral particle and allowing uncoating (Pinto *et al.* 1992). The action of the M2 as a proton pump provides an explanation for the earlier observation that rimantadine prevents the secondary uncoating stages (Bukrinskaya *et al.* 1982a,b). Amantadine and rimantadine both act by interfering with M2 protein activity, presumably by acting like a gate to obstruct the ion

channel. These important drugs and their mode of action is discussed in more detail in Chapter 35.

Influenza A virus M2 proton pump inhibitors other than amantadine

Studies of the role of M2 as a proton pump have emerged as a result of interest in the mode of action of amantadine. There is evidence that the pump may exert several important influences. For example, the demonstration of the H^+ conductance of the M2 channel provides direct evidence that the channel can acidify the interior of the virion as a prerequisite to viral uncoating and also in shunting the H^+ gradient of the trans-Golgi network. However, acidification of the virion would be incomplete if the only ion channel in the virion were a H^+ conducting channel. For example, in the absence of a counter ion only a few H^+ ions would enter the virion before an unacceptable membrane potential developed. It may turn out therefore that ions other than H^+, which would exert ion selectivity and antiviral properties on certain avian viruses, are also conducted by the M2 protein. M2 may prevent the pH of the trans-Golgi network dropping to a level which would inactivate HA prior to insertion into the plasma membrane Other compounds based on the structures of amantadine and rimantadine have been shown to inhibit influenza virus replication (Garcia Martinez *et al.* 1995). Compounds 1 and 11 in Table 37.1 have been shown to have a high therapeutic index (TI) against influenza (TI = 1000). Their anti-influenza activity appears to

Table 37.1 Biological properties of substituted 1-norbornylamines with antiviral activity (Garcia Martinez *et al.* 1995).

Compound in Fig. 37.2	MIC_{50} (µg/ml)	MTC_{50} (µg/ml)	Therapeutic index (ratio of MIC_{50} to MTC_{50})
1	0.1	100	1000
2	5	50	10
6	< 10	100	> 10
11	0.1	100	1000
12	5	200	40
13	1	100	10
Amantadine	0.5	300	600

MIC_{50}, minimum inhibitory concentration required to effect a 50% reduction in virus yield; MTC_{50}, minimum toxic concentration affecting 50% of the cells.

be favoured in the presence of a *gem*-dimethyl group at the C-2 (or C-7) positions of the 1-norbornylamine framework (Fig. 37.2).

A novel inhibitor of the influenza A virus M2 proton pump has recently been identified. This compound (2-[3-azaspiro (5,5) undecanol)]-2-imidazoline) is designated BL1743. This compound blocked the action of the M2 in *Xenopus laevis* oocytes (Tu *et al.* 1996). Interestingly the action of this compound, unlike that of amantadine, is reversible. However, amino acid substitutions in M2 that confer resistance to BL1743 also confer resistance to amantadine and vice versa.

Bafilomycin A1 (Baf-A1) is a novel and highly specific inhibitor for vacuolar-type proton (V-H$^+$) pumps and has also been shown to prevent influenza A and B infection in MDCK cells *in vitro* (Ochiai *et al.* 1995). Baf-A1 caused the disappearance of acidified compartments such as endosomes and lysosomes in both infected and uninfected cells after treatment with 0.1 μM inhi-

bitor for 1 h at 37 °C. After Baf-A1 is removed the acidified compartments reappear and this is correlated with the recovery of virus growth.

Protease inhibitors

In general terms viral proteases have been a focus of many studies with HIV (Mozen 1993; Garten *et al.* 1994; Wlodawer 1994; Boucher & Reedijk 1995; Deminie *et al.* 1996; Keulen *et al.* 1996; Moyle 1996) and rhinoviruses (Molla *et al.* 1993; Heinz *et al.* 1996). These enzymes are therefore of great interest to antiviral chemotherapists and the blockade of the cellular enzymes required to proteolytically cleave the influenza HA is a very valid target for antivirals. The requirement for cleavage of the HA for the influenza virus to be infective is demonstrated by the fact that only virions with cleaved HA have the ability to fuse with membrane and are infectious (Garten *et al.* 1981; Webster & Rott 1987). Importantly HA cleavage is required for all three

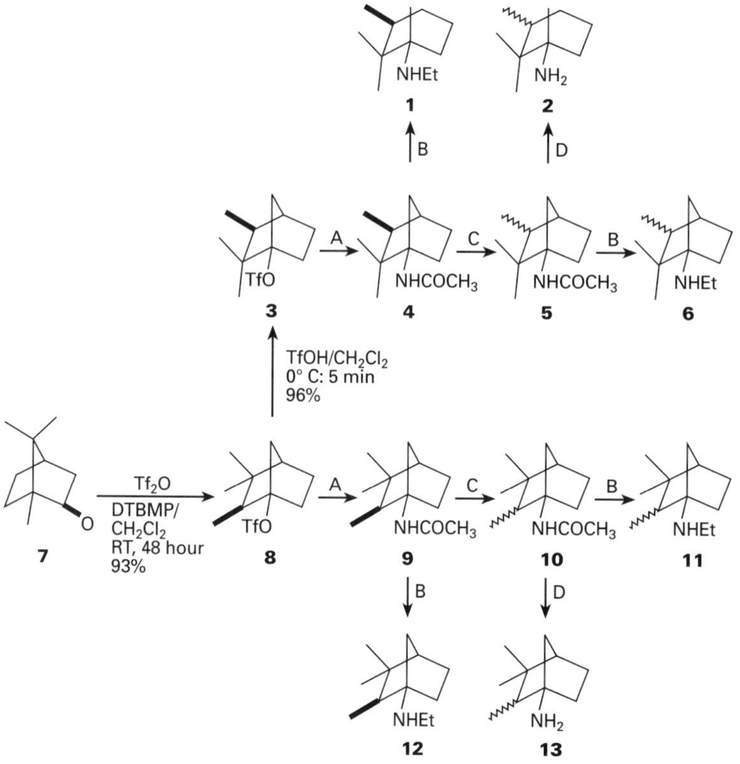

Fig. 37.2 Structures of substituted 1-norbornylamines with antiviral activity. The reaction of camphor (7) with triflic anhydride (Tf$_2$O) yields the bridgehead triflate (8). The Nametkin rearrangement of 8–3 was realized by treatment with triflic acid. The solvolysis of 3 and 8 in acetonitrile gives the AT-acetyl-1-norbornylamines 4 and 9. The hydrogenation of 4 and 9 gives the amides 5 and 10. The corresponding 1-norbornylamines 2 and 13 and the N-ethyl derivatives 1, 6, 11 and 12 were obtained by basic hydrolysis or reduction with LAiH$_{41}$, respectively, of the amides 4, 5, 9 and 10 (From Garcia Martinez *et al.* 1995, with permission from American Chemical Society.)

types of influenza (A, B and C); therefore a compound that is capable of inhibiting proteolytic cleavage of the HA may be active against all influenza viruses.

The protease inhibitors ε-aminocaproic acid and aprotinin have both been shown to suppress human influenza virus A replication in infected mice, presumably through prevention of HA cleavage at monobasic cleavage sites (Zhirnov *et al.* 1984). Another protease inhibitor, leupeptin, prevented replication of swine influenza A virus during a coinfection with *Staphylococcus aureus*, where the staphylococcal proteases catalysed the cleavage of the HA (Tashiro *et al.* 1987). The synthetic protease inhibitors, peptidyl choloralkyl ketones, have also been shown to inhibit influenza virus replication (fowl plague virus) at multibasic cleavage sites (Garten *et al.* 1989).

The trypsin inhibitor 6-amino-2-naphthyl-p-guanidinobenzoate (Futhan) completely blocks influenza A WSN virus-induced plaque formation in MDCK cells and uncleaved HA accumulates within the cells (Someya *et al.* 1990).

An anticathepsin B IgG antibody has also been shown to inhibit replication of influenza A WSN virus in MDCK cells (Someya *et al.* 1994). Unfortunately there are a large number of cellular enzymes with trypsin-like properties that are capable of catalysing this important cleavage of HA and it has so far proved difficult to identify suitable inhibitory compounds.

HA conformation stabilizing compounds

Studies of inhibitors of rhinovirus have uncovered a whole series of compounds that bind to structural virus proteins and stabilize the virion, preventing uncoating (Andries *et al.* 1988). Some low molecular weight compounds have been described which prevent conformational changes of HA (Bodian *et al.* 1993). These are small molecules that bind to the non-fusogenic form of HA and stabilize that conformation over all other fusogenic conformations. Using a computer-assisted technique a range of putative HA ligands were selected. One of these compounds (4A,5,8,8A-tetrahydro-5,8-methano-11,4-napthoquinone) prevented the conversion of

influenza A (X31) HA to a conformation recognized by α-fusion peptide antisera. In addition several derivatives of this compound including benzoquinones and hydroxyquinones also showed activity.

Stage 4: Primary transcription of input influenza vRNA to give mRNA

Within minutes of infection of a cell by influenza virus the negative-sense, single-stranded segmented RNA genome within the virus particle is transcribed and replicated by the trimeric virion transcriptase composed of PB1, PB2 and PA (Honda *et al.* 1988; Krug 1989) (see Fig. 37.3). The host cell transcriptional machinery is utilized for both viral RNA transcription and also methylation and splicing of viral mRNAs (Kelly *et al.* 1974). All influenza viral RNA synthesis is nuclear (Shapiro *et al.* 1987). Viral mRNA species are transcribed from the vRNA, transported to cellular ribosomes and translated into virus proteins (Shapiro *et al.* 1987). The mRNAs are shorter than the template and lack sequences complementary to the last 17–22 nucleotides of the 5′ end of the vRNA. Their primary transcripts are capped at the 5′ end and polyadenylated at the 3′ end. Influenza virus uses novel mechanisms for mRNA synthesis utilizing host cell capped mRNA (or pre-mRNA) as primers for virus transcription (Plotch *et al.* 1981). The viral protein PB2 acts as an endonuclease that recognizes and cleaves capped and methylated host RNAs at a purine residue 10–13 nucleotides from the cap (Shaw & Lamb 1984). These RNA fragments are then used as primers (Ulmanen *et al.* 1983; Braam-Markson *et al.* 1985). PB1 initiates transcription by catalysing the incorporation of a G residue and is then involved in elongation (Ulmanen *et al.* 1981; Blass *et al.* 1982; Penn *et al.* 1982; Ulmanen *et al.* 1983; Romanos & Hay 1984).

Antisense oligonucleotides

Sequence-specific antisense oligonucleotides can bind to and block the promoter recognition site of the RNA polymerase complex and should therefore inhibit the copying process of influenza virus, but

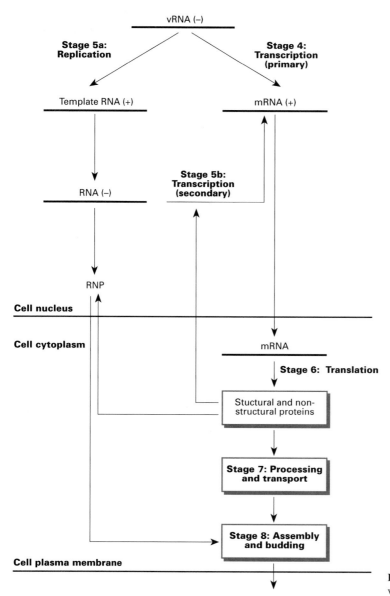

Fig. 37.3 Stages 4–8 of the influenza virus life cycle.

should not interfere with the host replication machinery. Also short oligonucleotides (4–9 nucleotides in length) can bind to influenza virus RNA polymerase and specifically inhibit cap-dependent mRNA synthesis.

Recently Fodor (1996) described oligoribonucleotides that may be useful as specific antiviral agents. These oligoribonucleotides bind to and block the promoter recognition site of the RNA polymerase complex and, in theory, they could inhibit the replication of influenza virus without interfering with the host cell's replicative machinery. A novel approach to the preparation of m^{7}Gppp-oligoribonucleotides for use as primers for influenza A virus RNA polymerase *in vitro* has also been described (Brownlee *et al.* 1995). These potential anti-influenza compounds are short, capped oligoribonucleotides in the range 4–9 nucleotides in length which can bind to influenza virus RNA polymerase and specifically inhibit cap-dependent mRNA synthesis *in vitro*.

Nucleoside analogues

For HIV and herpes viruses nucleoside analogues and dideoxy nucleoside analogues have proved to be a fruitful source of new drugs, but for influenza only a handful of nucleoside analogues have been identified. Ribavirin, a synthetic nucleoside analogue 1-β-D-ribofuranosyl-1,2,4-triazole-3-carboxamide, has shown anti-influenza A and B virus activity in cell culture, in animal models and in certain clinical situations. It is a guanosine analogue, broad-spectrum antiviral agent that is considered to decrease the available pool of guanosine triphosphate (GTP), thereby indirectly suppressing synthesis of viral nucleic acid. It achieves this by potently inhibiting inosine 5'-monophosphate dehydrogenase activity (Malinoski & Stollar 1981). It is suggested that the remaining cellular and viral enzymes compete for the depleted concentration of GTP. This hypothesis however, suffers from the observation that the 1,4,5-triazole derivative of ribavirin—which also depletes the cellular pool of GTP—has no antiviral activity (Smith 1984). However, it should be emphasized that other mechanisms of action have also been proposed and therefore this does not preclude depletion of GTP as being important in the activity of ribavirin. Thus it has been proposed that ribavirin may also act by causing the synthesis of RNA with an abnormal or no cap structure. This hypothesis is based upon observations with vaccinia virus (Katz *et al.* 1976). The compound was an effective direct competitive inhibitor of mRNA (guanine-N^7-)-methyltransferase (Gotch *et al.* 1987).

Finally, it may also act directly to suppress the action of the viral polymerase (Oxford 1975; Browne 1979; Burlington et al. 1983; Wray *et al.* 1985). Studies with the varicella zoster virus have shown that ribavirin does have a direct effect on the viral polymerase (Toltzis *et al.* 1988). It is suggested that ribavirin may be similar to the natural substrates of the enzyme including all four of the nucleoside triphosphates.

In clinical trials when used prophylactically at a dose of 1000 mg per day ribavirin can reduce the severity of the influenza illness and the level of virus shedding (Magnussen *et al.* 1977). However, this dose is not effective orally if onset of symptoms has occurred, even if given promptly, i.e. within 24 h (Smith *et al.* 1980). Ribavirin can however, be effective therapeutically if administered by aerosol in a nebulizer. In experiments with college students ribavirin administered by aerosol for 18 h on the first day and 12 h daily for the next 2–3 days was shown to be effective at reducing the duration of fever, virus shedding and general systemic symptoms. The total dose administered was 2.4 g over 48 h (Gilbert *et al.* 1985). Shorter-duration higher-dose aerosolized therapy with ribavirin has been shown to be effective in controlling respiratory syncytial virus (RSV) infection in infants (Knight *et al.* 1991); further human studies are now required with influenza virus. Generally, however, the use of aerosolized ribavirin would appear to be limited due to practicalities of administration, i.e. the long duration of therapy and the requirement for hospitalization. Pharmacokinetic data regarding ribavirin is limited. The plasma half-life is approximately 9 h (Van Dyke *et al.* 1982) and approximately 53% of the administered dose is excreted in the urine (Catlin *et al.* 1980).

A number of other nucleoside analogues have anti-influenza activity *in vitro* but have not progressed to studies in animal models or humans (Shigita *et al.* 1988).

Direct binding to the RNA transcriptase enzyme

Studies soon after the discovery of the influenza virion-associated transcriptase enzyme identified a series of molecules with powerful enzyme inhibitory activities. The compounds were strong chelators of heavy metals such as zinc and copper. This approach explored the possibility that the viral enzyme was a zinc metalloenzyme (Oxford & Perrin 1977). Subsequent studies have identified zinc finger motifs (Nasser *et al.* 1996). In general, at least two approaches are possible, the most straightforward being compounds to bind zinc and the transcriptase complex and hence to sterically hinder the enzymatic process. An alternative, but less appealing approach, would be to dissociate zinc from the enzyme complex. We were able to quantify zinc in the RNP complex of highly purified influenza viruses by sensitive atomic absorption and to identify a series of thiocarbazones as potent *in vitro* inhibitors of the viral RNA polymerase. However, these compounds failed to inhibit viral replication *in vitro*.

Stage 5: Replication of vRNA and secondary transcription

Synthesis of template RNA$^+$ is dependent on continued viral protein synthesis. Presumably a modified form of the viral transcriptase enzyme is used as a replicase. Both enzymes are unique viral enzymes and so represent excellent targets for inhibition. It is therefore somewhat surprising that more inhibitory compounds have not been discovered. Template RNA$^+$ represents a complete transcript of vRNA and lacks poly(A) (Lamb & Choppin 1983). Replication is under the control of the viral polymerase proteins, but there is no requirement for host cell capped mRNA to act as primers (Beaton & Krug 1984). Secondary transcription uses these newly synthesized vRNAs to produce more mRNAs.

Stimulation of host cell RNA synthesis

In view of all the considerations detailed above of specific virus-coded targets could alternative approaches be explored in the search for new anti-influenza drugs?

Inosine pranobex is a synthetic compound formed from the p-acetamido benzoate salt of N-N dimethylamino-2-propanol and inosine in a 3:1 molar ratio. Host cell RNA synthesis is stimulated by inosine pranobex, with a resulting decrease in viral RNA synthesis (Ohnishi *et al.* 1982). In addition it is believed to have an immunomodulating effect. It does not stimulate resting lymphocytes, but augments immunological processes by lymphocytes once triggered by mitogen or viral infection (Campoli-Richards *et al.* 1986).

One proposed mechanism of action is that a

component of the drug or the drug complex links itself to the ribosomes of the virus-infected cells. This provokes a steric modification that renders an advantage to cellular RNA over viral RNA in the competition for linkage with the ribosomal combining sites. The consequence would be a non-reading or incorrect transcription of the viral RNA.

In vivo experiments have shown that influenza virus shedding is reduced when the drug is used and there is a corresponding increase in survival of mice infected experimentally with influenza A or B viruses (Glasky *et al.* 1971; Muldoon *et al.* 1972; Ohinski *et al.* 1983).

There have only been limited clinical trials conducted with inosine pranobex to determine efficacy against influenza virus. In double-blind placebo-controlled studies in volunteers challenged intranasally with influenza A, doses as high as 4–5 g per day failed to reduce the incidence of illness or the rate of seroconversion. However, two of the studies did show a significant reduction in viral shedding (Longley *et al.* 1973; Betts *et al.* 1978) and in three of the studies a significant reduction in symptoms was also observed in those given the drug (Betts *et al.* 1978; Schiff *et al.* 1978; Khakoo *et al.* 1981). Generally inosine pranobex is well tolerated by patients and free of serious side-effects (Glasky *et al.* 1975).

Stage 6: Translation of mRNA

New influenza viral proteins can be detected in cells within 1 h of influenza virus infection. With some, but certainly not all, influenza A viruses there is a decrease in host cell protein synthesis soon after infection (Skehel 1972). Several groups have delineated an early phase of influenza virus replication where viral proteins NP and NS1 are preferentially synthesized. This is followed by a later phase where the synthesis of NS1 declines and that of M1, HA and NA increases (Skehel 1973; Meier-Ewert & Compans 1974; Hay *et al.* 1977; Inglis & Mahy 1979; Minor et al. 1979). Not unexpectedly, variations in this pattern have been reported which depend on the host cell. Synthesis of PB1, PB2 and PA continue at a low rate throughout the infectious cycle. At present no details have been presented of antivirals that may interfere with this closely controlled series of events.

Stage 7: Post-translational modification of viral proteins

The influenza HA and the NA glycoprotein spike proteins are cotranslationally inserted into the rough endoplasmic reticulum (RER). The N-terminal signal peptide is removed and the polypeptides are glycosylated (Lamb & Choppin 1983). The glycoproteins are then transported via the Golgi apparatus to the cell membrane. The HA trimer is believed to be formed in the RER, before the HA enters the Golgi apparatus (Copeland *et al.* 1986; Gething *et al.* 1986). At what stage the NA tetramers are formed is not yet clear.

Once assembled, the HA trimer is rapidly exported from the RER to the *cis* face of the Golgi apparatus. In the Golgi apparatus the oligosaccharides on the glycoproteins are enzymatically 'trimmed', that is, glucose and mannose residues are removed and N-acetylglucosamine, galactose and fucose are added (Keil *et al.* 1984). For some strains of influenza the cleavage of the HA into HA_1 and HA_2 can occur in the Golgi apparatus. In other strains cleavage occurs at the plasma membrane.

The other structural viral proteins are believed to reach the plasma membrane by diffusion. The viral M1 protein forms an electron-dense layer beneath the plasma membrane (Schulze 1972). Synthesis of this protein may be the rate-limiting stages for the formation of virus particles (Lazarowitz *et al.* 1971). No antiviral compounds have yet been described that act at this important stage of the virus life cycle.

Stage 8: Assembly of viral structural components and release of progeny virus

At the plasma membrane the influenza structural proteins are assembled into virions. Surprisingly, no host cell proteins are detected in the mature virus and presumably a mechanism exists to exclude them (Wang *et al.* 1976). The viral glycoproteins are inserted into the plasma membrane (Lenard & Compans 1974), and then the NP and M

proteins become attached to the cytoplasmic side of the membrane where there is a patch of spike proteins on the extracellular side. A 'tail' of AA may be a recognition factor for M1. The exact mechanism whereby influenza A virus particles bud from the plasma membrane is not understood. For viruses containing an M protein, such as influenza, it has been proposed that coupling of the nucleocapsid causes the M protein to polymerize. The plasma membrane then bulges outward. This is dependent on there being sufficient glycoprotein inserted into the plasma membrane to anchor the M protein layer (Simons & Garoff 1980).

The progeny virus particles are produced by budding from the cell membrane. The NA glycoprotein acts enzymatically to ensure the release of mature virus from the N-acetylneuraminic acid incorporated in the virus glycoproteins and on the cell surface. Thus anti-NA antibodies prevent release of progeny virus, causing them to aggregate at the cell surface (Dowdle *et al.* 1974; Webster *et al.* 1982). Likewise the new anti-NA compounds can act at this stage of the virus life cycle; see Chapter 36.

The viral NP and M1 proteins are found in association near the plasma membrane of an infected cell, but they are not found near virus particles which suggests that budding is rapid (Patterson *et al.* 1988). Virus assembly is clearly a potential target for chemotherapeutic intervention. The observations that a synthetic peptide mimicking the intracellular domain of the HA can prevent the release of progeny virions suggest that this may be a feasible approach to chemotherapy (Collier *et al.* 1991). This decapeptide contains the amino acids corresponding to the residues 213–222. It has been observed that between concentrations of 50 and 250 µg/ml a dose-dependent response is observed when the peptide is added to cultured cells for a 2-hour period during a one-cycle viral growth. The peptide was not found to have any effect on the formation of intracellular virus-specific proteins or assembly of nucleocapsids and did not inhibit replication of two unrelated enveloped RNA viruses (Sindbis and vesicular stomatitis virus). Peptides of a similar size, but not corresponding to the transmembrane domain, were not effective (Collier *et al.* 1991), suggesting that the peptide is a competitive inhibitor for virus-specific protein–protein interaction between the HA and the matrix protein or nucleocapsid during the assembly of the virion. It is important to emphasize that the synthesis of viral HA protein is unaffected and that therefore the immune response would still be maintained, adding in the *in vivo* situation to the antiviral effect of the peptide. However, the three influenza viruses (A, B and C) have different amino acid sequences in the intracellular domain which would make it difficult to design a single general anti-influenza virus peptide.

Conclusion

It is not surprising that the influenza virus NA protein, because of the detailed X-ray structure analysis already carried out, has recently been the primary antiviral target and that two drugs have been discovered with some realistic clinical potential. The viral RNA transcriptase, being constituted of several proteins, will be a much more complicated enzyme structure to solve. We can safely predict though that nucleotide sequence data of all the influenza genes could be exploited for new drug design. An excellent example is the M2 proton pump where, given data on amino acid sequence and the amino acid changes in drug-resistant variants, a reasonably clear functional picture can be reconstructed of the functional viral protein and possible inhibitors can be designed.

Of the immediate need for a new generation of antiviral drugs there can be no doubt. A new pandemic influenza A virus is expected, while in addition, the yearly epidemics take a surprisingly high toll even with new antibiotics and new vaccination campaigns directed at the vulnerable over 75-year-olds in the population.

In a broad sense, antiviral chemotherapy has been transformed beyond all recognition since the tentative beginnings with amantadine and influenza A virus in the late 1960s. Now leading pharmaceutical companies depend on antiviral drugs such as Zovirax against herpes (Cassidy & Whitley 1997) and Retrovir and a wide range of antiviral reverse transcriptase enzyme drugs (Oxford *et al.* 1996) to generate finance for further research into new antivirals. Influenza has benefited from this realization that viral disease can be prevented and also treated and that antivirals can be profitable pharmaceuticals. In addition, the simple idea of drug combinations against highly mutable RNA viruses has begun to prove its worth in HIV clinics and this has led to active cooperation between pharmaceutical companies which possess antiviral drugs acting at different targets during the viral life cycle. Basic scientific interest in the method of action of antivirals has led to exciting new discoveries, for example the work on M2 protein and amantadine resistance. The most difficult but probably the most satisfactory target for influenza remains the viral RNA transcriptase/replicase enzyme and we would predict that amongst the many 'other antivirals', this could generate the most exciting science and drugs over the next few years.

References

Andries, K., Dewindt, B., Brabander, M., Stokbroetex, R.W. & Jansen, P.A.J. (1988) In-vitro activity of R61837, a new anti-rhinovirus compound. *Arch Virol* **101**, 155–67.

Ashley, J., Smith, T. & Dunnel, K. (1991) In: *Population Trends: Office of Population Censuses and Surveys*, Vol. 65, pp. 16–20. HM Stationery Office, London.

Beaton, A.R. & Krug, R.M. (1984) Synthesis of templates for influenza virion RNA replication *in vitro*. *Proc Natl Acad Sci USA* **81**, 4682–6.

Betts, R., Douglas, R. Jr, George, S. & Rinehart, C. (1978) In: *67th Annual Meeting of the American Society for Microbiology*.

Bizebard, T., Gigant, B., Rigolet, P. *et al.* (1995) Structure of influenza virus haemagglutinin complexed with a neutralizing antibody. *Nature* **376**, 92–4.

Blass, D., Patezelk, E. & Kuecher, E. (1982) Identification of the cap binding protein of influenza virus. *Nucl Acids Res* **10**, 4803–12.

Bodian, D.L., Yamasaki, R.B., Buswell, R.L., Stearns, J.F., White, J.M. & Kuntz, I.D. (1993) Inhibition of the fusion-inducing conformational change of influenza hemagglutinin by benzoquinones and hydroquinones. *Biochem* **32**, 2967–78.

Boucher, C.A. & Reedijk, M. (1995) Viral resistance: a major challenge in managing HIV disease. *J Biol Regul Homeost* **9**, 91–4.

Braam-Markson, J., Jaudon, C. & Krug, R.M. (1985) Expression of a functional influenza viral cap-recognising protein by using a bovine papilloma virus vector. *Proc Natl Acad Sci USA* **82**, 4326–30.

Browne, M.J. (1979) Mechanism and specificity of action of ribavirin. *Antimicrobial Agents Chemother* **15**, 747–53.

Brownlee, G., Fodor, E. & Pritlove, D. (1995) Characterisation of the RNA-fork model of virion RNA in the initiation of transcription in influenza A virus. *Nucl Acids Res* **23**, 2641–7.

Bukrinskaya, A.G., Vorkunova, N.K., Kornilayeva, R., Narmanbetova, R.A. & Vorkunova, G.K. (1982a) Influenza virus uncoating in infected cells and effect of rimantadine. *J Gen Virol* **60**, 49–59.

Bukrinskaya, A.G., Vorkunova, N.K. & Pusharskaya, N.L. (1982b) Uncoating of a rimantadine-resistant variant of influenza virus in the presence of rimantadine. *J Gen Virol* **60**, 61–6.

Bullough, P.A., Hughson, F.M., Skehel, J.J. & Wiley, D.C. (1994) Structure of influenza haemagglutinin at the pH of membrane fusion. *Nature* **371**, 37–43.

Burlington, D.B., Meiklejohn, G. & Mostow, S.R. (1983) Anti-influenza A activity of combinations of amantadine and ribavirin in ferret tracheal ciliated epithelium. *J Antimicrobial Chemother* **11**, 7–14.

Campoli-Richards, D.M., Sorkin, E.M. & Heel, R.C. (1986) Inosine pranobex. A preliminary review of its pharmacodynamic and pharmacokinetic properties, and therapeutic efficacy. *Drugs* **32**, 383–424.

Cassidy, K.A. & Whitley, R.J. (1997) New therapeutic approaches to the alpha herpes virus infections. *J Antimicrobial Chemother* **39**, 119–28.

Catlin, D., Smith, R. & Samuels, A. (1980) In: Smith, R. & Kirkpatric, W. (eds) *Ribavirin – A Broad Spectrum Antiviral Agent*, pp. 83–98. Academic Press, New York.

Collier, N.C., Knox, K. & Schlesinger, M.J. (1991) Inhibition of influenza virus formation by a peptide that corresponds to sequences in the cytoplasmic domain of the hemagglutinin. *Virology* **183**, 769–72.

Copeland, C., Doms, R.W., Bolzau, E.M., Webster, R.G. & Helenius, A. (1986) Assembly of influenza haemagglutinin trimers and its role in intracellular transport. *J Cell Biol* **103**, 1179–84.

Daniels, R.S. (1985) Fusion mutants of the influenza virus hemagglutinin glycoprotein. *Cell* **40**, 431–9.

Davey, J., Hurtley, S.M. & Warren, G. (1985) Reconstitution of an endocytic fusion event in a cell-free system. *Cell* **43**, 643–52.

Deminie, C.A., Bechtold, C.M., Stock, D. *et al.* (1996) Evaluation of reverse transcriptase and protease inhibitors in two-drug combinations against human immunodeficiency virus replication. *Antimicrobial Agents Chemother* **40**, 1346–51.

Deng, W.P. & Nickoloff, J.A. (1994) Preferential repair of UV damage in highly transcribed DNA diminishes UV-induced intrachromosomal recombination in mammalian cells. *Mol Cell Biol* **14**, 391–9.

Doms, R.W., Helenius, A. & White, J. (1985) Membrane fusion activity of the influenza virus hemagglutinin. *J Biol Chem* **260**, 2973–81.

Dourmashkin, R.R. & Tyrrell, D.A.J. (1970) Attachment of two myxoviruses to ciliated epithelial cells. *J Gen Virol* **9**, 77–88.

Dowdle, W.R., Downie, J.C. & Laver, W.G. (1974) Inhibition of virus release by antibodies to surface antigens of influenza viruses. *J Virol* **13**, 269–75.

Ellens, H., Bentz, J., Mason, D., Zhang, F. & White, J.M. (1990) Fusion of influenza haemagglutinin-expressing fibroblasts with glycophorin-bearing liposomes: role of haemagglutinin surface density. *Biochem* **29**, 9697–707.

Fodor, E. (1996) In: *Options for the Control of Influenza III.* Cairns, Australia.

Garcia Martinez, A., Teso Vilar, E., Garcia Fraile, A. *et al.* (1995) Synthesis of substituted 1-norbornylamines with antiviral activity. *J Med Chem* **38**, 4474–7.

Garten, W., Bosch, F.X., Linder, D., Rott, R. & Klenk, H.D. (1981) Proteolytic activation of the influenza virus hemagglutinin: the structure of the cleavage site and the enzymes involved in cleavage. *Virology* **115**, 361–74.

Garten, W., Hallenberger, S., Ortmann, D. *et al.* (1994) Processing of viral glycoproteins by the subtilisin-like endoprotease furin and its inhibition by specific peptidylchloroalkylketones. *Biochimie* **76**, 217–25.

Gething, M.J., Doms, R.W., York, D. & White, J.M. (1986) Studies on the mechanism of membrane fusion: site-specific mutagenesis of the hemagglutinin of influenza virus. *J Cell Biol* **102**, 11–23.

Gilbert, B., Wilson, S. & Knight, V. (1985) Ribavirin small-particle aerosol treatment of infections caused by influenza virus strains A/Victoria/7/83 (H1N1) and B/Texas/1/84. *Antimicrobial Agents Chemother* **27**, 309.

Glasky, A., Settineri, R. & Lynes, T. (1975) In: Meuwissen (ed.) *Combined Immunodeficiency Disease and Adenosine Deficiency, a Molecular Defect*, pp. 156–72. Academic Press, London.

Glick, G. & Toogood, P. (1991) Molecular recognition of bivalent sialosides by influenza virus. *J Am Chem Soc* **113**, 4701–4701.

Glick, G.D., Toogood, P.L., Wiley, D.C., Skehel, J.J. & Knowles, J.R. (1991) Ligand recognition by influenza virus. The binding of bivalent sialosides. *J Biol Chem* **266**, 23660–9.

Gotch, F., Rothbard, J., Howland, K., Townsend, A. & McMichael, A. (1987) Cytotoxic T lymphocytes recognize a fragment of influenza virus matrix protein in association with HLA-A2. *Nature* **326**, 881–2.

Gottschalk, A. (1957) The specific enzyme of influenza virus and *Vibrio cholerae*. *Biochim Biophys Acta* **23**, 645–8.

Hay, A.J., Lomniczki, B., Bellamy, A.R. & Skehel, J.J. (1977) Transcription of the influenza virus genome. *Virology* **83**, 337–55.

Heinz, B.A., Tang, J., Labus, J.M., Chadwell, F.W., Kaldor, S.W. & Hammond, M. (1996) Simple *in vitro* translation assay to analyze inhibitors of rhinovirus proteases. *Antimicrobial Agents Chemother* **40**, 267–70.

Honda, A., Ueda, K., Nagata, K. & Ishihama, A. (1988) RNA polymerase of influenza virus: role of NP in RNA chain elongation. *J Biochem* **104**, 1021–6.

Ikeda, S., Neyts, J., Verma, S., Wickramasinghe, A., Mohan, P. & De Clercq, E. (1994) *In vitro* and *in vivo* inhibition of ortho- and paramyxovirus infections by a new class of sulfonic acid polymers interacting with virus-cell binding and/or fusion. *Antimicrobial Agents Chemother* **38**, 256–9.

Inglis, S.C. & Mahy, B.W.J. (1979) Polypeptides specified by the influenza virus genome. 3. Control of synthesis in infected cells. *Virology* **95**, 154–64.

Itoh, M., Hetterich, P., Isecke, R., Brossmer, R. & Klenk, H.D. (1995) Suppression of influenza virus infection by an N-thioacetylneuraminic acid acrylamide copolymer resistant to neuraminidase. *Virology* **212**, 340–7.

Katz, E., Margalith, E. & Winer, B. (1976) Inhibition of vaccinia virus growth by the nucleoside analogue 1-beta-D-ribofuranosyl-1,2,4-triazole-3-carboxamide (virazole, ribavirin). *J Gen Virol* **32**, 327–30.

Keil, W., Niemann, H. & Schwatz, R.T. (1984) Carbohydrates of influenza virus. V. Oligosaccharides attached to individual glycosylation sites of the haemagglutinin of fowl plaque virus. *Virology* **179**, 759–67.

Kelly, D.C., Avery, R.J. & Dimmock, N.J. (1974) Failure of an influenza virus to initiate infection in enucleate BHK cells. *J Virol* **13**, 1155–61.

Kemble, G.W., Daniels, T. & White, J.M. (1994) Lipid anchored influenza haemagglutinin promotes semi-fusion not complete fusion. *Cell* **76**, 383–91.

Keulen, W., Boucher, C. & Berkhout, B. (1996) Nucleotide substitution patterns can predict the requirements for drug-resistance of HIV-1 proteins. *Antiviral Res* **31**, 45–57.

Khakoo, R., Watson, G., Waldman, R. & Ganguly, R. (1981) Effect of inosiplex (isoprinosine) on induced human influenza A infection. *J Antimicrob Chemother* **7**, 389–97.

Knight, V., Gilbert, B.E., Wyde, P.R. & Englund, J.A. (1991) High dose–short duration ribavirin aerosol treatment—a review. *Bulletin of the International Union Against Tuberculosis & Lung Disease* **66**, 97–101.

Krug, R.M. (1989) *The Influenza Viruses*. Plenum Publishing Corporation, New York.

Krumbiegel, M., Dimitrov, D.S., Puri, A. & Blumenthal, R. (1992) Dextran sulfate inhibits fusion of influenza virus and cells expressing influenza hemagglutinin with red blood cells. *Biochim Biophys Acta* **1110**, 158–64.

Lamb, R.A. & Choppin, P.W. (1983) The gene structure and replication of influenza virus. *Annu Rev Biochem* **52**, 467–506.

Lambkin, R., Oxford, J., Lo, K., Biao, L. & Fleming, D. (1997) A proportion of those in high-risk groups vaccinated against influenza fail to respond to the vaccine. In preparation.

Lazarowitz, S.G., Compans, R.W. & Choppin, P.W. (1971) Influenza virus structural and nonstructural proteins in infected cells and their plasma membranes. *Virology* **46**, 830–43.

Lees, W.J., Spaltenstein, A., Kingery-Wood, J.E. & Whitesides, G.M. (1994) Polyacrylamides bearing pendant alpha-sialoside groups strongly inhibit agglutination of erythrocytes by influenza A virus: multivalency and steric stabilization of particulate biological systems. *J Med Chem* **37**, 3419–33.

Lenard, J. & Compans, R.W. (1974) The membrane structure of lipid-containing viruses. *Biochim Biophys Acta* **332**, 341–50.

Longley, S., Dunning, R. & Waldman, R. (1973) Effect of isoprinosine against challenge with A (H3N2)/Hong Kong influenza virus in volunteers. *Antimicrobial Agents Chemother* **3**, 506–9.

Magnussen, C., Douglas, R. & Betts, R. (1977) Double blind evaluation of oral ribavirin (virazole) in experimental influenza A infection in volunteers. *Antimicrobial Agents Chemother* **12**, 498.

Malinoski, F. & Stollar, V. (1981) Inhibitors of IMP dehydrogenase prevent Sindbis virus replication and reduce GTP levels in *Aedes albopictus* cells. *Virology* **110**, 281–91.

Mammen, M., Dahmann, G. & Whitesides, G.M. (1995) Effective inhibitors of hemagglutination by influenza virus synthesized from polymers having active ester groups. Insight into mechanism of inhibition. *J Med Chem* **38**, 4179–90.

Marsh, M. (1984) The entry of animal viruses into cells by endocytosis. *Biochem J* **218**, 1–10.

Martin, K. & Helenius, A. (1991a) Nuclear transport of influenza ribonuclear proteins: the viral matrix protein (M1) promotes export and inhibits import. *Cell* **67**, 117–30.

Martin, K. & Helenius, A. (1991b) Transport of incoming influenza virus nucleocapsids into the nucleus. *J Virol* **65**, 232–44.

Martin, R.R., Couch, R.B., Greenberg, S.B., Cate, T.R. & Warr, G.A. (1981) Effects of infection with influenza virus on the function of polymorphonuclear leukocytes. *J Infect Dis* **144**, 279–80.

Matlin, K.S., Reggio, H., Helenius, A. & Simons, K. (1981) Infectious entry pathway of influenza virus in a canine kidney cell line. *J Cell Biol* **91**, 601–13.

Meier-Ewert, H. & Compans, R.W. (1974) Time course of synthesis and assembly of influenza virus proteins. *J Virol* **14**, 1083–91.

Minor, P.D., Hart, J.G. & Dimmock, N.J. (1979) Influence of the host cell on proteins synthesized by different strains of influenza virus. *Virology* **97**, 482–7.

Molla, A., Hellen, C.U. & Wimmer, E. (1993) Inhibition of proteolytic activity of poliovirus and rhinovirus 2A proteinases by elastase-specific inhibitors. *J Virol* **67**, 4688–95.

Morens, D.M. & Rash, V.M. (1995) Lessons from a nursing home outbreak of influenza A. *Infect Control Hosp Epidemiol* **16**, 275–80.

Moyle, G.J. (1996) Use of viral resistance patterns to anti-retroviral drugs in optimising selection of drug combinations and sequences. *Drugs* **52**, 168–85.

Mozen, M.M. (1993) HIV inactivation in plasma products. *J Clin Apheresis* **8**, 126–30.

Nagai, T., Moriguchi, R., Suzuki, Y., Tomimori, T. & Yamada, H. (1995) Mode of action of the anti-influenza virus activity of plant flavonoid 5,7,4′-trihydroxy-8-methoxyflavone, from the roots of *Scutellaria baicalensis*. *Antiviral Res* **26**, 11–25.

Nasser, E.,H., Judd, A.K., Sanchex, A., Anastasiou, D. & Bucher, D.J. (1996) Antiviral activity of influenza virus M1 zinc finger peptides. *J Virol* **70**, 8639–44.

Ochiai, H., Sakai, S., Hirabayashi, T., Shimizu, Y. & Terasawa, K. (1995) Inhibitory effect of bafilomycin A1, a specific inhibitor of vacuolar-type proton pump, on the growth of influenza A and B viruses in MDCK cells. *Antiviral Res* **27**, 425–30.

Ohnishi, H., Kosuzume, H., Inaba, H., Ohura, M. & Morita, Y. (1982) Mechanism of host defense suppression induced by viral infection: mode of action of inosiplex as an anti-viral agent. *Infect Immun* **38**, 243–50.

Outlaw, M.C. & Dimmock, N.J. (1993) IgG neutralization of type A influenza viruses and the inhibition of the endosomal fusion stage of the infectious pathway in BHK cells. *Virology* **195**, 413–21.

Oxford, J.S. (1975) Inhibition of the replication of influenza A and B viruses by a nucleoside analogue (ribavirin). *J Gen Virol* **28**, 409–14.

Oxford, J.S. (1994) Sodium deoxycholate exerts a direct destructive effect on HIV and influenza viruses *in vitro* and inhibits retrovirus-induced pathology in an animal model. *Antiviral Chem Chemother* **5**, 176–81.

Oxford, J.S. & Perrin, D.D. (1977) Influenza RNA transcriptase inhibitors: studies *in vitro* and *in vivo*. *Ann NY Acad Sci* **284**, 613–23.

Oxford, J.S., Al-Jabri, A.A., Stein, C.A. & Levantis, P. (1996) In: Kuo, L.C., Olsend, D.B. & Carroll, S.S. (eds) *Viral Polymerases and Related Proteins*, Vol. 275, pp. 555–600. Academic Press, San Diego.

Patterson, S. & Oxford, J.S. (1986) Early interactions between animal viruses and the host cell: relevance to viral vaccines. *Vaccine* **4**, 79–90.

Patterson, S., Gross, J. & Oxford, J.S. (1988) The intracellular distribution of influenza virus matrix protein and nucleoprotein in infected cells and their relationship to haemagglutinin in the plasma membrane. *J Gen Virol* **69**, 1859–72.

Penn, C.R., Blaas, D., Kuechler, E. & Mahy, B.W.J. (1982) Identification of the cap-binding protein of two strains of influenza A/FPV. *J Gen Virol* **62**, 177–80.

Pinto, L.H., Holsinger, L.J. & Lamb, R.A. (1992) Influenza M2 protein has ion channel activity. *Cell* **69**, 517–28.

Plotch, S.J., Bouloy, M., Ulmanen, I. & Krug, R.M. (1981) A unique cap (m^{7}GpppXm)-dependent influenza virion endonuclease cleaves capped mRNAs to generate the primers that initiate viral mRNA transcription. *Cell* **23**, 847–58.

Romanos, M.A. & Hay, A.J. (1984) Identification of the influenza virus transcriptase by affinity-labelling with pyridoxal 5′-phosphate. *Virology* **132**, 110–17.

Roy, R., Pon, R.A., Tropper, F.D. & Andersson, F.O. (1993) Michael addition of poly L-lysine to N-acryloylated sialosides—syntheses of influenza A virus hemagglutinin inhibitor and group B meningococcal polysaccharide vaccines. *J Chem Soc Chem Comm* 264–5.

Ruigrok, R.W.H., Martin, S.R., Wharton, S.R. *et al.* (1986a) Conformational changes in the haemagglutinin of influenza virus which accompany heat-induced fusion of virus with liposomes. *Virology* **155**, 484–97.

Ruigrok, R.W.H., Wrigley, N.G., Calder, L.J. *et al.* (1986b) Electron microscopy of the low pH structure of influenza virus hemagglutinin. *EMBO J* **5**, 41–9.

Ruigrok, R.W., Aitken, A., Calder, L.J. *et al.* (1988) Studies on the structure of the influenza virus haemagglutinin at the pH of membrane fusion. *J Gen Virol* **69**, 2785–95.

Ryan, D.M., Ticehurst, J., Dempsey, M.H. & Penn, C.R. (1994) Inhibition of influenza virus replication in mice by GG167 (4-guanidino-2,4-dideoxy-2,3-dehydro-N-acetylneuraminic acid) is consistent with extracellular activity of viral neuraminidase (sialidase). *Antimicrobial Agents Chemother* **38**, 2270–5.

Ryan, D.M., Ticehurst, J. & Dempsey, M.H. (1995) GG167 (4-guanidino-2,4-dideoxy-2,3-dehydro-N-acetylneuraminic acid) is a potent inhibitor of influenza virus in ferrets. *Antimicrobial Agents Chemother* **39**, 2583–4.

Sabesan, S., Duus, J.O., Neira, S. *et al.* (1992) Cluster sialoside inhibitors for influenza virus—synthesis, NMR, and biological studies. *J Am Chem Soc* **114**, 8363–75.

Sauter, N.K., Bednarski, M.D., Wurzburg, B.A. *et al.* (1989) Hemagglutinins from two influenza-virus variants bind to sialic-acid derivatives with millimolar dissociation constants—a 500 MHz proton nuclear magnetic resonance study. *Biochemistry* **28**, 8388–96.

Scheid, A. & Choppin, P.W. (1977) Two disulphide-linked polypeptide chains constitute the active F protein of paramyxoviruses. *Virology* **80**, 54–7.

Schiff, G., Roselle, G., Young, B., May, D. & Rotte, T. (1978) Clinical evaluation of isoprinosine in artificially induced influenza in humans. In: *78th Annual Meeting of the American Society of Microbiology*, abstract no. A74.

Schulze, I.T. (1972) The structure of influenza virus. II. A model based on the morphology and the composition of subviral particles. *Virology* **47**, 181–96.

Shapiro, G.I., Gurney, T. & Krug, R.M. (1987) Influenza virus genome expression: control mechanisms at early and late times of infection and nuclear cytoplasmic transport of virus-specific RNAs. *J Virol* **61**, 764–73.

Shaw, M.W. & Lamb, R.A. (1984) A specific sub-set of host-cell mRNAs prime influenza virus mRNA synthesis. *Virus Res* **1**, 455–67.

Shibata, M., Aoki, H., Tsurumi, T. *et al.* (1983) Mechanism of uncoating of influenza B virus in MDCK cells: action of chloroquine. *J Gen Virol* **64**, 1149–56.

Simons, K. & Garoff, H. (1980) The budding mechanisms of enveloped animal viruses. *J Gen Virol* **50**, 1–21.

Skehel, J.J. (1972) Polypeptide synthesis in influenza virus-infected cells. *Virology* **49**, 23–36.

Skehel, J.J. (1973) Early polypeptide synthesis in influenza virus-infected cells. *Virology* **56**, 396–408.

Skehel, J.J. & Waterfield, M.D. (1975) Studies on the primary structure of the haemagglutinin of influenza virus. *Proc Natl Acad Sci USA* **72**, 93–6.

Smith, R.A. (1984) In: Smith, R.A., Knight, V. & Smith, J. (eds) *Clinical Applications of Actions of Ribavirin*, pp. 1–18. Academic Press, New York.

Smith, C., Charette, R. & Fox, J. (1980) Lack of effect of oral ribavirin in naturally occurring influenza A virus (H1N1) infection. *J Infect Dis* **141**, 548.

Someya, A., Tanaka, N. & Okuyama, A. (1990) Inhibition of influenza virus A/WSN replication by a trypsin inhibitor, 6-amidino-2-naphthyl p-guanidinobenzoate. *Biochem Biophys Res Commun* **169**, 148–52.

Someya, A., Tanaka, N. & Okuyama, A. (1994) Inhibition of influenza virus A/WSN replication by serine protease inhibitors and anti-protease antibodies. *Antiviral Chem Chemother* **5**, 187–90.

Spevak, W. (1993) *J Am Chem Soc.*

Spevak, W., Nagy, J.O., Charych, D.H., Schaefer, M.E., Gilbert, J.H. & Bednarski, M.D. (1993) Polymerized liposomes containing C-glycosides of sialic acid — potent inhibitors of influenza virus *in vitro* infectivity. *J Am Chem Soc* **115**, 1146–7.

Stegmann, T. (1994) Membrane fusion Anchors aweigh. *Curr Biol* **4**, 551–4.

Stegmann, T., Morselt, H.W., Booy, F.P., van Breemen, J.F., Scherphof, G. & Wilschut, J. (1987) Functional reconstitution of influenza virus envelopes. *EMBO J* **6**, 2651–9.

Stuart-Harris, C.H., Schild, G.C. & Oxford, J.S. (1984) *Influenza, the Viruses and the Disease.* Edward Arnold, London.

Tashiro, M., Ciborowski, P., Reinacher, M., Pulverer, G., Klenk, H.D. & Rott, R. (1987) Synergistic role of staphylococcal proteases in the induction of influenza virus pathogenicity. *Virology* **157**, 421–30.

Toltzis, P., O'Connell, K. & Patterson, J.L. (1988) Effects of phosphorylated ribavirin on vesicular stomatitis virus transcription. *Antimicrob Agents Chemother* **32**, 492–7.

Toogood, P.L., Galliker, P.K., Glick, G.D. & Knowles, J.R. (1991) Monovalent sialosides that bind tightly to influenza A virus. *J Med Chem* **34**, 3138–40.

Tu, Q., Pinto, L.H., Guangxiang, L. *et al.* (1996) Reversible inhibition of the influenza virus M2-ion channel by a spirene-containing compound, BL-1743. *J Virol* **70**, 822–9.

Ulmanen, I., Broni, B. & Krug, R.M. (1981) Role of two of the influenza virus core P proteins in recognising cap 1 structures (m7GpppNm) on RNAs and in initiating viral RNA transcription. *Proc Natl Acad Sci USA* **78**, 7355–9.

Ulmanen, I., Broni, B. & Krug, R.M. (1983) Influenza virus temperature-sensitive cap (m7gpppXm)-dependent endonuclease. *J Virol* **45**, 27–35.

Van Dyke, R., Hintz, M. & Connor, J. (1982) In: *Program and Abstracts of the Twenty Second Interscience Conference on Antimicrobial Agents And Chemotherapy.* American Society for Microbiology, Miami, Florida.

von Itzstein, M., Dyason, J.C., Oliver, S.W. *et al.* (1996) A study of the active site of influenza virus sialidase: an approach to the rational design of novel anti-influenza drugs. *J Med Chem* **39**, 388–91.

Wang, E., Wolf, B.A., Lamb, R.A., Choppin, P.W. & Goldberg, A.R. (1976) In: Goldman, R., Pollard, T. & Rosenbaum, J. (eds) *Cold Spring Harbor Symposium of Cell Motility*, Vol. 3, pp. 589–98. Cold Spring Harbor Laboratory, New York.

Watowich, S.J., Skehel, J.J. & Wiley, D.C. (1994) Crystal structures of influenza virus hemagglutinin in complex with high-affinity receptor analogs. *Structure* **2**, 719–31.

Webster, R.G. & Rott, R. (1987) Influenza virus A pathogenicity: the pivotal role of hemagglutinin. *Cell* **50**, 665–6.

Webster, R.G., Hinshaw, V.S. & Laver, W.G. (1982) Selection and analysis of antigenic variants of the neuraminidase of N2 influenza viruses with monoclonal antibodies. *Virology* **117**, 103–11.

Weiss, W., Brown, J.H., Cusack, S., Paulson, J.C., Skehel, J.J. & Wiley, D.C. (1988) Structure of the influenza virus haemagglutinin complexed with its receptor, sialic acid. *Nature* **333**, 426–31.

Wiley, D.C. & Skehel, J.J. (1987) The structure and function of the hemagglutinin membrane glycoprotein of influenza virus. *Annu Rev Biochem* **56**, 365–94.

Wiley, D.C., Wilson, I.A. & Skehel, J.J. (1981) Structural identification of the antibody-binding sites of Hong Kong influenza haemagglutinin and their involvement in antigenic variation. *Nature* **289**, 373–8.

Witirouw, M., Site, J.A., Mateu, M.Q. *et al.* (1994) Activity of a sulphated polysaccharide extracted from the red seaweed *Agharahiella tenera* against human immunodeficiency virus and other enveloped viruses. *Antiviral Chem Chemother* **5**, 297–303.

Wlodawer, A. (1994) Rational drug design: the proteinase inhibitors. *Pharmacotherapy* **14**, 9S–20S.

Woods, J.M., Bethell, R.C., Coates, J.A. *et al.* (1993) 4-Guanidino-2,4-dideoxy-2,3-dehydro-*N*-acetylneuraminic acid is a highly effective inhibitor both of the sialidase (neuraminidase) and of growth of a wide range of influenza A and B viruses *in vitro*. *Antimicrobial Agents Chemother* **37**, 1473–9.

Wray, S.K., Gilbert, B.E. & Knight, V. (1985) Effect of ribavirin triphosphate on primer generation and elongation during influenza virus transcription *in vitro*. *Antiviral Res* **5**, 39–48.

Yoshimura, A., Kuroda, K., Kawasaki, K., Yamashina, S., Maeda, T. & Ohnishi, S.-I. (1982) Infectious cell entry mechanism of influenza virus. *J Virol* **43**, 284–93.

Zhirnov, O.P. (1990) Solubilisation of membrane protein M1/M from virions occurs at different pH for orthomyxo- and paramyxoviruses. *Virology* **176**, 274–9.

Zhirnov, O.P., Ovcharenko, A.V., Bukrinskaia, A.G., Ursaki, L.P. & Ivanova, L.A. (1984) Antiviral and therapeutic action of protease inhibitors in viral infections: experimental and clinical observations. *Vopr Virusol* **29**, 491–7 [in Russian].

CHAPTER 38

Guidelines for the Clinical Use of Antivirals

Arnold S. Monto

Antivirals for use against influenza have been available in the USA almost continuously for 30 years, and in the former Soviet Union for nearly that long (Zlydnikov *et al.* 1981). However, in much of the rest of the developed world, experience with drugs which affect the replication of influenza virus is much more limited, and in some countries non-existent. New antivirals for influenza are currently in active development, and may be available in many countries relatively soon. Since methods for employing the newer anti-influenzal drugs should draw on past experience with amantadine and rimantadine, their appropriate use will be discussed first. This may only be directly relevant in those places where one or both of these drugs are available as antivirals, but will be helpful more globally in developing strategies for use of any new compounds that become available.

Amantadine and rimantadine

Properties affecting use

As discussed elsewhere in this volume, amantadine and rimantadine have similar chemical structures and mechanisms of action. While early *in vitro* studies suggested that there might be a broader spectrum of activity, only type A influenza viruses are affected at blood and tissue levels which can be safely achieved (Davies *et al.* 1964; Maassab & Cochran 1964). However, all known subtypes of type A influenza viruses are inhibited, as would, presumably, any new subtypes that might arise (Cochran *et al.* 1965). This observation was documented early in the laboratory but in the USA it was

initially not recognized by the regulatory authority. Amantadine had been licensed in 1966 for use only against influenza type A (H2N2) (American Medical Association 1967). The next year viruses of this subtype disappeared and pandemics of type A (H3N2) began, but the drug could not be used legally against those strains until 1976, when it was more realistically relicensed for all type A viruses. This timing was fortunate. When type A (H1N1) viruses appeared the following year in pandemic form in younger individuals, amantadine was available when there was no time to produce vaccine (Monto *et al.* 1979). Success in this episode has meant that antivirals such as amantadine and rimantadine have been a vital part of the plans developed to control pandemics in countries where they are available, caused as they invariably are by type A viruses (Patriarca & Cox 1997).

It was originally thought that the drugs prevented absorption of viruses into the host cells. It is now recognized that the action is more complex, with early and late effects. Of practical importance is the M_2 protein, which forms a transmembrane channel across the membrane of normally acidic cellular vesicles. Amantadine and rimantadine block the normal acidic flux through this ion channel. The primary sequence of the protein is critical, since antiviral resistance is associated with amino acid substitutions (Hay *et al.* 1979; Hay 1989; Sugrue & Hay 1991).

The most dramatic practical difference between the drugs relates to metabolism and excretion. Amantadine is mainly excreted unchanged by a mechanism of renal tubular secretion. Rimantadine is extensively metabolized by the liver, with up to

90% excreted in the form of hydroxylated and conjugated metabolites, some of which possess antiviral activity. From 2 to 20% of the rimantadine is excreted intact. This is in contrast to amantadine in which nearly all of the drug is excreted in an unmetabolized form (Aoki & Sitar 1988; Wills 1989). Thus, there is greater concern about use of amantadine in those people with decreased renal function and accumulation is undoubtedly related to some of the occurrence of reactions, especially in older individuals (Borison 1979; Horadam *et al.* 1981; Wu *et al.* 1982). It is particularly necessary to review individually each patient's renal status, especially when putting entire groups on drugs, such as in controlling outbreaks in nursing homes, a situation in which such issues may be overlooked (Capparelli *et al.* 1988).

In cell cultures, the drugs produce inhibition of type A strains at relatively low concentrations, with rimantadine slightly more active. This difference favouring rimantadine is more extreme in organ culture (Burlington *et al.* 1982; Browne *et al.* 1983). Both drugs are administered orally, and are well absorbed from the gastrointestinal tract, although the process can sometimes be slow. This is not typically a major problem based on their relatively long half-lives. The half-life of amantadine is 17 h and rimantadine is 37 h. There are no preparations for parenteral administration and aerosol use is possible, but has basically been limited to experimental situations (Hayden *et al.* 1980; Atmar *et al.* 1990). Concentrations of rimantadine in nasal mucus are approximately 50% higher for rimantadine than amantadine. This difference has lead to debate about whether it is appropriate to use the drugs at the same dosage, which has generally been done (Aoki *et al.* 1979; Hayden *et al.* 1985; Tominack & Hayden 1987).

Efficacy in prophylaxis and therapy

If is easier to quantify the efficacy of an antiviral in prophylaxis than in therapy, since the endpoint is dichotomous; individuals are either protected from infection and/or disease, or they are not. Two studies conducted some time ago, several years apart, definitively determined that both rimanta-dine and amantadine are at least 70% efficacious in preventing clinical disease confirmed as influenza by laboratory studies and suggested that efficacy increases if specific antibody is present in the population. The 70% figure was determined for amantadine in a study conducted during the first reappearance of type A (H1N1) virus following an absence of approximately 20 years. Thus, the young population at risk did not possess any antibody at that time (Monto *et al.* 1979). The second study conducted several years later identified the prophylactic efficacy of amantadine at 91% and rimantadine at 85%, highly significantly different from placebo but not significantly different from each other (Dolin *et al.* 1982). By that time, type A (H1N1) virus, the predominant strain in the outbreak, had circulated for several years, and individuals had developed considerable antibody to it. Overall, this puts the drugs at the same level of protective efficacy as inactivated vaccines. In both studies, protection against influenza infection with clinical disease was better than against total infection, that is, infection with or without an associated illness. Thus, some asymptomatic infections may continue to occur while on prophylaxis, producing antibody which may protect against a later infection.

The effectiveness of amantadine and rimantadine in therapy cannot be quantified as precisely as its efficacy in prophylaxis. Aside from fever, most of the signs or symptoms of influenza are subjective, and varying scales to estimate their severity have been used. In addition, treatment will have different effects depending on how long after infection it is given; most studies here require that illnesses being treated be within 48 h of onset. Among the current two circulating type A subtypes, A (H3N2) produces the more severe disease, and improvement with antiviral therapy is more dramatic especially when fever is present (Monto *et al.* 1985). Most of the studies demonstrating value of therapy of amantadine and rimantadine were rather small, partially a result of difficulty in identifying large numbers of infected ill individuals at single sites. One of the larger studies involved 45 individuals with confirmed A (H1N1) illness. Those on rimantadine or amantadine exhibited significantly faster resolution of fever. Symptom scores were reduced from entry levels by 50% in 48 h in treated individuals compared to somewhat under 72 h in placebo individuals. There was reduction in virus shedding for those with interpretable data and quicker return to normal activity in those on active therapy (Van Voris *et al.* 1981). Similar results were obtained comparing rimantadine alone to placebo in an A (H3N2) outbreak. There was also statistically significant reduction in virus shedding by day 2 (Hayden & Monto 1986).

At this point, some still questioned the use of the specific antiviral instead of traditional symptomatic therapy which, in general, was less expensive and which would be appropriate even when the diagnosis was not type A influenza. This issue was resolved by another study involving illnesses in young adults who were treated with the antiviral, with aspirin or placebo. As would be expected based on the 50% reduction of fever and symptoms at 48 h in the above studies, aspirin was superior to amantadine in the first day of the illness since its symptomatic effect was rapid. However, the antiviral was clearly advantageous in more rapid resolution of the overall illness, indicating the difference between symptomatic and specific therapy (Younkin *et al.* 1983).

Side-effects and resistance

Because of their different pharmacokinetics, amantadine and rimantadine exhibit quite different frequencies and types of side-effects (Hayden *et al.* 1983). Amantadine has clear central nervous system activity, which resulted in its being used in the therapy of Parkinson's disease (Parkes *et al.* 1970; Schwab *et al.* 1972). Rimantadine has no such activity. Side-effects are best quantified when the drugs are used in prophylaxis. In therapy, the characteristics of the viral illness makes evaluation of the side-effects difficult. In general, especially for rimantadine, the drugs have generally not produced single adverse symptoms significantly in excess of those seen with placebo. Only by examining clusters of symptoms or consequences of them, such as withdrawal from the study, could differences be detected. In two studies involving

amantadine prophylaxis, at least 6% of those on drugs had withdrawals which could be attributed to its use (Monto *et al.* 1979; Dolin *et al.* 1982). They were mostly related to the central nervous system, including insomnia, lack of concentration and jitteriness. Under the same study conditions there was no difference in withdrawals between rimantadine and placebo. Side-effects of amantadine have generally occurred early and have ceased with termination of use. They have only been a particular problem in elderly subjects, especially but not only when used in those with renal insufficiency, problems such as unsteadiness in gait and falls have been observed (Postma & Van Tilburg 1975; Degelau *et al.* 1990). With rimantadine, in elderly people, it has been difficult to show significant differences in potential side-effects when individual symptoms in placebo and drug recipients are compared (Dolin *et al.* 1983). However, in a 6-week study in nursing home populations, there were more frequent overall withdrawals in those on drug. This study also pointed out the necessity to study further possible drug interactions (Monto *et al.* 1995).

The potential of emergence of antiviral resistance to these drugs has been known for many years (Oxford *et al.* 1970). More recently, it has become clear that the reason resistance can develop so quickly under certain circumstances is that influenza viruses exist as mixtures with nearly all of the virions susceptible to the drugs, and others resistant. There is complete crossresistance between amantadine and rimantadine, and resistance is associated with amino acid substitutions in the M_2 protein of the virus (Lubeck *et al.* 1978; Belshe *et al.* 1988). Because the substitutions can occur in several different amino acids, it is possible to track the spread of a virus between individuals. However, the number of substitutions are low enough for the tracking not to be absolute. Resistance has not been associated with prophylaxis but rather with therapy. However, emergence of resistant virus does not result in treatment failure, as might be expected (Hayden *et al.* 1991). The practical consequence occurs only when transmission takes place from a person on therapy to another individual who is on prophylactic drugs. In that case, the drug will have no effect in preventing an infection caused by resistant virus (Hayden *et al.* 1989). Given the epidemic nature of influenza, the main public health concern then would be possible gradual replacement of susceptible viruses in the population by resistant ones. As yet there is no evidence that this has not taken place (Belshe *et al.* 1989). There has been much speculation to explain this observation, including the possibility that resistant viruses have a competitive disadvantage, and that is why in the natural situation they are present in only small numbers (Monto & Arden 1992). It is at least theoretically possible, if drug use increases over time, that infection caused by resistant virus could begin to be seen in situations where there is no direct involvement of the antivirals. Organizations such as the Centers for Disease Control and Prevention (CDC) in the USA are monitoring circulating viruses to guard against such a possibility.

Perspectives on the use of amantadine and rimantadine

These drugs are not extensively used outside North America except in a limited number of countries. There, much experience has accumulated on methods of employing the drugs. Both will be considered together, since, except for side-effects and reduction in dosage associated with renal insufficiency, their effects are similar. For prophylaxis, influenza vaccine remains the main line of defence on a population basis. Vaccine is inexpensive, and it gives protection over the entire season. There are vaccine failures, especially when there is not a good relationship between the virus in the vaccine and that circulating, but that phenomenon, termed lack of fit, has become relatively rare. Vaccine does not protect certain segments of the population as well as others and this is particularly true among elderly people in nursing homes. The current effort to produce improved vaccines is evidence of the fact that while effective, they are not ideal, especially compared to some of the newer vaccines in use to prevent various other infections. In addition, amantadine and rimantadine must be administered daily and their protection extends to all type A strains but does not include type B.

However, vaccine takes at least 2 weeks to take effect, but the antivirals show some prophylactic effect 1 day and full effect 2 days after administration begins. Thus, they can be used for prophylaxis when individuals who are recommended to receive vaccine come to medical attention only after an outbreak is underway. In this situation, vaccine can be administered at the same time the patient is started on antiviral prophylaxis. There are additional situations when vaccination is contraindicated such as patients in groups recommended for vaccination with egg hypersensitivity, which is uncommon, or more commonly when dealing with such a patient who does not wish to be vaccinated even though there are no specific medical contraindications. Prophylaxis may sometimes be used for an individual who, for personal reasons, does not want to chance acquiring type A influenza infection during a short period, for example on a business trip into an area where recognized type A influenza outbreaks are taking place. Postexposure prophylaxis in the family setting has also been attempted, usually involving placing other members on drugs for a limited time period after infection is recognized in an index case (Galbraith *et al.* 1969a,b.

It is in therapy that there is no alternative to use of the antivirals at present, except for drugs which only provide relief of symptoms. Some distinguish, as with vaccines, between younger healthy persons and those individuals in the traditional high-risk groups, older individuals and persons of all ages with specific chronic diseases. However, although it is possible to hypothesize, based on observations such as the more rapid resolution of small airways abnormalities on treatment, that complications of influenza would be prevented, there is as yet no evidence to that effect. In fact, no data exist to indicate that these antivirals are of value in treating influenzal pneumonia, although compassionate use in this situation has occurred at a frequency difficult to define. Thus, there are no medical reasons to restrict use of amantadine and rimantadine in any adult who has an influenza-like illness when encountered in the course of a recognized type A outbreak. Use in children is also possible for amantadine, although approval for that indication has not been given by the regulatory authority in the USA because of lack of sufficient numbers.

The questions, then, are how to define whether influenza is circulating and how to determine that a particular patient is suffering acutely from influenza. Ideally, a rapid detection test would be available that is both sensitive and specific and which can distinguish between type A and B infections. At present, the rapid tests are limited in their availability and add to the expense of treating a patient. Over the years, a method has developed, which might be termed the epidemiological diagnosis of infection. Initially, this has involved following the occurrence of influenza in a particular geographical area and then using standard clinical criteria for making a diagnosis of influenza. It has been shown that fever, cough and conjunctivitis distinguish between influenza-positive and influenza-negative illnesses (Monto & Ohmit 1996). Symptoms such as malaise and myalgias are common in influenza, but are also common in non-influenzal illnesses. Many doctors are able to make a diagnosis based on clinical experience which is quite accurate in recognizing the most severe and typical cases in an outbreak. New rapid diagnostic tests will be of help, especially in situations when type A and B viruses are cocirculating, which occurs periodically.

The value of using antivirals in therapy of uncomplicated influenza in the people not in the high-risk groups can be further documented by examining the course of untreated influenza. The most severe illness is caused by type A (H3N2) viruses, the least by type A (H1N1) and type B is intermediate. The illness is of relatively long duration, 12 days in children and 15 days in adults for type A (H3N2) as measured by median time to cessation of the last symptom (Monto *et al.* 1985). Specific treatment which shortens the length of an illness of this duration would be routinely applied if it were caused by a bacterium, in which situation an antibiotic would be prescribed. Thus, it seems paradoxical to propose that use of an active therapeutic antiviral agent be restricted, especially when data are available which indicate superiority long term over symptomatic therapy.

The issue of antiviral resistance has been raised as a barrier to more general use of these agents.

Again it should be remembered that the study which first demonstrated apparent transmission of resistant virus in the family setting showed that the treated individuals had the same significant reduction in the severity of illness whether they were shedding resistant virus or not (Hayden 1991). It was only in other persons in the family in contact with the treated cases, who were themselves on antiviral prophylaxis, where drug failure was demonstrated (Hayden *et al.* 1989). The major concern, then, is whether use of this class of antivirals will produce in a region or globally an increase in the occurrence of resistant viruses. As discussed above, this has not yet been observed, but surveillance is on-going. The ultimate test of this issue will be in the pandemic situation, where in all probability, antiviral use will be extensive limited mainly by drug availability.

A more substantive question is how long after onset of illness amantadine and rimantadine will still be effective. The recommendation for use within 48 h of onset of illness is based on lack of data beyond that time, since studies generally required cases to be of such duration to be admitted. As is apparent from the biology of influenza infection, the closer to onset, the better the response to any antiviral. Reducing of the therapeutic activity of the antivirals as time from onset of symptoms to beginning of administration increases will be a gradual one, and the 48-h time frame should be viewed as a guide, based on existing data.

Amantadine and rimantadine have had their most dramatic results in control of influenza in nursing homes. These institutions bring together highly susceptible individuals in close proximity. Outbreaks still occur in well-vaccinated homes, probably related to the difficulty in enforcing vaccination standards on staff, who in certain situations are transient, as well as less than ideal vaccine protection in the frail elderly. In the USA, whenever an outbreak of type A influenza in a nursing home is detected, it is strongly recommended by the Advisory Committee on Immunization Practices that all residents, whatever their vaccination status and, ideally, staff be placed on amantadine or rimantadine (Centers for Disease Control and Prevention 1994). This recommendation has not been based on controlled trials, which are not possible given the necessity of placing an entire home on a drug, but rather on the repeated observation of the success of the approach, and the fact that this success would be predicted based on the known effectiveness of the antiviral. The rationale has been discussed in detail elsewhere (Monto & Arden 1992). The doses of both should be no more than 100 mg daily, with appropriate further reductions, especially of amantadine, determined by overall renal and hepatic status. The antivirals, then, are used pragmatically, in the midst of the institutional outbreak, in some residents who are ill for treatment, in some for prophylaxis, and in a few who are in the incubation period. In general, the outbreaks terminate within 2 days. It is curious that in this situation, ideal for emergence and transmission of resistant strains, that this phenomenon has been observed to interfere with the strategy so rarely (Mast *et al.* 1991). The occasional failure of this approach has mainly been related to improper use of a drug, when only some residents are treated, often intermittently. Occasionally side-effects have been a problem, typically, but not always related to use of amantadine.

For this method to be effective, it is necessary for a system to be in place rapidly to detect the occurrence of influenza and to start therapy. It is rare for nursing home outbreaks to occur before transmission is identified in the surrounding population so attention to reports of regional viral transmission is helpful. The detection of influenza transmission is aided when there is an infection control system in place for identification and follow-up of cases of febrile illness. In many regions such a system is required by regulation. While influenza is often afebrile in the elderly population, fever still allows recognition of the more severe illness with acceptable loss of sensitivity and increased specificity. One method that has been successfully employed is to use the occurrence of 2% of residents with new febrile respiratory illness in a single week to alert the staff to the possibility that influenza is circulating; then rapid viral identification tests can be employed to confirm that influenza is involved. This also confirms that the virus is type A. If rapid tests are not available, the number of cases required

in a week may need to be increased. These tests need not be used in all illnesses, but rather to help in identifying the aetiology of the outbreak.

It has also been demonstrated that, in elderly vaccinated populations, use of rimantadine increases the protective effect of vaccination. This is in keeping with the observation that the antivirals and antibodies have an additive or synergistic effect (Dolin *et al.* 1983; Monto *et al.* 1995). Unlike the situations described above, especially involving therapy, in which decisions on use of the antivirals would not distinguish between risk groups, this sort of prophylaxis in the already vaccinated appears appropriate only for persons who would be exceedingly vulnerable should they be infected. Again, issues such as inevitable occurrence of some side-effects and of cost would have to be balanced against the resulting increased protection (Patriarca *et al.* 1984).

Newer antiviral drugs: the neuraminidase inhibitors

Just as our current inactivated influenza vaccines are effective but not ideal, amantadine and rimantadine could clearly be improved upon as antivirals. First, there is the limitation of efficacy to type A viruses. Additionally, side-effects, while manageable, do occur with some frequency, especially with respect to amantadine. Finally, there is the question of antiviral resistance, which, while not yet a practical problem, clearly is theoretically an issue and may currently inhibit use.

Another class of antivirals, the neuraminidase inhibitors, are in the course of development (Luo *et al.* 1996; von Itzstein *et al.* 1996). There is currently considerably more information available on zanamivir (GG167), the compound being developed by Glaxo Wellcome, than for GS4104 (RO 64-0796) the compound being developed by Gilead and Roche. Like amantadine and rimantadine, the compounds are similar in certain essential features of their activity, as discussed in Chapter 36, and the major difference is in their pharmacokinetics. Sufficient data have not accumulated to allow comparison of potential side-effects. Both drugs are active against type A and B influenza viruses, and antiviral resistance, while demonstrable in the laboratory for zanamivir, does not appear to be of consequence in human or even animal infections, unlike the situation with amantadine and rimantadine.

Only early data on efficacy in humans are available for GS4104 (RO64-0796) and therefore the discussion will be restricted to the limited published data on zanamivir. That drug was shown to be extremely effective in animals such as the ferret when administered intranasally or by aerosol. It was much less effective when given either orally or parenterally. These findings were in keeping with the poor oral bioavailability and tissue penetration of the drug (Hayden *et al.* 1996). Thus, the initial human investigations, a series of challenge experiments using a type A (H1N1) virus, were conducted using topical, intranasal administration of the drug. The studies were set up to mimic drug use in prophylaxis and therapy. In the prophylactic experiment, zanamivir was 82% efficacious in preventing infection, with or without symptoms and was 95% efficacious in preventing infection with clinical illness. Although the numbers are small these results suggest at least one similarity to rimantadine and amantadine, in which the prevention of clinical illnesses occurs more commonly than prevention of all infections. In the experiment to evaluate use in therapy, symptomatic benefit was equally dramatic, with duration of virus shedding, fever and overall duration significantly reduced. The recently published multicentre study evaluating treatment of naturally occurring type A and B influenza confirms the safety of the drug and the lack of production of resistant variants. Given either by inhalation or by inhalation and intranasal route combined, zanamivir shortened the time to a predefined alleviation of symptoms, when compared with placebo. The effect was greater among cases with laboratory confirmed influenza infection when the illness was treated within the first 30 hours of symptoms or when fever was present. The former suggests a biological phenomenon relating to the duration of infection at the time treatment was begun, while the latter may reflect the greater ability to show improvement when the initial symptoms are more severe. Viral replication was also affected by the drug. A total of 417 individuals participated in this study (Hayden *et al.* 1997).

Additional studies involving more than three times that number have been carried out with similar results in the overall treated groups. Comparison with prior investigations involving rimantadine or amantadine are not possible, because of different eligibility requirements and end-points employed. However, it should be noted that in those with fever and those with short duration of symptoms at the start of therapy, zanamivir shortened the median duration of illness from 7 days to 4 days.

Possible uses for the newer drugs

Based on these early data, and on prior knowledge of the characteristics of amantadine and rimantadine in prophylaxis and treatment, how might the neuraminidase inhibitors be used? The most conservative approach in planning would be to assume they are equally or slightly more effective than amantadine and rimantadine in both prophylaxis and therapy. Any further demonstrated efficacy might make recommendations more enthusiastic, but would not change the overall approach. Thus far, the drugs, especially zanamivir, of which there is most information, appear quite safe, so that they could be used without the careful monitoring which is now required, particularly with amantadine. Lack of demonstration of resistance would also increase the comfort level, especially when several individuals in a closed population are on treatment or prophylaxis at the same time. Probably the greatest advantage, in addition to safety, will be the effectiveness against type A and B viruses. In many years, transmission of the two types may overlap for part of the season, and sometimes for nearly the entire period. A drug which works against both types of influenza would be a distinct advantage in such years.

The greatest use of the drug would be in therapy, since vaccines would remain the first line of defence in prophylaxis. However, targeted use of the drugs in prophylaxis in special situations would occur, and would be an alternative or addition to vaccination, as described for amantadine and rimantadine. Again, if a potent and safe antiviral agent is available, it should not be restricted in treatment to those in any high-risk group, especially in the absence of a major question of resistance. Rather, given an appropriate safety profile, children and adults with clinical influenza, that is with fever, cough and systemic symptoms should be candidates. A neuraminadase inhibitor would be a welcome addition to the control of pandemic influenza. Here, issues of stockpiling and shelf-life become important. Use in the pandemic situation would likely be greater in those countries in which the neuraminidase inhibitor is the only licensed influenza antiviral, since it will be impossible to use amantadine and rimantadine if they are not already approved for use. A challenge in these countries, in or out of the pandemic period, will be to develop familiarity with the use of an anti-influenzal drug. For those already used to the concepts for employing amantadine and rimantadine, moving to the neuraminidase inhibitors will be more easily accomplished, since the overall principles in prophylaxis and therapy remain the same.

References

American Medical Association, Council on Drugs (1967) The amantadine controversy. *J Am Med Assoc* **201**, 372–3.

Aoki, F.Y. & Sitar, D.S. (1988) Clinical pharmacokinetics of amantadine hydrochloride. *Clin Pharmacokinet* **14**, 35–51.

Aoki, F.Y., Sitar, D.S. & Olgilvie, R.I. (1979) Amantadine kinetics in healthy young subjects after lterong-m dosing. *Clin Pharmacol Ther* **26**, 729–36.

Arden, N.H., Monto, A.S. & Ohmit, S.E. (1995) Vaccine use and the risk of outbreaks in a sample of nursing homes during an influenza epidemic. *Am J Public Health* **85**, 399–401.

Atmar, R.L., Greenberg, S.B., Quarles, J.M. *et al.* (1990) Safety and pharmacokinetics of rimantadine small-particle aerosol. *Antimicrobial Agents Chemother* **34**, 2228–33.

Belshe, R.B., Burk, B., Newman, F., Cerruti, R.L. & Sim, I.S. (1989) Resistance of influenza, A virus to amantadine and rimantadine, results of one decade of surveillance. *J Infect Dis* **159**, 430–5.

Belshe, R.B., Hall-Smith, M., Hall, C.B., Betts, R. & Hay, A.J. (1988) Genetic basis of resistance to rimantadine emerging during treatment of influenza virus infection. *J Virol* **5**, 1508–12.

Borison, R.L. (1979) Amantadine-induced psychosis in a geriatric patient with renal disease. *Am J Psychiatr* **136**, 111–12.

Browne, M.J., Moss, M.Y. & Boyd, M.K.R. (1983) Comparative activity of amantadine and ribavirin against influenza virus *in vitro*, possible clinical relevance. *Antimicrobial Agents Chemother* **23**, 503–5.

Burlington, D.B., Meikeljohn, G. & Mostow, S.R. (1982) Anti-influenza A virus activity of amantadine hydrochloride and rimantadine hydrochloride in ferret tracheal ciliated epithelium. *Antimicrobial Agents Chemother* **21**, 794–9.

Capparelli, E.V., Stevens, R.C., Chow, M.S., Izard, M. & Wills, R.J. (1988) Rimantadine pharmacokinetics in healthy subjects and patients with end-stage renal failure. *Clin Pharmacol Ther* **43**, 536–41.

Centers for Disease Control and Prevention (1994) Prevention and control of influenza. Part I. Antiviral agents—recommendations of the Advisory Committee on Immunization Practices (ACIP). *MMWR* **43**, 1–10.

Cochran, K.W., Maassab, H.F., Tsunoda, A. *et al.* (1965) Studies on the antiviral activity of amantadine hydrochloride. *Ann NY Acad Sci* **130**, 432–9.

Davies, W.L., Grunert, R.R., Haff, R.F. *et al.* (1964) Antiviral activity of, L-adamantanamine, HCl. *Science* **144**, 862–3.

Degelau, J., Somani, S., Cooper, S.L. & Irvine, P.W. (1990) Occurrence of adverse effects and high amantadine concentrations with influenza prophylaxis in the nursing home. *J Am Geriatr Soc* **38**, 428–32.

Dolin, R., Betts, R.F., Treanor, J.J. *et al.* (1983) Rimantadine prophylaxis of influenza in the elderly. In: *Program and Abstracts of the 23rd Interscience Conference on Antimicrobial Agents and Chemotherapy*, abstract 691, p. 210. American Society for Microbiology, Washington DC.

Dolin, R., Reichman, R.C., Madore, H.P. *et al.* (1982) A controlled trial of amantadine and rimantadine in the prophylaxis of influenza A infection. *N Engl J Med* **307**, 580–4.

Galbraith, A.W., Oxford, J.S., Schild, G.C. & Watson, G.I. (1969a) Protective effect of, 1-adamantanamine hydrochloride on influenza, A2 infections in the family environment. A controlled double-blind study. *Lancet* **2**, 1026–8.

Galbraith, A.W., Oxford, J.S., Schild, G.C. & Watson, G.I. (1969b) Study of, L-adamantanamine hydrochloride used prophylactically during the Hong Kong influenza epidemic in the family environment. *Bull WHO* **41**, 677–82.

Hay, A.J. (1989) The mechanism of action of amantadine and rimantadine against influenza viruses. In: Notkins, A.L. & Oldstone, M.B.A. (eds) *Concepts in Viral Pathogenesis*, Vol. 3, pp. 561–7. Springer, Berlin.

Hay, A.J., Kennedy, N.T.C., Skehel, J.J. & Appleyard, G. (1979) The matrix protein gene determines amantadine-sensitivity of influenza viruses. *J Gen Virol* **42**, 189–91.

Hayden, F.G., Belshe, R.B., Clover, R.D., Hay, A.J., Oakes, M.G. & Soo, W. (1989) Emergence and apparent transmission of rimantadine-resistant influenza A virus in families. *N Engl J Med* **321**, 1696–702.

Hayden, F.G., Hall, W.J. & Douglas, R.G. Jr (1980) Therapeutic effects of aerosolized amantadine in naturally acquired infection due to influenza A virus. *J Infect Dis* **141**, 535–42.

Hayden, F.G., Hoffman, H.E. & Spyker, D.A. (1983) Differences in side-effects of amantadine hydrochloride and rimantadine hydrochloride relate to differences in pharmacokinetics. *Antimicrobial Agents Chemother* **23**, 458–64.

Hayden, F.G., Minocha, A. Spyker, D.A. & Hoffman, H.E. (1985) Comparative single-dose pharmacokinetics of amantadine hydrochloride and rimantadine hydrochloride in young and elderly adults. *Antimicrobial Agents Chemother* **18**, 216–221.

Hayden, F.G. & Monto, A.S. (1986) Oral rimantadine hydrochloride therapy of influenza, A.virus, H3N2 subtype infection in adults. *Antimicrobial Agents Chemother* **29**, 339–41.

Hayden, F.G., Osterhaus, A.D.M.E., Treanor, J.J. *et al.* (1997) Efficacy and safety of the neuraminidase inhibitor zanamivir in the treatment of influenza virus infection. *N Engl J Med* **337**, 874–80.

Hayden, F., Sperber, S.J., Belshe, R., Clover, R., Hay, A. & Pyke, S. (1991) Recovery of drug-resistant influenza A virus during therapeutic use of rimantadine. *Antimicrobial Agents Chemother* **35**, 1741–7.

Hayden, F.G., Treanor, J.J., Betts, R.F., Lobo, M., Esinhart, J.D., Hussey, E.K. (1996) Safety and efficacy of the neuraminidase inhibitor, GG 167 in experimental human influenza. *J Am Med Assoc* **275**, 295–9.

Horadam, V.W., Sharp, J.G., Smilack, J.D. *et al.* (1981) Pharmacokinetics of amantadine hydrochloride in subjects with normal and impaired renal function. *Ann Intern Med* **94**, 454–8.

Lubeck, M.D., Schulman, J.L. & Palese, P. (1978) Susceptibility of influenza A viruses to amantadine is influenced by the gene coding for M protein. *J Virol* **28**, 710–16.

Luo, M., Air, G.M. & Brouillette, W.J. (1996) Design of aromatic inhibitors of influenza virus neuraminidase. In: Brown, L.E., Hampson, A.W. & Webster, R.G. (eds) *Options for the Control of Influenza*, Vol. 3, pp. 702–12. Elsevier Science, Amsterdam.

Maassab, H.F. & Cochran, K.W. (1964) Rubella virus inhibition *in vitro* by amantadine hydrochloride. *Science* **145**, 1443–4.

0Mast, E.E., Harmon, M.W., Gravenstein, S. *et al.* (1991) Emergence and possible transmission of amantadine-resistant viruses during nursing home outbreaks of influenza A (H3N2). *Am J Epidemiol* **134**, 988–97.

Monto, A.S. & Arden, N.H. (1992) Implications of viral resistance to amantadine in control of influenza A. *Clin Inf Dis* **15**, 362–7.

Monto, A.S., Gunn, R.A., Bandyk, M.G. *et al.* (1979) Prevention of Russian influenza by amantadine. *J Am Med Assoc* **241**, 1003–7.

Monto, A.S., Koopman, J.S., Longini, I.M. Jr (1985) Tecumseh study of illness. XIII. Influenza infection and disease, 1976–81. *Am J Epidemiol* **121**, 811–22.

Monto, A.S., Ohmit, S.E. (1996) The evolving epidemiology of influenza infection and disease. In: Brown, L.E., Hampson, A.W. & Webster, R.G. (eds) *Options for the Control of Influenza*, Vol. 3, pp. 45–9. Elsevier Science, Amsterdam.

Monto, A.S., Ohmit, S.E., Hornbuckle, K. & Pearce, C.L. (1995) Safety and efficacy of long-term use of rimantadine for prophylaxis of type A influenza in nursing homes. *Antimicrobial Agents Chemother* **39**, 2224–8.

Oxford, J.S., Logan, I.S. & Potter, C.W. (1970) *In vivo* selection of an influenza A2 strain resistant to amantadine. *Nature* **226**, 82–3.

Parkes, J.D., Zilkha, K.J., Marsden, P. *et al.* (1970) Amantadine dosage in treatment of Parkinson's disease. *Lancet* **i**, 1130–3.

Patriarca, P.A. & Cox, N.J. (1997) Influenza pandemic plan for the United States. *J Infect Dis* **176**, S4–7.

Patriarca, P.A., Kater, N.A., Kendal, A.P., Bregman, D.J., Smith, J.D. & Sikes, R.K. (1984) Safety of prolonged administration of rimantadine hydrochloride in the prophylaxis of influenza A virus infections in nursing homes. *Antimicrobial Agents Chemother* **26**, 101–3.

Postma, J.U. & Van Tilburg, W. (1975) Visual hallucinations and delirium during treatment with amantadine (Symmetrel). *J Am Geriatr Soc* **23**, 212–15.

Schwab, R.S., Poskanzer, D.C., England, A.C. Jr *et al.* (1972) Amantadine in Parkinson's disease. *J Am Med Assoc* **222**, 792–5.

Sugrue, R.J. & Hay, A.J. (1991) Structural characteristics of the M2 protein of influenza A viruses, evidence that it forms a tetrameric channel. *Virology* **180**, 617–24.

Tominack, R.L. & Hayden, F.G. (1987) Rimantadine hydrochloride and amantadine hydrochloride use in influenza A virus infections. *Infect Dis Clin N Am* **1**, 459–78.

Van Voris, L.P., Betts, R.G., Hayden, F.G. *et al.* (1981) Successful treatment of naturally occurring influenza A/USSR/77 H1N1. *J Am Med Assoc* **245**, 1128–31.

von Itzstein, M., Dyason, J.C., Oliver, S.W. *et al.* (1996) A study of the active site of influenza virus sialidase: an approach to the rational design of novel anti-influenza drugs. *J Med Chemother* **39**, 388–91.

Wills, R.J. (1989) Update on rimantadine's clinical pharmacokinetics. *J Resp Dis* **10** (suppl), 20–5.

Wu, M.J., Ing, T.S., Soung, L.S. *et al.* (1982) Amantadine hydrochloride pharmacokinetics in patients with impaired renal function. *Clin Nephrol* **17**, 19–23.

Younkin, S.W., Betts, R.F., Roth, F.K. *et al.* (1983) Reduction in fever and symptoms in young adults with influenza A/Brazil/78 H1N1 infection after treatment with aspirin or amantadine. *Antimicrobial Agents Chemother* **23**, 577–82.

Zlydnikov, D.M., Kubar, O.I., Kovaleva, T.P. *et al.* (1981) Study of rimantadine in the USSR a review of the literature. *Rev Infect Dis* **3**, 408–21.

Section 10
Virus Challenge
Studies

CHAPTER 39

Volunteer Challenge Studies

John J. Treanor and Frederick G. Hayden

As pointed out elsewhere in this textbook, influenza is perhaps unique among the common respiratory viral illnesses of adults in that epidemics are regularly associated with excess hospitalizations and deaths. However, for the vast majority of healthy adults, influenza is an occasionally severe and disabling, but ultimately self-limited illness from which complete recovery is to be expected. For this reason, the concept of intentionally infecting normal volunteers with the virus for purposes of intensive study of the infection and disease, was raised almost immediately upon its initial discovery. Since that time, experimental inoculation of susceptible healthy volunteers with live influenza virus, or so-called 'challenge' studies, has made a great contribution to the study of the physiological and immune response of humans to this virus, and particularly in the development of vaccines and antivirals for the control of infection. In the following chapter, general features of the human challenge model of influenza will be reviewed, and examples of the use of this model in understanding the pathophysiology of disease and development of control measures will be described briefly.

History

A viral aetiology for the clinical syndrome recognized as influenza was established in humans when it was demonstrated that a febrile respiratory illness with characteristic pathological findings in the lungs could be transmitted to ferrets by intranasal inoculation of the ferrets with bacteria-free filtrates of throat gargles from humans with typical influenza. Transmission of influenza to ferrets was first reported in England (Smith *et al.* 1933), with the isolation of the virus subsequently designated influenza A/WS/33, and by workers in the USA, with transmission to ferrets by secretions from individuals involved in a typical outbreak in Puerto Rico (Francis 1934); the prototypic virus from this outbreak was subsequently named A/PR/8/34. Illness could be serially transmitted from ferret to ferret by filtrates from the respiratory tract but not from other organs, and was also transmissible to mice, and eventually to hamsters and a variety of other animals. Ill animals developed an antibody response which could be demonstrated by the ability of postinfectious sera to neutralize the infectivity of filtrates for other animals. Postillness sera from humans experiencing typical influenza could also neutralize the infectivity of these inocula for mice and ferrets, and through the use of such *in vivo* neutralization techniques, it was determined that the WS and PR8 viruses were related to each other antigenically, and also to the virus of swine influenza, which had previously been identified by Shope and coworkers (Shope 1931a). Similar techniques were used several years later to identify a virus associated with acute influenza which was not neutralized by sera which neutralized previously identified influenza viruses, and by previous agreement the new virus was identified as influenza B virus (Francis 1940). Since the prototypic virus was isolated from a patient named Lee it was designated the influenza B/Lee/40 virus.

At the time these experiments were taking place, there was some uncertainty about whether influenza virus alone was sufficient to cause clinical influenza in humans, or whether coinfection with a bacterial agent would be required. Studies in swine, in which illness could only be produced by coadministration of swine influenza virus and the bacteria *Haemophilus suis* (Shope 1931b), suggested the latter hypothesis. However, the absence of known bacterial pathogens in the experimentally infected ferrets supported the role of virus alone. This view was strengthened by the observation of occasional cases of clinical influenza in laboratory workers who were exposed to the infected ferrets (Francis 1934; Smith & Stuart-Harris 1936). It was recognized with the initial identification of influenza virus that definitive determination of the role of the virus in this disease would require clinical studies in humans, but that such 'direct experiments on man [would be] fraught with difficulties' (Smith *et al.* 1933).

However, within 2 years of the first report of transmission of influenza to ferrets, transmission of disease to humans by intranasal administration of a suspension of nasal turbinate from an infected ferret was attempted (Andrewes *et al.* 1935). These experiments were initially unsuccessful, for reasons which were well recognized by the investigators, including the fact that the virus inocula had been multiply passaged in ferrets, and may have become somewhat attenuated for humans, and that the subjects had antibody to influenza and may not have been susceptible to experimental infection. In fact, the investigators had not been able to find subjects who did not possess antibody to the challenge virus as assessed by the *in vivo* neutralization test, and had therefore been forced to resort to challenge of subjects with known prechallenge antibody. Ironically, both the varying degrees of partial attenuation for humans of the highly passaged laboratory strains of influenza used for challenge studies, and the fortune of the investigator in finding sufficient numbers of serologically susceptible subjects, remain the two factors which make the greatest contributions to the success or failure of human influenza challenge experiments.

Studies of influenza virus challenge of humans continued to be done, with success first reported by Smorodintsev and colleagues who induced typical illness in approximately one-third of experimentally infected young subjects (Smorodintsev *et al.* 1937). These studies clearly identified prechallenge neutralizing antibody as protecting against illness, which was almost exclusively seen in those who lacked such antibody. Since infection was accompanied by the induction of high levels of antibody, it was suggested that intentional exposure to the virus, perhaps in attenuated form, could be an effective control measure for influenza, but this idea was rejected as overly 'heroic' by the editors of the journal in which it initially appeared (Smorodintsev *et al.* 1937).

Several laboratory advances occurred in the next few years which enhanced further research in influenza considerably, including the development of embryonated eggs as a substrate for the propagation of virus (Smith 1935), the recognition that infected allantoic fluids could agglutinate chick red blood cells (Hirst 1941), and the development of haemagglutination-inhibition (HAI) tests for influenza antibody (Hirst 1942). The HAI test was demonstrated to parallel the more cumbersome *in vivo* neutralization type tests very closely, and became the predominant method for assessing influenza immunity and for characterizing influenza viruses antigenically.

During this time, work continued towards the development of an effective influenza vaccine. Potential influenza vaccines were generated by concentration and chemical inactivation of infected allantoic fluids, and administered subcutaneously, by aerosol administration or by other routes (Taylor & Dreguss 1940; Eaton & Martin 1942; Hirst *et al.* 1942). Large numbers of subjects were immunized and immune responses to vaccination measured, but assessment of the potential protective effects of such vaccines was hampered by the relatively low levels of influenza activity observed during the winters following immunization. Therefore, challenge studies were among the first to demonstrate the induction of protective immunity against influenza by vaccination (Henle *et al.* 1943; Francis *et al.* 1944; Salk *et al.* 1944). Human challenge studies also evaluated the safety, immune response to and protective efficacy of live attenuated vaccines (Burnet & Foley 1940; Burnet 1942, 1943). Subsequently, such studies played an important role in the clinical development of cold-adapted influenza vaccines (Clements *et al.* 1984) as well as in the evaluation of antiviral drugs such as amantadine (Jackson *et al.* 1963), rimantadine (Simorondintsev *et al.* 1970), and ribavirin (Hall *et al.* 1983) as they became available.

The postwar period represented a 'golden age' of virology, with the development of *in vitro* cell culture systems and initial isolation of many important respiratory viruses including adenoviruses (Rowe *et al.* 1953), rhinoviruses (Price 1956), parainfluenza virus (Chanock 1956) and respiratory syncytial virus (Chanock *et al.* 1957), among others. Human challenge studies played a role in evaluating the human response to infection with these viruses as well, and centres for the conduct of such studies in which certain standard procedures were used were developed at several locations. With the Asian influenza pandemic of 1957, and the development of amantadine, there was renewed interest in challenge of human subjects with influenza. In a series of studies conducted at the National Institutes of Health (NIH) clinical centre and elsewhere (Knight 1964; Knight *et al.* 1965) the challenge model of influenza was refined, and by the early 1960s had been standardized essentially as such studies are conducted today. These refinements included the development of standard criteria for the inoculum, the methods of screening subjects for antibody against the specific challenge viruses being used, and the routine use of the intranasal route for administration of virus, as described below.

General features of the human influenza challenge model

The following section reviews the variables which need to be considered in designing and conducting human challenge studies with influenza. Generally, after selecting the specific strain of virus to be used for the study, one must select subjects based on relevant criteria, determine the outcome measure of interest, perform the study, and analyse the results appropriately. One is confronted with multiple decisions at each of these phases of a typical challenge study. The typical approach is described here

but individual investigators will have their own preferences, and study design should be flexible and focused on the primary outcome of interest.

Screening of volunteers

Among the features that determine the eventual outcome of influenza challenge in a particular individual, the prechallenge level of immunity to the challenge virus is one of the most important. Therefore, it is critical in designing such studies to ensure that the study groups are equivalent in the level of prechallenge immunity in order for the results to be interpretable (Sabin 1967). It is important to recognize in this regard, that in the interpandemic period adults have been infected with closely related influenza viruses on multiple occasions previously, and are therefore at least partially immune regardless of antibody titre. However, the very earliest studies of influenza challenge identified serum neutralizing antibody as highly predictive of infection in challenge studies. The development of the HAI test for determination of functional antibody to influenza simplified the task of screening for susceptibility significantly, and it is now routine to use subjects with relatively low levels of prechallenge HAI antibody to the challenge virus in such studies. By convention, a level of 1 to 8 or less is usually used as the threshold for enrolment.

The nuances of the HAI test are described elsewhere in this textbook (Chapter 22). However, several points are worth considering. Firstly, it is critical to pretreat sera to remove non-specific inhibitors of haemagglutination in order to find susceptibles. Several techniques exist for this purpose and it is worth trying more than one in the case of difficulties, as haemagglutinins may differ in the sensitivities of their inhibitors to treatment (Subbarao *et al.* 1992). Secondly, the reading of the endpoint in the HI test is somewhat subjective, and it is useful to designate an individual as the reader for the sake of consistency. Appropriate control sera should also be included with each run of the assay. It is especially helpful if a sera which is known to have a titre at about the breakpoint of susceptibility is available. Generally, the HAI test is felt to have a reproducibility of about 1 dilution, i.e. two-fold. Finally, it is important to measure antibody to the challenge virus itself, as HAI antibody to older antigenic variants within the same subtype does not predict susceptibility accurately. The predictability of susceptibility to influenza B virus is less precise by HAI, even when using ether-treated antigen, which increases the sensitity of the test. Thus, some investigators have advocated the use of the neutralization test to screen subjects for susceptibility to influenza B virus (Frank *et al.* 1985).

In addition to selection of subjects based on serological prediction of susceptibility, it is prudent to perform reasonable testing to ensure that the subjects do not possess previously unrecognized conditions that would render influenza challenge unsafe. There is no standard routine for this evaluation. At a minimum, a careful history and physical examination should be performed. The yield of other screening laboratory and radiological tests is obviously quite low in young adults who have no significant past medical history and normal physical examination. In most studies, a complete blood count and differential, and often chemical tests of liver and renal function are performed, but it is very rare to detect an unsuspected, clinically relevant abnormality in this way. There is currently little data to suggest that influenza is more severe or more likely to cause complications in individuals in the early stages of human immunodeficiency virus (HIV) infection. However, most challenge studies involve the obtaining and processing of multiple samples of blood, and it is reasonable to screen subjects for antibody to HIV and hepatitis B, and possibly hepatitis C as well.

In order to prevent the possible inadvertent transmission of the challenge virus to non-study participants, subjects will usually be housed in some form of isolation following challenge. It is therefore prudent to use good judgement in the selection of subjects in order to avoid entering those who will be unable to comply with this need. Depending on the level of experience one has in this regard, and also on the duration and arduousness of the projected isolation, formal psychological screening may be performed. Because influenza may be more severe in smokers, subjects are generally requested to refrain from smoking during the challenge period, and reasonable caution should be used to exclude subjects who would not be able to do so. Individuals who are current abusers of illicit drugs and/or alcohol also generally do not do well in the inpatient challenge setting.

Selection of challenge strains and safety testing of virus pools

The process for selection and safety of wild-type influenza viruses for use as human challenge strains generally follows the procedures described previously (Knight 1964) and can be summarized as in current use as follows (L. Potash, DynCorp 1997, personal communication). Wild-type viruses are derived from the same sources that are used to derive cadidate strains for generation of inactivated vaccines, such as the World Health Organization (WHO) Surveillance or the Centers for Disease Control. Ideally, these viruses would have been initially isolated from ill individuals directly in SPAFAS eggs. (These are fertilized hens' eggs derived from specific flocks of chickens which have been certified free of a large spectrum of avian pathogens and which undergo a frequent and stringent quality assurance programme.) However, this is often not possible and primary egg isolates from non-SPAFAS eggs must be used. The virus is subsequently biologically cloned by plaque to plaque passage in primary chick kidney cells before further expansion in SPAFAS eggs.

A crude harvest of the expanded pool is then subjected to extensive testing to detect the potential presence of adventitious agents, including microbial sterility testing for bacteria, fungi, mycobacteria and mycoplasmas, animal safety testing including intraperitoneal and intracerebral inoculation of adult and suckling mice, and two serial passages in suckling mice. The crude harvest is filtered through a 0.45-micron filter, and placed in the final containers. This 'final container' material is then subjected to retesting for microbial sterility, a general safety test consisting of intraperitoneal injection of mice and guinea-pigs to detect any unexpected untoward reactions, and a test for the presence of reverse transcriptase. At both the initial and final phase of the process, the identity of the virus is confirmed with specific antisera to the haemagglutinin and neuraminidase. In addition a test for virulence is ferrets is done prior to use in humans, and the titre of virus in the final material is determined by plaque and/or liquid cell culture titration.

Almost all recent influenza virus challenge studies have been performed using such inocula prepared in eggs, and generally represent viruses which have been multiply passaged and are somewhat laboratory adaped. It is widely recognized that there are multiple mutations which occur, particularly in the haemagglutinin, during this process (Katz & Webster 1988). The impact of such laboratory adaptation on the 'virulence' of the challenge viruses for humans has not been rigorously defined. Limited studies using inocula prepared in mammalian cell culture suggest that such viruses retain relatively greater virulence for humans (Douglas 1975). The cell lines currently acceptable for human vaccine production do not support influenza replication to high enough titre for routine use for this purpose, although additional cell lines are being explored (Govorkova *et al.* 1995). Importantly, there can be significant variability from virus to virus in the ability to infect and cause illness in subjects who appear to be equally susceptible by serological means, although this statement should be tempered by the knowledge that such pools are not generally tested in a comparative way.

Because of this variability in the infectivity of individual wild-type virus pools, it is usually prudent to perform a preliminary dose titration to determine the 50% human infectious dose (HID_{50}) and the level of clinical symptoms of new virus challenge pools in susceptible adults before proceeding to larger studies. If the susceptibility of the subjects to infection is reasonably uniform, then such a dose titration can take place in a small number of subjects, generally from four to 10 subjects per virus inoculation level. Conversely, the estimate of HID_{50} will not be very precise if there is substantial unaccounted difference from subject to subject.

Inoculum size and delivery

The early studies referred to above typically used some form of aerosolized administration of virus, although the average particle size of such aerosols is unclear, and it is likely that the majority of the inoculum in these studies was deposited in the upper respiratory tract. Subsequently, typical illness was also introduced in volunteers by intranasal inoculation of virus by drops or spray. Generally, symptoms produced by the two methods were similar, although the two methods of administration have rarely been directly compared. In dose-ranging studies with an inhaled aerosol having a mean particle diameter of 1.5 mm, the HID_{50} of influenza A/Bethesda/10/63 (H2N2) was estimated to be 0.6–3 50% tissue culture infectious doses ($TCID_{50}$) in volunteers with low HAI antibody titres (Alford *et al.* 1966). The results suggested that the lower respiratory tract exposure is 40–500 times more susceptible to infection than the other respiratory tract. Other evidence suggests that aerosol inoculation is associated with somewhat shorter incubation period (12–48 h compared to 36–72 h following nasopharyngeal inoculation) and with somewhat more protracted illness than nasal inoculation (Douglas 1975). Because nasal administration appears to have a greater safety profile, and because the total dose of virus administered is easier to control by this method, it has become the more commonly used method for inoculation.

Typical influenza challenge pools possess an HID_{50} titre of between 100 and 1000 $TCID_{50}$, and are generally administered to subjects at a dose of approximately 100 HID_{50} or slightly higher. Since egg-grown pools typically contain about 10^7 $TCID_{50}$/ml, this usually works out to a dose of about 0.5 ml of a 1/10–1/100 dilution of allantoic fluid, delivered by drops or coarse spray intranasally. The infectivity of influenza viruses for humans inoculated in the nasopharynx appears to vary from strain to strain. The HID_{50} was found to be 127 and 320 $TCID_{50}$ for an influenza A (H3N2) virus (Couch *et al.* 1971, 1974). The HID_{50} also varies with the antibody status of the host, and it has not been possible to assess this directly with truly seronegative individuals. Once infection occurs there appears to be little effect of viral inocula ranging from 10^3 to 10^9 TCID$_{50}$ on illness, except for shortening of incubation period at higher viral doses (Douglas 1975). There is no evidence that immunity to the virus can be overcome by the administration of a higher dose inoculum.

Outcome measurements

The choice of outcome measurements will depend somewhat on the nature of the questions being asked in the study. In a typical challenge study a combination of virological, immunological and clinical measurements are included. The most precise and predictable type of outcome in a typical challenge study is nasopharyngeal shedding of the challenge virus, and several studies have demonstrated significant positive correlations between the quantity of virus recovered and severity of illness (Couch *et al.* 1971; Murphy *et al.* 1973b). Sampling can be done by nasopharyngeal swabbing, nasal wash or by throat gargles. Nasal washes have been used most frequently to assess quantitative shedding patterns. These samples have been the most consistently positive ones, although it is possible that their high yield may reflect in part early nasopharyngeal replication following intranasal virus inoculation (Douglas 1975). In this procedure, 5–10 cm^3 of a sterile saline solution is instilled into the nares with the glottis closed, and secretions for virus culture are collected into a sterile container by gravity and placed in appropriate transport media. These secretions are evaluated for the presence of virus by inoculation of cell culture, and the quantity of virus determined in positive samples. Highest sensitivity can be achieved if samples are cultured within 24 h of collection without freezing. Types of outcomes which can be analysed include the frequency, level, and duration of virus shedding. It is usually not practical to assess lower respiratory shedding in these studies due to the difficulty of obtaining appropriate samples, so that lower respiratory tract replication of virus is difficult to evaluate other than by assessment of lower respiratory tract symptoms.

Immune responses to infection can be assessed by a variety of assays which are reviewed in detail elsewhere (Chapter 22). For the purposes of defining infection, most studies have used a four-fold or greater increase in serum HAI antibody against the challenge virus. Other types of techniques, particularly enzyme-linked immunoadsorbent assay (ELISA) type tests, may actually be more sensitive for serological detection of virus infection (Madore *et al.* 1983), but are not as well standardized for diagnosis as is HAI. As described below, other types of immune responses may also be of interest to measure, such as cell-mediated responses, including cytotoxic, lymphoproliferative or cytokine responses.

The clinical symptoms generally followed represent commonsense clinical endpoints associated with influenza. Such symptoms include those which represent upper respiratory tract illness, such as rhinitis, sore throat, earache, and hoarseness; those which represent lower respiratory tract illness, such as cough; and systemic symptoms, such as myalgias, headache and malaise. Several of these symptoms, particularly headache and malaise, can be more related to changes in sleep–wake cycles, and other changes to daily routine associated with the inpatient challenge setting, and are therefore not very specific indicators of influenza. There are many scales which have been devised for measurement of clinical symptoms scores, none of which have a clear-cut advantage over the others. The lack of standardization of clinical symptom scores and definitions of clinical illness between studies makes fine comparisons of the severity of illness from study to study difficult.

In most studies, a limited physical examination is performed daily. However, physical findings with the exception of fever, are minimal in the challenge setting. Subjects may exhibit rhinorrhoea, pharyngeal erythema or tracheal tenderness, but it is more typical to see no clear-cut objective findings on physical examination, even in symptomatic subjects who are shedding virus. Because of the subjective nature of the clinical measurements, additional efforts have been made to use more objective quantification markers of illness. These have included such measurements as nasal mucus weights, and middle ear pressure measured by tympanometry (Doyle *et al.* 1994). Such measurements often correlate well with other objective measurements of treatment effects in human challenge studies (Walker *et al.* 1997).

Typical rates of infection and illness

Typical rates of clinical illness, virus shedding and infection following intranasal inoculation of serosusceptible adults with recent, egg-grown strains of influenza A and B are shown in Tables 39.1–39.3. The data are drawn from the placebo groups of recently published challenge studies conducted over approximately the last 10 years. The majority of adults in each of these studies were infected by the challenge viruses, as manifested by the detection of virus shedding, HAI seroresponse to the challenge virus, or both. As shown in these tables, almost all subjects with any evidence of infection shed virus, and there are no significant differences between influenza types in infection frequency. In general virus is recovered in moderate quantities on the first day after inoculation. Peak viral concentrations (3.0–$7.0 \log_{10}$ $TCID_{50}$/ml) occur on the second or third days after infection and then fall off gradually, so that virus is no longer detectable typically after the fifth to seventh day after inoculation (Murphy *et al.* 1973b; Douglas 1975). There can be significant differences from study to study even using the same challenge virus, which makes comparison of viruses for virulence quite difficult unless such comparisons are done concurrently.

The rates of clinical illness are also shown in Tables 39.1–39.3. These rates are more difficult to compare between studies, as mentioned above, because investigators have not used a standard definition of illness or lower respiratory tract illness, and do not report results in a consistent fashion from study to study. With this caveat, however, it does appear that symptoms following influenza A H1N1 or A H3N2 are similar, while experimentally induced influenza B is typically more mild or asymptomatic in young individuals. In part, this may be related to the problems in

finding individuals who are truly susceptible to influenza B using the HAI test. Overall, illnesses in these challenge studies are quite mild, and mostly manifested by upper respiratory tract symptoms of sore throat and stuffy nose. Systemic or febrile illnesses are seen in a minority of subjects, and the disease is clearly less severe than classic symptomatic influenza in young adults. As described above, the reasons for the relatively attenuated nature of the illness, even in sero susceptible subjects, is unclear, but may be related both to the highly passaged nature of the inoculum as well as the route of administration.

Statistical considerations and study group sizes

Because of the variability in attack rates from study to study and the subjective nature of outcome measurements such as clinical symptoms in the challenge model, human challenge studies should employ a randomized, blinded, placebo-controlled study design whenever possible. Statistical methods to be used include comparisons of rates and proportions for outcomes such as virus shedding and illness. Clinical symptom scores are rarely normally distributed, and so are usually compared by non-parametric tests, such as the Mann–Whitney test. Such tests are also used to compare the peak titre of virus shed between groups, while the pattern of virus shedding can be compared using ANOVA techniques (analysis of variance).

An important consideration in the design of human challenge studies is the relatively small sample size that can be reasonably studied under these circumstances. Because of these small sample sizes, challenge studies in adults need to be realistic in terms of their goals, and involve relatively few numbers in each treatment group, so as to require exposure of the smallest number of subjects to the pathogen as practical. The high attack rates seen in the challenge setting can partially offset this disadvantage. For example, if 100% of the subjects can be expected to become infected after challenge, demonstration of 50% or greater protective efficacy at $\alpha = 0.05$ would require only 15 subjects in each group with 80% power.

Table 39.1 Clinical and virological response of young healthy adults with prechallenge serum antibody of 1 to 8 to the challenge virus to intranasal challenge with influenza A (H1N1) virus.

References	Dose (log$_{10}$ TCID$_{50}$)	Proportion of subjects*				Proportion of subjects with*		
		Infected†	Shedding virus	Mean peak titre virus shed (log$_{10}$ TCID$_{50}$ ± SE)	Mean duration of shedding (days ± SE)	Systemic or febrile illness	Respiratory illness	Lower respiratory illness‡
A/California/10/78								
Treanor et al. (1987)	4.5	8/9	8/9	1.98	NR	0/9	5/9	NR
Treanor et al. (1990)	4.5	8/8	8/8	2.4 ± 0.4	3.6 ± 0.6	2/8	3/8	NR
Clements et al. (1986)	4.0	11/15	11/15	3.8 ± 1.6	6.8 ± 1.5	5/15	3/15	1/15
A/Hong Kong/123/77								
Betts et al. (1985)	4.2	15/16	15/16	4.2 ± 2.1	4.7 ± 2.1	8/16	5/16	NR
A/Kawasaki/9/86								
Yougner et al. (1994)	7.0	NR	10/14	2.2 ± 0.4	NR	3/14	6/14	NR
Hayden et al. (1994)	7.0	16/16	16/16	2.8 ± 0.5	NR	1/16	NR	2/16
A/Texas/1/85								
Sears et al. (1988)	6.4	26/28	26/28	3.1 ± 1.9	4.5 ± 2.4	8/28	11/28	NR
Sears & Clements (1987)	6.7	20/22	18/22	3.0 ± 1.9	3.5 ± 1.7	5/22	9/22	1/22
A/Texas/91								
Hayden et al. (1996b)	5.0	26/26	24/26	3.2 ± 2.1	2 (0–6)§	10/26	21/26	7/26

NR, not reported.

* No. with finding/no. evaluated.

† Virus shedding, serum antibody response, or both.

‡ Reported as 'lower respiratory illness' or 'cough'.

§ Expressed as median (range).

Table 39.2 Clinical and virological response of young healthy adults with prechallenge serum antibody of 1 to 8 to the challenge virus to intranasal challenge with influenza A (H3N2) virus.

| References | Dose (log$_{10}$ TCID$_{50}$) | Proportion of subjects* | | Mean peak titre virus shed (log$_{10}$ TCID$_{50}$ ± SE) | Mean duration of shedding (days ± SE) | Proportion of subjects with* | | |
		Infected†	Shedding virus			Systemic or febrile illness	Respiratory illness	Lower respiratory illness‡
A/Bethesda/1/85								
Treanor *et al.* (1990)	4.5	5/5	4/5	2.4 ± 0.6	3.0 ± 1.0	2/5	2/5	NR
Sears *et al.* (1988)	7.0	10/10	10/10	4.2 ± 1.4	5.9 ± 1.3	3/10	1/10	NR
Reuman *et al.* (1989)	7.1	18/19	18/19	3.5 ± 0.5	6.5	NR	11/19	NR
A/England/40/83								
al/Nikib *et al.* (1986)	4.1	31/31	30/31	4.0	NR	NR	17/31	NR
A/Korea/1/82								
Snyder *et al.* (1988)	6.0	12/14	12/14	3.4 ± 0.5	5.1 ± 0.3	1/14	5/14	NR
A/Los Angeles/2/87								
Clements *et al.* (1992)	7.0	22/24	16/24	1.5 ± 0.3	2.6 ± 0.4	4/24	11/24	NR
A/Washington/897/80								
Clements *et al.* (1986)	6.0	25/27	22/27	3.8 ± 1.6	4.3 ± 2.0	10/27	7/27	3/27

NR, not reported.

* No. with finding/ no. evaluated.

† Virus shedding, serum antibody response, or both.

‡ Reported as 'lower respiratory illness' or 'cough'.

Table 39.3 Clinical and virological response of young healthy adults with prechallenge serum antibody of 1 to 8 to the challenge virus to intranasal challenge with influenza B virus.

References	Dose (log$_{10}$ TCID$_{50}$)	Proportion of subjects*		Mean peak titre virus shed (log$_{10}$ TCID$_{50}$ ± SE)	Mean duration of shedding (days ± SE)	Proportion of subjects with*		
		Infected†	Shedding virus			Systemic or febrile illness	Respiratory illness	Lower respiratory illness‡
B/Ann Airbor/1/86								
Clements *et al.* (1990)	7.0	10/12	8/12	4.0 ± 0.7	5.4 ± 1.0	2/12	5/12	
B/Texas/1/84								
Keitel *et al.* 1990)	7.1	6/6	6/6	2.2 ± 0.7	5.0 ± 0.6		3/6	
B/Yamagata/16/88								
Treanor & Betts (1993)	7.0	10/10	7/10	2.3		3/10	7/10	2/10

NR, not reported.
* No. with finding/no. evaluated.
† Virus shedding, serum antibody response, or both.
‡ Reported as 'lower respiratory illness' or 'cough'.

Advantages and limitations of the challenge model

There are several advantages and limitations to the use of human challenge studies for influenza. The greatest advantage of these studies is that the timing, dose, level of exposure and specific virus causing infection is under the control of the investigator, and that appropriate prechallenge specimens can be obtained at leisure. In addition, the timing of sample collection in relationship to virus exposure is under control. However, it must be considered that these studies are invariably performed in a partially immune population, which may impact on assessment of immune response. The challenge studies also require the availability of appropriate wild-type pools which are sufficiently infectious and virulent to cause illness in adults. In addition, assessment of virological response is limited to the upper respiratory tract, as is most of the clinical illness produced. Therefore, it is possible that these models tend to overemphasize measures which are active in the upper respiratory tract, while not reflecting the impact of control measures on the lower respiratory tract very accurately.

The advantage of this approach to vaccine evaluation is that the high attack rates that may be expected in the wild-type challenge study can allow estimates of vaccine protective efficacy in a relatively small number of subjects. However, the disadvantage of this approach is that limited numbers of subjects can be accommodated in such studies, and the cost per individual subject is often high. In addition, the degree to which the challenge model accurately reflects acquisition of the disease in the real world could be argued. However, challenge studies can provide the initial evidence that a new approach has promise, can provide an early indication that a particular strategy should be abandoned, and can act as a powerful catalyst for further studies, if indicated. In the following sections, the use of human challenge studies in the evaluation of immunity, vaccines, pathogenesis and antivirals will be reviewed, as well as the degree to which such challenge studies have predicted the utility of vaccine or antiviral agents in the field.

Applications of the human challenge model

Studies on influenza pathogenesis

Various investigators have used experimentally infected volunteers to study various pathogenic aspects of influenza. Unlike naturally occurring infections, the prospective design and carefully controlled conditions of experimentally induced influenza studies enable the collection of data before infection and sequentially thereafter. However, the interpretation of the findings is limited by the general good health and youth of the persons studied, the intranasal route of virus exposure, and the relatively modest severity of experimentally induced illness. In particular, the paucity of lower respiratory tract symptoms differs from the typical course of classic influenza.

Effects on peripheral blood leucocytes

The peripheral blood leucocyte responses to experimental influenza infection have been assessed in several studies. Among symptomatically infected volunteers, neutrophilia occurs on the second day after inoculation followed by neutropenia on the sixth day (Douglas *et al.* 1966). Lymphocyte counts decrease on the first day of illness and sometimes rise on the sixth day above the preinoculation level. Others have found modest early polymorphonuclear (PMN) leucocytosis and later impairment in PMN chemotaxis following experimental influenza. Douglas *et al.* (1966) also found that total leucocyte counts above $10\,000/$mm^3 were present at the onset of illness in approximately 38% of those who were ill and 12% of those who were not. Total leucocyte counts of less than 5000 were found later during illness in a few subjects. Significant changes in eosinophil, monocyte or red blood cell counts are generally not observed.

The lymphopenia that accompanies experimental influenza affects all lymphocyte subpopulations but primarily reflects decreases in T cells (Criswell *et al.* 1979). Subset analyses have found decreases in both CD4$^+$ and CD8$^+$ cells but increases in the proportion of activated T lymphocytes approximately 1 week after infection (Skoner *et al.* 1996c). These changes have been postulated to relate in part to increased cortisol elaboration (Criswell *et al.* 1979). Increased natural killer (NK) cell activity, decreased numbers of activated NK cells, and decreased blastogenic responses to mitogens have been reported following experimental infection (Skoner *et al.* 1996c). An associated decrease in the magnitude of delayed hypersensitivity reactions to intradermal antigens occurs during the first week after infection (Skoner *et al.* 1996a).

Homologous and heterosubtypic *in vitro* blastogenic responses are demonstrable following experimental infection (Dolin *et al.* 1978). These responses were lower than baseline values at 3 days after viral infection but were significantly increased by 6 days after challenge. Blastogenic responses were noted only in volunteers who were actively infected, as measured by virus shedding, but occurred in those who were asymptomatic as well as clinically ill. Other studies have reported more prolonged decreases in influenza-specific blastogenic responses (Skoner *et al.* 1996c). In humans inoculated with influenza virus, cytotoxic T-cell levels correlates with viral clearance independent of specific antibody levels (McMichael *et al.* 1983).

Effects on cytokine elaboration

Experimental infection is accompanied by interferon rises in respiratory secretions and serum samples (Jao *et al.* 1970). Following A/Bethesda/ 10/63 (H3N2) infection, 67% of 15 infected adults developed detectable interferon levels in nasal wash and/or serum samples, and 40% had rises at both sites. Viral shedding preceded interferon appearance at either site by 1–2 days, and there was a temporal correspondence between improvements in clinical symptoms and the peak of interferon levels. Other studies have confirmed significant interferon rises in nasal washings with peak titres on day 3 after challenge and detectability up to 8 days (Murphy *et al.* 1973a; Hayden *et al.* 1998).

More recent studies have identified other pro-inflammatory cytokine responses during experimental influenza. Following experimental influenza A/Texas/36/91 (H1N1) infection, nasal lavage IL-6 and interferon-α (IFN-α) levels peak early after infection and correlate with viral titres, fever, mucus weights and symptom severity scores (Hayden *et al.* 1998). Blood IL-6 levels also rise by day 2 after infection, whereas nasal wash TNF-α and IL-8 rise later in the course of illness.

Pulmonary and otological function

In general, cough is a relatively minor symptom and no significant spirometric changes are noted after experimental influenza in healthy volunteers. Histamine-induced bronchial hyperreactivity developed in asthmatic patients, but variably in previously healthy persons, following experimental infection with a live attenuated virus (Laitinen & Kava 1980; Laitinen *et al.* 1991). Recently, no significant changes in spirometry or methacholine-induced airway responsiveness were found in healthy persons or those with allergic rhinitis following experimental A/Kawasaki/86 (H1N1) infection (Skoner *et al.* 1996b).

Experimental influenza in adults is associated with increased mucociliary transit time, eustachian tube dysfunction, abnormal ear pressures, and less often acute otitis media (Doyle *et al.* 1994). Following experimental influenza A/Kawasaki/9/86 (H1N1) infection, assessments have found eustachian tube dysfunction in ~80% of subjects by sonotubometry, middle ear underpressures in ~70% by digital tympanometry, and otoscopic evidence of otitis media in up to 20% (Doyle *et al.* 1994; Buchman *et al.* 1995). Such changes provide objective measures of the responses to drug interventions. Interestingly, initiation of oral rimantadine at 48 h after virus challenge at a time when subjects are already symptomatic has not been associated with improvements in these function abnormalities (Doyle *et al.* 1998). In contrast, administration of the topical neuraminidase inhibitor zanamivir at approximately 30 h after experimental infection has been associated with a significant reduced frequency of middle ear pressure abnormalities following experimental influenza A/Texas/1/91 (H1N1) infection (Walker *et al.* 1997).

Effects on bacterial flora

Alterations to the bacterial flora of the upper respiratory tract have received limited study following experimental influenza infection. Smorodintsev *et al.* (1937) performed serial bacteriological studies before and at various days after infection with an influenza A (H1N1) virus. No quantitative or qualitative changes in flora were found. More recently, experimental influenza A/Kawasaki/86 (H1N1) infection was associated with trends towards increased rates of oropharyngeal colonization by *Streptococcus pneumoniae* (15% of volunteers on postchallenge day 6) but decreased rates of recovering *Haemophilus influenzae* and no changes in the commensal flora (Wadowsky *et al.* 1995). The interpretation of such results is complicated by the relatively small numbers of subjects involved, the lack of uninfected controls, and the semi-quantitative nature of the bacteriological data.

Studies of the immune response to infection and evaluation of vaccines

The human challenge model can be quite useful for measurement of immune responses to infection. Because the exposure to virus can be controlled, such studies can carefully define the kinetics of the response as well. This model has been used to assess both local and systemic antibody responses to influenza infection, as well as cellular responses.

Similarly, the challenge model is an excellent tool for testing hypotheses about the role of specific immune effector arms in mediating protection against infection, elimination of virus, and amelioration of illness. A unique feature for this purpose is the ability to the status of other immune factors in order to analyse one component at a time. As described earlier, challenge studies clearly showed the role of neutralizing, and later, HAI antibody in prevention of influenza, and demonstrated the relatively greater importance of antibody against specific antigenic variants rather than reference strains (Morris *et al.* 1966). Later challenge studies were used to demonstrate the protective effect of neuraminidase-inhibiting antibody (Clements *et al.* 1986b), and of mucosal haemagglutinin-specific

antibody measured by ELISA (Clements *et al.* 1986b), and the role of cytotoxic T lymphocytes in humans (McMichael *et al.* 1983).

The most direct test of a hypothesis about immunity is to intervene with a vaccine, and it is in the realm of vaccine testing that human challenge studies have played the greatest role. As mentioned above, human challenge studies were among the first to demonstrate the protective efficacy of inactivated influenza vaccines, and by varying the time interval between vaccination and challenge, these studies were used to determine the duration of the protective effect. Challenge studies have also been used extensively to evaluate live virus vaccines, including egg-adapted viruses (Burnet & Foley 1940), neuraminidase-deficient mutants (Betts *et al.* 1977), temperature-sensitive mutants (Douglas *et al.* 1979), avian-human influenza reassortant viruses (Sears *et al.* 1988) and cold-adapted influenza A and B reassortant vaccines.

If the appropriate wild-type virus is available, the human challenge model can also be used in demonstrating the attenuation of a live virus vaccine candidate by direct comparison to the corresponding wild-type virus in serosusceptible adults. There are no strict criteria for defining attenuation in this type of study, although an appropriately attenuated vaccine would be expected to at a minimum not cause fever or systemic symptoms, and would typically manifest significantly decreased replication in comparison to the wild-type virus. It should be noted, however, that if the wild-type virus does not induce significant symptoms in the model, attenuation of a candidate vaccine can probably not be assessed reliably.

A further development of this type of study design is to assess the contributions of each individual gene segment to the attenuation phenotype of a live influenza virus vaccine, through the generation and testing of single gene reassortant viruses. It is important in such a study to define before the study begins what criteria will be accepted as evidence of attenuation of the reassortants, as the level of replication of these viruses may be somewhat intermediate. This type of design has been used previously to determine the genetic basis of attenuation of the cold-adapted influenza A/

Ann Arbor/6/60 virus (Snyder *et al.* 1988) and the avian A/Mallard/NY/6750/78 virus (Clements *et al.* 1992). Two points are noteworthy regarding such studies: it is important to be aware that some findings may represent gene constellation effects that may not be seen consistently with reassortants in a different wild-type background (Subbarao *et al.* 1992), and findings in humans may not always be consistent with findings in animals, even primates (Tian *et al.* 1985).

Generally, studies such as these would be undertaken after the HID_{50} of the human challenge virus had been established, and would be performed in subjects who had been screened for susceptibility, if this is possible. If a live, attenuated virus vaccine is also being used, it is usually necessary to determine the HID_{50} of the vaccine virus as well. After performance of these preliminary studies, a typical study design would randomly assign subjects to receive vaccine or placebo. If there is concern that there might be significant variability in susceptibility, then this randomization might be stratified based on markers of immunity, if known. At some time point

after vaccination, subjects are brought to the isolation facility and challenged with the wild-type virus. The time between vaccination and challenge is variable. Generally, initial studies are done approximately 1 month postchallenge, in order to test the vaccine under ideal circumstances, if promising results are obtained, further studies can be done to evaluate the duration of protection (Clements *et al.* 1986a). Outcome measures of the wild-type challenge study are designed to evaluate the protection afforded by vaccination against infection (virus shedding or seroresponse), virus shedding, and clinical illness. In addition, if a live virus vaccine is being evaluated, the level and duration of virus shedding, and clinical response to challenge in placebo recipients can be compared with the responses to live virus vaccine as evidence of attenuation. An example of a recent study design in which the efficacy of a trivalent live attenuated vaccine was tested against each of the three corresponding wild-type viruses is shown in Fig. 39.1.

Studies of antiviral agents

Outcome measures

Human experimental influenza infection has been used to evaluate the potential efficacy of a wide range of influenza virus inhibitors. The endpoints

Fig. 39.1 Schematic diagram of a typical study design to test the efficacy of a trivalent live attenuated influenza vaccine against each of the three corresponding wild-type viruses in serosusceptible healthy adults.

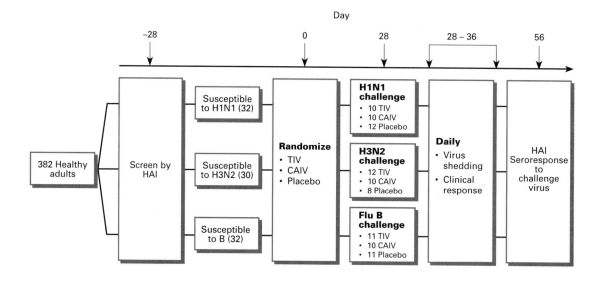

in such trials include both virological and clinical ones. Typical virological measures include overall rates of infection based on recovery of the challenge virus from the upper respiratory tract and/or development of four-fold or greater rise in specific antibody titres. In addition, the number of days and duration of virus recovery, the proportions of individuals shedding virus over time, and the quantity of the virus recovered from the upper respiratory tract have provided useful measures of the effects of antiviral agents on the virological course of infection. An integrated measure that provides a sensitive indicator of antiviral effects is the area under the viral shedding curve (Hayden *et al.* 1996b).

The clinical outcomes in such trials vary somewhat with the particular challenge strain but usually include the proportions of volunteers developing fever, upper respiratory tract illness, systemic illness manifested by myalgia, and sustained cough. Compared to naturally occurring infection, the frequency and duration of both fever and cough are generally lower in experimental infections. In addition to symptom scores, which can be integrated to provide a measure of symptom burden over time, objective measures of rhinorrhoea (nasal mucus weights) and middle ear function (middle pressures by digital tympanometry) have also been incorporated in certain trials.

Amantadine and rimantadine

The most frequently studied antiviral agents in experimental human infections have been amantadine and rimantadine. The initial efficacy studies of amantadine in humans were conducted by Jackson *et al.* (1963) and showed that initiation of amantadine beginning 18h before virus challenge was associated with a 46% protective efficacy against infection determined by antibody rise in seronegative individuals. This study also showed that serum HAI antibody provided a separate protective effect. No reductions in seroconversion rates were observed if the drug was begun immediately before or 3h after virus exposure. In contrast a study done several years later by Dawkins *et al.* (1968) found that rimantadine at a higher dose did not protect

against serologically documented infection but significantly reduced the proportion of individuals who had recoverable virus from throat swabs, as well as the proportions who had illness or fever (Table 39.4) (Jackson *et al.* 1963; Stanley *et al.* 1965; Dawkins *et al.* 1968; Smorodintsev *et al.* 1970; Sears & Clements 1987; Reuman *et al.* 1989). Smorodintsev *et al.* (1970) found that prophylaxis with amantadine provided an overall efficacy against infection based on serological rise of 55% and efficacy of 61% against febrile illness. Subsequent studies (Sears & Clements 1987; Reuman *et al.* 1989) confirmed protective effects against febrile illness although no clear-cut dose response was observed over a range of amantadine doses from 50 to 200 mg/day. Virological effects in these trials have been somewhat inconsistent (Table 39.4). Significant reductions in peak titres but variable effects on the duration of virus shedding have been reported. The protective efficacy against febrile illness has generally ranged from 60 to 100%. In summary, these studies have found significant protection against infection and/or illness for influenza A viruses of all three recognized human subtypes.

Several studies of experimentally induced infections have found evidence for therapeutic effects with these drugs. When rimantadine was begun 1 day after virus challenge either orally or by aerosol, significant reductions in the frequencies of fever and symptom scores were observed in either drug group compared to placebo (Hayden *et al.* 1982). More recently, treatment as late as 48h after inoculation of influenza A/Kawasaki/86 (H1N1) were associated with clinical benefits, although the frequency of fever in this study was so low as to make this a non-evaluable endpoint (Doyle *et al.* 1998).

Other antiviral agents

A variety of other antiviral agents have been screened for activity against experimental human influenza challenge. Prophylaxis studies have found clinical and virological benefit with congeners of amantadine (Beare *et al.* 1972; al-Nakib *et al.* 1986), the topical neuraminidase inhibitor

Table 39.4 Representative studies of oral amantadine and rimantadine for prophylaxis against experimental influenza A virus challenge.

Study (references)	Drug (number studied)	Virus (inoculum in TCID$_{50}$)	Antibody status	Drug dose (mg)	Initiation of therapy
Jackson et al. 1963 Stanley et al. 1965	Amantadine (n = 199)	A(H2N2)	50% HI $\leq$ 10	A 100/12 hours for 6 days	−18 hours
				A 100/12 hours for 6 days	+4 hours
				Placebo	−18 hours
				Placebo	+4 hours
Dawkins et al. 1968	Rimantadine (n = 55)	A/Rockville/1/65 (H2N2) 10$^{4.8}$	Nt $\leq$ 2	R 200 b.d. for 11 days	−1 day
				Placebo	
Smorodintsev et al. 1970	Amantadine (n = 404)	A(H2N2)	Unselected	A 100 or 200/day for 11 days	−1 day
				Placebo	
		A/HongKong (H3N2)		A 100 or 200/day	
				Placebo	
Sears & Clements 1987	Amantadine (n = 44)	A/Texas/1/85 (H1N1) 10$^{6.7}$	HI $\leq$ 8	A 100/day for 8 days	−3 days
				Placebo	
Reuman et al. 1989	Amantadine (n = 88)	A/Bethesda/1/85 (H3N2) 10$^{7.2}$	HI $\leq$ 8	A 50/day for 8 days	−3 days
				A 100/day for 8 days	
				A 200/day for 8 days	
				Placebo	

zanamivir (GG167) (Hayden *et al.* 1996a, 1996b), and to lesser extent with intranasal interferon-α (Phillpotts *et al.* 1984; Treanor *et al.* 1987). The protective efficacies of intranasal zanamivir against infection (~80%) and febrile illness (~95%) are the highest recognized to date. This agent has also been associated with protection against experimental influenza B (Hayden *et al.* 1996a) and with antiviral and therapeutic benefits when begun approximately 1 day after virus challenge. In contrast, no important prophylactic activity has been found with other agents like oral ribavirin at doses of 600–1000 mg/day (Cohen *et al.* 1976; Togo & McCracken 1976; Magnussen *et al.* 1977) or the thiobendazole LY217896 (Hayden *et al.* 1994).

Predictive value of challenge studies for antivirals

An important issue in regard to the use of experimentally induced influenza in humans to assess the potential value of antiviral agents and other interventions is the predictive value of the results. When specific agents have been tested sequentially in experimental and naturally occurring infections, the overall qualitative outcomes (benefit or no benefit) and the magnitude of the beneficial effects have generally corresponded (Table 39.5). This has been observed in studies of both prophylaxis and treatment. In general, it appears that studies in experimental influenza in humans provide useful positive and negative predictive results. Studies in experimentally infected volunteers can also be used

Fourfold antibody rise (%)	Infected (%)	Virus position (%) (mean days of shedding)	Ill (%)	Fever (%)	Comments
	37				Prophylactic efficacy = 46% for infection in
	72				seronegatives
	66				Strong protective affect of HI Ab
	72				No reduction in seroconversion rate if drug at −0.5 or +3 hours
93		0	26	11	Efficacy for fever = 84%
100		18 (throat swabs)	86	68	Efficacy for illness = 70%
18				25	
35				64	Efficacy for serological rise = 55%
					Efficacy for febrile illness = 61%
24				29	
88				75	
73	77	50 (1.6)	9	0	Efficacy for infection = 16%
91	91	82 (4.2)	41	23	Efficacy for fever = 100%
					Efficacy for illness = 78%
					Reduction peak titres ~1.7 $\log_{10}$
40	80	65 (5.3)	20	10	Efficacy for infection = 16%, 37%, 28%,
30	60	55 (5.7)	15	15	resp., at each dose level
37	68	63 (5.5)	11	11	Efficacy for febrile illness = 68%, 74%, 82%,
68	95	95 (6.5)	58	58	resp.
					Reduction in peak titres ~ 2 $\log_{10}$
					Efficacy for virus shedding = 32%, 42% 28%, resp.

to collect relevant pharmacokinetic and pharmacodynamic (e.g. quantitative viral shedding) data, but it remains to be determined how closely these experimental infections predict efficacious drug doses in the field.

The route of drug delivery is also an important variable, since experimental infections are induced by intranasal inoculation and are associated with a paucity of lower respiratory tract symptoms. These feature contrast with natural influenza and have important implications for administration of topical antiviral agents. For example, intranasal prophylaxis with interferon is protective against intranasal influenza challenge at higher doses (Phillpotts *et al.* 1984; Treanor *et al.* 1987), but intranasal interferon does not appear to be protective against natural influenza (Saito *et al.* 1985; Douglas *et al.* 1986; Foy *et al.* 1986; Hayden *et al.* 1986; Tannock *et al.* 1988).

References

Al-Nakib, W.P.G., Higgins, W, Willman J. *et al.* (1986) Prevention and treatment of experimental influenza A virus infection in volunteers with a new antiviral ICI 130,685. *J Antimicrobial Chemother* **18**, 119.

Alford, R.H., Kasel, J.A., Gerone, P.J. & Knight, V. (1966) Human influenza resulting from aerosol inhalation. *Proc Soc Exp Biol Med* **122**, 800.

Andrewes, C.H., Laidlaw, P.P. & Smith, W. (1935) Influenza: observations on the recovery of virus from man and on the antibody content of human sera. *Br J Exp Pathol* **16**, 566.

Beare, A.S., Hall, T.S. & Tyrrell, D.A. (1972) Protection of volunteers against challenge with A-Hong Kong-68

Table 39.5 Predictive value of human influenza virus challenge studies compared with studies in naturally occurring infections.

Intervention [references]	Route	Indication	Relative efficacy*	
			Experimental	Natural
Inactivated vaccine	Intramuscular	Prophylaxis	++++	++++
Cold adapted vaccine	Intranasal	Prophylaxis	++++	++++
Amantadine/rimantadine [Slepushkin & Zlydnikov 1987; Douglas 1990; Wintermeyer & Nahata 1995]	Oral	Prophylaxis	++++	++++
Rimantadine [Slepushkin & Zlydnikov 1987; Douglas 1990; Wintermeyer & Nahata 1995]	Oral	Treatment	++	++
Amantadine/rimantadine [Hayden et al. 1980; Hayden et al. 1982]	Aerosol inhalation	Treatment	++	+
Interferon [Merigan et al. 1973; Phillpotts et al. 1984; Treanor et al. 1987; Hayden et al. 1986; Douglas et al. 1986; Foy et al. 1986; Tannock et al. 1988]	Prophylaxis	Prophylaxis	+++ to 0†	0
Ribavirin‡ [Cohen et al. 1976; Togo & McCracken 1976; Magnussen et al. 1977; Smith et al. 1980; Stein et al. 1987]	Oral / Oral	Prophylaxis / Treatment	+/0 / Not determined	Not determined / 0 to +
Zanamivir [Hayden et al. 1996a,b; Hayden et al. 1997]	Intranasal/ aerosol	Treatment	++	++

* Estimated efficacy based on clinical and virological effects relative to placebo controls: ++++, $\geq 80\%$; +++, $\geq 60\%$; ++, $\geq 40\%$; +, $\geq 20\%$.
† Variable protection against illness depending, partly, on dose.
‡ Based on dose of 1 g/day for treating natural disease. Higher doses may have some beneficial effects in natural influenza [Stein et al. 1987]. Two prophylaxis studies were negative at dose of 600 mg/day and one found partial protection at 1 g/day starting at 6 hours after challenge.

influenza virus by a new adamantane compound. *Lancet* **i**, 1039.

Betts, R.F., Douglas, R.G. & Murphy, B.R. Jr (1985) Resistance to challenge with influenza A/Hong Kong/123/77 (H1N1) wild-type virus induced by live attenuated A/Hong Kong/123/77 (H1N1) cold-adapted reassortant virus. *J Infect Dis* **151**, 744.

Betts, R.F., Douglas, R.G., Roth, F.K. Jr, Little, J.W. (1977) Efficacy of live attenuated influenza A/Scotland/74 (H3N2) virus vaccine against challenge with influenza A/Victoria/3/75 (H3N2) virus. *J Infect Dis* **136**, 746–53.

Buchman, C.A., Doyle, W.J., Skoner D.P. *et al.* (1995) Influenza A virus-induced acute otitis media. *J Infect Dis* **172**, 1348.

Burnet, F.M. (1942) Influenza virus B: II immunization of human volunteers with living attenuated virus. *Med J Australia* **1**, 673.

Burnet, F.M. (1943) Immunization against influenza with living attenuated virus. *Med J Australia* **1**, 385.

Burnet, F.M. & Foley, M. (1940) The results of intranasal inoculation of modified and unmodified influenza

virus strains in human volunteers. *Med J Australia* **1**, 655.

Chanock, R.M. (1956) Association of a new type of cytopathogenic myxovirus with infantile croup. *J Exp Med* **104**, 555.

Chanock, R., Roizman, B. & Myers, R. (1957) Recovery from infants with respiratory illness of a virus related to chimpanzee coryza agent (CCA). I. Isolation, properities, and characterization. *Am J Hygeine* **66**, 291.

Clements, M.L., Betts, R.F. & Murphy, B.R. (1984) Advantage of live attenuated cold-adapted influenza A virus over inactivated vaccine for A/Washington/80 (H3N2) wild-type virus infection. *Lancet* **i**, 704.

Clements, M.L., Betts, R.F., Tierney, E.L. & Murphy, B.R. (1986a) Resistance of adults to challenge with influenza A wild-type virus after receiving live or inactivated virus vaccine. *J Clin Microbiol* **23**, 73.

Clements, M.L., Betts, R.F., Tierney, E.L. & Murphy, B.R. (1986b) Serum and nasal wash antibodies associated with resistance to experimental challenge with influenza A wild-type virus. *J Clin Microbiol* **24**, 157.

Clements, M.L., Snyder, M.H., Buckler-White A.J. *et al.* (1986c) Evaluation of avian-human reassortant influenza A/Washington/897/80 × A/Pintail/119/79 virus in monkeys and adult volunteers. *J Clin Microbiol* **24**, 47.

Clements, M.L., Snyder, M.H., Sears, S.D., Maassab, H.F. & Murphy, B.R. (1990) Evaluation of the infectivity, immunogenicity, and efficacy of live cold-adapted influenza B/Ann Arbor/1/86 reassortant virus in adult volunteers. *J Infect Dis* **161**, 869.

Clements, M.L., Subbarao, E.K., Fries L.F. *et al.* (1992) Use of single-gene reassortant viruses to study the role of avian influenza A virus genes in attenuation of wild-type human influenza A virus for squirrel monkeys and adult human volunteers. *J Clin Microbiol* **30**, 655.

Cohen, A., Togo, Y., Khakoo, R., Waldman, R. & Sigel, M. (1976) Comparative clinical and laboratory evaluation of the prophylactic capacity of ribavirin, amantadine hydrochloride and placebo in induced human influenza type A. *J Infect Dis* **133**: A114.

Couch, R.B., Douglas, R.G., Fedson, D.S. Jr & Kasel, J.A. (1971) Correlated studies of a recombinant influenza-virus vaccine. III Protection against experimental influenza in man. *J Infect Dis* **124**, 473.

Couch, R.B., Kasel, J.A., Gerin, J.L., Schulman, J.L. & Kilbourne, E.D. (1974) Induction of partial immunity to influenza by a neuraminidase-specific vaccine. *J Infect Dis* **129**, 411.

Criswell, B.S., Couch, R.B., Greenberg, S.B. & Kimzey, S.L. (1979) The lymphocyte response to influenza in humans. *Am Rev Respir Dis* **120**, 700.

Dawkins, A.T.J., Gallager, L.R., Togo, Y., Hornick, R.B. & Harris, B.A. (1968) Studies on induced influenza in man. II Double-blind study designed to assess the prophylactic efficacy of an analogue of amantadine hydrochloride. *J Am Med Assoc* **203**, 1095.

Dolin, R., Murphy, B.R. & Caplan, E.A. (1978) Lymphocyte blastogenic responses to influenza virus antigens after influenza infection and vaccination in humans. *Infect Immun* **19**, 867.

Douglas, R.G. Jr (1975) Influenza in man. *The Influenza Viruses and Influenza*, p. 395. New York, Academic Press.

Douglas, R.G. Jr (1990) Prophylaxis and treatment of influenza. *N Engl J Med* **322**, 443.

Douglas, R.G. Jr, Alford, R.H., Cate, T.R. & Couch, R.B. (1966) The leucocyte response during viral respiratory illness in man. *Ann Int Med* **64**, 521.

Douglas, R.G. Jr, Markoff, L.J., Murphy B.R. *et al.* (1979) Live Victoria/75-ts-1[E] influenza A virus vaccines in adult volunteers: role of hemagglutinin immunity in protection against illness and infection caused by influenza A virus. *Infect Immun* **26**, 274.

Douglas, R.M., Moore, B.W., Miles H.B. *et al.* (1986) Prophylactic efficacy of intranasal alpha$_2$-interferon against rhinovirus infections in the family setting. *N Engl J Med* **314**, 65.

Doyle, W.J., Skoner, D.P., Hayden F.G. *et al.* (1994) Nasal and otologic effects of experimental influenza A virus infection. *Ann Otol Rhinol Laryngol* **103**, 59.

Doyle, W.I., Skoner, D.P., Alper, C.M. *et al.* (1998) Effect of rimantadine treatment on clinical manifestations on otological complications in adults experimentally infected with influenza A (H1N1) virus. *J Infect Dis* (in press).

Eaton, M.D. & Martin, W.P. (1942) Immunization with inactive virus of influenza B: comparison of antibody response with that produced by infection. *Public Health Rep* **57**, 445.

Foy, H.M., Fox, J.P. & Cooney, M.K. (1986) Efficacy of alpha 2-interferon against the common cold (letter). *N Engl J Med* **315**, 513.

Francis, T. Jr (1934) Transmission of influenza by a filterable virus. *Science* **80**, 457.

Francis, T. Jr (1940) A new type of virus from epidemic influenza. *Science* **92**, 405.

Francis, T. Jr, Salk, J.E., Pearson, H.E. & Brown, P.N. (1944) Protective effect of vaccination against influenza A. *Proc Soc Exp Biol Med* **55**, 104.

Frank, A.L., Taber, L.H. & Wells, J.M. (1985) Comparison of infection rates and severity of illness for influenza A subtypes H1N2 and H3N2. *J Infect Dis* **151**, 73.

Govorkova, E.A., Kaverin, N.V., Gubareva, L.V., Meignier, B. & Webster, R.G. (1995) Replication of influenza A viruses in a green monkey continuous cell line (Vero). *J Infect Dis* **172**, 250.

Hall, C.B., Walsh, E.E., Hruska, J.F., Betts, R.F. & Hall, W.J. (1983) Ribavirin treatment of experimental respiratory syncytial viral infection. *J Am Med Assoc* **249**, 2668.

Hayden, F.G., Hall, W.J. Jr & Douglas, R.G. (1980) Therapeutic effects of aerosolized amantadine in naturally acquired infection due to influenza A virus. *J Infect Dis* **141**, 535.

Hayden, F.G., Zlydnikov, D.M., Iljenko, V.I. & Padolka, Y.V. (1982) Comparative therapeutic effect of aerosolized and oral rimantadine HCl in experimental human influenza A virus infection. *Antiviral Res* **2**, 147.

Hayden, F.G., Albrecht, J.K., Kaiser, D.L. & Gwaltney, J.M. (1986) Prevention of natural colds by contact prophylaxis with intranasal alpha-2 interferon. *New Engl J Med* **314**, 71.

Hayden, F.G., Tunkel, A.R., Treanor J.J. *et al.* (1994) Oral LY217896 for prevention of experimental influenza A virus infection and illness in humans. *Antimicrobial Agents Chemother* **38**, 1178.

Hayden, F.G., Lobo, M. Jr, Hussey, E.K. *et al.* (1996a) Efficacy of intranasal GG167 in experimental human-influenza A and B virus infection. In: Brown, L.E., Hampson, A.W., Webster, R.G. (eds). *Options for the Control of Influenza III*. Elsevier, Amsterdam, 718–25.

Hayden, F.G., Treanor, J.J., Betts R.F. *et al.* (1996b) Safety and efficacy of the neuraminidase inhibitor GG167 in experimental human influenza. *J Am Med Assoc* **275**, 295.

Hayden, F.G., Osterhaus, A., Treanor, J.J. *et al.* (1997) Efficacy and safety of the neuraminidase inhibitor zanamivir (GG167) in treatment of influenza virus infections. *N Engl J Med* **337**(13): 874–9.

Hayden, F.G., Fritz, R.S., Lobo, M.C., Alvord, W.G., Strober, W. & Straus, S.E. (1998) Local and systemic cytokine responses during experimental human influenza A virus infection: Relation to symptom formation and host defense. *J Clin Invest* (in press).

Henle, W., Henle, G. & Stokes, J. (1943) Demonstration of the efficacy of vaccination against influenza type A by experimental infection of human beings. *J Immunol* **46**, 163.

Hirst, G.K. Jr (1941) The agglutination of red cells by allantoic flid of chick embryos infected with influenza virus. *Science* **94**, 22.

Hirst, G.K. (1942) The quantitative determination of influenza virus and antibodies by means of red cell agglutination. *J Exp Med* **75**, 49.

Hirst, G.K., Rickard, E.R., Whitman, L. & Horsfall, F.L. (1942) Antibody response of human beings following vaccination with influenza viruses. *J Exp Med* **75**, 495.

Jackson, G.G., Muldoon, R.L. & Akers, L.W. (1963) Serologic evidence for prevention of influenza infections by an anti-influenzal drug adamantanamine hydrochloride. *Antimicrobial Agents Chemother* **1963**, 703.

Jao, R.L., Wheelock, E.F. & Jackson, G.G. (1970) Production of interferon in volunteers infected with Asian influenza. *J Infect Dis* **121**, 419.

Katz, J.M. & Webster, R.G. (1988) Antigenic and structural characterization of multiple subpopulations of H3N2 influenza virus from an individual. *Virology* **165**, 446.

Keitel, W.A., Couch, R.B., Cate, T.R., Six, H.R. & Baxter, B.D. (1990) Cold-recombinant influenza B/Texas/1/84 virus vaccine: attenuation, immunogenicity, and efficacy against homotypic challenge. *J Infect Dis* **161**, 22.

Knight, V. (1964) The use of volunteers in medical virology. *Progr Med Virol* **6**, 1.

Knight, V., Kasel, J.A., Alford R.H. *et al.* (1965) New Research on influenza: studies with normal volunteers. *Ann Int Med* **62**, 1307.

Laitinen, L.A. & Kava, T. (1980) Bronchial reactivity following uncomplicated influenza A infection in healthy subjects and in asthmatic patients. *Eur J Respir Dis* **106** (suppl).

Laitinen, L.A., Elkin, R.B., Empey D.W. *et al.* (1991) Bronchial hyperresponsiveness in normal subjects during attenuated influenza virus infection. *Am J Respir Dis* **143**, 358.

McMichael, A.J., Gotch, F.M., Noble, G.R. & Beare, P.A.S. (1983) Cytotoxic T-cell immunity to influenza. *N Engl J Med* **309**, 13.

Madore, H.P., Reichman, R.C. & Dolin, R. (1983) Serum antibody responses in naturally occurring influenza A virus infection determined by enzyme-linked immunosorbent assay, hemagglutination-inhibition, and complement fixation. *J Clin Microbiol* **18**, 1345.

Magnussen, C.R., Douglas, R.G., Betts, R.F. Jr, Roth, F.K. & Meagher, M.P. (1977) Double-blind evaluation of oral ribavirin (Virazole) in experimental influenza A virus infection in volunteers. *Antimicrobial Agents Chemother* **12**, 498.

Merigan, T.C., Reed, S.E., Hall, T.S. & Tyrrell, D.A. (1973) Inhibition of respiratory virus infection by locally applied interferon. *Lancet* **i**, 563.

Morris, J.A., Kasel, J.A., Saglam, M., Knight, V. & Loda, F.A. (1966) Immunity to influenza as related to antibody levels. *N Engl J Med* **274**, 527.

Murphy, B.R., Baron, S., Chalhub, E.G., Uhlendorf, C.P. & Chanock, R.M. (1973a) Temperature-sensitive mutants of influenza virus IV. Induction of interferon in the nasopharynx by wild-type and a temperature-sensitive recombinant virus. *J Infect Dis* **128**, 488.

Murphy, B.R., Chalhub, E.G., Nusinoff, S.R., Kasel, J. & Chanock, R.M. (1973b) Temperature-sensitive mutants of influenza virus III. Further characterization of the ts-1(E) influenza A recombinant (H3N2) in man. *J Infect Dis* **128**, 479.

Phillpotts, R.J., Higgins, P.G., Willman J.S. *et al.* (1984) Intranasal lymphoblastoid interferon ('Wellferon') prophylaxis against rhinovirus and influenza virus in volunteers. *J Interferon Res* **4**, 535.

Price, W.H. (1956) The isolation of a new virus associated with respiratory clinical disease in humans. *Proc Natl Acad Sci* **42**, 892.

Reuman, P.D., Bernstein, D.I., Keefer M.C. *et al.* (1989) Efficacy and safety of low dosage amantadine hydrochloride as prophylaxis for influenza A. *Antiviral Res* **11**, 27.

Rowe, W.P., Heubner, R.J., Gilmore, L.K., Parrott, R.H. & Ward, T.G. (1953) Isolation of a cytopathogenic agent from human adenoids undergoing spontaneous degeneration in tissue culture. *Proc Soc Exp Biol Med* **84**, 570.

Sabin, A.B. (1967) Amantadine hydrochloride: analysis of data related to its proposed use for prevention of A2 influenza virus disease in human beings. *J Am Med Assoc* **200**, 135.

Saito, H., Takenaka, H., Yoshida S. *et al.* (1985) Prevention from naturally acquired viral respiratory infection by interferon nasal spray. *Rhinology* **23**, 291.

Salk, J.E., Pearson, H.E., Brown, P.N. & Francis, T. (1944) Protective effect of vaccination against induced influenza B. *Proc Soc Exp Biol Med* **55**, 106.

Sears, S.D. & Clements, M.L. Jr (1987) Protective efficacy of low-dose amantadine in adults challenged with wild-type influenza A virus. *Antimicrobial Agents Chemother* **31**, 1470.

Sears, S.D., Clements, M.L., Betts R.F. *et al.* (1988) Comparison of live attenuated H1N1 and H3N2 cold-adapted and avian-human influenza A reassortant viruses and inactivated virus vaccine in adults. *J Infect Dis* **158**, 1209.

Shope, R.E. (1931a) Swine influenza I. Experimental transmission and pathology. *J Exp Med* **54**, 349.

Shope, R.E. (1931b) Swine influenza III. Filtration experiments and etiology. *J Exp Med* 373–85.

Skoner, D.P., Angelini, B.L., Jones A. *et al.* (1996a) Suppression of *in vivo* cell-mediated immunity during experimental infleunza A virus infection of adults. *Int J Pediatr Otorhinolaryngol* **38**, 143.

Skoner, D.P., Doyle, W.J., Seroky, J. & Fireman, P. (1996b) Lower airway responses to influenza A virus in healthy allergic and non-allergic subjects. *Am J Critical Care Med* **154**, 661.

Skoner, D.P., Whiteside, T.L., Wilson J.W. *et al.* (1996c) Effect of influenza A virus infection on natural and adaptive cellular immunity. *Clin Immunol Immunopathol* **79**, 294.

Slepushkin, A. & Zlydnikov, D.M. (1987) Safety and efficacy of rimantadine: the Russian experience. *J Respir Dis* **8** (suppl. 11A): S51.

Smith, C.B., Charette, R.P., Fox, J.P., Cooney, M.K. & Hall, C.E. (1980) Lack of effect of oral ribavirin in naturally occurring influenza A virus (H1N1) infection. *J Infect Dis* **141**, 548.

Smith, W. (1935) Cultivation of the virus of influenza. *Br J Exp Pathol* **16**, 508.

Smith, W., Andrewes, C.H. & Laidlaw, P.P. (1933) A virus obtained from influenza patients. *Lancet* **ii**, 66.

Smith, W. & Stuart-Harris, C.H. (1936) Influenza infection of man from the ferret. *Lancet* **ii**, 121.

Smorodintsev, A.A., Tushinsky, M.D., Drobyshevskaya, A.I., Korovin, A.A. & Osetroff, A.I. (1937) Investigation of volunteers infected with the influenza virus. *Am J Med Sci* **194**, 159.

Smorodintsev, A.A., Zlydnikov, D.M., Kiseleva A.M., Romanov, J.A., Kazantsev, A.P., Rumovsky, V.I. (1970) Evaluation of amantadine in artificially induced A2 and B influenza. *J Am Med Assoc* **213**, 1448–54.

Smorodintsev, A.A., Zlydnikov, D.M. Kiseleva A.M., Romanov, J.A., Kazantsev, A.P., Rumovsky, V.I. (1970) Evaluation of amantadine in artificially induced A2 and B influenza. *J Am Med Assoc* **245**, 1428.

Snyder, M.H., Betts, R.F., DeBorde D. *et al.* (1988) Four viral genes independently contribute to attenuation of live influenza A/Ann Arbor/6/60 (H2N2) cold-adapted reassortant virus vaccines. *J Virol* **62**, 488.

Stanley, E.D., Muldoon, R.L., Akers, L.W. & Jackson, G.G. (1965) Evaluation of antiviral drugs: the effect of amantadine on influenza in volunteers. *Ann NY Acad Sci* **130**, 44.

Stein, D.S., Creticos, C.M., Jackson, G.G. *et al.* (1987) Oral ribavirin treatment of influenza A and B. *Antimicrob Agent Chemother* **31**, 1285–7.

Subbarao, E.K., Kawaoka, Y., Ryan-Pourier, K., Clements, M.L. & Murphy, B.R. (1992) Comparison of different approaches to measuring influenza A virus-specific hemagglutination inhibition antibodies in the presence of serum inhibitors. *J Clin Microbiol* **30**, 996.

Subbarao, E.K., Perkins, M., Treanor, J.J. & Murphy, B.R. (1992) The attenuation phenotype conferred by the M gene of the influenza A/Ann Arbor/6/60 cold-adapted virus (H2N2) on the A/Korea/82 (H3N2) reassortant virus results from a gene constellation effect. *Virus Res* **25**, 37.

Tannock, G.A., Gillett, S.M., Gillett R.S. *et al.* (1988) A study of intranasally administered interferon-α (rIFN-α2A) for the seasonal prophylaxis of natural viral infections of the upper respiratory tract in healthy volunteers. *Epidemiol Infect* **101**, 611.

Taylor, R.M. & Dreguss, M. (1940) An experiment in immunization against influenza with a formaldehyde-inactivated virus. *Am J Hygeine* **31**, 31.

Tian, S.-F., Buckler-White, A.J., London W.T. *et al.* (1985) Nucleoprotein and membrane protein genes are associated with restriction of replication of influenza A/Mallard/NY/78 virus and its reassortants in squirrel monkey respiratory tract. *J Virol* **53**, 771.

Togo, Y. & McCracken, E.A. (1976) Double-blind clinical assessment of ribavirin (Virazole) in the prevention of induced infection with type B influenza virus. *J Infect Dis* **133** (suppl): A109.

Treanor, J.J. & Betts, R.F. (1993) Evaluation of live attenuated cold-adapted influenza B/Yamagata/16/88 reassortant virus vaccine in healthy adults. *J Infect Dis* **168**, 455.

Treanor, J., Dolin, R., Betts R.F. *et al.* (1987) Intranasal interferon as prophylaxis against experimentally induced influenza in humans. *J Infect Dis* **156**, 379.

Treanor, J.J., Roth, F.K. & Betts, R.F. (1990) Use of live cold-adapted influenza A H1N1 and H3N2 virus vaccines in seropositive adults. *J Clin Microbiol* **28**, 596.

Wadowsky, R.M., Mietzner, S.M., Skoner, D.P., Doyle, W.J. & Fireman, P. (1995) Effect of experimental influenza A infection on isolation of *Streptococcus pneumoniae* and other aerobic bacteria from the oropharynges of allergic and non-allergic adult subjects. *Infect Immun* **63**, 1153.

Walker, J.B., Hussey, E.K., Treanor, J.J., Montalvo, A. & Hayden, F.G. Jr (1997) Effects of the neuraminidase inhibitor Zanamivir on otologic manifestations of experimental human influenza. *J Infect Dis* **176**, 1417–22.

Wintermeyer, S.M. & Nahata, M.C. (1995) Rimantadine: a clinical perspective. *Ann Pharmacother* **29**, 299.

Youngner, J.S., Treanor, J.J., Betts, R.F. & Whitaker-Dowling, P. (1994) Effect of simultaneous administration of cold-adapted influenza A virus on clinical manifestations of experimental wild-type influenza A virus infection in humans. *J Clin Microbiol* **32**, 750.

Section 11
Economic Impact
of Influenza

CHAPTER 40

Socioeconomics of Influenza

Tom Jefferson and Vittorio Demicheli

Introduction

Health-care workers and policy-makers at all levels are usually interested in the socioeconomics of important diseases, such as influenza, in order to determine their impact on society and subsequently to analyse the consequences of the total or partial prevention of the diseases and their sequelae. A general practitioner's interest can be expressed in questions such as: 'If I vaccinate all my elderly population against influenza ahead of the announced epidemic, am I going to diminish morbidity and hence workload on my practice?' Similarly a policy-maker's view is echoed in a dilemma such as: 'Should I devote more resources to the problem of influenza, or should I invest in our breast screening programme?'

In this chapter we aim to give readers an idea of the methods which health economists employ to help answer such questions. The chapter is meant as an introduction and not as a 'hands-on' tutor. Readers should refer to an elementary textbook of economic evaluation for a more in-depth presentation of the methods (see Jefferson *et al.* 1996).

Traditionally science-based answers to the two questions are given in two phases:
• firstly a descriptive phase in which the burden of the disease to society is estimated; and
• secondly an analytical phase in which an estimation of the costs and consequences of removing such a burden, either in its entirety or in part, is made.

The description of the burden of influenza

The first phase is usually carried out through *cost-of-illness (COI) studies* (Rice 1994). The aim of COI studies is descriptive: to itemize, value and sum up the costs of a particular problem with the aim of giving an idea of its economic burden.

The first stage is the identification of all cases of influenza in a reference population. Usually this is done on the basis of national statistics, if available, or by extrapolating to the whole population from a smaller survey. Traditionally the process suffers from the limitations of the epidemiological data on which it is based, such as difficulty in case definition, undernotification of cases, and so on.

Next, costs generated by all the cases of the illness are identified and listed. These are traditionally classified as:

Direct costs — those borne by the health-care system, community and family in directly addressing the problem.

Indirect costs — mainly productivity losses caused by the problem or diseases, borne by the individual, family, society or employer.

Intangible costs — usually the costs of pain, grief and suffering and loss of leisure time. The cost of a life is usually included in the case of death.

Rarely are such costs calculated for all cases of influenza identified in the study, more often a sample of cases is costed and the results are extrapolated to the population of cases.

The incidence method (which estimates costs of cases from their onset to their disappearance for

541

whatever reason—usually cure or death) is the appropriate one for collecting cost data on influenza, a disease with relatively short duration and fluctuation of incidence. The COI approach is concerned with defining the value of resources directly used up by the illness. For example, one of the possible resource items in the burden of influenza is the number of days in hospital because of that illness. The total cost of such hospital stay, however, does not represent the real 'burden' of the illness to society since a part of the hospital costs is fixed and is independent from the onset of influenza cases. Thus *avoidable costs* should be used. For the purpose of this example these could be equated to marginal costs, i.e. the cost of producing an extra unit of a service (in this case the costs avoided by preventing x number of cases of influenza). *Marginal costs* express the value of the resources directly generated by cases of influenza and which would be avoided if the epidemic did not occur. An example of a possible template for the listing of resources used by an influenza epidemic in a reference population in a defined period is shown in Table 40.1. An extensive COI study on influenza, which has withstood the test of time, was carried out in the US by Kavet (1977) for his doctoral thesis in which he analysed influenza-related resource consumption for three epidemic years (1963, 1966 and 1969). Kavet applied his results to a reference population, and valued resources using 1968–1969 US prices, thus estimating influenza burden for that year. Table 40.2 shows Kavet's estimates for the three years (appropriately named models 63, 66 and 69).

An alternative way of assessing costs of illness could be the so-called *willingness to pay (WTP) approach* which estimates the burden of a disease by measuring what individuals would be prepared to pay in order to avoid that disease or problem. The practical application of WTP, however, is full of difficulties, mainly relating to the questions asked and the meaning of answers given.

Perhaps the greatest methodological limitation of COI studies, like other descriptive techniques, is their frequent use of average costs to estimate the value of resources, which often leads to unreliable and overinflated assessments of the burden of diseases. Such mistakes can lead to overestimation of benefits (costs avoided by interventions such as vaccination against influenza) when the economic convenience of interventions to diminish the burden of influenza is analysed in the second phase, that of analysis.

Table 40.1 Template for listing resource use during an influenza epidemic.

Number of cases (definition can be either clinical, i.e. persons who had clinical signs and symptoms of influence or its complications, or laboratory-based i.e. as above but accompanied by a rise in anti-influenza antibody titre)
Age profile of cases
Number of population at risk
Number of times a GP is involved per case
Number of times other community workers are involved per case (e.g. nurses)
Number and type of GP prescriptions per case
Number and type of GP investigations per case (e.g. chest X-ray, serology, etc.)
Number and destination of GP referrals (expressed as percentage of GP contacts for influenza). Referrals occur when patients are either sent to hospital or sent to a specialist
Number of hospital admissions for influenza
Percentage in facilities where a higher than normal level of care is required
Percentage of dead, expressed as percentage of admissions
Crude mortality rate and standardized mortality ratio for influenza and related illnesses
Average length of stay in hospital (in days)
Percentage of hospital discharges requiring follow-up
Days of sickness caused by influenza (expressed as working days lost in community-treated or hospital-treated populations
Likely social class distribution of illness

Table 40.2 Estimates of resource consumption in the USA during three influenza epidemic years (after Kavet 1977). Items marked * are counted in thousands.

Category	Model 63	Model 66	Model 69
Cases of influenza*	27 140	21 748	51 155
Percentage of cases medically attended	51.3	44.9	41.7
Physicians' services related to hospitalization*	3759	2637	5760
Diagnostic evaluations*	418	293	640
Routine follow-up visits*	3341	2344	5120
Hospital admissions*	418	293	640
Hospitalized days*	3759	2637	5760
Prescriptions issued*	13 923	9765	21 332

Analytical economic framework

These analyses, known as economic evaluations, list, value and compare the cost and consequences of different courses of action, each designed to answer questions such as the ones posed at the beginning of the chapter. Wider questions are likely to lead to the adoption of wider (societal) viewpoints. In these evaluations, known as cost–benefit analysis (CBA), both costs and outcomes are valued in monetary terms. CBA would be the technique of choice to answer our hypothetical policy-maker's question of whether to commit resources to influenza or to breast screening. If, however, a narrower question similar to the one posed by our hypothetical general practitioner is asked, then a cost-effectiveness analysis (CEA) is required. In CEA, costs of alternative ways of preventing influenza (e.g. by vaccination or with antivirals) are compared for the same outcome, usually expressed in natural units such as cost per case avoided. Thus, in addition to the COI-type listed information already gathered, we also need to assess the costs of vaccination or treatment campaigns. This allows estimation of the costs of these interventions and a comparison to be made with the consequences of each course of action, thus illustrating their pros and cons. Such a list is given in Table 40.3.

However, in an analytical framework there are a few more methodological elements that need to be applied, such as the use of effectiveness estimates of the vaccine, sensitivity analysis and discounting for the effects of time.

The choice of effectiveness estimates for the intervention being assessed is of crucial importance to the whole analytical framework. This is especially so for influenza vaccines which try to target a virus undergoing yearly changes with an unknown level of herd immunity. As a general rule, the results of large, well-designed studies are to be

Table 40.3 Template for listing resource use during a prevention campaign using vaccine against influenza.

Vaccine efficacy estimates
Yearly efficacy evidence of herd immunity
Number of doses per vaccine cycle
Extra resources likely to be needed for mounting the publicity for the vaccination campaign
Extra administration resources likely to be needed for mounting the vaccination campaign
Quantity of disposables needed for campaign (i.e. needles, syringes, swabs etc.)
Modality of vaccine administration (i.e., intramuscular, subcutaneous etc.)
Number and severity of side-effects
Quality and limitations of assessment of data (including assumptions and guesswork)

preferred to those of smaller ones. Some studies are full randomized controlled trials, but frequently cohort or case control studies, lower down the strength of evidence ladder, are all that is available for a particular vaccine configuration. The results of some of these can be pooled together in a so-called meta-analysis. Properly conducted meta-analyses give more powerful and less biased estimates of effectiveness of a vaccine, as in the case of the study by Gross *et al.* (1995). In this study, which pooled results of 20 observational (cohort) studies on elderly people, influenza vaccines were found to be 56% effective (with confidence intervals of between 39% and 68%) in preventing respiratory illness, 53% effective (35–66%) in preventing pneumonia, 48% effective (28–65%) in preventing hospitalization and 68% effective (56–76%) in preventing death. Estimates like these can be used to calculate the impact (number of avoided outcomes) of a vaccination campaign. Point estimates of effectiveness are likely to be misleading given the uncertainty over size of effects, as the confidence intervals around the estimates demonstrate. Additional uncertainty is present whenever extrapolation from one setting to another is attempted, and as a consequence it is common practice to examine the robustness of results of economic evaluations over a range of alternative estimates for uncertain parameters. These are usually varied one by one over a range of possible values. If the basic conclusions of the evaluation are not altered by changing a particular parameter, our confidence in the conclusions is increased. This formal procedure is called *sensitivity analysis*. According to the number of parameters which are simultaneously varied, sensitivity analysis is defined as 'one way' or 'two way'. A further refinement which is necessary when our analysis comprises events which are likely to take place over a period of time is *discounting*. This consists of decreasing annual values attached to resource consumption by a rate, called the discount rate, which (at least in theory) expresses society's preference and its strength. Discounted benefits and costs are given a lesser value the further into the future they accrue. It is accepted practice for evaluations to present results using a range of discount rates including both the current government

recommended discount rate for public expenditure programmes and no discounting. This allows the choice and use of a discount rate to be one of the variables in the sensitivity analysis. Traditionally, economic evaluations of influenza prevention have not consistently discounted costs or consequences because of the relatively short immunity conferred by the vaccines.

Secondary model

To give readers an idea of how an economic evaluation of influenza prevention is constructed, we have included in this chapter a model based on a systematic review of the studies on the economics of influenza vaccination. (As this is based on existing research, it is called a 'secondary model'.) Methods of search consisted of: a MEDLINE CD-ROM search in all European languages since 1966; a check of bibliographies of retrieved studies; correspondence with manufacturers of the vaccine; and contact with researchers active in the field. After studies had been retrieved, the screening criteria proposed by us in a systematic review of the economics of hepatitis B vaccine aimed at identifying reliable studies were used (Jefferson & Demicheli 1994). All studies which used resource or cost estimates derived from other works were eliminated. Data on quantities of resources used in the prevention and treatment of influenza were extracted from the primary studies in the review and used to construct a secondary model by using local unit costs and applying the data to a notional population. To construct the model, a 'resource costing approach' was used. This looks at the possibility of deriving data on resources from existing studies and estimating costs and cost-effectiveness from unit cost data specific to a particular setting. Thus, all those studies that did not contain a clear separation between resources used and unit costs or give enough data to allow calculation resource quantities were eliminated. As in all reviews, the use of sensitive criteria for inclusion of studies had the effect of reducing the numbers of observations in the analysis. For example, out of a total of 32 studies, 12 were excluded on the basis of methodological criteria, 9 studies contained data allowing extraction of estimates of resource use, but only 6 studies contained comparable resource estimates (for a complete bibliography see Jefferson & Demicheli 1996). Calculations of indirect benefits for the elderly were not included because of the methodological difficulty of valuing such costs. Rather than calculating an average value, ranges of estimates were pooled into an economic model based on a simulated general population cohort of 1 000 000 individuals. Costing of pooled resources was carried out with estimates of unit costs of hospital and other care and lost working time derived from a COI study on salmonella recently carried out in the Emilia region of Italy (Demicheli *et al.* 1995). Readers could, however, input their local unit costs data into the secondary resource model to carry out their own evaluation. The sensitivity of the resulting benefit-to-cost ratios (BCRs) is assessed using three levels of cost assumptions (high, medium and low) and high and low attack rates (250 and 100 per 1000 population). The efficacy of the vaccine is held at 80% throughout (although Gross's estimates can be used instead and the robustness of conclusions tested in a sensitivity analysis).

Table 40.4 sets out the distribution of costs estimates obtained from the included studies.

Table 40.5 shows the distribution of utilization of resources obtained from the included studies. High, medium and low estimates (when present) correspond to 75th percentile, median and 25th percentile values. Cost estimates were converted into 1995 US dollars by using the US Consumer Price Index (CPI) and the current exchange rates.

Figure 40.1 shows how BCRs change with the different resource estimates and attack rate used. The number of doctor-patient consultations and work days lost do not appear to greatly affect the BCR, whereas the model is sensitive to the estimate used for length of hospital stay. The BCR range from 0.3 to 1.2 for the low attack rate scenarios and from 1.1 to 3.6 for the high attack rate scenarios. Readers will note that there is a linear relationship between estimated incidence/attack rates and BCR, supporting the view that consistent methodology was used across the primary evaluations satisfying the entry criteria. Thus, available economic estimates pooled into an analytical model show that influenza vaccination is an efficient activity. This conclusion holds true when subgroup analysis is

Table 40.4 Distribution of estimates from studies of immunization against influenza derived from systematic review of economic evaluations. Monetary estimates are adjusted in US dollars to 1995 using US Consumer Price Index and appropriate exchange rates.

Variable	Number of observations	Unit	High	Medium	Low
Incidence					
Study group	14	%	26.6	10.1	4
General population	6	%	9.8	5.7	1.7
Vaccine effectiveness	16	%	90	60	30
Direct costs	16	US $ 1995	1102	712	95
Indirect costs	6	US $ 1995	1251	745	129
Intangible costs	2	US $ 1995	4677	2456	236
Vaccination cost					
Acquisition	15	US $ 1995	10	6	2
Administration	15	US $ 1995	17	13.5	8
Cost per avoided case	6	US $ 1995	321	266	40
Cost per healthy life-year gained	6	US $ 1995	145	143	133
Cost–benefit ratio	6	—	0.06	0.22	1.4

Table 40.5 Distribution of estimates of utilization of resources by influenza cases obtained from studies included in the review.

Variable	Number of studies	Unit	High	Medium	Low
Consultation	7	Number per case	2.3	2	0.2
Hospital admission	3	Number per case	0.05	0.03	0.012
Hospital length of stay	7	Days per episode	12	8	8
Laboratory tests	3	Number per case	1	0.6	0.3
Working days lost	8	Days per case	7	5.7	3

carried out for example on active workers or the elderly.

Conclusions

The economic evaluation of influenza prevention is an important decision-making tool. Traditionally the analytical stage is preceded by a descriptive stage which is useful in gaining more knowledge of the subject matter and good estimates of resource use. Models to address this

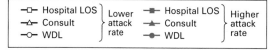

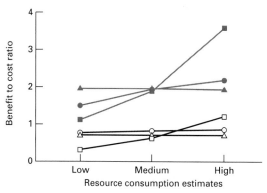

Fig. 40.1 Benefit to cost ratio model of influenza vaccination using resources consumption estimates derived from the literature, medium cost estimates and the two extreme estimates of influenza attack rates. LOS, length of stay; Consult, consultations; WDL, working days lost. (From Jefferson & Demicheli 1996, with permission from ADIS International Ltd.)

issue can be derived from economic literature and may be adapted to local needs. The secondary model shown in Fig. 40.1 tells us that whenever an epidemic is imminent and there is local pressure on the availability of beds, prevention of influenza is likely to be an efficient practice, especially if carried out through the means of an effective vaccine.

Curiously, however, such relatively strong evidence of both effectiveness and efficiency of influenza vaccines has not been translated into firm and clear preventive policies and vaccination coverage has remained variable. For example, in the 1980s there was a 10-fold variation in vaccine use in 18 different developed countries (ranging from the USA to Canada, countries in the EU, Australia and New Zealand). Although historical and cultural factors appeared to be important, the most important determinant appeared to be the existence of a reimbursement scheme for the vaccine (Fedson *et al.* 1995). In the USA an experimental community study showed that the linking of physician financial incentives with vaccination performance is likely to be a successful strategy for increasing levels of influenza immunization in the elderly (Kouides *et al.* 1993). It would appear that no programme of prevention against influenza can ignore such factors if it is to succeed.

Acknowledgement

The authors would like to gratefully acknowledge the many useful suggestions made by Professor Alan Maynard on reading a previous draft of this chapter.

References

Demicheli, V., Casadio, G.P., Lanciotti, G., Novaco, F. & Jefferson, T.O. (1995) The Emilia costing study: valutazione dell'impatto economico della salmonellosi umana. *Mecosan* **11**, 8–15 [in Italian].

Fedson, D.S., Hannoun, C., Leese, J. *et al.* (1995) Influenza vaccination in 18 developed countries, 1980–1992. *Vaccine* **13**, 623–27.

Gross, P.A., Hermogenes, A.W., Sacks, H.S., Lau, J. & Levandowski, R.A. (1995) The efficacy of influenza vaccine in elderly people. A meta-analysis and review of the literature. *Ann Intern Med* **123**, 518–27.

Jefferson, T.O. & Demicheli, V. (1994) Is vaccination against hepatitis B efficient?, A review of world literature. *Health Econ* **3**, 25–37.

Jefferson, T.O. & Demicheli, V. (1996) Economic evaluation of influenza vaccination and economic modelling. Can results be pooled? *Pharmacoeconomics* **9** (Suppl. 3), 67–72.

Jefferson, T.O., Demicheli, V. & Mugford, M. (1996) *Elementary Economic Evaluation in Health Care.* BMJ Books, London.

Kavet, J.A. (1977) Perspective on the significance of pandemic influenza. *Am J Public Health* **67**, 1063–70.

Kouides, R.W., Lewis, B., Bennett, N.M. *et al.* (1993) A performance-based incentive programme for influenza immunization in the elderly. *Am J Prevent Med* **9**, 250–55.

Rice, D.P. (1994) Cost-of-illness studies: fact or fiction? *Lancet* **344**, 1519.

Bibliography

Eono, P. & Desfontaine, M. (1993) Vaccinations en Milieau Militaire. Etude coût/efficacité (unpublished) [in French].

Gavira, F.J. & Lardinois, R. (1990) Analisis de rentabilidad de la vacunacion antigripal en una poblacion rural (La Victoria, Cordoba). *Med Clin (Barc)* **94**, 777–81 [in Spanish].

Helliwell, B.E. & Drummond, M.F. (1988) The costs and benefits of preventing influenza in Ontario's elderly. *Can J Public Health* **79**, 175–80.

Hocking, B. (1989) Benefits and costs of influenza immunization in the workforce. *Asia Pacific Human Resource Management* **November**, 87–93.

Koplin, A.N., Francis, B.J., Martin, R.J., Zimmerman, B.J. & Winegar, A. (1979) Administrative costs of the influenza control program of 1976–1977 in Illinois. *Med Care* **17**, 201–9.

Kumpulainen, V. & Makela, M. (1996) Influenza vaccination among healthy employees. A cost-benefit analysis (unpublished).

Levy, E. & Levy, P. (1992) La vaccination contre la grippe des personnes d'âge actif (25–64 ans): une étude coût–bénéfice. *Rev Epidémiol Santé Publique,* **40**, 285–95 [in French].

Makela, P.H., Jokinen, C., Koivula, I., Makela, M. & Pyhala, R. (1993) Pneumonia in the elderly and cost-effectiveness of influenza vaccination. In: Hannoun, C. Klenk, H.D. Kendal, A.P. & Ruben, F.L. (eds) *Options for the Control of Influenza,* pp. 63–68. Excerpta Medica, London.

Maucher, J.M. & Gambert, S.R. (1990) Cost-effective analysis of influenza vaccination in the elderly. *Age* **13**, 81–85.

Mullooly, J.P., Bennett, M.D., Hornbrook, M.R.P. *et al.* (1994) Influenza vaccination programs for elderly persons: cost-effectiveness in a health maintenance organization. *Ann Intern Med* **121**, 947–52.

Nichol, K.L., Margolis, K.L., Wuorenma, J. & VonSternberg, T. (1994) The efficacy and cost effectiveness of vaccination against influenza among elderly persons living in the community. *New Engl J Med* **331**, 778–83.

Nichol, K.L., Lind, A., Margolis, K.L. *et al.* (1995) The effectiveness of vaccination against influenza in health-working adults. *New Engl J Med* **333**, 889–93.

Office of Technology Assessment US Congress (1982) *Cost-Effectiveness of Influenza Vaccination.* Government Printing Office, Washington.

Patriarca, P.A., Arden, N.H., Koplan, J.P. & Goodman, R.A. (1987) Prevention and control of type A influenza infections in nursing homes. Benefits and costs of four approaches using vaccination and amantadine. *Ann Intern Med* **107**, 732–40.

Riddiough, M.A., Sisk, J.E. & Bell, J.C. (1983) Influenza vaccination: cost-effectiveness and public policy. *J Am Med Assoc* **249**, 3189–95.

Sauras, I.A. (1987) Analisis economico del coste de la gripa aplicado a la provincia de Huesca. *Revista Sanitaria Higiene Publica* **61**, 1017–28 [in Spanish].

Schoenbaum, S.C., McNeil, B.J. & Kavet, J. (1976) The swine-influenza decision. *New Engl J Med* **295**, 759–65.

Scott, W.G. & Scott, H.M. (1996) Economic evaluation of vaccination against influenza in New Zealand. *Pharmaeconomics* **9**, 51–60.

Smith, J.W.G. & Pollard, R. (1979) Vaccination against influenza: a five-year study in the Post Office. *J Hygiene.* **83**, 157–80.

Section 12
Pandemic Planning

CHAPTER 41

Pandemic Planning

Jane Leese and Susan E. Tamblyn

Introduction

Influenza viruses, by virtue of their ability to exchange genetic material with each other, are able to emerge, or re-emerge, as 'new' viruses with the potential to spread rapidly through susceptible populations and cause worldwide epidemics—pandemics—of influenza.

Records suggest that influenza pandemics have occurred at intervals for many centuries. Three have occurred in the 20th century: in 1918/19 ('Spanish' flu), now known to have been due to an A (H1N1) virus subtype related to swine influenza virus (Taubenberger *et al.* 1997); in 1957 ('Asian' flu), following a shift to an A (H2N2) subtype; and in 1968/69 ('Hong Kong' flu) when this subtype was replaced by an A (H3N2) subtype. The pandemic of 1918/19 remains one of the greatest scourges of modern times. It is estimated that by the end of the winter of 1918/19, two billion people around the world had suffered influenza infection and between 20 and 40 million people had died from influenza, a toll greater than that during the whole of the First World War. At least 150 000 people are estimated to have died from influenza in England and Wales.

For a pandemic to occur, the following criteria must coexist:

1 the appearance in humans of a genetically 'new' influenza virus;

2 the ability of that virus to infect and cause disease in humans; and

3 a large susceptible population worldwide, lacking immunity to the new virus.

It is generally agreed that the potential continues to exist for new strains both to emerge and to spread, and that future pandemics of influenza are likely, if not inevitable. When this might be, however, is unpredictable. Past pandemics have occurred at intervals varying from 11 to 42 years with no recognizable pattern and have occurred at varying times of the year.

When pandemics do occur, they spread rapidly, cause huge morbidity and mortality and put excessive demands on health services. They also threaten to disrupt other services through high absenteeism, and result in large economic losses. The only specific intervention currently available—influenza vaccine—cannot be prepared until the potentially pandemic strain of virus is known, and its availability as a preventive measure is likely to be restricted, at least in the early stages.

The scale of disruption is likely to be greater than that caused by most other emergencies for which the health sector develops contingency plans. Large geographical areas will be affected more or less simultaneously (so that support from neighbouring services is unlikely to be available) and the emergency is likely to last longer—at least 6–8 weeks in the first instance, with probable second and even third waves of illness a few months later. Past experience suggests that up to 25% of the population may develop clinical illness during this relatively short time, with asymptomatic infections also occurring (Miller *et al.* 1971); potentially, the whole population could be affected. The severity of illness is another unpredictable factor: it has varied between pandemics, and between different waves of the same pandemic, that of 1918 being particularly severe.

The need for greater pandemic preparedness, and what that should entail, has been the subject of discussion at several international fora in recent years (Tamblyn & Hinman 1993; Aymard *et al.* 1994; Rowe 1995; Ada *et al.* 1997). A broad consensus has emerged over the general approach, with recognition of the need for planning at international, national and local levels to facilitate a prompt and effective response. The World Health Organization (WHO) has announced plans to set up a Pandemic Influenza Task Force and several countries, including the USA, Canada, the UK and some other European countries and Japan, are reviewing and updating or developing national plans. The USA presented its draft conceptual plan to a meeting in Bethesda, Maryland in December 1995 (Monto 1997) and has since consulted on a draft planning guide containing a checklist for state and local health officials. The UK issued its national plan in March 1997 (UK Health Departments 1997). Weaknesses have already been identified in the global capacity to respond to a pandemic, some of which are now being addressed.

The aims of pandemic planning

The main aims of pandemic planning are:
1 to recognize promptly the emergence of a potential pandemic strain of virus and monitor its course;
2 to establish a formal mechanism to declare and manage a pandemic;
3 to reduce morbidity, mortality and hospitalization from influenza illness;
4 to be able to cope if necessary with large numbers of people ill and dying, both in the community and in hospital;
5 to ensure that essential services are maintained and reduce the disruption of normal daily life; and
6 to provide appropriate, timely, authoritative and up-to-date information for all those who require it, including health-care and other professionals, managers, the public and the media, at all stages of the pandemic.

A pandemic also offers opportunities for research, especially in areas which are difficult to study during interpandemic years because of the unpredictable and variable occurrence of influenza, the cocirculation of other respiratory viruses and the lack of specific markers of influenza infection as end points for clinical studies. Protocols for epidemiological, scientific and operational research, including international collaborations, should therefore ideally be prepared during the planning process, for activation should a pandemic occur. These should include arrangements for 'banking' of suitable laboratory samples for later research.

Development of plans

The overall responsibility for developing national pandemic influenza plans rests with national administrations. In addition, local plans, adapted to local needs and local organization of services, need to be developed by those who will be involved in their implementation, so that there is local 'ownership' of the plans. At all levels, a named coordinator is required, but a wide range of bodies and individuals need to be involved or consulted. At national level, this will include government departments, those responsible for national influenza surveillance and for the licensing and quality assurance of vaccines, vaccine manufacturers, health professionals, communications experts and finance officials. At local level, those involved may include a wide range of interests from the health sector and local government (e.g. public health officials, primary and secondary care physicians, microbiologists, virologists and epidemiologists, hospital and community nurses, infection control officers, pharmacists, communications experts), social service agencies, volunteer organizations, health education and information officers, the local media, emergency services, transport, large industries and employers in the area and finance and legal officers.

Phasing the response

Common to most pandemic influenza plans is an outline of the responsibilities of the principal bodies and organizations that would be involved in the response, which is conveniently divided into phases:

Phase 0 — The interpandemic period.

Phase 1 — The emergence of an influenza virus with a novel haemagglutinin and/or neuraminidase (a 'new virus') outside the country concerned.

Phase 2 — Outbreaks of influenza caused by the new influenza virus outside the country concerned.

Phase 3 — The new influenza virus isolated in the country concerned: pandemic imminent.

Phase 4 — Pandemic influenza in the country concerned.

Phase 5 — Return to background activity.

The phases are to some extent arbitrary but, broadly, phase 0 (the interpandemic period) is the preparatory planning phase. During this time deficiencies in current systems need to be identified and improved, and contingency plans refined and kept up to date. Phases 1–4 are implementation phases, phases 1–3 representing the time available for developing a vaccine and completing other preparations. This time may be short: although drifted strains of influenza in interpandemic years may take a year to 18 months to circulate worldwide, pandemic strains have previously circulated within 6 months. Increasing travel and shorter travel times, to the East particularly, are likely to shorten this time even further in future pandemics. Phase 4 may include more than one wave of illness. Phase 5 is the time for auditing the plan's implementation and effectiveness after the event in order to feed back into the planning process and refine the plans for the future.

The intervals between phases may or may not be distinct. Also, although most new viruses emerge in the East and spread westwards, it is possible that a new virus may emerge in the country concerned, in which case phases 1 and 2 would be bypassed.

International surveillance sometimes results in the identification of new viruses which do not subsequently fulfil their pandemic potential. This occurred in 1976 when an H1N1 swine influenza-like virus subtype was identified among military recruits at Fort Dix, Iowa. Plans were implemented to immunize the whole population of the USA, but the virus did not, in the event, spread beyond the base. Such false alarms are inevitable in a sensitive alert system. The phased response allows for plans to be activated, but later stood down, in the event

that a new virus does not become established in the way anticipated. Plans could be aborted at any stage, although certain commitments, for example to vaccine manufacturers, may have to be honoured.

Surveillance

Good surveillance is a prerequisite for planning — at global, national and local levels — to give the earliest possible warning of an influenza pandemic, and the required information about its impact and spread in order to make sound public health decisions.

Identification of a potentially pandemic virus

The World Health Organization routinely monitors influenza virus strains throughout the world through a network of national laboratories and its collaborating centres in London, Atlanta, Melbourne and Tokyo. Timely recognition of new variants has improved considerably in recent years, and has led to more accurate predictions of the likely prevalent circulating strains and improved matching of vaccines.

Weaknesses in global surveillance were identified early during the pandemic planning process. Of particular significance was the paucity of timely data from China. Many pandemic influenza virus strains — as indeed, drifted variants in interpandemic periods — appear to have originated in China. Increasing evidence suggests that major antigenic changes in influenza viruses result from reassortment of avian and mammalian subtypes, and that pigs — which serve as an intermediate host for both — act as a 'mixing vessel' for such reassortants (Webster *et al.* 1992). In rural China, avian species (particularly ducks), pigs and humans live in close proximity, increasing the probability of coinfection with different A subtypes and making China a continued likely source of genetically reassorted viruses (Shortridge 1995).

The WHO has strengthened its surveillance in China, but additional sites are needed in southern and western China and gaps in surveillance remain in other parts of the developing world. One suggestion for filling these gaps has been the concept of 'sister laboratories', a laboratory in a developing country being linked to, and supported by, one in a developed country. This would not only strengthen local laboratories, but also result in more timely shipping of isolates to reference centres. An important outcome of virological surveillance is the early provision of isolates in appropriate media as potential candidate vaccine strains.

Further study is required to determine the extent to which transmission of influenza strains already occurs between species without further spread. Collaborative surveillance of human and animal (particularly pig) influenza viruses in south-east Asia, and serological surveys of agricultural workers in rural areas of China for antibodies to non-human strains are needed.

Could a future pandemic strain be anticipated and what criteria could be used to assess the pandemic potential of a new virus? Previous strain mapping, together with serological archaeology, has suggested that few subtypes affect humans and that these may occur in cycles (Table 41.1) (Hope-Simpson 1992). In recent years H1N1 and H3N2 subtypes have cocirculated. It has been speculated that an A subtype containing an H2 or H7 component is likely to be the next new virus to emerge (Webster 1994). However, any of the 15 haemagglutinin and nine neuraminidase subtypes known to exist in nature could, in theory, emerge.

Monitoring the spread of the virus

Monitoring of the international spread of influenza viruses is coordinated by the WHO and requires local laboratory capacity and rapid communication. The identification of a potential pandemic virus should trigger enhanced national virological surveillance at least until the pandemic has become established (or the threat has disappeared). Thereafter, virological surveillance should continue at a level which allows monitoring of antiviral susceptibility and identification of variants that might be responsible for a second wave of illness.

Monitoring influenza infection

Clinical surveillance of influenza-like illness can give more timely information and also a more accurate picture of the true impact of influenza than virological surveillance, which requires laboratory diagnosis. In a pandemic, clinical surveillance should detect the arrival of influenza promptly and provide timely information on influenza activity at local and national level. It is particularly useful to have timely information on the numbers of people seeking medical attention, attack rates, the clinical characteristics of illness and its severity, the nature and severity of complications, hospitalizations and deaths.

There are large geographical gaps in disease-based surveillance, especially in areas such as China where it would be most useful, for early warning purposes, to know whether a new virus is causing human illness. Awareness of local outbreaks of illness in the area, for example in schools, would be particularly helpful.

Even among European countries, where 17 out of 25 countries in one survey had a reporting scheme,

Table 41.1 Major influenza A subtypes 1989–1997. From Hope-Simpson (1992).

Year	Major A serotype	
1889–1900	A (H2N2)	?Antigenically similar to the Asian H2N2 strains of 1957 which disappeared in 1968
1900–1918	A (H3N2)	
1908–1918	A (H1N1)	
1918–1928	A (H1 swine-like)	
1929–1946	A (H0N1)	
1946–1957	A (H1N1)	
1957–1968	A (H2N2)	
1968–	A (H3N2)	
1976	A (H1N1 swine-like)	
1977–	A (H1N1)	

comparison of data is hampered by differences in case definitions, methodology and denominator populations as well as by differences in the way health care is provided. Most surveillance systems are based on consultation data from sentinel general practitioners; a few include other markers of the impact of influenza in the community such as absenteeism and consumption of over-the-counter remedies. The interpandemic period presents an opportunity to standardize and develop complementary surveillance systems.

Other surveillance activities

Serosurveys enable an assessment of population susceptibility to a new virus, and monitoring of attack rates. Other surveillance activities required during a pandemic will include monitoring of vaccine uptake, adverse reactions to vaccine, antiviral susceptibility, and infections complicating influenza and their antibiotic susceptibility, as well as monitoring of sickness absence and hospital admissions. Enhanced surveillance may be appropriate in certain groups, for example, in particular age groups.

Review of the needs, and building and maintenance of the capability and capacity for disease-based surveillance, preferably linked to virological surveillance, is one of the tasks of the interpandemic period. Contingency plans should cover the arrangements for enhanced surveillance during the pandemic and identify the resources and personnel required for outbreak investigations and special field studies.

Pronouncement of a potential pandemic and the immediate response

In the event of the isolation of a new virus with pandemic potential, the WHO would be informed by one of its collaborating centres. The WHO would then send an investigation team to the area of origin of the virus, convene its influenza advisory committee and inform its counterparts in the member states, who would then activate their own plans. For most countries, this would entail convening a high-level influenza advisory committee with responsibility for collating the information available and advising on and coordinating the national response. Pandemic plans should outline the membership and reporting relationship, and clearly define the role, of this committee (along with clear definition of the role of other government bodies, including the licensing authority). In exceptional circumstances, an individual country might implement its plan independently after an assessment of the information available.

Pandemic influenza vaccine

Inactivated split virus influenza vaccines prepared from viruses related to the prevalent strains are now in routine use in annual influenza immunization programmes in most developed countries. The role of these programmes is to prevent morbidity and mortality by immunizing those most at risk of serious influenza-related illness, rather than to interrupt transmission of infection.

There remain questions about the minimum effective dose of vaccine in a pandemic, and whether this should be administered as one or two doses and at what interval. There is some evidence that in unprimed individuals—the pandemic situation—the immunogenicity of inactivated split virus vaccines is reduced (hence the current recommendation that young children who have neither been exposed to influenza viruses nor been previously immunized receive two doses of vaccine) (Nicholson *et al.* 1979).

In the longer term, the aim must be to produce more immunogenic vaccines, for example, using adjuvants. The role of DNA and cold-adapted live attenuated vaccines is also under investigation. Their use in a pandemic would depend on their prior evaluation: it would not normally be appropriate to use a new type of vaccine for the first time in a mass immunization campaign in an emergency.

Vaccine production

In the event of a pandemic, one role of national administrations will be to secure sufficient influenza vaccine for an expanded target population in the shortest possible time without any drop in standards of purity, potency, safety and efficacy. Manufacturers will work closely with governments and licensing agencies on quality control and on fast-tracking licence approval.

The manufacture of influenza vaccine is, however, a time consuming process, usually requiring 6–8 months from the time a new variant is identified before large numbers of doses are available for use. Rate-limiting factors in its production include:
1 the availability of embryonated hens' eggs from suitable flocks for growth of the viruses; they may not be readily available in large numbers, especially outside the normal production cycle (January–August), and flocks are susceptible to decimation by disease or other events beyond the control of the chicken farmer or vaccine manufacturers;
2 the availability of seed virus;
3 the availability of candidate vaccine virus strains which grow well in eggs;
4 the time taken to produce and standardize, and the availability of, test reagents;
5 the availability of production facilities—these may have been shut down at the end of one manufacturing season for cleaning;
6 the availability of personnel;
7 unforeseen problems with the manufacturing process; and
8 time required for packaging and labelling.
More advanced automation in the manufacturing process and improved testing and lot-release methods have already improved both the quality and quantity of influenza vaccines. Relatively simple measures such as the use of multidose vials rather than single-dose syringe presentations might save time. An increased number of doses would be available if the vaccine were presented as a monovalent preparation, although the benefit of this might be offset if it were found that two doses of vaccine were needed rather than one.

The technology for producing high growth reassortants has already improved; one possible area for further exploration is that of building up a bank of viruses of various subtypes with pandemic potential.

For the longer term, another aim is to develop alternative strategies for vaccine production that do not depend on eggs, such as the use of continuous cell lines for virus growth and DNA vaccines which could be readily stored and transported.

Liability for adverse reactions to a pandemic vaccine is another issue which needs to be addressed.

Vaccine supply and distribution

A pandemic produces a number of challenges for vaccine supply and delivery.

It is likely that, whatever the normal annual arrangements, the bulk of vaccine will be purchased centrally and plans should address funding of this. Distribution will also have to be overseen centrally and mechanisms will be needed to allocate and distribute limited supplies efficiently and equitably, for use in the agreed priority groups. Arrangements should allow for reallocation and redistribution if necessary.

How equitable distribution of vaccine is to be achieved internationally, especially to those countries without a domestic source of vaccine, requires further discussion with the manufacturers at both national and international levels. Ideally, appropriate agreements would be drawn up in advance.

Priority groups for immunization

A key strategy during the interpandemic period is the improvement of immunization levels in high-risk groups, with periodic reassessments of annual immunization programmes. In a pandemic, most countries will aim to immunize wider groups than those recommended for annual influenza immunization in interpandemic years. Some have chosen a selective strategy, which allows, however, for increasingly wide sections of the population to be immunized should vaccine supplies allow; others, such as the USA, aim to immunize everyone. Whatever the strategy chosen, as it is likely that supplies of vaccine will be limited, at least initially, priorities must be set for the groups to be offered vaccine and population estimates developed for each group. Initially, a balance has to be sought between the need to prevent mortality in high-risk groups and the need to keep key workers at work. Mortality can be expected to be mainly among the elderly, but some flexibility must be retained to take account of the evolving epidemiology of the pandemic and any particular risk groups which emerge (Table 41.2). Children play an important role in the transmission of influenza; if vaccine supplies permit, immunization of children might be considered in order to block transmission as well as to reduce morbidity in this group.

Organization of immunization

Most countries will need to make special arrangements to administer vaccine as rapidly as possible to persons in the target groups. Locally, arrangements will be necessary for temporary deployment of staff. Logistical difficulties will arise if a second dose of vaccine is needed for optimal protection and a strategy for securing compliance will be required. Consideration should be given to coordinated mass public health campaigns (similar to 'Sabin Sundays'), although local flexibility will be required.

Pneumococcal immunization

Pneumococci are a significant cause of secondary bacterial infection during an influenza pandemic. One of the tasks of the interpandemic period should be to assure a high uptake of pneumococcal vaccine in those at increased risk of pneumococcal infection. It is unlikely that large-scale 'catch-up' pneumococcal immunization would be feasible in the midst of a pandemic.

Antiviral agents

The antiviral agents amantadine and rimantadine, although active against influenza A (Smorodintsev *et al.* 1970), are little used in most countries for either the prevention or treatment of influenza. A number of factors, including their side-effect profile, emergence of resistance and limited supply, are likely to preclude their widespread use in a pandemic. The stockpiling of antiviral agents appears to be impractical. The limited circumstances for which they would be recommended need to be defined, and guidelines prepared for health professionals. When used for treatment, they shorten illness by a day or two. Their main application is therefore likely to be in prevention, as an adjunct to vaccine. Appropriate indications may include:
- short-term prevention in high-risk individuals while vaccine takes effect;
- short-term postexposure treatment in high-risk groups;
- longer-term prevention during the period of the pandemic in high-risk groups for whom vaccine is not available or contraindicated;
- prevention in health-care and other key workers, during the period of the pandemic if vaccine is not available, or until vaccine becomes available;
- possibly the treatment of severe influenza in hospitalized patients; and
- outbreak control in long-term care facilities.

Guidelines will need to take account of new antiviral agents as these become available.

Table 41.2 Priority groups for immunization (adapted from the UK Health Departments' Multiphase Contingency Plan for pandemic influenza, 1997). **NB** The order of priority to be finally decided in light of emerging data on the epidemiology of the evolving pandemic.

1 Groups at high risk of severe influenza-related morbidity and death who are currently recommended for annual immunization	5 Health-care assistants, care assistants, support staff, home helps
2 All aged over 65 or 75 years (if not already included in (1) above)	6 Pregnant women
3 Health-care providers	7 Household contacts of those in high-risk groups
4 Key personnel providing essential community services (e.g. in government departments, the police, fire service, ambulance service, undertakers, prisons, security, telephone, electricity and gas, military personnel)	8 Other selected industries
	9 Those aged 16–64 years
	10 Those aged 0–15 years

Emergency preparedness and response

Existing emergency plans will almost certainly require modification during the interpandemic period to take account of the circumstances of a pandemic. These will need to cover, and consider the resources for, the following:

• *The provision of primary and secondary health care for patients with influenza.* Health-care facilities will be overstretched. Cancellation of non-urgent admissions, and full use of community hospitals will help to relieve the pressure.

• *The provision of social and community services.* An increased demand for social and community services is inevitable, and will be an important measure for maintaining people in their homes as far as possible, and avoiding unnecessary hospital admissions. Ways of providing increased community support should be considered.

• *Mortuary arrangements*

• *Supplies.* Key supplies will need to be assured in each locality including vaccines and antiviral agents, over-the-counter medicines, prescription medicines, antibiotics, oxygen, needles and syringes and bedding. National planning is required over appropriate antibiotic choice and supplies if shortages are to be avoided.

• *Personnel.* Staff rotas, for health-care and other essential services, will need to cover essential work and augment areas where additional work is required; strategies may include redeployment of staff from non-essential areas, mobilizing additional staff such as recently retired health-care staff, and making full use of voluntary organizations and volunteers.

Prevention of spread of influenza

It is unlikely that the spread of pandemic influenza can be greatly influenced. Spread could possibly be slowed by reducing inessential, especially international, travel. Specific advice will be required about travel, curfews (for example, closing cinemas, theatres, clubs or sporting venues), and whether to close schools.

Attempts should be made by infection control teams in hospitals and nursing homes to limit the spread of infection by appropriate isolation, cohorting and discharge of patients who may still be shedding virus. Consideration should also be given, and guidance issued, about the advisability of closing residential homes and long-stay medical facilities to new admissions during the pandemic to prevent the introduction of infection.

Communication and coordination

Successful implementation of any strategy requires a clear chain of command and agreed lines and content for communications. These must be established at international, national and local level during the interpandemic period and any gaps identified and remedied, recognizing the different information needs of different groups. Some information exchange will need to be secure and restricted.

There will be an overwhelming demand for accurate and timely information on a number of different aspects of the pandemic. Conflicting information, misinformation and rumours will inevitably circulate, and public confidence will waver over the information being given and predictions being made. It will be important to collect and widely disseminate timely, accurate and consistent information about influenza activity and severity, epidemiological and laboratory findings, disease control efforts, including the availability of and recommendations for vaccine and antiviral agents, arrangements for immunization, other recommended health measures and any contingency arrangements. Designated contact points for information should be widely advertised. Professional societies can assist and add credibility by endorsing the national approach and communicating with their members.

The media can make an important contribution to communication and education and should be involved at the planning stage. Sources of facts may include question-and-answer briefing, leaflets, video tapes, telephone and fax helplines, and the internet. The needs of groups which are difficult to reach, for example because of language difficulties, need to be addressed. Much can be developed in advance, in several languages, for later completion and distribution as camera-ready copy that can be individualized.

Health-care and other workers will require educational programmes and material on influenza viruses, pandemic influenza, expected clinical disease and the recommended interventions.

After the pandemic

At the end of a pandemic, one of the functions of local and national pandemic committees should be to review the course of the pandemic and the effectiveness of the response, prepare a report and make recommendations for the future.

Conclusion

A future pandemic of influenza seems inevitable. Detailed advance planning will enable prompt detection and effective monitoring of the event, and help to ensure that contingency arrangements are in place for an effective response. Such planning is required at local, national and international levels.

References

Ada, G.L., Tannock, G.A. & Hampson, A.W. (1997) Options for the control of influenza III, conference report. *Vaccine* **15**, 245–7.

Aymard, M., Cox, N.J., Dubois, G. *et al.* (1994) Recommendations of the 7th European meeting on influenza and its prevention. *Eur J Epidemiol* **10**, 525–6.

Hope-Simpson, R.E. (1992) *The Transmission of Epidemic Influenza.* p. 56. Plenum Press, London.

Miller, D.L., Pereira, M.S. & Clarke, M. (1971) Epidemiology of the Hong Kong/68 variant of influenza A2 in Britain. *Brit Med J* **1**, 475–79.

Monto, A.S. (ed.) (1997) Pandemic influenza: confronting a re-emergent threat. *J Infect Dis* **176**, S1–S90.

Nicholson, K.G., Tyrrell, D.A.J., Harrison, P. *et al.* (1979) Clinical studies of monovalent inactivated whole virus and subunit A/USSR/77 (H1N1) vaccine: serological responses and clinical reactions. *J Biol Standard* **7**, 123–136.

Rowe, P.M. (1995) Pandemic influenza (un)preparedness described. *Lancet* **346**, 1699.

Shortridge, K.F. (1995) The next pandemic influenza virus? *Lancet* **346**, 1210–12.

Smorodintsev, A.A., Karpuhin, G.I., Zlydnikov, D.M. *et al.* (1970) The prophylactic effectiveness of amantadine hydrochloride in an epidemic of Hong Kong influenza in Leningrad in 1969. *Bull WHO* **42**, 865–72.

Tamblyn, S.E. & Hinman, A.R. (1993) Pandemic planning: conclusions and recommendations. In: Hannoun, C., Kendal, A.P., Klenk, H.D. & Ruben, F.L. (eds) *Options for the Control of Influenza II*, pp. 457–9. Elsevier Science Publishers, Amsterdam.

Taubenberger, J.K., Reid, A.H., Krafft, A.E., Bijwaard, K.E. & Fanning, T.G. (1997) Initial genetic characterisation of the. 1918 'Spanish' influenza virus. *Science* **275**, 1793–6.

UK Health Departments (1977) *Multiphase Contingency Plan for Pandemic Influenza.* Department of Health, London.

Webster, R.G. (1994) While awaiting the next pandemic of influenza A. [Editorial] *Brit Med J* **309**, 1179–80.

Webster, R.G., Bean, W.J., Gorman, O.T., Chambers, T.M. & Kawaoka, Y. (1992) Evolution and ecology of influenza A viruses. *Microbiol Rev* **56**, 152–79.

The H5N1 Influenza Outbreak in Hong Kong: A Test of Pandemic Preparedness

Robert G. Webster and Alan J. Hay

Influenza is an emerging disease and an extensive strategic plan has been developed over the past few years to deal with the next pandemic, which is imminent. During the final stages of preparing the initial plan, an H5N1 influenza outbreak occurred in chickens in Hong Kong and the virus was transmitted directly to humans. These events took place while this book was at the draft page-proof stage. This appendix documents the events of the H5N1 outbreak and establishes that the pandemic plan must be viewed as an evolving document that is updated regularly as influenza reveals how peripatetic it can be.

The index case

A 3-year-old boy who became ill with fever, sore throat and abdominal pain on 11th May 1997 was admitted to the Queen Elizabeth Hospital, Hong Kong on the 16th May and subsequently died on 21st May of multiple medical complications including pneumonia, ARDS, Reye's syndrome and multiple organ failure. A virus isolated from a tracheal aspirate was identified as H5N1 subtype influenza A (De Jong *et al.* 1997). This case is the first known infection of humans with an H5N1 influenza virus. The virus which infected the child originated from those responsible for a March–May 1997 outbreak of avian H5N1 influenza in chickens in the New Territories of Hong Kong; three chicken farms were affected, with an overall mortality of 70% among the 6800 chickens. On two of the farms the mortality was 100% (Claas *et al.* 1998). It is not known whether the child in the index case had contact with infected poultry, but chickens were kept as pets at the child's kindergarten.

The isolates from the index case and the earlier chicken H5N1 viruses have been characterized extensively (Subbarao *et al.* 1998, Claas *et al.* 1998), and there is no doubt that the chicken H5N1 virus was the precursor of the human H5N1 strain. The salient features are as follows:

- Both viruses belong to the H5 lineage of Eurasian avian influenza viruses.

- All gene segments are of Eurasian avian origin and were not derived by reassortment.

- The nucleotide sequence homology of the eight gene segments of the human and chicken H5N1 isolates varies from 98% for the polymerase A gene (PA) to 100% for the matrix (M) and non-structural (NS) genes. The haemagglutinin (HA) genes of the chicken and human isolates are 99.6% homologous, and the neuraminidase (NA) genes are 99.5% homologous.

- The HA1 of the avian H5N1 strains differs by only three amino acids from that of the human isolate. The index human strain lacks the carbohydrate at asparagine 156 that is present in the HA of chicken isolates. This residue is adjacent to the receptor-binding pocket and may influence antigenicity.

- The putative component residues of the receptor-binding site did not differ between the human and avian H5N1 viruses. It is likely, therefore, that the human H5 HA retains a preference for sialic acid receptors attached to the galactoside through an $\alpha2,3$ linkage. This specificity of binding is characteristic of avian viruses. The human H5N1 isolate has not acquired mutations leading to the preferential binding of $\alpha2,6$-linked receptors, as is typical for human viruses.

- Even after passage in mammalian cells the human virus remained highly pathogenic for chickens: all chickens inoculated intratracheally died within 3 days of a fulminating systemic infection with symptoms typical of fowl plague. The passaged human strain retained the series of basic amino acids (RERRRKKR) associated with high pathogenicity of avian influenza viruses (see Chapter 12).
- The NAs of both the avian and human H5N1 strains have a unique 19-amino acid deletion in the stalk region.
- Both viruses are closely related antigenically, but monoclonal antibodies and ferret antiserum can distinguish the avian from the human virus.
- Both the human and avian H5N1 isolates replicated in domestic pigs and ducks but caused no signs of disease. However, in Balb/c mice, both viruses replicated to high titres after intranasal inoculation and caused high mortality (R.G. Webster, unpublished results).
- Regarding the thermal stability of the H5N1 isolates in faecal droppings from chickens: if the samples were dried at ambient temperature (20°C) they lost infectivity in one day, whereas wet faeces retained infectivity for up to 3 days at ambient temperature, and at 4°C they retained complete infectivity for at least 4 days (R.G. Webster, unpublished results).
- Serological surveillance of humans in Hong Kong revealed evidence of H5N1 infection in 5 of 29 poultry workers but no evidence of detectable infection of 4 family contacts of the index case or among the general population, and infection of 1 of 54 healthcare workers who cared for the infected child (MMWR 1998).

The second wave

In the ensuing months it appeared that this was an isolated case of infection by an avian H5N1 virus. A second case in a 2-year-old boy (with a ventral septal defect) who developed flu-like symptoms on 11th November, however, heralded a cluster of a further 16 cases of H5N1 influenza. On this occasion the patient recovered completely and was discharged from hospital within 3 days. Of the 16

subsequent cases of confirmed H5N1 infection (total 18), who fell ill between 20th November and 28th December, 5 died. All cases were limited to the Hong Kong region, the patients living in different parts of the territory.

The patients ranged in age from 1 year to 60 years. The clinical features of the first 12 cases have been described by Yuen *et al.* (1998). The onset was typical of classic influenza, with fever and upper respiratory tract infection. However, these cases were associated with a high percentage of severe complications: pneumonia occurred in 7 of the 12 patients, and gastrointestinal complications, elevation in liver enzymes and renal failure were particularly prominent. Except for the index case, children faired better than adults. All patients over 13 years of age had severe disease (4 deaths), whereas children 5 years of age or younger (*n* = 6) had mild symptoms, with the exception of the child with Reye's syndrome associated with intake of aspirin. Systemic spread of the virus, as is found in chickens, was unconfirmed, but studies are still in progress. Therefore, humans infected with H5N1 influenza virus in Hong Kong were at risk of severe consequences, especially primary viral pneumonia, with high mortality in individuals over 13 years of age.

In early December 1997, H5N1 viruses were isolated from the live-bird market at which some of the families of patients did their shopping. More extensive virological surveillance of live-bird markets revealed that H5N1 influenza viruses were present in chickens in most of the markets tested and were also isolated from ducks and geese. In addition, multiple subtypes of influenza A virus, including H9N2, H6NX and H11NX were isolated, but the significance of this remains to be resolved. One possibility is that coinfection may have modulated the pathogenic potential of the H5N1 virus, for few of the markets had evidence of mortality in chickens. In contrast, each of the H5N1 viruses isolated in the live-bird markets was highly lethal in chickens after experimental oral inoculation. The absence of dead chickens in the markets and the presence of ducks and geese that shed H5N1 virus with no signs of disease probably perpetuated H5N1 in the live-bird markets in Hong Kong and created the conditions that permitted transmission to humans. An outbreak of H5N1 infection on a chicken farm in the New Territories in mid-December and deaths of chickens at one of the wholesale markets set the scene for disposal of all chickens in Hong Kong.

The H5N1 viruses from the live-bird markets and 18 patients are still being characterized. Preliminary information about these human and avian H5N1 isolates indicates the following:

• Two variants are distinguishable among the human isolates, which correspond to equivalent variants among viruses isolated from chickens in different locations. This provides further evidence that many of the human infections were the result of independent transmission from infected birds.

• The most notable difference was the presence or absence of a potential glycosylation site at asparagine 156 of the H5 haemagglutinin.

• Post-infection ferret antisera against viruses lacking this site (e.g. the initial isolate A/Hong Kong/156/97) reacted less well in haemagglutination–inhibition tests with those viruses possessing the additional glycosylation site and could distinguish between the two groups of variants. Antisera against viruses with the additional glycosylation site were more broadly cross-reactive, indicating that these viruses are potentially preferable vaccine candidates.

• The N1 neuraminidase of the H5N1 viruses was closely related antigenically and genetically to certain recent avian virus N1s (e.g. turkey/England/91) and also to those of recent European 'avian-like' swine H1N1 viruses. A prominent difference was the deletion of 19 amino acids in the stalk of the molecule, relative to NAs of, for example, the swine viruses. Since the length of the NA stalk is known to influence significantly the growth characteristics of viruses in different cells, this feature may well be an important determinant of the biological characteristics of these human H5N1 viruses. Antibodies to the NA of human H1N1 viruses did not inhibit the neuraminidase activity of the H5N1 viruses and thus antibody induced by the current influenza vaccine or by natural infection is unlikely to provide any significant level of protection.

• There is no evidence of genetic reassortment with current human H3N2 or H1N1 subtype viruses or with other avian influenza strains.

• There is little evidence of human-to-human transmission of the virus.

At present there is no explanation for the ability of the H5N1 viruses to infect and replicate efficiently in cells of the human respiratory tract but apparently fail to transmit effectively to other human contacts.

No additional cases of H5N1 in humans or poultry in Hong Kong have been reported since the slaughter of poultry in the live-bird markets and of chickens in the New Territories was initiated on 29th December 1997. However, the risk of transmission of H5N1 to humans continues. We may be in the second lag phase, for eradication of these H5N1 variants from all avian species in Asia is unlikely. The precursors of these viruses are still circulating in their wild-bird reservoirs.

Lessons in pandemic preparedness

The interspecies transmission of a highly pathogenic avian H5N1 to humans created a unique situation, and, in a number of ways, the then current pandemic plan was not designed to cope with several problem areas.

• If the Hong Kong H5N1 virus had become established in humans, with human-to-human transmission, all domestic chicken flocks in the world would have been in jeopardy. The threat would probably also have extended to turkeys, quail and other species. Thus, a leading protein source would have been threatened and chicken eggs could have been unavailable for the preparation of vaccine.

• The highly pathogenic H5N1 avian strain could not be used as a vaccine strain, because it is a human and veterinary biohazard. Suitable non-pathogenic H5N1 surrogate strains were sought, and few were available. The best match was A/duck/Singapore-Q/F119-3/97 (H5N3), but this isolate has an inappropriate NA necessitating separate surrogate strains for both the HA and the NA. Selection of the most appropriate donor strain (A/PR/8/34 [H1N1] or a non-pathogenic avian strain) for providing high growth potential for the preparation of conventional inactivated vaccines prompted environmental concerns. Alternative strategies for making vaccines included genetic modification of the H5N1 HA to eliminate the basic amino acids in the connecting peptide and the engineering of a non-pathogenic strain (see Chapter 32). Other strategies include production of the H5 HA in the baculovirus expression system, attenuated vaccines and DNA vaccine approaches. Each product would have a place in future control strategies.

• Suitable high containment BL3+ facilities for working with the H5N1 strains were very limited throughout the world, inhibiting virus characterization, vaccine development and testing of potential antiviral agents.

• Both amantadine and rimantadine were useful for therapy of humans in Hong Kong and for prophylaxis of laboratory workers. However, if the H5N1 virus had spread, there would not have been enough of these anti-influenza drugs available to make a useful impact. The new antiviral drugs that target the NA (zanamivir and GS4014) were efficacious in a mouse model of H5N1 infection and will have future potential in pandemic control when they are approved for human use.

One positive outcome of the H5N1 experience was that the slaughter of the chickens and other poultry interrupted the spread of the virus to humans; this shows that the reduction of interspecies transmission can influence the emergence of influenza viruses. In addition, the outbreak prompted changes in the live-bird markets, which have been described as the missing link in the epidemiology of avian influenza (Senne *et al.* 1992). The transmission of H5N1 viruses to humans in Hong Kong indicates that these markets are a risk factor in the transmission of avian strains to humans. The current practice of marketing chickens separate from other birds, especially aquatic species such as ducks and geese, potentially will reduce the spread of influenza A viruses between species.

An important lesson regarding pandemic preparedness is that huge gaps in our knowledge of influenza viruses remain. Why did these particular H5N1 viruses transmit directly to humans? Why did only a few people become infected when probably a high proportion of the Hong Kong population was exposed to the H5N1 virus in the live-bird markets? Any plan for dealing with the anticipated influenza pandemic is only as good as the knowledge upon which the plan is based. Gaps in knowledge will lead to an incomplete plan and any strategic plan must be updated as new findings emerge. Moreover, the real practical challenge remains – implementation of the recommended plan during the present interpandemic period so that we are better prepared when the next pandemic emerges.

In conclusion, this episode highlights once again the importance and effectiveness of the WHO network for surveillance and research on influenza in the early detection of novel viruses infecting the human population and in facilitating constructive collaboration between health authorities, medical scientists and veterinarians to meet the threat. On this occasion, however, the H5N1 virus has not become established within the human population, the 'outbreak' was contained and ceased with the removal of the source of the infection. It has not proved necessary to produce a vaccine, although work continues to identify suitable non-pathogenic vaccine strains. It is a reminder of the enigmatic behaviour of influenza A viruses and the unpredictability of the nature of the virus which will cause the next pandemic.

Acknowledgements

The studies in Hong Kong were supported by Public Health Research Grant AI29680 from the National Institute of Allergy and Infectious Diseases (USA), by Cancer Center support CORE grant CA-21765 and the American Lebanese Syrian Associated Charities, by the Health Department of Hong Kong and by the World Health Organization. The studies of H5N1 in Hong Kong were made possible by the outstanding collaboration of many organizations including the Health Department of Hong Kong, the Agricultural and Fisheries of Hong Kong, Hong Kong University, the National Influenza Center of the Netherlands, the Centers for Disease Control and Prevention, the World Health Organization, and the International Task Force on H5N1 (Hong Kong University). A special thank you is gratefully extended to Dr Margaret Chan,

Director of the Health Department, Hong Kong, and to Professor Kennedy F. Shortridge, Hong Kong University, for their insight and their understanding of Hong Kong. We thank Enid Bedford for rapid preparation of this manuscript.

References

Claas, E.C.J., Osterhaus, A.D.M.E., Van Beck, R. *et al.* (1998) Human influenza A (H5N1) virus related to a highly pathogenic avian influenza virus. *Lancet* **351**, 472–7.

De Jong. J.C., Claas, E.C.J., Osterhaus, A.D.M.E., Webster, R.G., Lim, W.L. (1997) A pandemic warning. *Nature* **389**, 554.

MMWR (1998) Update: isolation of avian influenza A (H5N1) viruses from humans – Hong Kong, 1997–98. *Morbid Mortal Weekly Rep* **46**, 1245–7.

Senne, D.A., Pearson, J.E., Panigraphy, B. (1992) Live poultry markets: a missing link in the epidemiology of avian influenza. In: *Proceedings of the Third Symposium on Avian Influenza, May 27–29 1992*, 50–8.

Subbarao, K., Kilmov, A., Katz, J. *et al.* (1998) Characterization of an avian influenza A (H5N1) virus isolated from a child with a fatal respiratory illness. *Science* **279**, 393–6.

Yuen, K.Y., Chan, P.K.S., Peiris, M. *et al.* (1998) Clinical features and rapid viral diagnosis of human disease associated with avian influenza A H5N1 virus. *Lancet* **351**, 467–71.

Index